DR P. HOLLAND

L.G.I Prediatric Dept.

£19.00

Pediatric Kidney Disease

Pediatric Kidney Disease

Chester M. Edelmann, Jr., M.D.
Editor

Associate Editors:
Henry L. Barnett, M.D.
Jay Bernstein, M.D.
Alfred F. Michael, M.D.
Adrian Spitzer, M.D.

Volume II

Little, Brown and Company Boston

Published November 1978

Copyright © 1978 by Little, Brown and Company (Inc.)

First Edition

Library of Congress Catalog Card No. 78-61278

ISBN 0-316-21071-4

Printed in the United States of America

Contents

Volume I

I. The Kidney and the Urinary Tract: Morphology and Physiology

Section One. The Normal Kidney and Urinary Tract

Section Two. Mechanisms of and Morphologic and Functional Responses to Injury

Section Three. Evaluation for Disease

Section Four. Major Manifestations of Renal Disease and Renal Insufficiency

Volume II

II. Diseases of the Kidney

Section One. Neonatal, Congenital, and Hereditary Disorders

Section Two. Glomerular Diseases

Section Three. Renal Abnormalities in Systemic Disease

II. Diseases of the Kidney

38. Diseases of the Kidney in the Newborn

Adrian Spitzer

It is characteristic of the seriously ill newborn to have nonspecific signs of illness such as fever, irritability, poor feeding, and failure to thrive. In these infants, disease of the kidneys and urinary tract must be considered in the differential diagnosis. Certain signs point directly toward urinary tract disease, and these are discussed in the following sections.

Disorders of Micturition

Within the first 24 hr after birth 92 percent of healthy infants pass urine, and 99 percent have done so by 48 hr [16, 20]. Often, however, the first micturition takes place in the delivery room and passes unnoticed. In the rare instance in which the newborn does not urinate within 72 hrs, serious consideration should be given to the possibility of bilateral renal agenesis, urinary tract obstruction, or a renovascular accident. Of these possibilities, the most important to diagnose is obstructive uropathy, since it is amenable to surgical correction.

Abnormalities in the volume of urine passed by the newborn during each 24-hr period are practically impossible to assess unless special attention is directed to the urinary system. The frequency of micturition varies from two to six times during the first and second days of life and from five to twenty-five times per 24 hr subsequently. The daily urinary volume is 30 to 60 ml during the first and second day, 100 to 300 ml during the following week, and between 200 and 400 for the rest of the first month.

Oliguria (urinary output below 15 to 20 ml/kg/24 hr) most often is a consequence of dehydration. Oliguria or anuria can also result from malformation, renovascular accident, or urinary tract obstruction. Oliguria of prerenal origin, as in association with diarrheal disease, maternal diabetes, or respiratory distress syndrome, usually can be identified by the high solute content of the urine, whereas in the oliguria of true renal insufficiency, urinary osmolality is low. Urinary retention can mimic anuria of renal origin. This retention can result from neurologic abnormalities, such as meningitis or disturbances in the innervation of the bladder (e.g., meningomyelocele), or from obstruction secondary to phimosis, posterior urethral valves, balanoposthitis, or vulvovaginitis. Palpation of the urinary bladder, which is easy to perform during the newborn period, and, if necessary, bladder catheterization establish the diagnosis.

Polyuria is most often the result of a defect in concentrating capacity, secondary to medullary abnormalities in renal dysplasia, to renal hypoplasia, or to nephronophthisis or medullary cystic disease. It is seen also in association with lack of antidiuretic hormone or with nephrogenic diabetes insipidus (Chap. 82).

Proteinuria

It is generally accepted that small amounts of protein ordinarily pass through the semipermeable glomerular basement membrane. De Luna and Hullet [4] reported a mean urinary excretion of 45 mg per day in newborns. However, we rarely find more than trace proteinuria in random urines from newborn infants. When protein is present in higher amounts, proteinuria suggests glomerular disease such as congenital nephrotic syndrome (Chap. 54) or glomerulonephritis (Chap. 43).

Hematuria

In the normal newborn, the excretion of erythrocytes in urine does not exceed 100 per minute or 75,000 per 12 hr. Reddish urine usually indicates hematuria [6], but it may also be caused by the presence of bile pigments, porphyrins, urate, or hemoglobin [1]. The differential diagnosis between hemoglobinuria and hematuria is easy to make if the urine is examined soon after collection. With standing, erythrocytes may hemolyze, especially in hypotonic urine, and no longer appear as formed elements. Hematuria in the newborn may result from a renovascular accident, cortical and medullary necrosis [2], neoplasia, obstructive uropathy, infection, nephritis, or coagulopathy.

Pyuria

The dividing line between a normal and an abnormal number of white blood cells in the urine is uncertain. We do not expect to find more than two to three leukocytes per high-power field in a centrifuged specimen of urine [9, 12]. Bag specimens of well-mixed, uncentrifuged urine obtained from 600 newborns on the sixth or seventh day of life contained five or fewer leukocytes per cubic millimeter in 98 percent of boys but in only 56 percent of girls. The percentage in girls increased to 94 when a clean-catch technique was used, suggesting perineal contamination of the bag specimens [13]. The most common cause of pyuria is urinary tract infection (Chap. 92). Increased rates of excretion of white blood cells also can accompany nephritis and nephrosis and can be indicative of any type of inflammatory process within the urinary tract, including those associated with drug reactions.

Edema

At an early stage, the retention of fluid can be detected only by repeated, accurate measurements of weight. Later, swelling becomes obvious. It is generally stated that the edema of renal disease involves primarily the face and is soft, whitish, and painless. None of these characteristics, however, is specific.

Edema is occasionally found in prematurely born infants during the first few days of life [7] and has been shown to be the result of shifts of fluid between body water compartments [14]. So-called late edema develops among some newborns with a birth weight below 1,300 gm and a short gestational age. The accumulation of fluid seems to correspond to the thirty-fifth to thirty-sixth week of gestational age. No other gross abnormalities are found in these babies, and the edema usually is transitory. Studies performed in infants with late edema and in healthy control subjects have not detected significant differences in external water and electrolyte balance. A difference was observed, however, in the distribution of fluids between various body compartments, with the extracellular compartment being larger than normal in the edematous babies [21]. The cause of this condition remains obscure, although some of these cases have been shown to be associated with vitamin E deficiency and anemia.

There are many extrarenal causes of edema in the newborn, such as primary lymphedema (Milroy's disease), congenital lymphedema with gonadal dysgenesis, the syndrome of inappropriate antidiuretic hormone secretion, hyperaldosteronism, congenital analbuminemia, severe protein deficiency, protein-losing gastroenteropathy, scleredema, syphilis, erythroblastosis fetalis, and hereditary angioneurotic edema. The differential diagnosis also should include maternal diabetes.

Ascites can occur in the congenital nephrotic syndrome, in which case the fluid has the character of an exudate with a protein content that usually does not exceed 500 mg per deciliter. A more common cause of ascites in the newborn is obstruction of the lower urinary tract, particularly in association with posterior urethral valves. At least 50 cases have been described in the literature, although this is an unusual complication of urinary tract obstruction. The ascitic fluid apparently represents urine that has leaked through a ruptured pelvis or calyx. The differential diagnosis includes chylous ascites, ascites caused by syphilis, hepatobiliary obstruction, ruptured intraabdominal cyst, meconium peritonitis, and bile ascites.

Abdominal Masses

Examination of the abdomen by palpation usually can be performed easily during the first 48 hr of extrauterine life because of the laxity of the abdominal muscles. The kidneys of the newborn are in a lower position than they are later in life, the right kidney usually being lower than the left. Using a very meticulous method of deep abdominal palpation in 10,000 infants, Mussels et al. [17] suspected renal anomalies in 77; 55 of these were confirmed by intravenous pyelography. The most common anomaly was a horseshoe-shaped, or fused, kidney, which occurred in 16 infants. Other conditions accounting for an apparently large kidney are hydronephrosis, tumor, thrombosis of the renal vein, and cystic disease. The possibility of an adrenal hemorrhage also should be kept in mind. A smooth mass is more likely to be the result of hydronephrosis or renal vein thrombosis, whereas an irregular surface suggests malformation or cystic disease.

Infection of the Urinary Tract

Asymptomatic bacteriuria has been found in less than 1 percent of apparently healthy full-term infants with equal frequency in males and females [5, 8, 11]. By contrast, studies in premature infants have demonstrated bacteriuria, confirmed by suprapubic puncture, in 2 to 5 percent [5] (see also Chap. 92).

In the majority of neonates with urinary tract infection, urologic-radiologic examination reveals structurally normal kidneys and collecting systems. This finding is in striking contrast to that in infants diagnosed as having urinary tract infection during the remainder of the first year of life and in whom the incidence of urologic malformation has been reported to be as high as 50 to 80 percent. The low incidence of asymptomatic bacteriuria in healthy full-term infants suggests that routine screening in this age group is not a profitable undertaking. In contrast, the infant with any evidence of illness is likely to have an otherwise silent urinary tract infection; accordingly, he should be examined appropriately.

Neonates with pyelonephritis may show relatively little evidence of serious infection, or they may appear as toxic, septic, desperately ill infants. A peculiar syndrome consisting of pyelonephritis, hepatomegaly, hemolytic anemia, and jaundice (direct- and indirect-reacting bilirubin) has been described [19]. Other features include poor feeding, lethargy, irritability, occasional vomiting and diarrhea, and azotemia. Hemolysis may be severe enough to require transfusion. The pathogenesis of this syndrome is unknown. The organisms most commonly cultured are the low-numbered serotypes of *Escherichia coli* (especially 04:115). As in presumptive septicemia, treatment is urgent and cannot await the results of cultures. The response to antibiotic therapy usually is prompt, with a return of the blood urea to normal, resolution of hepatomegaly, clearing of jaundice, and cessation of hemolysis.

Renal Insufficiency and Renal Failure

Inadequacy of renal function may be a consequence of any of the developmental anomalies, may arise from prerenal factors such as dehydration and shock, or may be the result of acquired disease of the kidneys. The recognition and treatment of renal insufficiency is discussed here without consideration of the nature of the specific underlying cause.

DIAGNOSIS

In the majority of cases the history reveals nonspecific signs such as lethargy, poor appetite, vomiting, and convulsions. Oliguria, although often present, is easily missed until other findings direct the attention toward the urinary system. Urinary output less than 15 to 20 ml/kg/24 hr in the newborn (beyond the first few days of life) is indicative of oliguria. It is vital to determine whether the cause of oliguria or anuria is prerenal (i.e., caused by inadequacy of the blood supply to the kidney), postrenal (i.e., urine being formed but not voided, because of obstructive uropathy or a neurogenic bladder), or true renal failure (i.e., malfunction of the kidneys caused by intrinsic disease, whether congenital or acquired) (Table 38-1). This differentiation usually is simple. In some instances, extensive radiologic or urologic investigation may be required to demonstrate the cause of postrenal failure.

The adequacy of the circulation must be assessed to rule out prerenal failure. If insufficiency of the

Table 38-1. Differentiation of Prerenal from True Renal Failure in Infancy

Measurement	Prerenal	True Renal
U_{Na}	<20 mEq/L	>70 mEq/L
U/P osmolality	>2	<1.1
U/P urea	>15	<5
U/P creatinine	>15	<5
Fractional excretion of sodium	<1.8%	>10%

vascular volume is suspected, the response to administration of fluid may be helpful. For this purpose, isotonic saline in a dose of 15 to 20 ml per kilogram of body weight, or mannitol (0.5 to 1.0 gm per kilogram in a 20% solution) can be given IV. A prompt increase in urinary output suggests that additional fluids may be needed. If there is no response, care must be taken to avoid administration of excessive amounts of fluids in order to "force" a diuresis.

CAUSES OF RENAL INSUFFICIENCY

Among 35 newborns with persistent renal insufficiency in one study, only 7 had normal kidneys [18]. The most common organic cause of renal failure in the newborn period is renal dysplasia, followed in frequency by urinary tract obstruction and cystic disease of the kidneys. Extrarenal causes are, in order of frequency, shock and dehydration, sepsis, and renal venous thrombosis. Perinatal anoxia [3] and respiratory distress syndrome [10] are additional causes of renal insufficiency.

TREATMENT

Treatment of renal insufficiency in the neonate is similar to treatment in the older child (see Chaps. 33, 34). Consideration must be given to maintenance of the balance of water, electrolytes, and hydrogen ions, and at the same time to provision of nutrition as near optimal as possible. Acute renal insufficiency is treated by providing a fluid intake equal to insensible water loss (25 to 40 ml/kg/24 hr) plus urinary output. In the anuric or severely oliguric patient, solute requiring urinary excretion is not given. In addition to withholding potassium, it may be necessary to reduce dangerously high plasma levels. When the concentration in plasma exceeds 6 mEq per liter, sodium or polystyrene sulfonate (Kayexalate) can be given (by enema or by mouth) in a starting dose of 0.5 to 1.5 gm per kilogram of body weight and is repeated as needed. Moderate or severe degrees of acidemia are treated by administration of sodium bicarbonate. Peritoneal dialysis may be indicated in the infant with total renal failure lasting more than 7 to 10 days or when severe metabolic disturbances cannot be managed with medical treatment alone.

In infants with chronic renal insufficiency, special attention must be paid to provision of adequate nutrition. Mild to moderate degrees of renal insufficiency usually can be managed by utilizing humanized milk such as Similac PM 60-40 or SMA as the sole source of nutrition. The usual dose of supplemental vitamins should be given.

With lesser degrees of function, other specific therapy may be required. Normal levels of pH and bicarbonate in the blood should be maintained by administration of sodium bicarbonate. The dose is adjusted to the patient, starting with 1 to 2 mEq/kg/day and increased as needed. Concentrations of calcium and inorganic phosphate in the blood should be measured frequently. Hyperphosphatemia usually does not develop in young infants fed low-phosphate diets until they reach advanced stages of renal failure. In such cases, phosphate-binding gels (such as aluminum hydroxide gel [Amphojel]) can be administered, although they are usually poorly tolerated. A dose of 50 to 150 mg/kg/day given PO is customary. If the plasma calcium level falls significantly below normal, supplemental calcium (such as calcium gluconate [Neo-Calglucon]) is given in a daily dose of 10 to 20 mg (of elemental calcium) per kilogram of body weight.

If these measures are not successful in maintaining normal blood levels of calcium, pharmacologic doses of vitamin D should be prescribed, starting with a dosage of 10,000 units per day. Recently, dihydrotachysterol has gained wide acceptance. This is an analogue of vitamin D that is activated in the absence of the kidneys. The drug is given PO. Care must be taken to avoid too-vigorous therapy and induction of hypercalcemia. The serum calcium × phosphate product should not be allowed to exceed 70.

In infants with severe uremia, vomiting may be a most troublesome symptom. Treatment with one of the phenothiazine drugs may be helpful.

Hypertension in infants is treated as in older children (Chap. 32). Every effort should be made to maintain normal levels of blood pressure. Treatment is usually initiated with reserpine (0.01 to 0.02 mg/kg/day) or hydralazine hydrochloride (1 to 2 mg/kg/day in four divided doses), or both. If these drugs are not successful, guanethidine sulfate can be added (0.2 to 0.3 mg/kg/day as a single dose). Diazoxide (Hyperstat), 5 mg per kilogram IV, is used whenever a prompt decrease in diastolic pressure is required.

Infants who cannot be maintained in a satisfactory metabolic state by dietary and medical therapy alone are candidates for dialysis (Chap. 35). Peritoneal dialysis can be used for short periods but probably is inadvisable if prolonged treatment is anticipated [15]. Special peritoneal catheters with perforations that are not more than 3 to 4 cm from the tip are required. Prior to the insertion of the catheter, the bladder, which is an intraabdominal organ in the newborn, should be emptied, and the abdominal cavity should be distended by injection of 30 to 40 ml of dialysis fluid per kilogram of body weight. A similar amount is usually well tolerated for each cycle. Care should be taken to avoid interference with the respiratory mechanism, which, in the newborn, is more dependent on diaphragmatic movements than in older children. Special attention should be given to the prevention of dehydration or overloading, which requires continuous monitoring of the baby's weight or the use of an automatic cycling dialysis machine. To avoid the development of hypothermia, the solution should be heated to 37°C.

Hemodialysis is technically difficult in infants and should be reserved for patients in whom peritoneal dialysis cannot be performed.

PROGNOSIS

The mortality among newborns with renal failure is high, being around 50 percent in several relatively large series [3, 15, 18]. Most of these infants have severe congenital renal and extrarenal anomalies, although the immediate cause of death often is sepsis or shock. Death usually occurs within a few days after birth.

Renal transplantation has not improved the outcome of patients of this age with end-stage renal disease (Chap. 36). To our knowledge, none of the newborns so far given transplants has survived.

References

1. Angella, J. J., Prieto, E. N., and Fogel, B. J. Hemoglobinuria associated with hemolytic disease of the newborn infant. *J. Pediatr.* 71:530, 1967.
2. Bernstein, J., and Meyer, R. Congenital abnormalities of the urinary system. II. Renal cortical and medullary necrosis. *J. Pediatr.* 59:657, 1961.
3. Dauber, I. M., Krauss, A. N., Symchych, P. S., and Auld, R. A. M. Renal failure following perinatal anoxia. *J. Pediatr.* 88:851, 1976.
4. DeLuna, M. B., and Hullet, W. H. Urinary protein excretion in healthy infants, children and adults. *Proc. Am. Soc. Nephrol.* 1967. P. 16.
5. Edelmann, C. M., Jr., Ogwo, J., and Fine, B. P. The prevalence of bacteriuria in full-term and premature infants. *J. Pediatr.* 82:125, 1973.
6. Emanuel, B., and Aronson, N. Neonatal hematuria. *Am. J. Dis. Child.* 128:204, 1974.
7. Fisher, D. A. Obscure and unusual edema. *Pediatrics* 37:506, 1966.
8. Gower, P. E., Husband, P., Coleman, J. C., and

Snodgrass, G. J. A. I. Urinary infection in two selected neonatal populations. *Arch. Dis. Child.* 45: 529, 1970.

9. Gruickshand, G., and Edmond, E. "Clean catch" urines in the newborn: Bacteriology and cell excretion patterns in first week of life. *Br. Med. J.* 4:705, 1967.

10. Guignard, J.-P., Torrado, A., Mazouni, S. M., and Gautier, E. Renal function in respiratory distress syndrome. *J. Pediatr.* 88:845, 1976.

11. Lincoln, K., and Winberg, J. Studies of urinary tract infection in infancy and childhood. II. Quantitative estimation of bacteriuria in unselected neonates with special reference to the occurrence of asymptomatic infections. *Acta Paediatr. Scand.* 53:307, 1964.

12. Lincoln, K., and Winberg, J. Studies of urinary tract infection in infancy and childhood. III. Quantitative estimation of cellular excretion in unselected neonates. *Acta Paediatr. Scand.* 53:447, 1964.

13. Littlewood, J. M. White cells and bacteria in voided urine of healthy newborn. *Arch. Dis. Child.* 46:167, 1971.

14. MacLaurin, J. C. Changes in body water distribution during the first two weeks of life. *Arch. Dis. Child.* 41:286, 1966.

15. Manley, G. L., and Collip, P. G. Renal failure in the newborn. Treatment with peritoneal dialysis. *Am. J. Child.* 115:107, 1968.

16. Moore, E. S., and Galvez, M. D. Delayed micturition in newborn period. *J. Pediatr.* 80:867, 1972.

17. Mussels, M., Gaudry, C. L., and Bason, W. M. Renal anomalies in the newborn found by deep palpation. *Pediatrics* 47:97, 1971.

18. Reimold, E. W., Don, T. D., and Worthen, H. G. Renal failure during the first year of life. *Pediatrics* 59:987, 1977.

19. Seeler, R. A., and Hahn, K. Jaundice in urinary tract infection in infancy. *Am. J. Dis. Child.* 118: 553, 1969.

20. Sherry, S. N., and Kramer, L. The time of passage of the first stool and first urine by the newborn infant. *J. Pediatr.* 46:158, 1955.

21. Wu, P. Y. K., Oh, W., Lubetkin, A., and Metcoff, J. "Late edema" in low birth weight infants. *Pediatrics* 47:97, 1971.

39. Renal Hypoplasia and Dysplasia

Jay Bernstein

Abnormal renal morphogenesis includes those processes leading to both deficient parenchyma and abnormally differentiated parenchyma [8]. A reduction in the number of nephrons results in a small kidney of otherwise normal gross and microscopic appearance, a condition known as *renal hypoplasia*. Altered structural differentiation of the metanephric components leads to incompletely and abnormally developed ducts and blastema, a condition known as *renal dysplasia*. Hypoplasia and dysplasia often coexist, but the two are separable in regard to both pathogenesis and ultimate morphologic appearance. The structural characterization of these renal malformations during the last 15 years has provided a morphologic basis for developing clinicopathologic correlations [8, 10, 12, 16, 43, 67].

Discussions of developmental renal abnormalities have customarily included cystic diseases [10]. The rationale for doing so is flawed, for there is some evidence that the major forms of polycystic disease are in fact not due to altered renal morphogenesis, despite their often being congenital. In the sense intended, the term *developmental* is applied to circumstances of nephrogenesis, metanephric differentiation, and growth. Hypoplasia and dysplasia are developmental abnormalities in which

nephrons are deficient or in which the architecture of the kidney is altered. Altered metanephric differentiation, the process by which the cells of the kidney became specialized and through which they achieve the structural and functional attributes of renal cells, is reflected in the presence of ductal and mesenchymal structures not normally found in the kidney. An important morphologic consideration in the function of the metanephric kidney is the spatial relationships of nephrons, ducts, and vessels to each other (renal architectonics), alterations of which result in impaired function. Reductions in numbers of renal lobes (reniculi) and nephrons are developmental abnormalities in the sense intended. That sense may be extended to include also retardation and arrest of postnatal renal growth and maturation.

In contradistinction to developmental abnormalities are those alterations that result from injury to the kidney [8]. An example of such injury might be intrauterine vascular occlusion, leading to atrophy and scarring. The lesion is not developmental, although it is congenital and affects the developing kidney. Certain heritable disorders fall into the same category of secondary renal injury, in that their effects on the kidney appear to be superimposed on normally developed nephrons. It is well recognized, for example, that the "swan-neck" deformity of the renal tubule in cystinosis is an acquired lesion and not an inherent feature of the syndrome. Similarly, heritable disorders that do not appear until adulthood or later childhood are likely not to be developmental, despite their genetic determinants. The renal lesion in adult polycystic disease, for example, is progressive, involving increasing numbers of nephrons and ducts. Even characterization of infantile polycystic disease in newborns as developmental is debatable, since microdissection shows a normal pattern of renal architectural development with apparently superimposed cystic change [63].

Most congenital malformations of the kidney appear to be sporadic rather than hereditary, certain exceptions granted. Both hypoplasia and dysplasia may be unilateral or bilateral, and bilateral, severe maldevelopment is obviously a cause of neonatal or early infantile death. Other congenital malformations include agenesis, a term signifying complete absence of the kidney, anomalies of form and shape, including renal duplication and supernumerary kidney, and anomalies of position, including ectopia and fusion.

Renal Hypoplasia

Renal hypoplasia is a condition in which the kidneys are small because of developmental parenchymal deficit [8]. Essential to this definition is the notion of normally developed and differentiated individual nephrons and ducts, although secondary changes commonly obscure the characteristic morphologic appearances. A conceptual distinction is implied, therefore, between smallness due to altered development and smallness due to acquired disease, although the practical criteria for differentiating hypoplasia from atrophy are imperfect.

The pathogenesis of hypoplastic kidneys may involve (1) a diminished number of nephrons and (2) diminished nephronic size [11]. The first circumstance may arise through either inadequate branching of the ureteric ducts or premature cessation of cortical nephrogenesis. A commonly encountered pattern is a diminished number of lobes (reniculi), which seems to be explained best by a primary defect in ductal branching. A localized inadequacy of metanephric blastema might be secondary to defective induction or to defective response, but the blastema ordinarily proliferates in response to ductal stimulation. Premature cessation of nephrogenesis in otherwise normally formed kidneys appears to be a hypothetical consideration, although certain patterns of malformation with thin cortices are best explained by curtailed nephrogenesis. Diminished nephronic size, on the other hand, is secondary to retarded growth, probably predominantly postnatal, which also may be regarded as a developmental abnormality. Small kidneys found in mentally retarded children, for example, contain glomeruli and tubules that are smaller than normal [69]. The factors responsible for abnormal ductal branching and for retarded nephronic growth remain unknown.

Renal hypoplasia can be regarded as a nongenetic malformation. Some cases are familial, but more than 90 percent are sporadic. Small kidneys are seen in association with malformations of other organ systems [74], and it is not established whether the renal abnormality is a primary component of the malformative syndrome or a secondary retardation of renal growth. Renal hypoplasia also occurs in genetically determined syndromes; it is listed, for example, as a relatively frequent component of the rare chromosome 13q- syndrome [44].

Small kidneys are common radiographic findings [19], and renal hypoplasia has been an abused diagnosis, arrived at uncritically and too readily. The radiographic appearances of renal shape and renal arterial size provide an uncertain basis for differentiating hypoplasia from atrophy, and radiographic criteria do not serve at all to differentiate hypoplasia from dysplasia. Both hypoplastic and dysplastic kidneys contain, for example, a diminished number of calyces, and both are supplied by small arteries. The demonstration of calyceal abnormalities and irregularities is more likely to indicate secondary scarring, as in reflux, rather than either of the two developmental abnormalities.

The radiographic diagnosis of renal hypoplasia requires appropriate standards for size and growth (Chap. 10). Data are now available showing that renal size correlates well with both age and body size in childhood [31, 39]. Radiographic indexes are also available for the evaluation of renal size in older patients [30, 50, 84]. Postmortem studies have shown that renal weight in childhood follows a predictable, allometric growth curve (Fig. 39-1), and that there is a high degree of correlation between renal weight and both age ($r = .937$) and height ($r = .881$) [46, 59]. The use of these data is based on the assumption that the kidney's functional capacity is related to its size and that the kidney's functional mass depends on the number of nephrons and reniculi [85].

The diagnosis of hypoplasia in the intended sense of a small kidney containing normally formed nephrons requires morphologic confirmation. The morphologic diagnosis of hypoplasia may be impaired by secondary changes that lead to atrophy

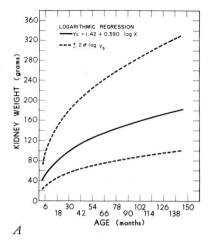

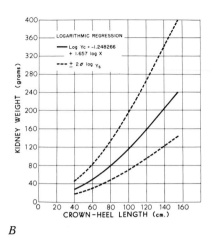

A   *B*

Figure 39-1. Renal growth in childhood. The logarithmic regression curve and range for kidney weight has been related to age (A) and to crown-heel length (B) in children 3 months to 12 years of age. (Fig. 39-1B from J. T. Oliver, M. Rubenstein, R. Meyer, and J. Bernstein. Congenital abnormalities of the urinary system. III. Growth of the kidney in childhood—determination of normal weight. J. Pediatr. 61:256, 1962.)

and scarring, but some of these secondary effects have been recognized and can be differentiated from the primary, underlying maldevelopment. Histologic examination is useful for quantifying glomerular diameter and tubular size, which are important in identifying the several types of hypoplasia. Morphologic examination is also necessary for the distinction between hypoplasia and dysplasia, which have often been completely confused and thoroughly intermingled [19]. The literature on hypoplasia has included small kidneys both with normally developed parenchyma and with abnormally developed parenchyma. Such distinctions are essential to the development of clinicopathologic correlations and to the determination of the natural history and prognosis of the conditions under discussion.

UNILATERAL HYPOPLASIA

Unilaterally small kidneys are relatively common findings in adults, with a postmortem frequency said to be approximately 1 : 500 [5]. The unilaterally small kidney is also recognized radiographically when there is a marked discrepancy in size between the two kidneys (Fig. 39-2). Such a kidney has been referred to as *miniature kidney, doll's kidney,* and *vest pocket kidney*—terms that give the impression of a kidney abnormal only in size. The differential diagnosis includes, as previously noted, renal dysplasia and renal atrophy—diagnoses that may be difficult to make in the absence of morphologic confirmation.

Unilateral hypoplasia appears to be a sporadic condition. It has been observed, however, in babies dying of multiple congenital malformations, some of which may constitute heritable syndromes. The condition in infants is nonetheless uncommon, an observation suggesting that "unilateral hypoplasia" in older persons is more often acquired than congenital.

A distinctive clinical pattern has not been delineated. The results of urinalysis and renal function tests are usually normal. The unilaterally small kidney is said to be prone to infection, lithiasis, and vascular disease. The most common symptom

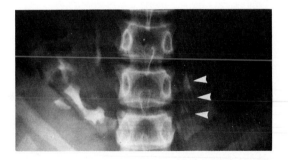

Figure 39-2. Unilateral hypoplasia. Excretory urogram in a 12-year-old girl showing a small left renal pelvis (arrowheads). The calyces appear to be deformed, suggesting parenchymal scarring, but there had been no clinical or radiographic evidence of vesicoureteric reflux. The differential diagnosis therefore lies between unilateral hypoplasia and unilateral dysplasia, and it cannot be resolved without morphologic examination. (Roentgenogram provided by Drs. Joseph O. Reed and Frederick B. Watts, Jr., Children's Hospital of Michigan.)

is pain, which may be related to any of the foregoing. Hypertension has been regarded as a major complication [5], although unilateral hypoplasia is only occasionally included in compilations of renal disease causing hypertension.

SEGMENTAL HYPOPLASIA

The condition known as segmental hypoplasia [38, 71], or Ask-Upmark kidney [18, 26], does not conform to the definition of hypoplasia previously given. These kidneys characteristically are small, with segmental and lobar areas of severe cortical and medullary abnormality [1]. Externally visible, transverse grooves mark the sites of thin segments that overlie dilated recesses of the renal pelvis (Fig. 39-3A). The affected segments contain atrophic tubules and thickened blood vessels, and glomeruli are either absent or exceedingly sparse (Fig. 39-4). Remnants of medulla are sometimes present, and microangiographic studies have shown that the hypoplastic segments often contain vascular patterns that indicate the presence of both cortex and medulla [49].

Many investigators have regarded the abnormality as congenital [38, 49], because the kidneys are small and because the abnormal cortical segments appear to lack glomeruli. This argument appears less than compelling, since similar changes could just as well result from acquired injury and secondary atrophy [8]. Current investigations into the renal effects of infantile vesicoureteral reflux suggest that many of these lesions may result from "reflux nephropathy." The frequency of demonstrable, anatomic abnormalities of the urinary tract, often with vesicoureteral reflux, is on the order of 20 percent [2, 71], perhaps higher, and females predominate by a large majority. Other causes of segmental renal scarring, for example local circulatory disturbances, must also be considered potential causative factors.

Clinical studies have been directed to the association of this lesion with hypertension [1, 23, 52, 71, 73]. The frequency of hypertension in any series depends on the basis of clinical selection: Series selected on morphologic grounds have shown a 50 percent incidence of hypertension [3], whereas other series consist principally of hypertensive patients. The cause of hypertension has remained in

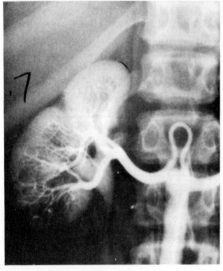
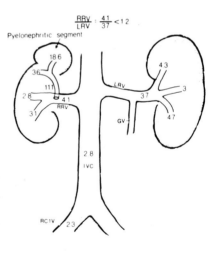

A   *B*

Figure 39-3. Segmental "hypoplasia." The patient was a 14-year-old girl with a history of recurrent urinary tract infection associated with vesicoureteric reflux. Her blood pressure was 200/150 mm Hg. A. Selective renal arteriogram demonstrates a lateral indentation corresponding to an area of scarring in the upper pole of the right kidney; the right kidney was 2 cm shorter than the left. The vascular pattern in the area of scarring appears to be partially obscured. B. Renin activity, determined by selective venous catheterization, was evaluated in the right upper pole as compared with other areas of both kidneys. The patient underwent resection of the right upper pole, which appeared to be scarred and contracted; microscopic examination revealed chronic inflammation. (Illustration provided by Dr. N. Javadpour, National Institutes of Health. From N. Javadpour et al. Segmental vein renin assay and segmental nephrectomy for correction of renal hypertension. J. Urol. 115:580, 1976. Copyright © 1976 by The Williams & Wilkins Co., Baltimore.)

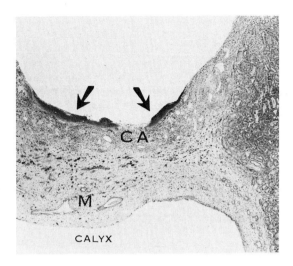

Figure 39-4. Segmental hypoplasia. Photomicrograph showing resected renal segment in an 11-year-old girl with hypertension. The cortex is indented (arrows). There are marked cortical attenuation (CA) and flattening of the medulla (M) in an area of atrophy. The involved segment contains atrophic tubules and occasional hyalinized glomeruli. The elongated calyceal recess is below it. The adjacent cortex contains normal tubules and glomeruli. (Trichrome, ×28 before 35% reduction.) (Specimen provided by Drs. C. Sotelo-Avila and B. S. Arant, Le Bonheur Children's Hospital, Memphis, Tennessee.)

doubt, partly because determinations of plasma renin have shown inconstant results [32]. Since hypersecretion of renin may be segmental (Fig. 39-3B), hyperreninemia may be missed in sampling from the main renal vein [41]. Hyperplasia of the juxtaglomerular apparatus in adjacent normal kidney has also been variable—at times inapparent [71], at times obvious [52], and at times demonstrable by cell count [32]. The hypoplastic segment contains neither intact glomeruli nor obvious juxtaglomerular cells, putting in question its ability to secrete renin, even though segmental nephrectomy has resulted in amelioration of the hypertension.

Urinalyses are negative in the absence of infection and hypertension. In the hypertensive child, the urine contains abnormal amounts of protein and red blood cells. Renal function varies from normal to severely reduced, depending on the degree of damage secondary to hypertension and infection. Excretory urography shows small, irregularly shaped kidneys with distorted calyces, and discrete areas of segmental scarring have been demonstrated by selective renal arteriography (Fig. 39-3A). Other clinical manifestations include infection and lithiasis [2], for which nephrectomy is also indicated [68]. The clinical aspects and medi-

cal management of hypertension are similar to those discussed elsewhere (Chap. 32). Pharmacologic control of hypertension may be exceedingly difficult, in which case surgical removal of the kidney or of the abnormal segment is necessary. Therapeutic failures may have been related to bilaterality of the lesion [8], which is relatively common, to multiple areas of involvement, and perhaps to secondary hypertensive vascular lesions in the kidneys that perpetuate the hypertension [38].

BILATERAL HYPOPLASIA

Bilateral renal hypoplasia is said to be the fourth most common cause of chronic renal failure in childhood, accounting for 20 percent of cases [13]. Two types have been observed: (1) simple hypoplasia [8], with histologically normal parenchyma, and (2) oligomeganephronia [72], with marked hypertrophy of individual nephrons. The kidneys in both types are, by definition, smaller in size and weight than normal, more markedly so in oligomeganephronia. The number of calyces and of renal pyramids are variably reduced in both types. Oligomeganephronia has been recognized as a clinicopathologic entity only within the last two decades [72]; cases reported earlier in the literature were designated as chronic nephritis because of the presence of secondary, atrophic glomerular and tubular changes [34]. The diagnosis of simple hypoplasia depends on a statistical concept of renal growth in childhood, and few cases have been recognized.

Simple Hypoplasia

Simple hypoplasia without dysplasia or nephronic hypertrophy, has been only rarely described [8, 11]. Clinical manifestations have included problems in salt and water metabolism, with difficulty in maintaining a state of adequate hydration and in conserving cations, particularly in the face of extrarenal disease or water deprivation. Patients also present with other evidence of tubular insufficiency, such as renal tubular acidosis [22] and refractory hypokalemia. Renal function may be moderately to severely reduced.

Despite the infrequency of clinically apparent cases, small kidneys are found in approximately 2.5 percent of pediatric autopsies [74]. Retrospective evaluation has shown that approximately 80 percent of autopsied children with kidney weights in the lowest 5 percent of the population also had anomalies or long-standing disease of the central nervous system. A similar association has been noted in histologic studies demonstrating that glomeruli and tubules in mentally defective children are smaller than normal [69]. A few patients with small kidneys had on retrospective evaluation circumstantial clinical evidence of renal impairment: dehydration, despite treatment or without apparent cause, and hyposthenuria [11]. Most of these children were also small for their ages, and a considerable number had been born prematurely. In many instances, microscopic examination disclosed focal tubular degeneration and disruption, with focal cortical scarring. The problem has not, however, been evaluated systematically or critically, and, except for the case with obvious renal functional impairment, clinical correlations are lacking.

Oligomeganephronia

Oligomeganephronia is more common than simple hypoplasia and is more easily recognized. The kidneys are extremely small and often contain an irregularly reduced number of lobes, sometimes only one or two pyramids [8]. Renal weight in middle childhood may be as little as 20 gm [70]. The number of nephrons has been estimated at approximately one-fifth of normal, and the individual nephrons are remarkably hypertrophied (Fig. 39-5), thereby accounting for the unusual, but generally accepted name of the condition. Measurements of glomeruli have shown an increase to approximately twice normal diameter, with a twelvefold increase in volume [25]. A more striking degree of enlargement takes place in the tubules, which seem in histologic sections to be cystic and which undergo a fourfold increase in length with a seventeenfold increase in proximal tubular volume [25]. The proximal convoluted tubules have been shown by microdissection to contain numerous diverticula [25]. As the result of tubular enlargement, the glomeruli in histologic sections appear to be unduly separated and scant [70]. Ultrastructural studies have shown thickening of the basement membrane and glomerular mesangial hypercellularity [20, 55]. The juxtaglomerular complexes are often prominent and enlarged, perhaps as a response to salt and water loss. Hypertension is uncommon.

The cause of oligomeganephronia is not known. It appears not to be hereditary and is rarely familial. It occurs usually as an isolated malformation, and other abnormalities of the urinary tract are only occasionally present, for example, ureteropelvic stricture and vesicoureteral reflux [14, 27]. Maternal abnormalities have not been identified, except that newborns with the condition are often of low birth weight [70]. The pathogenesis of oligomeganephronia may be related to hypertrophy of individual nephrons in compensation for a nephronic deficit. It does not occur unilaterally, except in solitary kidneys [36, 81].

Oligomeganephronia occurs more commonly in

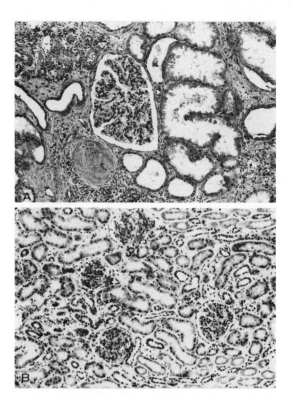

Figure 39-5. Oligomeganephronia. A. Kidney from a 12-year-old boy with renal failure. His kidneys appeared small on radiographic examination, and on bilateral nephrectomy in preparation for renal transplantation they weighed approximately 45 gm apiece. As shown, histopathologic examination disclosed extremely large glomeruli and large dilated tubules, with patchy tubular atrophy, focal glomerular obsolescence, and patchy cortical fibrosis. B. A normal kidney for comparison of glomerular and tubular size taken from a 13-year-old boy who died of a head injury following an automobile accident. (H&E, both at magnification ×120 before 44% reduction.) (Specimen provided by Drs. Chung-Ho Chang and A. Joseph Brough, Children's Hospital of Michigan.)

males than females, in a ratio of approximately 3 : 1. The principal manifestations, affecting almost all children, are polyuria and severe polydypsia, usually beginning within the first 2 years of life. The urinary specific gravity is customarily less than 1.012. The defect in urinary concentration is associated with a defect in sodium resorption, and the two abnormalities persist throughout life. Patients suffer from hyperchloremic metabolic acidosis [70]. Ammonia secretion is said to be impaired [75], although it may be normal when corrected for glomerular filtration rate [70]. Moderate proteinuria is usually present early in the disease, although it is rarely, if ever, of sufficient severity to cause the nephrotic syndrome. Excretion of cellular elements is normal until late in the course. Glomerular function also is impaired, remaining relatively stable in a state of moderately severe azotemia in early childhood and progressing ultimately to chronic renal insufficiency in late childhood. Early in the course there usually is sufficient function for radiographic visualization of the urinary system and for the evaluation of associated urinary tract malformations.

Young children suffer from frequent episodes of dehydration and unexplained fever, vomiting, anorexia, diarrhea, and failure to thrive. All children suffer from growth retardation, and renal rickets is seen as a late complication in the stage of renal failure. Most patients remain normotensive.

The condition undergoes a natural evolution to terminal renal insufficiency over a period of 10 to 12 years [72]. A major factor in the evolution may be progressive renal damage. Morphologic studies have shown progressive glomerular sclerosis, tubular atrophy, and interstitial fibrosis (see Fig. 39-5), a situation similar to that observed in experimental forms of severe renal reduction.

The differential diagnosis includes renal dysplasia and familial juvenile nephronophthisis (Chap. 42). Dysplasia is commonly associated with abnormalities of the lower urinary tract and with earlier deterioration of renal function. Nephronophthisis, which, like oligomeganephronia, is characterized by a concentrating defect and mild proteinuria, may be associated with more rapid deterioration of renal function and earlier onset of terminal renal failure. It is characterized also by anemia out of proportion to renal functional impairment. A familial incidence is common.

Treatment early in the course includes maintenance of fluid and electrolytye balance and correction of acidosis. Other therapeutic measures include maintenance of nutrition and correction of anemia. Management of the terminal stages follows the principles usually employed in treating chronic renal insufficiency. Affected children are regarded as excellent candidates for renal transplantation, since other anomalies are rare and since the slow progression of the disease allows survival into the second and third decades of life.

Renal Dysplasia

Abnormalities of metanephric development, with altered structural organization and abnormal nephronic and ductal differentiation, are known collectively as renal dysplasia [8, 21, 51, 65]. A distinction is made, as previously noted, between dysplasia and hypoplasia, although the two abnormalities often coexist. Dysplasia is also a different abnor-

mality than polycystic disease, even though dysplastic kidneys are often cystic.

Renal dysplasia is not a single, specific malformation, but rather a group of malformations with varying degrees of structural and functional impairment [6, 8, 65, 66]. Affected kidneys may be solid or cystic, large or small, and reniform or misshapen. Their capacity to excrete urine and to function is variable, depending in part on the severity of maldevelopment and in part on the severity of accompanying urinary tract malformation. Renal dysplasia is associated with other abnormalities of the ureters, bladder, and urethra with a frequency of approximately 90 percent [74], an association that appears to be of importance in its pathogenesis.

MORPHOLOGY AND PATHOGENESIS

The definition of renal dysplasia as an abnormality of development depends on certain histologic features, which serve also as diagnostic criteria [8, 21, 51]. Histologic examination of a typically dysplastic kidney (Fig. 39-6) discloses a degree of structural disorganization involving the cortex, the medulla, or both. The normal structural organization of the kidney includes its lobar configuration, the differentiation of medullary pyramids, and the development of certain structural interrelations among nephrons, ducts, and blood vessels. The integrity of these anatomic arrangements is presumably requisite to normal renal function. Abnormal nephronic and ductal differentiation in renal dysplasia may result from a developmental arrest, but it must be emphasized that the abnormalities do not correspond simply to early stages of normal development, and that dysplasia is not simply a retention of fetal form. Abnormalities of differentiation involve (1) the collecting system, in which the columnar epithelium remains undifferentiated and around which the connective tissue becomes fibromuscular to form *primitive ducts,* and (2) the mesenchymal metanephric blastema, in which altered cellular differentiation leads to *cartilaginous metaplasia.* Primitive ducts are found in both cortex and medulla, but are more numerous and prominent in the latter, where they are associated with excessive connective tissue, diminished tubules, and diminished blood vessels, a condition known as *deltalike medulla* [51]. The medulla may be incompletely differentiated from the surrounding pelvic mesenchyme, with concomitant calyceal underdevelopment. Columnar epithelium sometimes undergoes squamous metaplasia, and primitive ducts frequently undergo cystic dilatation, both as phenomena apparently coincidental to the dysplastic state. Metaplastic cartilage, as a deriva-

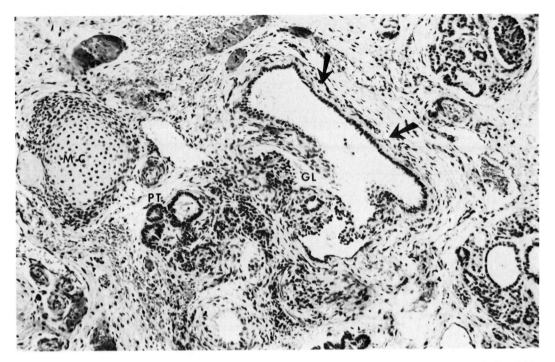

Figure 39-6. Renal dysplasia. Cortical structures are abnormal and in disarray. Clusters of tubules (PT) are lined by poorly differentiated "primitive" epithelium, and a cortical ductule is surrounded by a rim of fibromuscular tissue (arrows). The glomeruli (GL) have an immature appearance. Metaplastic cartilage (MC) represents abnormally differentiated, metanephric blastema. (H&E, ×150 before 14% reduction.)

tive of metanephric blastema, lies principally in the cortex, and the cartilaginous nests occasionally become ossified. Dysplastic kidneys also contain incompletely differentiated and immature glomeruli and tubules, which are frequently designated "primitive."

The histologic features of dysplastic kidneys have been subject to varying interpetation. Primitive ducts and cartilage are regarded as evidence of abnormal renal morphogenesis [8, 21, 65]. Immature, poorly differentiated, or "primitive" glomeruli, tubules, and cortical ductules, on the other hand, can almost certainly result from postnatal influences and cannot be regarded as sufficient or necessary evidence of renal maldevelopment. The evidence for this statement is circumstantial, but studies of renal injury in both clinical material and experimental animals have demonstrated that similarly altered structures can be induced by a number of agents, including urinary tract obstruction, ischemic injury, and local trauma [8]. The changes thus produced may constitute arrested development, but they appear to be predominantly retrogressive changes within previously normal nephrons. It has been speculated that cartilage is also a response to acquired inflammation and renal injury

[80]—perhaps, but metaplastic cartilage has not been demonstrated in experimentally damaged neonatal kidneys, indicating that it is an earlier response of undifferentiated mesenchyme [83]. Its presence in hydronephrotic or in severely inflamed kidneys would seem ·to be evidence of associated maldevelopment, and its presence in otherwise histologically normal kidneys, as observed occasionally in trisomy syndromes and rarely in normal subjects, would seem also to constitute evidence of focal metanephric maldevelopment. Dysplasia is neither the result nor the cause of chronic pyelonephritis—although the dysplastic kidney may be more susceptible to chronic infection—and inflammation develops only in those dysplastic kidneys with patent ureters and secondary urinary stasis or reflux [65].

Morphologic studies of dysplastic kidneys show several discernible patterns [6, 8, 65, 67]. All kidneys contain some evidence of corticomedullary differentiation. The nephronic structures (glomeruli and tubules) are often sparse, but metanephric tissue, no matter how rudimentary, is closely associated with primitive ducts in a manner resembling the relationship of cortex to medulla. The arrangement of ducts is often radial, demonstrating their origins in the branching collecting system. Almost all dysplastic kidneys contain atrophic and cystic, ductular, and nephronic elements in admixture with primitive and abnormally differentiated elements. The histologic similarities among them preclude sharp distinctions, and the admixture of overlapping forms has been interpreted as evidence that nephrogenesis continues, despite its alteration. The agent responsible for the abnormality must therefore act over a period of time. Furthermore, the commonly more severe involvement of the outer cortex suggests that the responsible agent becomes operative after the formation of the inner cortex and presumably after it has begun to excrete urine. The agent that seems most realistically to fulfill this role is urinary tract obstruction, which affects the kidney from the earliest secretion of urine through later stages of development.

The very frequent association of renal dysplasia with other abnormalities of the urinary tract is of significance because of the obstructive nature of most such anomalies. In a general sort of way, the more severe the obstruction, the more severe the dysplasia: Ureteropelvic occlusion is associated with severely deformed, multicystic kidneys; severe infravesical obstruction due to posterior urethral valves is associated with peripheral cortical dysplasia, whereas mild infravesical obstruction is rarely associated with dysplasia. Unilateral ureteral anomalies are associated with ipsilateral dysplasia and lower urinary tract anomalies with bilateral dysplasia. Segmental dysplasia in duplex kidneys relates to the obstruction of one of the two ureters by an ectopic ureterocele. These associations may be coincidental and may result from widespread abnormalities in urinary tract development, but they seem more likely to be causally related and to indicate that renal dysplasia is for the most part initiated by external factors during nephrogenesis.

However, not all renal dysplasia occurs in association with urinary tract obstruction. The most consistent examples of nonassociation are seen in heritable syndromes of multiple malformation [7], e.g., cystic dysplasia in the Meckel syndrome of posterior encephalocele, polydactyly, and cleft palate and lip. Medullary dysplasia associated with the Beckwith-Wiedemann syndrome of hyperplastic visceromegaly also occurs independently of urinary tract obstruction. Although there are exceptions to the rule, the association of dysplasia and urinary tract obstruction is a strong one, and the patterns of malformation in relationship to the types of obstruction indicate that the latter are of pathogenetic importance.

The classification of renal dysplasia is to a large degree descriptive. It may be divided into several broad clinicopathologic categories, but many specimens are still unclassifiable.

CLINICAL FORMS OF DYSPLASIA

Obstructive Renal Dysplasia

The patterns of dysplasia that occur in association with lower urinary tract obstruction constitute a major portion of the evidence that the altered renal development is secondary. Normal renal morphogenesis is partially dependent on the excretion of fluid by the developing kidney. Development of the pelvis and calyces and their transformation from branches of the ureteric bud depend on fluid pressure. In addition, nephrogenesis at the periphery of the kidney continues, even while nephrons in deeper portions of the cortex are producing urine. Abnormally increased hydrostatic or back pressure, whether from urinary stasis or reflux, leads to abnormal ductal growth and altered nephronic induction. The peripheral cortex often becomes cystic (Fig. 39-7), and microdissection studies have demonstrated distention of primitive subcapsular nephrons and of the terminal portions of the collecting tubules [63]. The medullary pyramids are often poorly differentiated from surrounding pelvic connective tissue, and they contain primitive ducts surrounded by increased fibrous tissue, a condition that, as noted, has been referred to as delta-like medulla [51].

Any form of congenital urinary tract obstruction may be associated with renal dysplasia. The renal lesion has been seen in association with the prune-belly syndrome, with vesical dysfunction due to spina bifida and meningomyelocele, with anterior urethral diverticulum, and with ectopic ureterocele [28, 57, 62, 66]. It is most common in male infants suffering from severe valvular obstruction of the posterior urethra [64] (Fig. 39-8); less severe valvular obstruction that remains clinically inapparent until later childhood is rarely associated with dysplasia. Renal dysplasia may be related to the concomitant presence of vesicoureteral reflux [17], which can be asymmetrical and can, therefore, account for the frequent asymmetry of the renal lesion.

The clinical significance of renal dysplasia lies in the reduced functional capacity of affected kidneys even after surgical correction of the urinary tract anomaly. Severe degrees of dysplasia may be associated with complete nonfunction, and milder degrees possibly increase susceptibility to bacterial infection. The kidneys are poorly visualized by excretory urography; the cystic abnormalities are probably too small to be visualized by sonography. The dysplastic kidneys are not always hydroneph-

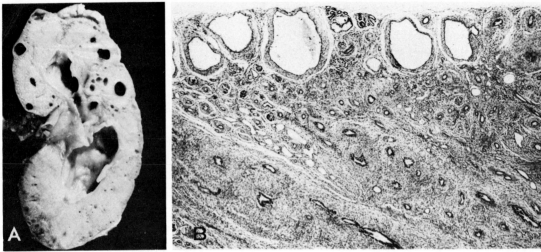

Figure 39-7. *Obstructive renal dysplasia. A. The kidney in a case of posterior urethral valves is moderately hydronephrotic. A line of cysts beneath the capsule and along the columns of Bertin represents peripheral cortical dysplasia. B. Microscopic examination of the renal tissue in a case of congenital urethral atresia discloses severe dysplasia with primitive ducts in the medulla and cysts in the peripheral cortex, both derived from collecting ducts. The inner cortex, lying between the two, is very narrow and contains irregularly sclerotic glomeruli and atrophic tubules. (H&E, ×30.)*

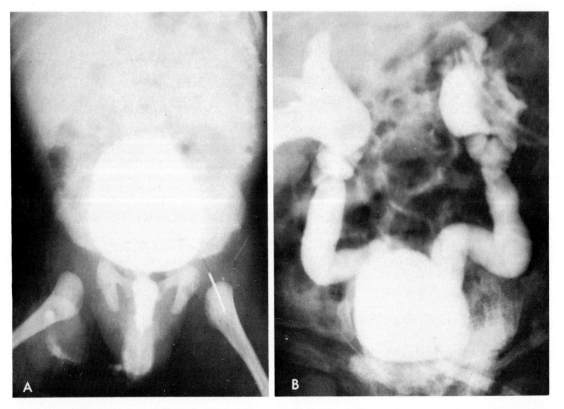

Figure 39-8. *Posterior urethral valve. A 2-week-old infant had palpable flank masses and a palpable suprapubic mass. Excretory urography disclosed poor visualization. A. A voiding film with a small catheter in the bladder demonstrated marked dilatation of the posterior urethra. B. Retrograde studies, carried out through a cystostomy, demonstrated bilateral hydronephrosis and bilateral hydroureter with marked redundancy. (Figure 39-8B from J. Bernstein. Renal Abnormalities in the Newborn. In H. L. Barnett [ed.], Pediatrics [15th ed.], 1972. Courtesy of Appleton-Century-Crofts Division of Prentice-Hall, Inc.)*

rotic; this variability presumably is due to variation in functional capacity and urinary output. Treatment is directed first toward relieving the obstruction and second toward preventing infection.

Multicystic and Aplastic Dysplasia

The terms *multicystic* [78] and *aplastic* [56] are applied to severely malformed kidneys that lack normal pyelocaliceal development. The usual lobar organization is frequently in disarray, and metanephric differentiation may be sparse or rudimentary. Both types of kidney are similar in structure, differing principally in the degree of cyst formation. Multicystic kidneys characteristically are enlarged and distorted by numerous cysts (Fig. 39-9); aplastic kidneys characteristically are small and solid. The typical forms of each can conveniently be regarded as the opposite ends of a spectrum that encompasses degrees of cyst formation. The usual lobar disorganization is often more apparent in multicystic kidneys than in aplastic kidneys, suggesting that the cysts contribute to apparent disorganization by distorting the structural relationships. Nonetheless, some evidence of metanephric differentiation is present [8, 82], and microangiographic studies have shown that corticomedullary differentiation is also present in altered form [48].

Both types of malformation are nonfunctioning and are characteristically associated with ureteropelvic occlusion. The significance of the obstruction in relation to renal dysplasia has been disputed. The combination might constitute a total maldevelopment of the urinary system, or it might, as indicated herein, reflect a causal relationship. The state of the ureter accompanying the multicystic kidney is the subject of mild disagreement in the literature, a confusion that results from frequent, loose application of the term *multicystic* in a descriptive way to several different forms of renal cystic disease. The multicystic kidney has, in the author's experience, been invariably associated with

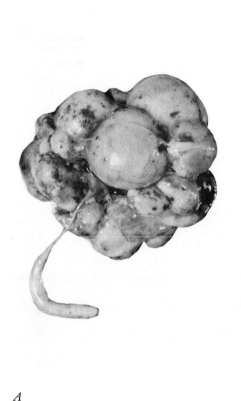

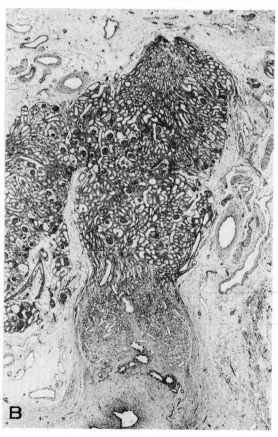

A

B

Figure 39-9. Unilateral multicystic dysplasia. A. The kidney is enlarged and grossly cystic, with sufficient irregularity in the size and arrangement of the cysts to obscure the usual reniform configuration. The ureter is atretic, and there is pyelocalyceal occlusion. B. Microscopic section shows that the septa among the cysts contain rudimentary lobules of metanephric tissue, in which glomeruli and tubules form a cap of metanephric tissue around a cluster of primitive ducts that correspond to medulla. (H&E, ×25.)

ureteropelvic atresia or ureteral absence. The occasional specimen with ureteral occlusion and pelvic patency [24] may constitute a subgroup, but its anatomic features have not been completely defined. The aplastic kidney is also often associated with ureteral atresia, and evaluation of this point is also hindered by imprecision and inconsistency of terminology and criteria. Part of the problem lies in separating aplastic kidneys from milder forms of dysplasia that allow for some functional capacity. Many small, dysplastic kidneys have patent pelves and ureters and show morphologic and radiographic evidence of excretory activity [6, 8]. The distinction between aplasia and milder dysplasia is conceptually simple and can be stated in terms of function versus nonfunction, but the application of this distinction in practice is more difficult. Extremely small kidneys with patent pelves and ureters show more clinical and radiographic evidence of excretory function than do larger kidneys with occluded pelves and ureters. Clinical studies [15, 37] of dysplasia obviously have been based on functioning kidneys with variable impairment and variable survival. The occurrence of morphologically intermediate and indeterminate forms that are still not classifiable makes it impossible to define strict categories [67].

Both aplastic and multicystic kidneys may be unilateral or bilateral. Bilateral multicystic dysplasia is probably the most common form of bilateral cystic disease in newborns. It is a lethal malformation and is associated with the intrauterine consequences of diminished urinary output and oligohydramnios [42], signs of which include amnion nodosum and Potter facies. Bilateral involvement is not necessarily symmetrical; one kidney can be large and cystic and the other small and solid.

Unilateral aplasia usually goes undetected until urologic evaluation leads to the demonstration of unilateral nonfunction. The aplastic kidney is said to be susceptible to chronic infection, but morphologic evidence of chronic inflammation is limited to those malformations with patent urinary tracts [65]. Hypertension is also said to be a serious complication. Symptoms include flank pain, urinary frequency, dysuria, and vague constitutional complaints, all of which could be related to infection and lithiasis. Critical evaluation of these clinical features has been hampered by the lack of precise criteria of morphologic and clinical diagnosis. Symptoms may also be related to contralateral abnormalities and vesicoureteral reflux.

Clinical recognition of unilateral multicystic dysplasia is earlier and more common than recognition of unilateral aplastic dysplasia, principally because the enlarged cystic kidney is palpable as a flank mass and has been recognized as a clinicopathologic entity [76]. It occurs more commonly on the left than on the right and slightly more often in males than in females. Because smaller masses go unnoticed in infants, the abnormality can persist into adult life. Older patients complain of pressure, abdominal or flank pain, and vague intestinal disorders. Both the aplastic and multicystic forms of dysplasia undergo progressive sclerosis, and cyst walls frequently become calcified. Hypertension is rare in childhood, having been described in one case in which an unusually severe degree of glomerular obsolescence and tubular atrophy was seen in the solid portions of the specimen [40]. Urinalysis is negative.

Radiography in infants reveals large masses that do not opacify on excretory urography. High-dose urography (total body opacification) may result in opacification of cyst walls [47, 58] (Fig. 39-10), and retention and puddling of contrast medium may be seen in delayed roentgenograms [87]. Septal opacification, when present, might be ex-

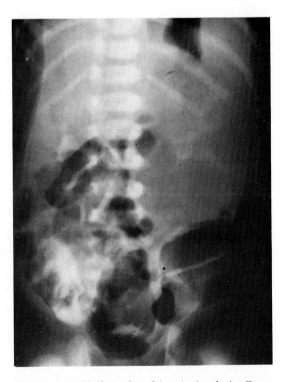

Figure 39-10. Unilateral multicystic dysplasia. Excretory urogram of an infant with a large flank mass discloses an irregularly septated mass in which there are cystic lucencies. The surgical specimen had the typical appearance of a multicystic kidney, and the proximal ureter was absent. (Roentgenogram provided by Dr. Walter E. Berdon, Columbia-Presbyterian Medical Center.)

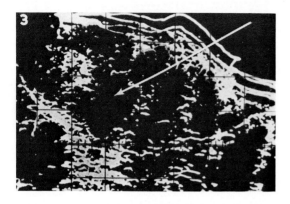

Figure 39-11. Unilateral multicystic disease. Ultrasonic scan of a kidney demonstrates a septated structure containing large cysts (arrow). (Illustration provided by Dr. Roger C. Sanders, Johns Hopkins Medical Institutions. From S. B. Bearman, P. L. Hine, and R. C. Sanders, Radiology 118:685, 1976.)

plained by the concentration of contrast medium in rudimentary metanephric lobules within the solid areas of the kidney. The renal artery is exceedingly hypoplastic and is usually not visualized by aortography [45]. Ultrasound scans demonstrate septated, cystic masses [4] (Fig. 39-11). Excretory urography in older patients also discloses unilateral nonfunction and occasional eggshell calcification of cyst walls [45].

The differential diagnosis of large, multicystic kidneys in young infants includes giant hydronephrosis (Fig. 39-12), which may be differentiated by sonography. Congenital Wilms' tumors, mesoblastic nephromas, and multilocular cystomas enter the differential diagnosis; they can usually be recognized by excretory urography and by their characteristic arteriographic appearances. Renal venous and arterial thrombosis causes renal enlargement and nonfunction, usually with hematuria. The differential diagnosis in older patients includes unilateral agenesis, a distinction that has no clinical implications, except possibly for hypertension.

Treatment of most cases in children has been surgical because of the theoretical danger of hypertension, the difficulty of differentiating masses from tumors, and unsupported speculation about potential malignant degeneration. The prognosis in both types of dysplasia depends on the state of the opposite kidney, which commonly undergoes compensatory hypertrophy, and of its ureter. A high incidence of contralateral abnormalities, including renal and ureteral ectopia and ureteral reflux, has been reported in some studies of multicystic kidney [35, 61], but patients identified clinically in childhood as having unilateral masses seem to have an excellent prognosis [58, 86]. Complete clinical and urographic evaluations are clearly indicated. It

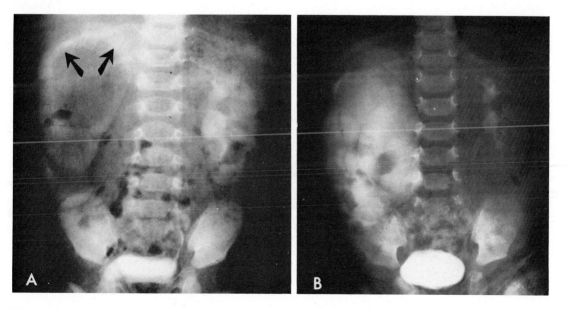

Figure 39-12. Giant congenital hydronephrosis. Excretory urography in a newborn infant with a unilateral mass shows (A) early (5 min) opacification of a parenchymal rim or crescent (arrows) surrounding a dilated pelvis and (B) subsequent (2 hr) filling of an irregularly outlined and dilated pelvis, secondary to ureteropelvic obstruction. (Roentgenograms provided by Dr. Walter E. Berdon, Columbia-Presbyterian Medical Center.)

seems certain, however, that unilateral dysplasia, whether solid or cystic, is not a progressive disorder that will eventually involve the other side.

General and Hereditary Cystic Dysplasia

A diffusely cystic form of renal dysplasia, unassociated with urinary tract obstruction, exists as a separate entity. The kidneys are enlarged and spongy, leading to confusion with polycystic disease, but histologic examination shows dysplastic structures and provides the basis for the distinction.

Cystic dysplasia occurs only occasionally as an isolated malformation, and then it is typically sporadic, without a family history of the disease. The rare instance of familial involvement has seemed to follow an autosomal recessive inheritance [15]. The degree of renal maldevelopment has been variable, with some affected kidneys apparently capable of supporting life and others associated with early neonatal death. The most severe examples have been enlarged and diffusely cystic, consisting almost entirely of dilated ductal elements with exceedingly scanty nephronic differentiation. Infants with very severe cystic dysplasia and enlarged kidneys have suffered from neonatal respiratory distress due to pulmonary hypoplasia and from early postnatal renal insufficiency.

Diffuse cystic dysplasia occurs more often in association with malformations of other organ systems. A particularly striking example is in the Meckel syndrome of microcephaly and posterior encephalocele [9]. The kidneys are usually large, sometimes large enough to cause fetal dystocia, although small kidneys have also been described [53, 60]. The cysts arise in dilated primitive ducts that represent branches of the collecting system, and nephrons are exceedingly sparse (Fig. 39-13). Thus, there appears to have been a remarkable defect in metanephric differentiation, despite the large size of the kidneys and the apparent development of a branched collecting system. Similar renal lesions have been described with other malformations of the central nervous system, for example, hydrocephalus [77] and anencephaly [29]; these abnormalities have been regarded as part of the spectrum of the Meckel syndrome. Still other patients have had apparently unrelated cerebral malformations [33, 54], thought to differ from those in the Meckel syndrome, but the similarity of renal malformations tempts one to suggest that these variations have at least a common, unifying thread [3]. Infants with the Meckel syndrome die shortly after birth, and their kidneys appear to be nonfunctional.

Cystic dysplasia occurs occasionally in certain other syndromes, notably the Jeune syndrome (asphyxiating thoracic dysplasia) and the Zellweger cerebrohepatorenal syndrome [9]. These associations have been confused by the frequent presence of small, scattered cortical cysts in the same syndromes [7]. The cysts, which may be accompanied by both involutional and proliferative epithelial changes, affect glomeruli, convoluted tubules, and collecting tubules. They appear morphologically to be trifling, and they have no functional significance. Cystic abnormalities in the Zellweger syndrome may, however, occasionally be sufficiently severe to affect the kidney in a form of diffuse dysplasia. The renal malformations have been overshadowed by other clinical features of the syndrome. Affected children have had mild azotemia and poor excretion of urographic contrast medium. The Jeune syndrome seems occasionally to include

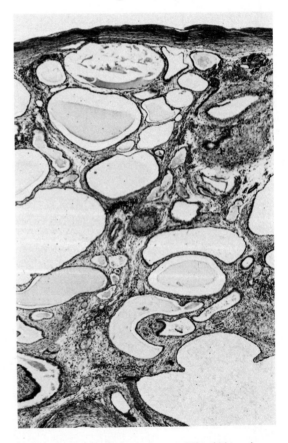

Figure 39-13. Meckel syndrome. The kidney is enlarged and irregularly cystic, although the reniform configuration is frequently preserved. The cysts are formed from dilated, abnormally differentiated collecting ducts, and there is an extraordinary deficiency of metanephric derivatives (glomeruli and convoluted tubules) within the cortex. (H&E, ×48.)

cystic dysplasia as part of a spectrum of tubular abnormality varying from trifling, focal, cystic degeneration at one end to diffuse cystic dysplasia at the other. Clinicopathologic correlations are confused further by the occurrence in the Jeune syndrome of a nephropathy comprising tubular dysfunction, cortical fibrosis, progressive glomerular obsolescence, and eventual renal failure. Common to all the renal manifestations in the Jeune syndrome are tubular damage and dysfunction with what appears to be secondary glomerular involvement. The variation in morphologic appearances may conceivably be related to a single metabolic abnormality which, when severe enough, interferes with nephronic development, resulting in cystic dysplasia, and which, when less severe, causes progressive tubular damage and the pattern of hereditary nephropathy [9]. The renal variants of these two syndromes might also result from genetic heterogeneity.

Noncystic medullary dysplasia has been observed in the Beckwith-Wiedemann syndrome of omphalocele, macroglossia, and hyperplastic visceromegaly [79]. Its functional implications are not known. The kidneys, which are larger than normal, contain a subcapsular zone of blastema and immature nephrons that persists well beyond the normal cessation of nephrogenesis; nephroblastomas are relatively common complications.

The renal lesion in some syndromes has been difficult to evaluate; in association with familial optic atrophy, for example, it appears more likely to be a form of hereditary nephropathy than dysplasia. The terminology and classification are limited by extreme variability in the severity of renal involvement, by the common practice of designating almost all cystic lesions as "polycystic disease," and by the use of the term *dysplasia* to encompass hereditary nephropathies. As a consequence, little can be said about functional and clinical correlations.

References

1. Ask-Upmark, E. Über juvenile maligne Nephrosklerose und ihr Verhaltnis zu Störungen in der Nierenentwicklung. *Acta Pathol. Microbiol. Scand.* 6:383, 1929.
2. Batzenschlager, A., Weill-Bousson, M., and Guerbaoui, M. L'hypoplasie segmentaire aglomérulaire du rein. I. Lésions rénales associées. *Sem. Hop. Paris* 50:601, 1974.
3. Batzenschlager, A., Weill-Bousson, M., and Guerbaoui, M. L'hypoplasie segmentaire aglomérulaire du rein. II. Complication hypertensive et résultats de la néphrectomie. *Sem. Hop. Paris* 50:609, 1974.
4. Bearman, S. B., Hine, P. L., and Sanders, R. C. Multicystic kidney: A sonographic pattern. *Radiology* 118:685, 1976.
5. Bengtsson, C., and Hood, B. The unilateral small kidney with special reference to the hypoplastic kidney. Review of the literature and authors' points of view. *Int. Urol. Nephrol.* 3:337, 1971.
6. Bernstein, J. The morphogenesis of renal parenchymal maldevelopment (renal dysplasia). *Pediatr. Clin. North Am.* 18:395, 1971.
7. Bernstein, J. Familial Renal Dysplasia and Renal Abnormalities Associated with Malformation Syndromes. In M. I. Rubin and T. M. Barratt (eds.), *Pediatric Nephrology*. Baltimore: Williams & Wilkins, 1975. P. 356.
8. Bernstein, J. Developmental Abnormalities of the Renal Parenchyma—Renal Hypoplasia and Dysplasia. In S. C. Sommers (ed.), *Kidney Pathology Decennial 1966–1975*. New York: Appleton-Century-Crofts, 1976. P. 1.
9. Bernstein, J., Brough, A. J., and McAdams, A. J. The Renal Lesions in Syndromes of Multiple Congenital Malformations. Cerebrohepatorenal Syndrome; Jeune's Asphyxiating Thoracic Dystrophy; Tuberous Sclerosis; Meckel's Syndrome. In D. Bergsma (ed.), *Birth Defects: Original Article Series*. New York: The National Foundation, 1974. Vol. X/4, p. 35.
10. Bernstein, J., and Kissane, J. M. Hereditary Disorders of the Kidney. In H. S. Rosenberg and R. P. Bolande (eds.), *Perspectives in Pediatric Pathology*. Chicago: Year Book, 1973. Vol. 1, p. 117.
11. Bernstein, J., and Meyer, R. Some speculations on the nature and significance of developmentally small kidneys (renal hypoplasia). *Nephron* 1:137, 1964.
12. Bois, E., Feingold, J., Benmaiz, H., and Briard, M. L. Congenital urinary tract malformations: Epidemiologic and genetic aspects. *Clin. Genet.* 8:37, 1975.
13. Broyer, M. Chronic Renal Failure. In P. Royer, R. Habib, H. Mathieu, M. Broyer, and A. Walsh (eds.), *Pediatric Nephrology*. Philadelphia: Saunders, 1974. P. 360.
14. Carter, J. E., and Lirenman, D. S. Bilateral renal hypoplasia with oligomeganephronia. Oligomeganephronic renal hypoplasia. *Am. J. Dis. Child.* 120:537, 1970.
15. Cole, B. R., Kaufman, R. L., McAlister, W. H., and Kissane, J. M. Bilateral renal dysplasia in three siblings: Report of a survivor. *Clin. Nephrol.* 5:83, 1976.
16. Currarino, G., and Allen, T. D. Congenital anomalies of the upper urinary tracts. *Prog. Pediatr. Radiol.* 3:179, 1970.
17. Cussen, J. J. Cystic kidneys in children with congenital urethral obstruction. *J. Urol.* 106:939, 1971.
18. Dein, R. W., Walker, D., and Hackett, R. L. The Ask-Upmark kidney: A case report. *Arch. Pathol.* 96:10, 1973.
19. Ekström, T. Renal hypoplasia. A clinical study of 179 cases. *Acta Chir. Scand.* [Suppl.] 203, 1955.
20. Elfenbein, I. B., Baluarte, H. J., and Gruskin, A. B. Renal hypoplasia with oligomeganephronia. Light, electron, fluorescent microscopic and quantitative studies. *Arch. Pathol.* 97:143, 1974.
21. Ericsson, N. O., and Ivemark, B. I. Renal dysplasia and pyelonephritis in infants and children. Part I; Part II. Primitive ductules and abnormal glomeruli. *Arch. Pathol.* 66:255, 264, 1958.
22. Fanconi, G., Calderali, E., Menano, H., and Cramer, R. Kongenitale Hypoplasie beider Nieren

mit Symptomen eines Morbus Cushing und eines Morbus Lightwood-Albright. *Helv. Paediatr. Acta* 7: 330, 1952.

23. Fay, R., Winer, R., Cohen, A., Brosman, S. A., and Bennett, C. Segmental renal hypoplasia and hypertension. *J. Urol.* 113:561, 1975.

24. Felson, B., and Cussen, L. J. The hydronephrotic type of unilateral congenital multicystic disease of the kidney. *Semin. Roentgenol.* 10:13, 1975.

25. Fetterman, G. H., and Habib, R. Congenital bilateral oligonephronic renal hypoplasia with hypertrophy of nephrons (oligoméganéphronie). Studies by microdissection. *Am. J. Clin. Pathol.* 52:199, 1969.

26. Fikri, E., Hanrahan, J. B., and Stept, L. A. Renovascular hypertension in a child: Ask-Upmark kidney. *J. Urol.* 110:728, 1973.

27. Fleischmann, L. E. Renal Agenesis and Hypoplasia. In M. I. Rubin, and T. M. Barratt (eds.), *Pediatric Nephrology.* Baltimore: Williams & Wilkins, 1975. P. 340.

28. Forbes, M. Renal dysplasia in infants with neurospinal dysraphism. *J. Pathol.* 107:13, 1972.

29. Fried, K., Liban, E., Lurie, M., Friedman, S., and Reisner, S. H. Polycystic kidneys associated with malformations of the brain, polydactyly, and other birth defects in newborn sibs. A lethal syndrome showing the autosomal-recessive pattern of inheritance. *J. Med. Genet.* 8:285, 1971.

30. Friedenberg, M. J., Walz, B. J., McAlister, W. H., Locksmith, J. P., and Gallagher, T. L. Roentgen size of normal kidneys. Computer analysis of 1,286 cases. *Radiology* 84:1022, 1965.

31. Gatewood, O. M. B., Glasser, R. J., and Vanhoutte, J. J. Roentgen evaluation of renal size in pediatric age groups. *Am. J. Dis. Child.* 110:162, 1965.

32. Godard, G., Vallotton, M. B., and Broyer, M. Plasma renin activity in segmental hypoplasia of the kidneys with hypertension. *Nephron* 11:308, 1973.

33. Goldston, A. S., Burke, E. C., D'Agostino, A., and McCaughey, W. T. C. Neonatal polycystic kidney with brain defect. *Am. J. Dis. Child.* 106:484, 1963.

34. Greene, C. H. Bilateral hypoplastic cystic kidneys. *Am. J. Dis. Child.* 24:1, 1922.

35. Greene, L. F., Feinzaig, W., and Dahlin, D. C. Multicystic dysplasia of the kidney, with special reference to the contralateral kidney. *J. Urol.* 105: 482, 1971.

36. Griffel, B., Pewzner, S., and Berandt, M. Unilateral "oligoméganéphronie" with agenesis of the contralateral kidney, studied by microdissection. *Virchows Arch. [Pathol. Anat.]* 357:179, 1972.

37. Gur, A., Siegel, N. J., Davis, C. A., Kashgarian, M., and Hayslett, J. P. Clinical aspects of bilateral renal dysplasia in children. *Nephron* 15:50, 1975.

38. Habib, R., Courtecuisse, V., Ehrensperger, J., and Royer, P. Hypoplasie segmentaire du rein avec hypertension artérielle chez l'enfant. *Ann. Pediatr. (Paris)* 12:262, 1965.

39. Hodgson, C. J., Drewe, J. A., Karn, M. N., and King, A. Renal size in normal children. *Arch. Dis. Child.* 37:616, 1962.

40. Javadpour, N., Chelouhy, E., Moncada, L., Rosenthal, I. M., and Bush, I. M. Hypertension in a child caused by a multicystic kidney. *J. Urol.* 104:918, 1970.

41. Javadpour, N., Doppman, J. L., Scardino, P. T., and Bartter, F. C. Segmental renal vein renin assay and

segmental nephrectomy for correction of renal hypertension. *J. Urol.* 115:580, 1976.

42. Johannessen, J. V., Haneberg, B., and Moe, P. J. Bilateral multicystic dysplasia of the kidneys. *Beitr. Pathol.* 148:290, 1973.

43. Kissane, J. M. Congenital Malformations. In R. H. Heptinstall (ed.), *Pathology of the Kidney.* Boston: Little, Brown, 1974. Vol. 1, chap. 3, p. 69.

44. Kravtzova, G. I., Lazjuk, G. I., and Lurie, I. W. The malformations of the urinary system in autosomal disorders. *Virchows Arch. [Pathol. Anat.]* 368:167, 1975.

45. Kyaw, M. M. Roentgenologic triad of congenital multicystic kidney. *Am. J. Roentgenol. Radium Ther. Nucl. Med.* 119:710, 1973.

46. Landing, B. H., and Hughes, M. L. Analysis of weight of kidneys in children. *Lab. Invest.* 11:452, 1962.

47. Leonidas, J. C., Strauss, L., and Krasna, I. H. Roentgen diagnosis of multicystic renal dysplasia in infancy by high dose urography. *J. Urol.* 108:936, 1972.

48. Ljungqvist, A. Arterial vasculature of the multicystic dysplastic kidney: A micro-angiographical and histological study. *Acta Pathol. Microbiol. Scand.* 64: 309, 1965.

49. Ljungqvist, A., and Lagergren, C. The Ask-Upmark kidney. A congenital renal anomaly studied by microangiography and histology. *Acta Pathol. Microbiol. Scand.* 56:277, 1962.

50. Lundin, H. Radiologic estimation of kidney weight. *Acta Radiol. [Diagn.] (Stockh.)* 6:561, 1967.

51. Marshall, A. G. The persistence of foetal structures in pyelonephritic kidneys. *Br. J. Surg.* 41:38, 1953.

52. Meares, E. M., Jr., and Gross, D. M. Hypertension owing to unilateral renal hypoplasia. *J. Urol.* 108: 197, 1972.

53. Mecke, S., and Passarge, E. Encephalocele, polycystic kidneys and polydactyly as an autosomal recessive trait simulating certain other disorders: The Meckel syndrome. *Ann. Genet. (Paris)* 14:97, 1971.

54. Miranda, D., Schinella, R. A., and Finegold, M. A. Familial renal dysplasia: Microdissection studies in siblings with associated central nervous system and hepatic malformations. *Arch. Pathol.* 93:483, 1972.

55. Morita, T., Wenzel, J., McCoy, J., Porch, J., and Kimmelstiel, P. Bilateral renal hypoplasia with oligomeganephronia: Quantitative and electron microscopic study. *Am. J. Clin. Pathol.* 59:104, 1973.

56. Nation, E. F. Renal aplasia: A study of sixteen cases. *J. Urol.* 51:579, 1944.

57. Newman, L., McAlister, W. H., and Kissane, J. Segmental renal dysplasia associated with ectopic ureteroceles in childhood. *Urology* 3:23, 1974.

58. Newman, L., Simms, K., Kissane, J., and McAlister, W. H. Unilateral total renal dysplasia in children. *Am. J. Roentgenol. Radium Ther. Nucl. Med.* 116: 778, 1972.

59. Oliver, J. T., Rubenstein, M., Meyer, R., and Bernstein, J. Congenital abnormalities of the urinary system. III. Growth of the kidney in childhood. Determination of normal weight. *J. Pediatr.* 61:256, 1962.

60. Opitz, J. M., and Howe, J. J. The Meckel Syndrome (Dysencephalia Splanchnocystica, the Gruber Syndrome). Proceedings of the First Conference on Clinical Delineation of Birth Defects. In D. Bergsma (ed.), *Birth Defects: Original Article Series.* New

York: The National Foundation, 1969. Vol. V/2, p. 167.

61. Pathak, I. G., and Williams, D. I. Multicystic and cystic dysplastic kidneys. *Br. J. Urol.* 36:318, 1974.

62. Perrin, E. V., Persky, L., Tucker, A., and Chrenka, B. Renal duplication and dysplasia. *Urology* 4:660, 1974.

63. Potter, E. L. *Normal and Abnormal Development of the Kidney.* Chicago: Year Book, 1972.

64. Rattner, W. H., Meyer, R., and Bernstein, J. Congenital abnormalities of the urinary system. IV. Valvular obstruction of posterior urethra. *J. Pediatr.* 63:84, 1963.

65. Risdon, R. A. Renal dysplasia. Part I. A clinicopathological study of 76 cases. Part II. A necropsy study of 41 cases. *J. Clin. Pathol.* 24:57, 65, 1971.

66. Risdon, R. A. Renal Dysplasia and Associated Abnormalities of the Urinary Tract. In M. I. Rubin and T. M. Barratt (eds.), *Pediatric Nephrology.* Baltimore: Williams & Wilkins, 1975. P. 346.

67. Risdon, R. A., Young, L. W., and Chrispin, A. R. Renal hypoplasia and dysplasia: A radiological and pathological correlation. *Pediatr. Radiol.* 3:213, 1975.

68. Reziciner, S., and Batzenschlager, A. Hypoplasie rénale segmentaire aglomérulaire. *Ann. Urol. (Paris)* 6:85, 1972.

69. Roosen-Runge, E. C. Retardation of postnatal development of kidneys in persons with early cerebral lesions. *Am. J. Dis. Child.* 77:185, 1949.

70. Royer, P. Malformations of the Kidney. In P. Royer, R. Habib, H. Mathieu, M. Broyer, and A. Walsh (eds.), *Pediatric Nephrology.* Philadelphia: Saunders, 1974. P. 9.

71. Royer, P., Habib, R., Broyer, M., and Nouaille, Y. Segmental hypoplasia of the kidney in children. *Adv. Nephrol.* 1:145, 1971.

72. Royer, P., Habib, R., Mathieu, H., and Courtecuisse, V. L'hypoplasie rénale bilatérale congénitale avec réduction du nombre et hypertrophie des néphrons chez l'enfant. *Ann. Pediatr. (Paris)* 38:753, 1962.

73. Rosenfeld, J. B., Cohen, L., Garty, I., and Ben-Bassat, M. Unilateral renal hypoplasia with hypertension (Ask-Upmark kidney). *Br. Med. J.* 2:217, 1973.

74. Rubenstein, M., Meyer, R., and Bernstein, J. Congenital abnormalities of the urinary system. I. A postmortem survey of developmental anomalies and acquired congenital lesions in a children's hospital. *J. Pediatr.* 35:259, 1936.

75. Scheinman, J. I., and Abelson, H. T. Bilateral renal hypoplasia with oligomeganephronia. *J. Pediatr.* 76:369, 1970.

76. Schröder, F. H., Fiedler, U., and Goodwin, W. E. Die multizystische Dysplasie der Niere—ein klinisches Syndrome. *Z. Urol. Nephrol.* 63:631, 1970.

77. Simopoulos, A. P., Brennan, G. G., Alwan, A., and Fidis, N. Polycystic kidneys, internal hydrocephalus and polydactylism in newborn siblings. *Pediatrics* 39:931, 1967.

78. Schwartz, J. An unusual unilateral multicystic kidney in an infant. *J. Urol.* 35:259, 1936.

79. Sotelo-Avila, C., and Singer, D. B. Syndrome of hyperplastic fetal visceromegaly and neonatal hypoglycemia (Beckwith's syndrome): A report of seven cases. *Pediatrics* 46:240, 1970.

80. Taxy, J. B., and Filmer, R. B. Metaplastic cartilage in nondysplastic kidneys. *Arch. Pathol.* 99:101, 1975.

81. Van Acker, K. J., Vincke, H., Quatacker, J., Senesael, L., and Van Den Brande, J. Congenital oligonephronic renal hypoplasia with hypertrophy of nephrons (oligonephronia). *Arch. Dis. Child.* 46:321, 1971.

82. Vellios, F., and Garrett, R. A. Congenital unilateral multicystic disease of the kidney: A clinical and anatomic study of 7 cases. *Am. J. Clin. Pathol.* 35:244, 1961.

83. Voth, D. Zur Genese des hyalinen Knorpelgewebes in hypoplastischen Nieren. *Zentralbl. Allg. Pathol.* 102:554, 1961.

84. Vuorinen, P., Antilla, P., Wegelius, U., Kauppila, A., and Koivisto, E. Renal cortical index and other roentgenographic measurements. *Acta Radiol. (Stockh.)* [Suppl.] 211, 1962.

85. Walter, F., and Addis, T. Organ work and organ weight. *J. Exp. Med.* 69:467, 1939.

86. Weinberg, S. R., O'Connor, W. J., and Senger, F. L. Unilateral multicystic renal diseases of the newborn. *Am. J. Dis. Child.* 92:576, 1956.

87. Young, L. W., Wood, B. P., Spohr, C. H., and Panner, B. Delayed excretory urographic opacification, a puddling effect, in multicystic renal dysplasia. *Ann. Radiol. (Paris)* 17:391, 1973.

40. Polycystic Disease

Jay Bernstein

The polycystic diseases of the kidney include two principal entities: *infantile polycystic disease* of autosomal recessive inheritance and *adult polycystic disease* of autosomal dominant inheritance. They differ clinically, radiographically, and morphologically, and within each category there is additional clinical and morphologic heterogeneity. The designations are faulty, because the two diseases are not age-specific, although the terms, *infantile polycystic disease* and *adult polycystic disease* are well established in current usage. The terms are herein used in the restricted sense indicated.

Not all renal cysts constitute polycystic disease [6]. A complete account of renal cysts extends beyond the two principal entities to encompass many other conditions, some found characteristically in children and others in adults. A major cystic abnormality of childhood is, for example, renal dysplasia (Chap. 39), and a miscellany of cysts is encountered also in syndromes of multiple malformation. The classification of cysts [8] (Table 40-1) leans strongly on morphologic and radiographic observations, modified by clinical and genetic factors. The clinicopathologic correlations that have been developed provide a suitable basis for investigation, prognostication, and genetic counseling. This classification, which has evolved over a period of years [7, 11, 24], shares with several others [30, 65] a similarity of terms and meanings.

Some cystic abnormalities are developmental and others acquired; some are heritable and others sporadic. Heritable diseases are not necessarily developmental, and cysts may form in normal tubules long after birth because of heritable, nephrotoxic, metabolic abnormalities. This distinction is of more than semantic importance if it can be

shown that cysts in polycystic disease are not themselves inherent but are secondary manifestations of some other heritable abnormality [22, 52]. It would be a reasonable therapeutic goal, for example, to mitigate the formation of cysts by pharmacologic intervention. This view is supported by the experimental production of cysts by a number of nephrotoxic agents that are capable of acting on mature kidneys [19, 61]. Their administration to laboratory animals long after the cessation of nephrogenesis precludes the possibility of a developmental disorder. Cysts can and do arise at any time during life, and they arise in any part of the nephron and collecting system. The differences in distribution and patterns of cysts are partly determined by the disease and partly by the age of the patient. The cystic renal manifestations of different disorders may therefore display great similarity, and the manifestations of a single disease may vary considerably with evolution over a span of time.

Polycystic disease is defined as a heritable disorder, with diffuse involvement of both kidneys. Renal dysplasia is excluded by definition. The group of medullary cystic diseases (Chap. 42), which includes uremic medullary cystic disease, familial juvenile nephronophthisis, and renal-retinal dysplasia, differs in several important respects from polycystic disease. Medullary sponge kidney (Chap. 72), despite certain resemblances to medullary cystic disease and to infantile polycystic disease, is also a separate entity.

Renal cysts are encountered in many hereditary syndromes (Table 40-2), usually in the form of peripheral cortical microcysts that lack clinical and functional significance [10]. Renal involvement of a severe degree, resembling that in adult polycystic disease (APCD), is seen in association with several other malformations and syndromes, for example Ehlers-Danlos syndrome. Other syndromes,

Table 40-1. Classification of Renal Parenchymal Cysts

Polycystic disease
  Infantile polycystic disease:
    Polycystic disease of the newborn
    Polycystic disease of infancy and childhood
    Congenital hepatic fibrosis
  Adult polycystic disease
Renal cysts in hereditary syndromes
  Diffuse cystic involvement in tuberous sclerosis
  Diffuse cystic involvement in von Hippel-Lindau disease
  Cystic dysplasia in Zellweger cerebrohepatorenal syndrome and Jeune asphyxiating thoracic dysplasia
  Severe cystic involvement in Ehlers-Danlos syndrome
  Cortical microcysts in syndromes of multiple malformation
Renal cortical cysts
  Diffuse glomerular cystic disease
  Juxtamedullary cortical microcysts (Finnish type congenital nephrotic syndrome)
  Solitary and multiple simple cysts
  Segmental and unilateral cystic disease
Renal medullary cysts
  Uremic medullary cystic disease complex:
    Familial juvenile nephronophthisis
    Medullary cystic disease
    Renal-retinal dysplasia
  Medullary sponge kidney
Renal dysplasia
  Cystic dysplasia associated with lower urinary tract obstruction
  Multicystic and aplastic dysplasia
  Hereditary cystic dysplasia
  Focal and segmental cystic dysplasia

Source: Modified from J. Bernstein and K. D. Gardner, Jr. Cystic Diseases of the Kidney and Renal Dysplasia. In J. H. Harrison, et al. (ed.), *Campbell's Urology* (4th ed.), Philadelphia: Saunders, 1979.

Table 40-2. Renal Cortical Cysts Associated with Syndromes of Multiple Malformation

Zellweger cerebrohepatorenal syndrome
Jeune asphyxiating thoracic dysplasia syndrome
Autosomal trisomy syndromes, D and E
Orodigitofacial syndrome
Lissencephaly syndrome
Goldenhar syndrome
Marden-Walker (Schwartz-Jampel) syndrome
Ehlers-Danlos syndrome
Congenital cutis laxa syndrome
Short rib–polydactyly syndrome
DiGeorge syndrome
Noonan syndrome
Turner syndrome
Chromosomal translocation syndromes

among them the Jeune and Zellweger syndromes, are occasionally associated with significant renal cystic disease that incorporates dysplastic elements (Chap. 39). A distinctive cystic abnormality occurring in the tuberous sclerosis syndrome is included in this chapter because of its importance in childhood.

Infantile Polycystic Disease

The term *infantile polycystic disease* (IPCD) is used to refer to a group of heritable conditions that occur predominantly in childhood. The term is, in a strict sense, inappropriate, since the disease also affects older children and adults. All forms of the disease are transmitted by autosomal recessive inheritance, and all forms are accompanied by hepatic abnormalities. The separation of IPCD from APCD is well established by genetic, clinical, radiographic, and morphologic studies. We have been unable to define IPCD in simple anatomic and clinical terms because of the clinical and morphologic variability of the condition, and there remains some disagreement about the genetic significance of that variability.

ETIOLOGY AND PATHOGENESIS

The hereditary nature of IPCD is undisputed. The means by which the disease is mediated is unknown. Most workers have thought the condition to be developmental, principally because of its relative frequency in newborns. Morphologic studies employing microdissection have shown, however, even in newborns with fully developed lesions, a pattern of normal ductal branching and normal nephronic induction [58], findings that indicate normal nephrogenesis and place in doubt the developmental nature of the disease. The essential abnormality appears to be enlargement or "gigantism" of the collecting tubules in association with cellular hyperplasia [58]. Morphologic studies have demonstrated normal pelvic and calyceal development. The evidence therefore points to an abnormality acquired later in gestation, perhaps superimposed on previously normal nephrons and ducts.

There is also reason to believe that the typical cysts are characteristic responses of fetal and neonatal kidneys. First, older infants with IPCD typically have less severe cyst formation than do newborns. Second, kidneys in children surviving the neonatal period may undergo diminution in radiographic size [49], suggesting resorption or collapse of cysts. Third, children have progressive renal impairment with tubular atrophy and cortical fibrosis rather than with an increase in cyst formation. It seems reasonable to suggest, therefore, that the pathogenesis of the condition lies in tubular injury and that cellular proliferation to produce tubular gigantism is a response predominantly of the immature kidney.

Even if we assume the validity of the preceding argument, the cause of tubular injury remains unknown. The progressive nature of the lesion makes it likely that the kidney is subject to continuing injury. The concomitant presence of hepatic involvement suggests a generalized abnormality. That the inheritance is recessive tends to implicate an enzymic abnormality, perhaps an epithelial protein in the kidney and liver, but a primary defect in renal ductular and hepatic ductal supporting structures cannot be excluded as a cause of secondary epithelial injury. The defect may well be an abnormal metabolic process or production of an abnormal metabolite whose identification could provide the basis of pharmacologic intervention. Despite these many uncertainties, this approach may also have heuristic value.

GENETICS

The inheritance of IPCD as an autosomal recessive condition was firmly established in studies of morphologically homogeneous neonates [37, 50]. The demonstration that IPCD extends beyond the neonatal period does not alter that interpretation.

There are at least two major clinical forms of IPCD, one in newborns and the other in older infants. A subclassification into four types has been proposed by Blyth and Ockenden [12] on the basis of clinicopathologic studies and genetic analysis. Each type is transmitted with autosomal recessive inheritance and has a typical clinical and morphologic appearance. They are characterized according to age at onset: (1) perinatal, with presentation at birth and with 90 percent of renal tubules dilated; (2) neonatal, with presentation within the first month and with 60 percent of renal tubules dilated; (3) infantile, with presentation between 3 and 6 months and with 25 percent of renal tubules dilated; and (4) juvenile, with presentation usually after the first year and with less than 10 percent of tubules dilated. The type of disease was found to be consistent among the members of any one family. Blyth and Ockenden [12] argued, therefore, for the existence of four separate mutant genes and thus for genetic heterogeneity within the syndrome of IPCD. The clinicopathologic correlations have been disputed, however, because the disease progresses to renal failure in older infants with only mild or minimal cyst formation [8]. The disease seems, therefore, to result from a process of continuing tubular damage rather than from a static malformation. Furthermore, a consistency within families in the age of onset has long been recognized in APCD [20] without necessarily carrying genetic implications.

A different outlook emerges from the studies published by Lieberman and colleagues [49], who also observed variability. They saw an age-related, changing clinical pattern that they regarded as the natural evolution of one disease. They did not find evidence of genetic heterogeneity within the group of patients designated as having IPCD.

Hepatic involvement was typically present in patients in both studies and also was more apparent in the older patients. The cases of IPCD that might be identified also as congenital hepatic fibrosis had variable, sometimes mild, impairment of renal function. Lieberman and colleagues [49] thought that congenital hepatic fibrosis, even with evidence of renal involvement, was clinically distinct from IPCD and that they were two separate diseases. The author [8] has disputed this view, taking the position that IPCD and congenital hepatic fibrosis with renal involvement are the same disease, with differences attributable to the progression of hepatic fibrosis and to the degree of renal involvement. Congenital hepatic fibrosis occurs in relatively older children, who may be predicted to have relatively mild renal involvement, and such differences do not necessarily constitute evidence of genetic heterogeneity. The validity of separating IPCD into several separate groups may turn out to be substantiated by additional studies, but the matter is currently unsettled.

CLINICAL MANIFESTATIONS

The most common clinical expression of IPCD is in the newborn with large kidneys and oliguria. The kidneys are greatly enlarged, at times causing abdominal distention severe enough to interfere with delivery of the fetus. The condition is commonly associated with oligohydramnios, which results from deficient fetal formation of urine, and many newborns have Potter facies with abnormal ears, small chin, beaked nose, and facial creases, a syndrome attributed to the oligohydramnios. Despite neonatal oliguria, death from renal failure is unusual. Infants suffer from respiratory distress and insufficiency secondary to pulmonary hypoplasia, which has also been attributed to oligohydramnios. Resuscitative measures frequently lead to interstitial pulmonary emphysema, pneumomediastinum, and pneumothorax. Some infants have enlarged livers, and hepatic involvement in polycystic disease is the rule. Other visceral cysts and malformations are rare in homogeneous populations of

IPCD, and their presence may be clues to other syndromes.

Radiographic examination in newborns shows poor function, and excretory urography demonstrates two characteristic patterns: (1) retention of contrast medium within cortical and medullary cysts to produce an irregularly mottled nephrogram [24, 34, 38] (Fig. 40-1), and (2) retention of contrast material in dilated medullary collecting ducts to produce linear, brushlike medullary opacifications [34, 64]. Opacification of dilated cortical ducts sometimes results in radiographic densities that are typically arranged as radial streaks in the outer portions of the kidney (Fig. 40-1). Renal opacification is often delayed, and material may be retained within kidneys for several days. The excretion of contrast medium is seldom sufficient for visualization of the pelvis and ureters, although ra-

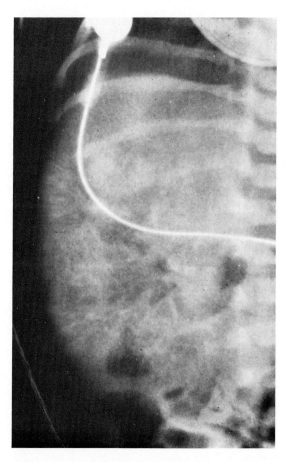

Figure 40-1. Excretory urography in a newborn infant with IPCD shows retention of contrast medium in a 12-hr film. There is a mottled nephrogram with radially oriented streaks corresponding to dilated cortical ducts. (Roentgenogram provided by Drs. J. O. Reed and Frederick B. Watts, Jr., Children's Hospital of Michigan.)

diographic material may be seen in delayed examinations to accumulate in the urinary bladder.

In older children, IPCD is attended by less severe renal enlargement, and the kidneys may actually become radiographically smaller during a period of several years, with stabilization at age 4 to 5 years [49]. Some degree of enlargement persists, however, and the kidneys usually remain palpable. Renal insufficiency begins in early childhood, but its progression is extremely variable. Urinalysis shows low specific gravity and mild proteinuria. The urinary sediment often contains an increased number of erythrocytes and white cells, but bacterial infection is infrequently demonstrated. Patients have elevated serum concentrations of urea and creatinine, and they are acidotic and moderately anemic. Hyperphosphatemia and hypocalcemia are late complications of renal failure. Systemic hypertension develops in almost all the children, and the clinical course is often complicated by congestive heart failure [49]. Other, nonspecific features include abdominal pain, nausea, vomiting, and growth retardation. Progressive hepatic fibrosis is associated with hepatomegaly and splenomegaly, and portal hypertension develops in some children. Liver function tests are usually negative, although hepatocellular dysfunction and hepatic insufficiency are seen occasionally. Progressive hepatic disease in older children with mild or inapparent renal involvement has been regarded as a separate entity by Lieberman and colleagues [49] and called "congenital hepatic fibrosis," although the point of differentiation from IPCD is unclear. It seems reasonably certain that hepatic fibrosis increases in the natural evolution of IPCD and that it leads to portal hypertension and its consequences.

Some patients may have minimal functional renal impairment, and the only radiographic evidence of renal involvement takes the form of medullary ductal ectasia. We have regarded such cases, even in adults with portal hypertension and asymptomatic renal involvement, to be part of the spectrum of IPCD. In other patients, portal hypertension and systemic hypertension coexist, and children have been known to suffer from both bleeding esophageal varices and chronic renal failure.

Radiographic examination in older children has shown variable renal enlargement and cyst formation. Excretory function is unpredictable. Excretory urography may show a mottled nephrogram or it may show a prompt excretion of contrast material, with delineation of calyces and pelvis [49, 70] (Fig. 40-2). Cyst formation may be apparent with newer techniques of magnified imaging. Pyelocalyceal deformities are usually mild. In several cases, Lieberman and colleagues [49] have

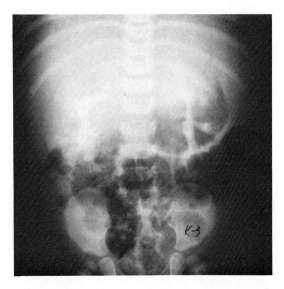

Figure 40-2. An excretory urogram in a 9-month-old child with IPCD shows bilateral renal enlargement with medullary ductal ectasia. Excretory function is sufficient for visualization of the pyelocalyceal system.

shown a diminution in renal size, apparently due to regression of renal cysts, over a period of years. Radiographic shrinkage should not, however, necessarily be taken as evidence of improvement, since progression of the disease to cortical atrophy and fibrosis may also be associated with shrinkage and with regression of cysts. The one characteristic radiographic finding in older infants, children, and adults is medullary ductal ectasia [59] (Fig. 40-2). It is the characteristic abnormality in all forms of IPCD, both in young children with progressive renal failure and in older patients with clinically inapparent renal disease. It is also the characteristic renal abnormality associated with congenital hepatic fibrosis [45, 64, 68]. The radiographic pattern is indistinguishable from that of medullary sponge kidney, a disease of different age incidence, different pathogenesis, and different genetic and clinical implications. The similarity has caused considerable confusion, and it emphasizes the need for employing other information in evaluating individual cases [27, 33, 71].

IPCD is usually fatal in childhood, but some children enjoy prolonged survival despite renal functional impairment [70]. The occurrence of the similar, though usually milder, renal impairment in patients with congenital hepatic fibrosis makes prognostication difficult. The categories proposed by Blyth and Ockenden [12], while of limited clinical applicability, confirm that siblings have similar diseases, a point of prognostic value.

RENAL FUNCTION

Newborns with severe cyst formation and greatly enlarged kidneys because of IPCD suffer from anuria or oliguria, but older children present a less consistent pattern. They typically have impaired concentrating ability and defective acidification [2]. Glomerular filtration rates and effective renal plasma flow are reduced. The concentrating defect, which is of variable severity, appears not to be dependent on reduced glomerular filtration rate, indicating that the abnormality resides either in tubules or in altered medullary pyramids; tubular abnormalities might also account for the reduced excretion of acid. Similar, though somewhat less severe, abnormalities are found in patients with congenital hepatic fibrosis, the majority of whom have a reduced ability to concentrate urine [2].

RENAL PATHOLOGY

The characteristic feature of IPCD, regardless of the patient's age and severity of involvement, is medullary ductal ectasia. It is seen grossly in newborns with enlarged kidneys, in older children with scattered cortical cysts, and in young adults with no other obvious impairment. The presence of medullary cysts in IPCD has resulted in confusion with medullary sponge kidney, which is an unrelated disorder (Chap. 72). The gross morphologic and radiographic differentiation may occasionally be difficult, but the histologic demonstration of cortical cysts, tubular atrophy, and interstitial fibrosis is indicative of IPCD [35].

The kidneys in newborns with severe involvement often have combined weights that exceed 300 gm (12 times normal). The kidneys are reniform in configuration, and they have a spongy appearance. Dilated peripheral ductules are visible through the attenuated capsule as tiny cysts that may measure 1 mm in diameter. The cortical collecting ducts are distended and are grossly visible as elongated cysts extending radially from the corticomedullary junctions to the subcapsular cortex (Fig. 40-3). The kidneys are usually edematous, a factor leading to much of the increase in renal weight. There is, however, little increase in cortical connective tissue. The lobar configuration of the kidney is preserved. The medullary pyramids, apart from being cystic, are normally formed, and the calyces and ureters are patent.

Microscopic examination and microdissection confirm that the dilated structures are collecting ducts [37, 58] (Fig. 40-4A). The epithelium lining the ducts is columnar or cuboidal, and the lack of atrophy or severe attenuation in distended cortical ducts has been taken as evidence of cellular

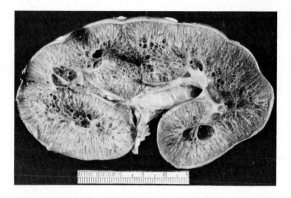

Figure 40-3. The kidney of a newborn infant with IPCD has a spongy appearance because of diffuse ductal dilatation. The kidney is edematous and enlarged, weighing slightly more than 200 gm. The dilated collecting ducts extend radially to the subcapsular cortex, and severe dilatation of the medullary ducts produces cysts that measure as much as 1 cm in diameter.

hyperplasia. The deeper, more severely distended medullary ducts are more often lined with flattened epithelium. Nephrons are present in normal numbers and have normal attachments to collecting tubules, which also show a normal pattern of branching in microdissected specimens [58]. The architecture of the kidney therefore appears to be normal with, perhaps, superimposed cystic change. The nephrons are often variably cystic by both light microscopy and microdissection, with dilatation of both tubules and glomerular spaces. Dysplastic elements are not present.

The degree of cyst formation is less severe in older than in younger children, a finding that Blyth and Ockenden [12] attribute to a genetically programmed difference between neonatal and childhood IPCD. The observations of Lieberman and colleagues [49] suggest that there may be a diminution in ductal dilatation. The cysts appear rounded rather than fusiform, and they are irregularly distributed within each kidney (Figs. 40-5A, 40-6A). Glomerular obsolescence, tubular atrophy, and cortical fibrosis are found in varying mixtures. The accompanying changes do suggest that cysts may have regressed and may have become more localized, perhaps with secondary, localized obstructions. The associated changes may also mean that nephronic damage is progressive without new cyst formation. Ultrastructural studies have shown peritubular fibrosis [67], which could be either primary or secondary in relation to tubular damage and progressive functional deterioration.

Hepatic involvement is almost invariably present

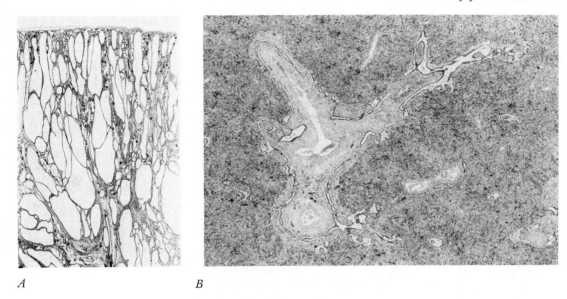

A   B

Figure 40-4. A. The dilated collecting ducts in neonatal IPCD involve the entire thickness of the cortex, and there is also mild dilatation of convoluted tubules and glomerular spaces. (H&E, ×15 before 38% reduction.) B. The liver in a newborn with IPCD contains enlarged portal areas, in which the biliary channels seem to be both enlarged and increased in number. They often encircle the portal areas and form anastomosing, almost continuous channels that are in fact flattened interconnecting cisterns. (H&E, ×24 before 18% enlargement.)

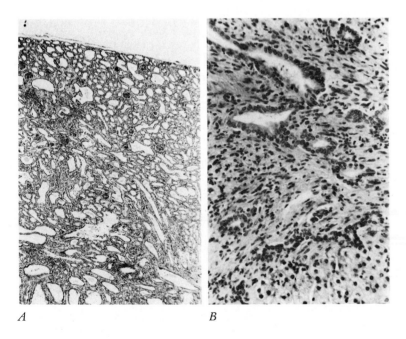

A   B

Figure 40-5. A. Kidney of a 9-month-old child with IPCD contains irregularly distributed cysts that often have a rounded configuration. There are also tubular atrophy and interstitial fibrosis. (H&E, ×36 before 29% reduction.) B. Increasing hepatic portal connective tissue leads to distortion of the biliary channels and to the histologic appearance of congenital hepatic fibrosis. (H&E, ×200 before 29% reduction.) (Renal and hepatic biopsy specimens from same patient whose roentgenogram appears in Fig. 40-2.)

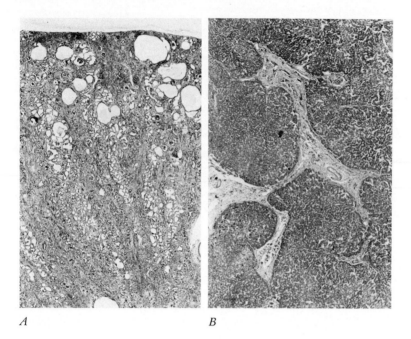

A   B

Figure 40-6. Severe renal cortical atrophy and hepatic portal fibrosis were seen on postmortem examination of a 5-year-old child with chronic renal failure due to IPCD. A. The renal cortex contains scattered small cysts that have a rounded configuration and are surrounded by increased interstitial connective tissue; tubules are atrophic, and occasional glomeruli are sclerotic. (Trichrome, ×16 before 14% reduction.) B. The portal areas are enlarged, containing compressed biliary channnels and ductules. (Trichrome, ×27 before 14% reduction.)

in IPCD, with few recorded exceptions [70]. The portal areas are enlarged and irregularly fibrotic, and they contain an increased number of bile ducts (Fig. 40-4B). The ducts seem, in the plane of section, to encircle the portal areas and to form anastomosing, almost continuous channels. The only reasonable explanation for these appearances is that the ducts are in fact flattened interconnecting sacs or cisterns, an interpretation supported by studies using techniques of serial reconstruction and stereology [41, 48]. The biliary passages therefore form an intercommunicating network that accounts for the lack of jaundice, despite the occasional occurrence of bile stasis. The main interlobular ducts within the portal areas are often lacking, indicating that differentiation of the ductal system, which follows the growth of liver cells, has been altered. There is an increase in periductal collagen [1, 67], contributing to the portal fibrosis (Figs. 40-5B, 40-6B). As the result of increased production of connective tissue, the abnormality leads to vascular obstruction and portal hypertension. Hepatic fibrosis with portal hypertension and with mild renal involvement is, as previously noted, often referred to as congenital hepatic fibrosis. The renal lesion is morphologically and functionally

the same as that in IPCD, though less severe, and the hepatic lesion in IPCD and congenital hepatic fibrosis is also the same by microdissection and in stereologic studies [41, 42, 48]. Congenital hepatic fibrosis, however, is not a specific or homogeneous condition [55], and in many patients with hepatic fibrosis there is no renal involvement. The ducts may become grossly dilated, despite free communication with the extrahepatic biliary tree, a condition sometimes referred to as Caroli disease. Caroli disease is also not synonymous with IPCD, and it apparently occurs as an isolated abnormality; neither the frequency of communicating ductal ectasia in IPCD nor the frequency of IPCD in intrahepatic ductal ectasia is known.

Cystic lesions of the pancreas are limited to mild dilatations of small ductules. Large pancreatic cysts and epididymal cysts are both associated with von Hippel-Lindau disease. Cystic lungs, which have sometimes been included in tabulations of visceral lesions in IPCD, appear also to represent misdiagnoses. The lungs in newborns are hypoplastic, sometimes less than one-half the expected weight for both body size and gestational age. Berry aneurysms of the cerebral arteries are uncommonly associated with IPCD; Lieberman and colleagues [49] found an aneurysm of the basilar artery in association with systemic hypertension in 1 of their 14 patients.

DIFFERENTIAL DIAGNOSIS

The differential diagnosis in newborns includes other causes of renal enlargement and cystic disease. An adequate family history is essential to exclude early infantile APCD and other heritable syndromes with renal involvement. Bilateral multicystic dysplasia with ureteral atresia is also associated with oligohydramnios and its consequences. It is ordinarily a sporadic malformation, and its differentiation from IPCD carries implications for genetic counseling. Other forms of diffuse cystic dysplasia are rare. The Meckel syndrome (Chap. 39) and other syndromes of multiple congenital malformations can be recognized by the nonrenal malformations. Bilateral hydronephrosis resulting from urinary tract obstruction produces flank masses; in this regard, the concomitant presence of enlarged kidneys and a suprapubic mass in male infants should suggest the diagnosis of posterior urethral valves rather than IPCD. Hydronephrosis may be recognized by ultrasonography. High-dose excretory urography and urography by direct puncture are helpful procedures in visualizing the urinary tract. Bilateral renal tumors are causes of renal enlargement, usually with relatively good opacification of adjacent parenchyma and pyelocalyceal systems. Circulatory disturbances, such as renal venous thrombosis, also cause considerable renal enlargement; significant hematuria is found, even in oliguric patients.

The differential diagnosis in older children includes other causes of progressive renal insufficiency with concentrating defect. A more common abnormality than IPCD is familial juvenile nephronophthisis (Chap. 42). The patients suffer from severe anemia and growth retardation. Renal function is usually inadequate for urographic studies, and the radiographic pattern of medullary ductal ectasia is not seen, despite the presence of medullary cysts. Hepatosplenomegaly is a strong clue to the diagnosis of IPCD, although a few cases with congenital hepatic fibrosis and a renal lesion designated as nephronophthisis have been reported [13].

THERAPY

Medical treatment of IPCD is supportive (Chap. 34). The risk of severe dehydration, due to concentrating defects, can be overcome by generous salt and water intake. Severe systemic hypertension requires the use of antihypertensive agents, and digitalization for the treatment of congestive heart failure may be necessary in young children. Chronic hemodialysis prolongs survival, and affected children are good candidates for renal allotransplantation.

Hepatic complications rarely cause hepatic dysfunction, the major problem being portal hypertension. Surgical portocaval shunt is the current, preferred form of therapy.

Adult Polycystic Disease in Childhood

The term *adult polycystic disease* refers to bilateral, diffuse cystic disease that occurs predominantly in adulthood. It is transmitted as an autosomal dominant trait, with high penetrance that approaches 100 percent in the eighth and ninth decades of life. The term is somewhat of a misnomer, since the disease may have its clinical onset in childhood. It is seldom, however, the cause of renal failure so early in life.

ETIOLOGY AND PATHOGENESIS

The etiology of APCD is unknown, except that its genetic transmission has been clearly established. The cause of nephronic dilatation and cyst formation is unknown; it may be related to the active transport of osmotically active solutes by the epithelium of the cysts [29, 32]. Grantham and colleagues [32] found two patterns of solute concentration, one characterized by isosmolar and the other by hyposmolar concentrations of sodium within the cyst fluid; the first pattern was thought to identify cysts arising in glomeruli and proximal tubules and the second, cysts arising in more distal portions of the nephron. The nature of the basic defect also remains unknown, and, just as with IPCD, there is disagreement between those who hypothesize a developmental abnormality and those who hypothesize a continuing metabolic abnormality. Nephronic obstruction seems not to play a role early in the evolution of the disease, but secondary tubular obstruction may contribute to the formation of cysts in later stages.

GENETICS

The longitudinal transmission, which is characteristic of an autosomal dominant inheritance, has been recognized in APCD for more than a half-century [14]. The frequent lack of a family history attests to a relatively high rate of spontaneous mutation, which has been estimated to be 6.5 to 12 $\times$ 10^{-5} mutations per gene per generation [20]. Although individual cases or families may seem to be exceptions, careful study of a large number of patients has confirmed the general rule of dominant inheritance [20].

Figures accumulated by the Michigan Kidney Registry [54] for end-stage renal disease indicate that APCD is relatively uncommon in blacks, although end-stage renal disease and hypertensive renal disease are both relatively more common in blacks than in whites in Michigan.

The occasional combination of APCD with other abnormalities is well known. Some of the hereditary conditions that have occurred in association with APCD include myotonic dystrophy [25], Peutz-Jeghers syndrome [46], orodigitofacial syndrome [36], lobster-claw deformity of the feet [15], and spherocytosis [16]. The association of renal cysts with Ehlers-Danlos syndrome [39, 47] and with von Hippel-Lindau disease [40] appears to be separate from and unrelated to APCD.

EPIDEMIOLOGY

In the United States, APCD is the third most common cause of renal failure in adults, accounting for approximately 6 percent of end-stage renal disease [54, 60]. Dalgaard's [21] data on incidence indicate a clinical frequency of approximately 1 : 3,500. This figure contrasts with a frequency at autopsy of 1 : 500, a difference that stems in part from clinical nonrecognition, in part from misdiagnosis, and in part from the widespread practice of labeling all renal cysts as "polycystic disease" [6].

The onset of disease (time of clinical recognition) is early in the fifth decade of life (average 40.7 years). Neonatal and childhood cases of adult-type autosomal dominant polycystic disease are rare. Only 1 patient in Dalgaard's series of 350 cases had the clinical onset of symptoms before the age of 10 years, and an additional 6 patients became symptomatic between 15 and 19 years [21].

The literature in the last few years has contained several reports of APCD in young infants [5, 12, 28, 44, 63, 66]. A childhood onset in a family with a previously more conventional clinical pattern raises questions about the pattern of inheritance in the affected infant, since Dalgaard [20] had found a consistency of age at onset within families, with a standard deviation of only 4 years. The observation means that all affected members of a family have a 95 percent chance of becoming symptomatic within a span of 16 years bracketing the mean age. One possible implication is that newborns or infants with precocious onset of APCD may be the victims of double-dose dominant homozygous inheritance, thereby having more severe disease that affects the kidneys earlier.

The sex distribution is equal. Nongenetic factors have not been identified in relation to human disease, although experimental cystic disease can be induced by chemical means in susceptible laboratory animals.

CLINICAL FEATURES

The earliest and most common symptom of APCD ordinarily is pain, which precedes the development of flank masses and renal impairment. However, very young infants usually have flank masses or palpable kidneys as the presenting abnormality. In some of them, excretory urography has demonstrated prompt visualization of the kidneys with pyelocalyceal distortion (Fig. 40-7). In other cases, visualization of the kidneys has been limited to a mottled nephrogram, and cysts can be demonstrated by tomography [57]. Sonography may show larger cysts, and smaller cysts are visualized better by arteriography and by magnified imaging techniques. Hypertension is a frequent feature of APCD, both in adults and in young children, and secondary cardiac complications have included myocardial infarction [53].

Laboratory studies in older children include elevated serum urea nitrogen and serum creatinine concentrations. Creatinine clearances are predictably reduced. Plasma renin concentrations may be high in hypertensive patients [44]. An early finding may be an inability to concentrate the urine maximally [51]. Sodium resorption appears to be unimpaired. Mild proteinuria may be present, and hematuria is common.

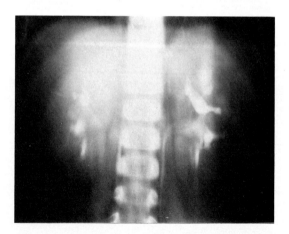

Figure 40-7. A nephrotomogram in a 1-year-old infant with enlarged kidneys discloses pyelocalyceal distortion by cysts. The pattern is compatible with APCD originating in early childhood. (Roentgenogram provided by Drs. J. O. Reed and Frederick B. Watts, Jr., Children's Hospital of Michigan.)

RENAL PATHOLOGY

Renal enlargement in infancy is bilateral, but it may, as in adults, be asymmetrical. The kidneys usually contain numerous, irregularly clustered, small cysts (Fig. 40-8), as opposed to the larger, scattered cysts in the typical adult pattern. Diffuse tubular dilatation occurs occasionally. Glomerular cysts are common and often dominate the histologic picture. Dilatation of Bowman's spaces may even be so striking as to obscure the histopathologic diagnosis, and glomerular cysts appear to be a characteristic feature of APCD in early life.

Older children and some younger children have the more conventional findings of irregularly sized cysts scattered in cortex and medulla, with intervening normal parenchyma. Microdissection in adults has shown that cysts may arise in any part of the nephron or collecting duct. Tubular cysts usually communicate with ducts, although occasional cysts may lack luminal connection. Glomerular cysts are often noncommunicating. The complications encountered in adults (hemorrhage, lithiasis, and infection) occur also in children, but they seem to be less frequent and less severe.

Hepatic involvement, which affects one-third of adults, is usually focal or unevenly distributed. The lesion consists of clusters of dilated ductules. The same lesion may be present in children, but its infrequency relative to hepatic involvement in IPCD makes liver biopsy a helpful procedure in identifying childhood cases. Berry aneurysms of the cerebral arteries, which affect approximately 10 percent of adults with APCD, are rare in children.

DIFFERENTIAL DIAGNOSIS

The differential diagnosis of APCD in early infancy includes IPCD and certain other forms of cystic disease. The diagnosis depends in large measure on an adequate family history—which should be unnecessary to say, but investigating the family history as part of a patient's clinical investigation is often done poorly. The proper diagnosis obviously carries genetic implications for both the parents and additional offspring; the recognition of cystic renal disease in an infant and the subsequent evaluation of the family has led to the recognition of APCD in an asymptomatic parent [66]. The lack of a positive family history, even after complete evaluation, does not negate the diagnosis because of the possibility of a new genetic mutation, even in cases of early onset.

The radiographic findings may be helpful, but some overlap occurs. Both IPCD and infantile APCD may be manifested on excretory urography either by a mottled nephrogram or by pyelocalyceal distortion and spreading. The finding of unequivocal medullary ductal ectasia would seem to be a strong point in favor of IPCD, although linear opacification within the kidney does not exclude APCD [28]. Renal tubular dysfunction (impaired acidification and Na resorption) could be regarded as evidence in favor of IPCD. Renal biopsies are extremely valuable in establishing the diagnosis, although the histologic pattern is not as well established or as easily recognized in APCD as in IPCD. Hepatic biopsies are also helpful, because involvement in APCD is at most focal, in contrast to the generalized and characteristic involvement in IPCD; there are but rare exceptions [70].

The diagnosis of other forms of renal cystic disease, usually in association with malformation syndromes, is based in large measure on recognizing other features of those syndromes. Cerebral maldevelopment may be a clue to the Meckel syndrome or one of its relatives (Chap. 39). A difficult point in differential diagnosis is raised by the occurrence of diffuse cystic disease in association with tuberous sclerosis, particularly since renal involvement may antedate other stigmata of the disease. Diagnosis then rests on recognizing its distinctive histopathologic pattern.

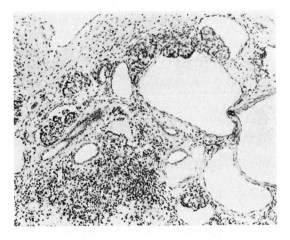

Figure 40-8. Renal biopsy in the child whose roentgenogram is shown in Fig. 40-7 discloses irregular glomerular and tubular dilatation, the pattern described in young infants with adult-type polycystic disease. (H&E stain, ×120 before 35% reduction.) (Specimen provided by Drs. A. Joseph Brough and Chung-Ho Chang, Children's Hospital of Michigan.)

TREATMENT

The treatment of APCD, like that of IPCD, is supportive, requiring adequate nutrition and correction of acidosis. Systemic hypertension is often severe enough to require antihypertensive medication, and digitalization is necessary for secondary congestive heart failure. Renal infection requires antibiotic therapy. Survival can be prolonged by chronic hemodialysis until allotransplantation is attempted.

Tuberous Sclerosis

Renal involvement is relatively common in tuberous sclerosis, usually in the form of angiomyolipoma, a benign hamartomatous tumor. The tumors are sometimes difficult to differentiate clinically from renal cysts [17, 56], which are usually small in size and few in number [4]. Diffuse cystic disease does occur, however, and it must be recognized as a cause of chronic renal insufficiency.

Severe cystic involvement in infancy (Fig. 40-9) is associated with renal enlargement, moderate azotemia, and hypertension [11, 24, 26, 43, 72]. Renal functional improvement has been observed following surgical decompression of the cysts, and follow-up examination 6 years after biopsy has not demonstrated recurrence of cysts or deterioration of renal function, indicating that the abnormality may be nonprogressive in some patients. It may differ, therefore, from APCD, in which progressive formation of cysts vitiates surgical decompression.

The clinical manifestations have been extremely variable, except for the early onset of severe hypertension [18, 43]. Adults with tuberous sclerosis and renal cysts have also suffered from hypertension [31] and progressive renal insufficiency [23, 62]. Renal impairment appears to result partially from replacement and partially from compression of renal parenchyma.

An interesting feature of the disease in children is that renal involvement often precedes the appearance of other stigmata of the syndrome. Early nonrenal manifestations have in several cases included mental retardation and convulsions, but other children have had only palpable flank masses. The cystic lesion is nonetheless sufficiently distinctive histologically to be diagnostic of tuberous sclerosis [9]. The cysts are lined with extraordinarily hyperplastic, eosinophilic epithelium that is thus far unique to this syndrome (Fig. 40-10). Microdissection in one newborn infant has revealed cysts of Henle's loops and subcapsular cysts within collecting tubules [58]. The renal tubular enlargement and cyst formation may be due to cellular hypertrophy and hyperplasia in a manner similar to that seen in other lesions of the syndrome. The cysts sometimes undergo enlargement as the result of intrarenal hemorrhage [23], and they appear also to have undergone collapse and sclerosis in one patient treated with chronic hemodialysis [62].

Renal impairment results from diffuse involvement by either hamartomas or cysts [3, 17]. The frequency of angiomyolipomas is said to be approximately 40 to 50 percent, and scattered, small cysts commonly coexist with the hamartomas. Extensive cyst formation, on the other hand, is rare, and the literature is limited to case reports. The two abnormalities, hamartomas and cysts, are not easily differentiated on clinical grounds, and the patient's condition cannot simply be attributed to hamartomas just because he is known to have tuberous sclerosis. Clinical recognition of renal involvement in the syndrome may be obtained from

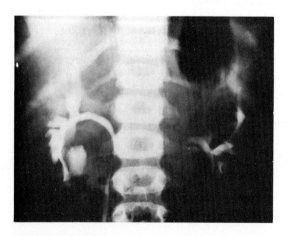

Figure 40-9. Excretory urogram in a child with tuberous sclerosis discloses pyelocalyceal distortion and irregular lucencies, compatible with cystic disease, which was confirmed by renal biopsy. (Roentgenogram provided by Dr. Walter E. Berdon, Columbia-Presbyterian Medical Center, New York.)

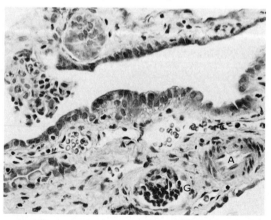

Figure 40-10. The cysts in tuberous sclerosis are lined with extremely hyperplastic, eosinophilic epithelium that is histologically unique. For comparison of size, note the adjacent glomerulus (G) and arteriole (A). (H&E, ×300 before 35% reduction.) (Specimen provided by Dr. A. B. Hamoudi, Children's Hospital, Columbus, Ohio.)

urographic studies, and sonography, nephrotomography, and selective arteriography [17, 69] help to differentiate tumors from cysts. In cases not recognized as tuberous sclerosis, the presence of typical cysts may be the first indication of that disease.

References

1. Albukerk, J., and Duffy, J. L. Fibrogenesis in congenital hepatic fibrosis. An electron and light microscopic study. *Arch. Pathol.* 92:126, 1971.
2. Anand, S. K., Chan, J. C., and Lieberman, E. Polycystic disease and hepatic fibrosis in children. Renal function studies. *Am. J. Dis. Child.* 129:810, 1975.
3. Anderson, D., and Tannen, R. L. Tuberous sclerosis and chronic renal failure. Potential confusion with polycystic kidney disease. *Am. J. Med.* 47:163, 1969.
4. Arey, J. B. Cystic lesions of the kidney in infants and children. *J. Pediatr.* 54:429, 1959.
5. Bengtsson, U., Hedman, L., and Svalander, C. Adult type of polycystic kidney disease in a new-born child. *Acta Med. Scand.* 197:447, 1975.
6. Bernstein, J. Heritable cystic disorders of the kidney: The mythology of polycystic disease. *Pediatr. Clin. North Am.* 18:435, 1971.
7. Bernstein, J. The classification of renal cysts. *Nephron* 11:91, 1973.
8. Bernstein, J. A Classification of Renal Cysts. In K. D. Gardner, Jr. (ed.), *Cystic Diseases of the Kidney.* New York: Wiley, 1976. Chap. 2, pp. 7–30.
9. Bernstein, J., Brough, A. J., and McAdams, A. J. The Renal Lesion in Syndromes of Multiple Congenital Malformations: Cerebrohepatorenal Syndrome; Jeune's Asphyxiating Thoracic Dystrophy; Tuberous Sclerosis; Meckel's Syndrome. In D. Bergsma (ed.), *Fifth Conference on the Clinical Delineation of Birth Defects. Birth Defects.* Original Article Series. New York: The National Foundation, 1974. Vol. X/4, p. 35.
10. Bernstein, J., and Kissane, J. M. Hereditary Disorders of the Kidney. In H. Rosenberg, and R. P. Bolande (eds.), *Perspectives in Pediatric Pathology.* Chicago: Year Book, 1973. Vol. 1, p. 435.
11. Bernstein, J., and Meyer, R. Parenchymal Maldevelopment of the Kidney. In V. C. Kelley (ed.), *Brennemann's Practice of Pediatrics.* Hagerstown, Md.: Harper & Row, 1967. Chap. 26.
12. Blyth, H., and Ockenden, B. G. Polycystic disease of kidneys and liver presenting in childhood. *J. Med. Genet.* 8:257, 1971.
13. Boichis, H., Passwell, J., David, R., and Miller, H. Congenital hepatic fibrosis and nephronophthisis. *Q. J. Med.* 42:221, 1973.
14. Cairns, H. W. B. Heredity in polycystic disease of the kidney. *Q. J. Med.* 18:359, 1925.
15. Cameron, J. R. Bilateral "hereditary" polycystic disease of the kidneys associated with bilateral teratodactyly of the feet. ("Pied en pince de homard") *Br. J. Urol.* 33:473, 1961.
16. Chanmugam, D., Rasaretnam, R., and Karunarathne, K. E. Genetic intelligence: Hereditary spherocytosis and polycystic disease of the kidneys in four members of a family. *Am. J. Hum. Genet.* 23:66, 1971.
17. Chonko, A. M., Weiss, S. M., Stein, J. H., and Ferris, T. F. Renal involvement in tuberous sclerosis. *Am. J. Med.* 56:124, 1974.
18. Cree, J. E. Tuberous sclerosis with polycystic kidneys. *Proc. R. Soc. Med.* 62:327, 1969.
19. Crocker, J. F. S., Brown, D. M., and Vernier, R. L. Developmental defects of the kidney: A review of renal development and experimental studies of maldevelopment. *Pediatr. Clin. North Am.* 18:355, 1971.
20. Dalgaard, O. Z. Bilateral polycystic disease of the kidneys: A follow-up study of 284 patients and their families. *Acta Med. Scand.* 158:[Suppl. 328], 1957.
21. Dalgaard, O. Z. Polycystic Disease of the Kidneys. In M. B. Strauss and L. G. Welt (eds.), *Diseases of the Kidney* (2nd ed.). Boston: Little, Brown, 1971. Chap. 35.
22. Darmady, E. M., Offer, J., and Woodhouse, M. A. Toxic metabolic defect in polycystic disease of the kidney: Evidence from microscopic studies. *Lancet* 1:547, 1970.
23. Dolder, E. Niereninsuffizienz bei tuberöser Sklerose (Morbus Bourneville). *Schweiz. Med. Wochenschr.* 105:406, 1975.
24. Elkin, M., and Bernstein, J. Cystic diseases of the kidney: Radiological and pathological considerations. *Clin. Radiol.* 20:65, 1969.
25. Emery, A. E. H., Oleesky, S., and Williams, R. T. Myotonic dystrophy and polycystic disease of the kidneys. *J. Med. Genet.* 4:26, 1967.
26. Engström, N., Ljungqvist, A., Persson, B., and Wetterfors, J. Tuberous sclerosis with a localized angiomatous malformation in the ileum and excessive albumin loss into the lower intestinal tract. Report of a case. *Pediatrics* 30:681, 1962.
27. Fairly, K. F., Leighton, P. W., and Kincaid-Smith, P. Familial visual defects associated with polycystic kidney and medullary sponge kidney. *Br. Med. J.* 1:1060, 1963.
28. Fellows, R. A., Leonidas, J. C., and Beatty, E. C., Jr. Radiologic features of "adult type" polycystic kidney disease in the neonate. *Pediatr. Radiol.* 4:87, 1976.
29. Gardner, K. D., Jr. Composition of fluid in twelve cysts in a polycystic kidney. *N. Engl. J. Med.* 281:985, 1969.
30. Gleason, D. C., McAlister, W. H., and Kissane, J. Cystic disease of the kidneys in children. *Am. J. Roentgenol. Radium Ther. Nucl. Med.* 100:135, 1967.
31. Gonzalez-Angulo, A., Alford, B. R., and Greenberg, S. D. Tuberous sclerosis. An otolaryngic diagnosis. *Arch. Otolaryngol.* 80:193, 1964.
32. Grantham, J. J., Grady, A., Welling, D., and Cuppage, F. Macropuncture study of human adult polycystic renal disease. *Clin. Res.* 23:541A, 1975.
33. Grossman, H., and Seed, W. Congenital hepatic fibrosis, bile duct dilatation and renal lesion resembling medullary sponge kidney. Congenital "cystic" disease of the liver and kidneys. *Radiology* 87:46, 1966.
34. Gwinn, J. L., and Landing, B. H. Cystic diseases of the kidneys in infants and children. *Radiol. Clin. North Am.* 6:191, 1968.
35. Habib, R., Mouzet Massa, M. T., and Courtecuisse, V. L'estasie tubulaire précalicielle chez l'enfant (Rein en éponge de Cacchi et Ricci). *Ann. Pediatr.* (Paris) 12:288, 1965.
36. Harrod, M. J. E., Stokes, J., Peede, L. F., and Goldstein, J. L. Polycystic kidney disease in a patient with the oral-facial-digital syndrome—type I. *Clin. Genet.* 9:183, 1976.
37. Heggö, O., and Natvig, J. B. Cystic disease of the kidneys. Autopsy report and family study. *Acta Pathol. Microbiol. Scand.* 64:459, 1965.

38. Hinkel, C. L., and Santini, L. C.   Polycystic disease of kidney in infants: Nephrograms following intravenous urography. *Am. J. Roentgenol. Radium Ther. Nucl. Med.* 76:153, 1956.

39. Imahori, S., Bannerman, R. M., Grof, C. J., and Brennan, J. C.   Ehlers-Danlos syndrome with multiple arterial lesions. *Am. J. Med.* 47:967, 1969.

40. Isaac, F., Schoen, I., and Walker, P.   An unusual case of Lindau's disease. Cystic disease of the kidneys and pancreas with renal and cerebellar tumors. *Am. J. Roentgenol. Radium Ther. Nucl. Med.* 75:912, 1956.

41. Jørgensen, M.   A stereological study of intrahepatic bile ducts. 3. Infantile polycystic disease. *Acta Pathol. Microbiol. Scand. [A]* 81:670, 1973.

42. Jørgensen, M.   A stereological study of intrahepatic bile ducts. 4. Congenital hepatic fibrosis. *Acta Pathol. Microbiol. Scand. [A]* 82:21, 1974.

43. Kawamura, J., Sawanishi, K., Miyake, Y., and Nishio, T.   Bourneville-Pringle phacomatosis with striking renal abnormality: Report of a case of four-year-old boy. *Acta Urol. Jap.* 15:91, 1969.

44. Kaye, C., and Lewy, P. R.   Congenital appearance of adult-type (autosomal dominant) polycystic kidney disease. Report of a case. *J. Pediatr.* 85:807, 1974.

45. Kerr, D. N. S., Warrick, C. K., and Hart-Mercer, J.   A lesion resembling medullary sponge kidney in patients with congenital hepatic fibrosis. *Clin. Radiol.* 13:85, 1962.

46. Kieselstein, M., Herman, G., Wahrman, J., Voss, R., Gitelson, S., Feuchtwanger M., and Kadar, S.   Mucocutaneous pigmentation and intestinal polyposis (Peutz-Jeghers syndrome) in a family of Iraqui Jews with polycystic kidney disease. With a chromosome study. *Is. J. Med. Sci.* 5:81, 1969.

47. Landing, B. H., Gwinn, J. L., and Lieberman, E.   Cystic Diseases of the Kidney in Children. In K. D. Gardner, Jr. (ed.), *Cystic Diseases of the Kidney.* New York: Wiley, 1976. Chap. 11, p. 187.

48. Landing, B. H., Wells, T. R., Reed, G. B., and Narayan, M. S.   Diseases of the Bile Ducts in Children. In E. A. Gall and F. K. Mostofi (eds.), *The Liver.* Baltimore: Williams & Wilkins, 1973. Chap. 22.

49. Lieberman, E., Salinas-Madrigal, L., Gwinn, J. L., Brennan, L. P., Fine, R. N., and Landing, B. H.   Infantile polycystic disease of the kidneys and liver: Clinical, pathological and radiological correlations and comparison with congenital hepatic fibrosis. *Medicine (Baltimore)* 50:277, 1971.

50. Lundin, P., and Olow, I.   Polycystic kidneys in newborns, infants and children. A clinical and pathological study. *Acta Paediatr.* 50:185, 1961.

51. Martinez-Maldonado, M., Yium, J. J., Eknoyan, G., and Suki, W. N.   Adult polycystic kidney disease: Studies of the defect in urine concentration. *Kidney Int.* 2:107, 1972.

52. McGeoch, J. E. M., and Darmady, E. M.   Polycystic disease of kidney, liver and pancreas; a possible pathogenesis. *J. Pathol.* 119:221, 1976.

53. Mehrizi, A., Rosenstein, B. J., Pusch, A., Askin, J. A., and Taussig, H. B.   Myocardial infarction and endocardial fibroelastosis in children with polycystic kidneys. *Johns Hopkins Med. J.* 115:92, 1964.

54. Michigan Kidney Registry.   Racial differences in the cause of end-stage renal disease. *The Record* 1(3), September, 1975.

55. Murray-Lyon, I. M., Ockenden, B. G., and Williams, R.   Congenital hepatic fibrosis—is it a single clinical entity? *Gastroenterology* 64:653, 1973.

56. O'Callaghan, T. J., Edwards, J. A., Tobin, M., and Moorkerjee, B. K.   Tuberous sclerosis with striking renal involvement in a family. *Arch. Intern. Med.* 135:1082, 1975.

57. Petereit, M. F.   Adult renal polycystic disease in the juvenile patient demonstrated by nephrotomography. Case report. *South Dakota Med. J.* 27:25, 1974.

58. Potter, E. L.   *Normal and Abnormal Development of the Kidney.* Chicago: Year Book, 1972.

59. Reilly, B. J., and Neuhauser, E. B. D.   Renal tubular ectasia in cystic disease of the kidneys and liver. *Am. J. Roentgenol. Radium Ther. Nucl. Med.* 84:546, 1960.

60. Renal Transplantation Registry, Advisory Committee.   The 12th report of the Human Renal Transplant Registry. *J.A.M.A.* 233:787, 1975.

61. Resnick, J. S., Brown, D. M., and Vernier, R. L.   Normal Development and Experimental Models of Cystic Renal Disease. In K. D. Gardner, Jr. (ed.), *Cystic Diseases of the Kidney.* New York: Wiley, 1976. Chap. 13, p. 221.

62. Rosenberg, J. C., Bernstein, J., and Rosenberg, B.   Renal cystic disease associated with tuberous sclerosis complex: Renal failure treated by cadaveric kidney transplantation. *Clin. Nephrol.* 4:109, 1975.

63. Ross, D. G., and Travers, H.   Infantile presentation of adult-type polycystic kidney disease in a large kindred. *J. Pediatr.* 87:760, 1975.

64. Six, R., Oliphant, M., and Grossman, H.   A spectrum of renal tubular ectasia and hepatic fibrosis. *Radiology* 117:117, 1975.

65. Spence, H. M., and Singleton, R.   What is sponge kidney disease and where does it fit in the spectrum of cystic disorders? *J. Urol.* 107:176, 1972.

66. Stickler, G. B., and Kelalis, P. P.   Polycystic kidney disease. Recognition of the "adult form" (autosomal dominant) in infancy. *Mayo Clin. Proc.* 50:547, 1975.

67. Thaler, M. M., Ogata, E. S., Goodman, J. R., Piel, C. F., and Korobkin, M. T.   Congenital fibrosis and polycystic disease of liver and kidneys. *Am. J. Dis. Child.* 126:374, 1973.

68. Unite, I., Maitem, A., Bagnasco, F. M., and Irwin, G. A. L.   Congenital hepatic fibrosis associated with renal tubular ectasia. *Radiology* 109:565, 1973.

69. Viamonte, M., Jr., Ravel, R., Politano, V., and Bridges, B.   Angiographic findings in a patient with tuberous sclerosis. *Am. J. Roentgenol. Radium Ther. Nucl. Med.* 98:723, 1966.

70. Vuthibhagdee, A., and Singleton, E. B.   Infantile polycystic disease of the kidney. *Am. J. Dis. Child.* 125:167, 1973.

71. Weiss, L., Reynolds, W. A., Saeed, S. M., and Cabal, L.   Congenital Hepatic Fibrosis and Polycystic Disease of Kidneys with the Roentgen Appearance of Medullary Sponge Kidney. In D. Bergsma (ed.), *Fifth Conference on the Clinical Delineation of Birth Defects. Birth Defects.* Original Article Series. New York: The National Foundation, 1974. Vol. X/4, p. 35.

72. Wenzl, J. E., Lagos, J. C., and Albers, D. D.   Tuberous sclerosis presenting as polycystic kidneys and seizures in an infant. *J. Pediatr.* 77:673, 1970.

41. Hereditary Nephritis

Jay Bernstein and John M. Kissane

The hereditary nephritides are a heterogeneous group of chronic renal diseases associated with recurrent hematuria and progressive renal failure. They are part of a larger group of genetically determined and familial nephropathies that have been recognized and identified with remarkably increasing frequency during the last decade. Although a satisfactory classification that meets all the requirements of morphology, physiology, and clinical medicine seems premature, the explosive proliferation of eponyms and syndromes has created an urgent need for ordering and grouping these conditions.

Hereditary nephritis should be differentiated from familial glomerulonephritis, in which glomerular injury is initiated by genetically triggered immune abnormalities, and from several other familial nephropathies in which primary tubular injury is initiated by genetically triggered metabolic abnormalities. An example of hereditary nephritis is the Alport syndrome, in which the structure of the glomerular basement membrane appears to be inherently abnormal. It is differentiated, for example, from the abnormality found in the syndrome of partial lipodystrophy, in which membranoproliferative glomerulonephritis seems to result from activation of the complement system with secondary glomerular injury. It is differentiated also from medullary cystic disease, in which a presumed metabolic defect leads to tubular dysfunction and renal atrophy. Other nosologic distinctions include the familial forms of nephrotic syndrome (e.g., the Finnish type of congenital nephrotic syndrome), the inherited metabolic diseases with incidental renal involvement (e.g., diabetes mellitus), and the heritable disorders of tubular transport (e.g., Lowe oculocerebrorenal syndrome).

Hereditary nephritis comprises several genetically unrelated and clinically dissimilar disorders with primary glomerular involvement. Its major categories are *hereditary progressive nephritis* (Alport syndrome) and *hereditary onycho-osteodysplasia* (nail-patella syndrome). The requirement that the condition be progressive may be stretched slightly in the instance of *familial recurrent hematuria,* in which renal failure is lacking or mild despite the histopathologic findings of focal glomerular sclerosis and tubular damage.

Alport Syndrome

Hereditary progressive nephritis, or Alport syndrome, is characterized by recurrent hematuria, progressive renal failure, and deafness. The renal manifestations are clinically somewhat variable, and extrarenal manifestations occur with varying frequency. Familial progressive renal disease was described by several writers in the late 19th century. In 1902 Guthrie [31] reported recurrent hematuria in a British family, in which a later study by Alport [1] demonstrated the association of renal failure and deafness. These papers are behind the common eponymic designations of hereditary progressive nephritis, but a distinction between Guthrie disease (hereditary nephritis alone) and Alport disease (hereditary nephritis with deafness) is meaningless, because both investigators studied and reported the same family.

ETIOLOGY AND GENETICS

The Alport syndrome is presumed to be secondary to a primary defect within the basement membrane. Ultrastructural studies show attenuation, disruption, and severe lamellation or duplication [13, 35, 72]. The primary abnormality may be a heritable metabolic defect that leads to abnormal synthesis and abnormal assembly of proteins in the basement membrane, perhaps in basement membrane collagen [70]. A similar defect in other basement membrane collagens could account for the abnormalities that are encountered in the ear and eye. Spear [70] has hypothesized that the abnormality may involve cross-linking through disulfide bonds, a point that relates to the characteristic presence of half-cystine in basement membrane collagen.

The disease appears to be transmitted through consecutive generations with autosomal dominant inheritance [11, 27, 55, 56, 58]. Studies of population genetics indicate that 18 percent of affected newborns suffer from new mutations [65]. There are, however, certain atypical features that need to be accounted for. Men are typically affected more severely than women, and afflicted men appear to father predominantly abnormal daughters and a deficient number of afflicted sons [57, 58]. Several alternative genetic mechanisms have been suggested, therefore, among them partial sex linkage [74] and preferential segregation with the X chromosome [14, 51, 59, 64], but neither hypothesis has been entirely satisfactory [58]. Variability in expression and penetrance of a dominant gene has also been proposed to account for the findings [32, 64]. The roles of nongenetic factors have not been adequately explored; if the same basement membrane lesion is present in both severely affected men and minimally affected women of the same family, as suggested by Churg and colleagues [13, 66], expression of the disease may be influenced by hormonal or other sex-related but nongenetic factors [7].

EPIDEMIOLOGY

The prevalence of Alport syndrome is not known. It accounts for approximately 3 percent of chronic renal failure in childhood [9]. The literature contains a large number of reported cases, but the incidence rate is not calculable. The condition is often apparent in early childhood, but other cases are not recognized until the second or third decade. Men may be affected earlier than women, and they are affected more severely, commonly dying before the age of 40. Women often have milder disease, perhaps microscopic hematuria or just deafness. There are, however, many exceptions to the rule, and it should be emphasized that the disease can be as severe in women as in men, particularly in prepubertal girls.

Differences in racial and ethnic distributions have not been well explored. The condition is said to be relatively uncommon in black Americans [26].

CLINICAL MANIFESTATIONS

The most common clinical feature of the Alport syndrome is persistent or recurrent hematuria, with frequent gross exacerbation following upper respiratory infection. The hematuria may be recognized early in childhood. Proteinuria is usually mild in the early stages, but it increases as the disease progresses. It is occasionally severe enough to result in the nephrotic syndrome [22, 39]. Urinary tract infection is an infrequent complication that appears to be unrelated to the main disease process. The course is commonly one of slowly progressive renal failure, often accompanied by hypertension, beginning in men late in the second and particularly in the third decade of life. Few affected men survive beyond the age of 40. Women have milder disease, often only episodes of hematuria related to stress or to pregnancy, and their longevity is often unaffected. However, renal failure early in life affects both sexes.

The majority of patients with Alport syndrome have neither deafness nor ocular defects, but loss of high-frequency auditory perception occurs frequently enough, in approximately 30 to 40 percent, to be used as a clinical marker in family studies. In reported family studies, some individuals may be deaf but lack evidence of renal disease and others may have severe renal disease without evidence of deafness. The acoustic loss is most often in the range of 4,000 to 8,000 Hz, and the defect may be detectable only by audiometric testing. Histopathologic studies of the inner ear have yielded inconsistent findings, among them loss of neurons, loss of hair cells, atrophy of the spiral ligaments, and degeneration of the stria vascularis [15, 17, 23, 28, 75], and it has been suggested that the morphologic variability reflects underlying heterogeneity [53]. The hearing loss may be asymmetric or even unilateral. Some patients develop a secondary conduction hearing loss late in the course of disease.

Ocular abnormalities are seen in approximately 15 percent, mostly in men [3, 8, 15, 69]. The abnormalities are usually lenticular, including cataracts, keratoconus, and spherophakia. Patients suffer from myopia and nystagmus.

RENAL PATHOLOGY

Histopathologic studies have shown little change early in the course of the Alport syndrome. The glomeruli appear to be normal, although there may be nonspecific focal mesangial hypercellularity and apparent thickening of the glomerular capillary walls [38]. The glomerular lesion is occasionally proliferative, both with mesangial hypercellularity and with severe extracapillary proliferation to form epithelial crescents [15]. Small glomeruli that appear to be unusually immature have also been described [2]. Later changes include more severe mesangial thickening and segmental sclerosis leading to glomerular obsolescence (Fig. 41-1).

Progressive glomerular disease leads to nephronic atrophy, but tubular atrophy may proceed as an independent abnormality and is sometimes relatively severe, disproportionate to the degree of glomerular alteration (Fig. 41-1). The resultant appearance is one of cortical atrophy, with interstitial fibrosis and interstitial cellular infiltration, that has sometimes been characterized as "mixed nephritis" [42]. Ultrastructural studies have shown that many of the small cells within the interstitium are tubular epithelial remnants and that infiltrates of inflammatory cells are commonly sparse. As the changes progress to involve the entire cortex, the kidneys become uniformly and symmetrically reduced in size, with pale and finely granular cortical surfaces. The cortex becomes thin, and yellow streaks corresponding to collections of interstitial

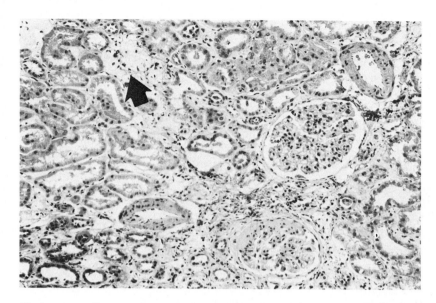

Figure 41-1. Alport syndrome. The glomerular capillary walls appear to be slightly thickened, and one glomerulus contains a segmental area of sclerosis. Bowman's capsules are slightly thickened, and there is periglomerular fibrosis. Tubular alterations, which are more severe than would be expected from the degree of glomerular sclerosis, include irregular dilatation and patchy atrophy (lower center.) Focal clusters of foam cells (arrow) are present in the interstitium, which contains increased connective tissue. The patient was a 16-year-old girl with a 12-year history of hematuria and proteinuria and with a serum creatinine concentration of 5 mg per deciliter. She had a unilateral loss of hearing; a younger sister also had hematuria and proteinuria. (H&E, ×120.)

foam cells appear at the corticomedullary junctions. The foam cells are not to be regarded as specific abnormalities of Alport syndrome, since they are found in other conditions, for example, membranoproliferative glomerulonephritis and membranous glomerulonephropathy with nephrotic syndrome. Arteriosclerosis also develops, often in association with clinical hypertension.

Immunofluorescent studies are usually negative [12]. Occasional localization of IgM and C3 may correspond to areas of sclerosis with nonspecific trapping of serum protein [24, 73]. Because exacerbations of disease follow clinical infection, occasional mesangial localization of immunoglobulin and complement may be detectable without being related to the primary glomerular defect. Ultrastructural studies have also shown accumulation of mesangial material that is suggestive of immune deposits [63], and the same limitations of interpretation apply.

Electron microscopic studies have shown alterations within the lamina densa of the glomerular capillary basement membrane [13, 24, 30, 35, 61, 71, 72]. The basement membranes are typically split and lamellated, containing within them numerous small, granular densities and fine lipid droplets (Fig. 41-2). The lesion is irregularly dis-

tributed and may be difficult to recognize. We have not observed it in several very young patients who were studied because of positive family histories and were clinically found to have hematuria, and the lesion may become more obvious with time [3a]. The lesion should, therefore, be looked for carefully in a suspected case, and silver methenamine stains of the ultrathin sections are helpful (Fig. 41-3). The abnormalities must, nonetheless, be clearly established for them to carry any weight, and simple duplication of the basement membrane cannot be taken as sufficient evidence of the disease. This problem in differential diagnosis may relate to the presence of resorbing intramembranous deposits within split basement membranes in children who have hematuria on the basis of resolving immune complex disease [34]. The characteristic lesion, with multiple lamellations, is a very helpful ultrastructural finding. In some studies the lesion has been found in all cases that were clinically diagnosed as hereditary progressive nephritis [24, 30, 72]. Churg and colleagues [13, 66] found it to be present in all affected members of a family, both male and female, but an affected sibling in another family has not had the lesion [3a]. It probably reflects defective turnover and repair of basement membrane,

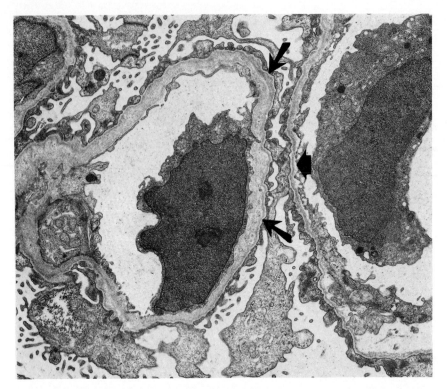

Figure 41-2. Alport syndrome. The basement membrane of the glomerular capillary wall is of irregular thickness. The basement membrane in the segment on the left is thicker than normal (long arrows), and it is lamellated, appearing to consist of multiple strands, among which there are granular densities. The basement membrane in the capillary segment on the right (wide arrow) is much thinner than normal. The patient was the 11-year-old sister of the patient whose biopsy is shown in Fig. 41-1; her renal function was normal, but she has since developed renal insufficiency. Electron micrograph. (×8,000.)

and in that sense it may be a genetic marker, but it does not serve to identify the patients destined to develop renal failure.

Another abnormality of the glomerular capillary basement membrane is marked attenuation (Fig. 41-2), often with discontinuity of the lamina densa [24, 30, 61, 71, 72]. The unusual thinness of the basement membrane, often between 150 and 200 nm, probably also reflects abnormal synthesis and maintenance of the lamina densa. A similar change is present in patients with familial recurrent hematuria [60], in which there is no progression to renal failure. Identification of this abnormality does not serve, therefore, to make the important clinical distinction between the Alport syndrome and familial recurrent hematuria.

Similar lesions are often present in the tubular basement membranes, which are also thickened and lamellated [7, 13]. The abnormality in the tubular basement membrane may precede the stage of tubular atrophy, but somewhat similar changes occur in the basement membranes of atrophic tubules in several forms of chronic nephritis. It is

conceivable, therefore, that damage to the tubular epithelium, which is often out of proportion to the severity of glomerular obsolescence, may result from a primary defect in the basement membrane. The tubular epithelial cells frequently contain lipid vacuoles, but rarely to the extent that they become foam cells. The abnormal basement membranes also contain numerous lipid droplets. These droplets have been interpreted to have diffused out of the tubular epithelial cells and are regarded as responsible for the interstitial foam cells, which are in close proximity. This explanation might account for the frequent occurrence of foam cells in Alport disease, and a similar diffusion of lipid from tubular epithelium might account for the development of foam cells in the nephrotic syndrome.

VARIANTS OF ALPORT SYNDROME

Hereditary progressive nephritis with deafness occurs in association with certain other inherited abnormalities. Because the renal lesions have not been clearly different from the renal lesions in Al-

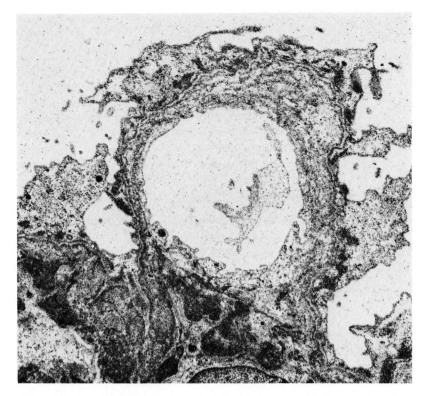

Figure 41-3. Alport syndrome. A silver methenamine impregnation of the glomerular basement membrane shows more clearly the splitting and lamellation. Same biopsy as Fig. 41-2. Electron micrograph. (×11,000.)

port syndrome, these associations are regarded as variants.

The most common association has been with hyperprolinemia [62], which has been reported in several related kindreds from different parts of the world. The relationship of hyperprolinemia to the renal disease is uncertain, but a review of reported cases [17, 19, 25, 31, 62] suggests that they are inherited separately.

The renal lesion in patients with hyperprolinemia and nephritis is said to be the same as the lesion in typical Alport syndrome, although some patients have had small and hypoplastic kidneys [62], perhaps the result of asymmetric atrophy, and in one case the kidney was replaced by cysts [19]. Other structural alterations have included chronic inflammatory lesions thought to represent chronic pyelonephritis. Most histologic studies have been carried out on end-stage kidneys in which the characteristic features could have been masked by secondary changes. Foam cells have been variably present. Electron micrographs of one biopsy have shown thickening of glomerular basement membranes [25], but in electron microscopic studies we have not been able to identify the characteristic changes of Alport syndrome.

Metabolic studies [19, 20] have shown that proline shares its transport mechanism in the renal tubule with hydroxyproline and glycine, and urinary concentrations of hydroxyproline and glycine are also increased in patients with hereditary hyperprolinemia. In support of the assumption that the two conditions are separable though associated, it must be pointed out that many carefully investigated patients with Alport syndrome have had neither hyperprolinemia nor abnormal urinary excretion of amino acids.

Other conditions have been less commonly associated with hereditary progressive nephritis and deafness. The members of one family with prolinuria also had severe ichthyosis [25]. Descriptions of some cases have included neurologic abnormalities, among them polyneuropathy [47] and a syndrome of photomyoclonus, diabetes, deafness, and cerebral dysfunction [33]. Myopathy secondary to hyaline vasculopathy has been described in association with familial nephritis [10]. Progressive nephropathy with focal glomerular sclerosis has been observed in several patients suffering from Charcot-Marie-Tooth disease [44], and electron microscopy of a renal biopsy has not disclosed typical changes in the glomerular basement membranes [45]. The clinical histories have not corresponded closely to typical Alport syndrome, and the relationship between the two syndromes is uncertain. A hematologic disorder consisting of thrombocytopenia with giant platelets has been associated with renal disease thought to be indistinguishable from Alport syndrome [6, 18, 21, 54]. In each of these instances renal disease has apparently been transmitted with an autosomal dominant inheritance.

DIFFERENTIAL DIAGNOSIS

The principal differential diagnosis of familial renal disease lies between hereditary progressive nephritis (Alport syndrome) and familial benign recurrent hematuria. Clinical differentiation before the stage of actual functional deterioration may be impossible in the absence of a family history of renal failure and deafness. The histopathologic findings of glomerular sclerosis, tubular atrophy, and interstitial foam cells constitute an important diagnostic constellation, but it must be recognized that focal glomerular sclerosis and tubular atrophy are also commonly encountered in patients with apparently nonprogressive familial disease. Finding the characteristic ultrastructural alteration of the glomerular basement membrane is an important factor in distinguishing between the two conditions [29, 36, 40].

The other hereditary condition from which the Alport syndrome should be separated is the nail-patella syndrome, in which the radiographic abnormalities include iliac horns, hypoplastic patellae, and malformed radial heads; the nails are dystrophic and hypoplastic. The evaluation of associated nonrenal abnormalities is essential, therefore, to the investigation of any patient.

Finally, Alport syndrome enters the differential diagnosis of all forms of chronic renal disease with hematuria, proteinuria, and renal failure. Many cases have gone unrecognized, having been regarded simply as chronic glomerulonephritis.

TREATMENT

No form of therapy is known to affect the basic course of disease. Intercurrent infections of the urinary tract require appropriate therapy. The care of patients in renal failure follows the accepted principles and practices. If prevention is an important part of treatment, then the major therapeutic approach takes the form of genetic counseling.

Familial Recurrent Hematuria

In some patients with persistent microscopic and recurrent gross hematuria, renal functional deteri-

oration is minimal or does not occur, and the patients are characterized as having "benign recurrent hematuria." Recurrent hematuria in the absence of progressive renal disease may be either sporadic or familial [44, 49]. Familial hematuria seems to be transmitted usually with an autosomal dominant inheritance [49, 60], but in some instances the inheritance appears to have followed a recessive pattern [48].

Clinical evaluation of such cases obviously includes an adequate family history, for the occurrence of renal insufficiency and deafness in relatives may be taken as strong indications of Alport disease. Histopathologic studies are also helpful in excluding other forms of glomerular disease, particularly glomerulonephritis, and immunofluorescent studies are essential features of a complete workup. Electron microscopic examination is important, as noted above, in excluding the characteristic basement membrane lesion of Alport syndrome, but it must be noted that the basement membrane in both conditions may be attenuated and disrupted [34, 60] (Fig. 41-4). The differential diagnosis in individual cases includes all causes of hematuria (Chaps. 9, 44).

The ultimate prognosis of so-called benign hematuria remains somewhat uncertain. Histopathologic examination often shows focal glomerular sclerosis and tubular atrophy, and mild or partial renal functional impairment may be present in patients at middle age.

Hereditary Onycho-osteodysplasia (Nail-Patella Syndrome)

Renal disease is found in approximately 30 to 40 percent of patients with the nail-patella syndrome, and it progresses to renal failure in approximately 25 percent [68]. It is estimated, therefore, that approximately 10 percent of patients with the nail-patella syndrome die of renal insufficiency. The clinical features, which serve also to differentiate the condition from Alport syndrome, include dystrophic and hypoplastic nails, iliac horns, malformed radial heads, and hypoplastic patellae [43, 52, 67]. These radiographic abnormalities have in the past been included in descriptions of Alport syndrome, but the two diseases are genetically separable. Cutaneous manifestations have occasionally been described, and ocular involvement takes the form of abnormal pigmentation of the iris.

The most characteristic clinical manifestation of renal involvement is proteinuria, which may be of sufficient severity to result in the nephrotic syndrome. Other patients have negligible clinical evidence of renal involvement despite characteristic

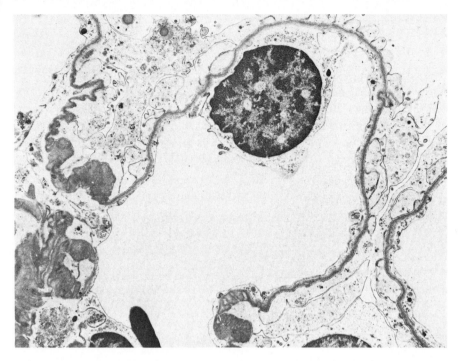

Figure 41-4. Familial recurrent hematuria. Uniformly thin basement membranes (average thickness 245 nm) are present in the glomerular capillary wall of a 29-year-old man with hematuria known to be of five years' duration; he also had mild proteinuria, but there was no clinical evidence of renal insufficiency. Electron micrograph. (×5,600.)

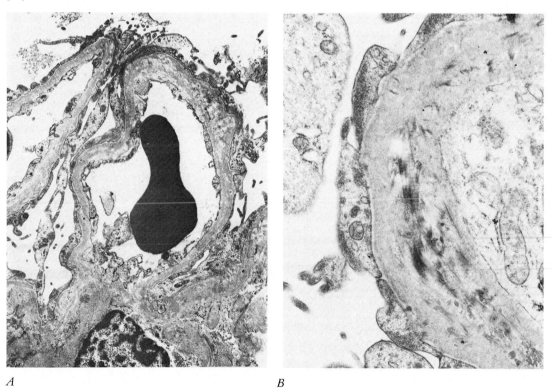

A   B

Figure 41-5. Nail-patella syndrome. The glomerular basement membrane is irregularly thickened by lucent areas (A) in which there are fibers that can be demonstrated to consist of collagen with regular structure and periodicity (B). (Electron micrographs: A, ×7,800 before 20% reduction; B, phosphotungstic acid impregnation, ×22,500 before 20% reduction.)

findings in renal biopsies [5]. Hypertension also occurs.

Histopathologic evaluation early in the course of nail-patella syndrome shows normal glomeruli, except that there may be thickening and irregularity of the capillary walls. The basement membranes proper appear to be thickened, an abnormality that is confirmed ultrastructurally [4, 5, 16, 37, 50]. The lamina densa is irregularly thickened and focally lucent [16], and collagen fibers can be demonstrated to reside within the basement membrane [4] (Fig. 41-5). The occurrence of collagen fibers with typical structure and periodicity within the lamina densa of the basement membrane has not been described in any other condition, as opposed to the presence of collagen fibers within the mesangium, which is a nonspecific reaction. Light microscopic studies show slowly progressive involvement leading to segmental sclerosis and obsolescence with tubular atrophy, cortical fibrosis, and the histologic features of chronic nephritis [46]. Immunofluorescent studies have shown focal deposits of IgM and complement [5, 37], presumably a nonspecific finding shared by other types of glomerular sclerosis.

The disease is transmitted with autosomal dominant inheritance, and the abnormality is linked to the gene locus for ABO blood groups.

References

1. Alport, A. C. Hereditary familial congenital haemorrhagic nephritis. *Br. Med. J.* 1:504, 1927.
2. Antonovych, T. T., Deasey, P. F., Tina, L. U., D'Albora, J. B., Hollerman, C. E., and Calcagno, P. L. Hereditary nephritis: Early clinical, functional, and morphological studies. *Pediatr. Res.* 3: 545, 1969.
3. Arnott, E. J., Crawfurd, M. D'A., and Toghill, P. J. Anterior lenticonus and Alport's syndrome. *Br. J. Ophthalmol.* 50:390, 1966.
3a. Beathard, G. A., and Granholm, N. A. Development of the characteristic ultrastructural lesion of hereditary nephritis during the course of the disease. *Am. J. Med.* 62:751, 1977.
4. Ben-Bassat, M., Cohen, L., and Rosenfeld, J. The glomerular basement membrane in the nail-patella syndrome. *Arch. Pathol.* 92:350, 1971.
5. Bennett, W. M., Musgrave, J. E., Campbell, R. A., Elliot, D., Cox, R., Brooks, R. E., Lovrien, E. W., Beals, R. K., and Porter, G. A. The nephropathy of the nail-patella syndrome: Clinicopathologic analysis of 11 kindred. *Am. J. Med.* 54:304, 1973.
6. Bernheim, J., Dechavanne, M., Byron, P. A., Lagarde, M., Colon, S., Pozet, N., and Traeger, J. Thrombocytopenia, macrothrombocytopathia, nephritis and deafness. *Am. J. Med.* 61:145, 1976.
7. Bernstein, J. The Pathology of the Hereditary Nephritides. In J. Strauss (ed.), *Pediatric Nephrology*, Vol. 2. Miami: Symposia Specialists, 1976. P. 301.
8. Brownell, R. D., and Wolter, J. R. Anterior lenticonus in familial hemorrhagic nephritis: Demonstra-
tion of lens pathology. *Arch. Ophthalmol.* 71:481, 1964.
9. Broyer, M. Chronic Renal Failure. In P. Royer, R. Habib, H. Mathieu, and M. Broyer (eds.), *Pediatric Nephrology*. Philadelphia: Saunders, 1974. Part IV, chap. 2.
10. Chazan, J. A., Ambler, M., Kalderon, A., Cohen, J. J., and Zacks, J. Vascular deposits causing ischemic myopathy in uremia: Two brothers with hereditary nephritis. *Ann. Intern. Med.* 73:73, 1970.
11. Chazan, J. A., Zacks, J., Cohen, J. J., and Garella, S. Hereditary nephritis: Clinical spectrum and mode of inheritance in five new kindreds. *Am. J. Med.* 50:764, 1971.
12. Chiricosta, A., Jindal, S. L., Metuzals, J., and Koch, B. Hereditary nephropathy with hematuria (Alport's syndrome). *Can. Med. Assoc. J.* 102:399, 1970.
13. Churg, J., and Sherman, R. L. Pathologic characteristics of hereditary nephritis. *Arch. Pathol.* 95:374, 1973.
14. Cohen, M. M., Cassady, G., and Hanna, B. L. Genetic study of hereditary renal dysfunction with associated nerve deafness. *Am. J. Hum. Genet.* 13:379, 1961.
15. Crawford, M. D'A., and Toghill, P. J. Alport's syndrome of hereditary nephritis and deafness. *Q. J. Med.* 37:563, 1968.
16. del Pozo, E., and Lapp, H. Ultrastructure of the kidney in the nephropathy of the nail-patella syndrome. *Am. J. Clin. Pathol.* 54:845, 1970.
17. Dubach, R. C., Minder, F. C., and Antener, I. Familial nephropathy and deafness: First observation of a family and close relatives in Switzerland. *Helv. Med. Acta* 33:36, 1966.
18. Eckstein, J. D., Filip, D. J., and Watts, J. C. Hereditary thrombocytopenia, deafness, and renal disease. *Ann. Intern. Med.* 82:639, 1975.
19. Efron, M. L. Familial hyperprolinemia: Report of a second case, associated with congenital renal malformations, hereditary hematuria and mild mental retardation, with demonstration of enzyme defect. *N. Engl. J. Med.* 272:1243, 1965.
20. Efron, M. L., Bixby, E. M., Palatto, L. G., and Pyles, K. V. Hydroxyprolinemia associated with mental deficiency. *N. Engl. J. Med.* 267:1193, 1962.
21. Epstein, C. J., Sahud, M. A., Piel, C. F., Goodman, J. R., Bernfield, M. R., Kushner, J. J., and Ablin, A. R. Hereditary macrothrombocytopathia, nephritis and deafness. *Am. J. Med.* 52:299, 1972.
22. Felts, J. W. Hereditary nephritis with the nephrotic syndrome. *Arch. Intern. Med.* 125:459, 1970.
23. Fujita, S., and Hayden, R. Alport's syndrome: Temporal bone report. *Arch. Otolaryngol.* 90:453, 1969.
24. Gaboardi, F., Edefonti, A., Imbasciati, E., Tarantino, A., Mihatsch, M. J., and Zollinger, H. U. Alport's syndrome (progressive hereditary nephritis). *Clin. Nephrol.* 2:143, 1974.
25. Goyer, R. A., Reynolds, J., Jr., Burke, J., and Burkholder, P. Hereditary renal disease. *Am. J. Med. Sci.* 256:166, 1968.
26. Grace, S. G., Suki, W. N., Spjut, H. J., Eknoyan, G., and Martinez-Maldonado, M. Hereditary nephritis in the Negro: Report of a kindred. *Arch. Intern. Med.* 125:451, 1970.
27. Graham, J. B. Chronic hereditary nephritis: Not shown to be partially sex-linked. *Am. J. Hum. Genet.* 12:382, 1960.
28. Gregg, J., and Becker, S. Concomitant progressive

deafness, chronic nephritis, and ocular lens disease. *Arch. Ophthalmol.* 69:293, 1963.

29. Grünfeld, J.-P., Bois, E. P., and Hinglais, N. Progressive and nonprogressive hereditary chronic nephritis. *Kidney Int.* 4:216, 1973.

30. Gubler, M. C., Gonzales-Burchard, G., Monnier, C., and Habib, R. Alport's Syndrome: Natural History and Ultrastructural Lesions of Glomerular and Tubular Basement Membranes. In G. B. Berlyne and S. Giovannetti (eds.), *Contributions to Nephrology.* Basel: Karger, 1976. Vol. 2, p. 163.

31. Guthrie, L. G. "Idiopathic" or congenital hereditary and familial haematuria. *Lancet* 1:1243, 1902.

32. Hallberg, A. Alport's syndrome: A report of three Swedish families. *Acta Paediatr. Scand.* 65:49, 1976.

33. Herrmann, C., Jr., Aguilar, M. J., and Sacks, O. W. Hereditary photomyoclonus associated with diabetes mellitus, deafness, nephropathy, and cerebral dysfunction. *Neurology* 14:212, 1964.

34. Hill, G. S., Jenis, E. H., and Goodloe, S., Jr. The nonspecificity of the ultrastructural alterations in hereditary nephritis: With additional observations on benign familial hematuria. *Lab. Invest.* 31:516, 1974.

35. Hinglais, N., Grünfeld, J.-P., and Bois, E. Characteristic ultrastructural lesion of the glomerular basement membrane in progressive hereditary nephritis (Alport's syndrome). *Lab. Invest.* 27:473, 1972.

36. Hinglais, N., Grünfeld, J.-P., Troconis, L., and Bois, E. Ultrastructural Lesions of the Glomerular Basement Membrane in Hereditary Chronic Nephritis. In J. Hamburger, J. Crosnier, and M. Maxwell (eds.), *Advances in Nephrology,* Vol. 3. Chicago: Year Book, 1974. P. 133.

37. Hoyer, J. R., Michael, A. F., and Vernier, R. L. Renal disease in nail-patella syndrome: Clinical and morphologic studies. *Kidney Int.* 2:231, 1972.

38. Kaufman, D. B., McIntosh, R. M., Smith, F. G., Jr., and Vernier, R. L. Diffuse familial nephropathy: A Clinicopathological study. *J. Pediatr.* 77:37, 1970.

39. Knepshield, J. H., Roberts, P. L., Davis, C. J., and Moser, R. H. Hereditary chronic nephritis complicated by nephrotic syndrome. *Arch. Intern. Med.* 122:156, 1968.

40. Kohaut, E. C., Singer, D. B., Nevels, B. K., and Hill, L. L. The specificity of split renal membranes in hereditary nephritis. *Arch. Pathol. Lab. Med.* 100:475, 1976.

41. Kopelman, H., Asatoor, A. M., and Milne, M. D. Hyperprolinaemia and hereditary nephritis. *Lancet* 2:1075, 1964.

42. Krickstein, H. I., Gloor, F. J., and Balogh, K., Jr. Renal pathology in hereditary nephritis with nerve deafness. *Arch. Pathol.* 82:506, 1966.

43. Leahy, M. S. The hereditary nephropathy of osteo-onychodysplasia. *Am. J. Dis. Child.* 112:237, 1966.

44. Lemieux, G., and Neemeh, J. A. Charcot-Marie-Tooth disease and nephritis. *Can. Med. Assoc. J.* 97:1193, 1967.

45. Lennert, T., Hanefeld, F., and Bernstein, J. Charcot-Marie-Tooth disease and chronic nephropathy. Presented at Program of the 10th Meeting of the European Society for Paediatric Nephrology, Barcelona, June 3–7, 1976.

46. Manigand, G., Auzepy, P., Paillas, A. J., Cohen de Lara, A., and Deparis, M. Ostéo-onycho-dysplasie avec néphropathie: Étude anatomo-clinique. *Sem. Hop. Paris* 47:2956, 1971.

47. Marin, O. S. M., and Tyler, H. R. Hereditary interstitial nephritis associated with polyneuropathy. *Neurology* 11:999, 1961.

48. Marks, M. I., and Drummond, K. N. Benign familial hematuria. *Pediatrics* 44:590, 1969.

49. McConville, J. M., West, C. C., and McAdams, A. J. Familial and nonfamilial benign hematuria. *J. Pediatr.* 69:207, 1966.

50. Morita, T., Laughlin, L. O., Kawano, K., Kimmelsteil, P., Suzuki, Y., and Churg, J. Nail-patella syndrome: Light and electron microscopic studies of the kidney. *Arch. Intern. Med.* 131:271, 1973.

51. Mulrow, P. J., Aron, A. M., Gathman, G. E., Yesner, R., and Lubs, H. A. Hereditary nephritis: Report of a kindred. *Am. J. Med.* 35:737, 1963.

52. Muth, R. G. The nephropathy of hereditary osteo-onychodysplasia. *Ann. Intern. Med.* 62:1279, 1965.

53. Myers, G. J., and Tyler, H. R. The etiology of deafness in Alport's syndrome. *Arch. Otolaryngol.* 96:333, 1972.

54. Parsa, K. P., Lee, D. B. N., Zamboni, L., and Glassock, R. J. Hereditary nephritis, deafness and abnormal thrombopoiesis: Study of a new kindred. *Am. J. Med.* 60:665, 1976.

55. Pashayan, J., Fraser, F. C., and Goldbloom, R. B. A family showing hereditary nephropathy. *Am. J. Hum. Genet.* 23:555, 1971.

56. Perkoff, G. T. Familial aspects of diffuse renal disease. *Annu. Rev. Med.* 15:115, 1964.

57. Perkoff, G. T., Nugent, C. A., Jr., Dolowitz, D. A., Stephens, F. E., Carnes, W. H., and Tyler, F. H. A follow-up study of hereditary chronic nephritis. *Arch. Intern. Med.* 102:733, 1958.

58. Preus, M., and Fraser, F. C. Genetics of hereditary nephropathy with deafness (Alport's disease). *Clin. Genet.* 2:331, 1971.

59. Purriel, P., Drets, M., Pascale, E., Sánchez-Cestau, R., Borrás, A., Ferreira, W. A., De Lucca, A., and Fernández, L. Familial hereditary nephropathy (Alport's syndrome). *Am. J. Med.* 49:753, 1970.

60. Rogers, P. W., Kurtzman, N. A., Bunn, S. M., Jr., and White, M. G. Familial benign essential hematuria. *Arch. Intern. Med.* 131:257, 1973.

61. Rumpelt, H. J., Langer, K. H., Schärer, K., Straub, E., and Thoenes, W. Split and extremely thin glomerular basement membranes in hereditary nephropathy (Alport's syndrome). *Virchows Arch. [Pathol. Anat.]* 364:225, 1974.

62. Schafer, I. A., Scriver, C. R., and Efron, M. L. Familial hyperprolinemia, cerebral dysfunction and renal anomalies occurring in a family with hereditary nephropathy and deafness. *N. Engl. J. Med.* 267:51, 1962.

63. Sessa, A., Cioffi, A., Conte, F., and D'Amico, G. Hereditary nephropathy with nerve deafness (Alport's syndrome): Electron microscopic studies on the renal glomerulus. *Nephron* 13:404, 1974.

64. Shaw, R. F., and Glover, R. A. Abnormal segregation in hereditary renal disease with deafness. *Am. J. Human Genet.* 13:89, 1961.

65. Shaw, R. F., and Kallen, R. J. Population genetics of Alport's syndrome: Hypothesis of abnormal segregation and the necessary existence of mutation. *Nephron* 16:427, 1976.

66. Sherman, R. L., Churg, J., and Yudis, M. Hereditary nephritis with a characteristic renal lesion. *Am. J. Med.* 56:44, 1974.

67. Silverman, M. E., Goodman, R. M., and Cuppage,

F. E.   The nail-patella syndrome: Clinical findings and ultrastructural observations in the kidney. *Arch. Intern. Med.* 120:68, 1967.

68. Similä, S., Vesa, L., and Wasz-Höckert, O.   Hereditary onycho-osteodysplasia (the nail-patella syndrome) with nephrosis-like renal disease in a newborn boy. *Pediatrics* 46:61, 1970.

69. Sohar, E.   Renal disease, inner ear deafness, and ocular changes: New heredo-familial syndrome. *Arch. Intern. Med.* 97:627, 1956.

70. Spear, G. S.   Alport's syndrome: A consideration of pathogenesis. *Clin. Nephrol.* 1:336, 1973.

71. Spear, G. S.   Pathology of the Kidney in Alport's Syndrome. In S. C. Sommers (ed.), *Pathology Annual 1974.* New York: Appleton-Century-Crofts, 1974. P. 93.

72. Spear, G. S., and Slusser, R. J.   Alport's syndrome: Emphasizing electron microscopic studies of the glomerulus. *Am. J. Pathol.* 69:213, 1972.

73. Spear, G. S., Whitworth, J. M., and Konigsmark, B. W.   Hereditary nephritis with nerve deafness: Immunofluorescent studies on the kidney, with a consideration of discordant immunoglobulin-complement immunofluorescent reactions. *Am. J. Med.* 49:52, 1970.

74. Stephens, F. E., Perkoff, G. T., Dolowitz, D. A., and Tyler, F. H.   Partially sex-linked dominant inheritance of interstitial pyelonephritis. *Am. J. Hum. Genet.* 3:303, 1951.

75. Winter, L., Cram, B., and Banovetz, J.   Hearing loss in hereditary renal disease. *Arch. Otolaryngol.* 88:238, 1968.

42. Familial Juvenile Nephronophthisis— Medullary Cystic Disease

Jay Bernstein and Kenneth D. Gardner, Jr.

A chronic form of renal disease in childhood that is characterized clinically by polyuria, growth failure, and progressive renal failure has been designated *familial juvenile nephronophthisis* (FJN) [10]. Renal medullary cysts, which were demonstrated in the early postmortem studies [44], are present in the majority of patients. The morphologic findings are similar to those found in a disorder that occurs predominantly in older patients and has been designated *medullary cystic disease* (MCD) [45]; its clinical manifestations also include a urinary concentrating defect and progressive azotemia. The morphologic and clinical similarities led several workers to unify these conditions under a single heading [19, 28, 46], but subsequent studies have clearly shown genetic heterogeneity within the group. Differences in genetic transmission and differences in characteristic age at onset have led to the separation of the syndrome into at least two diseases [12], as follows: (1) familial juvenile nephronophthisis, an autosomal recessive disorder with onset typically in childhood and with the occasional association of nonrenal abnormalities; and (2) medullary cystic disease, an autosomal dominant disorder (or one of indeterminate heredity) with an onset typically in adult life. Isolated cases, which possibly result from new, dominant mutations, are designated as sporadic MCD.

Because of nosologic confusion, the literature contains several different terms that have been used synonymously with FJN and MCD: cystic disease of the renal medulla, uremic medullary cystic disease, uremic sponge kidney, salt-losing nephritis, polycystic disease of medullary type, and Fanconi's nephronophthisis. The term *renal-retinal dysplasia* designates a variant of FJN with associated retinal degeneration [40], and it will be used in that sense in this discussion.

Pathogenesis and Genetics

Although some cases of renal disease with the morphologic and clinical features described above are sporadic, the genetic background of the FJN-MCD complex is clearly established. Medullary cystic disease has been defined as an autosomal dominant condition that occurs predominantly in adulthood [12]. Familial juvenile nephronophthisis has been defined as an autosomal recessive condition that occurs predominantly in childhood, as originally reported by Fanconi and his colleagues [10]. This childhood form of the syndrome accounts for two-thirds of the reported cases. A history of consanguinity is unusually frequent. The ratio of affected to unaffected siblings is, however, unexpectedly high, a point that might be explained by the difficulty in recognizing individual isolated cases and by the relative ease of arriving at the diagnosis when there is involvement of several siblings. It might also be explained by a general tendency to report cases with good family histories, in which case the literature would be biased.

The issue of recessive inheritance could be clarified were it possible to identify the heterozygous state. In several families a urinary concentrating defect has been documented in otherwise normal parents or siblings. We have also seen a family in which uncertain and incompletely defined renal abnormalities were present in one parent. In general, however, evidence of an abnormality in heterozygous carriers is inconclusive.

Gardner, in analyzing differences between reported cases having a dominant inheritance and those having a recessive inheritance, has identified a clear difference in age at onset and at time of death [12]. Patients with dominantly inherited disease have a mean age at onset in the third decade of life, in contrast to a mean onset within the first decade among patients with recessively determined disease (Fig. 42-1). The relationship between age and inheritance resembles that found in polycystic disease, although the discrepancy in age and the morphologic and clinical differences between the infantile recessive and adult dominant forms are much greater in polycystic disease than in the FJN-MCD complex.

The occurrence of sporadic adult cases probably results from new dominant mutations. The occurrence of disease in only one young child of a family probably reflects the odds of acquiring an autosomal recessive condition.

The pathogenesis of FJN-MCD, apart from these genetic considerations, is unknown. The primary renal defect appears on both functional and morphologic grounds to be tubular, and it has been assumed, therefore, that the genetic abnormality affects tubular function, that tubular damage is progressive, and that glomerular and interstitial alterations are secondary. It is an attractive theory that these diseases are mediated through

hereditary metabolic defects that result in nephrotoxic metabolic products, but the theory lacks supporting evidence. Some support has come from the circumstantial evidence provided by experiments in which renal cysts can be induced by feeding rats cystogenic nephrotoxic agents [35]. The possibility of a heritable defect in structural protein, either within the tubular cell or in its basement membrane, cannot be excluded, particularly in dominantly transmitted disease. There is no evidence for a circulating nephrotoxic agent; it should be noted that the disease has not recurred in transplanted kidneys. It seems unlikely, therefore, that a simple deficiency or excess of a normal metabolite accounts for the renal abnormalities that have been observed.

Epidemiology

Figures for the incidence and prevalance of FJN-MCD are unavailable, and the diseases appear to be uncommon. Familial juvenile nephronophthisis may, however, account for as much as 10 to 20 percent of renal failure in children [3, 38]. There is probably, as noted above, a strong bias in the reporting of familial cases, and it is also likely that sporadic cases have gone unrecognized.

Gardner reviewed and summarized 238 reported cases [13]. Males and females were equally affected. The reports included 67 propositi with positive and 29 with negative family histories. Differences in ages at onset and death were demonstrated in relation to the pattern of inheritance, giving a bimodal distribution (see Fig. 42-1). Patients with adequately documented, recessively inherited disease had a mean age of onset of 10.0 ± 1.2 years, whereas patients with adequately documented, dominantly inherited disease had a mean age at onset of 28.4 ± 2.4 years ($p < .001$). The duration of disease was approximately the same in both groups, and ages at death showed, therefore, the same bimodal distribution.

The most significant socioeconomic factor that has been identified in the study of patients with FJN is the frequency of consanguineous marriages among the parents of affected children, a point that also strongly supports the interpretation of genetically recessive inheritance. Most reports in which race is mentioned identified the patient as white; a few cases in black and Japanese patients have been reported.

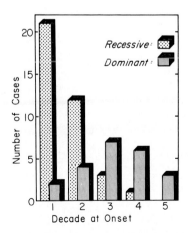

Figure 42-1. Ages at onset by decade among 37 recessively inherited and 22 dominantly inherited cases of the nephronophthisis–medullary cystic complex selected from the literature by virtue of detailed clinical, familial, and pathologic descriptions. Bimodality is clear-cut and statistically significant [13].

Clinical Manifestations

The clinical features of FJN and MCD are similar [5, 14, 18, 19, 28, 38, 46, 47]. Children with FJN have as presenting signs and symptoms polyuria and polydypsia (>80 percent), anemia and weakness (>60 percent), and growth retardation (>40 percent) [13]. Most patients (75 percent) suffer from azotemia at the time of initial evaluation. Hypertension has been variable; a pressure greater than 140/90 mm Hg has been observed in approximately 30 percent of cases [13]. The frequency of red or blond hair in patients with MCD is very high [34], although the rate needs to be determined and verified from several sources.

The anemia may or may not be related solely to renal failure, but its severity parallels the degree of renal insufficiency. Anemia has been present in about one-third of patients not in renal failure. No mechanism other than azotemia has been identified as a possible cause of anemia, but the matter has received relatively little study.

The urinary concentrating defect occurs independently of renal failure, and we have observed it to be present in children with very little morphologic evidence of renal damage. Its basis appears, therefore, to be independent of the glomerular filtration rate, and it has been attributed to a primary tubular defect. A reduction in maximal urinary concentrating ability can be encountered early in the course of disease, but the presence of renal insufficiency in so many patients at the time of initial evaluation may make evaluation of tubular function difficult. Patients commonly suffer also from increased urinary loss of sodium, which is additional evidence of a defect in tubular function. Sodium wasting may account for the relatively low frequency of hypertension in the late stages of renal failure. The frequency of salt wasting remains unsettled; it has been demonstrated in two out of every three patients in whom specific studies of renal handling of sodium have been done [13]. Persistent hypokalemia has also been described [25]. Urinary acidification is occasionally abnormal [15], and aminoaciduria is rare. Urinary findings are minor; proteinuria is minimal (1+ to 2+), and erythrocytes and leukocytes are rarely present in significant numbers. Bacteriuria is also uncommon.

The end stage of renal failure in FJN-MCD is associated with its usual manifestations, including secondary hyperparathyroidism and abnormal bone metabolism. Parathyroid hyperplasia of a moderate degree does occur in children.

Radiographic studies have been of limited value because renal function is usually so poor at the time of clinical evaluation. Renal arteriograms [27] have shown small kidneys with diminished blood flow; cysts appear as lucencies in the nephrographic phase, and the renal arteries are distorted. Sonography has been inconclusive.

Apparent variants of FJN have been observed in variable combination with ocular, cerebellar, skeletal, and hepatic abnormalities. The best known of these rare syndromes combines renal disease with tapetoretinal degeneration [23, 30, 42] and is known as renal-retinal dysplasia [40]. The renal lesion is similar both clinically and morphologically to that seen in FJN without ocular involvement. The ocular lesion in young infants with presumably severe involvement often takes the form of congenital blindness of Leber with retinal aplasia and other developmental abnormalities; older patients characteristically develop retinitis pigmentosa. The renal and retinal abnormalities are both transmitted with recessive inheritance. The complex has been attributed to a pleiotropic genetic defect [40], although mild pigmentary degeneration has been described in a patient's relatives who did not have clinical evidence of renal disease [2]. Similar renal and ocular abnormalities have been associated with cerebral and cerebellar abnormalities [7], with cerebellar dysfunction [24, 31], and with mental retardation [23, 33, 37]. Incidentally, renal disease when associated with familial cerebral and retinal abnormalities usually corresponds to FJN; the renal disease associated with familial lenticular abnormalities, on the other hand, usually corresponds to Alport syndrome. Some patients have also had skeletal abnormalities [24, 31], but the combination of FJN and skeletal dysostosis is not always associated with ocular involvement [36]. There has been one report of chromosomal abnormalities [39]. Several patients have been found to have increased urinary excretion of proline and hydroxyproline [2, 11, 37], but the significance of iminoaciduria is not known. These complex variants, like prototypic renal-retinal dysplasia, may be the effects of a single abnormal gene, but that interpretation has yet to be proved [41].

The other combinations are even less common than renal-retinal dysplasia, and they have presented some nosologic difficulty. Among the variants of FJN, only some of those patients with retinal involvement have thus far had typical renal medullary cysts [2, 11, 19, 26, 32]. One child with congenital blindness was described as having cortical cysts [7]. A renal abnormality similar to that in FJN has been seen in association with hepatic fibrosis [4, 33, 36], but only a child who also had tapetoretinal degeneration and mental retardation had medullary cysts [33]. The renal lesion has consisted otherwise of tubular involvement leading to cortical atrophy, with impaired urinary concentrating ability and progressive renal failure; the histopathology in one family of three siblings [4] was marked by numerous glomerular cysts, which cannot be regarded as an established characteristic of FJN-MCD. Patients having skeletal involvement, a form of chondrodysplasia with cone-shaped phalangeal epiphyses and mild femoral dysostosis, have all had retinal degeneration, although none has had medullary cysts [24, 31, 36]. Medullary cysts are admittedly not a requirement of the diagnosis of FJN, and the relatively high frequency of "acystic" cases among the variants of FJN may reflect only the availability of some other, readily recognizable clinical characteristic, a finding other than cysts, that serves to identify cases. The obverse of this problem is the difficulty of classifying cases of familial "interstitial nephritis" [6] when there are no related clinical findings or when medullary cysts are lacking. It is noteworthy that none of the variants has been reported to have a dominant inheritance.

A rare syndrome of obesity, diabetes mellitus, blindness, and deafness known as Alström syndrome has been associated with a nephropathy characterized by tubular dysfunction and a concentrating defect [17]. The appearance of the kidney is similar to that in FJN, except that cysts have not been described. A similar renal lesion has also been described in the Laurence-Moon-Bardet-Biedl syndrome, and some patients have had medullary cysts [20]. The observation that many patients with FJN-MCD have red or blond hair [34] may reflect genetic linkage.

Pathology

Renal biopsies early in the disease may show little or no change, an observation that emphasizes the functional nature of the renal tubular defect. The characteristic morphologic abnormality in more advanced cases is tubular atrophy out of proportion to glomerular damage (Fig. 42-2). In the terminal stages of disease, the kidneys are shrunken and the cortices are thin and atrophic, observations that account for the term *nephronophthisis* (Fig. 42-3). Findings include tubular atrophy with basement membrane thickening, periglomerular fibrosis, interstitial fibrosis and inflammatory cell infiltration, and patchy glomerular obsolescence [21, 29, 45]. A correlation between cortical atrophy and renal insufficiency probably holds in general, although we have seen biopsies that show only focal tubular atrophy in patients with significant degrees of clinical renal failure.

A striking morphologic feature of both FJN and MCD is renal medullary cysts (see Fig. 42-3). The cysts have been shown by microdissection to be located within the distal convolutions and collecting tubules, and they usually communicate freely with other portions of the nephron [43].

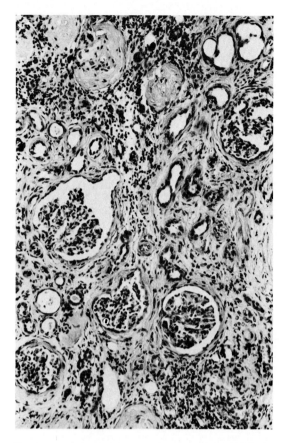

Figure 42-2. A renal biopsy of a young boy with polydypsia, polyuria, growth retardation, and anemia shows severe tubular atrophy with interstitial fibrosis and an irregular infiltrate of chronic inflammatory cells. The fibrous tissue is accentuated around glomeruli, and many glomeruli have undergone obsolescence and sclerosis. The appearance is characteristic of nephronophthisis in an advanced stage. (H&E, ×120.)

Their epithelial lining is flattened, and the cysts are surrounded by thickened basement membranes [9, 29]. Occasional cortical cysts may be found [16], but a large number suggests the diagnosis of infantile polycystic disease, in which medullary cysts are characteristically present (Chap. 40) The cysts are, on one hand, a diagnostic criterion, and in sporadic cases microscopic cysts have been present and confirmed by tissue examination at autopsy. Cysts are not, on the other hand, invariably present, and cases identified because of sibling involvement have not always had renal medullary cysts. Some reported cases have been correctly recognized in advance of any morphologic evidence of renal cysts through identification of such characteristic clinical findings as a positive family history, renal salt wasting, and progressive renal fail-

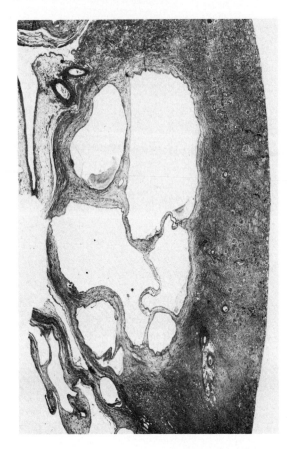

Figure 42-3. Postmortem specimen 6 months later from the patient whose biopsy is shown in Fig. 42-2, demonstrating severe cortical atrophy and large medullary cysts. (H&E, ×6.)

ure of unknown etiology in preadolescence or early adolescence.

If "acystic" disease proves ultimately to be otherwise identical to the "cystic" disorder (as it now appears to be on the bases of functional, morphologic, and genetic criteria), one might expect the prevalence of medullary cysts to decline from its current figure of 75 percent [13] as more cases of the acystic variety are recognized and reported. Cysts, by virtue of their presence alone, do not explain all of the clinical manifestations or functional defects, and they often are less striking than the accompanying cortical tubular atrophy. It appears, therefore, that medullary cysts are not necessary either to the inception of FJN-MCD or to its progression to renal failure.

Differential Diagnosis
The differential diagnosis of FJN-MCD includes other forms of chronic renal failure and other renal diseases that bear morphologic similarities.

The evaluation of a patient with azotemia, anemia, and a concentrating defect is obviously difficult, and a clear understanding of the original, basic renal disease may never be achieved. Since so many patients are not seen until after the onset of renal failure, family histories and postmortem examinations have been and continue to be of paramount importance in identifying the syndrome. Recognition of early clinical features, particularly a urinary concentrating defect, polyuria, polydypsia, and growth retardation in childhood, increases the index of suspicion in any case.

The differential diagnosis of FJN-MCD in childhood includes, therefore, oligomeganephronia, which is a form of renal hypoplasia (Chap. 39) with a severe reduction in the number of nephrons. The clinical manifestations, as in FJN-MCD, include a concentrating defect and growth retardation. Renal failure in oligomeganephronia progresses less rapidly than in FJN, and the children enjoy a longer period of relative stability. Oligomeganephronia is also rarely familial, in contrast to the high frequency of familial involvement in FJN.

Infantile polycystic disease is an important differential consideration in children, and there is some evidence that it enters into the differential diagnosis in adults. Infantile polycystic disease (polycystic disease of autosomal recessive type) affects both older children and adults with varying degrees of renal impairment (Chap. 40). Its cardinal features include early renal tubular dysfunction, impaired concentrating ability, and progressive renal insufficiency. Excretory urography in infantile polycystic disease shows a pattern of medullary ductal ectasia that is radiographically indistinguishable from medullary sponge kidney, and similar appearances in adults with congenital hepatic fibrosis and mild degrees of renal tubular dysfunction indicate that so-called infantile polycystic disease actually extends well beyond the confines of infancy and even beyond childhood.

The differential diagnosis of FJN-MCD in adults includes, in addition to nonspecific renal failure, medullary sponge kidney. Medullary sponge kidney (MSK) is a condition of different genetic background with different clinical features and with almost no impairment of renal function. The point is raised because both it and MCD feature renal medullary cysts, which are sometimes recognized radiographically and which can be seen morphologically. The point should be made that excretory urography does not succeed in demonstrating the medullary cysts in most cases of FJN-MCD, because renal function is inadequate for good concentration of the contrast medium, because the cysts rarely exceed 1 cm in diameter, and because the cysts are corticomedullary and intramedullary rather than papillary in location. Neither nephrocalcinosis, even microscopic, nor urolithiasis has been described in FJN-MCD, in contrast to their incidence of 50 percent or more in medullary sponge kidney [8]. The radiographic diagnosis of medullary sponge kidney in relatives of patients with MCD raises questions about an association between the two conditions [1, 22]. The questions remain incompletely answered, because it is still not clear if the two diseases (MSK and MCD) have been associated coincidentally or if all the afflicted family members have been suffering from the same disease.

Treatment

The treatment of FJN-MCD is nonspecific and supportive. There is no known method of preventing progression of renal failure. Salt wasting requires replacement therapy; the use of sodium bicarbonate is effective in combatting metabolic acidosis. Renal failure is managed by maintenance dialysis, and patients are acceptable candidates for renal transplantation, providing care is exercised in the selection of living related donors.

Prognosis

The prognosis is uniformly poor. Gardner's figures on the duration of the disease indicate a progression from clinical recognition to death in approximately 4 years, with no difference between the recessive and dominant types of disease [13]. Renal failure is accompanied by a worsening of the anemia and by renal osteodystrophy.

Genetic counseling for patients with positive family histories is relatively straightforward. More challenging can be the evaluation of apparently sporadic cases and the determination of their hereditary background.

References

1. Bennett, W. B. Kindred coexistence of medullary sponge kidney and medullary cystic disease. *Ann. Intern. Med.* 85:829, 1976.
2. Bennett, W. M., Simon, N. M., Krill, A. E., Weinstein, R. F., and Carone, F. A. Cystic disease of the renal medulla associated with retinitis pigmentosa and imino acid abnormalities. *Clin. Nephrol.* 4:25, 1975.
3. Betts, P. R., and Forrest-Hay, I. Juvenile nephronophthisis. *Lancet* 2:473, 1973.
4. Boichis, H., Passwell, J., David, R., and Miller, H. Congenital hepatic fibrosis and nephronophthisis. *Q. J. Med.* 42:221, 1973.
5. Broberger, O., Winberg, J., and Zetterström, R. Juvenile nephronophthisis: Part I. A genetically determined nephropathy, with hypotonic polyuria and azotaemia. *Acta Paediatr.* 49:470, 1960.
6. Coles, G. A., Robinson, K., and Branch, R. A. Familial interstitial nephritis. *Clin. Nephrol.* 6:513, 1976.
7. Dekaban, A. S. Hereditary syndrome of congenital retinal blindness (Leber), polycystic kidneys and maldevelopment of the brain. *Am. J. Ophthalmol.* 68:1029, 1969.
8. Ekström, T., Engfeldt, B., Lagergren, C., and Lindvall, N. *Medullary Sponge Kidney: A Roentgenologic, Clinical, Histopathologic and Biophysical Study.* Stockholm: Almqvist and Wiksell, 1959.
9. Evan, A. P., and Gardner, K. D., Jr. Comparison of human polycystic and medullary cystic kidney disease with diphenylamine-induced cystic disease. *Lab. Invest.* 35:93, 1976.
10. Fanconi, G., Hanhart, E., von Albertini, A., Uhlinger, E., Dolivo, G., and Prader, A. Die familiäre juvenile Nephronophthise. *Helv. Paediatr. Acta* 6:1, 1951.
11. Fillastre, J. P., Guenel, J., Riberi, P., Marx, P., Whitworth, J. A., and Kuhn, J. M. Senior-Loken syndrome (nephronophthisis and tapeto-retinal degeneration): A study of 8 cases from 5 families. *Clin. Nephrol.* 5:14, 1976.
12. Gardner, K. D., Jr. Evolution of clinical signs in adult-onset cystic disease of the renal medulla. *Ann. Intern. Med.* 74:47, 1971.
13. Gardner, K. D., Jr. Juvenile Nephronophthisis and Renal Medullary Cystic Disease. In K. D. Gardner, Jr. (ed.), *Cystic Diseases of the Kidney.* New York: Wiley, 1976.
14. Gibson, A. A., and Arneil, G. C. Nephronophthisis: Report of 8 cases from Britain. *Arch. Dis. Child.* 47:84, 1972.
15. Giselson, N., Heinegard, D., Holmberg, C.-G., Lindberg, L.-G., Lindstedt, E., Lindstedt, G., and Schersten, B. Renal medullary cystic disease or familial juvenile nephronophthisis: A renal tubular disease. Biochemical findings in two siblings. *Am. J. Med.* 48:174, 1970.
16. Goldman, S. H., Walker, S. R., Merigan, T. C., Jr., Gardner, K. D., Jr., and Bull, J. M. C. Hereditary occurrence of cystic disease of the renal medulla. *N. Engl. J. Med.* 274:984, 1966.
17. Goldstein, J. L., and Fialkow, P. J. The Alström syndrome: Report of three cases with further delineation of the clinical, pathophysiological, and genetic aspects of the disorder. *Medicine* 52:53, 1973.
18. Hackzell, G., and Lundmark, C. Familial juvenile nephronophthisis. *Acta Paediatr.* 47:428, 1958.
19. Herdman, R. C., Good, R. A., and Vernier, R. L. Medullary cystic disease in two siblings. *Am. J. Med.* 43:335, 1967.
20. Hurley, R. M., Dery, P., Nogrady, M. B., and Drummond, K. N. The renal lesion of the Laurence-Moon-Biedl syndrome. *J. Pediatr.* 87:206, 1975.
21. Ivemark, B. I., Ljungqvist, A., and Barry, A. Juvenile nephronophthisis: Part II. A histologic and microangiographic study. *Acta Paediatr.* 49:480, 1960.
22. Kliger, A. S., and Scheer, R. L. Familial disease of the renal medulla: A study of progeny in a family with medullary cystic disease. *Ann. Intern. Med.* 85:190, 1976.
23. Løken, A. C., Hanssen, O., Halvorsen, S., and Jølster, N. J. Hereditary renal dysplasia and blindness. *Acta Paediatr.* 50:177, 1961.
24. Mainzer, F., Saldino, R. M., Ozonoff, M. D., and

Minagi, H. Familial nephropathy associated with retinitis pigmentosa, cerebellar ataxia and skeletal abnormalities. *Am. J. Med.* 49:556, 1970.

25. Mangos, J. A., Opitz, J. M., Lobeck, C. C., and Cookson, D. U. Familial juvenile nephronophthisis: An unrecognized renal disease in the United States. *Pediatrics* 34:337, 1964.

26. Meier, D. A., and Hess, J. W. Familial nephropathy with retinitis pigmentosa: A new oculorenal syndrome in adults. *Am. J. Med.* 39:58, 1965.

27. Mena, E., Bookstein, J. J., McDonald, F. D., and Gikas, P. W. Angiographic findings in renal medullary cystic disease. *Radiology* 110:277, 1973.

28. Mongeau, J.-G., and Worthen, H. G. Nephronophthisis and medullary cystic disease. *Am. J. Med.* 43:345, 1967.

29. Pascal, R. R. Medullary cystic disease of the kidney: Study of a case with scanning and transmission electron microscopy and light microscopy. *Am. J. Clin. Pathol.* 59:659, 1973.

30. Pierson, M., Cordier, J., Hervouët, F., and Rauber, G. Une curieuse association malformative congénitale et familiale atteignant l'oeil et le rein. *J. Genet. Hum.* 12:184, 1963.

31. Popović-Rolović, M., Čalic-Perišič, N., Bunjevački, G., and Negovanovič, D. Juvenile nephronophthisis associated with retinal pigmentary dystrophy, cerebellar ataxia, and skeletal abnormalities. *Arch. Dis. Child.* 51:801, 1976.

32. Price, J. D. E., and Pratt-Johnson, J. A. Medullary cystic disease with degeneration. *Can. Med. Assoc. J.* 102:165, 1970.

33. Proesmans, W., Van Damme, B., and Macken, J. Nephronophthisis and tapetoretinal degeneration associated with liver fibrosis. *Clin. Nephrol.* 3:160, 1975.

34. Rayfield, E. J., and McDonald, F. D. Red and blond hair in renal medullary cystic disease. *Arch. Intern. Med.* 130:72, 1972.

35. Resnick, J. S., Brown, D. M., and Vernier, R. L. Normal Development and Experimental Models of Cystic Renal Disease. In K. D. Gardner, Jr. (ed.), *Cystic Diseases of the Kidney.* New York: Wiley, 1976.

36. Robins, D. G., French, T. A., and Chakera, T. M. H. Juvenile nephronophthisis associated with skeletal abnormalities and hepatic fibrosis. *Arch. Dis. Child.* 51:799, 1976.

37. Rokkones, T., and Løken, A. C. Congenital renal dysplasia, retinal dysplasia and mental retardation associated with hyperprolinuria and hyper-OH-prolinuria. *Acta Paediatr.* 57:225, 1968.

38. Royer, P., Habib, R., Mathieu, H., and Broyer, M. *Pediatric Nephrology.* Philadelphia: Saunders, 1974. Part I, chap. 4; and part IV, chap. 2.

39. Sarles, H. E., Rodin, A. E., Poduska, P. R., Smith, G. H., Fish, J. C., and Remmers, A. R., Jr. Hereditary nephritis, retinitis pigmentosa and chromosomal abnormalities. *Am. J. Med.* 45:312, 1968.

40. Schimke, R. N. Hereditary renal-retinal dysplasia. *Ann. Intern. Med.* 70:735, 1969.

41. Senior, B. Familial renal-retinal dystrophy. *Am. J. Dis. Child.* 125:442, 1973.

42. Senior, B., Friedman, A. I., and Braudo, J. L. Juvenile familial nephropathy with tapetoretinal degeneration. *Am. J. Ophthalmol.* 52:625, 1961.

43. Sherman, F. E., Studnicki, F. M., and Fetterman, G. H. Renal lesions of familial juvenile nephronophthisis examined by microdissection. *Am. J. Clin. Pathol.* 55:391, 1971.

44. Smith, C. H., and Graham, J. B. Congenital medullary cysts of the kidneys with severe refractory anemia. *Am. J. Dis. Child.* 69:369, 1945.

45. Strauss, M. B. Clinical and pathologic aspects of cystic disease of the renal medulla: An analysis of eighteen cases. *Ann. Intern. Med.* 57:373, 1962.

46. Strauss, M. B., and Sommers, S. C. Medullary cystic disease and familial juvenile nephronophthisis: Clinical and pathological entity. *N. Engl. J. Med.* 277:863, 1967.

47. Von Sydow, G., and Ranström, S. Familial juvenile nephronophthisis. *Acta Paediatr.* 51:561, 1962.

Section Two. Glomerular Diseases

43. Glomerular Diseases: Introduction and Classification

Jay Bernstein, Henry L. Barnett and Chester M. Edelmann, Jr.

The effective clinical application of information gained from recent advances in the understanding of glomerular diseases requires precise nosologic definitions. The term *glomerular disease* is used here to indicate that the initial and major point of impact is in the glomerulus rather than in any of the other three basic components of renal tissue—tubules, interstitial tissue, or vasculature. The concept that diseases of the kidney may be confined to the glomerulus is a relatively recent one. Its elaboration followed the development and widespread use of renal biopsy, which showed that early abnormalities could become obscured by the diffuse and advanced changes seen in postmortem studies of terminal renal disease. The major exception to this situation was in children with the nephrotic syndrome, many of whom died of infection before the introduction of effective antibacterial drugs just prior to 1940. The changes in these kidneys were described as involving not the glomeruli, but principally the tubules [18], which were infiltrated by birefringent lipid. The concept of isolated glomerular disease must therefore be considered to be one of the many important advances stemming from (1) the availability of renal tissue obtained by biopsy from patients early in the course of disease and (2) the development of ultrastructural and immunopathologic techniques that permit accurate localization of the disease.

Glomerular diseases, like other disorders or syndromes of unknown cause, can be classified by their clinical and laboratory characteristics observable at the onset, by their course (natural history) and ultimate outcome (prognosis), and by their response to medical intervention. Such clinical classifications have several important purposes. They can, by defining homogeneous subgroups within diseases that have multiple causes, refine the background information used to predict outcome and to assess the effects of treatment. The greater the degree of homogeneity, the greater the likelihood that correlations between various characteristics of the disease will yield clues to pathogenesis and etiology.

Present classifications [1–15, 17, 18] of glomerular disease are based on either clinical or pathologic characteristics or on correlations between them. There is, however, no unitarian classification linking separate, well-defined clinical states with single histopathologic or immunopathologic lesions. Thus, what appear to be identical clinical states may be associated with several very different pathologic lesions. Conversely, what appear to be distinct pathologic lesions may be associated with several very different clinical states. All classifications must be considered tentative, since significant advances are still being made, especially in the field of immunology [2, 7, 15, 16, 19]. Despite these deficiencies, classifications are required to meet the needs that have been stated.

It is often said that the ultimate goal is an etiologic classification; certainly, one would be highly desirable, especially for possible prevention of disease. Nonetheless, even greater knowledge of etiology will not necessarily provide a unifying classification with complete clinical relevance, since the same apparent etiologic agent can result in very different clinical diseases [3]. For example, a variety of histopathologic lesions and clinical manifestations can result from a single agent, such as the DNA-antiDNA complex or hepatitis B virus.

The major categories of primary glomerular disease* have been classified in general terms on the basis of observable clinical characteristics (Table 43-1). In one instance the same term, *glomerulonephritis*, is used both to define a clinical state and to identify a histopathologic entity. This double usage is unavoidable, unless one is prepared—which we are not—to invent and to sponsor a new designation for either the clinical state or the histopathologic entity. The histopathologic and immunofluorescent correlates of the major clinical categories are shown in Table 43-2, thus completing the classification. The variety of glomerular abnormalities accompanying different systemic diseases is presented in Table 43-3. The classifications are neither complete nor final; certainly, future modifications must be considered desirable. They do, however, approach the stated purpose of providing a nosologic basis for making judgments and decisions concerning the diagnosis, prognosis, and assessment of treatment and course of the major glomerular diseases associated with primary renal disorders in children.

The foregoing classifications and clinicopathologic correlations still do not provide the information required to recognize (1) the morphologic heterogeneity of glomerular lesions associated with clinical renal syndromes in children and (2) the clinical heterogeneity of renal disease associated with distinctive morphologic patterns.

Table 43-1. Clinical Classification of Primary Glomerular Diseases

I. Isolated hematuria and proteinuria
   A. Recurrent gross hematuria
   B. Postural proteinuria
   C. Persistent hematuria and proteinuria
II. Glomerulonephritis
   A. Acute glomerulonephritis
   B. Rapidly progressive glomerulonephritis
   C. Chronic glomerulonephritis
III. Primary nephrotic syndrome
   A. Congenital nephrotic syndrome
   B. Corticosteroid-responsive nephrotic syndrome
   C. Corticosteroid-nonresponsive nephrotic syndrome
IV. Familial nephritis
   A. Hereditary progressive nephritis
   B. Familial recurrent hematuria
   C. Nail-patella syndrome

* The term *primary glomerular disease* refers here to disorders that occur solely or primarily in the kidney, in contrast to those associated with systemic diseases.

Table 43-2. Clinical Classification with Histopathologic and Immunofluorescent Correlations: Glomerular Abnormalities in Primary Renal Disorders

Clinical Diagnosis	Light Microscopy	Immunofluorescence
I. Isolated hematuria and proteinuria		

A. Recurrent gross hematuria	1. Normal histologic findings
	2. Focal and mesangial glomerulonephritis
	3. Focal and necrotizing glomerulonephritis
		1. Negative
		2. a. Mesangial IgA, IgG, C3
		   b. Mesangial IgM, IgG, C3, C1q
		3. a. Mesangial IgA, IgG, C3, properdin
		   b. Linear IgG, linear or granular C3, fibrin

B. Postural proteinuria	Variable mild mesangial proliferation	
C. Persistent hematuria and proteinuria	1. Normal histologic findings 2. Any type of glomerular lesion	Presence and distribution variable
II. Glomerulonephritis		
A. Acute glomerulonephritis	1. Diffuse exudative and proliferative glomerulonephritis 2. Membranoproliferative glomerulonephritis (subendothelial deposit) 3. Membranoproliferative glomerulonephritis (dense deposit)	Peripheral granular IgG, variable IgM, C3, C4, C1q, properdin Peripheral subendothelial and mesangial granular C3, IgG, C1q, C4, occasional IgM, properdin Linear (faint) capillary and granular mesangial C3
B. Rapidly progressive glomerulonephritis	Crescentic and necrotizing glomerulonephritis	1. Linear IgG, linear or granular C3, C4, C1q; extracapillary fibrin 2. Peripheral and mesangial granular IgG, C3, C4, C1q; variable IgA and IgM, extracapillary fibrin

C. Chronic glomerulonephritis
    1. Prior to end stage
    2. End-stage kidney
	Any type of glomerular lesion
	Glomerular obsolescence and hyalinization
		Variable IgG, IgM, C3

III. Primary nephrotic syndrome		
A. Congenital nephrotic syndrome	1. Microcystic (Finnish) disease 2. Diffuse mesangial sclerosis	Negative Negative
B. Steroid-responsive nephrotic syndrome	Minimal change*	Negative; occasional late IgM
C. Steroid-nonresponsive nephrotic syndrome 1. Normocomplementemic	a. Focal segmental glomerulosclerosis* b. Membranous glomerulonephropathy* c. Mesangial nephritis* d. Proliferative and sclerosing* glomerulonephritis e. Crescentic glomerulonephritis* f. Membranoproliferative glomerulonephritis (subendothelial deposit)	Segmental IgM, C3 Peripheral, finely granular IgG, C3, C4, C1q, occasional IgM and IgA Occasional mesangial IgA, C3 Presence and distribution variable Extracapillary fibrin, ? IgG and C3 Peripheral subendothelial and mesangial granular C3, IgG, occasional IgM, properdin
2. Hypocomplementemic	Membranoproliferative glomerulonephritis (dense deposit)	Linear (faint) capillary and granular mesangial C3
IV. Familial nephritis		
A. Hereditary progressive nephritis (Alport)	1. Focal glomerular sclerosis 2. Proliferative and crescentic glomerulopathy	Negative
B. Familial recurrent hematuria	Negative	Negative
C. Nail-patella syndrome	Focal glomerular sclerosis	Negative

* Although there are occasional exceptions, the predominant clinical patterns are given here.

Table 43-3. Clinical Classification with Histopathologic and Immunofluorescent Correlations: Glomerular Abnormalities in Systemic Disorders

Clinical Diagnosis	Light Microscopy	Immunofluorescence
I. Systemic diseases of immune origin		
A. Schönlein-Henoch purpura	Focal and diffuse, proliferative and crescentic glomerulonephritis	Mesangial IgA, IgG, C3, properdin, focal fibrin
B. Systemic lupus erythematosus	1. Focal and diffuse proliferative glomerulonephritis	Mesangial and subendothelial IgG, IgM, IgA, C3, C4, C1q, DNA, properdin, focal fibrin
	2. Membranous glomerulonephropathy	Extramembranous IgG, C3, IgM, IgA
C. Goodpasture syndrome	Focal and diffuse crescentic glomerulonephritis	Linear IgG, occasionally granular IgG; linear and granular C3; extracapillary fibrin
D. Periarteritis and hypersensitivity angiitis	Focal and diffuse, necrotizing and proliferative glomerulonephritis	Focal fibrin; variable IgG, IgA, and C3
E. Wegener granulomatosis	Focal and diffuse, necrotizing and crescentic glomerulonephritis	Extracapillary fibrin; variable IgG, IgM, C3
F. Mixed essential cryoglobulinemia	Diffuse proliferative glomerulonephritis	Subendothelial and endocapillary IgG, IgM or IgA, C3
G. Rheumatic fever	Proliferative and sclerosing glomerulonephritis	Endomembranous C3, IgG
II. Systemic disease with presumed secondary immune disturbance[a]		
A. Sickle cell disease[b]	Membranoproliferative glomerulonephritis	Subendothelial IgG, C3, C1q
B. Progressive lipodystrophy	Membranoproliferative glomerulonephritis (dense deposit)	Linear C3; variable subendothelial IgG
C. Hereditary deficiency of complement	1. Focal proliferative glomerulonephritis	Focal IgG, IgM, IgA, C3, properdin
	2. Membranoproliferative glomerulonephritis	Subendothelial IgG, C3
D. Neoplasia	1. Minimal change	Negative
	2. Proliferative glomerulonephritis	
	3. Membranous glomerulonephropathy	Subepithelial IgG, IgM, C3
E. Sarcoidosis	1. Membranous glomerulonephropathy	Subepithelial IgG, IgM, IgA, C3 (variable)
	2. Proliferative glomerulonephritis	Linear IgG, mesangial IgG and IgM
F. Drug-induced nephropathy		
1. Trimethadione, d-penicillamine, gold, mercury	a. Minimal change	Negative
	b. Membranous glomerulonephropathy	Subepithelial IgG, IgM, C3 (variable)
2. Narcotic addiction	a. Proliferative and sclerosing glomerulonephritis	Variable IgG, IgM, C3
	b. Focal glomerular sclerosis	Linear IgG
G. Chronic infection[c]		
1. Chronic staphylococcal bacteremia (infected ventriculoatrial shunt)	Membranoproliferative glomerulonephritis	Subendothelial fibrin, C3, variable IgG and IgM
2. Bacterial endocarditis	Focal and diffuse, proliferative glomerulonephritis	Peripheral and mesangial IgG, C3
3. Quartan malaria	Subendothelial membranous glomerulonephropathy	Peripheral and subendothelial IgG, IgM, C3
4. Hepatitis B antigenemia	a. Membranoproliferative glomerulonephritis	Peripheral and mesangial IgG, IgM, C3, HbAg
	b. Membranous glomerulonephropathy	Subepithelial IgG, IgM, C3, HbAg
5. Congenital syphilis	Mixed membranous and proliferative glomerulonephritis	Peripheral IgG, IgM, C3

Table 43-3. (Continued)

Clinical Diagnosis	Light Microscopy	Immunofluorescence
III. Miscellaneous		
A. Hemolytic-uremic syndrome	Thrombotic microangiopathy	Subendothelial fibrin
B. Diabetes mellitus	1. Diffuse and nodular mesangial sclerosis	Variable endocapillary and mesangial IgM, C3, IgG, fibrin
	2. Hyaline insudative glomerular and arteriolar lesions	– – – –
C. Amyloidosis	Mesangial amyloidosis and glomerular sclerosis	Variable mesangial IgG, IgM, ?C3
D. Metabolic storage diseases		
1. Fabry disease	Epithelial foam cells and glomerular sclerosis	(Ceramide trihexoside storage)
2. Familial lecithin-cholesterol acyltransferase	Mesangial foam cells and glomerular sclerosis	(Phospholipid and cholesterol storage)
E. Renal vein thrombosis	1. Membranous glomerulonephropathy	Subepithelial IgG, IgM, C3
	2. Minimal change nephrotic syndrome	Negative

[a] Glomerulonephritis is occasionally encountered in certain nonrenal disorders, possibly as an immunologic complication: proliferative glomerulonephritis following a bee sting; proliferative glomerulonephritis and membranous glomerulonephropathy accompanying poison oak dermatitis; membranous glomerulonephropathy complicating several bullous dermatoses.

[b] Light microscopy in patients with sickle cell disease and the nephrotic syndrome also shows minimal change with negligible immunofluorescence, and occasional patients have membranous glomerulonephropathy.

[c] A few other examples of glomerulonephritis occasionally associated with infectious disease include: proliferative glomerulonephritis in varicella and infectious mononucleosis; focal sclerosing glomerulonephritis in falciparum malaria; membranous glomerulonephropathy in Guillain-Barré syndrome, subacute sclerosing panencephalitis, filarial loiasis, and schistosomiasis.

Table 43-4. Morphologic Heterogeneity of Glomerular Lesions within Clinical Syndromes

Recurrent Gross Hematuria
Normal glomerular histology
Diffuse proliferative glomerulonephritis
Focal glomerulonephritis
IgA-IgG and IgM-IgG mesangial glomerulonephritis
Membranoproliferative glomerulonephritis
Focal segmental glomerulosclerosis
Disseminated glomerular obsolescence, sclerosis and hyalinization (chronic glomerulonephritis)
Glomerular sclerosis with basement membrane lamellation (Alport syndrome)
Lupus nephropathy

Acute Glomerulonephritis
Diffuse exudative and proliferative glomerulonephritis
Crescentic glomerulonephritis
Focal and necrotizing glomerulonephritis
IgA-IgG and IgM-IgG mesangial glomerulonephritis
Membranoproliferative glomerulonephritis
Lupus nephritis
Glomerular sclerosis with basement membrane lamellation (Alport syndrome)
Disseminated glomerular obsolescence, sclerosis and hyalinization (chronic glomerulonephritis)

Rapidly Progressive Glomerulonephritis
Crescentic glomerulonephritis
Necrotizing glomerulonephritis
Proliferative glomerulonephritis
Membranoproliferative glomerulonephritis
Thrombotic microangiopathy

Chronic Glomerulonephritis
Focal segmental glomerulosclerosis
Disseminated glomerular obsolescence, sclerosis and hyalinization (chronic glomerulonephritis)
Proliferative and sclerosing glomerulonephritis
Membranoproliferative glomerulonephritis
Membranous glomerulonephropathy
Mesangial and nodular intercapillary glomerulosclerosis (diabetic nephropathy)
Glomerular sclerosis with basement membrane lamellation (Alport syndrome)
Glomerular sclerosis with basement membrane collagenosis (nail-patella syndrome)
Lupus nephropathy

Nephrotic Syndrome
Minimal change nephrotic syndrome
Focal segmental glomerulosclerosis
Membranoproliferative glomerulonephritis (subendothelial and dense deposit)
Proliferative glomerulonephritis (mesangial, exudative, sclerosing and crescentic)
Membranous glomerulonephropathy
Disseminated glomerular obsolescence, sclerosis, and hyalinization (chronic glomerulonephritis)
Microcystic disease (congenital nephrotic syndrome)
Diffuse mesangial sclerosis (congenital nephrotic syndrome)

Table 43-5. Clinical Heterogeneity within Histopathologic Categories

Proliferative Glomerulonephritis
Nephrotic syndrome
Acute glomerulonephritis
Rapidly progressive (oliguric) glomerulonephritis
Chronic glomerulonephritis
Persistent hematuria and proteinuria
Schönlein-Henoch purpura
Systemic lupus erythematosus
Periarteritis nodosa and hypersensitivity angiitis
Bacterial endocarditis
Mixed essential cryoglobulinemia
Rheumatic fever
Narcotic abuse
Hereditary progressive nephritis (Alport syndrome)
Hereditary deficiency of complement
Tumor-associated nephropathy
Sarcoidosis
Bee-sting nephrotic syndrome

Membranoproliferative Glomerulonephritis
Nephrotic syndrome
Acute glomerulonephritis
Rapidly progressive (oliguric) glomerulonephritis
Chronic glomerulonephritis
Slowly progressive glomerulonephritis
Persistent hematuria and proteinuria
Schönlein-Henoch purpura
Systemic lupus erythematosus
Allograft rejection
Progressive and partial lipodystrophy
Sickle cell disease
Hereditary deficiency of complement
Hepatic cirrhosis and chronic hepatitis
Quartan malaria
Chronic staphylococcal bacteremia ("shunt nephritis")

Necrotizing and Crescentic Glomerulonephritis
Acute glomerulonephritis
Rapidly progressive glomerulonephritis
Membranoproliferative glomerulonephritis
Chronic glomerulonephritis
Schönlein-Henoch purpura
Periarteritis nodosa and hypersensitivity angiitis
Goodpasture syndrome
Wegener granulomatosis
Systemic lupus erythematosus
Mixed essential cryoglobulinemia
Bacterial endocarditis
Hereditary progressive nephritis (Alport syndrome)

Focal Glomerulonephritis
Nephrotic syndrome
Acute glomerulonephritis
Chronic glomerulonephritis
Chronic hematuria
Bacterial endocarditis
Schönlein-Henoch purpura
Systemic lupus erythematosus
Goodpasture syndrome
Periarteritis nodosa and hypersensitivity angiitis
Wegener granulomatosis
Hereditary deficiency of complement

Membranous Glomerulonephropathy
Nephrotic syndrome
Chronic glomerulonephritis
Renal vein thrombosis
Systemic lupus erythematosus
Diabetes mellitus
Tumor-associated nephropathy
Sarcoidosis
Rheumatoid arthritis
Bullous dermatoses
Chronic infection
  Syphilis, schistosomiasis
  Filariasis, Guillain-Barré
  Hepatitis B antigenemia
Drug-associated nephrotic syndrome
  Trimethadione, D-penicillamine
  Gold, mercury
Slowly progressive glomerulonephritis

Focal Segmental Glomerulosclerosis
Nephrotic syndrome
Chronic glomerulonephritis
Persistent hematuria
Asymptomatic proteinuria
Rheumatoid arthritis
Narcotic abuse (heroin)
Hereditary progressive nephritis (Alport and nail-patella
  syndromes)
Sickle cell disease
Massive obesity
Allograft rejection

Table 43-6. Principal Differential Diagnoses of Clinical Syndromes

Persistent Microscopic and Recurrent Gross Hematuria	*Nephrotic Syndrome*
Benign recurrent hematuria	Corticosteroid-sensitive minimal change nephrotic
Hereditary progressive nephritis (Alport)	syndrome
IgA nephropathy (Berger)	Corticosteroid-resistant nephrotic syndrome with focal
Schönlein-Henoch purpura	segmental glomerulosclerosis
Systemic lupus erythematosus	Corticosteroid-resistant nephrotic syndrome with
Membranoproliferative glomerulonephritis	membranous glomerulonephropathy
Postinfectious glomerulonephritis	Corticosteroid-resistant nephrotic syndrome with
Chronic glomerulonephritis	membranoproliferative glomerulonephritis
Sickle cell disease	Congenital nephrotic syndrome
	Acute postinfectious glomerulonephritis
Acute glomerulonephritis	Schönlein-Henoch purpura
Acute postinfectious glomerulonephritis	Systemic lupus erythematosus
Following streptococcal infection	Narcotic addiction
Following other infections (staphylococcal, viral)	Sickle cell disease
Membranoproliferative glomerulonephritis	Familial nephritis (Alport)
Exacerbation of persistent glomerulonephritis	Diabetes mellitus
Recurrent hematuria and IgA nephropathy	Amyloidosis
Schönlein-Henoch purpura	Renal vein thrombosis
Systemic lupus erythematosus	Quartan malaria
Familial nephritis (Alport)	Congenital syphilis
	Drug reaction
Rapidly Progressive Glomerulonephritis	Neoplasia
Idiopathic crescentic and necrotizing glomerulonephritis	Bee stings
Acute postinfectious glomerulonephritis	Poison oak dermatitis
Membranoproliferative glomerulonephritis	Bullous dermatoses
Goodpasture syndrome	
Hemolytic-uremic syndrome	
Schönlein-Henoch purpura	
Systemic lupus erythematosus	
Hypersensitivity angiitis	

The different morphologic patterns that may be encountered on renal biopsy in association with five major clinical syndromes are listed in Table 43-4. The various clinical diseases that may be associated with recognizable patterns of glomerular abnormality are listed in Table 43-5. To complete the picture, the clinical differential diagnosis of several major clinical syndromes is given in Table 43-6. The lists in these two tables are not classifications and are not necessarily exhaustive, but they include conditions that are thought to be important because of either frequency or clinical significance in the context of pediatric renal disease. These tables, then, should provide in a concise and accessible manner the best available answers to the following questions:

1. Which morphologic form of glomerular disease may be present in a child with the characteristic clinical manifestations of recurrent hematuria or acute glomerulonephritis or rapidly progressive glomerulonephritis or chronic glomerulonephritis or the nephrotic syndrome? (Table 43-4)
2. Which diseases and syndromes may be present in a child whose renal biopsy has shown proliferative glomerulonephritis or membranoproliferative glomerulonephritis or necrotizing and crescentic glomerulonephritis or focal glomerulonephritis or membranous glomerulonephropathy or focal segmental glomerular sclerosis? (Table 43-5)
3. Which diseases may be present in a child with the characteristic clinical manifestations of recurrent hematuria or acute glomerulonephritis or rapidly progressive glomerulonephritis or the nephrotic syndrome? (Table 43-6)

An understanding of these associations and of the overlapping between clinical disease and morphologic lesion is required to arrive at the proper diagnosis and treatment and to assess the natural and treatment histories of glomerular disease in childhood. Individual syndromes and diseases will be discussed in the subsequent chapters.

References

1. Bohle, A., Eichenseher, N., Fischbach, H., Neild, G. H., Wehner, H., Edel, H. H., Losse, H., Renner, E., Reichel, W., and Schütterle, G. The different forms of glomerulonephritis. Morphological and clinical aspects, analyzed in 2500 patients. *Klin. Wochenschr.* 54:59, 1976.

2. Burkholder, P. M. *Atlas of Human Glomerular Pathology*. Hagerstown, Md.: Harper & Row, 1974. Chap. 3.
3. Cameron, J. S. A Clinician's View of the Classification of Glomerulonephritis. In P. Kincaid-Smith, T. H. Mathew, and E. L. Becker (eds.), *Glomerulonephritis*. New York: Wiley, 1973. Pp. 66–79.
4. Churg, J., and Duffy, J. L. Classification of Glomerulonephritis Based on Morphology. In P. Kincaid-Smith, T. H. Mathew, and E. L. Becker (eds.), *Glomerulonephritis*. New York: Wiley, 1973. Pp. 43–61.
5. Churg, J., Habib, R., and White, R. H. R. Pathology of the nephrotic syndrome in children. A report for the International Study of Kidney Disease in Children. *Lancet* 1:1299, 1970.
6. Fischbach, H., Bohle, A., Meyer, D., Edel, H. H., Frotscher, U., Kluthe, R., Renner, D., Rinsche, K., and Scheler, F. The morphological and clinical course of the different forms of glomerulonephritis. *Klin. Wochenschr.* 54:105, 1976.
7. Germuth, F. G., and Rodriguez, E. *Immunopathology of the Renal Glomerulus*. Boston: Little, Brown, 1973. Chap. 4.
8. Habib, R. Classification of Glomerulonephritis Based on Morphology. In P. Kincaid-Smith, T. H. Mathew, and E. L. Becker (eds.), *Glomerulonephritis*. New York: Wiley, 1973. Pp. 17–41.
9. Habib, R. Classification of Glomerular Nephropathies. In M. I. Rubin and T. M. Barratt (eds.), *Pediatric Nephrology*. Baltimore: Williams & Wilkins, 1975. Chap. 22.
10. Habib, R., and Kleinknecht, C. The Primary Nephrotic Syndrome of Childhood. Classification and Clinicopathologic Study of 406 Cases. In S. C. Sommers (ed.), *Pathology Annual*. New York: Appleton-Century-Crofts, 1971. Pp. 417–474.
11. Hayslett, J. P., Siegel, N. J., and Kashgarian, M. Glomerulonephropathy. *Adv. Intern. Med.* 20:215, 1975.
12. Heptinstall, R. H. *Pathology of The Kidney* (2nd ed.). Boston: Little, Brown, 1974. Chap. 8.
13. Hyman, L. R., and Walker, P. F. Progressive renal failure and nephrotic syndrome in children: A spectrum of glomerulonephropathies. *Milit. Med.* 140:608, 1975.
14. Kincaid-Smith, P., and Hobbs, J. B. Glomerulonephritis: A classification based on morphology with comments on the significance of vessel lesions. *Med. J. Aust.* 2:1397, 1972.
15. McCluskey, R. T., and Klassen, J. Immunologically mediated glomerular, tubular and interstitial renal disease. *N. Engl. J. Med.* 288:564, 1973.
16. Morel-Maroger, L., Leathem, A., and Richet, G. Glomerular abnormalities in nonsystemic diseases: Relationship between findings by light microscopy and immunofluorescence in 433 renal biopsy specimens. *Am. J. Med.* 53:170, 1972.
17. Schreiner, G. E. The Nephrotic Syndrome. In M. B. Strauss and L. G. Welt (eds.), *Diseases of the Kidney* (2nd ed.). Boston: Little, Brown, 1971. Chap. 16.
18. Volhard, F., and Fahr, T. *Die Brightsche Nierenkrankheit*. Berlin: Springer, 1914.
19. Wilson, C. B., and Dixon, F. J. Diagnosis of immunopathologic renal disease. *Kidney Int.* 5:389, 1974.

44. Persistent Hematuria and Proteinuria

Henry L. Barnett, Chester M. Edelmann, Jr., and Jay Bernstein

The occurrence of hematuria and proteinuria in a child with no urologic disease and no clinical, immunologic, or other biochemical evidence of renal disease is a frequent problem in pediatric nephrology. The term *isolated hematuria and proteinuria* is used here to describe this important group of patients. The group is heterogeneous and the urinary findings are variable (Table 44-1). Among the patterns encountered are recurrent gross hematuria with insignificant proteinuria, and postural proteinuria unaccompanied by hematuria, both of which are discussed elsewhere (Chaps. 46, 45). The occurrence of transient or nonrepetitive proteinuria and microscopic

hematuria is of no known clinical importance, except insofar as such children must be identified in interpreting the results of clinical screening studies. Persistent or recurrent microscopic hematuria and persistent nonpostural proteinuria in most instances also appear to be benign; however, they may reflect the presence of serious, organic and progressive renal disease.

The defining characteristics of persistent hematuria and proteinuria, a subgroup of isolated hematuria and proteinuria, are that at the time of detection and for an indeterminant period thereafter, the hematuria, which is either persistent or recurrent, is microscopic, and the proteinuria, also

Table 44-1. Clinical Patterns in Isolated Hematuria and Proteinuria

Recurrent gross hematuria

Postural proteinuria

Persistent or recurrent hematuria and proteinuria
   Persistent or recurrent microscopic hematuria
   Persistent or recurrent nonpostural proteinuria
   Persistent or recurrent microscopic hematuria and non-
     postural proteinuria

Transient hematuria and proteinuria

either persistent or recurrent, is nonpostural. The absence of other clinical or laboratory findings of renal disease does not exclude organic renal disease as a cause of persistent hematuria and proteinuria. A renal biopsy done at the time the urinary abnormalities are first detected may reveal normal glomerular histologic findings or any one of the glomerular diseases listed in Table 43-1 of Chap. 43. In addition, some children eventually manifest other evidence of renal disease, although most apparently never do.

Other diagnostic terms have been used to describe similar groups of children. Some terms (*asymptomatic hematuria and proteinuria* [24]) include the condition described, but do not exclude transient urinary abnormalities, recurrent gross hematuria, postural proteinuria, or organic renal disease. Other terms (*benign* [1] or *benign essential* [17, 21] *hematuria, benign persistent asymptomatic proteinuria* [16], *primary hematuria* [11, 12], and *recurrent* [13] or *symptomless* [6] *hematuria of childhood*) are only partially inclusive. The terms *permanent isolated proteinuria* [8] and *isolated hematuria* used by Habib and her colleagues [10] coincide most closely with the concept intended here.

The major clinical questions are first, whether or not these children have organic glomerular disease, and second, whether or not this information is sufficiently important to recommend a renal biopsy, which is the only means of obtaining it. The knowledge needed to answer these questions is the distribution of patients with persistent hematuria and proteinuria among the histopathologic categories of renal disease. For example, if it were known that a very high proportion of patients had either normal glomerular histology or lesions indicative of resolving acute postinfectious glomerulonephritis, a renal biopsy probably would not be recommended unless other clinical, biochemical, or immunologic evidence of renal disease were to appear subsequently. Because of the lack of such basic information, recommendations

about renal biopsies have varied greatly (see Indications for Biopsy).

Incidence and Demographic Aspects

Epidemiologic screening for proteinuria and hematuria in large populations of school children provides the only available data from which estimates of incidence can be made. The difficulty is in estimating the proportion of those children who would fulfill the present criteria. In three major studies of populations of school children ranging from 4,000 to over 12,000 [4, 20, 24], the incidence of proteinuria and hematuria on initial screening was found to be about 50 to 60 per 1,000. It would appear that roughly one-half to one-third of these children had transient, nonrepetitive urinary abnormalities and that as many as two-thirds of those with proteinuria may have had postural proteinuria [4]. The proportion of children with hematuria who might also have had recurrent gross hematuria cannot be determined, but the figure is probably very low. Starting with an estimated incidence rate of hematuria and proteinuria of 50 per 1,000 on initial screening and reducing it by one-half for children with transient abnormalities and arbitrarily by one-fourth for those with postural proteinuria, it would appear that a rate of about 15 to 20 per 1,000 would not be an overestimation of the incidence of persistent hematuria and proteinuria in children. This estimate, if valid, emphasizes the importance of this clinical state in pediatric nephrology. For example, the rate is some 100 times greater than the 15.7 per 100,000 estimated for children with the nephrotic syndrome (Chap. 52).

The demography of persistent hematuria and proteinuria can be surmised only from estimates of the proportion of children in screening studies who fulfill the diagnostic criteria set forth. Even this supposition assumes that the demographic characteristics of children with persistent hematuria and proteinuria are similar to those of the entire group of children screened. With this reservation, it appears that the incidence of both proteinuria and hematuria increases progressively with age in children from 6 to 12 years, and that for each age the rate is higher for girls than for boys, especially after age 8 or 10 years. In at least one large screening study, no consistent difference was found among different ethnic or socioeconomic groups [4].

Criteria for Diagnosis of
Hematuria and Proteinuria

The pathophysiologic features of hematuria and of proteinuria are considered in Chaps. 16 and 15 respectively, and rates of excretion of red blood cells and protein are discussed there. Unfortunately, data based on the distribution of values obtained in large populations of normal children are not available to define the upper limits of normal. Even then, such data would be difficult to interpret, since the clinical significance of, for example, excretion rate greater than two SDs above the mean would still need to be determined. Also, careful differentiation between children with transient or nonrepetitive hematuria and proteinuria and those with persistent abnormalities has not been made.

It is therefore apparent that criteria used for defining rates of excretion of red blood cells and protein need further study. Those used to establish a "case" in the screening studies have been based on the results of a dipstick test and semiquantitative measurements of the concentrations of red blood cells and protein in standardized specimens, usually overnight or early morning specimens. In most studies using chemically impregnated strips, a 1+ value for protein and a positive test for red blood cells were considered diagnostic. Dodge et al. [4] made careful comparisons between screening and more precise methods and found that, except for specimens showing trace amounts of protein by the stick method, the quantity of protein by the screening and sulfosalicylic acid methods was comparable. Only one-half the specimens found to contain trace amounts of protein by the stick method were subsequently found to contain 10 mg per deciliter or more of protein by the sulfosalicylic acid test. Almost 100 percent of the urine specimens positive for red blood cells by the stick method were observed to contain at least a few ghost cells on microscopic examination of centrifuged urinary sediment. However, only 80 percent of the stick-positive urines contained 5 to 10 red blood cells per high-power field, and slightly more than 90 percent contained 3 to 5. No urine specimens found to be negative by the stick method were demonstrated to contain protein or red blood cells when tested by other methods.

Distribution of Patients Among Histopathologic Categories

Information about the distribution of patients among histopathologic categories with which persistent hematuria and proteinuria may be associated is very limited. Habib and her associates [8] examined tissue obtained from renal biopsies in 65 children with permanent isolated proteinuria and found no glomerular abnormalities in 55. In the remaining 10 patients, segmental and focal

hyalinosis (focal segmental glomerulosclerosis) was found in biopsy sections taken between 9 months and 9 years after discovery of the proteinuria.

Renal biopsies in 6 children with persistent asymptomatic proteinuria reported by McLaine and Drummond [18] showed no glomerular abnormalities, except for minor focal mesangial changes in one. No evidence of progressive glomerulopathy was detected in a follow-up period averaging 4.6 years.

Urizar et al. [23] examined tissue obtained from renal biopsies in 17 children with persistent asymptomatic proteinuria. They found no abnormalities on light and fluorescent microscopy, although there was slight but significant thickening of the glomerular basement membrane on electron microscopy in 9 patients.

Sinniah and coworkers [22] described the histopathologic findings in renal biopsy specimens from 145 adults with asymptomatic microscopic hematuria and associated proteinuria. These patients appear to fulfill the diagnostic criteria for persistent hematuria and proteinuria; however, their ages ranged from 14 to 48 years. The morphologic patterns of glomerular disease found in these patients were reported as follows: minimal change ("nil"), 6.9 percent; minimal change with increased mesangial matrix or cells, 35.9 percent; diffuse proliferative glomerulonephritis (mesangial hypercellularity), 51.7 percent; focal segmental proliferative glomerulonephritis, 3.4 percent; membranous glomerulonephritis, 0.7 percent; and mesangiocapillary glomerulonephritis, 1.4 percent. These findings suggest that histopathologic categories may be distributed differently in adults than in children.

Clinical Care

The only clinical care required by these asymptomatic children is a clear explanation to them and their families of the nature of the problem and the prognosis. The way in which this is done by individual clinicians is subject to their own interpretation of the condition and to their own ability to deal with uncertainty. The capacity of the children and their families to deal with uncertainty is also an important consideration, often ignored. A major question is whether or not a renal biopsy should be done. Its risks are low when the procedure is done by experienced personnel (see Chap. 12), but as with any diagnostic procedure that has any risk and is disturbing to patients and their families, it should be done only if the expected benefit exceeds the risk. If the clinician believes the wisest course is to assume, at least for a period of time, that there is either no organic glomerular disease or a resolving acute postinfectious glomerulonephritis and that the patient and the family can accept his judgment with tolerable anxiety, he will reassure them and recommend that the patient be followed without performing a biopsy. His knowing that there is no known effective treatment at this stage, even if organic glomerular disease is present, would strengthen this position. If, on the other hand, the physician himself is uneasy about the uncertainty, or if he honestly believes that the family cannot tolerate it, he may recommend that a biopsy be done soon after the clinical diagnosis is made. It is important for clinicians to realize that their own tolerance for uncertainty influences such decisions, which often must be made on tenuous evidence.

Indications for Biopsy

Acute postinfectious glomerulonephritis is probably the most frequent of the identifiable glomerular abnormalities in children with persistent hematuria and proteinuria who have organic glomerular lesions. It is generally held that these patients have an excellent prognosis, especially those whose initial attack was asymptomatic, a factor that would hold, by definition, for those with persistent hematuria and proteinuria. Most clinicians would therefore agree that if these patients could be identified, they should not have a biopsy. The clinical feature of acute postinfectious glomerulonephritis most helpful in this regard is that the abnormal urinary findings disappear over a period of weeks or months. Thus, a major reason for not recommending a biopsy at the time urinary abnormalities are first detected in a patient with persistent hematuria and proteinuria is to avoid doing a biopsy in children with acute postinfectious glomerulonephritis. It is generally stated that in a large proportion of patients the urine becomes normal within periods ranging from 6 weeks to 6 months of the onset of postinfectious glomerulonephritis. The urines of patients who are initially asymptomatic, and who might be included in the group with persistent hematuria and proteinuria, would be expected to become normal in even a shorter period of time. On the other hand, the proportion of children whose urinary abnormalities persist for a year or more may be greater than generally thought [14, 15]. In a prospective study of 41 children initially assigned a morphologic diagnosis of acute postinfectious glomerulonephritis, Dodge et al. [3] reported persistence or recurrence of proteinuria, usually unaccompanied by hematuria, for 12

months or longer in 25 (61 percent) and for 24 months or longer in 14 (36 percent).

It is understandable that recommendations concerning renal biopsies in children with persistent hematuria and proteinuria vary widely. Many authors agree that a renal biopsy should not be recommended for those who have hematuria with no proteinuria [2, 10, 11, 15, 25]. There is less agreement concerning children with proteinuria. Recommendations concerning children with persistent proteinuria without hematuria take into account both the duration and severity of the proteinuria. It has been recommended, for example, that a biopsy be done in patients whose proteinuria has persisted for periods of 6 months [5] or 1 or 2 years [9] and in patients whose proteinuria exceeds 1.5 gm per 24 hr [9]. Among patients with both hematuria and proteinuria, some authors recommend that biopsies be done in those who have small amounts of protein [19, 25], whereas others believe they should be done only if the proteinuria is greater than 300 [5] or 500 mg per day [11].

At present, the authors and their colleagues [7] recommend that biopsies be done when proteinuria with or without hematuria has persisted for 6 to 12 months. Although more information is required before confident decisions can be made about patients with persistent microscopic hematuria and no proteinuria, we recommend at present that biopsies be done only if other evidence of renal disease appears or if the physician, after evaluating his own feelings and those of the patient and the family, concludes that the uncertainty about the prognosis cannot be tolerated.

References

1. Ayoub, E. M., and Vernier, R. L. Benign recurrent hematuria. *Am. J. Dis. Child.* 109:217, 1965.
2. Barratt, T. M. Renal Biopsy. In M. I. Rubin and T. M. Barratt (eds.), *Pediatric Nephrology.* Baltimore: Williams & Wilkins, 1975. P. 886.
3. Dodge, W. F., Spargo, B. H., Travis, L. B., Srivastava, R. N., Carrajal, H. F., De Beukelaer, M. M., Longley, M. P., and Menchaca, J. A. Poststreptococcal glomerulonephritis. *N. Engl. J. Med.* 286:273, 1972.
4. Dodge, W. F., West, E. F., Smith, E. H., and Bunce, H. III. Proteinuria and hematuria in schoolchildren: Epidemiology and early natural history. *J. Pediatr.* 88:327, 1976.
5. Ettenger, R. B. Workshop of the Child with Proteinuria. In E. Lieberman (ed.), *Clinical Pediatric Nephrology.* Philadelphia: Lippincott, 1976. P. 27.
6. Glasgow, E. F., Moncrieff, M. W., and White, R. H. R. Symptomless haematuria in childhood. *Br. Med. J.* 2:687, 1970.
7. Greifer, I. The Diagnosis and Evolution of Sus-

pected Renal Disease. In J. Strauss (ed.), *Pediatric Nephrology*. New York: Stratton Intercontinental, 1974. Vol. 1, p. 150.

8. Habib, R. The Major Syndromes. In P. Royer, R. Habib, H. Mathieu, and M. Broyer, *Pediatric Nephrology*. Philadelphia: Saunders, 1974. P. 249.

9. Habib, R. The Major Syndromes. In P. Royer, R. Habib, H. Mathieu, and M. Broyer, *Pediatric Nephrology*. Philadelphia: Saunders, 1974. P. 250.

10. Habib, R. The Major Syndromes. In P. Royer, R. Habib, H. Mathieu, and M. Broyer, *Pediatric Nephrology*. Philadelphia: Saunders, 1974. P. 252.

11. Hayslett, J. P. Primary hematuria. *Kidney,* 9:11, 1976.

12. Hendler, E. D., Kashgarian, M., and Hayslett, J. P. Clinicopathological correlations of primary haematuria. *Lancet* 1:458, 1972.

13. Johnston, C., and Shuler, S. Recurrent haematuria in childhood. *Arch. Dis. Child.* 44:483, 1969.

14. Lewy, J. E., Salinas-Madrigal, L., Herdson, P. B., Pirami, C. L., and Metcoff, J. Clinico-pathologic correlations in acute poststreptococcal glomerulonephritis. *Medicine (Baltimore)* 50:453, 1971.

15. Lieberman, E. Workup of the Child With Hematuria. In E. Lieberman (ed.), *Clinical Pediatric Nephrology*. Philadelphia: Lippincott, 1976. P. 12.

16. Lieberman, E., and Donnell, G. N. Recovery of children with acute glomerulonephritis. *Am. J. Dis. Child.* 109:398, 1965.

17. Marks, M. I., and Drummond, K. N. Benign familial hematuria. *Pediatrics.* 44:590, 1969.

18. McLaine, P. N., and Drummond, K. N. Benign persistent asymptomatic proteinuria in childhood. *Pediatrics* 46:548, 1970.

19. Northway, J. D. Hematuria in children. *J. Pediatr.* 78:381, 1971.

20. Randolph, M. F., and Greenfield, M. Proteinuria. *Am. J. Dis. Child.* 114:631, 1967.

21. Rogers, P. W., Kurtzman, N. A., Bunn, S. M., Jr., and White, M. G. Familial benign essential hematuria. *Arch. Intern., Med.* 131:257, 1973.

22. Sinniah, R., Pwee, H. S., and Lim, C. H. Glomerular lesions in asymptomatic microscopic hematuria discovered on routine medical examination. *Clin. Nephrol.* 5:216, 1976.

23. Urizar, R. E., Tinglof, B. O., Smith, F. G., Jr., and McIntosh, R. M. Persistent asymptomatic proteinuria in children. *Am. J. Clin. Pathol.* 62:461, 1974.

24. Wagner, M. G., Smith, F. G., Jr., Tinglof, B. O., and Cornberg, E. Epidemiology of proteinuria. *J. Pediatr.* 73:825, 1968.

25. West, C. D. Asymptomatic hematuria and proteinuria in children: Causes and appropriate diagnostic studies. *J. Pediatr.* 89:173, 1976.

45. Postural Proteinuria

Roscoe R. Robinson and Ronald P. Krueger

The exact clinical significance of postural or orthostatic proteinuria is controversial. Traditionally, it has been regarded as a benign condition that is not associated with underlying renal disease [1, 5, 19]. This concept of the disorder may well be true in many children, perhaps even in the majority. However, other observations have suggested that, rather than being uniformly benign, postural proteinuria may reflect the presence of early or incipient renal disease, at least in some patients [9, 28]. A final statement concerning the clinical significance of postural proteinuria, especially in terms of subsequent morbidity or mortality in individual patients, has been restricted by complex clinical and physiologic issues that have not yet been resolved.

In contemporary clinical practice, a diagnosis of postural proteinuria is established most commonly by using qualitative tests for urinary protein under appropriate conditions of body posture. This practice ignores the relationship between rates of protein excretion measured quantitatively and the results of qualitative testing. However, it does provide a clinical definition of postural proteinuria based on the results of qualitative testing. Accordingly, in qualitative terms, postural proteinuria can be defined most broadly as a laboratory syndrome that requires complete qualitative absence of proteinuria during recumbency and its presence during quiet upright ambulation or standing. It may be intermittent, transient, continuous, or "fixed" in its appearance. The diagnosis cannot be made when proteinuria is detected during routine urinalysis, when body posture is uncontrolled. For this reason, it has been difficult to establish the relationship between postural proteinuria and other qualitative patterns of proteinuria described by terms such as *intermittent, trace, transient, physiologic,* or *benign.*

Some observers have restricted the diagnosis of postural proteinuria further to patients of a particular age group or to those who are asymptomatic and show no evidence of systemic disease, impaired renal function, abnormalities of urinary sediment, abnormal findings on physical examination, or radiographic abnormalities of the genitourinary tract. In such a setting, postural proteinuria has been described as "isolated," indicating that it represents a single and isolated clinical finding. Such patients undoubtedly constitute a large and important group, perhaps even the majority of all patients. It is also possible that under such circumstances the clinical significance of the disorder may differ from that of a clinical picture in which postural proteinuria is accompanied by one or more additional abnormal findings, however subtle. Nevertheless, restrictive criteria such as these are obviously arbitrary, and their use may tend to obscure the identification of all conditions that may be associated with this laboratory syndrome.

Unfortunately, despite a suspicion that postural proteinuria occurs most often as an isolated finding, reliable data on this point are lacking, and the relative frequency of isolated postural proteinuria as opposed to its occurrence in association with other possible alterations has not been established. For these reasons, the present discussion will consider postural proteinuria in asymptomatic and apparently healthy patients with qualitative proteinuria during quiet upright ambulation alone, irrespective of the presence or absence of other associated signs or symptoms. Whenever possible, observations on patients with isolated postural proteinuria will be distinguished from those in which the disorder is accompanied by other evidences of renal disease or altered function. Cases in which upright proteinuria is induced solely by exposure to unusual postural attitudes, such as exaggerated lordosis, or to transient environmental conditions, such as exposure to heat or cold, or exercise, will not be discussed.

Clinical Classification and Evaluation of the Patient

A uniform method for the clinical classification of proteinuria is essential. The serial urine collection test of Derow [3] has proven useful in this regard. This test requires the timed and sequential collection of urine specimens in recumbent and quiet ambulatory postures during moderate antidiuresis. A measurement of specific gravity and a qualitative test for protein are performed on each specimen.

Three major patterns of proteinuria can be identified by this test: (1) "persistent" proteinuria during *both* the recumbent and upright postures; (2) "transient" postural proteinuria that is present inconstantly from day to day; (3) "fixed" postural proteinuria that is demonstrable consistently on separate days. King [7] reported that in young and asymptomatic adult males with proteinuria on routine urinalysis, 5 to 10 percent exhibited persistent

proteinuria, whereas fixed postural proteinuria was noted in perhaps 15 percent. It is likely that the remainder showed qualitative proteinuria either transiently or intermittently, and that it was persistent or orthostatic for only a short period of time. Overall, transient postural proteinuria is probably much more frequent than the fixed variety. Unfortunately, similar figures are not available for other age groups. It must also be emphasized that repetitive testing must be performed if these criteria are to be applied, and that claims for reproducibility of a given pattern in a single patient have only been established over relatively short periods of time. It is possible, and even likely, that an ever-changing appearance of differing types of proteinuria might well be observed in the same patient over longer periods of observation. Finally, it must be emphasized strongly that these so-called types or patterns of proteinuria represent nothing more than an arbitrary clinical description. It is illogical to view them as specific entities or syndromes as is sometimes done, particularly if this implies that one or another type of proteinuria is due to a single cause.

Even with these reservations, the serial collection test provides no more than a first approximation to an ideal classification of asymptomatic patients with proteinuria. Continued reliance on qualitative testing alone has retarded the possible recognition of characteristic quantitative excretory patterns for specific proteins that might prove to be of diagnostic usefulness. Furthermore, it is already known that a "trace" reaction in highly concentrated urine is of dubious clinical significance, since protein excretion by some upright healthy subjects may be sufficiently high to be detectable by qualitative tests during marked antidiuresis [23]. Similarly, at least in some subjects with fixed postural proteinuria, the rate of protein excretion during recumbency may be higher than that observed in normal subjects, yet still be insufficiently high to permit qualitative detection [25]. In other patients, quantitative measurements of protein excretion during recumbency have been said to be within the range of normal. Further efforts are needed to quantify the excretory rates of specific proteins in patients whose proteinuria has also been classified qualitatively.

Once it has been established that proteinuria is postural in nature, it is convenient to distinguish between patients whose postural proteinuria is isolated and those in whom it is accompanied by other possible evidences of altered function. Accordingly, the minimal initial evaluation should include a thorough history and physical examination in which evidences of antecedent renal or systemic disease are sought, including examination of the urinary sediment, quantification of urinary protein excretion, excretory urography, and a measurement of creatinine clearance. Renal biopsy is not performed routinely, particularly in patients in whom postural proteinuria represents an isolated finding.

Quantity and Character of the Urine Proteins

Total daily protein excretion is usually below 1.5 gm, but amounts as high as 10 gm per day have been described. Most, or virtually all, of this amount probably is excreted during upright ambulation. The fact that fractional daily protein excretion may be similarly high in healthy subjects during upright ambulation [23] suggests that postural proteinuria in some patients may reflect nothing more than the upper range of the normal distribution curve for upright protein excretion. If so, quantitative measurements of total protein excretion per se cannot be used with confidence to distinguish patients with possible renal disease from those who are normal. Diagnostic aid may yet be provided by electrophoretic or immunophoretic characterization of the excretory patterns of specific proteins. The excretion of B_2-microglobulin, a low-molecular-weight indicator of possible "tubular" proteinuria, is said to be normal [18]. Unfortunately, measurements of specific proteins are still limited in number, and most, but not all, of them have revealed the existence of concentration patterns for individual proteins that resemble those of normal urine, including a relatively large percentage of proteins of higher molecular weight [15, 17, 26]. Such excretory patterns have been said to be "non-selective" or "physiologic," in contrast to the "selectivity" that has been observed in other patients with comparable degrees of proteinuria and documented glomerular alterations of minimal severity. In simplest terms, this finding could imply that (1) postural proteinuria is a variant of normal or (2) it is a condition in which glomerular permeability, or tubular resorption, is altered differently from that in patients with minimal glomerular lesions and proteinuria.

Clinical Presentation

Postural proteinuria is usually discovered during a routine health examination or an acute intercurrent illness in children who are more than 5 to 10 years of age. Both sexes are affected equally, and the syndrome appears to be especially common in adolescents or young adults; its incidence in older age groups has not yet been established reliably. Its documented occurrence during subsiding acute glomerulonephritis, the subsiding nephrotic syndrome, or active pyelonephritis [3, 9] illustrates that it can and does occur in association with renal disease. Nevertheless, in most patients, the clinical examination is nonrevealing and renal function is normal, although abnormalities of the urinary sediment, or urographic abnormalities, or both have been described in variable proportions [1, 13, 16]. With respect to associated urographic alterations, there is no evidence that they occur with any greater frequency than in the healthy nonproteinuric population. The practical clinical problem generally is to differentiate between proteinuria accompanying underlying renal disease and postural proteinuria in the absence of any other signs, symptoms, or laboratory abnormalities, i.e., isolated postural proteinuria.

Renal Histologic Findings

Light-microscopic studies of the biopsy specimens from young adult patients with fixed postural proteinuria revealed that 8 percent had unequivocal evidence of well-defined disease, 45 percent had subtle but definite alterations of glomerular structure (focal or diffuse capillary-wall thickening without alteration of the true basement membrane, or focal hypercellularity), and 47 percent exhibited a histologic pattern that could not be differentiated from that of normal tissue [22, 24]. Observations in children are more limited, but similar alterations have since been observed both in children and adults [4, 27]. Still other investigators have reported that renal tissue in children is perfectly normal, at least in small series of patients [2]. A limited number of electron-microscopic observations have confirmed the presence of subtle and focal glomerular alterations [22, 27], and immunohistologic studies have shown that both immunoglobulin and complement can be localized within such foci [12]. Histologic observations from patients with transient postural proteinuria are so few that definite conclusions cannot be drawn.

The clinical significance of these glomerular alterations is far from clear. Their existence has given rise to the suggestion that postural proteinuria may reflect the presence of early or incipient renal disease. However, it is still uncertain whether they are the cause or the effect of proteinuria or perhaps nothing more than an incidental finding. If they are the cause, it is possible that they have been induced by more than one etiologic agent, and it is thus illogical to assume that the subsequent clinical course should be identical in all patients. Therefore, in some instances, the glomerular alterations may represent the healed or recovery phase of a previous episode of renal disease; in others, the earliest manifestation of a future form of renal disease; and in still others, nothing more than a subtle variation of normal architecture.

Regardless of the exact nature of these changes, their very existence may provide a reasonable explanation for the proteinuria; i.e., an underlying defect of the capillary wall that permits an increased transglomerular passage of plasma proteins. However, in itself, the existence of an altered capillary wall is not sufficient to explain an apparent rise of protein excretion only during quiet ambulation, a phenomenon that has been well documented [16] in at least some patients with postural proteinuria on qualitative testing.

Possible Mechanism of Fixed Postural Proteinuria

The mechanism by which assumption of the upright posture effects an increased excretion of protein in these patients is still uncertain. Earlier concepts postulated that any one of the several renal hemodynamic alterations in the upright posture might serve as the *primary* cause of postural proteinuria: renal venous congestion or ischemia and reduction in glomerular filtration rate have been implicated [1, 6]. This hypothesis became suspect when it was shown that the upright renal hemodynamic response in these patients was no different from that in healthy subjects [10]. A quantitatively similar upright reduction of renal blood flow and filtration rate and an elevation of filtration fraction were observed. Of these three possible hemodynamic determinants of transglomerular protein transfer, the results of clearance studies suggested that the normal and usual upright reduction of blood flow was of greatest importance, and that it might secondarily facilitate or "permit" an increased transfer of protein across the altered capillary wall via some unknown mechanism [25]. According to this view, the combination of an altered capillary wall and a normal upright reduction of blood flow might be sufficient to effect an increased transglomerular passage of protein during standing that readily exceeds the normal tubular resorptive capacity. Conversely, transglomerular protein passage might be less during recumbency (but still higher than normal) since blood flow is higher, and the kinetics of protein resorption might be such that the normal resorptive capacity would be exceeded very little, if at all.

This hypothesis is tentative. For example, an upright alteration of renal tubular resorption of protein has not yet been excluded. Alternatively,

increased capillary permeability to protein during standing might be mediated via a direct effect of certain humoral agents (whose release is also increased by postural changes) on the altered capillary wall. Such a role has been suggested for renin or angiotensin, or both, because of the known ability of these substances to produce proteinuria in experimental animals [29].

Clinical Significance and Natural History

Final determination of the cause and clinical significance of postural proteinuria is particularly obscure when it occurs in the absence of the following: (1) the nephrotic syndrome or a systemic disease such as diabetes mellitus or hypertension; (2) impaired renal function; (3) an abnormal urinary sediment; (4) anatomic alteration on excretory urography; or (5) a past history of renal disease, i.e., when postural proteinuria is isolated. Resolution of this problem may rest eventually on the results of long-term prospective follow-up studies of patients who have undergone a thorough initial examination. The early results of a few such studies are available.

In one 10-year follow-up study of young men with an initial diagnosis of isolated and fixed orthostatic proteinuria, Thompson et al. [28] found that 49 percent still exhibited a qualitative pattern of proteinuria. No evidence of renal functional impairment or progressive renal disease had yet developed in any of the patients. Furthermore, there was no relationship between the initial "normalcy" or "abnormalcy" of the renal histologic findings and any subsequent pattern of renal function or the continued presence of proteinuria. In short, the 10-year prognosis for these young men with fixed orthostatic proteinuria was excellent.

The exact significance of the subtle glomerular alterations that were described initially in 45 percent of the patients remains uncertain, but the decreasing presence of proteinuria of any type and the maintenance of normal renal function suggest that their presence did not reflect an incipient manifestation of progressive renal disease, at least in some patients. However, the eventual appearance of altered renal function has yet to be excluded in an equal number of patients who were still proteinuric after 10 years. These results are not surprising in view of the heterogeneity of the initial histologic observations. It seems illogical to expect that all of them would lead to overt illness even after a long period of time. Subtle or minimal alterations may represent no more than nonpathologic structural defects; even among those representing definite pathologic lesions and undoubtedly reflecting the impact of multiple causes, some may have already begun to heal, some may begin to heal eventually, whereas others may progress with such indolence that clinical significance as a cause of morbidity or mortality is never achieved within a lifetime. A similarly benign intermediate-term course of 5 to 10 years or so has been described by other observers [2, 11, 16]. However, in 531 young men, King [8, 9] observed that persistent proteinuria developed in 18 percent, and 14 percent later exhibited diastolic hypertension.

Taken together, these findings suggest that fixed postural proteinuria does not represent a transient condition of adolescence, and that it may still reflect the earliest expression of a future form of renal disease in some patients. Continued observation is necessary to establish the validity of this suspicion, although it must be acknowledged that the 10-year prognosis does appear to be excellent in almost all subjects.

Similar information is less available from patients with transient postural proteinuria, although this condition is more common by far. It is this type of postural proteinuria that probably is present in most patients who are said without further amplification to have orthostatic proteinuria. Most observers have felt that it is largely benign [14] and that its prognosis is excellent. In many patients, transient episodes of postural proteinuria may well reflect nothing more than transient exposure to such environmental factors as heat, cold, fever, or exercise. Even so, in view of the suggestion that the persistence or repetitive occurrence of any qualitative pattern of proteinuria may be of greater predictive value (in terms of definite morphologic evidence of underlying kidney disease) than the actual nature of the pattern itself [14, 20, 21], it may be wise to regard the significance of transient episodes of postural proteinuria with at least modest suspicion if such episodes recur over a long period of time.

Treatment

Treatment for isolated postural proteinuria is not required, and restriction of physical activity is not beneficial. Immunization can be carried out without harm. The greatest emphasis should be placed on modulated follow-up evaluation at relatively infrequent intervals of once or twice yearly; more frequent observation is indicated in patients with any associated findings, such as hypertension or abnormalities of the urinary sediment, even though renal function may be entirely normal on initial evaluation. Renal biopsy usually is not indicated unless there is a distinct change in the clinical course, such as an abrupt and definite increase in daily protein excretion, the appearance of distinct and persistent abnormalities of the urinary sediment, or impairment of renal function.

References

1. Bull, G. M. Postural proteinuria. *Clin. Sci.* 7:77, 1948.
2. Chaptal, J., Jean, R., Bonnet, H., and Pages, A. Etude histologique du rein dans 33 cas de proteinurie isolée de l'enfant. *Arch. Fr. Pediatr.* 23:385, 1966.
3. Derow, H. A. The diagnostic value of serial measurements of albuminuria in ambulatory patients. *N. Engl. J. Med.* 227:827, 1942.
4. Dodge, W. F., Daeschner, C. W., Brennan, J. C., Rosenberg, H. S., Travis, L. B., and Hopps, H. C. Percutaneous renal biopsy in children. *Pediatrics* 30:477, 1962.
5. Fishberg, A. M. Orthostatic Proteinuria. In *Hypertension and Nephritis* (5th ed.). Philadelphia: Lea & Febiger, 1954. Pp. 396–407.
6. Greiner, T., and Henry, J. P. Mechanism of postural proteinuria. *J.A.M.A.* 157:1373, 1955.
7. King, S. E. Patterns of protein excretion by the kidney. *Ann. Intern. Med.* 42:296, 1955.
8. King, S. E. Albuminuria (proteinuria) in renal disease. II. Preliminary observations on the clinical course of patients with orthostatic albuminuria. *N.Y. State J. Med.* 59:825, 1959.
9. King, S. E. Diastolic hypertension and chronic proteinuria. *Am. J. Cardiol.* 9:669, 1962.
10. King, S. E., and Baldwin, D. S. Renal hemodynamics during erect lordosis in normal man and subjects with orthostatic proteinuria. *Proc. Soc. Exp. Biol. Med.* 86:634, 1954.
11. Lagrue, G., Bariety, J., Druet, P. H., and Milliez, P. Les divers types de proteinuries. In *Les Proteinuries*. Paris: Sandoz, 1969.
12. Lange, K., Treser, G., Sagel, I., Ty, A., and Wasserman, E. Routine immunohistology in renal diseases. *Ann. Intern. Med.* 64:25, 1966.
13. Lecocq, F. R., McPhaul, J. J., and Robinson, R. R. Fixed and reproducible orthostatic proteinuria. V. Results of a five year follow-up evaluation. *Ann. Intern. Med.* 64:557, 1966.
14. Levitt, J. I. The prognostic significance of proteinuria in young college students. *Ann. Intern. Med.* 66:685, 1967.
15. Manuel, Y., Revillard, J. P., Francois, R., Traeger, J., Gaillard, L., Salle, B., Freycon, M. T., and Borenstein, I. Trace Proteinuria. In Y. Manuel, J. P. Revillard, and H. Betuel (eds.), *Proteins in Normal and Pathological Urine*. Basel: Karger, 1970. Pp. 198–208.
16. Mery, J. P., Berger, J., Milhaud, A., and Crosnier, J. La proteinurie orthostatique. A propos de 300 observations. *Rev. Prat. (Paris)* 11:3115, 1961.
17. McKay, E., Slater, R. J., and Brown, B. Studies on human proteinuria. II. Some characteristics of the γ globulins excreted in normal, exercise, postural and nephrotic proteinuria. *J. Clin. Invest.* 41:1638, 1962.
18. Peterson, P. A., Evrin, P. E., and Berggord, I. Differentiation of glomerular, tubular and normal pro-

teinuria: Determinations of urinary excretion of B$_2$-microglobulin, albumin, and total protein. *J. Clin. Invest.* 48:1189, 1969.

19. Prince, C. L. Orthostatic albuminuria. *J. Urol.* 50: 608, 1954.

20. Robinson, R. R. Idiopathic proteinuria. *Ann. Intern. Med.* 71:1019, 1969.

21. Robinson, R. R. Proteinuria in Asymptomatic Patients. In *Proceedings of the Fifth International Congress of Nephrology.* Basel: Karger, 1974. Vol. 3, pp. 27–33.

22. Robinson, R. R., Ashworth, C. T., Glover, S. N., Phillippi, P. J., Lecocq, F. R., and Langelier, P. R. Fixed and reproducible orthostatic proteinuria. II. Electron microscopic study of renal biopsy specimens from five cases. *Am. J. Pathol.* 39:405, 1961.

23. Robinson, R. R., and Glenn, W. G. Fixed and reproducible orthostatic proteinuria. IV. Urinary albumin excretion by healthy human subjects in the recumbent and upright positions. *J. Lab. Clin. Med.* 64:717, 1964.

24. Robinson, R. R., Glover, S. N., Phillippi, P. S., Lecocq, F. R., and Langelier, P. R. Fixed and re-

producible orthostatic proteinuria. I. Light microscopic studies of the kidney. *Am. J. Pathol.* 39:291, 1961.

25. Robinson, R. R., Lecocq, F. R., Phillippi, P. J., and Glenn, W. G. Fixed and reproducible orthostatic proteinuria. III. Effect of induced renal hemodynamic alterations upon urinary protein excretion. *J. Clin. Invest.* 42:100, 1963.

26. Rowe, D. S., and Soothill, J. F. The proteins of postural and exercise proteinuria. *Clin. Sci.* 21:87, 1961.

27. Ruckley, V. A., MacDonald, M. K., MacLean, P. R., and Robson, J. S. Glomerular ultrastructure and function in postural proteinuria. *Nephron* 3:153, 1966.

28. Thompson, A. L., Durrett, R. R., and Robinson, R. R. Fixed and reproducible orthostatic proteinuria. VI. Results of a 10-year follow-up evaluation. *Ann. Intern. Med.* 73:235, 1970.

29. Tobian, L., and Nason, P. The augmentation of proteinuria by an acute sodium depletion that stimulates the secretion of renin. *J. Clin. Invest.* 43:1301, 1964.

46. Recurrent Hematuria—Focal Glomerulonephritis: Inflammation of the Mesangium

Robert L. Vernier

The terms *focal nephritis* and *focal glomerulonephritis* have been used interchangeably to describe both clinical conditions *and* a histopathologic lesion commonly seen in several well-defined syndromes. Volhard and Fahr [36] used the term *focal nephritis* as a clinical diagnosis to describe patients with gross hematuria occurring at the height of a respiratory infection. The use of percutaneous needle biopsy has, in the 20 years since its introduction, greatly increased the number of clinical conditions found to be associated with this abnormality. For example, Heptinstall and Joekes [13] encountered thirteen examples of focal glomerulonephritis in one hundred consecutive renal biopsy specimens in adult patients with systemic lupus erythematosus, periarteritis nodosa, Schönlein-Henoch purpura, and the nephrotic syndrome. Thus, it should be understood that focal glomerulonephritis is used herein as a descriptive pathologic term. The term is useful, since there are good correlations between this pathologic lesion and the prognosis or outcome of the associated diseases.

The purpose of this chapter is to describe the syndrome of recurrent hematuria, a relatively common clinical problem in children. Although other lesions or no abnormalities may be found by light microscopy, most patients with recurrent hematuria have focal proliferative glomerulonephritis. The probable pathogenetic mechanisms involved in the development of this lesion will be discussed in an attempt to relate it to certain other diseases and processes, briefly mentioned. Finally, an analysis of the current knowledge of the function, immunology, and morphology of the glomerular mesangial cell system will be presented.

Recurrent Hematuria

CLINICAL MANIFESTATIONS

The syndrome of recurrent gross or persistent microscopic hematuria is relatively common in both children and adults. It has been estimated to occur in 5 to 8 percent [2, 16] of patients seen by urologists. Unfortunately, these patients are often subjected to many unnecessary urologic investigations and therapeutic programs. In one series [17], 36 patients were subjected to 28 procedures, including cystoscopy, retrograde pyelography, and arteriography. We have seen a 7-year-old boy who was subjected to cystoscopy on seven occasions

The research on which this review was in part based was supported by Public Health Service grants HL-06314, AI-10,704, and AM-TI-05671.

over a period of 2 years in a useless and dangerous search for the cause of recurrent gross hematuria. The widespread recognition of the syndrome and of its clinical characteristics and pathologic manifestations will perhaps result in reduced trauma to this population of patients.

The syndrome is characterized by recurrent episodes of gross hematuria, which often begin at the onset or at the height of an upper respiratory infection. The absence of a delay between the infection and the symptom of hematuria contrasts sharply with the history usually obtained in acute poststreptococcal glomerulonephritis and is one of the most striking clinical features of the syndrome. Other patients have persistent microscopic hematuria without episodes of gross hematuria, but otherwise appear to be similar. Dark urine, red blood cell casts, and hematuria typically appear on the day of, or within 2 to 3 days of, onset of an infection. The macroscopic hematuria rarely lasts longer than 2 to 5 days and is usually accompanied by low-grade proteinuria (< 1 gm per 24 hr). Occasional patients suffer transient reduction of renal function during episodes of gross hematuria, but renal function is usually normal between attacks. Several reports have emphasized the relationship of hematuria and strenuous exercise [9, 11].

The association of the presenting sign, hematuria, with upper respiratory infection has resulted in numerous reports that focus on the bacterial flora of the upper respiratory tract. Although positive throat cultures or serologic evidence of recent infection with beta-hemolytic streptococci has been found in 30 to 40 percent of hospitalized children in some studies [1], it has been shown that this incidence of presumed streptococcal infection closely approximates the average experience in hospitalized children. A clear relationship has not been documented between streptococcal or other infectious agents and recurrent hematuria. It seems likely that the syndrome is the result of a variety of etiologic agents operating through a common pathogenetic mechanism [29].

This syndrome more often affects males than females, and in most series the male-female ratio is about 2 : 1. Several reports describe an incidence of recurrent macroscopic hematuria in other family members [1, 10, 30]. Although familial nephritis, such as the Alport syndrome, is usually recognizable by virtue of overt nephritic manifestations and deafness in relatives, this important differential diagnostic problem must always be considered in patients with symptomless hematuria.

Urinalysis is helpful in identifying red blood cell casts, which may establish the existence of parenchymal disease as the cause of hematuria, thus obviating extensive urologic investigation. If the patient is a child, if the voiding pattern is normal, without hesitation or straining, and if a normal stream is present, the presence of red blood cell casts obviates the need for cystoscopy. Cellular casts (either red or white blood cells or tubular cells) were present in 29 of 30 patients in one series [17]. Hematuria may continue for many years.

Proteinuria is usually minimal, except occasionally during episodes of gross hematuria. Proteinuria in excess of 1 gm per 24 hr, in association with focal sclerotic lesions in a kidney biopsy specimen, has been shown by Roy et al. [29] to indicate a poor prognosis and ultimate development of renal failure. Hypertension is uncommon in this group of patients and, when present, suggests some type of diffuse glomerulonephritis.

An additional important characteristic of patients with recurrent hematuria is the consistently normal value of serum complement [9, 18, 29]. Since complement levels are low in the majority of patients with acute poststreptococcal glomerulonephritis, persistently normal complement levels are of great value in reducing the likelihood of that diagnosis, especially in patients who have positive throat cultures for beta-hemolytic streptococci. Serum cryoglobulins are usually not found [17], providing another contrast with acute poststreptococcal glomerulonephritis. In addition, antinuclear factors and latex fixation tests show negative findings.

RENAL PATHOLOGIC AND IMMUNOPATHOLOGIC FEATURES

Patients with typical recurrent gross or persistent microscopic hematuria should have a renal biopsy to identify the histopathologic abnormality, to rule out more ominous forms of glomerulonephritis, and to avoid further invasive procedures. The study of tissue specimens by the fluorescent-antibody method, improved understanding of renal morphology and experimental pathology, and the developments in clinical immunology of the past 10 years have provided considerable insight into the probable mechanisms involved in the pathogenesis of this well-known syndrome.

Ross [28], in 1960, described focal proliferative glomerular lesions in renal biopsy specimens from 5 patients with recurrent macroscopic hematuria. Although many patients will have focal proliferative lesions, several other glomerular lesions have been described. The most common lesion involves only a portion of the glomerulus in one or more discrete centrolobular areas and consists of increased numbers of mesangial cells and increased

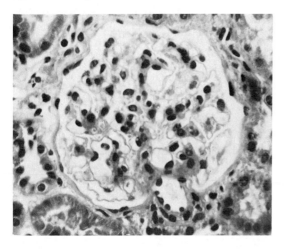

Figure 46-1. Typical minimal changes of mesangial cell proliferation and matrix increase in scattered lobules of a glomerulus from a patient with recurrent hematuria. (H&E, ×612 before 21% reduction.) (From R. L. Vernier et al., Kidney Int. 7:224, 1975.)

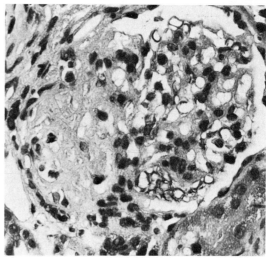

Figure 46-2. An area of glomerular focal sclerosis. This lesion may have prognostic significance when accompanied by proteinuria. (H&E, ×582 before 17% reduction.) (From R. L. Vernier et al., Kidney Int. 7: 224, 1975.)

mesangial matrix (Fig. 46-1). The glomeruli are often irregularly involved, some glomeruli within the same microscopic field being normal or showing only an increase of mesangial matrix without proliferation. Other patients with an identical clinical syndrome will have normal glomeruli or minimal increase in mesangial matrix without proliferation. A minority of patients have diffuse proliferative glomerulonephritis with focal crescent formation, and focal sclerotic lesions appear to develop in a few patients (Fig. 46-2). For example, in a study of 36 children with recurrent macroscopic hematuria, Levy et al. [18] found minimal lesions in 12, focal gomerulonephritis in 17, and diffuse proliferative glomerulonephritis with focal crescents in 7. Roy et al. [29] observed that the appearance of focal glomerular sclerosis *and* proteinuria in excess of 1 gm per day was associated with progressive renal failure in 5 of 16 children observed over 3 to 16 years. Levy et al. [18] presented evidence that children with diffuse proliferative glomerulonephritis and recurrent hematuria have more severe proteinuria (more than 1 gm per day in 4 of their 7 patients) and may also have a higher risk of progressive renal failure than the other groups. It is clear that a small percentage of patients have slowly progressive renal failure and that the process is not always benign. The prognostic and therapeutic significance of proteinuria, other clinical findings, or the pathologic lesions found in a given patient are difficult to assess, since few long-term observations are available.

Electron microscopy of the focal glomerular lesions usually demonstrates an increase in mesangial cells and matrix in the centrolobular regions (Fig. 46-3), associated with granular, electron-dense "deposits" in the mesangium. The deposits are usually more dense than either glomerular basement membrane or mesangial matrix. They occupy the area between the glomerular basement membrane and the mesangial cytoplasm and lie in the expanded spaces between mesangial cells. The quantity of deposited material varies from region to region within a glomerulus—and among glomeruli in patients with focal glomerulonephritis. This observation suggests that the deposits contribute in a major way to the expansion of the mesangial volume in some patients, whereas in others the expansion is more related to an increase in mesangial matrix and cellularity.

Although most authors have commented on the absence of subepithelial deposits (humps) in patients with recurrent hematuria [10, 17, 18, 19], Singer et al. [30] described 6 patients with glomerular subepithelial deposits seen on electron microscopy. They speculated that these patients, who were not otherwise different from a larger population without these lesions, might have had resolving acute glomerulonephritis. Unfortunately the methods that might help to differentiate these entities, such as streptococcal serology, serum complement levels, and fluorescence microscopy, were not used.

Perhaps the most intriguing and consistent abnormality in the recurrent hematuria syndrome is provided by fluorescence microscopy. Bodian et al.

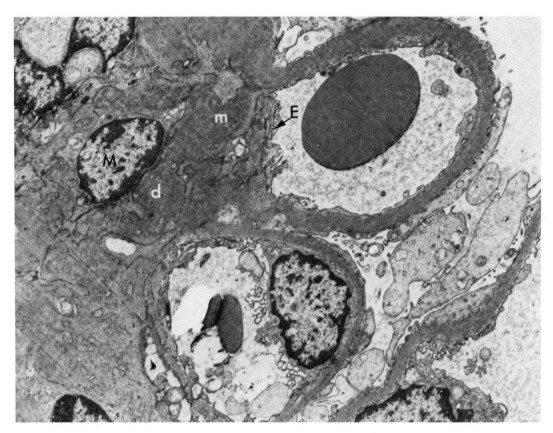

Figure 46-3. Electron micrograph of a portion of a glomerular lobule in a patient with recurrent hematuria. The principal abnormality consists of an increase in the mesangial matrix (m) associated with an increased density (d) of the matrix near the mesangial nucleus (M). E = endothelium. (×7,800 before 14% reduction.) (From R. L. Vernier et al., Kidney Int. *7:224, 1975.)*

[5] studied 14 patients with fluorescein-labeled antisera to human gamma globulin and remarked on the contrast between the generalized mesangial distribution of the antibody and the focal glomerular abnormalities observed by light microscopy. Berger [3] described biopsy specimens from 55 patients (children and adults), who demonstrated generalized mesangial deposits of IgA, IgG, and C3, all of whom had microscopic hematuria as the major clinical manifestation; 22 patients also had one or more episodes of gross hematuria, usually occurring with a sore throat. He commented on the striking uniformity of the glomerular deposits of IgA and IgG, which were intense even in those glomeruli that were normal by light microscopy. These observations have now been confirmed in many laboratories [10, 18, 19, 25, 29]. The impressive concentrations of IgA and the inconstant presence of IgG have raised important questions regarding the possible role of IgA in the pathogenesis of this rather common syndrome. However, in some series, IgM has been found in a mes-

angial distribution more frequently than IgA [17]. There is much evidence to suggest that the condition is an example of immune complex injury, in which complexes of IgA and IgM antibody, often with IgG and complement components, localize within the glomerular mesangium.

Following Berger's [3] description of diffuse mesangial IgA-IgG deposits, and the retrospective association with recurrent hematuria in about 50 percent of his patients, several clinicopathologic reports have suggested that this immunofluorescent pattern is diagnostic. The typical findings consist of fixation of antibody to human IgA, IgG, and C3 in a characteristic granular and interrupted linear mesangial pattern (Fig. 46-4). The finding of immune deposition in histologically normal glomeruli (Fig. 46-5) remains unexplained. Rarely is IgA found alone, unassociated with IgG and C3 [19]. Properdin, a component of the alternate pathway of complement activation [26], has recently been shown to be present in glomeruli in more than 50 percent of cases [7, 25, 26, 29].

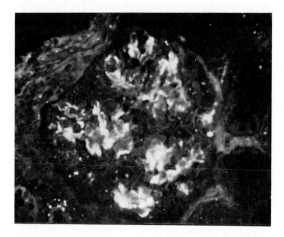

Figure 46-4. Fluorescent photomicrograph demonstrating the typical mesangial pattern of localization of labeled antibody to IgA in a glomerulus in recurrent hematuria. (×764 before 20% reduction.) (From R. L. Vernier et al., Kidney Int. *7:224, 1975.)*

Mesangial deposits of IgA and IgG are not unique to the syndrome of recurrent hematuria, since a similar pattern of fluorescence is frequently observed in anaphylactoid purpura (Schönlein-Henoch purpura) [3, 7, 33] and in an occasional patient with systemic lupus erythematosus [3]. The importance of IgA in the pathogenesis of the glomerular lesions is supported by Berger's [3] observation of recurrence of similar deposits in a biopsy specimen from a kidney transplanted into a patient with this disease.

The critical unanswered questions relate to the mechanism of the injury and the specific role of IgA in the pathogenesis of the disease. Although IgA is recognized as a principal effector of local immunity in external secretions [32], there is no evidence of the participation of intact secretory IgA in the renal injury, since complete secretory IgA has not been demonstrated within the deposits [19]. Although the normal serum immunoglobulin levels, normal serum electrophoretic patterns, and the absence of cryoprecipitates in these patients [17, 19] argue against the concept of a paraproteinemia or perversion of the IgA system, Lagrue et al. [14] and Berger [4] have described significant elevations of serum IgA levels. Further studies of this controversial matter may confirm the concept proposed by the latter authors, that the glomerular injury results from deposition within the mesangium of complexes of abnormal IgA.

DIFFERENTIAL DIAGNOSIS

Hematuria may be a presenting sign or symptom in many circumstances, including renal trauma, various bleeding disorders, sickle cell disease, tumors of the renal pelvis and bladder, renal stones, and, rarely urinary tract infection, including tuberculosis. These diagnoses do not often present a problem, since a careful history and physical examination, repeated analysis of concentrated urine specimens, urine culture, renal function studies, excretory urography, and studies of coagulation effectively exclude these diagnoses. Rarely, hematu-

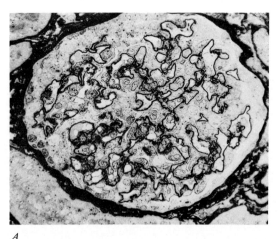

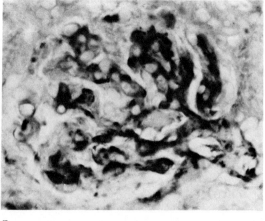

A

B

Figure 46-5. A. Photomicrograph of a silver methenamine–stained, 0.5-μ section of a glomerulus illustrating the minimal but definite increase in silver-positive mesangial matrix in several lobules. (×651 before 20% reduction.) B. Adjacent glomerulus from the same kidney biopsy demonstrating the diffuse mesangial distribution of C3 globulin by the peroxidase-labeled antibody technique. All glomeruli in the specimen showed a similar pattern of staining for IgA, IgG, and C3, although the pathologic changes seen by light microscopy were minimal. (×595 before 20% reduction.) (From R. L. Vernier et al., Kidney Int. *7:224, 1975.)*

ria may be associated with an apparently nonbacterial interstitial nephritis [17, 28], but in these instances the patients were not studied by fluorescence microscopy, and thus it is not clear whether or not they also had an associated mesangial lesion.

An additional form of familial hematuria has been described that differs from hereditary nephritis (the Alport syndrome and its variants) and is associated with an excellent prognosis [20, 24, 27]. Electron microscopy demonstrated unusually thin glomerular capillary walls in renal biopsy sections from affected family members [27]. Immunofluorescent studies in this form of familial hematuria and in hereditary glomerulonephritis are negative for immunoglobulins and complement, which is another important distinction between these syndromes and recurrent hematuria.

TREATMENT

No specific therapy is available for recurrent hematuria, and treatment with potentially toxic drugs is not warranted, since the prognosis is very good. Similarly, the available evidence does not support treatment with antibiotics, corticosteroids, epsilon-aminocaproic acid, and other compounds that have been utilized in the past. Although bed rest has been advocated, there is no evidence that it is beneficial, and it is clear that prolonged bed rest in itself is harmful, since it removes the child from his peer group and encourages excessive patient and parental concern.

PROGNOSIS

The syndrome of recurrent hematuria has been termed *recurrent benign* [1], *idiopathic* [31], *unexplained* [2], *symptomless* [10], and *primary* [11] *hematuria*. Such a list reveals our ignorance about the etiology and pathogenesis of this problem, but cannot convey the concern that the symptoms invoke in the parents of affected children. Once the diagnosis has been established, the family needs reassurance that the vast majority of patients maintain normal renal function even after years of hematuria and eventually recover completely. Nevertheless, as mentioned earlier, renal failure occasionally develops [29], and the disease has recurred in renal transplants [3].

Inflammation of the Mesangial Cells

The lesion found most often in recurrent hematuria is a typical inflammatory response of the glomerular mesangial cells, namely, focal glomerulonephritis. Renewed interest in this common pathologic lesion dates from the description of Heptinstall and Joekes [12, 13], who observed these changes in renal biopsy specimens from patients with certain systemic diseases (systemic lupus erythematosus, bacterial endocarditis, polyarteritis, and Schönlein-Henoch purpura), hereditary nephritis (Alport syndrome), and in certain patients with nephrotic syndrome and recurrent hematuria. There is now considerable evidence to suggest that focal glomerulonephritis represents the response of the mesangial cell system to a variety of stimuli [34, 35].

The mesangium normally consists of two to three cells that occupy the central region of each glomerular lobule (Fig. 46-6). The cells are intercapillary, bounded on their outer aspects by basement membrane and separated from the capillary lumens by an attenuated endothelium. The mesangial cells have numerous cytoplasmic processes and are separated from one another by narrow bands of fibrillar and amorphous, dense, basement-membrane-like matrix material. Studies of kidney biopsy specimens from normal kidney donors frequently reveal variations in mesangial cell morphology. These are shown schematically in Fig. 46-6. Processes of mesangial cytoplasm may be seen projecting through the endothelium into the capillary lumen, often forming blebs of considerable size. Mesangial processes may also extend between the endothelium and the basement membrane of the capillary loops for short distances. Denser masses of matrix of varying size may be found within broadened regions of the mesangial matrix. It is probable that these morphologic changes represent normal responses of the mesangial cells to changes in the capillary blood and in their immediate environment.

Many studies demonstrate that macromolecules injected into the bloodstream gain access to the mesangial zone [34]. The pathway of entry of larger particles into the mesangium has, for example, been clearly revealed by examination of rat glomeruli a few minutes after injection of colloidal carbon into the circulation [6]. Carbon entered the matrical spaces between mesangial cells (Fig. 46-7), demonstrating the potential channels originally proposed by Latta et al. [15]. Subsequently, carbon particles were found within phagocytic vacuoles of mesangial cells.

The potential importance of the mesangial cell system in glomerulonephritis and in other glomerular diseases involving immune mechanisms has been emphasized by several recent studies. Mauer et al. [21, 22] examined the kinetics of the phagocytic function of mesangial cells in experimental kidney disease. Injected macromolecules, such as heat-aggregated IgG, were readily taken up by the mesangium of normal rats; greatly increased quantities entered the mesangium in experimental ne-

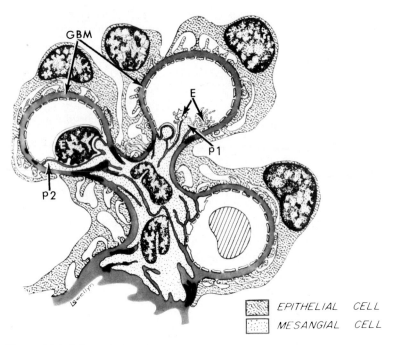

Figure 46-6. Schematic drawing of a glomerular lobule with three capillary loops. The central loop illustrates a common response of mesangial cells; pseudopod formation, with one process (p-1) projecting into the capillary lumen, between segments of the endothelial cells (E), which show microvillus formation. The loop to the left portrays a pseudopod (p-2) projecting between the endothelium and the glomerular basement membrane (GBM). The dark lines within the mesangium represent matrix channels in which deposits are often found in disease (see text). (From R. L. Vernier et al., Kidney Int. 7:224, 1975.)

phrotic syndrome and nephrotoxic serum nephritis. The evidence suggested that glomerular injury associated with proteinuria was also associated with increased mesangial permeability. Germuth and Rodriquez [8] have demonstrated a consistent relationship between the size of the immune complexes formed in chronic "serum sickness" nephritis in rabbits and the pattern of localization of the complexes. Rabbits responded to repeated injections of bovine serum albumin by formation of antibody-antigen complexes with a molecular weight of 1×10^6 daltons or greater, and such complexes were shown by immunofluorescence to localize primarily within the glomerular mesangium. Microscopic study demonstrated relatively minor histologic changes, consisting of cellular proliferation and hypertrophy of the mesangial matrix without inflammatory exudate, and these rabbits did not have significant proteinuria. In contrast, more severe diffuse proliferative glomerulonephritis, granular capillary loop deposits of IgG and C3, and heavy proteinuria developed in rabbits shown to have formed smaller immune complexes (less than 1×10^6 daltons).

An additional experimental model of renal injury in rabbits that is of special relevance to the syndrome of recurrent hematuria in man has recently been described by Mauer et al. [23] (Fig. 46-8). Antigen (aggregated human IgG [AHIgG] or albumin [AHSA]) was injected IV, and 10 hours later, when the aggregates were shown to be within the glomerular mesangium, a kidney was removed and transplanted into a normal rabbit. The recipient rabbit then received an IV injection of rabbit antibody to either AHIgG or AHSA. Within minutes of infusion of antibody there was a fall in serum complement, an infiltration of polymorphonuclear cells into the kidney, and swelling of glomerular cells. Proliferation of mesangial cells and increase in mesangial matrix occurred progressively over the next 3 days, to result in typical focal glomerulonephritis, which progressed to focal sclerosis in some animals by the eighth day. These experiments clearly demonstrated that antigen present within the mesangium was accessible to and reacted with circulating antibody and complement, with resultant severe glomerular injury.

Assuming that the functions of the mesangial cell system in man are similar to that of the rabbits and rats, several possible explanations for the pathophysiology of focal glomerulonephritis are

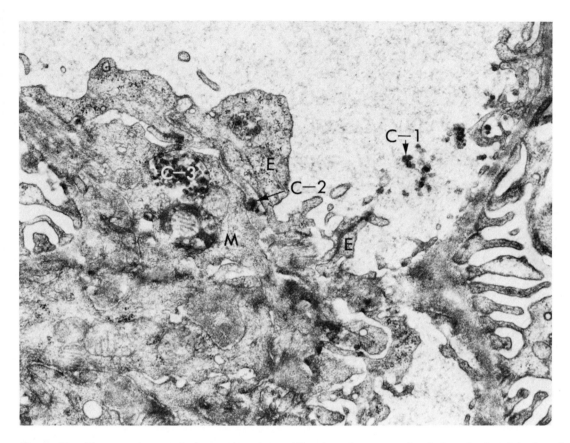

Figure 46-7. Electron micrograph of a portion of a capillary loop from a rat that had received an injection of colloidal carbon 15 minutes earlier. Carbon particles are seen within the lumen (C-1), within a channel containing mesangial matrix, between the endothelium (E) and mesangial cell cytoplasm (M) (C-2), and within a phagosome of a mesangial cell (C-3). We propose that the particles indicate the pathway of entry of large macromolecules into the mesangial cell system (see text). (×29,000 before 14% reduction.) (From R. L. Vernier et al., Kidney Int. *7:224, 1975.)*

MESANGIAL INFLAMMATION – FIXED ANTIGEN EXPERIMENTS

IgG Aggregates   Passive Antibody

Transplant →

Results

1) Severe Mesangitis

2) Prompt Fall Complement

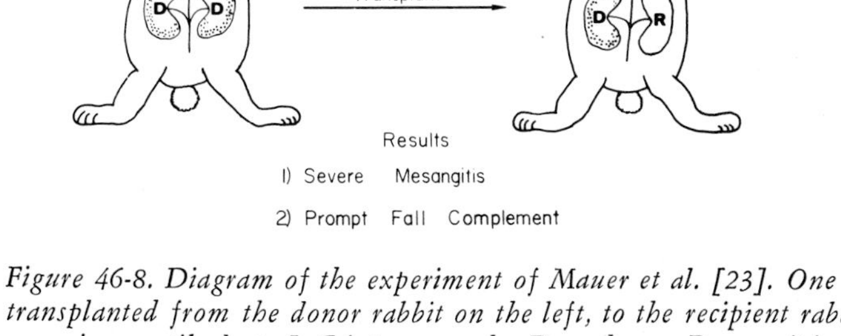

Figure 46-8. Diagram of the experiment of Mauer et al. [23]. One kidney containing aggregates of IgG was transplanted from the donor rabbit on the left, to the recipient rabbit, on the right. The recipient rabbit then was given antibody to IgG intravenously. D = donor, R = recipient. (From R. L. Vernier et al., Kidney Int. *7:224, 1975.)*

apparent. In theory, any large circulating macromolecule, antigen or other, might enter the glomerular mesangial cell system and incite a local inflammatory reaction, through various mediators. On the other hand, excessive amounts of noninflammatory, nonantigenic materials could overload the degrading system of the mesangium (the efferent limb) and accumulate as increased "matrix" material, without apparent inflammation.

As indicated previously, antibody, especially IgM and IgA, is frequently found in the mesangium in a variety of kidney diseases, which are also associated with focal glomerulonephritic lesions. These diseases are probably examples of immunologic injury of the glomerulus, in which either larger circulating antigen-antibody complexes (e.g., IgA–viral complex or aggregated IgM complexes) are selectively taken up by the mesangium, or, perhaps, antibody reacts with antigens fixed within the mesangium (e.g., virus-platelet aggregates, bacterial cell wall, or other debris). These and other hypotheses must be evaluated in man before the precise role of the mesangial cell system in human kidney disease can be firmly established. More effective mechanisms for prevention and cure of these challenging problems may then evolve.

Acknowledgments

The author is grateful to Ms. Susan Sisson, Jeanette Lewellyn, and Mr. Marshall Hoff for preparation of the illustrations and to Ms. Rita Kyle for preparation of the manuscript.

References

1. Ayoub, E. M., and Vernier, R. L.   Benign recurrent hematuria. *Am. J. Dis. Child.* 109:217, 1965.
2. Burkholder, G. V., Dotin, L. N., Thomason, W. B., and Beach, P. D.   Unexplained hematuria. *J.A.M.A.* 210:1729, 1969.
3. Berger, J.   IgA glomerular deposits in renal disease. *Transplant Proc.* 1:939, 1969.
4. Berger, J.   Immunopathology of the mesangium. Report presented to the American Society of Nephrology, Washington, D.C., November, 1973.
5. Bodian, M., Black, J. A., Koboyashi, N., Lake, B. D., and Shuler, S. E.   Recurrent hematuria in childhood. *Q. J. Med.* 34:359, 1965.
6. Elema, J. D., Hoyer, J. R., and Vernier, R. L.   The glomerular mesangium: Uptake and transport of intravenously injected colloidal carbon in rats. *Kidney Int.* 9:395, 1976.
7. Evans, D. S., Williams, D. G., Peters, D. K., Sissons, J. G. P., Boulton-Jones, J. M., Ogg, C. S., Camaron, J. S., and Boffbrand, B. I.   Glomerular deposition of properdin in Henoch-Schönlein syndrome and idiopathic focal nephritis. *Br. Med. J.* 3:326, 1973.
8. Germuth, F. G., and Rodriquez, E.   Immunopathology of the Renal Glomerulus. In *Immune Complex Deposit and Antibasement Membrane Disease.* Boston: Little Brown, 1973. Pp. 22–44.
9. Gervais, M., and Drummond, K. N.   L'hematurie récidivante chez l'enfant. *Union Med. Can.* 99:1232, 1970.
10. Glasgow, E. F., Mancrieff, M. W., and White, R. H. R.   Symptomless hematuria in childhood. *Br. Med. J.* 2:687, 1970.
11. Hendler, E. D., Kashgarian, M., and Hayslett, J. P.   Clinico-pathological correlations of primary hematuria. *Lancet* 1:458, 1972.
12. Heptinstall, R. H.   Focal Glomerulonephritis. In M. D. Strauss and L. G. Welt (eds.), *Diseases of the Kidney.* Boston: Little Brown, 1971. P. 463.
13. Heptinstall, R. H., and Joekes, H. M.   Focal glomerulonephritis. A study based on renal biopsies. *Q. J. Med.* 28:329, 1959.
14. Lagrue, G., Hirbec, G., Fournel, M., and Intrator, L.   Glomerulonephrite mésangiale á depôts d'IgA: Etude des immunoglobulines sériques. *J. Urol. Nephrol. (Paris)* 4:385, 1974.
15. Latta, H., Maunsbach, A. B., and Madden, S. C.   The centrolobular region of the renal glomerulus studied by electron microscopy. *J. Ultrastruct. Res.* 4:455, 1960.
16. Lee, L. W., and Davis, E., Jr.   Gross urinary hemorrhage: A symptom not a disease. *J.A.M.A.* 153:782, 1953.
17. Levinus, B. A., Rivjere, G. B., and Van Breda Vriesman, P. J. C.   Recurrent or persistent hematuria: Sign of mesangial immune-complex deposition. *N. Engl. J. Med.* 290:1165, 1974.
18. Levy, M., Beaufils, H., Gubler, M. D., and Habib, R.   Idiopathic recurrent hematuria and mesangial IgA-IgG deposits in children (Berger's disease). *Clin. Nephrol.* 1:63, 1973.
19. Lowance, D. C., Mullins, J. D., and McPhaul, J. J., Jr.   Immunoglobulin A (IgA) associated glomerulonephritis. *Kidney Int.* 3:167, 1973.
20. Marks, M. I., and Drummond, K. N.   Benign familial hematuria. *Pediatrics* 44:590, 1969.
21. Mauer, S. M., Fish, A. J., Blau, E. B., and Michael, A. F.   The glomerular mesangium. I. Kinetic studies of macromolecular uptake in normal and nephrotic rats. *J. Clin. Invest.* 51:1092, 1971.
22. Mauer, S. M., Fish, A. J., Day, N. K., and Michael, A. F.   The glomerular mesangium. II. Studies of macromolecular uptake in nephrotoxic nephritis in rats. *J. Clin. Invest.* 53:431, 1974.
23. Mauer, S. M., Sutherland, D. E. R., Howard, R. J., Fish, A. J., Najarian, J. S., and Michael, A. F.   The glomerular mesangium. III. Acute immune mesangial injury: A new model of glomerulonephritis. *J. Exp. Med.* 137:553, 1973.
24. McConville, J. M., West, C. D., and McAdams, A. J.   Familial and non-familial benign hematuria. *J. Pediatr.* 69:207, 1966.
25. McCoy, R. C., Abramowsky, C. R., and Tisher, C. C.   IgA nephropathy. *Am. J. Pathol.* 76:123, 1974.
26. Michael, A. F., and McLean, R. H.   Evidence for Activation of the Alternate Pathway in Glomerulonephritis. In J. Hamburger, J. Crosnier, and M. H. Maxwell (eds.), *Advances in Nephrology.* Chicago: Year Book, 1974. Vol. 4, pp. 49–66.
27. Rogers, P. W., Kurtzman, N. A., Bunn, S. M., and White, M. G.   Familial benign essential hematuria. *Arch. Intern. Med.* 131:257, 1973.
28. Ross, J. H.   Recurrent focal nephritis. *Q. J. Med.* 29:391, 1960.
29. Roy, L. P., Fish, A. J., Vernier, R. L., and Michael,

A. F. Recurrent macroscopic hematuria, focal nephritis, and mesangial deposition of immunoglobulin and complement. *J. Pediatr.* 82:767, 1973.

30. Singer, D. B., Hill, L. L., Rosenberg, H. S., Marshall, J., and Swenson, R. Recurrent hematuria in childhood. *N. Engl. J. Med.* 279:7, 1968.

31. Spear, G. S., Roskes, S. D., Slusser, R. J., and Alsruhe, J. P. Idiopathic hematuria in childhood. *Hum. Pathol.* 4:349, 1973.

32. Tomasi, T. B., Jr., and Bienstock, J. Secretory immunoglobulins. *Adv. Immunol.* 9:1, 1968.

33. Urizar, R. D., Michael, A., Sisson, S., and Vernier, R. L. Anaphylactoid purpura. II. Immunofluorescent

and electron microscopic studies of the glomerular lesions. *Lab. Invest.* 19:437, 1968.

34. Vernier, R., Mauer, S., Fish, A., and Michael, A. F. The mesangial cell in glomerulonephritis. In J. Hamburger, J. Crosnier, and M. H. Maxwell (eds.), *Advances in Nephrology*. Chicago: Year Book, 1971. Vol. 1, pp. 31–46.

35. Vernier, R. L., Resnick, J. S., and Mauer, S. M. Recurrent hematuria and focal glomerulonephritis. *Kidney Int.* 7:224, 1975.

36. Volhard, F., and Fahr, T. *Die Brightische Nierenkrankheit: Klinik Pathologie und Atlas*. Berlin: Springer, 1914.

47. Acute Postinfectious Glomerulonephritis

Luther B. Travis

Glomerulonephritis is the term generally reserved for that variety of renal disease in which the proliferation and inflammation of the glomerulus is secondary to an immunologic mechanism. The modification of this term by the adjective *acute* (acute glomerulonephritis, AGN) has imposed temporal restrictions and, as most commonly used, has defined an almost characteristic clinicopathologic correlation. The term has also implied certain distinctive features concerning etiology, pathogenesis, course, and prognosis (Chap. 43).

The majority of instances of AGN appear to be postinfectious, and a number of bacterial and viral infections have been etiologically incriminated. The most commonly recognized clinical picture appears following infections with the group A, beta-hemolytic streptococcus, and the term *acute glomerulonephritis* has become almost synonymous with this etiologic agent. Throughout this chapter, AGN will be used to signify the broad manifestations of the disease, while PSAGN (poststreptococcal acute glomerulonephritis) will be used when considering those manifestations that are clearly related to the nephritogenic streptococcus.

Acute glomerulonephritis is the most common, nonsuppurative renal disease of childhood. Although this diagnosis accounts for approximately 0.5 percent of all hospital admissions for children, the true incidence of the disease is unknown. It is undoubtedly much higher than such statistics would indicate, due to the large number of affected children with mild, and often unrecognized, disease. Kaplan et al. [81] found that approximately one-half the patients discovered to have PSAGN during an epidemic were asymptomatic.

Additionally, in studies of sibling contacts of children with PSAGN, only 16 percent of those discovered to have either clinical or laboratory evidence of nephritis had been considered to be ill by their parents [40]. The highest incidence is in the early school years, and the clinical disease is uncommon in children under 3 years of age. It has, however, been well documented even in the first few months of life [56]. In most reported series, there is a male-to-female ratio of approximately 2 : 1 [98, 128], the reasons for which are not clear.

Pathogenesis

There is a vast array of epidemiologic, pathologic, and immunologic data to support the proposition that most instances of AGN are primarily immunologic in nature. In the most common variety of AGN, that related to a prior streptococcal infection, evidence suggests that immune complexes are formed with streptococcal antigens, localize on the glomerular capillary wall, and initiate a proliferative and inflammatory response.

EPIDEMIOLOGIC CHARACTERISTICS

It has long been known that most cases of AGN are etiologically related to infection with the group A, beta-hemolytic streptococcus, but it was not until the early 1950s that the association of type 12 streptococcal infections with AGN was established [121, 122]. It was this finding of a "nephritogenic" strain that partially explained the differences in attack rate that occurred between AGN and acute rheumatic fever. Initial and subsequent reports of epidemic streptococcal pharyngitis–

related AGN demonstrated frequent association with M-type 12 and occasional associations with M-type 1 and 4 streptococci. Other studies subsequently suggested that, although several types of streptococci were responsible for epidemics of PSAGN, the sporadic variety almost always followed a type 12 infection of the nasopharynx. In such instances, there was a definite seasonal pattern (winter-spring), a well-defined latent period (about 10 days), and clear evidence (in over 80 percent of the cases) of a prior streptococcal infection, suggested by a rise in the titer of antistreptolysin O [155].

In contrast to this winter-spring variety of pharyngitis-related AGN, there were reports as early as 1940 from tropical climates of sporadic cases of AGN following skin infections [20, 26, 32, 59]. The first recognized major epidemic of impetigo-related AGN occurred at the Red Lake Indian Reservation in 1953 and led to the discovery of a previously unrecognized serotype, type 49 [88, 147]. Subsequently, this serotype has been isolated during some stage of almost all epidemics of impetigo-related AGN and has been found to be the most common type of streptococcus isolated from the sporadic form of pyoderma-related AGN [32, 38, 73, 81, 100, 114, 116, 155]. Pyoderma-related AGN is typically seen in the more southern regions of the United States and may account for as many as 60 to 70 percent of the cases of PSAGN. Characteristically, pyoderma-related PSAGN reaches its peak incidence in the summer and fall. Careful analysis of patient data from large centers in the southern United States reveal two peaks of AGN admissions, one corresponding with the peak of respiratory illness and the other, with the peak of skin infections. Although type 49 is discovered most often, a variety of other serotypes of streptococci have also been isolated from small groups of patients with AGN, and evidence suggests an etiologic relationship [6, 12, 35, 37, 65, 138]. It has been demonstrated that cutaneous streptococcal infections often evoke a poor antibody response to streptolysin O [33, 81], which has previously led to some difficulty with confirmation of a cause and effect relationship.

The actual incidence of AGN is hard to ascertain, even when one knows the incidence of streptococcal infection. In part, this is due to the relatively large percentage of cases of PSAGN that are subclinical in nature and therefore unrecognized. It appears likely that host factors, as well as the possibility of varying "immunologic virulence" of the organism, account for a marked variability in attack rate [4]. Valkenburg et al.

[148] reported an annual incidence of AGN of 20 per 100,000 population in their studies from the Netherlands. Several studies have shown the incidence of AGN following pyoderma to be in the range of 1 to 2 percent [5, 27, 29, 65]. This figure is similar to the incidence of AGN said to follow scarlet fever [97]. In contrast, attack rates up to 20 percent have been reported [14, 154], and a recent report by Sagel and his associates [129] showed that 14 percent of 248 children with proved streptococcal disease had an abnormal urine, while 8 percent had both an abnormal urine and a lowering of serum complement activity. The prospective studies by Anthony, et al. [4] relative to the 1966 epidemic of type 49 streptococcal infection at the Red Lake Indian Reservation revealed an 8 percent incidence of nephritis (plus a 7 percent incidence of "unexplained" hematuria). Of considerable interest was the development of hematuria in 24 percent of the children following type 49 pyoderma but in only 4.5 percent after type 49 pharyngitis. These figures were not distinctly different from those obtained in an earlier controlled study of patients who had had type 12 streptococcal pharyngitis [136].

Acute glomerulonephritis has been reported in association with a number of other infectious illnesses. Transient and mild hematuria has been seen rather commonly at the height of illness in both streptococcal and nonstreptococcal infections. Proved glomerulonephritis has been observed following staphylococcal and pneumococcal infections [18, 70, 109, 132] and certain viral illnesses: coxsackievirus B_4 [13], echovirus type 9 [162], influenza [3, 126], mumps [135], and others [58, 76]. At times, the clinical picture of AGN is indistinguishable from that usually associated with PSAGN. Only the absence of a prior streptococcal illness, as evidenced by bacteriologic and serologic studies, and the temporal association with the viral syndrome, distinguish such a patient. Since the immediate and long-term prognosis of nonstreptococcal AGN is unknown and may be significantly different from that of PSAGN, a diligent effort should be made to identify the etiologic agent.

SEROLOGIC RESPONSE TO STREPTOCOCCAL INFECTION

Extracellular antigens of the infecting streptococcus stimulate an antibody response in the host, and their measurement can provide a valuable indication of such an infection. The most commonly measured antibody titer used clinically to detect the streptococcus is antistreptolysin O (ASO). Following streptococcal pharyngitis, a significant rise in ASO titer occurs in 70 to 80 percent of cases [101, 156], and there is strong evidence that patients who have PSAGN (following pharyngitis) have higher titers than control subjects who do not [9, 136, 155]. In such patients the ASO titer begins to rise about 10 to 14 days after the streptococcal infection, reaches its peak levels in 3 to 5 weeks, and then slowly declines over a variable period of 1 to 6 months. Treatment with penicillin early in the course of the infection prevents this characteristic rise in the ASO titer [84, 156]. A similar response probably occurs following other antistreptococcal agents.

Contrary to the high level of responsiveness of the ASO titer following respiratory tract infections, the response following skin infections has been disappointing. A number of studies have now shown that the rise in ASO titer following pyoderma-related AGN is poor [6, 12, 17, 33, 37, 65, 80, 99, 138, 148, 155]. Although the cause for this poor ASO response remains obscure, some studies have demonstrated that skin lipids interfere with the antigenicity of streptolysin O [68, 82]. In contrast to the sluggish response of the ASO titer, there are brisk and significant rises in the titers of antihyaluronidase and antideoxyribonuclease B (anti-DNase B) [9, 17, 36, 37, 80, 144, 155]. Most investigators agree that the anti-DNase B is the single most sensitive indicator of prior streptococcal infection, and that a combination of the three measurements will detect virtually 100 percent of persons with recent streptococcal illness.

Recent studies by Dillon and Reeves [37] have demonstrated a significantly greater immunologic response (to both anti-DNase B and ASO) in patients with PSAGN than in patients with comparable clinical and bacteriologic evidence of streptococcal infection without AGN. Their studies also demonstrated a more striking antibody response in children under 9 years of age. There is no direct correlation between the magnitude of the serologic response and either the severity of the initial illness or the eventual prognosis. Since the serologic responsiveness is a measure of antibody response, and thus of immunity to that particular strain of streptococcus, an absent or sluggish response might suggest a failure to achieve immunity.

IMMUNOLOGIC CHARACTERISTICS

Although there is clear evidence that streptococcal infections are intimately associated with AGN, the exact mechanism by which renal injury occurs is still under investigation. Current evidence suggests that the inflammatory lesion in the glomerulus is associated with the fixation of soluble streptococcal antigen-antibody complexes. Several investigators have detected streptococcal antigens in renal biopsy material obtained from patients early in the course of AGN [91, 108, 131, 146], but the major evidence supporting an immune complex type of nephritis has been the finding of nodular deposits of immunoglobulin G (IgG) and the third component of complement (C3) on the capillary basement membrane [54, 55, 92, 102, 108]. Not all investigators have been able to detect the streptococcal antigen, and others have been able to find it in only a minority of cases. Since it has not been possible to isolate circulating streptococcal antigen-antibody complexes from the patients' sera, the evidence remains circumstantial.

It has been known for a number of years that serum complement activity is depressed in the acute phase of PSAGN, and more recent studies have shown that serum C3 levels are similarly reduced [7, 27, 32, 34, 60, 63, 115, 117, 157]. Initially, it was assumed that the depression of the late components of complement (C3 through C9) depended on activation of early complement components (C1, C4, C2). However, various investigators [27, 60] have demonstrated inconsistent decreases in C4, whereas C3 levels have been found depressed in 80 to 90 percent of cases; studies in our laboratory have demonstrated a depression in 92 percent of patients. Götze and Müller-Eberhard [64] have demonstrated an alternate pathway by which the "early-reacting" components of complement can be bypassed. This alternate pathway appears to prevail in PSAGN [107, 113, 149, 160], and in the early stages of this disease there is depression of properdin and C3 proactivator levels. The C3 levels are markedly depressed [27] in most patients with PSAGN, but many show rapid returns to normal. Potter and her associates [117] demonstrated two major patterns of return of C3 to normal levels: (1) a return to normal within 1 month and (2) a return to normal delayed until after 1 month. In their first category, there were some patients in whom the rebound to normal was rapid, i.e., within 2 weeks. Of interest was the fact that all their patients with early return had nephritis secondary to impetigo, while only 42 percent of their "late returns" had impetigo. There was also a marked sex difference, with 77 percent of the early group but only 17 percent of the latter group being female. The significance of these differences is not clear. Cameron et al. [27] have demonstrated a return to normal C3 levels by 8 weeks in 94 percent of children with PSAGN. A patient whose C3 has not returned to normal by this time should be strongly suspected of having some other condition.

IMMUNOPATHOLOGIC FEATURES

Deposits of immunoglobulin G (IgG) and C3 are detected by immunofluorescence microscopy in the majority of patients with PSAGN [54, 55, 92, 102, 108, 131, 146, 153, 158, 161], and it is on this basis that this disease is considered a clinical example of an immune complex nephritis. IgG and C3 are generally seen in close association with one another along the peripheral capillary loops. The typical picture is shown in Fig. 47-1, in which the immunoglobulins are seen in a granular pattern. Whenever streptococcal antigen has been detected within the glomerulus, it has always been in the mesangium [91, 108, 131, 146]. It is in this mesangial area that fibrin generally is detected [24, 90, 102], occasionally in association with C3 but virtually never with IgG. Biopsy sections from patients with PSAGN have also been shown to contain properdin [158] and, very early, may contain C3 activator. Only on rare occasions is there deposition of C4. The presence of com-bined deposits of fibrin and fibrinoid material, coupled with the detection of fibrin degradation products in blood and urine [21, 117, 137], suggests the presence of intravascular clotting, as occurs in experimental glomerulonephritis. The work of Kantor [79] has demonstrated deposition of fibrinogen by streptococcal M-protein, and this may have considerable importance in the pathogenesis of glomerular injury. The work of several investigators suggests that local activation of the clotting mechanism might provide a partial explanation for the increased capillary permeability as well as for the mesangial deposition of fibrin [74, 102, 150, 163].

Pathologic Findings

Only in the past decade has it been possible to correlate the clinical features of PSAGN with the renal histopathologic findings. Prior to this time, the pathologic characteristics of PSAGN were rarely observed except in that small percentage of patients whose disease progressed to death. The availability of percutaneous renal biopsy has dramatically changed concepts about the disease by

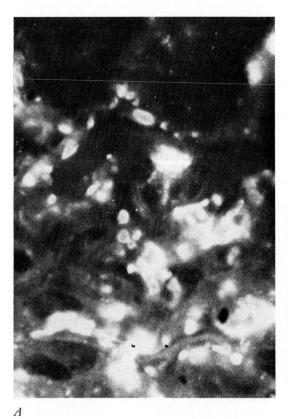 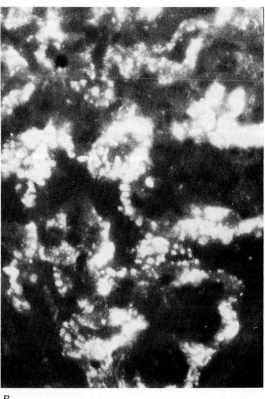

A   B

Figure 47-1. Immunofluorescent photomicrograph of a renal biopsy specimen from a 7-year-old girl with typical PSAGN. A. Staining for C3. B. Marked granular pattern of IgG.

providing the opportunity to observe the kidney serially, from onset through resolution. Extensive studies have been carried out on the histopathologic features of the early disease and will not be reviewed here in depth. The interested reader is referred to a recent article or text for a more comprehensive review [24, 39, 41, 54, 55, 66, 67, 95, 102, 108].

Although the degree of severity of the initial inflammatory response varies, the overall histologic pattern is very consistent. Generally, the glomerular tufts appear enlarged and swollen, often filling Bowman's space. The capillary lumens appear closed, and the entire tuft may appear almost bloodless. A moderate to marked increase in cell nuclei is evident, and this is primarily due to proliferation of mesangial and epithelial cells (Fig. 47-2). In the very early stage, there is often an increase in nonglomerular cells, i.e., polymorphonuclear leukocytes, eosinophils, and macrophages. The increase in polymorphonuclear leukocytes may be marked and they may occasionally be seen in

adherence to capillary walls. In such areas the cell wall may show disruption and dissolution (Fig. 47-3). The increased cell mass expands the central lobular area in a centrifugal pattern, leading to further narrowing in adjacent capillary lumens. The capillary basement membrane of the tuft is usually not thickened, but there may be aggregates of amorphous material and scattered debris from necrotic cells. Bowman's space contains increased granular debris, many red blood cells, and occasional neutrophils. With extensive inflammatory changes, the epithelial cells of Bowman's capsule proliferate, forming a crescent. Fibrin aggregates may be conspicuous between the cells of crescents as well as in Bowman's space. The tubular pattern is usually regular, with only minimal distortion.

With the use of special stains, small nodules are seen along the outer surface of the capillary basement membrane (Fig. 47-4). The nodules correspond to the electron-dense deposits seen by electron microscopy [66, 85, 86, 144] and with the

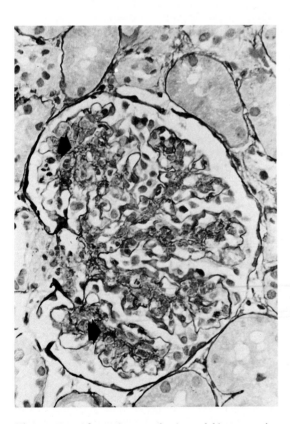

Figure 47-2. Photomicrograph of renal biopsy section from a 5-year-old boy with PSAGN, obtained approximately 2 weeks after onset of clinical disease. There is a generalized increase in cellularity, most marked in the mesangium. Note the expanded, hypercellular mesangium (arrows) in two areas.

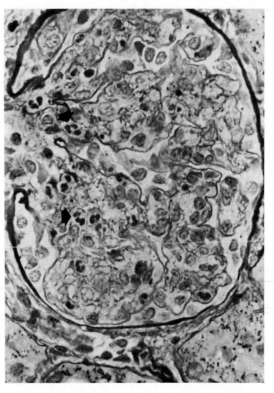

Figure 47-3. Photomicrograph of a renal biopsy specimen from an 8-year-old boy with severe PSAGN. The glomerular tuft is swollen, almost filling Bowman's space. There is extensive increase in cellularity, and, as in Fig. 47-2, this is primarily an increase in the number of mesangial cells. Exudation with large numbers of polymorphonuclear leukocytes is in evidence, however. The arrows point to two leukocytes.

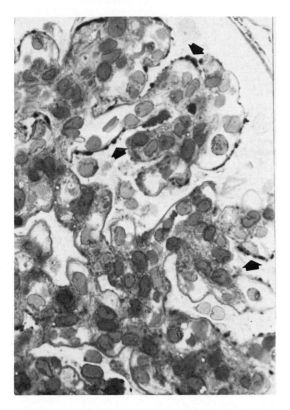

Figure 47-4. Photomicrograph of renal histologic section from the child in Fig. 47-3. The specimen has been sectioned at 1 μ and stained with methylene blue. Marked mesangial proliferation is seen throughout. Dense deposits (arrows) are seen external to the capillary basement membrane. These are the same "humps" that are seen by electron microscopy.

nodular collections of C3 and IgG seen on immunofluorescence microscopy. Under examination by the electron microscope, the dense deposits are most often seen to be located in the subepithelial space (Fig. 47-5) and are regularly observed in the early stages. The humps are usually discrete and often in close proximity to the mesangium. Occasionally, deposits may be seen within the lamina densa, as well as in the subendothelial space. Kobayashi et al. [89] observed these characteristic humps in 25 of 26 instances of AGN when the examination was performed within 3 weeks of clinical onset. Hinglais and coworkers [71] have presented detailed pathologic data on 50 patients with a histologic diagnosis of endocapillary glomerulonephritis (i.e., clinical diagnosis of AGN) and could demonstrate humps in only 35. However, the duration of disease at the time of biopsy was variable and may have exceeded the time necessary for resolution of the deposits. After 3 weeks, the deposits are less commonly observed, but in some instances they are still in evidence up

to 3 to 5 months after clinical onset. This contrasts with the findings of others, who rarely are able to demonstrate humps after a duration of more than 6 weeks [67].

The severity of the histologic lesion correlates relatively well with the severity of the early clinical illness, the degree of depression of the glomerular filtration rate and tubular function, and perhaps with ultimate prognosis [41, 44, 71, 89, 95, 111]. Kobayashi et al. [89] suggested that the severity and duration of the clinical disease relates linearly to the number of deposits observed by electron microscopy, and support for this contention is found in several other studies. It is not an unexpected finding, since the deposits are thought to be aggregates of antigen-antibody complexes: the more circulating complexes, the more glomerular basement membrane deposition and the more intense the glomerular lesion. Epithelial crescents are usually considered to suggest a poorer prognosis, but their significance depends on the extent of involvement. Crescents that affect only a few glomeruli, or are focal and segmental in nature, are consistent with complete recovery.

It is well recognized that PSAGN undergoes a period of histologic resolution that may or may not parallel clinical resolution [41, 66]. Jennings and Earle in 1961 [75] and Callis et al. in 1967 [25] were the first to document that histologic "healing" may be delayed for as much as 2 years after onset. More recent studies [42, 144] have even documented histologic healing after a period of over 3 years.

Physiologic Response to Acute Glomerulonephritis

There is ample evidence that the patient with moderate to severe AGN has a diminished capacity to excrete water and solute and consequently has an expanded extracellular fluid volume (ECF) [31, 44, 50, 53, 57, 130]. In most of these patients there is a measurable reduction in glomerular filtration (GFR) by any of the standard clearance techniques [41, 44, 47, 53, 95]; the reduction in GFR is always more marked than that of renal plasma flow. As might be expected, the disruption of glomerular function is always more marked than that of tubular function.

The expansion of ECF volume is secondary to salt and water retention, but the mechanism by which this retention occurs cannot be adequately explained only by the reduction in GFR. The hormonal factors that might conceivably be operable in the genesis of this ECF expansion do not appear to play an important role. There are no physiologic stimuli to the secretion of antidiuretic hor-

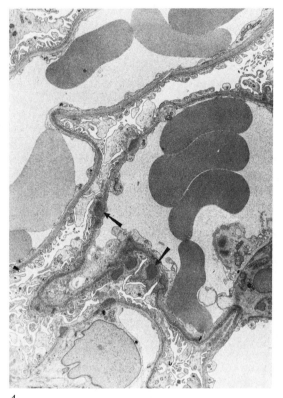
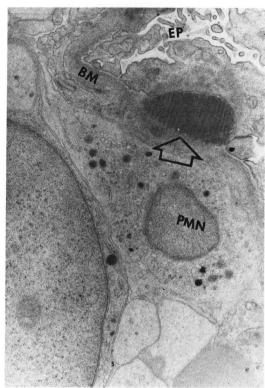

A

B

Figure 47-5. Electron micrograph of renal biopsy specimen taken from the child in Figs. 47-3 and 47-4. A. Arrows indicate the deposits on the epithelial side of the basement membrane. B. Polymorphonuclear leukocyte (PMN) is seen adjacent to the basement membrane (BM). A typical electron-dense hump (arrow) projects outward from the basement membrane into the urinary space. Epithelial cell processes (EP) are normal.

mone and aldosterone, and no rationale for activation of the renin-angiotensin system is apparent. In addition, aldosterone excretion has been shown to be normal [44], and most studies have demonstrated normal or low renin levels [62, 93]. Other studies of renin are somewhat inconclusive [19], but, as noted, there does not appear to be a suitable stimulus. It is therefore highly likely that other factors, perhaps physical in nature, are partially responsible for the salt and water retention.

The sodium and water retention not only leads to clinical edema but is also responsible for the generalized circulatory congestion. This circulatory congestion is similar to that produced by primary fluid overload, and the bulk of evidence does not suggest any associated inflammatory disease of the heart or blood vessels. When the circulatory congestion is marked, clinical signs and symptoms include dyspnea, orthopnea, pulmonary congestion, increased venous pressure, and cardiac enlargement. In most instances, definitive evidence

of congestive heart failure does not exist, and several studies have demonstrated a normal cardiac output and arteriovenous oxygen difference [28, 31, 57].

The expanded ECF volume is in part responsible for various other aspects of the clinical syndrome of AGN, including hypertension, anemia, and encephalopathy. These aspects will be discussed more fully later.

Clinical Characteristics

The typical case of PSAGN is difficult to define because of the varied and diverse nature of the individual presentation. At one extreme is the child who is incidentally discovered to have PSAGN. As noted previously, PSAGN occurs asymptomatically in at least 50 percent of patients showing subclinical and laboratory evidence of involvement [40, 49, 81]. At the other extreme is the child who presents with severe systemic manifestations with or without significant urinary abnormalities [2, 29, 61, 159]. Somewhere between these two extremes lies the so-called typical case, and, although somewhat artificial, it is perhaps prudent to consider and define the features of the typical case before considering the other variations.

TYPICAL CASE

Latent Period

A latent period varying from a few days to approximately 3 weeks is characteristically observed between the onset of the streptococcal infection and the development of clinical glomerulonephritis. This latent period, more easily observed and timed following pharyngeal infections, averages approximately 10 days [119]. Latent periods in excess of 3 weeks are uncommon, and an interval of 4 weeks suggests a doubtful association. The development of clinical nephritis within 1 to 4 days of the onset of the streptococcal infection should suggest that there is preexisting glomerulonephritis, with an acute exacerbation of symptomatic disease [42, 133, 144]. Additionally, such an early onset of symptoms referable to the kidney (usually hematuria) might suggest the syndrome of recurrent (idiopathic or "benign") hematuria [8, 15, 143, 127, 134]. During the latent period, the child is usually asymptomatic, but microscopic hematuria and proteinuria are occasionally observed.

Initial Symptoms

The initial symptoms usually have an abrupt onset, with the two most common presenting complaints being *edema* and *hematuria*. Accompanying these two features may be varying degrees of nonspecific symptomatology: malaise, lethargy, anorexia, fever, abdominal pain, weakness, and headaches. Some children, however, have none of these systemic manifestations.

Edema

Edema is the most frequent presenting symptom, and most often involves the face, with particular involvement of the periorbital area. The predilection for the periorbital area appears related primarily to the lack of tissue resistance in this area. In the majority of patients the edema is mild and appears confined to the face, but in others the degree of involvement is so marked as to suggest a nephrotic picture. The degree of edema is dependent on a number of factors, including the extent of glomerular involvement (i.e., reduction in glomerular filtration), the intake of oral fluids, the degree of proteinuria, and perhaps other factors mentioned previously. Occasional children with otherwise typical PSAGN have such heavy proteinuria (usually in excess of 4 gm/m² body surface area/day) that marked hypoalbuminemia and anasarca develop. Characteristically, the edema in AGN is dependent and therefore "shifting" in nature. While the patient is in bed, the edema centers about the face and trunk, but it becomes dependent with standing (scrotal, pretibial, and pedal). On occasion, there may be a significant increase in ECF volume without clinical evidence of edema. In such instances, the subclinical edema becomes apparent when the glomerular inflammatory response subsides and diuresis or weight loss occurs.

Gross Hematuria

Gross hematuria occurs at the onset in 30 to 50 percent of those children with AGN who require hospitalization and is therefore often the presenting symptom. Microscopic hematuria is, of course, present in almost all children with PSAGN. When the hematuria is gross, it is often described as smoky, coke-colored, tea-colored, rusty, or reddish-brown. In most instances, the gross hematuria clears within a few days, but it has been observed for up to 4 weeks. Once it has cleared, recurrences may be associated with increased activity or infections, both streptococcal and nonstreptococcal.

Hypertension

Hypertension is the third of the cardinal features of AGN and, once again, occurs in most children who require hospitalization. The pathogenesis of the hypertension is unknown, but is probably multifactorial and related only in part to volume expansion. The work of Repetto et al. [123] has demonstrated that diuresis (induced by diuretics) does not necessarily lead to reduction in the level of hypertension, suggesting other pathogenetic factors. Studies in our laboratory have led to similar observations and are more fully discussed in the therapy section. The blood pressure elevation in PSAGN is highly variable and may be mild or severe. It is not uncommon to detect systolic pressures in excess of 200 mm Hg and diastolic pressures in excess of 120 mm Hg. The blood pressure often has a biphasic character [142]. The first phase occurs early, lasts 3 to 5 days, and is the most severe. After a brief period of 2 to 5 days, when the pressure elevation is less marked, a less severe but more persistent blood pressure elevation occurs, which may last for an additional period of 1 to 2 weeks. Persistence of hypertension past the first 3 to 4 weeks usually indicates chronic disease or rapid progression of the AGN.

The syndrome of *hypertensive encephalopathy*

has been reported in about 5 percent of hospitalized children with AGN [22, 23, 72, 118] and is the most serious of the early consequences of the nephritic syndrome. Recent evidence suggests that the very high blood pressures induce cerebral vasodilatation with consequent damage to the blood brain barrier. Brain edema then forms, due to focal plasma leakage through the walls of the overstretched arterioles [77]. The hypertension is usually severe and may be accompanied by one or more signs of central nervous system dysfunction, such as headaches, vomiting, depression of sensorium, confusion, visual disturbances, aphasia, memory loss, coma, and convulsions. Hypertensive encephalopathy is most often seen when the hypertension is severe; it appears to occur more often in the child who is minimally to moderately edematous than in those with massive edema.

Circulatory Congestion

Circulatory congestion is apparent on careful examination in the majority of children admitted to the hospital, but only rarely is it responsible for significant early symptomatology. There may be dyspnea and orthopnea, and cough occasionally is bothersome. Pulmonary rales are often audible in the lung bases at onset. Percussion dullness is not uncommonly found and suggests the accumulation of pleural fluid. As noted previously, this congestion is related to an increase in plasma and ECF volume; in the presence of a previously normal cardiovascular system, cardiac failure and pulmonary edema are unusual.

Pallor

Pallor is commonly observed at the onset, and its pathogenesis is not entirely explained on the basis of the frequent anemia, which most often appears dilutional. It has been suggested that this pallor is related to the skin edema and its compression of skin capillaries. Reduced urine output is observed in the majority of hospitalized children with AGN and anuria has been described, but uncommonly. Almost characteristic by their absence are signs and symptoms such as arthralgia, arthritis, rash (other than residua from impetigo or the occasional association with scarlatina), purpura, severe abdominal pain, evidence of carditis, evidence of hepatic involvement, and gastrointestinal bleeding.

Patient A.F., a 5-year-old Mexican-American male, was well until the day prior to admission, when facial edema first became apparent. Later that day he complained that his shoes were "too tight." The facial swelling was more marked the next morning, and dark, "coke-colored" urine was passed. The child was taken to his physician, who confirmed the edema, detected a blood pressure of 164/108 mm Hg, and found gross hematuria, red cell casts, and 3+ proteinuria. There was no prior history of respiratory or skin infection, but the boy's 8-year-old sibling had had a "throat infection" 3 weeks earlier and had been treated with penicillin.

Significant laboratory studies revealed the following: ASO titer, 650 Todd units; C3, 2 mg per deciliter (normal, 55 to 120); C4, 16 mg per deciliter (normal, 20 to 50); BUN, 28 mg per deciliter; serum creatinine, 0.7 mg per deciliter; hemoglobin, 10 gms per deciliter; hematocrit, 31 percent. Streptococci were not isolated from the nasopharynx.

A.F. was hospitalized and required antihypertensive medications on three occasions over the first 48 hr. Oliguria was present for approximately 3 days before diuresis occurred, and he lost 5½ pounds over the next 3 days. Three months later he was asymptomatic, normotensive, and had neither hematuria nor proteinuria on concentrated samples. The C3 was normal (125 mg per deciliter), and the ASO was 250 Todd units. Blood urea nitrogen was 11 mg per deciliter.

The clinical presentation and initial course in this 5-year-old are almost classic. Although he had no clinical symptoms suggesting a prior infection, the elevated ASO titer and significant lowering of the C3 provide strong circumstantial evidence of a streptotoccus-related immune complex nephritis.

Patient D.A., a 9-year-old white male, had experienced "chronic" impetigo for about 3 months before the clinical onset of facial edema, 1 day prior to admission. On the morning of admission, he complained of headaches, nausea, and blurring of vision and was lethargic. Generalized clonic and tonic seizures suddenly occurred, and he was transported to the emergency room. Examination revealed a mildly edematous and pale boy who was comatose but having intermittent and generalized convulsive jerks. His blood pressure was 240/160 mm Hg, and his optic disc margins were not distinct. He was given IV injections of phenobarbital and 2 mg of reserpine. His seizures stopped as his blood pressure declined over the first hour to 150/100 mm Hg.

Subsequent laboratory studies revealed the following: ASO titers of 250 Todd units both at the onset and 2 weeks later; anti-DNase B titers three times normal at onset, with a "two-tube" dilutional rise at 2 weeks; a C3 of 12 mg per deciliter; red cells and red cell casts in the urine; evidence of decreased renal function (BUN, 32 mg per deciliter); and beta-hemolytic streptococcus from both the impetiginous lesions and the posterior pharynx.

D.A. required only one injection of antihypertensive medications and did not have a significant return of the hypertension. Diuresis brought about only a 3-pound weight loss over the first week. The subsequent course was uneventful.

The illness of Patient D.A. was a more severe version of the typical picture. Several notable items are apparent in this boy's case: (1) His ASO titer was not elevated, but the anti-DNase titers indicated recent streptococcal invasion, and the C3 suggested an immune complex disease; (2) the severe hypertension was adequately controlled with a single injection of antihypertensive medication; and (3) the expansion of ECF volume (as indicated by a 3-pound weight loss) was not marked.

OTHER CLINICAL PRESENTATIONS

Asymptomatic children may have PSAGN, as noted earlier in this section. When it is known that a sibling or close contact has AGN or that there is a nephritogenic streptococcus prevalent in the community, it is relatively easy to consider the asymptomatic child who is discovered to have microscopic hematuria as an example of AGN. However, the same child discovered to have hematuria without the accompanying history of contact presents a more difficult diagnostic problem. Since AGN, taken in the broadest context, is the most common cause of hematuria in children, the recognition of an asymptomatic hematuria should first lead one to exclude this diagnosis whenever possible.

It is now well known that *AGN with minimal urinary findings* occurs [2, 29, 61, 159], but the precise etiology of the patient's illness may be overlooked unless there is a high index of suspicion. In many of the reported cases, the clinical symptomatology has been extreme, with presentations such as hypertensive encephalopathy, pulmonary edema, and generalized peripheral edema. Eliciting a history of a prior streptococcal infection or a positive family history coupled with evidence of an immune complex disease (i.e., depression of C3) is usually sufficient to suggest the diagnosis.

Patient R.M., an 11-year-old white female, showed generalized edema and had some respiratory difficulty 2 weeks following a "sore throat." Blood pressure was 154/98 mm Hg, and there was marked generalized edema. The cardiac rhythm was regular, with only a grade II systolic ejection murmur. There were rales in both lung bases and radiographic evidence of pulmonary congestion and bilateral pleural fluid. The admitting diagnosis was "acute carditis and congestive heart failure." The ECG was normal.

The urine had a specific gravity of 1.025, and there was neither proteinuria nor hematuria. There were five to eight polymorphonuclear leukocytes and four to five renal epithelial cells per high-power microscopic field of urinary sediment. Red blood cell excretion was only 3,600 cells per hour on a 4-hr timed sample, and 12-hr protein excretion was less than 250 mg. The BUN was 18 mg per deciliter; the C3, 18 mg per deciliter; and the ASO titer, 333 Todd units, with a rise to 600 units at 2 weeks. Renal histologic examination revealed a proliferative glomerulonephritis, and on immunofluorescence microscopy, nodular deposition of C3, IgG, IgA, and fibrinogen was seen. Electron-microscopic examination revealed subepithelial electron-dense deposits.

Drug-induced diuresis began on the second hospital day, and R.M. subsequently lost 23 pounds of edema fluid, representing over 25 percent of her admission weight.

This girl presented without significant urinary abnormalities and thus confused the initial evaluators. The initial diagnosis was directed toward the possibility of acute rheumatic fever, but the absence of ECG evidence of carditis and the hypertension led to the determination of serum C3. Despite the normal urine, the low C3 dictated a renal histologic appraisal and "confirmation" of AGN, presumably related to a streptococcal infection.

A relatively "typical" *nephrotic syndrome,* simulating lipoid or minimal lesion nephrosis is occasionally the presenting symptom. In such children there is a less abrupt (almost insidious) onset of edema, which may progress to anasarca. Proteinuria is massive and hypoalbuminemia marked. In many patients the only suggestion of PSAGN is the presence of microscopic hematuria. More commonly, the child with a more typical PSAGN and severe nephrotic component also has hypertension and azotemia.

Patient E.B., an 8-year-old black male, was well until about 15 days prior to admission, when his mother noted periorbital edema. Because this was not marked and was assumed to be a normal weight gain, medical advice was not sought. The edema was intermittent during the next 10 days, but finally became persistent and progressed during the last few days prior to hospitalization. On admission, E.B. was markedly edematous, with ascites, pleural fluid, and scrotal edema. Blood pressure was 100/70 mm Hg, and the only other finding was the presence of multiple impetiginous lesions over the lower extremities. The initial diagnosis was lipoid nephrosis.

Significant laboratory studies revealed the following: 40 to 50 red blood cells per microscopic field, with 4+ proteinuria; 12-hr urine protein excretion, 3.6 gm; serum albumin, 2.1 gm per deciliter, with a total protein of 5.5 gm per deciliter; hemoglobin, 12 gm per deciliter; C3, 80 mg per deciliter; ASO titer of 125 Todd units; antihyaluronidase titer of 1 : 256, with a three-tube rise over the next 2 weeks;

cholesterol, 402 mg per deciliter; BUN, 18 mg per deciliter. Renal biopsy was performed and revealed a marked proliferative glomerulonephritis. On immunofluorescence microscopy, granular deposits of IgG and C3 were seen lining the capillary loops; on electron microscopy, "typical" humps were seen on the epithelial side of the basement membrane. No splitting of the basement membrane was observed.

Diuresis occurred, with a loss of 13 pounds of edema fluid and reduction in the 12-hr urine protein excretion to 0.8 gm by 4 weeks. Repeat determinations of C3 did not show a lowering below 80 mg per deciliter. Six weeks after hospitalization, the urine showed only 1+ proteinuria, with 60 to 80 red blood cells and serum albumin had risen to 3.6 gm per deciliter, with reduction of the cholesterol to 250 mg per deciliter. By 6 months, the urine was clear of both protein and cells.

This boy's early clinical course was almost typical for minimal change nephrotic syndrome, and only the presence of microscopic hematuria strongly suggested otherwise. The histologic picture, however, was characteristic of PSAGN, and the subsequent course has been typical of AGN.

Laboratory Investigations

URINALYSIS

In AGN the urine is most often reduced in volume and concentrated. The specific gravity commonly exceeds 1.020 and the osmolality 700 mOsm per kilogram in the early or oliguric phase of the disease. The urine pH is low, accounting for the reddish-brown or rusty color that the grossly hematuric urine assumes, as hemoglobin is converted to acid hematin. Glucosuria occurs occasionally, but ketonuria is rare. Proteinuria is usually present in direct proportion to the degree of hematuria. Qualitatively, it rarely exceeds a 3+ reaction and most often is between trace and 2+. Quantitatively, there is usually less than 2 gm/m²/24 hr, but amounts in excess of this are still compatible with the diagnosis.

Hematuria is the most consistent urinary abnormality. Polymorphonuclear leukocytes and renal epithelial cells may be seen in large numbers—particularly, early in the disease process—and may, on occasion, outnumber the red cells. These white cells do not necessarily suggest an infection, although bacteriuria is a not infrequent complication. Cylindruria is virtually always present and ranges from hyaline casts to cellular casts. Red blood cell casts should be sought meticulously, for their presence localizes the site of bleeding to the glomerulus. Red cell casts are reported to be found in from 60 to 85 percent of children hospitalized

with AGN. Faulty urine acquisition technique and examination probably prevent these figures from being much higher.

Urinary abnormalities return to normal at varying durations after onset. Proteinuria may disappear within the first 2 to 3 months or may be present in decreasing amounts for up to 6 months. Intermittent proteinuria and postural proteinuria have been noted to be present occasionally, even after the first year [42]. Microscopic hematuria has usually disappeared by 6 months, but may be present for up to a year without eliciting undue concern, and even more prolonged hematuria has been observed. However, when hematuria is present for a period exceeding 1 year, the specter of chronic nephritis is raised. If this hematuria is accompanied by persistent proteinuria, the suggestion is even stronger, and biopsy should be considered.

During the first few weeks following clinical onset, there may be a dramatic recurrence of the gross hematuria or an impressive increase in the degree of microscopic hematuria. These recurrences usually do not suggest reactivation of the nephritis, but they do occur most commonly following viral or bacterial infections of the upper respiratory tract. The increase in the degree of hematuria may also be observed with a sudden increase in level of physical activity [105].

BACTERIOLOGIC AND SEROLOGIC EXAMINATIONS

Group A, beta-hemolytic streptococci can usually be cultured either from the nasopharynx or from the impetiginous sites in children who have not received prior antimicrobial therapy [16, 155]. Sometimes, however, the interval between the original infection and the onset of nephritis will have been sufficiently long to make the cultures meaningless. Further, the mere presence of group A streptococci on culture indicates no more than a temporal association.

In most instances, and particularly in situations in which cultural proof of a streptococcal infection is lacking, the measurement of streptococcal antibody titers is helpful. As noted earlier, the anti-DNase B titer is the most helpful of the serologic tests, whereas the ASO titer is least helpful, particularly following pyoderma. The combined assessment of the ASO, antihyaluronidase, and anti-DNase B titers will detect a prior streptococcal disease in almost 100 percent of affected persons. Whatever the test utilized, serial measurements at 2-week to 3-week intervals are more meaningful than a single measurement. Measurement of serum complement activity is also of diagnostic significance, as discussed previously.

RENAL FUNCTIONAL TESTS

The GFR may show varying degrees of depression, the degree of reduction usually corresponding to the degree of histologic injury. In most instances, the reduction in GFR is not sufficient to raise the BUN and serum creatinine levels above the range of normal. In a small percentage of children, there is extreme azotemia, with elevations of BUN and serum creatinine and even elevation of serum phosphorus, the latter signifying a reduction of approximately 80 percent in glomerular filtration. In such patients there may be hyperkalemia and metabolic acidosis, with depression of the plasma bicarbonate concentration.

HEMOGRAM

Anemia is common in the early phase of AGN; the degree parallels the degree of expansion of the ECF. Thus, the major cause for reduction in the hemoglobin and hematocrit is dilutional [44, 125], and both values tend to return toward normal levels as diuresis occurs. Although not marked, there is a secondary fall in hemoglobin, hematocrit, and red cell count that occurs somewhat later [44], and there is some evidence to suggest augmented erythrocyte destruction, decreased iron uptake, and delayed erythrocyte production and maturation [44, 51, 151].

The white blood cell count usually is normal or slightly increased, and the platelet count is usually normal. The erythrocyte sedimentation rate is usually elevated in the acute phase and returns toward normal as the activity of the disease lessens.

OTHER LABORATORY STUDIES

The total serum protein concentration is slightly decreased in the majority of edematous patients with AGN, and there is a uniform reduction in the concentration of each of the plasma proteins. Like the anemia, this appears to result mainly from the retention of water and solute in the extracellular space. On occasion, when the degree of proteinuria is massive, there will be lowering of the serum albumin and gamma globulins, with increases in alpha-2 and beta globulins. Heyman and Wilson [69] have demonstrated that approximately 40 percent of children with a clinical diagnosis of AGN have elevated serum lipids. This contrasts with an elevation in about 25 percent in another series [125]. The pathogenesis of hyperlipemia is not understood and does not correlate with the level of albumin, degree of edema, or clinical severity of the initial illness.

RADIOGRAPHIC STUDIES

The roentgenographic findings in the chest are sometimes considered almost pathognomonic of AGN. There is usually evidence of pulmonary congestion in the hilar area, radiating outward in a "sunburst" manner [87, 140]. On occasion, there is generalized cardiomegaly and pulmonary edema. It is not unusual to find pleural fluid. The changes quickly revert to normal as diuresis occurs. Radiographic examination of the abdomen may reveal evidence of ascites. Intravenous pyelography may demonstrate delayed visualization of the collecting system, particularly during the early stages. The kidneys are normal to increased in size.

INDICATIONS FOR RENAL BIOPSY

As noted previously, the histologic pattern in the early stages of PSAGN is fairly typical and, in doubtful cases, is of diagnostic assistance. At the same time, it should be recognized that there is nothing that is *absolutely* diagnostic about the histologic features of PSAGN and that the changes become less diagnostic as the interval between onset and biopsy lengthens. Consequently, the renal biopsy will be most helpful in the diagnosis early in the course. After the first few months, the changes are often confused with chronic nephritis.

In the vast majority of children hospitalized for AGN, the clinical picture appears characteristic enough to suggest that renal biopsy is rarely indicated. However, it should be pointed out that an acute exacerbation of a previously existing (chronic) nephritis may closely mimic AGN [42, 48, 133, 144, 152]. In three different studies, approximately 10 percent of patients presenting with relatively typical clinical features of AGN were found to have "old" histologic lesions [42, 48, 144, 152]. In these instances, the nephritis had been exacerbated by a recent streptococcal infection. There are also instances in which AGN is confirmed by biopsy examination when some other condition was suspected on the basis of the clinical examination.

It is perhaps justifiable to consider the use of renal biopsy in AGN in two broad categories of patients: (1) children whose presentation or laboratory data differ significantly from the "typical" PSAGN and (2) children in whom there is a significant delay in the rate of resolution of one or more clinical or laboratory features. Table 47-1 lists some indications for *considering* renal biopsy; in most instances, two or more of these findings should mandate a histologic evaluation.

*Table 47-1. Indications for Considering Renal Biopsy in Acute Glomerulonephritis**

"Atypical" presentation
 Etiology:
  Absence of infection prior to onset
  Onset of renal symptoms coincident with infection
  Absence of serologic evidence of streptococcal etiology (using appropriate tests)
  Absence of depression of serum complement, or C3
 Early clinical course:
  Anuria
  Presence of nephrotic syndrome
  Azotemia out of proportion to other clinical findings
 Miscellaneous factors:
  Age less than 2 years and over 12 years
  Prior history of renal disease
  Abnormal growth data
  Family history of nephritis
  Significant systemic symptomatology
Delay in rate of "resolution"
 Early:
  Oliguria and/or azotemia persisting past 2 weeks
  Hypertension persisting past 3 weeks
  Gross hematuria persisting past 3 weeks
  C3 continues low beyond 6 weeks
 Late:
  Persistent proteinuria and hematuria past 6 months
  Persistent proteinuria past 6 months
  Persistent hematuria past 12 months

* One or more of these indications may cause the physician to *consider* whether biopsy is, or is not, indicated.

Differential Diagnosis

A number of renal diseases share certain similarities with PSAGN and should be considered in the differential diagnosis. Already mentioned are the broad array of bacterial and viral illnesses in which coincident glomerulonephritis has been observed [3, 13, 18, 58, 70, 76, 109, 126, 132, 135, 162]. These will not be considered further except to restate that care should be taken in identifying the presence or absence of a streptococcal etiology. Course and prognosis may depend on the inciting infectious agent, as well as the host response. Although many other renal syndromes may mimic the early picture of AGN, only four conditions do so commonly: (1) a chronic glomerulonephritis with an acute exacerbation, (2) anaphylactoid purpura with nephritis, (3) idiopathic hematuria (e.g., focal nephritis, benign hematuria, recurrent hematuria, IgA nephropathy), and (4) familial nephritis. Renal biopsy is often necessary to distinguish similar presentations.

ACUTE EXACERBATION OF CHRONIC GLOMERULONEPHRITIS

Acute exacerbation of chronic glomerulonephritis (CGN) is perhaps the condition most commonly confused with AGN and, as mentioned previously, may cause perplexity in as many as 10 percent of hospitalized patients [48, 144, 152]. It is important to distinguish these conditions from AGN because the prognoses differ so dramatically. The presence of bacteriologic and serologic evidence of streptococcal disease does not exclude the possibility of exacerbation of CGN, which commonly follows acute illnesses of any type. A high index of suspicion and a diligent search for evidence of chronic disease often will lead to the correct diagnosis.

A prior history of similar renal symptoms should suggest chronic nephritis, and a search should be made of existing records for prior evaluations of blood pressure and urinalysis. Careful assessment of growth data may indicate a prior falloff in linear growth and suggest the earlier presence of renal disease. The onset of nephritis coincident with an infection and thus without a latent period does not support the diagnosis of PSAGN and should alert one to the possibility of exacerbation of chronic disease.

The presence of significant anemia at the onset of symptoms provides evidence of CGN, and azotemia that is more marked than expected on the basis of other findings (edema, hypertension) adds weight to the evidence. A nephrotic syndrome associated with other findings of nephritis suggests membranoproliferative glomerulonephritis, which becomes even more likely if the C3 level fails to return to normal within 4 to 6 weeks.

Patient C.C., a 10-year-old white female, was apparently in normal health until 3 days following onset of a "sore throat," when generalized edema and gross hematuria developed. On examination she was found to have a blood pressure of 170/120 mm Hg. Her height was at the 5th percentile, but there was no prior history of illness. Initial laboratory studies revealed the following: 3+ proteinuria and gross hematuria; hemoglobin, 7 gm per deciliter; BUN, 68 mg per deciliter; creatinine, 1.9 mg per deciliter; ASO titer, 333 Todd units, with an eventual rise to 720 units; beta-hemolytic streptococcus cultured from the throat; C3, 35 mg per deciliter; antinuclear antibody titer, negative.

Renal biopsy, performed 10 days after clinical onset, revealed an acute proliferative glomerulonephritis, and immunofluorescent microscopy revealed 3+ granular staining for IgG and C3, associated with mesangial staining of fibrinogen. Occasional humps were seen by electron microscopy, but there were numerous smaller electron-dense deposits, both epimembranous and intramembranous. Approximately one-third of the glomeruli were sclerotic, and there was associated tubular atrophy and interstitial fibrosis. Still another one-third of the glomeruli had marked mesangial sclerosis.

This girl is an example of how closely an acute exacerbation of CGN can mimic PSAGN. The only clinical features that suggested a chronic process were the early onset of renal symptoms and the minimal growth retardation. A further suggestion of chronic disease was based on the degree of anemia and the considerable reduction in renal function. The renal biopsy revealed chronic glomerulonephritis with extensive tubulo-interstitial changes and a superimposed acute process suggesting PSAGN. This girl's subsequent history has been one of slow but progressive deterioration in renal function.

ANAPHYLACTOID PURPURA WITH NEPHRITIS

Glomerulonephritis occurs in approximately 50 percent of children with anaphylactoid purpura [43, 145] (Chap. 61), and the "nephritis" may overshadow the other features and cause confusion in diagnosis. In most instances an associated history of abdominal pain or arthralgia and the finding of the characteristic rash confirm the diagnosis. In some patients, however, the rash may not be typical, the abdominal pain be questionable, and the arthralgia only transient. To add to the confusion, the symptoms and signs of nephritis may precede the onset of other clinical features. Anaphylactoid purpura is often associated with a respiratory infection, but rarely is it streptococcal. Consequently, serologic evidence of a prior streptococcal illness usually is missing, and C3 levels are not depressed. Renal biopsy is most often diagnostic [39, 145].

IDIOPATHIC HEMATURIA

Hematuria of unknown etiology is well recognized and is not uncommonly confused with AGN. Idiopathic hematuria probably occurs as a consequence of a number of etiologic agents and is often referred to as "benign" hematuria, recurrent hematuria, focal nephritis, IgA-IgG nephropathy, and glomerulitis [8, 15, 143] (Chaps. 44, 46).

In most instances the differentiation from PSAGN is easy, since only one of the cardinal features is commonly present, namely, gross hematuria. Characteristically, edema and hypertension are absent, and it is unusual to see a reduction in renal function. The onset of hematuria is often associated with the onset of a respiratory infection or with exercise. Not uncommonly, there is a history of previous episodes of hematuria, each occurring following a similar event and subsiding without apparent consequence. Streptococcal association is missing, and complement levels are not depressed.

FAMILIAL NEPHRITIS

Like any other form of chronic nephritis, familial nephritis may be exacerbated by a streptococcal infection. Careful evaluation of the family usually reveals other affected members. The associated finding of hearing deficit of the neurologic type in either the patient or family members aids in the diagnosis. The severity of the azotemia and hypertension at the time of the acute exacerbation often is more marked than would be anticipated in PSAGN.

Treatment

By the time the child with PSAGN presents with symptomatic disease, it is much too late for any therapeutic measure to influence the course. On the other hand, morbidity and early mortality are considerably influenced by appropriate medical therapy and are therefore of the greatest importance.

HYPERTENSION AND HYPERTENSIVE ENCEPHALOPATHY

Hypertension of mild to moderate severity does not usually warrant emergency management unless there are associated cerebral signs. On the other hand, severe hypertension (pressures in the range of 180 to 220 mm Hg systolic and 110 to 150 mm Hg diastolic) or hypertension associated with signs of cerebral dysfunction demands immediate treatment.

Hypertensive encephalopathy is a medical emergency and all attempts should be made to lower the pressure as rapidly as possible. The most effective agent currently available for such an acute crisis appears to be diazoxide [90a, 106a]. Kohaut and associates [90a] demonstrated the effectiveness and safety of this drug in 26 patients with AGN who had moderate to severe hypertension. Thirteen of these patients had clinical evidence of hypertensive encephalopathy and in each the symptoms rapidly abated, which is consistent with the author's experience. Diazoxide should be given intravenously by rapid, bolus injection and doses of 5 mg per kilogram body weight are recommended. In instances of AGN with an associated severe nephrotic component (with hypoproteinemia), the bolus dose might be reduced to 3 mg per kilogram body weight. Occasionally, hyperglycemia is a consequence of repeated diazoxide administration, and the patient should be closely monitored. It is the author's practice to administer intravenous furosemide (2 mg/kg body weight) along with the bolus injection of diazoxide.

Severe hypertension without signs of encephalopathy should also be treated promptly with parenteral medications; of those commonly used, reserpine has proved to be the most effective [30, 52, 142]. It is administered in a dosage of 0.03 to 0.10 mg per kilogram of body weight (1 to 3 mg per square meter of body surface area) and, depending on the severity of the hypertension, may be given IM or IV. Reserpine should not be given PO because of its delayed therapeutic action. Following IV administration, the blood pressure begins to decline within one-half hour, and the effect may be prolonged. Intramuscular reserpine can be administered as often as every 8 to 12 hr; more frequent administration will lead to the development of basal ganglia symptoms suggestive of parkinsonism. Unexplained "chills" and "shivers" commonly occur after acute administration, but are not accompanied by an alteration in body temperature. The antihypertensive effect of reserpine is augmented by the simultaneous use of hydralazine [52, 142]. This drug is administered parenterally in doses of approximately 0.15 to 0.30 mg per kilogram of body weight and may be repeated every 2 to 4 hr as needed to control the blood pressure. Headache, nausea, vomiting, dizziness, and significant tachycardia are occasional complications of hydralazine therapy.

Methyldopa has been recommended by some [83], but others have found it to be a poor antihypertensive in PSAGN [140]. Diuretics are not particularly effective in the treatment of the hypertension of PSAGN [123]. However, Retan and Dillon [124] have suggested that less antihypertensives are required in those patients treated with furosemide.

Mild to moderate hypertension should be treated with bed rest, fluid restriction, and one or more of the drugs mentioned previously. With mild hypertension, the antihypertensive agents (other than reserpine) usually can be administered by mouth and in smaller amounts.

CIRCULATORY CONGESTION AND EDEMA
In most children with AGN, the edema and circulatory congestion are not sufficiently marked to produce more than minimal discomfort. In these children, the most effective therapy is restriction of salt and water intake.

Fluid administration should be by the oral route whenever possible and, until the status of renal function is known, should be limited to an amount necessary to replace insensible losses. Since there is often central nervous system depression and peripheral edema—both reducing the amount of insensible losses—the estimate for replacement is at or near basal requirements. Details of management are given in Chap. 33. If circulatory congestion is

marked, it is appropriate to use potent diuretic agents such as furosemide; response to this drug has been generally good and toxicity minimal [15, 39, 110, 117a, 124]. In the rare child with severe and life-threatening cardiopulmonary complications, more dramatic therapy to reduce plasma volume is indicated. The use of phlebotomy, "bloodless" phlebotomy (rotating tourniquets), or peritoneal dialysis with hypertonic dialysis fluids all are effective.

ANURIA OR SEVERE AND PERSISTENT OLIGURIA
Approximately 10 percent of hospitalized patients with AGN have anuria or severe oliguria [94–96]. Improvement in the therapy of the complications of acute renal failure over the last 20 years has contributed to a great extent to the marked decrease in mortality from AGN. Fortunately, the severe oliguria is most often transient, and every attempt should be made to support life and maintain electrolyte balance until diuresis occurs. Dietary management and the use of dialysis are discussed in Chaps. 33 and 35.

OTHER THERAPY
Antibiotics
In any patient found to have PSAGN, it is appropriate to assure eradication of the infecting streptococcus by antibiotic therapy. If the person is not allergic, a course of penicillin should be administered either orally or parenterally, although there is no indication that such a course of therapy has any influence on the course of the disease. Some clinicians have advocated penicillin prophylaxis during the early convalescent period [130] in the hope of decreasing streptococcus-related exacerbations, but this practice is not widely followed. There are sufficient epidemiologic data to suggest that prolonged prophylactic therapy is unwarranted.

Bed Rest
Bed rest has long been recommended for the convalescent period of AGN, in the belief that health and recovery would be benefited and that the probability of progression to chronic nephritis would be lessened. Three separate studies [1, 78, 105] have failed to document any beneficial results of prolonged bed rest, and it is well known that there are considerable emotional and psychological penalties associated with prolonged social isolation. Consequently, as a general rule, bed rest is utilized only during the acute phase, when there is hypertension, gross hematuria, and significant edema.

Family Screening

Family screening for streptococcal disease is appropriate, since studies have confirmed a high incidence of the nephritogenic strain in household contacts [33, 40, 65]. If clinical or bacteriologic evidence of streptococcal infection is found, penicillin treatment is indicated. Additionally, the author recommends that household contacts have a blood pressure determination and a urine examination to detect those with subclinical disease.

Follow-up

A plan for follow-up of the child with nephritis should be clearly outlined and discussed with the family. The actual plan will depend on many factors, but should take into consideration the relatively slow rate of clinical recovery that is usually observed. Blood pressure measurement and examination of the urine for protein and blood constitute the hallmarks of follow-up. Examinations should be done at 4-week to 6-week intervals during the first 6 months and at 3-month to 6-month intervals thereafter, until there has been persistent absence of both hematuria and proteinuria for 1 year. Afterward, a urinalysis once yearly appears sufficient.

Course and Prognosis

Epidemic PSAGN appears to undergo virtually complete resolution and healing in all patients, and this is particularly true in children, in whom recovery approaches 100 percent [45, 112, 120]. The outcome in patients of all ages is less certain following the sporadic form of PSAGN. In adult subjects, from 15 to 30 percent of patients with sporadic AGN have been reported to progress to a chronic state [45, 46], while estimates in children have generally ranged from approximately 5 to 10 percent [42, 103, 104, 106, 144]. Three reports [10, 11, 71] that included both adults and children have suggested a progression to chronic nephritis in as many as one-half the hospitalized cases. The author has presented an analysis of the differences in these studies [139–141].

The ultimate prognosis in PSAGN is in major part due to the severity of the initial insult. The initial glomerular inflammation may be so marked that the involved glomerulus undergoes fibrosis and sclerosis, with death of the nephron unit. In severe clinical disease, this marked degree of glomerular involvement is so uniform as to produce irreversible changes in a significant proportion of the nephrons. There is either persistent or progressive renal failure culminating in death of the kidney within a variable but relatively short period of time. This course is seen in from 0.5 to 2.0 percent of patients with AGN who are admitted to the hospital. In the more typical patient, glomerular involvement is not uniformly severe, and in only a small percentage of the glomeruli are there progressive sclerosis and obsolescence. In these instances, varying degrees of resolution can be expected; the clinical course is characterized by subsidence of the acute process within 1 to 3 weeks and apparent resolution of the disease within 6 to 12 months. As previously indicated, existing data conflict as to how often resolution is complete and how frequently progression to chronic nephritis occurs.

Poststreptococcal acute glomerulonephritis undergoes a period of histologic resolution that may or may not parallel clinical resolution. A 2-year delay in complete histologic resolution was observed initially by Jennings and Earle [75] and has been confirmed subsequently [42, 71]. As suggested previously, the individual glomerulus may undergo one of at least three possible courses. Glomeruli that are mildly to moderately involved may have complete histologic reversal to a normal glomerulus. In one investigation [42, 144], 50 percent of the children studied had normal glomeruli on repeat biopsy. The glomeruli that initially show more severe involvement in the proliferative process cannot be expected to undergo complete reversal, and residual changes are found on subsequent biopsy. These residual changes may consist only of mesangial sclerosis, but there are often synechiae, and focal areas of sclerosis can be observed. Still more severely involved glomeruli may have had partial or complete obliteration. The majority of these sclerotic lesions appear static and show no apparent tendency to progression. In the study just mentioned [42, 144], an additional 42 percent of the patients showed these varying degrees of "healing" with residual changes. Thus, 92 percent of the patients in this well-controlled study had histologic resolution of their disease.

It is still impossible to answer the ultimate question as to whether there might be either slow progression in some of these patients or a true "latency" period, with its implication of subclinical and subpathologic disease, followed by spontaneous reactivation at some later date. It is felt by most investigators, however, that the likelihood of a recrudescence of nephritis, with progressive deterioration in renal function, is unlikely. It is thus probable that the eventual recovery from PSAGN is assured in over 95 percent of the patients. No such statement can be made concerning AGN from other causes.

Acknowledgment

The photomicrographs of renal histology were kindly supplied by Dr. Gerald A. Beathard, Associate Professor of Pathology, University of Texas Medical Branch, Galveston, Texas.

References

1. Akerren, Y., and Lindgren, M. Investigation concerning early rising in acute haemorrhagic nephritis. *Acta Med. Scand.* 151:419, 1955.
2. Albert, M. S., Leeming, J. M., and Scaglione, P. R. Acute glomerulonephritis without abnormality of the urine. *J. Pediatr.* 68:525, 1966.
3. Alexander, E. A. Recurrent hemorrhagic nephritis with exacerbation related to influenza A. *Ann. Intern. Med.* 62:1002, 1965.
4. Anthony, B. F., Kaplan, E. L., Wannamaker, L. W., Briese, F. W., and Chapman, S. S. Attack rates of acute nephritis after type 49 streptococcal infection of the skin and of the respiratory tract. *J. Clin. Invest.* 48:1697, 1969.
5. Anthony, B. F., Perlman, L. V., and Wannamaker, L. W. Skin infection and acute nephritis in American Indian children. *Pediatrics* 39:263, 1967.
6. Anthony, B. F., Yamauchi, T., Penso, J. S., Kamei, I., and Chapman, S. S. Classroom outbreak of scarlet fever and acute glomerulonephritis related to type-2 (M-2, T-2) group A streptococcus. *J. Infect. Dis.* 129:336, 1974.
7. Arisz, L., Bretjens, R. H., Van der Ham, G. K., and Madema, E. Clinical value of serum B_1A and B_1E globulin levels in adult patients with renal disease. *Acta Med. Scand.* 192:255, 1972.
8. Ayoub, E. M., and Vernier, R. L. Benign recurrent hematuria. *Am. J. Dis. Child.* 109:217, 1965.
9. Ayoub, E. M., and Wannamaker, L. W. Evaluation of the streptococcal deoxyribonuclease B and diphosphopyridine B and diphosphopyridine nucleotidase antibody tests in acute rheumatic fever and acute glomerulonephritis. *Pediatrics* 29:527, 1962.
10. Baldwin, D. S., Gluck, M. C., Schacht, R. G., and Gallo, G. The long-term course of poststreptococcal glomerulonephritis. *Ann. Intern. Med.* 80:342, 1974.
11. Baldwin, D. S., Gluck, M. C., Schacht, R. G., Moussallii, A., and Gallo, G. F. Long-term Follow-up of Poststreptococcal Glomerulonephritis. In P. Kincaid-Smith, T. H. Mathew, and E. L. Becker (eds.), *Glomerulonephritis: Morphology, Natural History and Treatment.* New York: Wiley, 1972. P. 327.
12. Bassett, D. C. J. Streptococcal pyoderma and acute nephritis in Trinidad. *Br. J. Dermatol.* 86:55, 1972.
13. Bayatpour, M., Zbitnew, A., Dempster, G., and Miller, K. B. Role of Coxsackie virus B-4 in the pathogenesis of acute glomerulonephritis. *Can. Med. Assoc. J.* 109:873, 1973.
14. Bengtsson, U., Ekedahl, C., and Holm, S. E. Acute poststreptococcal glomerulonephritis. A retrospective study. *Scand. J. Infect. Dis.* 5:111, 1973.
15. Berger, J. IgA glomerular deposits in renal disease. *Transplant. Proc.* 1:939, 1969.
16. Bernstein, S. H., and Stillerman, M. A. A study of the association of group A streptococci and acute glomerulonephritis. *Ann. Intern. Med.* 52:1026, 1960.
17. Bisno, A. L., Nelson, K. E., Waytz, P., and Brant, J. Factors influencing serum antibody response in streptococcal pyoderma. *J. Lab. Clin. Med.* 81:410, 1973.
18. Black, J. A., Callacombe, D. N., and Ockenden, B. G. Nephritic syndrome associated with bacteremia after shunt operations for hydrocephalus. *Lancet* 2:921, 1965.
19. Blumberg, A., Nelp, W. B., and Hegstrom, R. M. Extracellular volume in patients with chronic renal disease treated for hypertension by sodium restriction. *Lancet* 2:69, 1967.
20. Blumberg, R. W., and Feldman, D. B. Observations on acute glomerulonephritis associated with impetigo. *J. Pediatr.* 60:677, 1962.
21. Braun, W. E., and Merrill, J. P. Urine fibrinogen fragments in human renal allografts. A possible mechanism of renal injury. *N. Engl. J. Med.* 278:1366, 1968.
22. Brod, J. Acute diffuse glomerulonephritis. *Am. J. Med.* 7:317, 1949.
23. Burke, F. G., and Ross, S. Acute glomerulonephritis: A review of ninety cases. *J. Pediatr.* 30:157, 1947.
24. Burkholder, P. M., and Bradford, W. D. Proliferative glomerulonephritis in children. A correlation of varied clinical and pathologic patterns utilizing light, immunofluorescence, and electron microscopy. *Am. J. Pathol.* 56:423, 1969.
25. Callis, L., Castello, F., and Garcia, L. Histopathological aspects of acute diffuse glomerulonephritis in children. *Helv. Paediat. Acta* 22:3, 1967.
26. Calloway, J. L., and O'Rear, H. B. Pyogenic infections of skin. *Arch. Dermatol.* 64:159, 1951.
27. Cameron, J. S., Vick, R. M., Ogg, C. S., Seymour, W. M., Chantler, C., and Turner, D. R. Plasma C_3 and C_4 concentrations in the management of glomerulonephritis. *Br. Med. J.* 3:668, 1973.
28. Catt, K. J., Cran, E., Zimmet, P. Z., Best, J. B., Cain, M. D., and Coghlan, J. P. Angiotensin. II. Blood levels in human hypertension. *Lancet* 1:459, 1971.
29. Cohen, J. A., and Levit, M. F. Acute glomerulonephritis with few urinary abnormalities. Report of two cases proved by renal biopsy. *N. Engl. J. Med.* 268:749, 1963.
30. Daeschner, C. W., Moyer, J. H., Bell, W. R., and Clark, J. Parenteral administration of reserpine in the treatment of hypertension due to acute and chronic nephritis. Clinical and renal hemodynamic studies. *Pediatrics* 19:566, 1957.
31. Defazio, V., Christensen, R. C., Regan, T. J., Baer, L. J., Mortia, Y., and Hellems, H. K. Circulatory changes in acute glomerulonephritis. *Circulation* 20:190, 1959.
32. Derrick, C. W., Reeves, M. S., and Dillon, H. C., Jr. Complement in overt and asymptomatic nephritis after skin infection. *J. Clin. Invest.* 49:1178, 1970.
33. Dillon, H. C., Jr. Streptococcal skin infection and acute glomerulonephritis. *Postgrad. Med. J.* 46:641, 1970.
34. Dillon, H. C., Jr., and Derrick, C. W. Streptococcal complications: The outlook for prevention. *Hosp. Pract.* 3:93, 1972.
35. Dillon, H. C., and Dillon, M. S. A. New streptococcal serotypes causing pyoderma and acute glomerulonephritis; types 59, 60, and 61. *Infect. Immun.* 9:1070, 1974.
36. Dillon, H. C., and Reeves, M. S. Streptococcal

antibody titers in skin infection and AGN. *Pediatr. Res.* 3:362, 1969.

37. Dillon, H. C., and Reeves, M. S. A. Streptococcal immune responses in nephritis after skin infections. *Am. J. Med.* 56:333, 1974.

38. Dillon, H. C., Reeves, M. S., and Maxted, W. R. Acute glomerulonephritis following skin infection due to streptococci of M-type 2. *Lancet* 1:543, 1968.

39. Dodge, W. F., Daeschner, C. W., Jr., Brennan, J. C., Rosenberg, H. S., Travis, L. B., and Hopps, H. C. Percutaneous renal biopsy in children. II. Acute glomerulonephritis, chronic glomerulonephritis, and nephritis of anaphylactoid purpura. *Pediatrics* 30:297, 1962.

40. Dodge, W. F., Spargo, B. F., and Travis, L. B. Occurrence of acute glomerulonephritis in sibling contacts of children with sporadic acute glomerulonephritis. *Pediatrics* 40:1029, 1967.

41. Dodge, W. F., Spargo, B. F., Bass, J. A., and Travis, L. B. The relationship between the clinical and pathologic features of post-streptococcal glomerulonephritis. A study of the early natural history. *Medicine (Baltimore)* 47:227, 1968.

42. Dodge, W. F., Spargo, B. F., Travis, L. B., Srivastiva, R. N., Carvajal, H. F., DeBeukelaer, M. M., Longley, M. P., and Menchaca, J. A. Poststreptococcal glomerulonephritis. A prospective study in children. *N. Engl. J. Med.* 286:273, 1972.

43. Dodge, W. F., Travis, L. B., and Daeschner, C. W., Jr. Anaphylactoid purpura, polyarteritis nodosa and purpura fulminans. *Pediatr. Clin. North Am.* 10:879, 1963.

44. Dodge, W. F., Travis, L. B., Haggard, M. E., Harris, L. C., Bryan, G. T., and Daeschner, C. W., Jr. Studies of Physiology during the Early Stage of Acute Glomerulonephritis in Children. In J. Metcoff (ed.), *Acute Glomerulonephritis.* Boston: Little, Brown, 1967. Pp. 319–331.

45. Earle, D. P. Natural History of Acute Glomerulonephritis in Adults. In J. Metcoff (ed.), *Acute Glomerulonephritis.* Boston: Little, Brown, 1967. P. 3.

46. Earle, D. P. Glomerulonephritis: Clinical aspects. *Bull. N.Y. Acad. Med.* 46:749, 1970.

47. Earle, D. P., Farber, S. J., Alexander, J. D., and Pellegrino, E. D. Renal function and electrolyte metabolism in acute glomerulonephritis. *J. Clin. Invest.* 30:421, 1951.

48. Edelmann, C. M., Jr., Greifer, I., and Barnett, H. L. The nature of kidney disease in children who fail to recover from apparent acute glomerulonephritis. *J. Pediatr.* 64:879, 1964.

49. Eichna, L. W. Circulatory congestion and heart failure. The George E. Brown Memorial Lecture. *Circulation* 22:864, 1960.

50. Eisenberg, S. Blood volume in patients with acute glomerulonephritis as determined by radioactive chromium tagged red cells. *Am. J. Med.* 27:241, 1959.

51. Emerson, C. P. The pathogenesis of anemia in acute glomerulonephritis: Estimation of blood production and blood destruction in a case receiving massive transfusions. *Blood* 3:363, 1948.

52. Etteldorf, J. N., Smith, J. D., and Johnson, C. The effect of reserpine and its combination and hydralazine on blood pressure and renal hemodynamics during the hypertensive phase of acute nephritis in children. *J. Pediatr.* 48:129, 1956.

53. Farber, S. J. Physiologic aspects of glomerulonephritis. *J. Chronic Dis.* 5:87, 1957.

54. Feldman, J. O., Mardiney, M. R., and Shuler, S. E. Immunology and morphology of acute post-streptococcal glomerulonephritis. *Lab. Invest.* 15:283, 1966.

55. Fish, A. J., Herdman, R. C., Michael, A. F., Pickering, R. J., and Good, R. A. Epidemic acute glomerulonephritis associated with type 49 streptococcal pyoderma II. Correlative study of light, immunofluorescent and electron microscopic findings. *Am. J. Med.* 48:28, 1970.

56. Fison, T. N. Acute glomerulonephritis in infancy. *Arch. Dis. Child.* 31:101, 1956.

57. Fleisher, D. S., Voci, G., Garfunkel, J., Puragganan, H., Kirkpatrick, J., Jr., Wells, C. R., and McElfresh, A. E. Hemodynamic fundings in acute glomerulonephritis. *J. Pediatr.* 69:1054, 1966.

58. Formijne, P. On an epidemic of acute glomerulonephritis in Amsterdam. *Acta Med. Scand.* 129:509, 1948.

59. Futcher, P. H. Glomerular nephritis following infections of the skin. *Arch. Intern. Med.* 65:1192, 1940.

60. Gewurz, H., Pickering, R. J., Mergenhogen, S. E., and Good, R. A. The complement profile in acute glomerulonephritis, systemic lupus erythematosus and hypocomplementemic chronic glomerulonephritis. *Int. Arch. Allergy* 34:556, 1968.

61. Goorno, W., Ashworth, C. T., and Carter, N. W. Acute glomerulonephritis with absence of abnormal urinary findings. Diagnosis by light and electron microscopy. *Ann. Intern. Med.* 66:345, 1967.

62. Goorno, W. E., and Kaplan, N. M. Renal pressor material in various hypertensive diseases. *Ann. Intern. Med.* 63:745, 1965.

63. Gotoff, S. P., Fellers, F. X., Valoter, G. F., Janeway, C. A., and Rosen, F. S. The beta IC globulin in childhood nephrotic syndrome. *N. Engl. J. Med.* 273:524, 1965.

64. Götze, O., and Müller-Eberhard, H. J. The C3-activator system: An alternate pathway of complement activation. *J. Exp. Med.* 134:91, 1971.

65. Hall, W. D., Blumberg, R. W., and Moody, M. D. Studies in children with impetigo; bacteriology, serology, and incidence of glomerulonephritis. *Am. J. Dis. Child.* 125:800, 1973.

66. Heptinstall, R. H. Acute Glomerulonephritis. In R. H. Heptinstall (ed.), *Pathology of the Kidney* (2nd ed.). Boston: Little, Brown, 1974. Pp. 331–369.

67. Herdson, P. B., Jennings, R. B., and Earle, D. P. Glomerular fine structure in post-streptococcal acute glomerulonephritis. *Arch. Pathol.* 81:117, 1966.

68. Hewitt, L. F., and Todd, E. W. The effect of cholesterol and of sera contaminated with bacteria on the hemolysins produced by hemolytic streptococci. *J. Pathol. Bact.* 49:45, 1939.

69. Heyman, W., and Wilson, S. G. F. Hyperlipemia in early stages of acute glomerular nephritis. *J. Clin. Invest.* 38:186, 1959.

70. Hill, L. L., Guerra, S., and Rosenberg, H. Acute glomerulonephritis secondary to pneumoncoccal infection. *J. Pediatr.* 67:904, 1965.

71. Hinglais, N., Garcia-Torres, R., and Kleinknecht, D. Long-term prognosis in acute glomerulonephritis. *Am. J. Med.* 56:52, 1974.

72. Hoyer, J. R., Michael, A. F., Fish, A. J., and Good,

R. A. Acute poststreptococcal glomerulonephritis presenting as hypertensive encephalopathy with minimal urinary abnormalities. *Pediatrics* 39:412, 1967.

73. Hughes, W. T., and Wan, R. T. Impetigo contagiosa: Etiology, complications, and comparison of therapeutic effectiveness of erythromycin and antibiotic ointment. *Am. J. Dis. Child.* 113:449, 1967.

74. Humair, L., Potter, E. V., and Kwaan, H. C. The role of fibrinogen in renal disease. I. Production of experimental lesions in mice. *J. Lab. Clin. Med.* 74: 60, 1969.

75. Jennings, R. B., and Earle, D. P. Poststreptococcal glomerulonephritis. *J. Clin. Invest.* 40:1525, 1961.

76. Jensen, M. M. Viruses and kidney disease. *Am. J. Med.* 43:897, 1969.

77. Johansson, B., Strandgaard, S., and Lassen, N. A. On the pathogenesis of hypertensive encephalopathy. *Circ. Res.* [Suppl. 1] 34–35:167, 1974.

78. Joseph, M. C., and Polani, P. E. The effect of bed rest on acute hemorrhagic nephritis in children. *Guys Hosp. Rep.* 107:500, 1958.

79. Kantor, F. S. Fibrinogen precipitation by streptococcal M-protein. *J. Exp. Med.* 121:849, 861, 1965.

80. Kaplan, E. L., Anthony, B. F., Chapman, S. S., Ayoub, E. M., and Wannamaker, L. W. The influence of the site of infection on the immune response to group A streptococci. *J. Clin. Invest.* 49:1405, 1970.

81. Kaplan, E. L., Anthony, B. F., Chapman, S. S., and Wannamaker, L. W. Epidemic acute glomerulonephritis associated with type 49 streptococcal pyoderma. *Am. J. Med.* 48:9, 1970.

82. Kaplan, E. L., and Wannamaker, L. W. Suppression of host response to streptolysin O by skin lipids and its clinical implications. *Pediatr. Res.* 7:375, 1973.

83. Kassirer, J. P. The treatment of acute poststreptococcal glomerulonephritis. *Kidney* 4:1, 1971.

84. Kilbourne, E. D., and Loge, S. P. The comparative effect of continuous and intermittent penicillin therapy on the formation of antistreptolysin in hemolytic streptococcal pharyngitis. *J. Clin. Invest.* 27:418, 1948.

85. Kimmelstiel, P. The hump—a lesion of acute glomerulonephritis. *Bull. Pathol.* 6:187, 1965.

86. Kimmelstiel, P., Kim, O. J., and Beres, J. Studies on renal biopsy specimens with the aid of the electron microscope: II. Glomerulonephritis and glomerulonephrosis. *Am. J. Clin. Pathol.* 38:280, 1962.

87. Kirkpatrick, J. A., Jr., and Fleisher, D. S. The roentgen appearance of the chest in acute glomerulonephritis in children. *J. Pediatr.* 64:492, 1964.

88. Kleinman, H. Epidemic acute glomerulonephritis at Red Lake. *Minn. Med.* 37:479, 1954.

89. Kobayashi, O., Okawa, K., Kamiyama, T., and Wada, H. Electron microscopic alterations of the glomerular capillaries in children with poststreptococcal glomerulonephritis. *Acta Med. Biol.* 19:75, 1971.

90. Koffler, D., and Paronetta, F. Immunofluorescent localization of immunoglobulins, complement and fibrinogen in human disease. II. Acute, subacute and chronic glomerulonephritis. *J. Clin. Invest.* 44:1665, 1965.

90a. Kohaut, E. C., Wilson, C. J., and Hill, L. L. Intravenous diazoxide in acute poststreptococcal glomerulonephritis. *J. Pediatr.* 87:797, 1975.

91. Lange, K. Role of Streptococcal Antigen in Pathogenesis of AGN. Proceedings of the Third International Congress on Pediatric Nephrology, Washington, 1974.

92. Lange, K., Treser, G., Sagel, I., Ty, A., and Wasserman, E. Routine immunohistology in renal disease. *Ann. Intern. Med.* 64:25, 1966.

93. Laragh, J. H., Baer, L., Braner, H. R., Buhler, F. R., Sealey, J. E., and Vaughn, E. D. The Renin-Angiotensin-Aldosterone System in Pathogenesis and Management of Hypertensive Vascular Disease. In J. H. Laragh (ed.), *Hypertension Manual.* New York: Yorke Medical Books, 1974. Pp. 313–351.

94. Lewy, J., Cruz, H., and Metcoff, J. Acute Renal Failure and Some Renal Functions in Acute Glomerulonephritis. In J. Metcoff (ed.), *Acute Glomerulonephritis.* Boston: Little, Brown, 1967. P. 339.

95. Lewy, J. E., Salinas-Madrigal, L., Herdson, P. B., Pirani, C. L., and Metcoff, J. Clinico-pathologic correlations in acute post-streptococcal glomerulonephritis. *Medicine (Baltimore)* 50:453, 1971.

96. Lieberman, E. Critical Analysis of Therapy of Acute Glomerulonephritis Exclusive of Immunosuppressive Drugs. In J. Metcoff (ed.), *Acute Glomerulonephritis.* Boston: Little, Brown, 1967. P. 367.

97. Lyttle, J. D. Addis sediment count in scarlet fever. *J. Clin. Invest.* 12:95, 1933.

98. Lyttle, J. D., and Rosenberg, L. The prognosis of acute nephritis in childhood. *Am. J. Dis. Child.* 38: 1052, 1929.

99. Markowitz, A., Bruton, H. D., Kuttner, A. G., and Cluff, L. E. The bacteriologic findings, streptococcal immune response and renal complications in children with impetigo. *Pediatrics* 35:393, 1965.

100. Maxted, W. R., Fraser, C. A. M., and Parker, M. T. Streptococcus pyogenes type 49: A nephritogenic streptococcus with a wide geographical distribution. *Lancet* 1:641, 1967.

101. McCarty, M. The Antibody Response to Streptococcal infection. In M. McCarty (ed.), *Streptococcal Infections.* New York: Columbia University Press, 1954. Pp. 130–142.

102. McCluskey, R. T., Vassalli, P., Gallo, G., and Baldwin, D. S. An immunofluorescent study of pathogenic mechanisms in glomerular disease. *N. Engl. J. Med.* 274:695, 1966.

103. McCrory, W. W. Natural History of Acute Glomerulonephritis in Children. In J. Metcoff (ed.), *Acute Glomerulonephritis.* Boston: Little, Brown, 1967. P. 15.

104. McCrory, W. W. Glomerulonephritis: Pediatric aspects. *Bull. N.Y. Acad. Med.* 46:789, 1970.

105. McCrory, W. W., Fleisher, D. S., and Sohn, W. B. Effects of early ambulation on the course of nephritis in children. *Pediatrics* 24:395, 1959.

106. McCrory, W. W., and Shibuya, M. Acute glomerulonephritis in childhood. *N.Y. State J. Med.* 68: 2416, 1968.

106a. McLaine, P. N., and Drummond, K. N. Intravenous diazoxide for severe hypertension in childhood. *J. Pediatr.* 79:829, 1971.

107. McLean, R. H., and Michael, A. F. Properdin and C3 proactivator: Alternate pathway components in human glomerulonephritis. *J. Clin. Invest.* 52:634, 1973.

108. Michael, A. F., Jr., Drummond, K. N., Good, R. A., and Vernier, R. L. Acute post-streptococcal glomerulonephritis: Immune deposit disease. *J. Clin. Invest.* 45:237, 1966.

109. Moncrief, M. W., Glasgow, E. F., Arthur, J. H., and Hargraves, H. M. Glomerulonephritis associated with *Staphylococcus albus* in a Spitz Holter valve. *Arch. Dis. Child.* 48:69, 1973.

110. Murth, R. G. Diuretic properties of furosemide in renal disease. *Ann. Intern. Med.* 69:249, 1968.

111. Parrish, A. E. A Relation Between Renal Function and Histology in Glomerulonephritis. In J. Metcoff (ed.), *Acute Glomerulonephritis*. Boston: Little, Brown, 1967. Pp. 291–299.

112. Perlman, L. V., Herdman, R. C., Kleinman, H., and Vernier, R. L. Poststreptococcal glomerulonephritis. A ten year follow-up of an epidemic. *J.A.M.A.* 194:175, 1965.

113. Perrin, L. H., Lambeth, P. H., Nydegger, U. E., and Miescher, P. A. Quantitation of C3PA (properdin factor B) and other complement components in diseases associated with a low C3 level. *Clin. Immunol. Immunopathol.* 2:16, 1973.

114. Poon-King, T., Mohammed, I., Cox, R., Potter, E. V., Simon, N. M., Siegel, A. C., and Earle, D. P. Recurrent epidemic nephritis in South Trinidad. *N. Engl. J. Med.* 277:728, 1967.

115. Popović-Rolović, M. Serum C3 levels in acute glomerulonephritis and postnephritic children. *Arch. Dis. Child.* 48:622, 1973.

116. Potter, E. V., Moran, A. F., Poon-King, T., and Earle, D. P. Characteristics of beta-hemolytic streptococci associated with acute glomerulonephritis in Trinidad, West Indies. *J. Lab. Med.* 71:126, 1967.

117. Potter, E. V., O'Keefe, T. J., Svartman, M., Poon-King, T., and Earle, D. B. Relationship of serum B_1C globulin to fibrinolysis in patients with post-streptococcal acute glomerulonephritis. *J. Lab. Clin. Med.* 82:776, 1973.

117a. Pruit, A. W., and Boles, A. N. N. Diuretic effect of furosemide in acute glomerulonephritis. *J. Pediatr.* 89:306, 1976.

118. Ramberg, R. The prognosis for acute nephritis. *Acta Med. Scand.* 127:396, 1947.

119. Rammelkamp, C. H., Jr. Glomerulonephritis. Frank Billings Lecture. *Proc. Inst. Med. Chic.* 19:371, 1953.

120. Rammelkamp, C. H., Jr. The Streptococcus and Chronic Glomerulonephritis. In F. Ingelfinger, A. Reman, and M. Finland (eds.), *Controversy in Medicine*. Philadelphia: Saunders, 1966. P. 342.

121. Rammelkamp, C. H., Jr., Wannamaker, L. W., and Denny, F. W. The epidemiology and prevention of rheumatic fever. *Bull. N.Y. Acad. Med.* 28:321, 1952.

122. Rammelkamp, C. H., Jr., and Weaver, R. S. Acute glomerulonephritis. *J. Clin. Invest.* 32:359, 1953.

123. Repetto, H. A., Lewy, J. E., Brando, J. L., and Metcoff, J. The renal functional response to furosemide in children with acute glomerulonephritis. *J. Pediatr.* 80:660, 1972.

124. Retan, J. W., and Dillon, H. C., Jr. Furosemide in the treatment of acute poststreptococcal glomerulonephritis. *South. Med. J.* 62:157, 1969.

125. Roscoe, M. H. Biochemical and hematological changes in type 1 and type 2 nephritis. *Q. J. Med.* 19:161, 1950.

126. Rousev, L., Nikolov, G., and Franz, S. Particu-larities in the clinical picture of the acute nephritis by influenza. *Suvr. Med.* 10:54, 1959.

127. Roy, L. P., Fish, A. J., Vernier, R. L., and Michael, A. F. Recurrent macroscopic hematuria, focal nephritis, and mesangial deposition of immunoglobulin and complement. *J. Pediatr.* 82:767, 1973.

128. Rudebeck, J. Clinical and prognostic aspects of acute glomerulonephritis. *Acta Med. Scand.* [Suppl.] 173:1, 1946.

129. Sagel, I., Treser, G., Ty, A., Yoshizarva, N., Kleinberger, H., Yuccoglu, A. M., Wassermann, E., and Lange, K. Occurrence and nature of glomerular lesions after group A streptococci infections in children. *Ann. Intern. Med.* 79:492, 1973.

130. Schwartz, W. B., and Kassirer, J. P. Clinical Aspects of Acute Poststreptococcal Glomerulonephritis. In M. B. Strauss and L. G. Welt (eds.), *Diseases of the Kidney*. Boston: Little, Brown, 1971. Pp. 419–462.

131. Seegal, B. C., Andres, G. A., Hsu, K. C., and Zabriskie, J. B. Studies on the pathogenesis of acute and progressive glomerulonephritis in many by immunofluorescein and immunoferritin techniques. *Fed. Proc.* 24:100, 1965.

132. Seegal, D. Acute glomerulonephritis following pneumococci lobar pneumonia: Analysis of 7 cases. *Arch. Intern. Med.* 56:912, 1935.

133. Seegal, D., Lyttle, J. D., Loeb, E. N., Jost, E. L., and Davis, G. On the exacerbation in chronic glomerulonephritis. *J. Clin. Invest.* 19:569, 1940.

134. Singer, D. B., Hill, L. L., Rosenberg, H. S., Marshall, J., and Swenson, R. Recurrent hematuria in childhood. *N. Engl. J. Med.* 279:7, 1968.

135. Steigman, A. J., Hughes, W. T., and deLong, H. Mumps 1961 and severe nephritis. *Lancet* 2:827, 1961.

136. Stetson, C. A., Rammelkamp, C. H., Jr., Krause, R. M., Kohen, R. J., and Perry, W. D. Epidemic acute nephritis: Studies on etiology, natural history, and prevention. *Medicine (Baltimore)* 34:431, 1955.

137. Stiehm, E. R., and Trygstad, C. W. Split products of fibrin in human renal disease. *Am. J. Med.* 46:774, 1969.

138. Svartman, M., Potter, E. V., Poon-King, T., and Earle, D. P. Streptococcal infection of scabetic lesions related to acute glomerulonephritis in Trinidad. *J. Lab. Clin. Med.* 81:182, 1973.

139. Travis, L. B. Course and prognosis of children with PSAGN. Report presented to the Third International Congress of Pediatric Nephrology, Washington, D.C., October, 1974.

140. Travis, L. B. Personal observations, unpublished.

141. Travis, L. B. Prognosis of acute glomerulonephritis in children. *South. Med. J.* 67:1396, 1974.

142. Travis, L. B., and Daeschner, C. W., Jr. Hypertension Associated with Acute Glomerulonephritis. In A. Brest and J. Moyer (eds.), *Hyptertension, Recent Advances*. Philadelphia: Lea & Febiger, 1961. P. 540.

143. Travis, L. B., Daeschner, C. W., Jr., Dodge, W. F., Hopps, H. C., and Rosenberg, H. S. "Idiopathic" hematuria. *J. Pediatr.* 50:24, 1962.

144. Travis, L. B., Dodge, W. F., Beathard, G. A., Spargo, B. H., Lorentz, W. B., Carvajal, H. F., and Berger, M. Acute glomerulonephritis in children: A review of the natural history with emphasis on prognosis. *Clin. Nephrol.* 1:169, 1973.

145. Travis, L. B., Street, L., Smith, E. H., and Chipps, B. E. Renal Involvement in Systemic Diseases in Childhood. In W. N. Suki and G. Eknoyan (eds.), *The Kidney in Systemic Disease*. New York: Wiley, 1976. P. 275.

146. Treser, G., Semar, M., McVicar, M., Franklin, M., Ty, A., Sagel, I., and Lange, K. Antigenic streptococcal components in acute glomerulonephritis. *Science* 163:676, 1969.

147. Updyke, E. L., Moore, M. S., and Conroy, E. Provisional new type of group A streptococci associated with nephritis. *Science* 121:171, 1955.

148. Valkenburg, H. A., Haverborn, M. J., Goslings, W. R. O., Lorrier, J. C., deMoor, C. E., and Maxted, W. R. Streptococcal pharyngitis in the general population. II. The attack rate of rheumatic fever and acute glomerulonephritis in patients not treated with penicillin. *J. Infect. Dis.* 124:348, 1971.

149. Vallota, E. H., Forristal, J., Spitzer, R. E., Davis, N. C., and West, C. D. Characteristics of non-complement dependent C3 reactive complex formed from factors in nephritic and normal serum. *J. Exp. Med.* 131:1306, 1970.

150. Vassalli, P., and McClusky, R. T. The Pathogenetic Role of the Coagulation Process in Glomerular Diseases of Immunologic Origin. In J. Hamburger, J. Crosnier, and M. H. Maxwell (eds.), *Advances in Nephrology*. Chicago: Year Book, 1971. P. 47.

151. Verel, D., Turnbull, A., Tudhope, G. R., and Ross, J. H. Anemia in Bright's disease. *Q. J. Med.* 28:491, 1959.

152. Vernier, R. L., Worthen, H. G., Wannamaker, L. W., and Good, R. A. Renal biopsy studies of the acute exacerbation in glomerulonephritis. *Am. J. Dis. Child.* 98:653, 1959.

153. Verroust, P. J., Wilson, C. B., Cooper, N. R., Edgington, T. S., and Dixon, F. J. Glomerular complement components in human glomerulonephritis. *J. Clin. Invest.* 53:77, 1974.

154. Wahrer, C. F. An epidemic of hemorrhagic nephritis following scarlet fever. *J.A.M.A.* 51:1410, 1908.

155. Wannamaker, L. W. Medical progress: Difference between streptococcal infections of the throat and of the skin. *N. Engl. J. Med.* 282:23, 78, 1970.

156. Weinstein, L., and Tsao, C. C. L. Effect of types of treatment on development of antistreptolysin in patients with scarlet fever. *Proc. Soc. Exp. Biol. Med.* 63:449, 1946.

157. West, C. D., Northway, J. D., and Davis, N. C. Serum levels of B1C globulin, a complement component in the nephritides, lipoid nephrosis, and other conditions. *J. Clin. Invest.* 43:507, 1964.

158. Westberg, N. G., Naff, G. B., Boyer, J. T., and Michael, A. F. Glomerular deposition of properdin in acute and chronic glomerulonephritis with hypocomplementemia. *J. Clin. Invest.* 50:642, 1971.

159. White, R. H. R. "Silent nephritis." A study based on renal biopsies. *Guys Hosp. Rep.* 113:190, 1964.

160. Williams, D. G., Charlesworth, J. A., Lachmann, P. J., and Peters, D. K. Role of C3b in the breakdown of C3 in hypocomplementaemic mesangiocapillary glomerulonephritis. *Lancet* 1:447, 1973.

161. Wilson, C. B., and Dixon, F. J. Diagnosis of immunopathologic renal disease. *Kidney Int.* 5:389, 1974.

162. Yuceoglu, A. M., Berkovich, S., and Minkowitz, S. Acute glomerulonephritis associated with ECHO virus type 9 infection. *J. Pediatr.* 69:903, 1966.

163. Zabriskie, J. B., Utermohlen, V., Read, S. E., and Fishetti, V. A. Streptococcus-related glomerulonephritis. *Kidney Int.* 3:100, 1973.

48. Rapidly Progressive Glomerulonephritis

Edmund J. Lewis and Melvin M. Schwartz

The clinical term *rapidly progressive glomerulonephritis* (RPGN) applies to patients with a particularly fulminant form of inflammatory glomerular disease. These patients present with a syndrome of acute onset and pursue a progressive course to renal failure in weeks or months. The historic origin of the term *RPGN* is credited to Ellis [19], who called attention to that small percentage (4 percent) of his patients with glomerulonephritis of acute onset (Ellis's type 1) whose clinical course was "rapidly progressive with persistence of symptoms and a fatal issue within a period of months." He correlated this clinical course with a typical histologic picture at au-

topsy.* The characteristic feature of the renal lesion is the abundant formation of glomerular crescents that may not be accompanied by severe cellular proliferation within the glomerular tuft, hence the term *extracapillary glomerulonephritis* suggested by Fahr [20]. Literature on the subject of RPGN is sometimes confusing due to the descrip-

* "When death occurs after the rapidly progressive course, the outstanding feature is the formation of large epithelial crescents and associated hemorrhage into Bowman's space; acute fibrinoid necrosis of arterioles is common and a few cases show an intense inflammatory infiltration of the interstitial tissue with 'explosive' lesions of the glomeruli and definite periglomerular inflammatory reaction [19]."

tive clinical nature of the term. This reflects the fact that a wide variety of diseases involving several pathogenetic mechanisms may result in a similar clinical and histopathologic constellation. The diagnostic categorization of RPGN, therefore, applies only after poststreptococcal glomerulonephritis and several systemic illnesses are ruled out. Other designations such as crescentic glomerulonephritis, malignant glomerulonephritis, severe fibrin and crescent glomerulonephritis, and subacute glomerulonephritis are among the terms that have also been used to describe the RPGN syndrome.

Clinical and Laboratory Features

Rapidly progressive glomerulonephritis is seen most commonly in adults, the mean age in several of the reported series being in the fourth decade [5, 31, 45]; however, it can occur at any age. The most frequently reported cases in the pediatric age group are in older children and adolescents (Table 48-1) [2, 13, 52, 56]. There does not appear to be any difference in the course and prognosis of the syndrome based upon the age of the patient; children fare as poorly as adults. In the typical case the onset is acute and the patient has felt ill for less than 3 weeks. A preceding upper respiratory or flulike illness has been described in up to one-half the cases in some series. There is usually no serologic evidence of viral or streptococcal infection (and strictly speaking, a documented, antecedent streptococcal infection excludes the patient from the diagnosis of RPGN). Acute poststreptococcal glomerulonephritis, which may present in an identical manner, is thus differentiated as a separate entity.

The patient is usually oliguric or anuric at the time of admission to the hospital. If elevation of the blood pressure does occur, it is usually not a prominent finding. Proteinuria, microscopic hematuria, and red cell casts are evident. The patient's renal function is usually markedly compromised at the time of hospitalization. Recovery is rare [31]. Serum C3 and C4 levels are normal or elevated. Immunoglobulins that precipitate at 4°C. (cryoglobulins) have been reported in some patients. While cryoglobulins have been characterized as immunoglobulins that are participating in an antigen-antibody reaction in systemic lupus erythematosus, essential IgG-IgM cryoglobulinemia, and serum sickness, the pathogenetic significance of this phenomenon in RPGN is unclear [1]. Circulating anti–glomerular basement membrane (anti-GBM) antibodies have been noted in many patients in several series of RPGN [30, 31, 35].

Pathology

The most striking lesion in RPGN is extracapillary proliferative glomerulonephritis, which, by definition, predominantly involves the epithelial cells [8, 9, 31, 42, 45]. Frequently exuberant cellular crescent formation appears to be compressing a collapsed glomerular capillary tuft (Fig. 48-1). The cellular composition of the crescent is classically believed to be proliferating parietal epithelial cells [42, 43]. Mitotic figures may be evident in the actively hyperplastic tissue of the crescent (Fig. 48-2). Evidence has been presented that supports the point of view that some of the cellular elements of the crescents in human RPGN are macrophages; this remains a controversial area

Table 48-1. Rapidly Progressive Glomerulonephritis in Children and Adolescents

Series	No. of Patients	Age (yr)	Males	Females	Recent Antecedent Illness	Oligoanuria	Hypertension
Anand et al. [2]	7	Range, 0–17	2	5	*	3	6
Berlyne and Baker [8]	3	10, 10, 17	0	3	0	3	1
Burkholder and Bradford [13]	4	1, 5, 10, 15	1	3	3	*	*
Lewis et al. [31]	2	18, 20	1	1	2	2	1
Sonsino et al. [52]	3	5, 14, 15	1	2	3	3	1
Striker et al. [56]	6	Range, 0–10	2	4	1	4	1
	14	Range, 11–20	5	9	8	13	3
TOTAL	39		12	27	17(53%)	28(80%)	13(37%)

* Data not available in report.

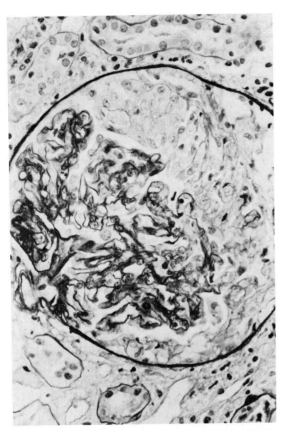

Figure 48-1. A representative glomerulus from a patient with rapidly progressive glomerulonephritis associated with anti–glomerular basement membrane antibodies. The "extracapillary" lesion is characterized by a crescent of epithelial cells that fill Bowman's space and surround the collapsed glomerulus. The glomerular basement membrane is well preserved, and there is little proliferation of cells intrinsic to the tuft. Periodic acid–Schiff reaction. (×350.)

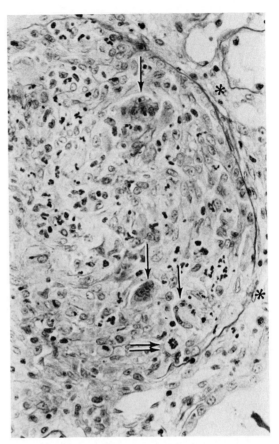

Figure 48-2. The cellular makeup of the glomerular crescent includes actively dividing cells; note the mitotic figure (double arrow). In addition, multinucleated giant cells are present (single arrows). Polymorphonuclear leukocytes are present in abundance in this crescent. Whereas the crescent has been considered to be composed of hyperplastic epithelial cells, some evidence supports the possibility that macrophages derived from blood monocytes are also present. Bowman's capsule (asterisks) shows focal dissolution. Periodic acid–Schiff reaction. (×350.)

[4, 27]. The pathologic diagnosis requires that a clear majority of glomeruli be involved by crescent formation.

The glomerular tuft can also be involved by a proliferative lesion; the cellular elements involved in this reaction appear to include the epithelial cells (Fig. 48-3). The lesion may be diffuse or it may be focal, with the glomerular architecture in a given biopsy ranging from normal to total destruction (Fig. 48-4). Disruption of the continuity of the glomerular capillary wall can sometimes be demonstrated using routine histologic stains (Fig. 48-5). In some cases of RPGN there is a dramatic cellular proliferation with complete destruction of the glomerular architecture and the production of giant cells, causing formation of a "pseudogranuloma" (Fig. 48-6) [31]. Neutrophils are often a prominent feature within the glomerulus and in crescents (Figs. 48-2, 48-3). The lesion is to be distinguished from that of acute poststreptococcal glomerulonephritis (see under Differential Diagnosis).

Lymphoid cells are noted in the interstitium of the cortex, and they frequently appear to have a periglomerular distribution. Acute vasculitis has been described in small renal arteries, making the distinction between the lesion of RPGN and that of microscopic polyarteritis nodosa difficult or impossible (Fig. 48-7) [22, 31]. It should be noted that vasculitis has been described in patients in whom anti-GBM antibodies are involved in the mediation of the glomerular damage. The pathogenesis of arteriolitis in these patients is unclear.

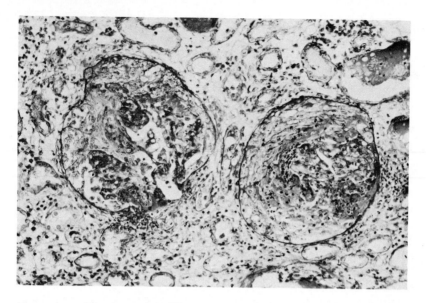

Figure 48-3. A pronounced proliferative and necrotizing lesion affects these two glomeruli. The endocapillary proliferation and necrosis are accompanied by extracapillary crescent formation. In addition, many polymorphonuclear leukocytes are seen in the tuft on the left of the photograph. Periodic acid–Schiff reaction. (×250.)

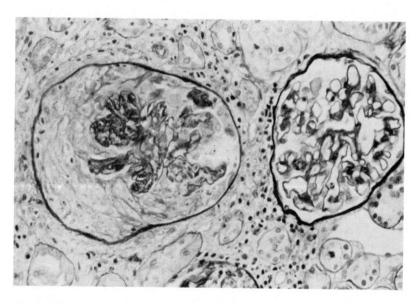

Figure 48-4. Variability in glomerulonephritis mediated by anti–glomerular basement membrane antibody. The glomerulus on the left has a large crescent, within which rests a partially collapsed capillary tuft. Note the virtually normal glomerulus on the right. Linear deposits of IgG were deposited on all the glomeruli in this biopsy. Periodic acid–Schiff reaction. (×250.)

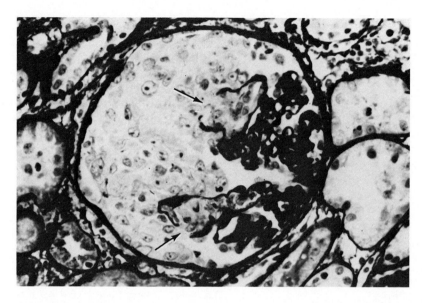

Figure 48-5. Glomerulus with obvious defects in the continuity of some capillary walls (arrows). The cells of the glomerular crescent, which occupy the entire left-hand portion of Bowman's space, appear contiguous with cellular elements that extend from these disrupted capillary loops. Methenamine silver, periodic acid–Schiff reaction. (×350.)

Immunopathology

Three varieties of RPGN may be distinguished according to the presence of IgG in the glomeruli and its pattern of deposition. The majority of patients with RPGN have evidence of anti-GBM antibodies deposited in glomeruli and responsible for the inflammatory glomerular damage. A second group of patients with identical clinical and histologic pictures has evidence of deposits of antigen-antibody complexes on the GBM. The third subtype has no evident IgG deposited on glomeruli or the deposited IgG is in an irregular, sparse, or focal pattern analogous to neither anti-GBM–mediated injury nor immune complex disease. Presumably this last type represents a separate pathogenetic subgroup.

RAPIDLY PROGRESSIVE GLOMERULONEPHRITIS WITH ANTI–GLOMERULAR BASEMENT MEMBRANE ANTIBODIES

The terms *continuous, ribbon-like,* or *linear* have been used to describe the immunofluorescent pattern of deposition of IgG along the GBM in RPGN with anti-GBM antibodies (Fig. 48-8) [30, 31, 38, 46]. A large proportion of these patients have demonstrable anti-GBM antibodies in their serum [31, 35, 39]. Immunoglobulins other than IgG may be found in the glomerular deposits associated with anti-GBM disease. Immunoglobulin M has been described in an interrupted,

patchy, linear pattern, and IgA and IgE have occasionally been noted. C3 is present in one-half to two-thirds of patients with anti-GBM–mediated nephritis [31, 40, 46]. There has been no adequate explanation for the absence of complement in some glomerular deposits [61, 62]. Proliferative glomerulonephritis is a prominent finding despite the inability to demonstrate deposited complement components, suggesting that some other mechanism is mediating glomerular damage. Further, patients with severe focal glomerular lesions (see Fig. 48-4) can have an identical deposition of IgG and C3 in both affected and unaffected glomeruli.

Fibrin is consistently found in the areas of crescent formation (Fig. 48-9) [31]. Experimental models of anti-GBM–mediated glomerulonephritis have been utilized to demonstrate the importance of fibrin deposition in the genesis of crescents. The interruption of the clotting system by heparin or fibrinogen depletion with ancrod (Malayan pit-viper venom coagulation factor) effectively prevents crescent formation in the heterologous anti-GBM (nephrotoxic) glomerulonephritis model [44, 57, 59]. It seems likely that the leakage of proteins of the clotting system through severely damaged glomerular capillary walls leads to fibrin deposition along Bowman's capsule. The mechanism whereby this deposition triggers crescent formation is not understood. Perhaps fibrin deposition along Bowman's capsule stimulates the

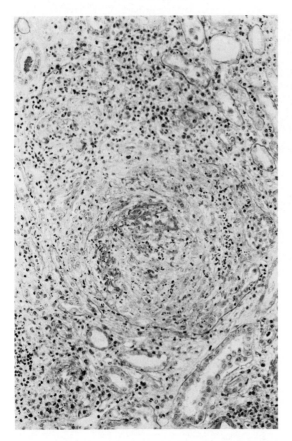

Figure 48-6. A destroyed glomerulus typical of the biopsy findings in glomerular injury mediated by anti–glomerular basement membrane antibody. The collapsed glomerulus is represented by the remnants of the glomerular basement membrane, which is compressed by epithelial cells forming a crescent completely encircling the capillary tuft. Bowman's capsule has been breached in many places as the crescent extends into the surrounding interstitium. Lymphoid cells plentifully surround this glomerulus, and multinucleated giant cells, which were present in other glomeruli, contribute to the histologic appearance of a so-called glomerular pseudogranuloma. Periodic acid–Schiff reaction. (×350.)

migration and proliferation of cells with phagocytic properties capable of the removal of this material [4, 27].

Electron Microscopy

No consistent ultrastructural lesion has been associated with RPGN with anti-GBM antibodies. A lucency and widening of the lamina rara interna may be noted, and in some areas the endothelium may appear to be detached from the GBM; however, these do not appear to constitute a specific lesion [5]. Usually there are no electron-dense de-

posits in the subepithelial or subendothelial areas. Nondiscrete intramembranous deposits may be present. "Gaps" or defects in the continuity of the GBM have been described, perhaps explaining the leakage of large proteins such as fibrinogen into Bowman's space. This abnormality has been termed the *focal disruptive lesion* of RPGN [55]. Fibrin extravasation can be demonstrated in Bowman's space. With time the epithelial crescent evolves into a fibrous crescent containing collagen [5, 10, 14].

Formation of Anti–Glomerular Basement Membrane Antibodies

The mechanism whereby antibody to native GBM antigens forms is a matter of great interest and speculation. While many patients have reported nonspecific illnesses prior to the onset of renal disease, common epidemiologic factors have not been identified. Several patients have had a concurrent history of cardiovascular pathology, including bacterial endocarditis, rheumatic fever, myocardial infarction, and aortic aneurysm [31]. However, the possible relationship between these diseases and the formation of anti-GBM antibody is unclear. Several general mechanisms for autosensitization to GBM have been suggested:

1. Immunization of an experimental animal with GBM antigens can lead to the development of pathogenetic anti-GBM antibodies [29, 53]. Therefore, a condition that is associated with the exposure to the immune system of an otherwise inaccessible GBM antigen may trigger the abnormal immune response. Presumably Klassen's case of membranous glomerulopathy that evolved into anti-GBM–associated RPGN could be explained on the basis of autosensitization due to antigen release from diseased glomeruli [26]. Reports of in vitro evidence of humoral and cellular immunity to GBM antigens in diseases such as renal cortical necrosis and thrombotic microangiopathy may also reflect the occurrence of this immune mechanism as a secondary phenomenon [33, 34].

2. The immunization of an animal with basement membrane material from another organ such as lung can initiate RPGN due to the development of antibodies that cross-react with the GBM [54]. In a model of passively induced nephrotoxic nephritis, heterologous antiserum to alveolar basement membrane deposits on GBM and causes glomerulonephritis, emphasizing the antigenic similarity of these two organs [41]. Hence the systemic release of an endogenous nonrenal basement membrane antigen could

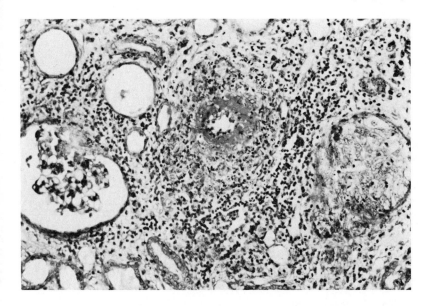

Figure 48-7. Acute vasculitis in rapidly progressive glomerulonephritis mediated by anti–glomerular basement membrane antibodies. The necrotic artery in the center of this illustration is involved by an acute inflammatory reaction throughout its wall. Fibrinoid necrosis is noted in the circumferential zone surrounding the swollen endothelium. Polymorphonuclear leukocytes infiltrate the muscular wall and the surrounding interstitium. The glomerulus on the left is relatively normal, while that on the right is entirely necrotic. (H&E, ×250.)

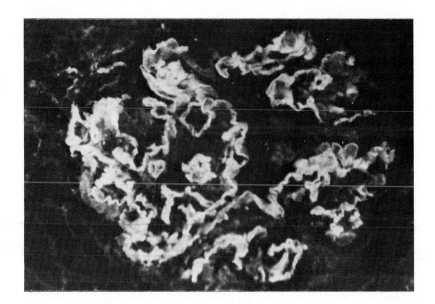

Figure 48-8. Rapidly progressive glomerulonephritis with anti–glomerular basement membrane antibodies. The typical distribution of immunoglobulin G is noted along the glomerular capillary basement membranes of this partially collapsed tuft. Goat antihuman IgG. (×350.)

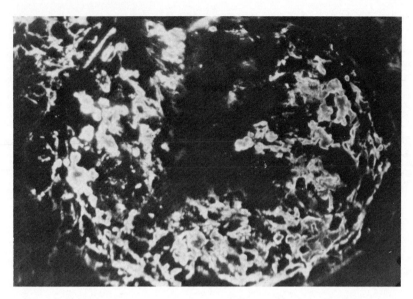

Figure 48-9. Antifibrinogen antiserum stains the cells and interstitial spaces of this glomerular crescent. The glomerular tuft is negative and appears as a central black arrowhead-shaped image pointed toward the left lower corner of the illustration (▶); it is embedded in the fibrinogen-rich crescent. Goat antihuman fibrinogen. (×350.)

elicit an immune response that would be capable of causing anti-GBM–mediated nephritis.

3. Some microorganisms have antigens that are similar in composition to GBM and could conceivably be capable of inducing cross-reacting antibodies to human GBM antigens [37].

4. It is possible that an alteration of the chemical structure of normal GBM could lead to antibody formation and subsequent cross-reaction with normal GBM. Curtis et al. have described a patient with nail-patella syndrome with its characteristic ultrastructural abnormality of GBM, and this patient developed anti-GBM antibodies and Goodpasture's syndrome [17]. It was hypothesized that an abnormality in the antigenic structure of the GBM ultimately led to antibody formation.

Pathogenicity of Anti–Glomerular Basement Membrane Antibodies

Attention to the significance of anti-GBM antibodies in clinical material was originally noted by Lerner et al., who demonstrated that these antibodies satisfied a modified form of Koch's postulates for pathogenicity [30]. Deposited antibodies could be transferred to normal glomeruli in vitro, indicating antibody specificity for fixed normal GBM antigen. When injected into the squirrel monkey, anti-GBM antibodies fixed to GBM in vivo and caused glomerular inflammation [30].

When a patient with anti-GBM antibody–mediated glomerulonephritis underwent renal transplantation, recurrent glomerulonephritis appeared concomitantly with deposition of antibodies in the allograft [6, 30]. Since these first observations, it has been pointed out that the deposition of anti-GBM antibodies in human glomeruli does not necessarily lead to severe extracapillary glomerulonephritis; indeed, such deposition may be associated with very mild disease [40]. The deposition of anti-GBM antibodies in renal allografts has not always led to recurrent nephritis, even when the original lesion was that of RPGN [16]. While reasons for the clinical variability of anti-GBM antibody expression remain unclear, the documented reports of recurrent glomerulonephritis in some transplants has established the potential pathogenicity of these antibodies [6].

Tests for Disease Mediated by Anti–Glomerular Basement Antibody

Direct Glomerular Immunofluorescence. Direct immunofluorescence revealing the presence and distribution of IgG on renal biopsy material usually is the initial laboratory observation that suggests anti-GBM–mediated nephritis (see Fig. 48-8) [30, 31]. While this test is readily performed on biopsy specimens, it is emphasized that there are many pitfalls to the technique. Nonspecific linear staining of the GBM with fluorescein-tagged antibody to human IgG is a common artifact of the direct immunofluorescent technique and does not necessarily indicate specific deposition of anti-GBM antibodies [18, 62]. Many technical factors related to handling and storage of frozen tissue and fluorescein conjugation of the antibody reagent can be responsible for nonspecific staining of the GBM. In addition, staining for IgG may be positive because IgG is present within an abnormally permeable GBM. Presumably this explains positive linear fluorescence in some biopsies from patients with systemic lupus erythematosus, diabetes mellitus, and amyloid in whom there is no demonstrable evidence that the IgG has anti-GBM activity [18, 21]. Because of the lack of specificity of the finding of a linear IgG deposit, other evidence of deposited or circulating anti-GBM antibody should be required in order to establish the diagnosis of anti-GBM–mediated nephritis. In addition, examination of the biopsy material by electron microscopy can help further differentiate the pathogenesis of the lesion.

Serum Anti-GBM Antibodies. INDIRECT IMMU-NOFLUORESCENCE. Immunofluorescence examination can be carried out after the incubation of serum with frozen sections from fresh normal kidney in order to determine whether there has been specific fixation of IgG in the specimen to normal GBM [30, 35, 39, 40, 62]. This reaction must be carefully controlled, however, and even under the most rigorous circumstances some nonspecific staining of the GBM can occur.

OTHER ANTIBODY DETECTION TECHNIQUES. Numerous serologic methods have been applied to determine serum anti-GBM activity. Passive hemagglutination [33–35], radioimmunoassay [35, 63] and the precipitin-in-gel reaction [30] have been successfully applied.

Cellular Hypersensitivity to GBM. Cellular techniques have been applied to the determination of GBM hypersensitivity. The standard guinea pig macrophage assay for migration inhibitory factor has been utilized in order to determine GBM sensitization [49]. Bendixen has used peripheral blood leukocytes in order to determine sensitization to kidney antigens [7, 51]. Mahieu [34] and others [33, 36] have observed that the leukocyte migration test for GBM sensitivity may be positive in patients with or without glomerular anti-GBM deposition. It is possible that cellular hypersensitivity to GBM can be an epiphenomenon in certain patients with severe glomerular damage [36]. The reactivity of some cellular tests for anti-GBM sensitivity is therefore not specific for humoral anti-GBM–mediated glomerulonephritis.

RAPIDLY PROGRESSIVE GLOMERULONEPHRITIS WITH ANTIGEN-ANTIBODY COMPLEXES

In the biopsies from some RPGN patients, granular deposits of IgG are found along the glomerular capillary wall [31, 49]. It is assumed that these granules represent aggregated immune complexes. Antigen-antibody complexes therefore have the potential to initiate the same histologic lesion as anti-GBM antibodies. As granules of IgG are also found on the GBM of glomeruli from biopsies of acute poststreptococcal glomerulonephritis, the latter diagnosis must be carefully ruled out by bacteriologic and serologic means.

RAPIDLY PROGRESSIVE GLOMERULONEPHRITIS WITH SCANTY OR NO GLOMERULAR IgG DEPOSITION

Cases of RPGN have been described with no characteristic pattern of immunoglobulin deposition [46]. The glomerular lesion appears to be mediated by some mechanism alternative to the classic immune pathways described above. These patients fall into a similar diagnostic category to those with microscopic periarteritis nodosa who may also have notable glomerular pathology and negative immunofluorescence findings.

Differential Diagnosis of Rapidly Progressive Glomerulonephritis

At the time of presentation, the patient with the acute onset of severe renal failure presents a puzzling diagnostic problem. Rapidly progressive glomerulonephritis must be differentiated from severe acute poststreptococcal glomerulonephritis and other inflammatory glomerulopathies, such as microscopic polyarteritis nodosa, Goodpasture's syndrome, membranoproliferative glomerulonephritis, systemic lupus erythematosus, essential cryoglobulinemia, Schönlein-Henoch purpura, and acute bacterial endocarditis (Table 48-2). Disorders that can simulate the clinical pattern of RPGN syndrome because they present with the insidious onset of acute renal insufficiency include the hemolytic-uremic syndrome, acute tubular necrosis (acute vasomotor nephropathy), and acute interstitial nephritis.

DIFFERENTIATION BETWEEN RAPIDLY PROGRESSIVE GLOMERULONEPHRITIS AND ACUTE POSTSTREPTOCOCCAL GLOMERULONEPHRITIS

Differentiation between RPGN and poststreptococcal acute glomerulonephritis (PSAGN) can be extremely difficult, as the clinical presentation of

Table 48-2. Differential Features among Syndromes with Extracapillary Glomerulonephritis

Feature	Pulmonary Hemorrhage	Histologic Vasculitis	Depressed C3	Anti-GBM	Cryo-globulins	ANA	Glomerular Immuno-fluorescence (IgG)
Rapidly progressive GN							
1.	0	±	0	+	±	0	Linear
2.	0	±	0	0	±	0	Granular
3.	0	±	0	0	±	0	None
Acute post-streptococcal GN	0	0–±	+	0	+	0	Granular
Microscopic periarteritis nodosa	±	+	0	0	+	0	Negative or granular
Goodpasture's syndrome	+	±	0	+	0	0	Linear
Membrano-proliferative glomerulonephritis	0	0	+	0	±	0	Peripheral lobular IgG, C3
Systemic lupus erythematosus	±	±	+	0	+	+	Granular
Schönlein-Henoch purpura	0	+	0	0	0	0	Mesangial IgA, IgG, fibrin
Essential cryoglobulinemia	0	+	+	0	+	±	Granular
Acute bacterial endocarditis	0	±	+	0	+	±	Granular

Note: GN = glomerulonephritis; GBM = glomerular basement membrane; ANA = antinuclear antibodies; 0 = not associated; ± = rare or uncharacteristic finding; + = characteristically associated.

patients with PSAGN may be identical with that of RPGN [28, 48, 50]. Severe hypertension and accompanying generalized edema, while unusual in RPGN, are consistent features of PSAGN. The antistreptolysin O, antistreptococcal hyaluronidase, and anti-DNase B titers are elevated in PSAGN. Serum C3 levels characteristically are depressed in PSAGN, while this is rarely the case in RPGN.

While the renal biopsy may reveal features similar to RPGN, there being extensive crescent formation in the more severe cases of PSAGN, several differential points have been cited. The cellular makeup of the glomerular lesion in PSAGN more often includes a prominent endocapillary component, and the proliferating cells in the tuft are primarily endothelial, mesangial, and possibly monocytic. This contrasts with the extracapillary epithelial cell proliferation of RPGN. In addition, glomerular changes in PSAGN are diffuse; all glomeruli appear equally affected and at the same stage of disease development. In contrast, RPGN is frequently a focal lesion with variation in the stage and degree of involvement among glomeruli.

Immunofluorescence microscopy may also help differentiate PSAGN and RPGN, revealing a granular deposition of IgG and C3 along the glomerular capillary loops and within the mesangium in PSAGN. However, when anti-GBM antibodies are not involved, the RPGN syndrome can be associated with granular IgG deposits.

The prognosis of PSAGN, even when it is associated with prolonged oliguria and many crescentic lesions, is statistically better than that of RPGN [28, 50], although precise separation of PSAGN from RPGN is still not possible.

DIFFERENTIATION BETWEEN RAPIDLY PROGRESSIVE GLOMERULONEPHRITIS AND MICROSCOPIC POLYARTERITIS NODOSA
There are many identical clinical and histologic features between the renal lesion of microscopic polyarteritis nodosa and RPGN [22, 31, 60]. Clinically the renal lesion in microscopic polyarteritis nodosa can overshadow other evidence of systemic disease. In addition, histologic evidence of vasculitis and circulating cryoglobulins has been reported in patients with both syndromes.

The linear deposition of IgG on the GBM has been taken as a differential feature for RPGN; the glomeruli in periarteritis nodosa frequently have no evidence of immunoglobulin deposition in the glomerulus or in affected vessels. To further emphasize the pathologic and immunologic overlap between microscopic polyarteritis nodosa and RPGN, patients with polyarteritis nodosa have been shown to have low-affinity anti-GBM antibodies in serum. Leukocyte migration tests for cellular sensitivity to GBM have also been positive in polyarteritis nodosa. The same findings have been noted also in diseases associated with severe glomerular necrosis, such as renal cortical necrosis and thrombotic microangiopathy. Therefore, it is possible that when in vitro anti-GBM reactivity occurs in polyarteritis nodosa, it is secondary to tissue damage rather than a primary pathogenetic process [33, 34].

In view of the clinical, pathologic, and immunologic overlap of microscopic polyarteritis nodosa and RPGN, it would appear appropriate to reserve the diagnosis of microscopic polyarteritis nodosa for patients who manifest clinical or pathologic evidence of microvascular inflammation in organs other than the kidney.

DIFFERENTIATION BETWEEN GOODPASTURE'S SYNDROME AND RAPIDLY PROGRESSIVE GLOMERULONEPHRITIS

The presentation and clinical course of the renal lesions in Goodpasture's syndrome and RPGN are often similar, although the prognosis in Goodpasture's syndrome does not appear to be as uniformly catastrophic as is that of RPGN. While pulmonary hemorrhage usually precedes or occurs at the same time as the renal abnormalities of Goodpasture's syndrome, there are occasional instances of a renal presentation of the disease. Therefore even the slightest complaint of hemoptysis or finding of minimal alveolar infiltrates on chest x-ray should be looked upon with suspicion in a patient initially diagnosed as having RPGN with anti-GBM antibodies.

OTHER DISORDERS IN THE DIFFERENTIAL DIAGNOSIS

Systemic Lupus Erythematosus. Occasionally patients with systemic lupus erythematosus will present with severe progressive glomerulonephritis and few systemic abnormalities. Positive tests for antibodies to native DNA and a low serum complement are noted in these patients. The histopathologic lesion may reveal diffuse proliferative glomerulonephritis with many glomeruli having crescents; however, prominent deposits of immunoglobulins and complement components in the capillary loops and mesangium and electron-dense subendothelial deposits differentiate this glomerular lesion from that of RPGN.

Schönlein-Henoch Purpura. Differential features are based upon the characteristic systemic involvement of gut, skin, and joints in Schönlein-Henoch purpura. While the histopathology of the kidney in Schönlein-Henoch purpura can be identical to that of RPGN, the immunopathologic features of this disease are quite different. Characteristically, IgA, IgG, and fibrin are deposited in the mesangium in Schönlein-Henoch purpura; the immunofluorescence lesion is therefore quite distinctive from that of RPGN with anti-GBM antibodies. The presence of large quantities of mesangial IgA therefore distinguishes Schönlein-Henoch purpura from other varieties of RPGN. Deposits of IgA in blood vessels of the skin may also occur in Schönlein-Henoch purpura.

Essential Cryoglobulinemia. Differentiation of these patients from those with RPGN is based upon the more characteristic multisystem involvement in patients with essential cryoglobulinemia [1]. The circulating cryoglobulin is usually composed of IgG and IgM. Rheumatoid factor is usually present. Antinuclear antibodies have been reported in some patients. Immunohistology of the glomerular lesion reveals deposition of IgG, IgM, and C3 in a granular pattern.

Bacterial Endocarditis. This entity must be included in the differential diagnosis of an acutely ill patient with severe renal disease and the biopsy finding of diffuse proliferative glomerulonephritis. In addition to the clinically differentiating features of the acutely ill patient with febrile disease and a cardiac lesion, the serologic and immunopathologic picture is somewhat distinct from that of RPGN. Serum C3 levels are usually depressed; rheumatoid factor may be present; cryoglobulins and antinuclear antibodies may also be in evidence. The renal biopsy reveals granular deposits of IgG, IgM, and C3, all of which are believed to represent the deposition of antigen-antibody complexes related to the bacterial infection.

Prognosis and Therapy

Several criteria have been assessed in determining the prognosis of patients with the RPGN syndrome. These include (1) clinical or serologic evidence of a preceding streptococcal infection; (2) the percentage of glomeruli involved by epithelial cell crescents; (3) the presence or absence of proliferation in the glomerular tuft; (4) the presence of endocapillary proliferation; and (5) the pattern of deposition of IgG in the glomeruli or serologic evidence of anti-GBM antibodies. The results in most series indicate that patients with evidence of preceding streptococcal infection have a much better prognosis than those with no apparent etiology for their disease [28, 50]. While there is no absolute percentage of crescentic glomeruli that would indicate a poor prognosis, it would appear that when more than two-thirds of glomeruli have crescents and there is no proliferation in the glomerular tuft, the prognosis is very poor [8, 10, 42]. If there is endocapillary proliferation accompanying the crescents, even when greater than 67 percent of glomeruli have these crescents, spontaneous resolution can occur [50]. This latter group presumably includes many patients with PSAGN. The finding of linear deposits of IgG in glomeruli and other evidence of anti-GBM antibodies has been associated with a poor prognosis [31].

Reports of therapeutic attempts aimed at amelioration of the immune and inflammatory lesions using corticosteroids and immunosuppressives and cytotoxic alkylating agents have been variable [25]. In general, the results have been poor. The role of anticoagulants in the treatment of the lesions has been the subject of controversy. Good responses to therapy [3, 12, 17, 23, 25, 54] have been categorized by the finding of fewer crescents when another biopsy is performed. The rigorous exclusion of patients who tend to go into remission spontaneously, particularly those with PSAGN, is required before the effectiveness of anticoagulants can be evaluated [11, 28, 47]. Nevertheless, experimental models of anti-GBM–mediated RPGN have provided support for the concept that fibrin polymerization appears to be an important factor in the development of the crescentic lesion. The prevention of crescent formation by anticoagulation or defibrination has been established in certain experimental circumstances [44, 57, 59].

Recently plasmapheresis has been used for the therapy of severe glomerulonephritis due to either immune complex [24, 32] or anti-GBM antibody mediation. Jones et al. described the value of the procedure in severe lupus vasculitis [24]. They suggested that removal of circulating immune complexes by this physical method may allow the reticuloendothelial system to begin functioning more efficiently and to remove whichever complexes remained in the circulation. Lockwood et al. have utilized plasmapheresis in 9 patients with RPGN that apparently was of an immune complex pathogenesis and did not appear to be post-streptococcal [32]. The success of these investigators will undoubtedly stimulate further evaluation

of the plasmapheresis technique. Similarly, the use of plasmapheresis in Goodpasture's syndrome has resulted in some positive clinical responses and is deserving of an appropriately controlled clinical trial (see Chap. 57).

In view of the lack of established response of the malignant glomerular lesion of RPGN to available therapies, supportive regimens that permit survival of the patient to a stage of stable chronic renal failure are presently the key to the care of these patients.

References

1. Adam, C., Morel-Maroger, L., and Richet, G. Cryoglobulins in glomerulonephritis not related to systemic disease. *Kidney Int.* 3:334, 1973.
2. Anand, S. K., Trygstad, C. W., Sharma, H. M., and Northway, J. D. Extracapillary proliferative glomerulonephritis in children. *Pediatrics,* 56:434, 1975.
3. Arieff, A. I., and Pinggera, W. F. Rapidly progressive glomerulonephritis treated with anticoagulants. *Arch. Intern. Med.* 129:77, 1972.
4. Atkins, R. C., Holdsworth, S. R., Glascow, E. F., and Matthews, F. The macrophage in human rapidly progressive nephritis. *Lancet* 1:830, 1976.
5. Bacani, R. A., Velasquez, F., Kanter, A., Pirani, C. L., and Pollak, V. E. Rapidly progressive (non-streptococcal) glomerulonephritis. *Ann. Intern. Med.* 69: 463, 1968.
6. Beleil, O. M., Coburn, J. W., Shinaberger, J. H., and Glassock, R. J. Recurrent glomerulonephritis due to anti-glomerular basement membrane-antibodies in two successive allografts. *Clin. Nephrol.* 1:377, 1973.
7. Bendixen, G. Organ specific inhibition of the in vitro migration of leukocytes in human glomerulonephritis. *Acta Med. Scand.* 184:99, 1968.
8. Berlyne, G. M., and Baker, S. B. de C. Acute anuric glomerulonephritis. *Q. J. Med.* 33:105, 1964.
9. Bialestock, D., and Tange, J. D. Acute necrotizing glomerulonephritis. The clinical features and pathology in nine cases. *Australas. Ann. Med.* 8:281, 1959.
10. Bohman, S.-O., Olsen, S., and Petersen, V. P. Glomerular ultrastructure in extracapillary glomerulonephritis. *Acta Pathol. Microbiol. Scand.* [Suppl.] 249:29, 1974.
11. Booth, L. J., and Aber, G. M. Immunosuppressive therapy in adults with proliferative glomerulonephritis. *Lancet* 2:1010, 1970.
12. Brown, C. B., Wilson, D., Turner, D., Cameron, J. S., Ogg, C. S., Chantler, C., and Gill, D. Combined immunosuppression and anticoagulation in rapidly progressive glomerulonephritis. *Lancet* 2: 1166, 1974.
13. Burkholder, P. M., and Bradford, W. D. Proliferative glomerulonephritis in children: A correlation of varied clinical and pathological patterns utilizing light, immunofluorescence and electron microscopy. *Am. J. Pathol.* 56:423, 1969.
14. Chirawong, P., Nanra, R. S., and Kincaid-Smith, P. Fibrin degradation products and the role of coagulation in "persistent" glomerulonephritis. *Ann. Intern. Med.* 74:853, 1971.
15. Churg, J., and Grishman, E. Ultrastructure of glomerular disease: A review. *Kidney Int.* 7:254, 1975.
16. Couser, W. G., Wallace, A., Monaco, A. P., and

Lewis, E. J. Successful renal transplantation in patients with circulating antibody to golmerular basement membrane: Report of two cases. *Clin. Nephrol.* 1:381, 1973.

17. Curtis, J. J., Bhathena, D., Leach, R. P., Galla, J. H., Lucas, B. A., and Luke, Ř. G. Goodpasture's syndrome in a patient with the nail-patella syndrome. *Am. J. Med.* 61:401, 1976.

18. Dupont, E., Mendes da Costa, R. C., and Dupuis, F. Linear deposits of immunoglobulins on glomerular basement membrane of human stored kidneys. *Transplantation* 18:458, 1974.

19. Ellis, A. Natural history of Bright's disease: Clinical, histological and experimental observations. *Lancet* 1:1, 1942.

20. Fahr, T. Pathologische Anatomie des Morbus Brightii. In F. Henke and O. Lubarsch (eds.), *Handbuch der Speziellen Pathologischen Anatomie und Histologie.* Berlin: Springer, 1925. Vol. 6, part. 1, p. 156.

21. Gallo, G. R. Elution studies in kidneys with linear deposition of immunoglobulin in glomeruli. *Am. J. Pathol.* 61:377, 1970.

22. Heptinstall, R. H. *Pathology of the Kidney* (2nd ed.). Boston: Little, Brown, 1974. P. 387.

23. Jensen, H., Olgaard, K., and Faarup, P. Successful immunosuppressive therapy of oliguric extracapillary glomerulonephritis. *Acta Med. Scand.* 196:383, 1974.

24. Jones, J. V., Cumming, R. H., Bucknall, R. C., Asplin, C. M., Fraser, I. D., Bothamley, J., Davis, P., and Hamblin, T. J. Plasmapheresis in the management of acute systemic lupus erythematosus? *Lancet* 1:709, 1976.

25. Kincaid-Smith, P., Saker, B. M., and Fairley, K. F. Anticoagulants in "irreversible" acute renal failure. *Lancet* 2:1360, 1968.

26. Klassen, J., Elwood, C., Grossberg, A. L., Milgrom, F., Montes, M., Sepulveda, M., and Andres, G. Evolution of membranous nephropathy into antiglomerular-basement-membrane glomerulonephritis. *N. Engl. J. Med.* 290:1340, 1974.

27. Kondo, Y., Shigematsu, H., and Kobayashi, Y. Cellular aspects of rabbit Masugi nephritis: II. Progressive glomerular injuries with crescent formation. *Lab. Invest.* 27:260, 1972.

28. Leonard, C. D., Nagle, R. B., Striker, G. E., Cutler, R. E., and Scribner, B. H. Acute glomerulonephritis with prolonged anuria: Analysis of 29 cases. *Ann. Intern. Med.* 73:703, 1970.

29. Lerner, R. A., and Dixon, F. J. The induction of acute glomerulonephritis in rabbits with soluble antigens isolated from normal, homologous and autologous urine. *J. Immunol.* 100:1277, 1968.

30. Lerner, R. A., Glassock, R. J., and Dixon, F. J. The role of antiglomerular basement membrane antibody in the pathogenesis of human glomerulonephritis. *J. Exp. Med.* 126:989, 1967.

31. Lewis, E. J., Cavallo, T., Harrington, J. T., and Cotran, R. S. An immunopathologic study of rapidly progressive glomerulonephritis in the adult. *Hum. Pathol.* 2:185, 1971.

32. Lockwood, C. M., Rees, A. J., Pinching, A. J., Pussell, B., Sweny, P., Uff, J., and Peters, D. K. Plasma-exchange and immunosuppression in the treatment of fulminating immune-complex crescentic nephritis. *Lancet* 1:63, 1977.

33. Macanovic, M., Evans, D. J., and Peters, D. K. Allergic response to glomerular basement membrane in patients with glomerulonephritis. *Lancet* 2:207, 1972.

34. Mahieu, P., Dardenne, M., and Bach, J. F. Detection of humoral and cell-mediated immunity to kidney basement membranes in human renal diseases. *Am. J. Med.* 53:185, 1972.

35. Mahieu, P., Lambert, P. H., and Miescher, P. A. Detection of anti-glomerular basement membrane antibodies by radioimmunological technique: Clinical application in human nephropathies. *J. Clin. Invest.* 54:128, 1974.

36. Mallick, N. P., Williams, R. J., and McFarlane, H. Cell mediated immunity in nephrotic syndrome. *Lancet* 1:507, 1972.

37. Markowitz, A. S., and Lange, C. F. Streptococcal related glomerulonephritis: I. Isolation, immunochemistry and comparative chemistry of soluble fractions from Type 12 nephritogenic streptococci and human glomeruli. *J. Immunol.* 92:565, 1964.

38. McCluskey, R. T. The value of immunofluorescence in the study of human renal disease. *J. Exp. Med.* 134:2425, 1971.

39. McPhaul, J. J., Jr., and Dixon, F. J. The presence of anti-glomerular basement membrane antibodies in peripheral blood. *J. Immunol.* 103:1168, 1969.

40. McPhaul, J. J., Jr., and Mullins, J. D. Glomerulonephritis mediated by antibody to glomerular basement membrane: Immunologic, clinical and histopathologic characteristics. *J. Clin. Invest.* 57:351, 1976.

41. Mercola, K. E., and Hagadorn, J. E. Complement-dependant acute immunologic lung injury in an experimental model resembling Goodpasture's syndrome. *Exp. Mol. Pathol.* 19:230, 1973.

42. Min, K. W., Györkey, F., Györkey, P., Yium, J. J., and Eknoyan, G. The morphogenesis of glomerular crescents in rapidly progressive glomerulonephritis. *Kidney Int.* 5:47, 1974.

43. Morita, T., Suzuki, Y., and Churg, J. Structure and development of the glomerular crescent. *Am. J. Pathol.* 72:349, 1973.

44. Naish, P., Penn, G. B., Evans, D. J., and Peters, D. K. The effect of defibrination in nephrotoxic serum nephritis in rabbits. *Clin. Sci.* 42:643, 1972.

45. Olsen, S. Extracapillary glomerulonephritis: A semiquantitative light microscopical study of 59 patients. *Acta Pathol. Microbiol. Scand.* [Suppl.] 249:7, 1974.

46. Olsen, S., Petersen, V. P., and Hansen, E. S. Immunofluorescent studies of extracapillary glomerulonephritis. *Acta Pathol. Microbiol. Scand.* [Suppl.] 249:20, 1974.

47. Richards, P., Evans, D. J., and Wrong, D. M. Recovery from acute renal failure due to "irreversible" glomerular disease. *Br. Med. J.* 2:459, 1968.

48. Richardson, J. A., Rosenau, W., Lee, J. C., and Hopper, J. Kidney transplantation for rapidly progressive glomerular nephritis. *Lancet* 2:180, 1970.

49. Rocklin, R. E., Lewis, E. J., and David, J. R. In vitro evidence for cellular hypersensitivity to glomerular-basement-membrane antigens in human glomerulonephritis. *N. Engl. J. Med.* 283:497, 1970.

50. Schreiner, G. E., Rakowski, T. A., Argy, W. D., Jr., Marc-Aurele, J., Maher, J. F., and Bauer, H. Natural History of Oliguric Glomerulonephritis. In P. Kincaid-Smith, T. H. Mathew, and E. L. Becker (eds.), *Glomerulonephritis: Morphology, Natural*

History and Treatment. New York: Wiley, 1973. Part II, p. 711.

51. Soborg, M., and Bendixen, G. Human lymphocyte migration as a parameter of hypersensitivity. *Acta Med. Scand.* 111:247, 1967.

52. Sonsino, E., Nabarra, B., Kazatchkine, M., Hinglais, N., and Kreis, H. Extracapillary Proliferative Glomerulonephritis—So-called Malignant Glomerulonephritis. In J. Hamburger, J. Crosnier, and M. H. Maxwell (eds.), *Advances in Nephrology.* Chicago: Year Book, 1972. Vol. 2, p. 121.

53. Steblay, R. W. Glomerulonephritis induced in sheep by injections of heterologous glomerular basement membrane and Freund's complete adjuvant. *J. Exp. Med.* 116:253, 1962.

54. Steblay, R. W., and Rudofsky, U. Autoimmune glomerulonephritis induced in sheep by injections of human lung and Freund's adjuvant. *Science* 160:204, 1968.

55. Stejskal, J., Pirani, C. L., Okada, M., Madelanakis, N., and Pollak, V. E. Discontinuities (gaps) of the glomerular capillary wall and basement membrane in renal disease. *Lab. Invest.* 28:149, 1973.

56. Striker, G. E., Cutler, R. E., Huang, T. W., and Benditt, E. P. Renal Failure Glomerulonephritis and Glomerular Epithelial Cell Hyperplasia. In P. Kincaid-Smith, T. H. Mathew, and E. L. Becker (eds.),

Glomerulonephritis: Morphology, Natural History and Treatment. New York: Wiley, 1973. Part II, p. 657.

57. Thomson, N. M., Moran, J., Simpson, I. J., and Peters, D. K. Defibrination with ancrod in nephrotoxic nephritis in rabbits. *Kidney Int.* 10:343, 1976.

58. Urizar, R. E., Tinglof, B., McIntosh, R., Litman, N., Barnett, E., Wilkerson, J., Smith, F., Jr., and Vernier, R. L. Immunosuppressive therapy of proliferative glomerulonephritis in children. *Am. J. Dis. Child.* 118:411, 1969.

59. Vassalli, P., and McCluskey, R. T. The pathogenic role of the coagulation process in rabbit Masugi nephritis. *Am. J. Pathol.* 45:653, 1964.

60. Wainwright, J., and Dawson, J. The renal appearances of the microscopic form of periarteritis nodosa. *J. Pathol. Bacteriol.* 62:189, 1950.

61. Wilson, C. B., and Dixon, F. J. Anti-glomerular basement membrane antibody-induced glomerulonephritis. *Kidney Int.* 3:74, 1973.

62. Wilson, C. B., and Dixon, F. J. Diagnosis of immunopathologic renal disease (editorial). *Kidney Int.* 5:389, 1974.

63. Wilson, C. B., Marquardt, H., and Dixon, F. J. Radioimmunoassay (RIA) for circulating antiglomerular basement membrane (GBM) antibodies (abstract). *Kidney Int.* 6:114a, 1974.

49. Chronic Glomerulonephritis

Chester M. Edelmann, Jr., Henry L. Barnett, and Jay Bernstein

The term *chronic glomerulonephritis* is used to designate a heterogeneous group of primary glomerular diseases characterized clinically by irreversibility and histopathologically by glomerular obsolescence and sclerosis. It commonly runs a protracted course, is often asymptomatic for long periods, and is associated with a relentless loss of nephrons, progressive reduction in renal function, and, ultimately, terminal renal insufficiency [2, 4]. According to Habib et al. [3], glomerular diseases are the single most frequent cause of chronic renal failure, accounting for 26 percent of cases in their series.

Glascock and Bennet [1] have replaced the venerable term *chronic glomerulonephritis* with the term *chronic nephritic syndrome.* Although their term indicates that a syndrome rather than a single disease is implicated, it does not help remove the confusion associated with the concept of chronic glomerulonephritis.

Pathogenesis

Chronic glomerulonephritis may develop either in the absence of any manifestations of previous renal disease or be recognized during the course of any of the primary or secondary glomerular diseases described in Chap. 43. Thus, it may develop and progress insidiously and be first recognized in the child with manifestations of renal insufficiency, or it may present initially as acute glomerulonephritis, asymptomatic hematuria, or the nephrotic syndrome. It is now clear that it is not the mode of presentation but the potential for progression to end-stage renal failure that defines chronic glomerulonephritis.

The relationship, if any, between acute poststreptococcal glomerulonephritis and chronic glomerulonephritis has been and continues to be a subject of vigorous controversy, as discussed elsewhere (Chap. 47). Whatever the final answer, it would appear that, contrary to previous opinion, acute poststreptococcal glomerulonephritis is an infrequent antecedent of chronic glomerulonephritis either in children or in adults.

Histopathologic Findings

The morphologic heterogeneity of glomerular lesions in chronic glomerulonephritis is indicated in

Chap. 43. In children, the most common lesions are focal segmental glomerulosclerosis and membranoproliferative glomerulonephritis, accounting for almost half the total [3]. Other lesions include proliferative and sclerosing glomerulonephritis, membranous glomerulonephropathy, diabetic nephropathy, the Alport syndrome, the nail-patella syndrome, lupus nephropathy, and Schönlein-Henoch nephritis.

Clinical Manifestations

The striking clinical feature in many children with chronic glomerulonephritis, whatever the origin, is the prolonged period during which they may remain asymptomatic, even to the extent that they grow and develop normally. In children with no prior manifestations of an active glomerular disease, early symptoms of uremia may be the first recognizable manifestation of chronic glomerulonephritis. In many children these symptoms first appear at the time of the adolescent growth spurt. As the disease progresses, it is accompanied by a complex series of biochemical and metabolic disturbances that are discussed in detail in Chaps. 17 to 30.

Diagnosis

The diagnosis depends on the demonstration of persistent urinary abnormalities and a slowly progressive reduction in glomerular filtration rate. The increased rates of excretion of protein and red blood cells may be very slight, and there are often long periods during which renal function is reduced but stable.

No fixed periods of time or degrees of reduction in glomerular filtration rate can be assigned. The diagnosis is usually not made until the abnormalities, especially reduced glomerular filtration rate, have persisted for periods of 6 months to a year or more.

Differential Diagnosis

The diagnosis of chronic glomerulonephritis should not be made without a careful search for other diseases, especially treatable ones, such as pyelonephritis, obstructive uropathy, and hypertensive disease. The latter two accounted for 21

and 10 percent respectively of the causes of chronic renal failure in the series of Habib et al. [3].

Treatment

Whether or not the process of progressive destruction of nephrons may be slowed by treatment with corticosteroids or immunosuppressive cytoxic agents in patients with any type of chronic glomerulonephritis remains to be demonstrated (see Chap. 70). At present, it must be doubted that any form of treatment favorably affects the underlying glomerular disease. Until renal insufficiency ensues, with symptoms of uremia or biochemical disturbances, no treatment is indicated. Severe restrictions of activity or changes in the diet in an asymptomatic patient have no discernible benefit and serve only to heighten concern about the condition. Avoiding overexertion from competitive sports during the asymptomatic period is often recommended and seems judicious.

Early recognition and prompt treatment of the signs and symptoms or uremia are of great importance clinically. These measures are discussed in Chap. 34.

Prognosis

The diagnosis of chronic glomerulonephritis by definition precludes the possibility of full recovery. However, the period from time of diagnosis until chronic hemodialysis or transplantation is required is variable. The major determinants appear to be the type of glomerular disease present and age at onset.

References

1. Glascock, R. J., and Bennett, C. M. Chronic Nephrotic Syndrome. In B. M. Brenner, and F. C. Rector, Jr. (eds.), *The Kidney.* Philadelphia: Saunders, 1966. Vol. 1, p. 981.
2. Habib, R. Prolonged or Chronic Glomerulonephritis. In P. Royer, R. Habib, H. Mathieu, and M. Broyer (eds.), *Pediatric Nephrology.* Philadelphia: Saunders, 1974. P. 281.
3. Habib, R., Broyer, M., and Benmatz, H. Chronic renal failure in children. *Nephron* 11:209, 1973.
4. Rubin, M. I. Chronic Glomerulonephritis. In M. I. Rubin and R. M. Barratt (eds.), *Pediatric Neprology.* Baltimore: Williams & Wilkins, 1973. P. 558.

50. Membranous Glomerulonephropathy in Children

Renée Habib, Claire Kleinknecht, Marie-Claire Gübler, and Micheline Lévy

Among the various forms of glomerulopathy defined by histologic pattern, there is a distinct type characterized by the presence of subepithelial deposits and the absence of mesangial proliferation. *Membranous nephropathy* and *membranous glomerulonephropathy* (MGN) are now the most widely accepted terms for this pattern, although other terms, such as *extramembranous* [37], *perimembranous* [13, 33], *epimembranous* [76], and *transmembranous* [34] GN have the advantage of being more precise in designating the location of the deposits in relation to the basement membrane.

Membranous glomerulonephropathy had long been considered to be a disease occurring only in adults, although 3 cases in children aged 11 months, 24 months, and 12 years were reported as early as 1962 by Royer et al. [65]. During the past few years, reports on more than 1,000 patients with MGN have been published, including approximately 100 children [8, 10, 22–25, 27, 30, 31, 33, 35, 37, 45, 49, 57, 59a, 60–62, 64, 73, 76].

The actual incidence of MGN in childhood is difficult to assess. Row et al. [64] found MGN in 2.7 percent of their nephrotic child patients and in 20 percent of their nephrotic adult patients. The International Study of Kidney Disease in children [16] reported that 2 of 127 nephrotic children had membranous glomerulonephropathy. In a more selected group of patients, Habib and Kleinknecht [36], found 37 children with MGN among 406 with nephrotic syndrome (NS). Analyzing all available published data, Pollak et al. [60] concluded that MGN occurred in 6 percent of nephrotic children and in 19 percent of nephrotic adults. However, it must be emphasized that MGN may be found in the absence of a nephrotic syndrome.

Pathogenesis

Because of its close morphologic and immunopathologic similarity to some experimental models, it seems likely that the glomerular lesions of MGN result from prolonged deposition of circulating antigen-antibody complexes [29].

The first extensively studied models were those produced by foreign serum proteins (experimental serum sickness) [21, 34]. In the last few years it has been demonstrated that autologous immune complexes can produce the same histologic pattern, two autologous antigens being the lipoprotein present in the brush border of the proximal tubular epithelium [3] and native thyroglobulin [42a, 50].

Membranous glomerulonephropathy may be associated with a few diseases in which the presence of circulating soluble antigen-antibody complexes is certain or likely, although circulating immune complexes have rarely been demonstrated, and only a few responsible antigens have been found in the deposits.

A tumor-specific antibody has been demonstrated in the glomeruli of 1 patient with carcinoma of the bronchus [47] and in 2 patients with carcinoma of the colon [18, 19]. The presence of hepatitis B surface antigen (HB_sAg) has been demonstrated by immunofluorescent techniques within the subepithelial deposits of patients with MGN [1, 13, 15, 17], but has been reported in other histologic types of glomerulonephropathy as well [15]; MGN is frequently observed in lupus nephritis [4]. The presence of DNA antigen and of anti-DNA antibodies has been demonstrated within the glomeruli of patients with systemic lupus erythematosus (SLE) nephropathy [43], but, to our knowledge, none of these patients had documented MGN. The first attempts to demonstrate *antitreponemal* antibodies [14] or treponemal antigen [11, 39, 42] in the deposits were unsuccessful. Recently, evidence for the presence of antitreponemal antibody within the deposits has been provided by Gamble and Reardan [32], and the presence of antitreponemal antigen has been documented by Tourville et al. [71]. The presence of renal tubular epithelial antigen in the subepithelial deposits of apparently primary MGN has been reported by Naruse et al. [55], but this finding has not been confirmed by other authors [77].

Clinical Manifestations

Differences in clinical manifestations and urinary findings between adults and children with MGN have not been clearly established, except that the disease is known to have a more favorable prognosis in children. Only three series have dealt exclusively with children: our own series of 50 patients [37], the 14 patients of Tsao et al. [73], and the 14 patients of Olbing et al. [57] and Trainin et al. [72]. Precise data for 19 additional children can be obtained from the reports of Ehrenreich et al. [25] (12 cases), and Row et al. [64] (7 cases).

Our experience, described here, is based on 73

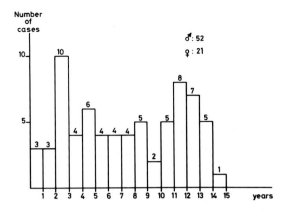

Figure 50-1. Age at clinical onset.

cases, including the 50 previously reported. The disease occurred in children in all age groups, including infants (Fig. 50-1). The youngest child was 2 months of age (No. 8). Males were significantly more often affected than females, as observed in adult series.

Clinical onset often was insidious. In our patients, drawn from a population that is frequently screened for proteinuria, the disease was discovered more often by routine urinalysis (57 percent) than by edema (36 percent) or gross hematuria (7 percent).

Proteinuria was always present, but extremely variable, both in its range of intensity from one patient to another and its daily fluctuations in individual patients. Proteinuria usually has been reported as being nonselective [64], but it was selective in half our patients. Proteinuria is often associated with NS.* In our series it was present at onset in 53 patients and developed subsequently in 10 patients. The NS was persistent in 14 patients and it remitted in 49, usually within 1 year.

Hematuria was often present in association with proteinuria and more frequent in our series than has been previously reported. It was found in 85 percent of our patients during the first months of the disease, and was macroscopic in 21 percent. It usually decreased or disappeared during the course of the disease.

Hypertension and azotemia at onset have been observed less frequently in children [37] than in adults [24]. Signs of proximal tubular dysfunction associated with chronic renal failure were found in 2 of our patients. These are discussed in detail in the next section.

---

* Nephrotic syndrome has been defined according to the following criteria: proteinuria higher than 50 mg/kg/day; hypoproteinemia below 6 gm per deciliter, and hypo-albuminemia below 3 gm per deciliter.

Associated Diseases

Several conditions have been described in association with MGN. In some, the role of a definite antigen can be considered as established; in others, this role is likely but remains to be demonstrated.

The main conditions coexisting with MGN have been extensively reviewed by Row et al. [64]. The more common, at least in adults, are *malignant* diseases, mainly carcinomas. Row et al. [64] found 26 such associations in the literature, and Eagen and Lewis [23a] compiled 19 cases with carcinomas, 3 with Hodgkin's disease, 1 with other malignant lymphoma, 2 with leukemia, and 2 with benign solid tumors. Tumor antigen has been identified in only 4 cases. Association with malignancy is rare in children; a single case with Wilms' tumor has been reported by Row et al. [64].

Hepatitis B antigenemia, either asymptomatic or associated with chronic hepatitis, has been reported by several authors [1, 13, 15, 17]. Moreover, Eknoyan et al. [26] demonstrated by electron microscopy the presence of tiny subepithelial deposits in patients with acute hepatitis. According to Libit et al. [48], *SLE* is the main cause of MGN in children. These authors, as well as others [41], emphasize that the nephropathy may precede serologic evidence of SLE by several years. Congenital and secondary *syphilis* is often associated with MGN. The prompt recovery usually obtained after specific therapy provides evidence that *Treponema* is responsible.

Other diseases that occasionally have been described in association with MGN are filariasis [5], malaria [2], Sjögren's syndrome [66], sarcoidosis [44, 67], autoimmune thyroiditis [57a], and bullous pemphigoid [28]. In none of these conditions has the responsible antigen been detected in the kidney, although these diseases are likely to be related to immunologic disorders.

Membranous glomerulonephropathy may result from the administration of *drugs,* particularly mercury [64], gold [64, 68, 70, 75], and D-penicillamine [38, 40]. Trimethadione has been claimed as a possible cause of MGN, but evidence for such an association is scant. By electron microscopy, Bar-Khayim et al. [9] found subepithelial deposits in 1 patient treated with trimethadione, but failed to demonstrate the typical pattern by immunofluorescence. Membranous glomerulonephropathy has been experimentally produced following injections of mercury [7] or gold [54]. Whether these drugs induce immune complexes by releasing tubular antigens, or act as haptens, or have other toxic effects remains unknown. Evidence for the former hypothesis has been provided in experimental

MGN by Kelchner et al. [42a]. Following administration of mercuric chloride, rats developed MGN and renal tubular basement membrane and renal tubular epithelial antibodies. Complexes of renal tubular epithelial antigen and antibody apparently were involved since both were present in the subepithelial deposits, and fluorescence was no longer observed after absorption with tubular epithelium but not with tubular basement membrane. In human subjects, Whitworth et al. [77] did not find renal tubular epithelial deposits in gold-induced (1 case) or penicillamine-induced (2 cases) MGN. In gold nephropathy, various investigators failed to demonstrate the presence of gold in the deposits, indicating that its action as a hapten is unlikely [75].

Another condition often reported in association with MGN is *renal venous thrombosis* [49]. In most cases thrombosis appears as a complication of MGN with severe nephrotic syndrome. Whether or not thrombosis is the primary event and triggers an immune disease remains unsettled. The study of Ozawa et al. [57b] suggests that thrombosis may lead to tubular epithelial antigen-antibody formation, since both have been found in the cryoproteins and in the glomerular deposits of a patient with unilateral venous thrombosis and MGN.

Of our 73 patients, 10 had a specific disease considered as a possible cause of MGN, and 16 had associated symptoms suggesting the concurrent involvement of other organs. These are recorded in Table 50-1.

Hepatitis was discovered in 3 of these patients (Nos. 4, 5, 26), and in all 3, proteinuria disappeared within several months. Australia antigen was detected in the only patient investigated for it. Two additional patients were found to be healthy carriers of the antigen (Nos. 31, 66). Further investigations have enabled us to detect Australia antigen in 11 of 22 patients with MGN and in only 1 of 45 patients with other types of glomerulonephritis. One patient had SLE with circulating antinuclear antibodies (No. 69), and one patient had congenital syphilis (No. 8) and recovered within a few weeks after penicillin therapy.

One patient (No. 58) had sickle cell disease and two (Nos. 52, 68) had sickle cell trait. The relationship between the hemoglobinopathy and the renal disease has not been documented, but the role of renal tubular epithelial antigen may be hypothesized, as in the patient described by Ozawa et al. [58] and as in other types of glomerulopathies [69, 78].

Polyarthralgias were present in 7 of our patients. They were associated with severe but transient hypertension and a purpuric rash (No. 9), rheumatic fever with cardiac involvement (No. 34), prolonged fever (No. 43), and skin rash (Nos. 27, 50). Five patients had extensive skin rash at the onset of their nephropathy (Nos. 6, 11, 13, 25, 35). A mild nephrotic syndrome developed in patient 24 at the age of 8, in the course of a disease characterized by polyarthralgia and recurrent purpura, 7 years after the onset of a myelomonocytic leukemia. He subsequently had a favorable outcome. Patient 47 had idiopathic thrombocytopenia without circulating antibodies.

To date, SLE has not developed in any of these patients, even though 8 have been followed for more than 5 years.

Two of our patients had a *Fanconi syndrome.* A severe nephrotic syndrome developed in patient 56 when he was 11 months old, and signs of tubular dysfunction associated with renal insufficiency developed 1 year later. He died from renal failure at the age of 8 years. Renal biopsy showed MGN and marked cellular infiltration of the interstitial tissue. Immunofluorescent studies were not performed. Patient 49 presented with a complete Fanconi syndrome, moderate renal failure, and mild proteinuria [46]. Renal biopsy showed the same glomerular and interstitial lesions as in patient 56. Immunofluorescence demonstrated the typical pattern of MGN, as well as linear and granular IgG deposits along the tubular basement membranes. Circulating antitubular antibodies were detected. Severe pneumonia developed, and anti–alveolar basement membrane antibodies were found in the plasma. Subsequently, the patient progressed to terminal renal failure, and anti–alveolar and anti–tubular basement membrane antibodies disappeared. A similar case has been reported by Tung and Black [74].

Table 50-1. *Findings Associated with Membranous Glomerulonephropathy in 26 Patients*

Associated Disease	Number of Patients
Conditions suggesting a definite etiology	
Hepatitis	3
Asymptomatic HBs antigenemia	2
SLE	1
Syphilis	1
Sickle cell disease or trait	3
Other associated diseases or symptoms	
Polyarthralgias	7
Rash	5
Polyarthralgias and purpura	1
Idiopathic thrombocytopenia	1
Tubular dysfunction	2

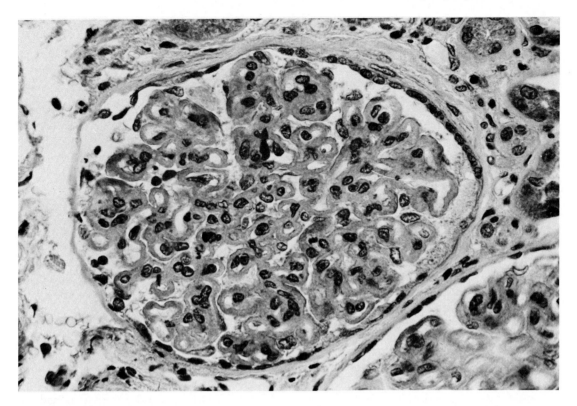

Figure 50-2. Advanced stage of MN. Note the diffuse thickening of the capillary walls and the absence of mesangial proliferation. (×900.)

Pathologic Features

By light microscopy the glomerular lesion is characterized by diffuse thickening of all capillary walls (Fig. 50-2), with widely patent lumens and hypertrophy of the epithelial cells. There is usually little mesangial proliferation, although mild hypercellularity can be demonstrated morphometrically [33]. In some instances, trichrome stains show this thickening to be due to the presence of abnormal deposits located more or less continuously along the epithelial side of the basement membrane (Fig. 50-3). These deposits are not argyrophilic, but spiky argyrophilic projections arising from the glomerular basement membrane can be demonstrated with silver stains (Fig. 50-4). The spikes, when numerous, give a comblike, hatched appearance to the capillary walls; however, in some instances they may be scanty or affect only some loops. In advanced cases the spikes may not be conspicuous, and capillary walls then have the appearance of twisted chains. Crescent formation is extremely rare [52, 56]. The interstitium and tubules are usually normal, but atrophic lesions of the tubules may be seen in advanced cases, together with sclerotic glomeruli. In

3 of our patients, in an early biopsy specimen, we found marked cellular infiltration of the interstitium associated with tubular atrophy, in the absence of severe glomerular changes (patients 49, 56, 66).

Some investigators have been able to distinguish three [6, 23] or four [24, 34, 63] patterns by electron microscopy and consider these to be phases in the histologic evolution of the disease. The earliest lesion is the presence of more or less numerous electron-dense deposits under the foot processes of epithelial cells (Fig. 50-5). The deposits are in close apposition to the foot processes and lie outside the basement membrane, as demonstrated by silver stains (Fig. 50-6). Later, projections of variable shape arise from the basement membrane between adjacent deposits (Fig. 50-6). Many of these spikes have lateral extensions that surround the deposits, often forming a new layer of basement membrane. Finally, the deposits are progressively incorporated into the basement membrane, where they lose their density and become difficult to distinguish from the basement membrane itself. At this stage the capillary walls are irregularly thickened.

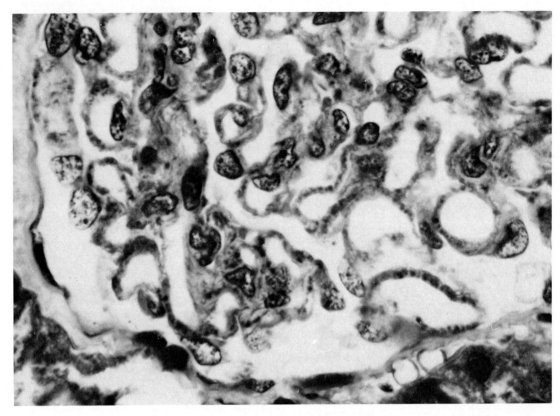

Figure 50-3. With trichrome stain, granules are visible on the epithelial side of the basement membrane. (×1,900.)

A reparative phase has been described in a few patients who have gone into remission [8, 30, 57]. The contour of the epithelial border becomes smooth, and a new lamina densa appears to have formed. On the uneven endothelial aspect of the basement membrane there are irregular electron-lucent areas that are believed to represent deposits that have undergone structural changes following their incorporation into the wall.

The pattern of immunofluorescence microscopy most often described in the literature is characterized by the presence of granules fixing mainly IgG, widespread along the capillary walls (Fig. 50-7) and having the appearance of pearls. In some instances, the granules are so small that the deposits seem to be linear. In our own experience, different patterns may be observed. The granules may be contiguous and of similar size or irregularly spaced and of different size. In some cases, multiple layers of granules may be seen. Although in most instances they are diffuse in all capillary walls, they may affect only some loops. We have observed a decrease in the amount of deposits over the years in patients with a favorable course. The results of immunofluorescence microscopy in 40

cases in our series is summarized in Table 50-2. The granules always contained IgG, frequently IgM, and in some instances IgA. The finding of IgA in isolated MGN does not, however, support the suggestion [48] that its presence is a clue to the diagnosis of lupus. Granular deposits of C3 are often observed, but this does not occur as consistently as for IgG. C1q and C4 may be found in some patients with or without extrarenal manifestations.

Germuth and Rodriguez [34] have reported the exclusive fixation of C3, mostly in patients in clinical recovery, and have concluded by analogy with the recovery state in the chronic bovine serum albumin–rabbit system that complexes are no longer being actively deposited in the glomeruli. This conclusion is supported by electron-microscopic data indicating that remission of MGN is characterized by the absence of newly formed subepithelial deposits. Various antigens have been demonstrated along the capillary walls in a granular pattern (see Pathogenesis).

In addition to granular deposits along the capillary walls of the glomeruli, granular deposits of IgG, C1q, and C3 have been reported (mainly in

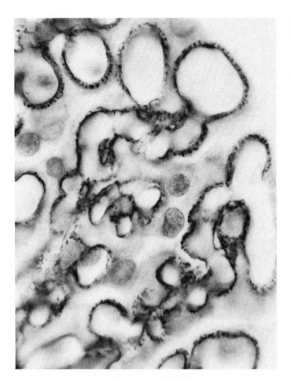

Figure 50-4. With silver stain, silver-positive spikes projecting outward from the basement membrane are visible on all the capillary walls. (×2,000 before 38% reduction.)

SLE) along the tubular basement membranes, the peritubular capillaries, and in the interstitium, where they represent deposition of immune complexes. However, in one of our patients without SLE we found granular deposits of IgG, C1q, and C3 along tubular basement membranes, together with a marked interstitial cellular infiltration.

Linear deposits of IgG and C3 along the tubular basement membranes associated with circulating antitubular anti–basement membrane antibodies were observed in one of our patients presenting with the Fanconi syndrome, mild proteinuria, and the characteristic histologic pattern of MGN. In addition, marked interstitial cellular infiltration and lesions of tubular atrophy were present [46].

Complement Studies

Plasma C3 levels have been normal in all the published series, including our own. Except for 2 patients reported by Row et al. [64] as having a normal plasma C4, there are no published data concerning the other complement components. The results of the first determinations of C1q, C4, and C3PA performed in our patients are shown in Fig. 50-8; values are significantly reduced when compared with controls.

Course

The clinical course is extremely variable. It was severe in only 10 percent of our patients, who progressed to renal failure. At last examination, with a mean follow-up of 5 years, half our patients were protein-free. Data concerning 69 children followed for more than 1 year are shown graphically in Figs. 50-9 and 50-10. Two patterns of evolution were observed.

1. Forty patients initially underwent complete remission, with or without subsequent relapse (Fig. 50-9). In this group, the NS was either absent or of short duration (less than 1 year), and proteinuria usually disappeared within 2 years after onset. There were no relapses in 27 children for periods up to 10 years. The remaining 13 relapsed, but their relapses were usually transient and characterized by asymptomatic proteinuria rather than by NS. None of these 40 patients progressed to renal failure.

2. Persistent proteinuria occurred in 29 patients (Fig. 50-10), 14 with unremitting NS. Of these 14, chronic renal failure developed in 6, 18 months to 5 years after onset. Nephrotic syndrome was present transiently in 10 patients, none of whom had renal failure. The final 5 never demonstrated NS. Of these, only 1 child, who presented with a Fanconi syndrome, had decreased renal function and a poor outcome.

Thus, the persistence of NS appears to be an ominous sign in children, as in adults [65], while its absence or rapid disappearance seems indicative of a good prognosis.

The outcome of the disease is much more favorable in children than that reported in most series of adults. In the series of 14 patients reported by Trainin et al. [72], 4 patients less than 6 years of age at onset were in remission, whereas 4 over 12 years of age when MGN was diagnosed were in renal failure or showed evidence of progressive renal disease. However, we failed to find any relationship between age at onset and outcome. The incidence of renal failure varies widely in the few children's series previously reported (Table 50-3); none of 14 reported by Tsao et al. [73], 1 of 7 in the series of Row et al. [64], 4 of 14 reported by Trainin et al. [72], and 7 of 12 reported by Ehrenreich et al. [25]. Similar differences have been observed in adults, with renal failure ranging from 10 percent [23] to 60 percent [31] and with remission ranging from 0 percent [27] to 30 percent [23, 45]. In fact, no reliable comparisons can be made among the published series in light of the differences in the patient selection and follow-up. Some series deal mainly with patients presenting with severe NS [24, 25, 30, 31], while

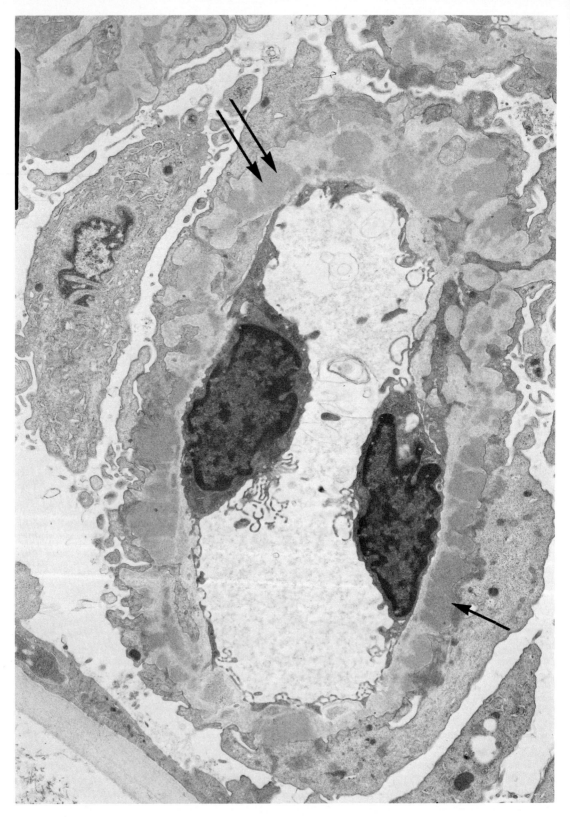

Figure 50-5. Electron micrograph showing thickening of the glomerular basement membrane by osmiophilic deposits. Most of them are located on the epithelial side between lamina densa and podocytes (single arrow). Some are included in the basement membrane (double arrow). (Lead citrate and uranyl acetate, ×10,500.)

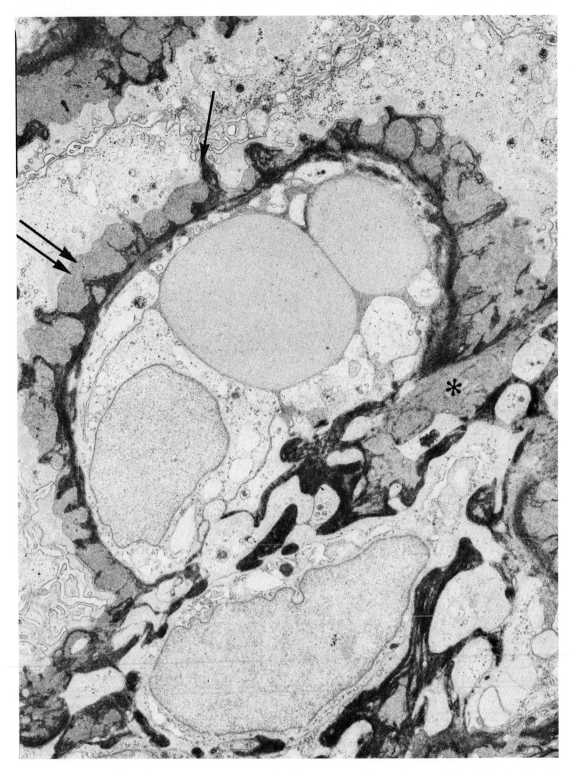

Figure 50-6. Electron micrograph showing presence of diffuse osmiophilic, nonargyrophilic deposits (double arrow) located on the epithelial side of the basement membrane. They are separated by spiky projections (single arrow) arising from the lamina densa and associated with mesangial deposits (asterisk). (Silver methenamine impregnation, ×12,000.)

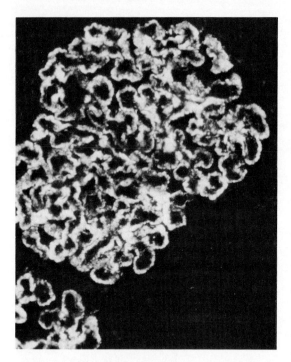

Figure 50-7. Fluorescent micrograph. Anti-IgG serum. A diffuse granular type of fluorescence is seen along the capillary walls. (×450 before 34% reduction.)

others are concerned primarily with patients presenting with asymptomatic proteinuria [23]. Since it is well established that the presence of NS is an ominous feature, it is not surprising that analysis of series dealing mainly with patients having asymptomatic proteinuria demonstrates a better prognosis.

Therapy

Since remissions were believed to be rare, some authors have claimed the beneficial effects of various treatments, including adrenocortical steroids [62], immunosuppressant agents [8], and anticoagulants in combination with immunosuppressants [45]. Recently, Ehrenreich et al. [25] em-

phasized the better long-term prognosis of patients treated with adrenocortical steroids. Most authors [37, 42b, 59a, 65], however, consider that none of the treatments used affect the course of the disease. The effect of drugs is difficult to assess in retrospective studies because of the possibility of spontaneous remissions and the lack of similarity at onset between the treated and the untreated groups. Furthermore, the clinical course varies widely in the different published series, irrespective of therapy. In our experience, remissions occurred during or after administration of corticosteroids or immunosuppressants, used either alone or in combination (Table 50-4). However, remissions were much more frequent in patients who had never been treated or had received no therapy for more than 1 year.

Controlled trials performed in adults have led to the conclusion that neither corticosteroids alone [12] nor with azathioprine [51] or cyclophosphamide [22] have a beneficial effect on proteinuria. No controlled trial has compared long-term survival with and without treatment. Laver and Kincaid-Smith [45] reported a high remission rate using anticoagulants in combination with immunosuppressive agents, but the frequency of remission (30 percent) was not higher than in some untreated series [23, 64], including our own.

In our opinion, the low mortality of the disease does not justify the use of drugs with potentially severe side effects, unless it becomes possible to identify the few patients who are at risk of renal failure.

Membranous glomerulonephropathy recurs rarely after transplantation. To our knowledge, only two cases have been reported [20, 59]. This statistic is surprising, considering the suggested pathogenesis. Even more surprising is the frequent occurrence of MGN in transplanted kidneys when the primary disease was not glomerulonephritis [53, 59, 63]. The possibility that Australia antigen could be responsible for the development of MGN in these patients cannot be excluded in all cases.

Table 50-2. Protein Deposits in Membranous Glomerulonephropathy Seen by Immunofluorescence Miscroscopy

Type of Membranous Glomerulonephropathy	IgA	IgG	IgM	C1q	C4	C3	Fibrinogen	Properdin	Albumin
Isolated	8/23	23/23	16/23	7/12	3/14	21/23	5/23	1/5	0/23
Membranous glomerulonephropathy with associated disorders	4/17	17/17	11/17	5/10	3/10	11/17	5/17	2/4	0/17

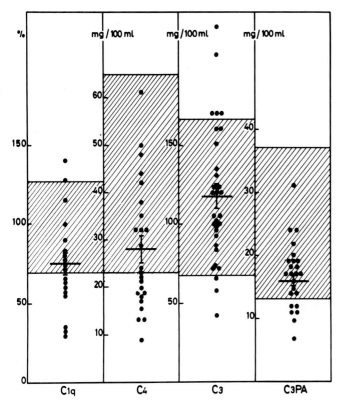

Figure 50-8. *Complement component determinations. C3 is normal, but the mean levels of C1q, C4, and C3PA are significantly reduced.*

Table 50-3. *Outcome in Membranous Glomerulonephropathy*

Study	Number of Patients	Renal Failure	Nonrenal Death	Active Disease	Remission
Adult Series					
Bariety et al. [8]	25	2		17	6
Pollak et al. [60]	19	9	1	6	3
Forland and Spargo [30]	21	6	1	8	6
Ducrot et al. [23]	42	4	2	24	12
Laver and Kincaid-Smith [45]	38	7	4	16	11
Gluck et al. [35]	38	14	5	14	5
Franklin et al. [31]	32	19	3	3	7
Erwing et al. [27]	48	17	4	27	0
Row et al. [64]	55	16	6	22	11
Ehrenreich et al. [25]	92	22	3	55	12
Pierides et al. [59a]	37	9	3	17	8
Total	447	125 (28%)	32 (7%)	209 (47%)	81 (18%)
Children series					
Tsao et al. [73]	14	0	0	10	4
Trainin et al. [72]	14	4	0	4	6
Row et al. [64]	7	1	0	1	5
Ehrenreich et al. [25]	12	7	0	2	3
Habib et al. [37 and un-published cases]	69	7	0	28	34
Total	116	19 (16%)	0	45 (39%)	52 (45%)

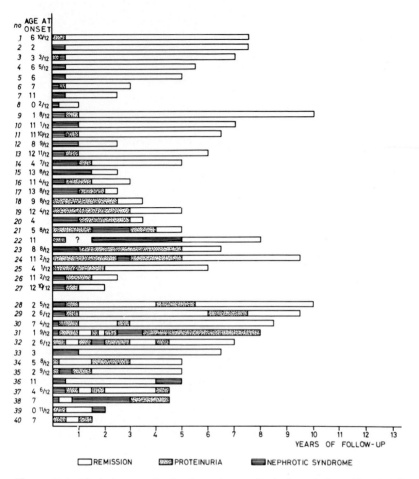

Figure 50-9. Clinical course in the 40 patients who had remissions. Renal failure did not develop in any of the patients.

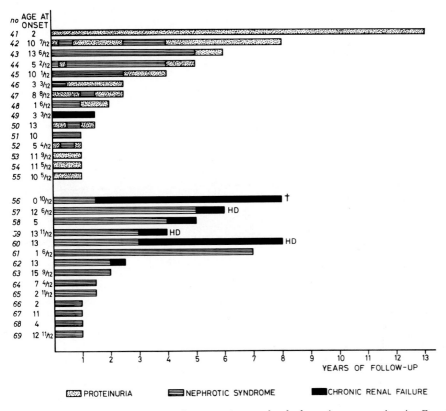

Figure 50-10. Clinical course in the 29 patients who had persistent proteinuria. Except for Patient 49, who presented with the Fanconi syndrome, all the unfavorable evolutions occurred in patients with a persistent nephrotic syndrome.

Table 50-4. Effects of Treatment in Membranous Glomerulonephropathy

Treatment	Number of Patients	Remission[a] Number	Remission[a] Percent
Corticosteroids	33	9	27
Chlorambucil	16	4	25
Corticosteroids and chlorambucil	11	6	54
No treatment[b]	42	30	71

[a] Disappearance of proteinuria during treatment or within one year after withdrawal of treatment.
[b] Evolution of patients either never treated (n = 21) or having received no drug for more than one year (n = 21).

References

1. Ainsworth, S. K., Brackett, N. C., Hennigar, G. R., and Givens, L. B. Glomerulonephritis with deposition of Australia antigen antibody complexes in the glomerular basement membrane (abstract). *Lab. Invest.* 30:369, 1974.
2. Allison, A. C., Hendrickse, R. G., Edington, G. M., Houba, V., Depetris, S., and Adeniyi A. Immune complexes in the nephrotic syndrome of African children. *Lancet* 1:1232, 1969.
3. Alousi, M. A., Post, R. S., and Heymann, W. Experimental auto-immune nephrosis in rats. *Am. J. Pathol.* 54:47, 1969.
4. Baldwin, D. S., Lowenstein, J., Rothfield, N. F., Gallo, G., and McCluskey, R. T. The clinical course of the proliferative and membranous forms of lupus nephritis. *Ann. Intern. Med.* 73:929, 1970.
5. Bariety, J., Barbier, M., Laigre, M. C., Tchernia, G., Lagrue, G., Samarcq, P., Freitel, D., and Milliez, P. Proteinurie et loase. Etude histologique, optique et électronique. *Bull. Soc. Med. Paris* 118:1015, 1967.
6. Bariety, J., Druet, P., Lagrue, G., Samarcq, P., and Milliez, P. Les glomérulonéphrites extramembraneuses. Etude morphologique en microscopie optique, électronique et immunofluorescence. *Pathol. Biol. (Paris)* 18:5, 1970.
7. Bariety, J., Druet, P., Laliberte, F., and Sapin, C. Glomerulonephritis with gamma and B1C-globulin deposits induced in rats by mercuric chloride. *Am. J. Pathol.* 65:293, 1971.
8. Bariety, J., Samarcq, P., Lagrue, G., Fritel, D., and Milliez, P. Evolution ultrastructurale favorable de deux cas de glomérulopathies primitives à dépôts extramembraneux diffus. *Presse Med.* 76:2179, 1968.
9. Bar-Khayim, Y., Teplitz, C., Garella, S., and Chazan, J. A. Trimethadione (Tridione [R])-induced nephrotic syndrome. A report of a case with unique ultrastructural renal pathology. *Am. J. Med.* 54:272, 1973.
10. Beregi, E., and Varga, I. Analysis of 260 cases of membranous glomerulonephritis in renal biopsy material. *Clin. Nephrol.* 2:215, 1974.
11. Bhorade, M. S., Carag, H. B., Lee, H. J., Potter, E. V,. and Dunea, G. Nephropathy of secondary syphilis: A clinical and pathological spectrum. *J.A.M.A.* 216:1159, 1971.
12. Black, D. A. K., Rose, G., and Brewer, D. B. Controlled trial of prednisone in adult patients with the nephrotic syndrome. *Br. Med. J.* 3:421, 1970.
13. Bläker, F., Hellwege, H., Kramer, U., and Thoenes, W. Perimembranose Glomerulonephritis bei chronisher Hepatitis mit persistierenden Hepatitis B antigen. *Dtsch. Med. Wochenschr.* 100:790, 1975.
14. Braunstein, G. D., Lewis, E. J., Galvanek, E. G., Hamilton, A., and Bell, W. R. The nephrotic syndrome associated with secondary syphilis. An immune deposit disease. *Am. J. Med.* 48:643, 1970.
15. Brzósko, W. J., Krawczynski, K., Nazarewicz, T., Morzycka, M., and Nowoslawski, A. Glomerulonephritis associated with hepatitis-B surface antigen immune complexes in children. *Lancet* 2:477, 1974.
16. Churg, J., Habib, R., and White, R. H. R. Pathology of the nephrotic syndrome in children. *Lancet* 1: 1299, 1970.
17. Combes, B., Stastny, P., Shorey, J., Eigrenbrodt, E. H., Barrera, A., Hull, A. R., and Carter, N. W. Glomerulonephritis with deposition of Australia antigen-antibody complexes in glomerular basement membrane. *Lancet* 2, 234, 1971.
18. Costanza, M. E., Pinn, V., Schwartz, R. S., and Nathanson, L. Carcinoembryonic antigen-antibody complexes in a patient with colonic carcinoma and nephrotic syndrome. *N. Engl. J. Med.* 289:520, 1973.
19. Couser, W. G., Wagonfield, J., Spargo, B. J., and Lewis, E J. Glomerular deposition of tumor antigen in membranous nephropathy associated with colonic carcinoma. *Am. J. Med.* 57:962, 1974.
20. Crosson, J. T., Wathen, R. L., Raij, L., Andersen, R. C., and Anderson, W. R. Recurrence of idiopathic membranous nephropathy in a renal allograft. *Arch. Intern. Med.* 135:1101, 1975.
21. Dixon, F. J., Feldman, J. D., and Vasquez, J. Y. Experimental glomerulonephritis: The pathogenesis of a laboratory model resembling the spectrum of glomerulonephritis. *J. Exp. Med.* 113:899, 1961.
22. Donadio, J. V., Holley, K. E., Anderson, C. F., and Taylor, W. G. Controlled trial of cyclophosphamide in idiopathic membranous nephropathy. *Kidney Int.* 6:431, 1974.
23. Ducrot, H., Tsomi, C., Jungers, P., de Montera, H., Hinglais, N., and Giromini, M. Étude anatomoclinique des glomérulonéphrites extramembraneuses. *Act. Nephrol. Hop. Necker* 1:115, 1969.
23a. Eagen, J. W., and Lewis, E. J. Glomerulopathies of neoplasia. *Kidney Int.* 11:297, 1977.
24. Ehrenreich, T., and Churg, J. Pathology of Membranous Nephropathy. In S. C. Sommers (ed.), *Pathology Annual.* New York: Appleton-Century-Crofts, 1968. Vol. 3, p. 145.
25. Ehrenreich, T., Porush, J. G., Churg, J., Garfinkel, L., Glabman, S., Goldstein, M. H., Grishman, E., and Yunis, S. L. Treatment of idiopathic membranous nephropathy. *N. Engl. J. Med.* 295:741, 1976.
26. Eknoyan, G., Györkey, F., Dischoso, C., Martinez-Maldonado, M., Suki, W. N., and Györkey, P. Renal morphological and immunological changes associated with acute viral hepatitis. *Kidney Int.* 1:413, 1972.
27. Erwing, D. T., Donadio, J. V., and Holley, K. E. The clinical course of idiopathic membranous nephropathy. *Mayo Clin. Proc.* 48:697, 1973.
28. Esterly, N. B., Gotoff, S. P., Lolekha, S., Moore, E. S., Smith, R. D., Medenica, M., and Furey, N. L. Bullous pemphigoid and membranous glomerulonephropathy in a child. *J. Pediatr.* 83:466, 1973.

29. Evans, D. J. Pathogenesis of membranous glomerulonephritis. *Lancet* 1:1143, 1974.
30. Forland, M., and Spargo, B. H. Clinicopathological correlations in idiopathic nephrotic syndrome with membranous nephropathy. *Nephron* 6:498, 1969.
31. Franklin, W. A., Jennings, R. B., and Earle, D. P. Membranous glomerulonephritis: Long-term serial observations on clinical course and morphology. *Kidney Int.* 4:36, 1973.
32. Gamble, C. N., and Reardan, J. B. Immunopathogenesis of syphilitic glomerulonephritis. *N. Engl. J. Med.* 292:449, 1975.
33. Gärtner, H. V., Fischback, H., Wehner, H., Bohle, A., Edel, H. H., Kluthe, R., Scheler, F., and Schmulling, R. M. Comparison of clinical and morphological features of peri (epi-extra) membranous glomerulonephritis. *Nephron* 13:288, 1974.
34. Germuth, F. G., and Rodriguez, E. *Immunopathology of the Renal Glomerulus.* Boston: Little, Brown, 1973. P. 81.
35. Gluck, M. C., Gallo, G., Lowenstein, J., and Baldwin, D. S. Membranous glomerulonephritis. Evolution of clinical and pathologic features. *Ann. Intern. Med.* 78:1, 1973.
36. Habib, R., and Kleinknecht, C. The primary nephrotic syndrome of childhood—classification and clinicopathology study of 406 cases. In S. C. Sommers (ed.), *Pathology Annual.* New York: Appleton-Century-Crofts, 1971. P. 414.
37. Habib, R., Kleinknecht, C., and Gübler, M. C. Extramembranous glomerulonephritis in children: Report of 50 cases. *J. Pediatr.* 82:754, 1973.
38. Hallauer, W., Gärtner, H. V., Kronenberg, K. H., and Manz, G. Immunkomplexnephritis mit nephrotischem Syndrome unter Therapie mit D-Penizillamin. *Schweiz Med. Wochenschr.* 104:434, 1974.
39. Hill, L. L., Singer, D. B., Falleta, J., and Stasney, R. The nephrotic syndrome in congenital syphilis: An immunopathy. *Pediatrics* 49:260, 1972.
40. Jaffe, I. A., Treser, G., Suzuki, Y., and Ehrenreich, T. Nephropathy induced by D-penicillamine. *Ann. Intern. Med.* 69:549, 1968.
41. Kallen, R. J., Lee, S. K., Aronson, A. J., and Spargo, B. H. Idiopathic membranous glomerulopathy preceding the emergence of systemic lupus erythematosus in 2 children. *J. Pediatr.* 90:72, 1977.
42. Kaplan, B. S., Wiglesworth, F. W., Marks, M. I., and Drummond, K. N. The glomerulopathy of congenital syphilis: An immune deposit disease. *J. Pediatr.* 81:1154, 1972.
42a. Kelchner, J., McIntosh, J. R., Boedecker, E., Guggenheim, S., and McIntosh, R. M. Experimental autologous immune deposit nephritis in rats associated with mercuric chloride administration. *Experientia* 32:1204, 1976.
42b. Kleinknecht, C., Broyer, M., and Habib, R. Steroids for idiopathic membranous nephropathy. *N. Engl. J. Med.* 296:49, 1977.
43. Koffler, D., Agnello, V., Thoburn, R., and Kunkel, H. G. Systemic lupus erythematosus: Prototype of immune complex nephritis in man. *J. Exp. Med.* 134:169S, 1971.
44. Laroche, C., Merillon, H., Morel-Maroger, L., Turpi, G., Uro, Y., and Darrain, F. Syndrome néphrotique avec glomérulite extramembraneuse associée à une sarcoïdose. *J. Urol. Nephrol.* 74:995, 1968.
45. Laver, M. C., and Kincaid-Smith, P. The Natural History and Treatment of Membranous Glomerulonephritis. In P. Kincaid-Smith, T. H. Mathew, and E. L. Becker (eds.), *Glomerulonephritis.* New York: Wiley, 1973. Vol. I, pp. 461–472.
46. Levy, M., Gagnadoux, M. F., and Habib, R. An immunologic Fanconi syndrome (abstract). *Third International Symposium of Pediatric Nephrology,* Washington, D.C., 1974. P. 13.
47. Lewis, M. G., Loughridge, L. W., and Phillips, T. M. Immunological studies in nephrotic syndrome associated with extrarenal malignant diseases. *Lancet* 2:134, 1971.
48. Libit, S. A., Burke, B., Michael, A. F., and Vernier, R. L. Extramembranous glomerulonephritis in childhood: Relationship to systemic lupus erythematosus. *J. Pediatr.* 88:394, 1976.
49. Llach, F., Arieff, A. I., and Massry, S. G. Renal vein thrombosis and nephrotic syndrome. A prospective study of 36 adult patients. *Ann. Intern. Med.* 83:8, 1975.
50. McIntosh, R. H., Griswold, W. R., Chernack, W., and Koss, M. N. The glomerulonephropathies—etiopathogenesis. In J. Strauss (ed.), *Pediatric Nephrology I.* Miami, Fla.: Symposia Specialists, 1974. Pp. 89–113.
51. Medical Research Council Working Party. Controlled trial of azathioprine and prednisone in chronic renal disease. *Br. Med. J.* 2:239, 1971.
52. Moorthy, A. V., Zimmermann, W., Burkholder, P. M., and Harrington, A. R. Association of crescentic glomerulonephritis and membranous glomerulopathy: Report of three cases. *Clin. Nephrol.* 6:319, 1976.
53. Murphy, W. M., Deodhar, S. D., McCormack, L. J., and Osborne, D. G. Immunopathologic studies in glomerular diseases with membranous lesions. *Am. J. Clin. Pathol.* 60:364, 1973.
54. Nagi, A. H., Alexander, F., and Barabas, A. Z. Gold nephropathy in rats. Light and electron microscopic studies. *Exp. Mol. Pathol.* 15:354, 1971.
55. Naruse, J., Kitamura, K., Miyakawa, Y., and Shibata, S. Deposition of renal tubular epithelial antigen along the glomerular capillary walls of patients with membranous glomerulonephritis. *J. Immunol.* 110:1163, 1973.
56. Nicholson, G. D., Amin, U. F., and Alleyne, C. A. O. Membranous glomerulopathy with crescents. *Clin. Nephrol.* 5:198, 1975.
57. Olbing, H., Greifer, I., Bennet, B. P., Bernstein, J., and Spitzer, A. Idiopathic membranous nephropathy in children. *Kidney Int.* 3:381, 1973.
57a. O'Regan, S., Fong, J. S. C., Kaplan, B. S., de Chadarevian, J. P., Lapointe, N., and Drummond, K. N. Thyroid antigen-antibody nephritis. *Clin. Immunol. Immunopathol.* 6:341, 1976.
57b. Ozawa, T., Boedecker, E. A., Schorr, W., Guggenheim, S., and McIntosh, R. M. Immune-complex disease with unilateral vein thrombosis. *Arch. Pathol. Lab. Med.* 100:279, 1976.
58. Ozawa, T., Mass, M. F., Guggenheim, S., Strauss, J., and McIntosh, R. M. Autologous immune complex nephritis associated with sickle cell trait: Diagnosis of the hemoglobinopathy after renal structural and immunological studies. *Br. Med. J.* 1:369, 1976.
59. Petersen, V. P., Olsen, T. S., Kissmeyer-Nielsen, F., Bohman, S. O., Hansen, H. E., Hansen, E. S., Skou, D. E., and Sølling, K. Late failure of human renal transplant. *Medicine (Baltimore)* 54:45, 1975.
59a. Pierides, A. M., Malasit, P., Morley, A. R., Wilkin-

son, R., Uldall, P. R., and Kerr, D. N. S. Idiopathic membranous nephropathy. *Q. J. Med.* 46:163, 1977.

60. Pollak, V. E., Pirani, C. L., and Clyne, D. H. The Natural History of Membranous Glomerulonephropathy. In P. Kincaid-Smith, T. H. Mathew, and E. L. Becker (eds.), *Glomerulonephritis.* New York: Wiley, 1973. Vol. 1, pp. 429–448.

61. Pollak, V. E., Rosen, S., Pirani, C. L., Muehercke, R. C., and Kark, R. M. Natural history of lipoid nephrosis and membranous glomerulonephritis. *Ann. Intern. Med.* 69:1171, 1968.

62. Rastogi, S. P., Hart-Mercer, J., and Kerr, D. N. S. Idiopathic membranous glomerulonephritis in adults: Remission following steroid therapy. *Q. J. Med.* 38: 335, 1969.

63. Rosen, S. Membranous glomerulonephritis: Current status. *Hum. Pathol.* 3:209, 1971.

64. Row, P. G., Cameron, J. S., Turner, D. R., Evans, D. J., White, R. H. R., Ogg, C. S., Chantler, C., and Brown, C. B. Membranous nephropathy. *Q. J. Med.* 44:207, 1975.

65. Royer, P., Habib, R., Vermeil, G., Mathieu, H., and Alizon, M. Les glomérulonéphrits prolongées de l'enfant. *Ann. Pediatr.* 38:793, 1962.

66. Safar, M., Bariety, J., Lagrue, G., Samarcq, P., and Milliez, P. Association d'un syndrome néphrotique et d'un syndrome de Gougerot-Sjøgren. *Sem. Hop. Paris* 40:1423, 1964.

67. Salomon, M. I., Poon, T. P., Hsu, K. C., King, E. J., and Tchertkoff, V. Membranous glomerulopathy in a patient with sarcoidosis. *Arch. Pathol.* 99:479, 1975.

68. Silverberg, D. S., Kidd, E. G., Shnitka, T. K., and Ulan, R. A. Gold nephropathy. A clinical and pathologic study. *Arch. Rheumatol.* 13:812, 1970.

69. Strauss, J., Pardo, V., Koss, M. N., Griswold, W., and McIntosh, R. M. Nephropathy associated with

sickle cell anemia: An autologous immune complex nephritis. *Am. J. Med.* 58:382, 1975.

70. Törnroth, T., and Skrifvars, R. Gold nephropathy prototype of membranous glomerulonephritis. *Am. J. Pathol.* 75:573, 1974.

71. Tourville, D. R., Byrd, L. H., Kim, D. V., Zajd, D., Lee, J., Reichman, L. B., and Baskin, S. Treponemal antigen in immunopathogenesis of syphilitic glomerulonephritis. *Am. J. Pathol.* 82:479, 1976.

72. Trainin, E. B., Boichis, H., Spitzer, A., and Greifer, I. Idiopathic membranous nephropathy. Clinical course in children. *New York State J. Med.* 76:357, 1976.

73. Tsao, Y. C., Chan, W. C., and Gibson, J. B. Persistent proteinuria in children. *Arch. Dis. Child.* 44: 443, 1969.

74. Tung, K. S. K., and Black, W. C. Association of renal glomerular and tubular immune complex disease and antitubular basement membrane antibody. *Lab. Invest.* 32:696, 1975.

75. Viol, G. W., Miniell, J. A., and Bistrichi, R. J. Gold nephropathy. A clinical and structural analysis (abstract). *Sixth International Congress of Nephrology,* Florence, 1975. P. 309.

76. White, R. H. R., Glasgow, E. F., and Mills, R. J. Clinicopathological study of nephrotic syndrome in childhood. *Lancet* 1:1353, 1970.

77. Whitworth, J. A., Leibowitz, S., Kennedy, M. C., Cameron, J. S., Evans, D. J., Glassock, R. J., and Schoenfeld, L. S. Absence of glomerular renal tubular epithelial antigen in membranous glomerulonephritis. *Clin. Nephrol.* 5:159, 1976.

78. Wong, W. C., Urizar, R. E., and McIntosh, R. Autologous immune-complex glomerulopathy in sickle cell disease (abstract). *Third International Symposium of Pediatric Nephrology,* Washington, D.C., 1974. P. 11.

51. Membranoproliferative Glomerulonephritis

Richard H. R. White

The term *membranoproliferative glomerulonephritis* was first applied by Habib and her colleagues [29, 54] to a form of persistent glomerulonephritis occurring in children in whom renal biopsy specimens showed, in addition to mesangial cellular proliferation, diffuse thickening of the glomerular capillary walls. They described identical capillary wall changes in biopsy specimens showing what had previously been called lobular glomerulonephritis [2, 37]. Although they classified these two groups separately, they reported associated reduction of serum B_{1A}-globulin (C3c) levels with both types of lesion [54]; in the light of subsequent studies of complement abnormalities, this suggests an etiologic similarity. Cameron et al. [13] provided evidence from clinical and labora-

tory data and repeat renal biopsies that the two were merely varieties of the same disease, and this view is now generally accepted [27].

Gotoff et al. [24] drew attention to the persistence of low serum C3 levels in children with chronic glomerulonephritis. They did not give detailed histologic descriptions but remarked on the presence of endocapillary cellular proliferation, with prominent lobulation of the tufts, polymorphonuclear leukocytic infiltration, and "basement membrane thickening." In the same year, West and coworkers [70] characterized the morphologic features of a similar group of children with "hypocomplementemic persistent glomerulonephritis," laying particular emphasis on the thickening of the capillary walls, due, apparently, to the splitting of the basement membrane by the progressive accumulation of nonargyrophilic material. Cameron et al. [13] reported their findings in 50 children and adults with membranoproliferative glomerulonephritis (MPGN) and demonstrated by electron microscopy that the capillary-wall changes were due to the interposition of cells, basement membrane–like fibrils, and electron-dense deposits between the true capillary basement membrane and the endothelial cytoplasm.

A major contribution of the study by Cameron et al. [13] was to unify under a common morphologic description a group of patients with widely differing clinical presentations at onset but a uniformly progressive course, of whom 16 percent never showed lowering of serum C3 levels, thus establishing a preference for the term *membranoproliferative glomerulonephritis* over *hypocomplementemic glomerulonephritis*. The more recent term *mesangiocapillary glomerulonephritis* [18] has merit as an anatomic description of the disease; it has not yet gained universal acceptance and is at risk of confusion with an altogether different lesion, *mesangial proliferative glomerulonephritis* [77], and with what Thoenes [58] has

called *mesangioproliferative glomerulonephritis.* Reference to the earlier literature reveals a variety of incomplete descriptions of the disease under terms such as *chronic latent* and *subacute nephritis* [1, 7], *chronic lobular glomerulonephritis* [2, 37], and *mixed membranous and proliferative glomerulonephritis* [38]. The recent reappraisal of three postmortem kidneys originally described by Richard Bright [10, 11] and left in the museum at Guy's Hospital, London, is of considerable historic interest in that it established two of them as the earliest known examples of MPGN [67].

Pathologic Features
GENERAL ASPECTS

The morphologic features of MPGN have been described in detail by a number of workers [5, 13, 14, 26, 27, 31, 70] and are illustrated in Figs. 51-1 to 51-10. The disease involves primarily the glomeruli, all of which are enlarged owing to diffuse endocapillary cellular proliferation (Figs. 51-1, 51-2, 51-6). Although electron microscopy demonstrates endothelial proliferation, the mesangial cells are predominantly affected. This mesangial hypercellularity varies considerably in de-

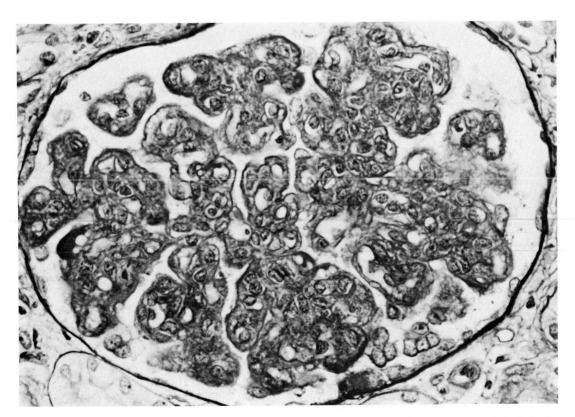

Figure 51-1. An enlarged glomerulus from type I MPGN showing moderately severe mesangial thickening and proliferation, together with a striking double contour of the capillary walls. (PAS, ×690.)

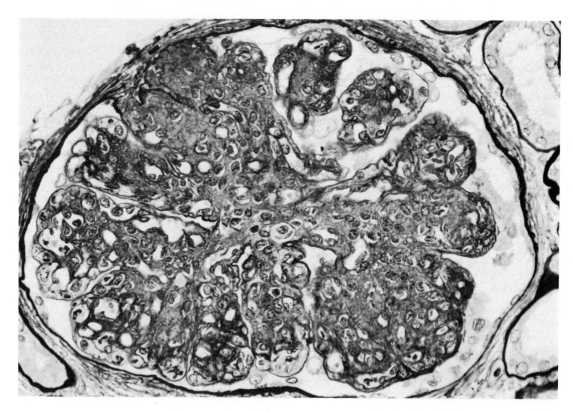

Figure 51-2. An extremely lobulated glomerulus (type I) owing to greatly increased mesangial matrix and cellularity. Note the infiltration with polymorphonuclear leukocytes, and the segmental sclerosis with adhesion to Bowman's capsule at 10 o'clock. (PASM, ×430.)

gree and is accompanied by a more or less commensurate increase of mesangial matrix, which, when marked, exaggerates the lobular pattern of the glomeruli (Fig. 51-2). Early descriptions [29] suggested lobular and nonlobular entities, but subsequent evidence [13] indicated that these merely represented the extremes of a continuous spectrum of mesangial reaction. Careful examination of renal biopsy specimens reveals that the degree of lobulation in individual glomeruli varies, while serial biopsy specimens may demonstrate changes in the amount of proliferation of both cells and matrix—and consequently in lobularity—with the passage of time. Small numbers of polymorphonuclear leukocytes are frequently observed in the glomerular tufts, and in some cases this infiltration is marked. On electron microscopy, polymorphs can sometimes be seen in the subendothelial region, in contact with the capillary basement membrane. Epithelial crescents may be found in about 15 percent of cases [27] and adversely affect the prognosis when they involve a high proportion of glomeruli.

CAPILLARY-WALL CHANGES

The disease is distinguished from other forms of proliferative glomerulonephritis by the presence of irregular thickening of the capillary walls. In the commoner variety (type I) the primary abnormality is the presence of immune deposits in the subendothelial region. It is presumably these that stimulate the nonspecific reaction referred to as "circumferential mesangial interposition" [6], in which mesangial matrix and cells extend between the true capillary basement membrane and the endothelium, causing them to separate and thereby producing the double contour (Fig. 51-3) that characterizes this lesion morphologically. It is not always possible to distinguish clearly between subendothelial deposits and cytoplasm in routine light microscopy preparations, and the former may be better visualized using trichrome stains. The structural alterations to the capillary wall are particularly well demonstrated by means of the periodic acid–silver methanamine (PASM) technique, which selectively stains the capillary basement membrane as well as mesangial fibrils.

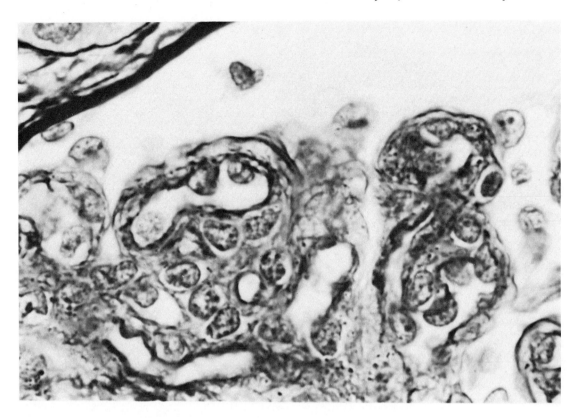

Figure 51-3. Detail of the capillary wall changes in type I MPGN showing the apparent duplication due to circumferential mesangial interposition. (PASM, ×1,730.)

On electron microscopy the true capillary basement membrane shows little or no thickening (Fig. 51-4) and occasional thin segments, giving its inner surface an irregular contour. The endothelial cytoplasm is separated from the basement membrane by a meshwork of membranous fibrils enclosing islands of mesangial cytoplasm and a variable number of electron-dense subendothelial deposits (Fig. 51-5). Subepithelial deposits similar to the "humps" observed characteristically in poststreptococcal glomerulonephritis (Chap. 47) are often present although sparse. Occasionally, a capillary loop may contain a larger number of subepithelial deposits separated by projections from the basement membrane ("spikes"), as in membranous glomerulonephropathy [27] (Chap. 50).

In type II MPGN, which was first described as an entity by Berger and Galle [8] and is generally referred to as "dense intramembranous deposit disease" [26], the capillary basement membrane is diffusely thickened, giving a ribbonlike appearance on light microscopy (Fig. 51-6). This is not always obvious in periodic acid–Schiff

(PAS) stains, particularly when the biopsy sections are thin, and may be better demonstrated with trichrome stains (Fig. 51-7). Although in more than half the cases a double contour of segmental distribution is seen in PASM stains, the capillary basement membrane is represented by a thickened and frequently scalloped band of a "washed-out" grayish-brown color (Fig. 51-8) instead of the crisp, thin black line seen in the subendothelial type. The reason for this is apparent on electron microscopy (Fig. 51-9); the lamina densa is more or less completely replaced by extremely dense, homogeneous material that causes variable and sometimes marked thickening of the basement membrane. The continuity of the dense deposits is interrupted in places by segments of normal basement membrane or occasionally by electron-lucent aggregates. Sparse subepithelial humps also may be found. Mesangial interposition tends to be focal and segmental and occasionally is absent. Similar dense intramembranous deposits may be seen focally in Bowman's capsule (Fig. 51-10) and tubules on both light and electron microscopy.

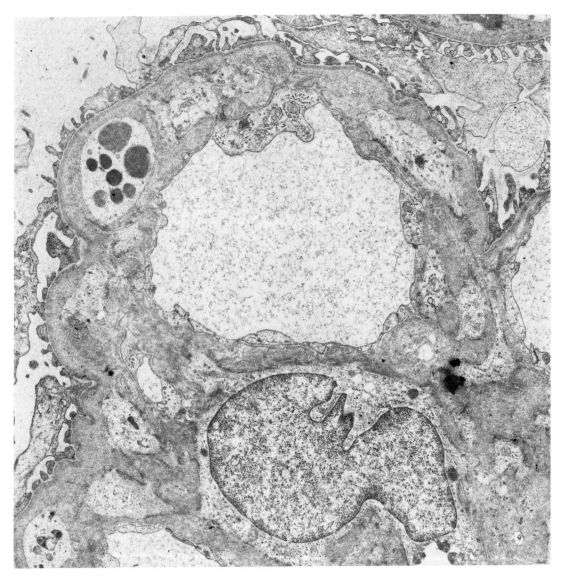

Figure 51-4. Electron micrograph of type I MPGN demonstrating the interposition of mesangial cytoplasm and matrix between the endothelium and the true capillary basement membrane. Note the polymorphonuclear leukocyte in contact with the basement membrane at top left. (×11,000.)

Burkholder et al. [11a] described a third morphologic variety, similar to type I MPGN on light microscopy, but with the addition of numerous subepithelial deposits, separated by "spikes" of basement membrane, as in membranous nephropathy (Chap. 50), as well as discrete intramembranous aggregates. Immunofluorescence gave particularly heavy, granular, peripheral deposits of IgG and IgM. There were no recognizable clinical or etiologic differences between the two varieties. More recently Strife et al. [57] have described a further variety (type III) in which the clinical

characteristic is persistent hypocomplementemia. Both subendothelial and subepithelial deposits were extensive. Whereas Burkholder et al. [11a] described these two layers of deposits as distinct, Strife et al. [57] observed that they were contiguous, and associated with disruption and lamination of the lamina densa. Possibly the latter is a more severe degree of the former. New basement membrane–like material often appeared to encircle the subepithelial deposits, as opposed to merely separating them with spikes. One of the cases illustrated by Anders and Thoenes [5] ap-

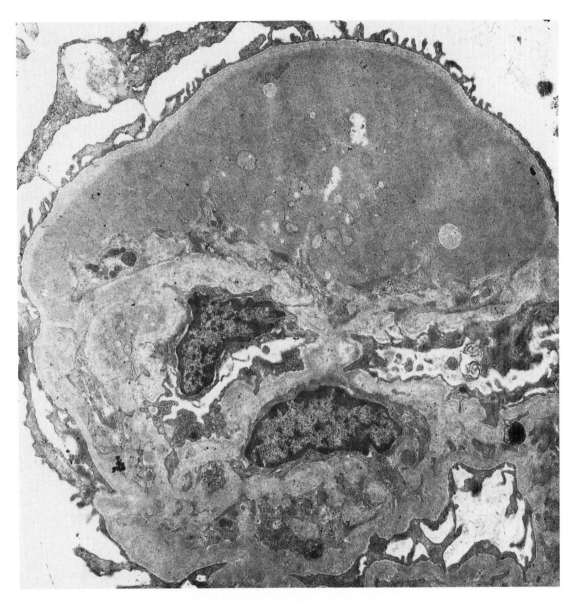

Figure 51-5. Another view of the same glomerulus showing a large subendothelial deposit. (×3,000.)

pears to be similar. The light microscopic appearances of type III MPGN were extremely variable, sometimes resembling the lobular form but more often superficially mimicking membranous nephropathy, although typical spikes were never seen on PASM stains. There were no clinical or etiologic features distinctive to the third varieties described by either Burkholder et al. [11a] or Strife et al. [57]. It has yet to be determined whether they constitute an entity or are extreme versions of type I MPGN, in which small numbers of subepithelial deposits are often seen.

OTHER GLOMERULAR ABNORMALITIES

The mesangial and other glomerular changes are similar in all varieties of MPGN, although on electron microscopy, finely granular deposits in the mesangium appear more numerous in type II disease. Mesangial hyperplasia, when marked, displaces the capillaries toward the periphery of the lobules and accentuates the lobular pattern of the tufts; in long-standing cases, sclerotic nodules develop as hypercellularity diminishes. Mesangial interposition leads to progressive narrowing of capillary lumens, and the end result is total glo-

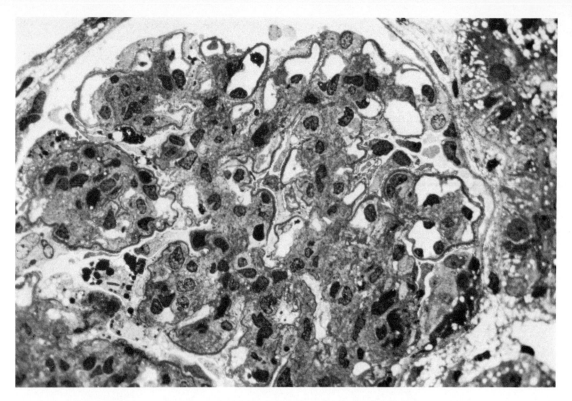

Figure 51-6. *Type II MPGN. There is moderate mesangial thickening and proliferation. The capillary walls lack a double contour showing instead slight but uniform thickening. A section from a repeat biopsy from the same child is shown in Fig. 51-10. (Epon, 1μ, Movat's silver stain, ×690.)*

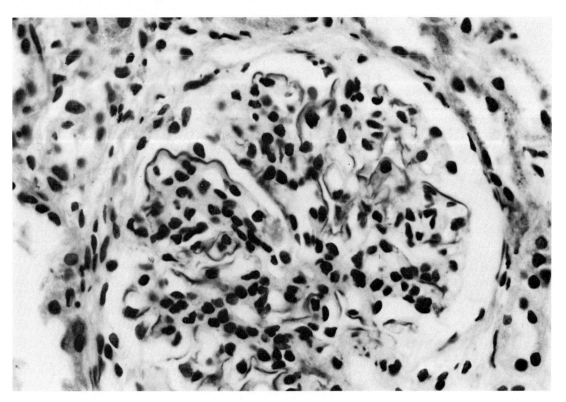

Figure 51-7. *The ribbonlike appearance of the dense intramembranous deposits is well demonstrated in this trichrome stain. (Martius scarlet-blue, ×690.)*

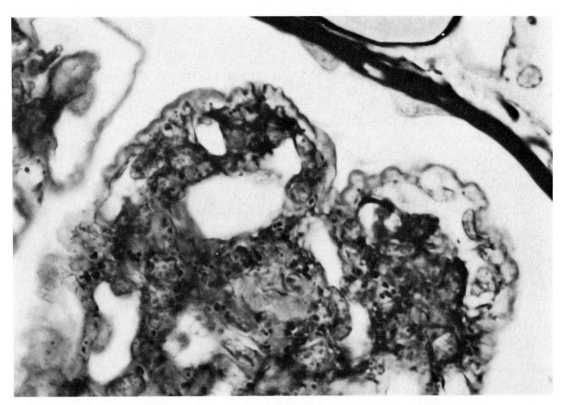

Figure 51-8. Detail of the capillary wall changes in type II MPGN. Note the "washed-out" appearance of the basement membrane in silver-stained paraffin sections. In this instance there is mesangial interposition, with a double contour. (PASM, ×1,730.)

merular sclerosis. The sclerosing process proceeds irregularly, however, and glomeruli showing segmental sclerosis with local capsular adhesion are often seen in biopsy specimens (see Fig. 51-2).

TUBULAR AND INTERSTITIAL CHANGES
In type II disease, dense deposits may be seen focally within the tubular basement membrane. Otherwise, the tubular and interstitial changes occurring in MPGN are of secondary significance. Tubular atrophy and interstitial fibrosis roughly parallel the extent of glomerular sclerosis. Interstitial edema and infiltration with chronic inflammatory cells may occur in the early phase of the disease but are generally patchy except in cases with numerous epithelial crescents, when they are likely to be extensive. Small foci of interstitial form cells are often observed.

Immunopathologic Features
The most constant finding on immunofluorescence microscopy (Fig. 51-11) of renal biopsy tissue is the glomerular deposition of C3 [26, 27, 31]. Michael and coworkers [45, 74] also demonstrated deposits of properdin in all the hypocomplemen-

temic patients whom they investigated and deposits of C1q and C4 in some two-thirds of biopsy specimens examined. Deposits of IgG are not infrequently found, whereas IgM and fibrin are not prominent, and IgA is rarely seen [31, 44, 45]. More recent studies correlating the immunofluorescence findings with morphologic subdivisions suggest basically different patterns of deposition in types I and II MPGN [26–28, 50, 66]. In the former, deposits are predominantly subendothelial, coarsely granular, and contain not only C3 but also C1q, C4, properdin, and sometimes IgG. Occasionally, deposits are also present in the mesangium, but these appear to be confined to C3 and properdin, C1q and C4 being absent. In type II MPGN, faint linear deposits of C3 are distributed segmentally on the capillary walls, while coarse granular deposits of C3 are prominent in the mesangium. IgG is observed rarely, and early-reacting complement components and properdin are not seen.

Etiology
In the majority of cases of MPGN there are no recognizable antecedents, and little is known

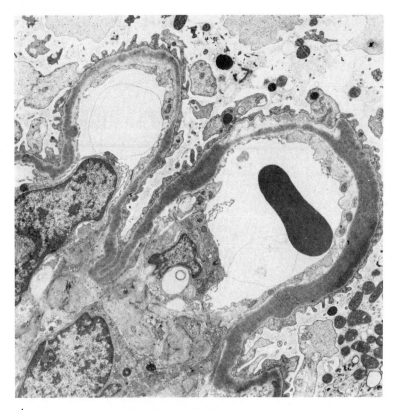

A

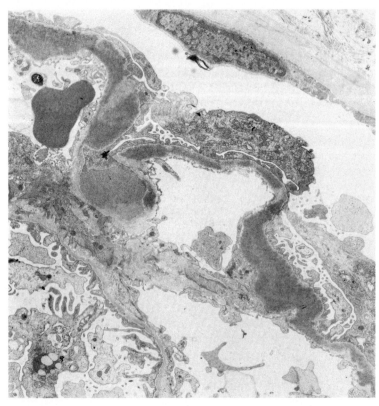

B

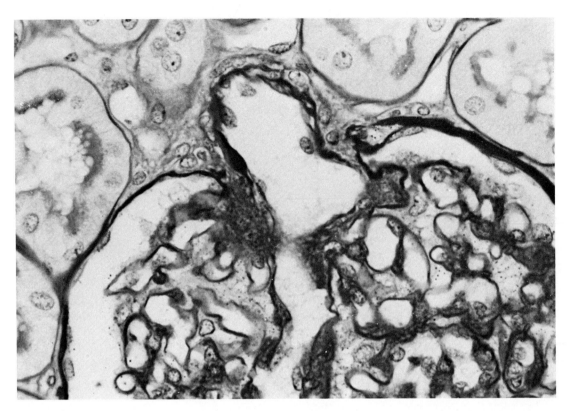

Figure 51-10. Part of a glomerulus from the same biopsy as in Fig. 51-9 showing dense intramembranous deposits in Bowman's capsule at top right. Note the lack of mesangial interposition. This biopsy specimen was obtained from a 10-year-old girl with asymptomatic, minimal proteinuria and persistent hypocomplementemia, 5 years after an acute nephritic onset. A section from her first biopsy is shown in Fig. 51-6. (PAS, ×690.)

about the etiology. Typical lesions have been observed on biopsy in a small number of patients with bacteremia due to *Staphylococcus albus* from infected ventriculoatrial shunts [9, 27, 44–46]. There is evidence that the lesion may resolve following eradication of infection, and its behavior is thus quite different from that of the idiopathic variety. Habib and her associates [27] also mentioned having seen MPGN in systemic lupus erythematosus, polyarteritis nodosa, and Schönlein-Henoch nephritis, but gave no details. A case was reported recently in association with rheumatoid arthritis [61a]. Although mesangial interposition and subendothelial immune deposits are undoubtedly seen in these disorders, their distribution is generally less diffuse than in MPGN, while additional features characteristic of the underlying disease are usually present. Moreover, these condi-

tions are usually distinguishable by different patterns of glomerular immune deposits in addition to either normal serum complement or, in the case of lupus, marked depression of C1q and C4. It is therefore questionable whether or not the term *membranoproliferative glomerulonephritis* should be used to describe such changes occurring in multisystem disorders.

There is no clear-cut relationship with poststreptococcal glomerulonephritis. In their original report, West et al. [70] favored the idea that this was the initiating event in hypocomplementemic MPGN, but later provided evidence to the contrary [49]. Admittedly, the sequence of an acute nephritic syndrome followed immediately or after an interval of months or years by a nephrotic syndrome [13, 41] is suggestive, although biopsies have rarely been performed in such patients dur-

Figure 51-9. Electron-microscopic appearance of type II MPGN. A. The dense intramembranous deposit is interrupted at the top of the right-hand capillary by electron-lucent aggregates. B. At the mesangiocapillary junction (left-center), there is a short segment of normal basement membrane incompletely surrounding a subepithelial "hump" that lies in the cleft between the two capillaries. (×8,000 before 32.5% reduction.)

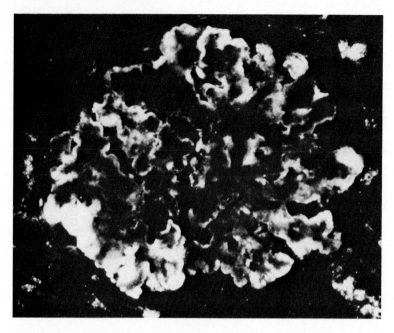

Figure 51-11. Immunofluorescent appearance of type I MPGN showing coarse, granular capillary-wall deposits of C3c (β1A globulin). (Courtesy of Dr. A. J. McAdams University of Cincinnati College of Medicine.) (×690 before 21% reduction.)

ing the initial episode. Although both conditions show broadly similar complement profiles [14, 16], the hypocomplementemia of poststreptococcal nephritis is transient [14, 16, 23, 56, 71], while a "nephritic factor" capable of breaking down C3 in normal human serum in vitro, comparable with that found in MPGN, has not been demonstrated [72]. While Habib et al. [26] observed raised antistreptolysin (ASO) titers more frequently in type II than type I MPGN, the proportion of all patients with MPGN exhibiting raised titers probably does not exceed that of a normal population [13]. Jenis et al. [36] have reported the cases of 3 children with an acute nephritic syndrome following upper respiratory infection associated with raised ASO titers and positive throat cultures for hemolytic streptococci that were identified as non–group A in 2 cases; biopsy sections from all 3 children showed type II MPGN, with frequent subepithelial humps. A somewhat more convincing case of transition from poststreptococcal nephritis to MPGN, supported by acceptable serologic and morphologic criteria, was described by Glasgow and White [23], but even in this patient there were patchy dense intramembranous deposits in the initial biopsy specimen, so that such a relationship must at present be regarded as unproved.

Van Acker et al. [65] reported the occurrence of MPGN in a pair of siblings, but there are no other reported examples of familial incidence, and it is not possible to draw conclusions regarding a genetic origin. However, the writer has seen a morphologically typical example of MPGN, with infantile onset of nephrotic syndrome and a fatal outcome, associated with normal serum C3 levels, in a boy whose two stepbrothers by the same mother, of Chinese origin, had previously died from uninvestigated nephritis, leaving two surviving, healthy stepsisters. Moreover, several of the mother's brothers had died, allegedly from "kidney trouble." This suggests the possibility of an X-linked recessive mode of inheritance.

Of considerable interest is the reported association between MPGN and partial lipodystrophy [30, 52, 80]. Reports indicate that the associated renal lesion is confined to type II MPGN [26, 52, 66], as suggested also by the electron micrographs illustrating a paper by Eisinger et al. [19]. Peters et al. [52] demonstrated persistently low C3 levels in their patients, together with circulating nephritic factor (C3NeF), while Alper and co-workers [3] and Thompson and White [61] showed that the complement defects can exist in the absence of renal disease. Thus, prospective studies of children with partial lipodystrophy may possibly shed further light on the etiology of MPGN.

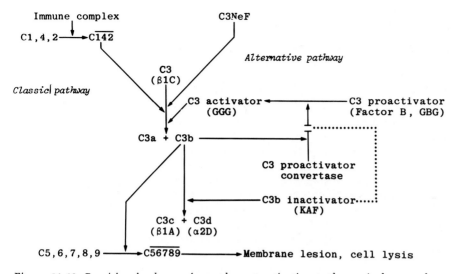

Figure 51-12. Provisional scheme of complement activation pathways in human glomerulonephritis.

Pathogenesis

The most characteristic immunologic finding is persistent hypocomplementemia. The complement lytic system and its relation to glomerulonephritis is described in detail in Chap. 3, and only a few of the more important landmarks in the study of this complex subject will be mentioned here. A provisional scheme of the complement activation pathways relevant to human glomerulonephritis is given in Fig. 51-12.

It is well known that serum C3 levels are reduced in most cases of MPGN [13, 14, 16, 24, 27, 28, 31, 44, 45, 47, 48, 50, 51, 55, 64, 66, 68–70, 72, 73, 78, 79, 82] and it has been generally accepted, until recently, that levels of the early-reacting components C1q, C4, and C2 fall within the normal range [14, 16, 21, 31, 33, 34, 42, 55], suggesting that C3 is activated via the alternative pathway [25]. The serum of patients with MPGN and hypocomplementemia frequently contains an anticomplementary substance, the C3 nephritic factor (C3NeF); this was demonstrated by Vallota et al. [63], who observed accelerated in vitro breakdown of C3 in normal serum when MPGN serum was added to it. The observation that purified C3 was not similarly split indicated that one or more serum cofactors were required for the reaction to take place.

The nature and origin of C3NeF is uncertain; Thompson [59, 60] has provided evidence that it is an IgG of subclass 3. It is clearly not the result of glomerulonephritis, since its activity has been shown to continue in the serum after bilateral nephrectomy [1, 51]. Moreover, the demonstra-

tion of its presence in nonnephritic children with partial lipodystrophy [61] indicates that, at least in that condition, it can precede the development of nephritis. The mechanism by which C3NeF activates C3 is unknown [72]. There is no conclusive evidence that properdin is involved [68], as it appears to be when the alternative pathway is activated by other substances, such as complex polysaccharides [53].

The catabolism of C3 takes place in two phases, whether it is activated via the classic or alternative pathway. It is initially cleaved to C3a and C3b; the latter activates C5 and thence the terminal components of complement. Experiments have shown that cleavage of C3 to C3a and C3b is dependent on the activation of glycine-rich beta-glycoprotein (GBG), also known as properdin factor B and C3 proactivator (C3PA), which changes to a gammaglycoprotein (GGG), the C3 activator or nephritic C3 convertase [55, 72]. This conversion is initiated by the enzyme C3PA convertase after it has been activated by C3b; it has been shown conclusively that the conversion of GBG to GGG will not take place in an in vitro mixture that does not contain C3b [78]. It is thus evident that once C3b has been formed, the cyclic portion of the alternative pathway (Fig. 51-12) will become autoactivated, unless inhibited, until the supply of the essential reactant, C3, is exhausted. However, C3b formed in vivo is rapidly inactivated by the conglutinogen activating factor, giving rise to C3c and C3d. The former is rapidly cleared from the circulation, whereas the latter accumulates; the presence of circulating C3d is evidence that in vivo breakdown of C3 occurs in MPGN [55, 73].

The disappearance rate of radiolabeled C3 observed in vivo in patients with MPGN is normal [4, 51]. Increased catabolism is therefore unlikely to be the sole explanation of the low serum C3 levels observed. The metabolic studies of Charlesworth et al. [17] have demonstrated that diminished synthesis also plays a major role. Vallota et al. [63] had shown that the rate of C3 breakdown by C3NeF was related to the initial C3 concentration, being extremely rapid when C3 was present in normal concentration and slow at low levels. On the basis of the published evidence and their own careful experiments, Williams et al. [78] proposed that depletion of C3b, as a result of diminished C3 synthesis, is the ultimate limiting factor in determining the catabolic rate; and further, that in the early stage of the disease, there is accelerated C3 catabolism, which slows down to a normal rate, balanced by reduced synthesis, when a new equilibrium is reached at low C3 levels. This reduced synthesis might thus be conceived as a protective mechanism to limit C3 activation; and although nothing is known of the way in which it is brought about, it is possibly related to the presence in the circulation of C3b or its catabolic products, C3c and C3d [78].

Closer examination of serum complement profiles in patients with MPGN reveals that the observed range of C1q and C4 levels not infrequently extends appreciably below normal. This complex picture has been to some extent clarified by studies that have related complement component levels to the morphologic variants [14, 16, 28, 50, 79, 82]. In summary, it appears that (1) C3 levels are almost invariably reduced in type II but may be normal in type I MPGN; (2) circulating C3NeF is found more frequently in type II than type I; (3) properdin factor B (GBG) levels are significantly lower in type II than type I; and (4) C1q, C4, and properdin levels are significantly lower in type I than in type II MPGN. Considered alongside recent immunofluorescence microscopy findings, these observations confirm that alternative pathway activation is the main defect in type II MPGN, but suggest that classic pathway activation plays a role in type I disease. Until the type III lesion has been more fully studied, its pathogenesis will not be known, but the evidence suggests similarity to type I.

The link between hypocomplementemia and the glomerular lesion is as yet undetermined. Ooi et al. [50a] reported that, although the presence of serum immune complexes, as determined by C1q-binding activity, correlated well with the clinical status, there was no correlation with serum levels of C3. Peters et al. [52] have commented on the apparent susceptibility to infection observed in some patients with partial lipodystrophy and have suggested that subjects depleted of C3 might suffer from defective elimination of immune complexes, which instead become trapped in the glomerular capillary walls. On the other hand, by no means all lipodystrophic patients experience recurrent infections [61]; moreover, the facts that C3 levels may be normal at some time during the course of the illness [13, 69] and that 16 percent of MPGN patients never become hypocomplementemic [13–15] have yet to be explained.

Clinical and Laboratory Findings at Onset

Membranoproliferative glomerulonephritis is essentially a disorder affecting older children and young adults [13, 14, 27, 31]; its onset before 5 or after 40 years of age is exceptional. There is a slight predominance of females in most reported series that is more marked during early adolescence. About one-third of patients may give a history of preceding upper respiratory infection, although it is doubtful that the incidence of raised ASO titers is significantly higher than that found in a normal population [13].

The commonest presenting symptoms are edema and hematuria. About one-third of patients are found to be hypertensive, and an equal number show impaired renal function at onset. The urine almost invariably contains a large amount of protein and erythrocytes and usually contains granular casts as well. In the majority of cases the proteinuria is poorly selective [14]. Assembling the various combinations of clinical and laboratory findings into recognizable syndromes, Cameron and associates [14] found that 44 percent of patients presented with a nephrotic syndrome, 26 percent with an acute nephritic syndrome, and 7 percent with recurrent hematuria; MPGN was diagnosed in the remaining 23 percent following the discovery of proteinuria on routine urinalysis. Habib et al. [27] reported a much higher incidence of symptomless proteinuria, perhaps reflecting the more extensive employment of routine urinalysis in French children. There are recorded instances of symptomless proteinuria and microscopic hematuria preceding the onset of clinical manifestations by months or years [31, 70].

Hypoproteinemia is a common finding, although, as Habib et al. [27] indicated, it is exceptional to find the extremely low serum albumin levels (i.e., less than 1.0 gm per deciliter) that are characteristic of corticosteroid-responsive nephrotic children. Serum gamma-globulin levels are generally reduced, while the cholesterol is increased in some two-thirds of patients, though rarely to very high levels. Nitrogen retention with a measurably impaired glomerular filtration rate (GFR) is observed initially in one-third of children and nearly half of adult patients with MPGN [13]. In most cases, renal function returns to normal within 4 to 8 weeks, and the impairment probably represents an acute phase of the disease, with much capillary obliteration due to cellular proliferation, although nephrotic hypovolemia may be an additional factor. Severe reduction of GFR is unusual and generally associated with hypertension; when present, it tends to persist and signifies a steadily downhill course [13]. Normochromic anemia is observed in half the patients and appears unrelated to azotemia [13]. Positive tests for lupus erythematosus and antinuclear factor are never obtained.

Total serum hemolytic complement activity frequently is reduced. The most consistent finding is a reduction of serum C3 concentration; this occurs in about two-thirds of patients when the disease is first diagnosed, but develops later in some patients, so that ultimately only one-sixth remain normocomplementemic [13–15]. The presence of nephritic factor (C3NeF) may be revealed in patients with low C3 levels by incubating their serum with normal human serum at 37°C and demonstrating C3 breakdown products (C3c and C3d) in the mixture by immunoelectrophoresis [63]. The activation of the complement system that accompanies C3 reduction is demonstrated in some patients by lowering of the serum levels of later-reacting components: C5 [72], C6 and C7 [14, 52, 59], and C$\overline{89}$ [14, 51]. However, these determinations have little diagnostic significance and are not established procedures in routine laboratories. Although, as mentioned earlier, recent studies have demonstrated lower mean levels of C1q and C4 in type I than type II MPGN, the degree of overlap observed seriously limits the usefulness of these measurements as clinical discriminators in individual patients. Thus, determination of the serum C3 level remains the most useful clinical test and is within the reach of most hospital laboratories.

Differential Diagnosis

In patients presenting with a nephrotic syndrome the first step is to separate those who might have MPGN from those likely to show "minimal changes." Corticosteroids, given in high daily dosage, may lead to deteriorating renal function and accelerated hypertension in patients with severe proliferative glomerulonephritis [76], and the use of a therapeutic trial as a diagnostic test is regarded as unacceptable today. The clinical and laboratory findings that are considered most useful in differential diagnosis of the nephrotic syndrome [75, 77] are summarized in Table 51-1. From this, it would appear that the minimal change group can be differentiated with a high degree of confidence without resort to renal biopsy, whereas the distinction between MPGN and other structural lesions such as focal glomerulosclerosis (Chap. 55) can be made with confidence only in those patients who show hypocomplementemia at onset. Before treatment is initiated, renal biopsy is therefore recommended in all patients in whom a structural lesion appears likely. These differentiations are discussed in greater detail in Chap. 52, in which the results of the prospective study of the nephrotic syndrome in children done by the International Study of Kidney Disease in Children are presented.

An acute nephritic onset of MPGN is more likely to occur in children than in adults [13] and may mimic poststreptococcal glomerulonephritis. The differential diagnosis of these two conditions is shown in Table 51-2. There are no appreciable differences in age and sex distribution.

Table 51-1. Differential Diagnosis of Membranoproliferative Glomerulonephritis in Patients Presenting with a Nephrotic Syndrome

Clinical or Laboratory Characteristics	Morphology		
	MPGN	Other Lesions	Minimal Changes
Male-female ratio	<1	1	2 : 1
Peak age incidence	Late childhood and adolescence	Variable	Preschool child
Hypertension	Variable	Variable	Absent or transient
Hematuria	Frequent	Frequent	Absent or transient
Protein selectivity	Moderate to low	Moderate to low	High to moderate
Hypoalbuminemia	Moderate	Moderate	Severe
Serum C3	Low in two-thirds	Normal	Normal

Table 51-2. Differential Diagnosis of Membrano-proliferative Glomerulonephritis in Patients Presenting with an Acute Nephritic Syndrome

Clinical or Laboratory Characteristics	MPGN	Poststreptococcal Glomerulonephritis
Hypertension	Present in half; usually persists	Present in half; always transient
Proteinuria	Persistent, heavy	Transient
Hypoalbuminemia	Frequent	Unusual, transient
ASOT ≧250 units	<40%	>90%
Serum C3 level	Persistently low	Low, rising to normal

Hematuria and proteinuria occur almost invariably in both conditions, and hypertension is common. However, in poststreptococcal glomerulonephritis, proteinuria and hypertension are less persistent, as is hypoalbuminemia when it occurs. A raised ASO titer is not helpful for diagnosis, but a normal titer favors a diagnosis of MPGN. The most reliable signs of MPGN are persistent heavy proteinuria and failure of the C3 level to return toward normal 4 to 6 weeks after onset of symptoms. Renal biopsy should be performed in such patients.

Patients with MPGN found to have symptomless proteinuria generally show biochemical evidence of a nephrotic state, although they are clinically free from edema. Microscopic hematuria is almost invariably present [13]; when absent, it probably represents long-standing, symptomless disease. The differential diagnosis is similar to that for patients with a nephrotic syndrome. Recurrent macroscopic hematuria is an unusual presentation for MPGN [13, 14, 22], and the diagnosis is suggested when proteinuria persists between attacks and hypocomplementemia is present.

Treatment and Prognosis
SUPPORTIVE MEASURES

Patients presenting with an acute nephritic onset with significant azotemia from reduction of GFR may require restriction of dietary protein and fluids as well as salt restriction, diuretics such as furosemide, and hypotensive agents for the control of hypertension, which is mainly sodium-dependent. In the absence of good evidence of a streptococcal etiology, penicillin is not indicated, although many patients will have been given antibiotics on the basis of an assumed but erroneous diagnosis of poststreptococcal nephritis before referral to a nephrologist for further evaluation. As in the case of poststreptococcal nephritis, a diuresis generally occurs within 1 to 2 weeks of onset, and renal function improves. However, heavy proteinuria continues in most cases, often with moderate hypoproteinemia. Patients presenting with recurrent macroscopic hematuria, and those found to have symptomless proteinuria, require no particular supportive therapy.

Persistent hypertension should be treated without delay in order to minimize the development of secondary renal vascular changes (Chap. 32).

Approximately half the patients present with a nephrotic syndrome, or it develops following a nephritic onset. Since a nephrotic syndrome is corticosteroid-resistant, it may run a protracted course, requiring dietary sodium restriction and the use of diuretics to control edema. The associated negative nitrogen balance may, if prolonged, lead to generalized muscle wasting. Although a high-protein diet may seem logical, there is no good evidence that it is effective, and, indeed, it is difficult to achieve with natural foods without risking sodium overload. The parents and family physician should be warned about the patient's increased susceptibility to infections, so that infections will be less likely to be overlooked. The current practice is to treat infections vigorously as they occur rather than to depend on chemoprophylaxis.

With time, proteinuria usually lessens in amount, and plasma protein levels return to normal, allowing edema to subside. In a minority of children—especially those in whom the renal lesion is complicated by the presence of numerous epithelial crescents—deterioration of renal function is comparatively rapid and associated with a nephrotic state until terminal renal failure supervenes. The renal tubular avidity for sodium that results from hypoproteinemic contraction of the plasma volume, together with the falling GFR and increasingly severe hypertension, poses an extremely taxing therapeutic problem. In spite of massive doses of furosemide or ethacrynic acid, edema and ascites may continue to increase; and although sodium depletion can be produced by an extremely unpalatable salt-poor diet, this may be achieved only at the cost of further reduction of GFR, through uncompensated hypovolemia, with consequent increased retention of nitrogen, phosphate, and potassium. If all these measures fail, peritoneal dialysis may afford temporary relief, but in these circumstances it may be advisable to start regular hemodialysis at a higher level of GFR than usual.

SPECIFIC DRUG THERAPY

It appears to be widely known among pediatric nephrologists that children with MPGN, treated with corticosteroids in high daily dosage, may show rapid deterioration of renal function and become severely hypertensive, although published reports of such occurrences [76] are rare. McAdams et al. [43] have reported the results of a retrospective study of alternate-day prednisone therapy in 8 patients followed up for periods of 3 to 9 years. They initially gave 1.5 to 2.0 mg per kilogram of body weight as a single dose on alternate mornings, followed by a gradual reduction after periods of 5 to 32 months to a maintenance dosage ranging from 0.4 to 1.0 mg per kilogram. Additionally, 5 of these children received either short courses of cyclophosphamide or courses of azathioprine lasting 1 to 2½ years; in three instances both drugs were employed. The improvement that they reported achieving was based on lessening of mesangial interposition and proliferation, giving rise to decreased lobulation, increased patency of capillary lumens, and thinner capillary walls, as well as maintenance of normal renal function, reduction of proteinuria, and increased levels of plasma protein. However, their conclusions were reached in spite of increased glomerular sclerosis and tubular atrophy in most patients. In the International Study of Kidney Disease in Children [35] identical changes with time have been observed in patients allocated to a lactose placebo in a double-blind controlled trial of alternate-day prednisone therapy. Indeed, the results showed greater deterioration among patients in the test group, while analysis of changes in renal function showed no significant differences. It must therefore be concluded that a role for corticosteroids in the treatment of MPGN has not yet been established.

The results of cytotoxic drugs are even less impressive. Although the literature contains no published reports of controlled trials, there is general agreement that neither cyclophosphamide nor azathioprine affords any benefit [13, 14, 32, 43, 66]; similarly, Habib et al. [26, 27] found chlorambucil unhelpful. However, Kincaid-Smith [39, 40] combined cyclophosphamide with dipyridamole and anticoagulants in 16 patients with impaired renal function for periods of up to 3½ years and observed an improved survival rate when compared with that of a group of patients who prior to 1967 (when the study began) had received only a brief course of corticosteroids or cytotoxic drugs. Serial renal biopsy sections showed diminution of mesangial interposition and proliferation in the glomeruli, but no reference was made to changes in the extent of glomerular sclerosis and tubular atrophy. Although these results are somewhat suggestive of a beneficial effect due to combined therapy, their real significance is necessarily limited by the major difference between the period of years during which they and the control patients were treated, which does not take into account factors such as improved general management and case selection. Vargas et al. [66] used a combination of prednisolone, azathioprine, dipyridamole, and anticoagulants to treat 2 patients with type II MPGN who had numerous crescents; one continued to deteriorate, while the other showed only temporary improvement.

PROGNOSIS

The problem of evaluating the results of therapy is best appreciated by examining the actuarial survival curves for MPGN (Fig. 51-13), which show that 50 percent mortality is reached at about 11 years in type I and at 8 years in type II MPGN. Clearly, studies designed to assess the effect of a drug on mortality would be valueless unless their duration was at least 10 years—hence the need to examine multiple prognostic criteria, such as serial changes in renal function and biopsy appearances in both treated cases and controls, in order to obtain an answer more quickly. From the larger reported series of children and adults with MPGN [13, 14, 26, 27, 39, 40, 45] the disease appears to be uniformly fatal, although the rate of decline of renal function is enormously variable. The disease occasionally may enter a silent phase [23, 31, 47], in which urinary abnormalities disappear intermittently and the only detectable defect is persistent hypocomplementemia.

Three factors are now well documented as having an influence on longevity. First, deterioration is more rapid when the lesion is characterized by abundant crescents [27]. Second, as indicated in Fig. 51-13, the survival curves are less favorable for patients with type II MPGN than for those with type I [12, 26, 27, 66]. Third, patients in whom a nephrotic syndrome never develops, either initially or during the course of their illness, survive for long periods with normal renal function [15, 26]. Additionally, Habib et al. [27] included initial macroscopic hematuria and nitrogen retention as unfavorable prognostic features. Conversely, Cameron et al. [15] found little difference in outcome between patients with initial hypocomplementemia at onset and those with normal levels of serum C3.

Thus, many children with MPGN ultimately will become candidates for dialysis and transplantation, and the prospect of recurrence of the origi-

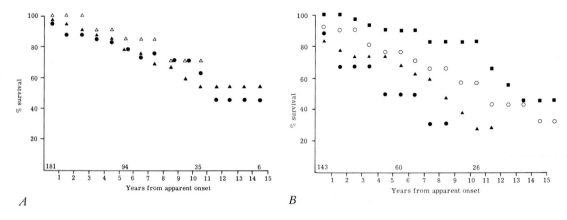

Figure 51-13. Actuarial survival curves in patients with MPGN. A. Type I, with subendothelial deposits, derived from three series of patients, as represented by the various symbols. B. Type II, with intramembranous dense deposits, from four series (13). (From J. S. Cameron. The Natural History of Glomerulonephritis. In D. A. K. Black [ed.], Renal Disease [4th ed.]. Oxford: Blackwell. To be published.)

nal disease in the renal allograft needs to be carefully elucidated. There are a number of reports of such recurrences [14, 20, 26, 31, 62, 66, 68, 81], and the evidence presented indicates that type II MPGN recurs with greater consistency than type I, suggesting the possibility of mediation of this lesion by humoral factors. However, the available evidence [6a, 62] suggests that recurrence of intramembranous dense deposit disease is not usually accompanied by overt signs of glomerulonephritis or reduced graft survival. In our present state of knowledge, it is therefore doubtful that a diagnosis of type II MPGN should be regarded as a contraindication to transplantation.

ACKNOWLEDGMENT
The author wishes to thank Dr. A. H. Cameron for permission to publish the photomicrographs. The electron micrographs were kindly supplied by Miss Dorothy Standring.

References
1. Addis, T. *Glomerular Nephritis.* New York: Macmillan, 1948.
2. Allen, A. C. The clinicopathologic meaning of the nephrotic syndrome. *Am. J. Med.* 18:277, 1955.
3. Alper, C. A., Bloch, K. J., and Rosen, F. S. Increased susceptibility to infection in a patient with type II essential hypercatabolism of C3. *N. Engl. J. Med.* 288:601, 1973.
4. Alper, C. A., and Rosen, F. S. Studies of the *in vivo* behaviour of human C3 in normal subjects and patients. *J. Clin. Invest.* 46:2021, 1967.
5. Anders, D., and Thoenes, W. Basement membrane changes in membranoproliferative glomerulonephritis. A light and electron microscopic study. *Virchows Arch. [Pathol. Anat.]* 369:87, 1975.
6. Arakawa, M., and Kimmelstiel, P. Circumferential mesangial interposition. *Lab. Invest.* 21:276, 1969.

6a. Beaufils, H., Gubler, M. C., Karam, J., Gluckman, J. C., Legrain, M., and Küss, R. Dense deposit disease: Long-term follow-up of three cases of recurrence after transplantation. *Clin. Nephrol.* 7:31, 1977.
7. Bell, E. T. A clinical and pathological study of subacute and chronic glomerulo-nephritis including lipoid nephrosis. *Am. J. Pathol.* 14:691, 1938.
8. Berger, J., and Galle, P. Dépôts denses au sein des basales du rein. *Presse Med.* 71:2351, 1963.
9. Black, J. A., Challacombe, D. N., and Ockenden, B. G. Nephrotic syndrome associated with bacteraemia after shunt operations for hydrocephalus. *Lancet* 2:921, 1965.
10. Bright, R. *Reports of Medical Cases Selected with a View of Illustrating the Symptoms and Cure of Diseases with a Reference to Morbid Anatomy.* London: Longmans, 1827. Vol. 1.
11. Bright, R. Cases and observations illustrative of renal disease accompanied with the secretion of albuminous urine. *Guys Hosp. Rep.* 1:380, 1836.
11a. Burkholder, P. M., Hyman, L. R., and Krueger, R. P. Characterization of Mixed Membranous and Poliferative Glomerulonephritis: Recognition of Three Varieties. In P. Kincaid-Smith, T. H. Mathew, and E. L. Becker (eds.), *Glomerulonephritis.* New York: Wiley, 1973. Pp. 557–589.
12. Cameron, J. S. The Natural History of Glomerulonephritis. In D. A. K. Black (ed.), *Renal Disease* (4th ed.). Oxford: Blackwell. To be published.
13. Cameron, J. S., Glasgow, E. F., Ogg, C. S., and White, R. H. R. Membranoproliferative glomerulonephritis and persistent hypocomplementaemia. *Br. Med. J.* 4:7, 1970.
14. Cameron, J. S., Ogg, C. S., Turner, D. R., Weller, R. O., White, R. H. R., Glasgow, E. F., Peters, D. K., and Martin, A. Mesangiocapillary Glomerulonephritis and Persistent Hypocomplementemia. In P. Kincaid-Smith, T. H. Mathews, and E. L. Becker (eds.), *Glomerulonephritis.* New York: Wiley, 1973. Pp. 541–556.
15. Cameron, J. S., Ogg, C. S., White, R. H. R., and Glasgow, E. F. The clinical features and prognosis of patients with normocomplementemic mesangio-

capillary glomerulonephritis. *Clin. Nephrol.* 1:2, 1973.

16. Cameron, J. S., Vick, R. M., Ogg, C. S., Seymour, W. M., Chantler, C., and Turner, D. R. Plasma C3 and C4 concentrations in management of glomerulonephritis. *Br. Med. J.* 3:668, 1973.

17. Charlesworth, J. A., Williams, D. G., Sherington, E., Lachmann, P. J., and Peters, D. K. Metabolic studies of the third component of complement and the glycine-rich beta-glycoprotein in patients with hypocomplementemia. *J. Clin. Invest.* 53:1578, 1974.

18. Churg, J., Habib, R., and White, R. H. R. Pathology of the nephrotic syndrome in children. *Lancet* 1:1299, 1970.

19. Eisinger, A. J., Shortland, J. R., and Moorhead, P. J. Renal disease in partial lipodystrophy. *Q. J. Med.* 41: 343, 1972.

20. Galle, P., Hinglais, N., and Crosnier, N. Evolution of recurrent lobular glomerulonephritis in a human kidney allotransplant: Combined light-, immunofluorescence- and electronmicroscopic studies of serial biopsies. *Transplant. Proc.* 3:368, 1971.

21. Gewurz, H., Pickering, R. J., Naff, G., Snyderman, R., Merganhagen, S. E., and Good, R. A. Decreased properdin activity in acute glomerulonephritis. *Int. Arch. Allergy Appl. Immunol.* 36:592, 1969.

22. Glasgow, E. F., Moncrieff, M. W., and White, R. H. R. Symptomless haematuria in childhood. *Br. Med. J.* 2:687, 1970.

23. Glasgow, E. F., and White, R. H. R. Acute, Poststreptococcal Glomerulonephritis with Failure to Resolve. P. Kincaid-Smith, T. H. Mathew, and E. L. Becker (eds.), *Glomerulonephritis.* New York: Wiley, 1973. Pp. 345–361.

24. Gotoff, S. P., Fellers, F. X., Vawter, G. F., Janeway, C. A., and Rosen, F. S. The beta$_{1C}$ globulin in childhood nephrotic syndrome. *N. Engl. J. Med.* 273: 524, 1965.

25. Gotze, O., and Müller-Eberhard, H. J. The C3-activator system: an alternate pathway of complement activation. *J. Exp. Med.* 134:905, 1971.

26. Habib, R., Gubler, M.-C., Loirat, C., Ben Maïz, H., and Levy, M. Dense deposit disease: A variant of membranoproliferative glomerulonephritis. *Kidney Int.* 7:204, 1975.

27. Habib, R., Kleinknecht, C., Gubler, M.-C., and Levy, M. Idiopathic membranoproliferative glomerulonephritis in children. Report of 105 cases. *Clin. Nephrol.* 4:194, 1973.

28. Habib, R., Loirat, C., Gubler, M.-C., and Levy, M. Morphology and Serum Complement Levels in Membranoproliferative Glomerulonephritis. In J. Crosnier and M. Maxwell (eds.), *Advances in Nephrology.* Chicago: Year Book, 1974. Pp. 109–136.

29. Habib, R., Michielsen, P., de Montera, H., Hinglais, N., Galle, P., and Hamburger, J. Clinical, Microscopic and Electron Microscopic Data in the Nephrotic Syndrome of Unknown Origin. G. E. W. Wolstenholme and M. P. Cameron (eds.), *Ciba Symposium on Renal Biopsy.* London: Churchill, 1961. Pp. 70–92.

30. Hamza, M., Levy, M., Broyer, M., and Habib, R. Deux cas de glomérulonéphrite membrano-proliférative avec lipodystrophie partielle de type faciotronculaire. *J. Urol. Nephrol.* 56:1032, 1970.

31. Herdman, R. C., Pickering, R. J., Michael, A. F., Vernier, R. L., Fish, A. J., Gerwurz, H., and Good, R. A. Chronic glomerulonephritis associated with low serum complement activity (chronic hypocomplementemic glomerulonephritis). *Medicine (Baltimore)* 49:207, 1970.

32. Holland, N. H., and Bennett, N. M. Hypocomplementemic (membranoproliferative) glomerulonephritis. Immunosuppressive therapy. *Am. J. Dis. Child.* 123:439, 1972.

33. Holland, N. H., de Bracco, M. M. E., and Christian, C. L. Pathways of complement activation in glomerulonephritis. *Kidney Int.* 1:106, 1972.

34. Hunsicker, L. G., Ruddy, S., Carpenter, C. B., Schur, P. H., Merrill, J. P., Müller-Eberhard, H. J., and Austin, K. F. Metabolism of third complement component (C3) in nephritis. *N. Engl. J. Med.* 287:837, 1972.

35. International Study of Kidney Disease in Children. Controlled trial of alternate-day prednisone therapy. In preparation.

36. Jenis, E. H., Sandler, P., Hill, G. S., Knieser, M. R., Jensen, G. E., and Roskes, S. D. Glomerulonephritis with basement membrane dense deposits. *Arch. Pathol.* 97:84, 1974.

37. Jones, D. B. Nephrotic glomerulonephritis. *Am. J. Pathol.* 33:313, 1957.

38. Kark, R. M., Pirani, C. L., Pollak, V. E., Muehrcke, R. C., and Blainey, J. D. The nephrotic syndrome in adults: A common disorder with many causes. *Ann. Intern. Med.* 49:751, 1958.

39. Kincaid-Smith, P. The treatment of chronic mesangiocapillary (membranoproliferative) glomerulonephritis with impaired renal function. *Med. J. Aust.* 2:587, 1972.

40. Kincaid-Smith, P. The Natural History and Treatment of Mesangiocapillary Glomerulonephritis. P. Kincaid-Smith, T. H. Mathew, and E. L. Becker (eds.), *Glomerulonephritis.* New York: Wiley, 1973. Pp. 591–609.

41. Lawrence, J. R., Pollak, V. E., Pirani, C. L., and Kark, R. M. Histologic and clinical evidence of post-streptococcal glomerulonephritis in patients with the nephrotic syndrome. *Medicine (Baltimore)* 42:1, 1963.

42. Lewis, E. J., Carpenter, C. B., and Schur, P. H. Serum complement component levels in human glomerulonephritis. *Ann. Intern. Med.* 75:555, 1971.

43. McAdams, A. J., McEnery, P. T., and West, C. D. Mesangiocapillary glomerulonephritis: Changes in glomerular morphology with long-term alternate-day prednisone therapy. *J. Pediatr.* 86:23, 1975.

44. Michael, A. F., Herdman, R. C., Fish, A. J., Pickering, R. J., and Vernier, R. L. Chronic membranoproliferative glomerulonephritis with hypocomplementemia. *Transplant. Proc.* 1:925, 1969.

45. Michael, A. F., Westberg, N. G., Fish, A. J., and Vernier, R. L. Studies on chronic membranoproliferative glomerulonephritis with hypocomplementemia. *J. Exp. Med.* 134:208, 1971.

46. Moncrieff, M. W., Glasgow, E. F., Arthur, L. J. H., and Hargreaves, H. M. Glomerulonephritis associated with *Staphylococcus albus* in a Spitz Holter valve. *Arch. Dis. Child.* 48:69, 1973.

47. Northway, J. D., McAdams, A. J., Forristal, J., and West, C. D. A "silent" phase of hypocomplementemic persistent nephritis detectable by reduced serum β_{1C}-globulin levels. *J. Pediatr.* 74:28, 1969.

48. Ogg, C. S., Cameron, J. S., and White, R. H. R. The C'3 component of complement (β_{1C}-globulin)

in patients with heavy proteinuria. *Lancet* 2:78, 1968.

49. Okuda, R., Watanabe, Y., Yamamoto, Y., and West, C. D.   The origin of membranoproliferative nephritis. Evidence against an origin from acute poststreptococcal nephritis. *Am. J. Dis. Child.* 119:291, 1970.

50. Ooi, Y. M., Vallota, E. H., and West, C. D.   Classical complement pathway activation in membranoproliferative glomerulonephritis. *Kidney Int.* 9:46, 1976.

50a. Ooi, Y. M., Vallota, E. H., and West, C. D.   Serum immune complexes in membranoproliferative and other glomerulonephritides. *Kidney Int.* 11:275, 1977.

51. Peters, D. K., Martin, A., Weinstein, A., Cameron, J. S., Barratt, T. M., Ogg, C. S., and Lachmann, P. J.   Complement studies in membranoproliferative glomerulonephritis. *Clin. Exp. Immunol.* 11:311, 1972.

52. Peters, D. K., Williams, D. G., Charlesworth, J. A., Boulton-Jones, J. M., Sissons, J. G. P., Evans, D. J., Kourilsky, O., and Morel-Maroger, L.   Mesangiocapillary nephritis, partial lipodystrophy, and hypocomplementaemia. *Lancet* 2:535, 1973.

53. Pillemer, L., Schoenberg, M. D., Blum, L., and Wurz, L.   Properdin system and immunity; interaction of properdin system with polysaccharides. *Science* 122:545, 1955.

54. Royer, P., Habib, R., Vermeil, G., Mathieu, H., and Alizon, M.   Les glomérulonéphritis prolongées de l'enfant. A propos de quatre aspects anatomiques révélés par la biopsie rénale. *Ann. Pediatr.* 38:173, 1962.

55. Ruley, E. J., Forristal, J., Davis, N. C., Andres, C., and West, C. D.   Hypocomplementemia of membranoproliferative glomerulonephritis. *J. Clin. Invest.* 52:896, 1973.

56. Strife, C. F., McAdams, A. J., McEnery, P. T., Bove, K. E., and West, C. D.   Hypocomplementemic and normocomplementemic acute nephritis in children; a comparison with respect to etiology, clinical manifestions and glomerular morphology. *J. Pediatr.* 84: 29, 1974.

57. Strife, C. F., McEnery, P. T., McAdams, A. J., and West, C. D.   A third type of membranoproliferative glomerulonephritis. *Clin. Nephrol.* 7:65, 1977.

58. Thoenes, G. H.   The immunohistology of glomerulonephritis—distinctive marks and variability. *Curr. Top. Pathol.* 61:61, 1976.

59. Thompson, R. A.   C3 inactivating factor in the serum of a patient with chronic hypocomplementaemic proliferative glomerulonephritis. *Immunology* 22: 147, 1972.

60. Thompson, R. A.   IgG3 levels in patients with chronic membranoproliferative glomerulonephritis. *Br. Med. J.* 1:282, 1972.

61. Thompson, R. A., and White, R. H. R.   Partial lipodystrophy and hypocomplementaemic nephritis. *Lancet* 2:679, 1973.

61a. Ting, H. C., and Wang, F.   Mesangiocapillary (membranoproliferative) glomerulonephritis and rheumatoid arthritis. *Br. Med. J.* 1:270, 1977.

62. Turner, D. R., Cameron, J. S., Bewick, M., Sharpstone, P., Melcher, D., Ogg, C. S., Evans, D. J., Trafford, A. J., and Leibowitz, S.   Transplantation in mesangiocapillary glomerulonephritis with intramembranous dense "deposits": Recurrence of disease. *Kidney Int.* 9:439, 1976.

63. Vallota, E. H., Forristal, J., Spitzer, R. E., Davis, N. C., and West, C. D.   Characteristics of a noncomplement-dependent C3-reactive complex formed from factors in nephritic and normal serum. *J. Exp. Med.* 131:1306, 1970.

64. Vallota, E. H., Forristal, J., Spitzer, R. E., Davis, N. C., and West, C. D.   Continuing C3 breakdown after bilateral nephrectomy in patients with membrano-proliferative glomerulonephritis. *J. Clin. Invest.* 50:552, 1971.

65. van Acker, K. J., van den Brande, J., and Vincke, H.   Membranoproliferative glomerulonephritis. *Helv. Paediatr. Acta* 25:204, 1970.

66. Vargas, A. R., Thompson, K. J., Wilson, D., Cameron, J. S., Turner, D. R., Gill, D., Chantler, C., and Ogg, C. S.   Mesangiocapillary glomerulonephritis with dense "deposits" in the basement membranes of the kidney. *Clin. Nephrol.* 5:73, 1976.

67. Weller, R. O., and Nester, B.   Histological reassessment of three kidneys originally described by Richard Bright in 1827–1836. *Br. Med. J.* 2:761, 1972.

68. West, C. D.   Membranoproliferative hypocomplementemic glomerulonephritis. *Nephron* 11:134, 1973.

69. West, C. D., and McAdams, A. J.   Serum β_{1C}-globulin levels in persistent glomerulonephritis with low serum complement: Variability unrelated to clinical course. *Nephron* 7:193, 1970.

70. West, C. D., McAdams, A. J., McConville, J. M., Davis, N. C., and Holland, N. H.   Hypocomplementemic and normocomplementemic persistent (chronic) glomerulonephritis: Clinical and pathologic characteristics. *J. Pediatr.* 67:1089, 1965.

71. West, C. D., Northway, J. D., and Davis, N. C.   Serum levels of β_{1C} globulin, a complement component, in the nephritides, lipoid nephrosis, and other conditions. *J. Clin. Invest.* 43:1507, 1964.

72. West, C. D., Ruley, E. J., Forristal, J., and Davis, N. C.   Mechanisms of hypocomplementemia in glomerulonephritis. *Kidney Int.* 3:116, 1973.

73. West, C. D., Winter, S., Forristal, J., McConville, J., and Davis, N. C.   Evidence for *in vivo* breakdown of β_{1C}-globulin in hypocomplementemic glomerulonephritis. *J. Clin. Invest.* 46:539, 1967.

74. Westberg, N. G., Naff, G. B., Boyer, J. T., and Michael, A. F.   Glomerular deposition of properdin in acute and chronic glomerulonephritis with hypocomplementemia. *J. Clin. Invest.* 50:642, 1971.

75. White, R. H. R.   The Nephrotic Syndrome. In D. Gairdner and D. Hull (eds.), *Recent Advances in Paediatrics* (4th ed.). London: Churchill, 1971. Pp. 281–315.

76. White, R. H. R., Cameron, J. S., and Trounce, J. R.   Immunosuppressive therapy in steroid-resistant proliferative glomerulonephritis accompanied by the nephrotic syndrome. *Br. Med. J.* 2:853, 1966.

77. White, R. H. R., Glasgow, E. F., and Mills, R. J.   Clinicopathological study of nephrotic syndrome in childhood. *Lancet* 1:1353, 1970.

78. Williams, D. G., Charlesworth, J. A., Lachmann, P. J., and Peters, D. K.   Role of C3b in the breakdown of C3 in hypocomplementaemic mesangiocapillary glomerulonephritis. *Lancet* 1:447, 1973.

79. Williams, D. G., Peters, D. K., Fallows, J., Petrie, A., Kourilsky, O., Morel-Maroger, L., and Cameron, J. S.   Studies of serum complement in hypocomplementaemic nephritides. *Clin. Exp. Immunol.* 18:391, 1974.

80. Williams, D. G., Scopes, J. W., and Peters, D. K.

Hypocomplementaemic membranoproliferative glomerulonephritis and nephrotic syndrome associated with partial lipodystrophy of the face and trunk. *Proc. R. Soc. Med.* 65:591, 1972.

81. Zimmerman, S. W., Hyman, L. R., Uehling, D. T., and Burkholder, P. M. Recurrent membranoproliferative glomerulonephritis with glomerular properdin deposition in allografts. *Ann. Intern. Med.* 80:169, 1974.

82. Zucchelli, P., Sasdelli, M., Cagnoli, L., Donini, U., Casanova, S., and Rovinetti, C. Membranoproliferative glomerulonephritis: Correlations between immunological and histological findings. *Nephron* 17:449, 1976.

52. The Nephrotic Syndrome

Henry L. Barnett, Morris Schoeneman,
Jay Bernstein, and Chester M. Edelmann, Jr.

The nephrotic syndrome is an arbitrarily defined clinical state characterized by proteinuria and hypoalbuminemia, usually accompanied by edema and hypercholesterolemia with generalized hyperlipidemia and sometimes accompanied by hematuria, hypertension, and reduced glomerular filtration rate. It may occur at any time in the course of many different primary and secondary glomerular diseases [3, 4, 26, 36, 37, 85, 92]. This definition discards the concept that the nephrotic syndrome represents a heterogeneous but related group of glomerular diseases. Rather, it considers it to be conceptually and practically a functional state that is associated with many different glomerular diseases. The nephrotic syndrome is associated only occasionally with some glomerular diseases, such as proliferative glomerulonephritis and the nephritis of lupus erythematosus and anaphylactoid purpura. It is usually present in others, such as focal segmental sclerosis, membranoproliferative glomerulonephritis, and membranous glomerulonephropathy; and, in minimal change nephrotic syndrome, in which a primary glomerular abnormality has been conceptualized, despite the lack of obvious histopathologic abnormality, the nephrotic syndrome is, by definition, invariably present.

Historic Aspects

The earlier historical aspects of the nephrotic syndrome are described in detail in Leiter's classic monograph [58]. Working in the Department of Pathology under Professor Theodore Fahr in Hamburg in 1927, Dr. Leiter (personal communication) had the opportunity to make histologic studies of autopsies of Dr. Volhard's patients and thus had firsthand information about the cases that established nephrosis as a clinical entity. His description of the origin of the term *nephrosis* and of its early travels through Europe and the United States is worthy of repetition, especially in view of current efforts to establish an acceptable world-wide terminology for renal disease.

"Nephrosis" began its existence in medical nomenclature as a point of view. The original views of Virchow in regard to parenchymatous inflammation proved inadequate and were replaced by the concepts of exudation and proliferation in the vascular and supporting systems. This made it desirable to have a general term for these changes in renal epithelium so commonly found but not properly belonging under the term "nephritis" which connotes "inflammation of the kidney." It was Friedrich Muller [71] who first saw the opportunity of clarifying the situation and in 1905 suggested the term "nephrosis" for the purely degenerative conditions of the kidney; meaning, presumably, although not expressly stating it at that time, the tubular nephropathies, and not the equally degenerative vascular changes of arterio and arteriolosclerosis. Friedrich Muller realized the difficulty of absolutely distinguishing, in some instances, between purely degenerative and partly inflammatory renal diseases, even in morphological studies. Hence, he was justly conservative in making no claims for clinical differentiation, although he had the possibility clearly in mind. "Nephrosis," therefore, was for the time being largely an anatomical term.

In less than ten years after its introduction the term "nephrosis" was to take the German medical world by storm and this time on a bold clinical footing with solid pathological background. As one of the trinity of Volhard and Fahr's [100] classical division of bilateral hematogenous renal disease—nephrosis, nephritis and nephrosclerosis—it became rapidly popular among most German clinicians, while stirring up a host of antagonists in the camp of pathologists. A few years later, nephrosis made its appearance in the United States as "Epstein's nephrosis," was translated on a somewhat shaky basis to Great Britain where it has only recently achieved any real recognition, and invaded France on occasions without making any serious impression upon the physiological classification of renal diseases prevailing there. Somewhat before the publication of Volhard and Fahr's monograph in 1914, Munk [72] established the unique

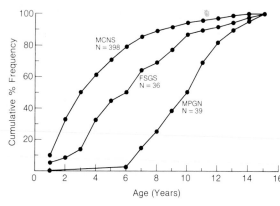

Figure 52-1. Age at time of diagnosis of the nephrotic syndrome in patients with minimal change nephrotic syndrome, focal and segmental glomerulosclerosis, and membranoproliferative glomerulonephritis, and cumulative percentage frequencies.

significance of "lipoid droplets in the urinary sediments of patients with "chronic parenchymatous nephritis" especially on a luetic basis. He quickly adopted the term "nephrosis," prefixing the word "lipoid," and thus gave the name "lipoid nephrosis" to the class of patients under discussion—a name that was far more accurately descriptive than any hitherto proposed. With Munk [73] the disease spread beyond the organic confines of the kidneys to become a general constitutional disturbance of all the colloids of the body. His views were widely accepted. Epstein [27] took a less mysterious, rather more logical view of the situation, particularly in regard to nephrotic edema. He reverted to Starling's [94] pioneer work on the role of colloid osmotic pressure of the serum proteins in the exchange of fluids between the vascular and tissue spaces in normal and edematous states, and built up a superstructure of fact and theory. . . . These developments in our knowledge of nephrosis came rather rapidly, thanks to the enormously stimulating effect of the new classification and terminology upon the morphological, clinical and biochemical studies of renal disease.

Major advances were made during this same period in elucidating some of the pathogenetic mechanisms of albuminuria, hypoproteinemia, edema, and disturbances in lipid metabolism. These are reviewed in detail by Leiter [58]. The introduction by Homer Smith [92] and others of methods of measuring discrete renal functions in man led to further advances in understanding the pathogenesis of edema. The data on this subject, together with other developments during the next two decades, were summarized by Barnett et al. [9] in 1953. Experimental models, exhibiting many of the characteristics of the nephrotic syndrome, were also developed during this period.

Since 1950, the ability to examine renal tissue from living patients by the techniques of light, electron, and immunofluorescence microscopy and the development of animal models and sophisticated techniques for studying them (see Chaps. 3, 6) have provided a firm basis for the present nosologic concept of the nephrotic syndrome [22, 37, 64, 104].

Clinical Classification

A classification of glomerular diseases, including those that may be associated with the nephrotic syndrome, is presented in Chap. 43.

The nephrotic syndrome associated with primary glomerular diseases is termed *primary nephrotic syndrome* (replacing the term *idiopathic nephrotic syndrome*). When it occurs as part of a recognized systemic disease or results from some evident cause, it is termed *secondary nephrotic syndrome.*

Primary nephrotic syndrome (Fig. 52-1) may be (1) congenital, (2) corticosteroid responsive, usually with minimal change nephrotic syndrome (MCNS), or (3) corticosteroid nonresponsive, usually with focal segmental glomerulosclerosis (FSGS), proliferative glomerulonephritis (PGN), membranoproliferative glomerulonephritis (MPGN), or membranous glomerulonephropathy (MGN). Secondary nephrotic syndrome in children is associated most often with systemic lupus erythematosus, anaphylactoid purpura, or sickle cell disease. It occurs less frequently with renal vein thrombosis, hereditary progressive nephritis, amyloidosis, diabetes mellitus, lymphoma, malaria, syphilis, varicella, and as a reaction to bee sting and a number of drugs. Other diseases that are associated with the nephrotic syndrome in adults but occur rarely, if ever, in children have been listed by Schreiner [89] and include the following: other metabolic diseases such as myxedema; other systemic diseases such as polyarteritis, dermatomyositis, the Goodpasture syndrome, and erythema multiforme; neoplastic diseases such as lymphocytic leukemia, pheochromocytoma, and carcinoma; other circulatory disturbances, such as spherocytosis, renal artery stenosis, pulmonary artery thrombosis, constructive pericarditis, congestive heart failure, tricuspid valvular insufficiency, and pulseless disease; other infections, such as tuberculosis, subacute bacterial endocarditis, herpes zoster; and miscellaneous conditions, such as chronic jejunoileitis, pregnancy, transplantation, intestinal lymphangiectasia, and central pontine myelinolysis.

The specific characteristics of the nephrotic syndrome in most of these primary and secondary glomerular diseases are discussed in separate chapters. The general characteristics of the nephrotic syndrome and specific aspects of miscellaneous conditions not considered elsewhere are discussed here.

Histopathologic Classification

The histopathologic classification of glomerular abnormalities associated with the nephrotic syndrome is given in Table 52-1. It is based on several reports [22, 37] that use similar terms with similar meanings. Despite a high degree of accord, a few points of contention and uncertainty remain about the nosologic and clinical implications of several categories. The problem areas may be identified as follows: (1) the limits of "minimal glomerular change" and the types of abnormality that the category encompasses; (2) the relationships and differences between early-onset and late-onset FSGS; and (3) the significance of mesangial proliferation either as a complication of early FSGS or as an isolated finding. With these reservations in mind, the major categories of glomerular disease are defined by light-microscopic criteria, which are, in turn, supplemented by certain immunofluorescence- and electron-microscopic observations.

Minimal Change Nephrotic Syndrome

In MCNS, the glomeruli are histologically almost normal, with abnormalities not exceeding minimal mesangial thickening, focal mesangial hypercellularity, and basement membrane thickening; immunofluorescence microscopy usually reveals nothing positive; electron microscopy shows epithelial hypertrophy with fusion of foot processes (see Chap. 53).

Focal Segmental Glomerulosclerosis

In FSGS, some glomeruli, often those in the juxtamedullary region, contain segmental areas of cap-

illary collapse and obliteration, with increased matrix and occasional deposits of hyalin. The essential feature is partial involvement, sometimes limited to a lobule, of at least some glomeruli, but severe, diffuse involvement is characteristic of advanced disease (see Chap. 55).

Proliferative Glomerulonephritis

In PGN, a moderate or marked increase in the density of mesangial cells (mesangial proliferation) may be accompanied by leukocytic infiltration (exudation), increased mesangial matrix with obliteration of capillary loops (sclerosis), and fibroepithelial proliferation within the urinary space (crescents and adhesions). Immunofluorescent studies have shown that this group is exceedingly heterogeneous, encompassing postinfectious glomerulonephritis, IgA nephropathy, glomerulonephritis secondary to systemic disease, and glomerulonephritis without evidence of immune complex deposition. The differentiation between proliferative and sclerosing glomerulonephritis and segmental sclerosis with mesangial hypercellularity is arbitrary, but it is clear that PGN with immune deposits can progress to FSGS; focal and segmental proliferative glomerulonephritis with nephrotic syndrome is usually a manifestation of systemic disease and is rarely an isolated lesion.

Membranoproliferative Glomerulonephritis

The category MPGN encompasses two types of disease. In one, the basic lesion appears to be subendothelial deposits of IgG and complement, leading to mesangial interposition and duplication (double contour) of the basement membrane. In the other, the capillary basement membrane is infiltrated and thickened by intramembranous dense deposits. Both types are associated with mesangial proliferation and with variable crescents, hyperlobulation, and epimembranous deposits (see Chap. 51).

Membranous Glomerulonephropathy

In MGN, subepithelial deposits are distributed on the basement membrane, frequently in a uniform and occasionally in an irregular fashion. They become separated by argyrophilic protrusions of basement membrane that form the characteristic "spikes" seen by light microscopy, and they penetrate the lamina densa, leading to a lacy pattern in tangential sections of the capillary wall. The deposits are associated with only mild mesangial proliferation, and the significance of the occasional case in which there is severe proliferation is not known (see Chap. 50).

Table 52-1. Classification of Glomerular Lesions Associated with Primary and Secondary Nephrotic Syndrome

Minimal change nephrotic syndrome
Focal segmental glomerulosclerosis
Proliferative glomerulonephritis:
    Pure diffuse mesangial proliferation
    Focal glomerulonephritis
    Sclerosing glomerulonephritis
Membranoproliferative glomerulonephritis
Membranous glomerulonephropathy
Chronic glomerulonephritis

Chronic Glomerulonephritis

In chronic glomerulonephritis, extensive glomerular obsolescence and hyalinization are usually associated with tubular atrophy and interstitial fibrosis (see Chap. 49).

Summary

It is apparent from this presentation that the category of MCNS is clearly conceptualized, despite the necessity of making a value judgment about the permissible degree of mesangial cellularity or mesangial thickening. It is apparent also that the lesion of FSGS is clearly defined, despite the occasional late evolution of MCNS to FSGS and despite the occasional evolution of PGN to FSGS. In that regard, segmental sclerosis occurs nonspecifically during the evolution of all forms of chronic renal glomerular diseases. Similarly, the categories of MPGN and MGN appear to be clearly established. The category that is least understood in relation to the nephrotic syndrome is that of proliferative glomerulonephritis, in which the inconstant evidence of immune complex deposition and the variability of proliferation and progression to sclerosis make generalizations exceedingly tenuous.

Frequency of Glomerular Diseases in the Primary Nephrotic Syndrome

Patients with primary nephrotic syndrome account for over 90 percent of all children with the nephrotic syndrome [17, 37]. The distribution of patients with primary nephrotic syndrome by histopathologic findings is given in Table 52-2. These data, and subsequent descriptions of the clinical and laboratory characteristics of the syndrome, are based on observations made in three separate studies of large numbers of children in whom a histopathologic diagnosis was made from a renal biopsy. Most of the data are from the *prospective* study of the International Study of Kidney Disease in Children (ISKDC) [42] of almost 500 *unselected* and previously *untreated* children observed between 1967 and 1974 in 19 clinics in 10 countries in Europe and North America and 1 clinic each in Israel and Japan. The second study is that reported by Habib and Kleinknecht [37] of 406 children referred between 1957 and 1967 to the Unité de Recherches sur les Maladies du Métabolisme chez L'enfant in the Hôpital des Enfants-Malades in Paris. The third study is that of White and coworkers [104], which involved 75 *unselected* and 70 *referred* patients at Guy's Hospital in London and the Children's Hospital in Birmingham from 1962 to 1965.

The proportion of all children with MCNS in the two groups of unselected cases is 77.9 percent. The lower values in the two series of referred cases are probably due to selective referral of a higher proportion of patients with FSGS, MPGN, PGN, and MGN, diseases in which problems of

Table 52-2. Distribution of Unselected and Referred Patients with Primary Nephrotic Syndrome by Histopathologic Findings

Histopathologic Finding	Unselected Cases						Referred Cases			
	ISKDC [42]		White, et al. [104]		Total		White et al. [104]		Habib and Kleinknecht [37]	
	N	%	N	%	N	%	N	%	N	%
Minimal change nephrotic syndrome	398	76.4	66	88.0	464	77.9	45	64.3	209	51.5
Focal global sclerosis	9	1.7							12	
Focal segmental glomerulosclerosis	36	6.9	4	5.4	40	6.7	8	11.4	35	8.6
Membranoproliferative glomerulonephritis	39	7.5	1	1.3	40	6.7	8	11.4	53	9.4
Pure mesangial proliferation	12	2.3								
Proliferative glomerulonephritis	12	2.3	4	5.3	16	2.7	7	10.0	41	13.8
Membranous glomerulonephropathy	8	1.5			8	1.3	2	2.9	37	9.1
Chronic glomerulonephritis	3	0.6			7	1.2				
Unclassified	4	0.8			21	3.5			13	6.5
Total	521	100.0	75	100.0	596	100.0	70	100.0	400	100.0

diagnosis or management would more often require consultation in a nephrology center. Although children in the ISKDC were unselected, the proportion with MCNS in different centers ranged from 68 percent (35 of 50) to 88 percent (32 of 36) and the proportion with MPGN, from none (of 71) to 11 percent (5 of 45). It would thus appear that there may very well be unknown geographic determinants of the distribution of patients among histopathologic categories.

Disorders Associated with the Secondary Nephrotic Syndrome
INCIDENCE

There are few published data on the frequency of identified general diseases or of exposure to known precipating agents in children with the nephrotic syndrome. The clinical diagnoses in 41 patients with secondary nephrotic syndrome reported by Habib and Kleinknecht [37] and of 22 patients seen at the Hospital of the Albert Einstein College of Medicine [35] are shown in Table 52-3. The frequency of these causes of secondary nephrotic syndrome would be expected to vary in different countries. Thus, systemic lupus erythematosus is apparently less frequent throughout Europe than it is in the United States, as can be seen in Table 52-3. Malaria, which does not appear in Table 52-3, provides a more striking example, accounting for about four-fifths of the cases of the nephrotic syndrome in Nigerian children [39].

Table 52-3. Distribution of Patients with Secondary Nephrotic Syndrome by Clinical Diagnosis

Clinical Diagnosis	Habib and Kleinknecht [37] N	Habib and Kleinknecht [37] %	Greifer [35] N	Greifer [35] %
Systemic lupus erythematosus	4	9.8	5	22.7
Anaphylactoid purpura	26	63.4	4	18.2
Sickle cell disease			3	13.6
Bee sting			2	9.1
Renal vein thrombosis	1	2.4	2	9.1
Syphilis			2	9.1
Alport syndrome	3	7.3	1	4.5
Amyloidosis			1	4.5
Hemolytic uremic syndrome	6	14.6	1	4.5
Heroin addiction			1	4.5
Nephroblastoma	1	2.4		
Total	41	100.0	22	100.0

MISCELLANEOUS FORMS OF SECONDARY NEPHROTIC SYNDROME INFECTIONS
Infections

Both *congenital* and *acquired secondary syphilis* are well recognized causes of the nephrotic syndrome [30, 79, 96, 109]. The histopathology is that of membranous nephropathy with immune deposits; the disease may occur in the absence of overt signs of lues. Complete recovery usually follows antisyphilitic therapy [11].

In West Africa, particularly in Nigeria, the nephrotic syndrome in children is frequently associated with *quartan malarial infection* (*Plasmodium malariae*) [2, 39, 49, 93]. Renal involvement is thought to be caused by immune complexes containing *P. malariae* antigen; proliferative and sclerosing lesions are seen on biopsy. Corticosteroid or other immunosuppressive therapy is rarely successful. Severe hypertension is a serious toxic effect of corticosteroids in these patients, and many die of complications of the treatment.

Certain *viruses,* such as coxsackievirus, echovirus, and mumps virus are occasionally associated with renal abnormalities. *Varicella* has been reported in association with the nephrotic syndrome, with PGN seen on biopsy [55]; the renal abnormalities disappeared completely as the varicella resolved. The nephrotic syndrome has been reported more commonly in association with *hepatitis B* [24, 52, 53]. It appears to be an immune complex disease involving the hepatitis B surface antigen (HGsAg); the histopathology seen most commonly is that of MGN; occasionally, FSGS or MPGN is seen. The course of the renal disease is not uniformly benign; in some patients the disease progresses to chronic renal failure.

Toxins

The nephrotic syndrome has been reported as a reaction to *bee stings* and *poison oak* [86, 87], due presumably to hypersensitivity. Many patients in whom the nephrotic syndrome is associated with bee stings have a relapsing course, with no evidence of the development of renal failure. The association of nephrotic syndrome with exposure to poison oak is much more tenuous and may not reflect a causal relationship. The clinical course in the cases reported ranges from that of a relapsing nephrotic syndrome to that of severe glomerulonephritis, with heavy proteinuria and death in uremia.

Drugs

Other toxic causes of the nephrotic syndrome include *penicillamine* and heavy metals, particularly organic compounds of *mercury* and *gold;* these are discussed in detail in Chap. 79. In addition, there is a report of the nephrotic syndrome occurring in a 6½-year-old girl as a complication of perchlorate treatment of thyrotoxicosis [57]. This patient improved after the medication was discontinued, but she still had mild proteinuria 6 months later. A renal biopsy at the time of nephrotic syndrome showed mild to moderate endothelial hypercellularity and focal basement membrane thickening.

A much more common pediatric problem has been the development of the nephrotic syndrome during treatment of petit mal epilepsy with *trimethadione* [6, 10, 38, 75, 103] or *paramethadione* [108], a chemically related drug. The first case was described by Barnett et al. in 1948 [10] in a 14-year-old girl, in whom the nephrotic syndrome developed during trimethadione treatment and in whom proteinuria disappeared promptly after the drug was discontinued. Proteinuria recurred and disappeared concomitantly with reinstitution and discontinuation of treatment with the drug on two additional occasions. The cases of approximately 24 patients in whom the nephrotic syndrome developed during trimethadione therapy have been described subsequently. In all cases the drug was stopped after appearance of the nephrotic syndrome, and, in many cases, proteinuria disappeared within the next 3 weeks to 6 months without requiring specific treatment.

The renal pathologic findings associated with trimethadione-induced nephrotic syndrome have not been well defined because of the few cases examined. Light microscopy in these cases has shown either normal glomeruli or only minor glomerular abnormalities, such as minimal focal mesangial hypercellularity [41, 78, 82] and irregular basement-membrane thickening resembling MGN [6]. Immunofluorescent staining for globulins and complement has produced negative results [6]. Although both corticosteroids and immunosuppressive therapy have been used in the treatment of trimethadione-induced nephrotic syndrome [77, 97], their efficacy has not been established.

Pathophysiologic Mechanisms in the Nephrotic Syndrome

The pathophysiologic mechanisms underlying the major metabolic alterations in the nephrotic syndrome are discussed in separate chapters referred to in each of the following sections, in which only summaries of the mechanisms involved are presented.

PROTEINURIA

Proteinuria (see Chap. 15) is generally accepted as the primary abnormality in children with the nephrotic syndrome. The rate of excretion generally considered diagnostic is about 1 gm per 24 hr; values of 50 mg/kg/24 hr [37] and 40 mg/hr/m² [42] have been used to standardize for body size. However, rates of excretion of 5 gm per 24 hr are not unusual before treatment, even in young children [37].

The major protein in the urine is albumin. Ratios of concentrations of various proteins (selectivity indexes) have been used to assess the severity of glomerular damage. However, these have proved less useful than initially suggested (see Chap. 9).

The alterations in the pathways whereby abnormal amounts of protein may enter the urine in disease states are also discussed in detail in Chap. 15. The major, if not the only, alteration in patients with the nephrotic syndrome is an increase in the permeability of the glomerular capillary wall to normal plasma proteins. There is no evidence that either reduced tubular resorption or tubular secretion plays any role.

Investigations of proteinuria in the nephrotic syndrome in both human subjects and experimental animals have contributed much of the present knowledge concerning increased glomerular permeability to plasma proteins. As early as 1961, Farquhar and Palade [28] suggested that the defect in the glomerular filtration membrane was due to a diffuse lesion in the basement membrane at the level of macromolecular organization. The fusion of the foot processes of the glomerular epithelial cells lining the basement membrane was thought to be a secondary phenomenon, due to the increased filtration of protein. One factor thought to be partly responsible for maintaining the gel filtration properties of the basement membrane is glomerular polyanion [102]. Sialic acid is the only glomerular polyanion identified histochemically. It is found in the glomerular basement membrane and on the cell membrane of the glomerular epithelial cell and its foot process [67]. Studies in pediatric patients with proteinuria secondary to glomerular disease have indicated a decrease in the sialic acid content of the glomerular epithelial cell membrane, perhaps accounting for the increased permeability of the filter [16]. A decrease in glomerular sialic acid has also been shown to occur concomitantly with an increase in glomerular capillary permeability in aminonucleoside nephrosis in rats [67]. Whether this decrease in sialic acid content is a primary event, causing the observed fusion of the epithelial foot processes, or is secondary to the changes in the foot processes is still unknown. Robson et al. [80] have shown in nephrotic children that glomerular permeability to molecules of uncharged polyvinyl pyrrolidone 40A° was reduced to 20 percent or less of normal at the same time that permeability to albumin was apparently increased. Reversal of the nephrotic syndrome resulted in return of permeability to normal, suggesting that the loss of glomerular polyanion from surfaces of the epithelial cells allows increased passage of albumin that normally is excluded from the epithelial slit pores by the sialic acid anions. In contrast, loss of glomerular polyanion would not modify the passage of uncharged polyvinyl pyrrolidone. Its transport, instead, might be hindered by the swelling of the epithelial foot processes, with obliteration of the epithelial slit pores, which would reduce the ability of small uncharged particles to enter the urine.

PLASMA PROTEIN ABNORMALITIES

The classic pattern of plasma protein abnormalities involves marked *hypoalbuminemia,* one of the major characteristics of the nephrotic syndrome. There is also a decrease in alpha globulin, a normal or low alpha-1-globulin, and a relative or absolute increase of alpha-2-globulins, beta globulin, and fibrinogen [31]. This increase in alpha-2-globulins was attributed by Kluthe et al. [51] to selective retention of this high-molecular-weight protein by the kidney in the presence of a normal rate of synthesis of alpha-2-macroglobulin.

Several mechanisms could be responsible for the hypoalbuminemia: massive urinary loss, diminished synthesis, increased catabolism, and extrarenal loss. Although massive urinary loss is undoubtedly the major cause, its role as the sole cause has been questioned because the capacity for protein synthesis by the adult has been estimated to be as high as 50 gm per day [101]. It thus seems unlikely that a urinary loss of only a fraction of this amount could cause persistent hypoproteinemia. However, Chinard et al. [20] have pointed out that albumin excretion is proportional to its concentration in plasma. As a consequence, if in a nephrotic child with a plasma albumin concentration of 0.3 gm per deciliter and albumin excretion of 3 gm per day, synthesis could be speeded up sufficiently to maintain the plasma albumin concentration at a normal value of 4 gm per deciliter, albumin excretion would increase to about 40 gm per day; and to maintain a steady state, the rate of synthesis would have to be increased equally. This feat is probably beyond the capacity of a nephrotic child, and it is therefore

understandable that hypoalbuminemia persists in spite of comparatively small urinary protein losses.

There is conflicting evidence regarding an abnormality of albumin synthesis as a contributing cause to the hypoalbuminemia. The rate of production of plasma albumin, when turnover rate is studied by tracer techniques, has been shown in some studies to be normal [32] and in others to be diminished [46]. The rate of albumin synthesis has also been shown to be directly related to the amount of protein intake [15], so that a stringent low-protein diet may have a depressant effect on albumin synthesis. There is also controversy about the rate of catabolism of albumin in the nephrotic syndrome. Using the disappearance rate of infused labeled albumin, albumin catabolism has been reported both to be normal [46] and to be increased [32]. Katz et al. [47] reported that the catabolic rate of albumin fell by about 50 percent after bilateral nephrectomy in rats made nephrotic by aminonucleoside, suggesting that the kidney plays an important role in albumin catabolism even in proteinuric states.

Alimentary losses of albumin and gamma globulin have been demonstrated during exacerbations of the nephrotic syndrome, with reversal during remission [84]. Also, a small degree of salivary loss of plasma proteins has been demonstrated in nonedematous nephrotic patients [14].

HYPERLIPIDEMIA

Increased concentrations of very low density lipoproteins, or low density lipoproteins, or both occur very frequently in children with the primary nephrotic syndrome [21, 76], the increase being most frequent and most marked in patients with MCNS.

There is, in general, an inverse relationship between concentrations of serum cholesterol and serum albumin [13]. The level of triglyceride, however, usually does not increase until the serum albumin falls to levels below 1 gm per deciliter. The mechanisms responsible for these alterations in serum lipids and lipoproteins are not known. Two possible mechanisms have been suggested: (1) that decreased concentrations of plasma albumin result in increased synthesis in the liver, not only of albumin but also of lipids, lipoproteins, and triglycerides [12, 91]; and (2) that the activity of lipoprotein lipase is decreased [65].

EDEMA

The pathogenesis of nephrotic edema (see Chap. 17) has stimulated a host of inquiries by many workers. The explanations currently accepted involve two factors. The first relates to the Starling hypothesis proposed in 1896 [95]. It explains the initiation of nephrotic edema on the basis of hypoalbuminemia, a decrease in intravascular oncotic pressure, and a resulting contraction of plasma volume. The second involves excessive renal tubular resorption of salt and water as a response to the depletion of plasma volume and explains the persistence of edema on the basis of various stimuli to continued salt and water retention [60]. One of the major stimuli is aldosterone—and, in fact, rates of aldosterone secretion and aldosterone excretion in the urine have both been shown to be elevated in the nephrotic syndrome [62].

Clinical Manifestations

In the past it was true that "To the child with the disease and to his parents the nephrotic syndrome is *edema*. Poor appetite, irritability, gastrointestinal upsets, and frequently severe infections are so closely related to the presence and severity of edema that they appear to be consequences of it" [9]. Treatment with corticosteroids, however, has altered the clinical course of the nephrotic syndrome drastically, and at present it might be said that to the child, the parents, and the physician, the nephrotic syndrome is no longer a problem of edema, but rather one of side reactions to drugs. About 80 percent of all children with the nephrotic syndrome have MCNS [42, 104], and, as will be discussed, over 90 percent of these children become free of edema and proteinuria within 8 weeks after the beginning of treatment with corticosteroids. Although proteinuria recurs in almost two-thirds of these patients, recurrence of edema can be prevented in most of them by prompt treatment. Persistent edema, however, with its disturbing complications, may be a major clinical problem in almost one-fourth of all patients with the primary nephrotic syndrome who are or become nonresponders and in whom edema cannot be readily controlled.

Edema is usually noted first about the eyes. Such minimal edema may be apparent to parents or to older patients themselves before a physician seeing the patient for the first time can be certain of its presence. The edema may persist and progress, either slowly or rapidly, or it may subside and reappear. During this period the periorbital edema is often attributed to a "cold" or to "allergy." Sooner or later, however, the edema becomes generalized, the waist size changes, the shoes become tight, and the true nature of the disease becomes apparent. Just prior to this stage, it is not uncommon for parents, worried about poor weight gain in their 2- to 3-year-old child, to be pleased with a sudden weight gain, but perplexed that it is occurring in the presence of a decrease rather than an increase in the child's appetite.

The onset of edema in the children with the nephrotic syndrome has typically been described as "insidious," without reference to the type of glomerular disease present. It now appears that the pattern of onset of edema varies in patients with different glomerular diseases. It tends to develop progressively and more rapidly over periods of days or weeks in children with MCNS, and more insidiously and intermittently in children with other glomerular diseases, especially MPGN.

Edema in children early in the course of the nephrotic syndrome is usually described as soft and pitting in contrast to the firm edema in children with acute nephritis. Pitting of the skin and subcutaneous tissue usually can be demonstrated, although the edema may be firm and the tissues feel tight early in the disease. Persistence of impressions made by binding clothes, such as socks or shorts, may be the only evidence of minimal edema. If the edema becomes massive, there may actually be spontaneous breaks in the skin, with escape of edema fluid. At this stage, edema tends to be distributed generally throughout all tissues, producing ascites, labial and scrotal swelling, and, less constantly for some unexplained reason, pleural effusion. With persistence of generalized edema, which occurs only rarely now, its distribution changes, so that it tends to localize as ascites. The face and extremities in these patients may be free of edema and may reveal the tissue malnutrition concealed earlier by more generalized edema.

Gastrointestinal disturbances are encountered frequently in the course of the nephrotic syndrome. Diarrhea is especially common during periods of massive edema. It does not seem to be associated with infection, and it has been attributed to edema of the intestinal mucosa.

Poor appetite is so closely related to the presence and severity of edema that it appears to be a consequence of it. Anorexia and loss of protein in the urine account for the severe degree of malnutrition seen occasionally in children with persistent nonresponsive diseases.

There are other physical abnormalities related to persistent edema, especially to massive ascites: umbilical hernias are common, the veins of the anterior abdominal wall may be dilated, and rectal prolapse may occur.

Respiratory difficulty resulting from abdominal distention, with or without pleural effusion, may be disturbing and occasionally alarming. The use of intravenous albumin and furosemide as described under Diuretics may be necessary to relieve this symptom.

Decreased elasticity of the auricular cartilage has been described [40] in a majority of children with the nephrotic syndrome, regardless of the presence or absence of edema. The cause of the phenomenon is unknown.

Other disturbances, discussed under Complications, may be due to persistent disease, treatment, or both. They include increased *susceptibilty to infections, hypercoagulability,* and *impairment of growth.*

Marked *disturbances in psychosocial functioning* are common in the children with the nephrotic syndrome [54] as in any serious illness that acts as a nonspecific stress on the developing child and his family. The personalities of the patient and the parents will all determine the psychological reactions to the child's illness. Anxiety and guilt are frequent emotional responses, not only in the parents, who are more likely to express them, but also in the children. "Why did my child get this disease?" "What did I do wrong?" "What did I fail to do?" These questions require discussion and reassurance. Latent problems in family relationships may become manifest. In some instances the disease serves as a common enemy and strengthens parents' support of each other.

Parental anxiety and frequent or prolonged hospitalizations may deprive the sick child of normal progression toward independence and the taking of responsibility for his own body and his own fate. The expansion of the child's social world may be limited. Finally, the nephrotic child is in danger of forming a greatly distorted concept of body image. The physician who is aware of these problems can contribute greatly toward fostering optimal development and adjustment in patient and family and can help minimize disability and unnecessary anxiety and distress.

Children with the nephrotic syndrome may progress to the stage of chronic renal insufficiency, and signs and symptoms of *uremia* may develop. Almost all of such patients have glomerular dis-

eases other than MCNS; they are discussed in the appropriate chapters.

Differential Diagnosis and Indications for Biopsy

Clinical differentiation between primary and secondary nephrotic syndrome depends on documenting the presence of other evidence of a generalized disease with which the syndrome may be associated. Although the nephrotic syndrome may be the presenting manifestation in the secondary forms, it is usually preceded by other evidence of the disease. Secondary nephrotic syndrome due to exposure to agents such as drugs or other nephrotoxins may be suspected from the history and in some cases from accompanying clinical manifestations, such as skin rashes from drugs or poisonous plants.

The single most important variable in discriminating among patients with glomerular diseases associated with the primary nephrotic syndrome is their response to an initial intensive course of treatment with corticosteroids. In this discussion, the terms *responder* and initial *nonresponder* are used to describe the clinical status following initial treatment with prednisone in a dosage of 60 $mg/m^2/day$ *given in divided doses for 4 weeks, followed by 40 $mg/m^2/day$ given in divided doses on 3 consecutive days out of 7 for an additional 4 weeks.* Patients in whom the rate of excretion of urinary protein has decreased to 4 $mg/m^2/hr$ or less (zero or trace on strip tests) on 3 consecutive days during the initial 8 weeks of therapy are classified as responders; those who have not responded by the end of 8 weeks are nonresponders.

The clinical responses of patients with different forms of histopathology in the ISKDC [42] and in the series of White et al. [104] are shown in Table 52-4. It can be seen that the proportion of responders among patients with MCNS is much greater than that among patients with other forms of glomerular disease. However, because such a

Table 52-4. Distribution of Responders and Initial Nonresponders Among Major Histopathologic Categories (Unselected Patients)

Histologic Category	ISKDC [42]			White et al. [104]			Total		
	Number of Patients	Resp. (%)	Nonresp. (%)	Number of Patients	Resp. (%)	Nonresp. (%)	Number of Patients	Resp. (%)	Nonresp. (%)
MCNS	335	92.8	7.2	95	97.9	2.1	430	94.0	6.0
FSGS	29	20.7	79.3	12	16.7	83.3	41	19.5	80.5
MPGN	27	7.4	92.6	9	0	100.0	36	5.6	94.4
Other	42	40.5	59.5	12	8.3	91.7	54	33.3	66.7
Total	433	77.6	27.4	128	75.0	25.0	561	77.0	23.0

Table 52-5. Proportion of Responders and Nonresponders with MCNS and Other Glomerular Diseases

Group	ISKDC [42]			White et al. [104]			Total		
	Number of Patients	MCNS (%)	Other (%)	Number of Patients	MCNS (%)	Other (%)	Number of Patients	MCNS (%)	Other (%)
Responders	336	92.6	7.4	96	96.9	3.1	432	93.5	6.5
Initial non-responders	97	24.7	75.3	32	6.3	93.7	129	20.2	79.8

high proportion of children with primary nephrotic syndrome have MCNS, about 20 percent of initial nonresponders are in that category (Table 52-5).

The decision about recommending a biopsy should be based on whether or not the information to be gained warrants the minimal risk involved (see Chap. 12). Present experience suggests that biopsies should be done in all patients with secondary nephrotic syndrome and in those with the primary forms who have glomerular histopathology *other than those of MCNS*. From the distribution of these glomerular diseases (see Table 52-2), it can be estimated that about 80 percent of all children with the nephrotic syndrome have MCNS. Thus, if these patients could be identified at the time of diagnosis, only one-fifth of children with the nephrotic syndrome would need to have biopsies. It might be suggested that all patients with primary nephrotic syndrome be treated first and that biopsies be done only on nonresponders. If this were the practice, biopsies would be done in only about 6 percent of patients with MCNS (see Table 52-4). The major objection to this approach is that patients with MPGN would be treated initially with large dosages of prednisone, which should be avoided, since they appear to be at greater risk than others of severe corticosteroid side reactions, including hypertension and convulsions (see Chap. 51).

It remains important therefore in deciding whether or not to do a biopsy to know how accurately the glomerular disease present can be predicted from the clinical and laboratory characteristics observable at the time of diagnosis.

It has been known for many years, long before percutaneous biopsies were done, that the prognosis in children who had no hematuria, hypertension, or reduction in glomerular filtration rate was better than in those in whom these findings were present [9, 63]. Since information from biopsies has been available, it has been believed that the absence of these abnormalities makes it likely that the patient has MCNS. This supposition is, in general, correct. The proportion of patients in

the ISKDC with these abnormalities among the major forms of the primary nephrotic syndrome is shown in Table 52-6. Among patients with MCNS, hypertension was present in 13.5 percent. Habib and Kleinknecht [37] reported similar findings: 5.7 percent for hypertension; 29.1 percent for hematuria; and 20.6 percent for blood urea levels greater than 60 mg per deciliter. As expected, the proportions of patients with FSGS and MPGN who have abnormal values for these characteristics are considerably higher than the proportions of patients with MCNS.

Examination of Table 52-6 reveals that children with MCNS differ from those with MPGN in almost every variable listed, whereas some characteristics of patients with FSGS are similar to those of MCNS (sex and serum C3) while others are similar to those of patients with MPGN (hypertension and hematuria), and still others are intermediate (serum creatinine, protein selectivity).

Knowledge of these various relationships has given many clinicians confidence that they can differentiate fairly well between patients with these three glomerular diseases associated with the nephrotic syndrome, especially between those with MCNS and MPGN. However, further analyses of data in Table 52-6 reveal how inaccurate such predictions would have been. For example, in this series, predicting that a child did not have MCNS because he had a low C3 would almost always have been correct since only 1.5 percent of patients with MCNS had low values. However, predicting that he did *not* have MPGN because he had a normal C3 would have been incorrect in about one-fourth of the cases with MPGN. Similarly, predicting that a patient did *not* have MCNS because he had hematuria would have been incorrect in more than one-fifth of the cases with MCNS, whereas predicting that a patient did *not* have MPGN because there was no hematuria would have been incorrect in more than two-fifths of patients with MPGN.

Predictive formulas obtained from multivariate analysis of the data collected by the ISKDC [42] permit more accurate prebiopsy identification of

Table 52-6. Proportion of Patients in the ISKDC with Clinical and Laboratory Characteristics Used Commonly at Time of Diagnosis to Differentiate Among the Major Forms of Primary Glomerular Disease Associated with the Nephrotic Syndrome in Children

Characteristic	MCNS n/N	MCNS %	FSGS n/N	FSGS %	MPGN n/N	MPGN %
Age ≦6[a, b, c]	317/398	79.6	18/36	50.0	1/39	2.6
Sex: female[a, c]	135/398	39.9	11/36	30.6	25/39	64.1
B.P. >98th percentile:						
Systolic[a, b]	72/347	20.7	16/33	48.5	19/37	51.4
Diastolic[b]	47/347	13.5	11/33	33.3	10/37	27.0
Hematuria:[a, b]						
RBC >100,000 m²/hr	80/352	22.7	15/31	48.4	20/34	58.8
Serum C3[a, c] <90 mg/dl	4/275	1.5	1/27	3.7	26/35	74.3
Serum cholesterol[a] <250 mg/dl	21/387	5.4	3/35	8.6	7/36	19.4
Selectivity index:						
Highly selective <.01[a, b]	110/208	52.9	3/23	13.0	1/10	10.0
Nonselective ≧.02[a, b]	32/208	15.4	13/23	56.5	6/10	60.0
Serum creatinine 98th percentile	112/345	32.5	13/32	40.6	19/38	50.0

n = number with characteristics; N = total number
[a] MCNS versus MPGN, p<.01
[b] MCNS versus FSGS, p<.01
[c] FSGS versus MPGN, p<.01

Source: International Study of Kidney Disease in Children. The nephrotic syndrome in children. Prediction of histopathology from clinical and laboratory characteristics at the time of diagnosis. *Kidney Int.* 13:43, 1978.

the underlying glomerular disease, especially in the clinically important *identification of patients with MPGN, to whom large doses of corticosteroids should not be given* (Chap. 51).

One formula used to predict whether a patient with the primary nephrotic syndrome has MPGN or some other primary glomerular disease uses the following readily observable variables: edema, hematuria, serum C3, creatinine, and albumin. Values for these variables are multiplied by the following coefficients and the sum of the products added to the constant, .9295 to yield a predictive Y value, $\hat{Y}$:

Edema (present = 1; absent = 0)
$$(1 \text{ or } 0) \times (+.2239) = \underline{\hspace{1cm}}$$
Hematuria (present = 1; absent = 0)
$$(1 \text{ or } 0) \times (-.0721) = \underline{\hspace{1cm}}$$
Serum C3 (<90 mg/dl = 1; ≧90 mg/dl = 0)
$$(1 \text{ or } 0) \times (-.6511) = \underline{\hspace{1cm}}$$
Serum creatinine (mg/dl)
$$(\text{value}) \times (-.0990) = \underline{\hspace{1cm}}$$
Serum albumin (gm/dl)
$$(\text{value}) \times (-.0580) = \underline{\hspace{1cm}}$$
$$+ .9295$$
$$\hat{Y} = \underline{\hspace{1cm}}$$

If a biopsy had been recommended before giving intensive corticosteroid treatment in all patients with Y value of 0.85 or less in the ISKDC series, there would have been very little chance of missing a case of MPGN, and a biopsy would have been done in less than about 8 percent of patients with MCNS. Conversely, if patients with Y values above 0.85 had been treated without doing a biopsy, there would have been very little chance that a patient with MPGN would have been included. Thus, using the same characteristics on which the clinician usually bases his clinical judgment, with the assistance of the formula, his decision concerning whether or not to do a biopsy before starting treatment would be made with a quantitative estimate of the accuracy of his prediction.

General Management
The most important factors in the nonspecific treatment of children with the nephrotic syndrome include diet, activity, and diuretic therapy. A guiding principle in treating these children is that they should be permitted to lead lives as normal as possible.

DIET
In general, it is recommended that the diet be normal for the child's age and that he be fed according to his appetite, without coaxing. When edema is present, *salt restriction* is advised, but only to the extent that it does not interfere markedly with the child's appetite. This usually means excluding foods with very high salt content and not adding salt to food at the table. *Fluids* are given as desired. No attempt is made to alter the *protein* content of the diet, either by restricting it or by encouraging increased intake.

ACTIVITY
Although diuresis is observed occasionally in previously ambulatory patients when they are sub-

jected to strict bed rest, and the rate of excretion of protein may decrease, there is no evidence that restriction of general activity favorably influences the course or outcome of the disease. For this reason, and because of the difficulty of enforcing bed rest in young children, no attempt should be made to restrict activity. During periods of extensive edema there is a certain amount of self-imposed limitation of activity in some children, although many remain remarkably active during these periods. It seems clear that the psychological benefits of permitting relatively normal activity are of greater importance than any known factors against it.

DIURETICS

Diuretic therapy of the nephrotic syndrome does not alter the natural history of the disease. When combined with moderate sodium restriction, however, it can help counteract the dangers of severe acute edema and ascites, and it can aid in relieving the discomfort, inconvenience, and danger of chronic edema.

Treatment with diuretics is indicated in patients with massive edema, especially in the presence of respiratory or gastrointestinal symptoms, visual abnormalities, severely restricted activity, or irritation of adjacent edematous skin surfaces. Diuretics are used in the presence of less extensive edema in preparation for renal biopsy and in patients with chronic or recurrent infections, especially peritonitis and skin infections, that may be directly related to edema. Diuretic agents are also indicated for the treatment of persistent edema in patients whose renal lesion is unresponsive to specific therapy.

Diuresis has been initiated by dextran, whole blood, plasma, and albumin, which presumably induce diuresis by increasing the oncotic pressure of the plasma and increasing plasma volume, with a resultant elevation of glomerular filtration rate and an inhibition of fractional resorption of sodium and water [25, 34, 45, 61, 66]. Other agents promote diuresis and natriuresis by directly inhibiting the renal tubular resorption of salt and water. These include osmotic diuretics such as urea [89] and mannitol [50], the organic mercurial diuretics, and the more potent diuretics, such as the thiazides, furosemide, and ethacrynic acid.

Mercurial diuretics are no longer recommended, both because they are relatively ineffective and because nephrotoxicity has been reported in adults with the nephrotic syndrome.

Thiazides, which are derivatives of chlorothiazide, are effective by mouth and can be given at home [90]. Hydrochlorothiazide is given in a dosage of 2 to 5 mg/kg/day in two divided doses. Because this diuretic may produce potassium depletion, supplemental potassium may be given in the form of potassium chloride or a mixture of potassium salts. Side effects of the thiazides include increases of serum uric acid and, more rarely, thrombocytopenia, hyperglycemia, rashes, jaundice, and pancreatitis.

Spironolactone is only moderately effective as a diuretic. It is usually not used alone, but it may be given with a thiazide for its potassium-sparing effect [107].

Furosemide and ethacrynic acid are more potent agents that act by increasing the excreted fraction of the filtered sodium load. Short courses of intravenous treatment with these drugs are often very effective in relieving edema [43, 74]. Injudicious use, however, may produce severe volume contraction, with hypokalemia, alkalosis, and azotemia. These agents should therefore be used only in the hospital, with careful monitoring of weight and blood pressure. Excessive dosages may cause elevation of serum uric acid and deafness.

It is often extremely difficult to achieve a satisfactory diuresis and elimination of edema with the usual doses of the common diuretics when the serum albumin is less than 1.5 gm per deciliter [89] and the patient is severely edematous. In these instances the following regimen has been used: *salt-poor human albumin* is given IV in a dose of 0.5 to 1.0 gm per kilogram over a period of 30 to 60 min, monitoring carefully for hypertension. After 30 to 60 min, furosemide is given IV in a dose of 1 to 2 mg per kilogram. A diuresis usually ensues, and the same regimen may be repeated every 4 to 6 hr as needed.

The response to this diuretic treatment is not entirely predictable; some patients lose a significant amount of edema fluid, while others do not. Grausz et al. [33] showed that sodium retention and formation of edema in hypoalbuminemic patients occur despite decreased fractional resorption of sodium proximally, thus the increased fractional sodium resorption must occur distally. Since distal sites are locations where furosemide and ethacrynic acid are supposed to act [23], one would expect a more consistent response than is usually seen with these agents in hypoalbuminemic patients. The evidence for increased fractional resorption of sodium distally is also difficult to reconcile with the poor response to aldosterone antagonists, which is thought to be due to such avid fractional resorption of sodium proximally that a reduced amount of sodium is delivered to the distal sites of action of aldosterone and aldosterone antagonist. The mechanisms responsible for the lack of diuretic response in some of these patients therefore remains unexplained.

Complications

HYPERCOAGULABILITY

An increased tendency to thrombosis in the nephrotic syndrome was first reported by Addis [1] in 1949. Since then, there have been frequent reports of arterial and venous thromboses, both in nonresponsive patients and when a massive diuresis follows therapy with corticosteroids or diuretics [48, 59]. Thromboses have occurred in the pulmonary, coronary, and mesenteric arteries and especially in the femoral artery following femoral punctures, and thromboses have occurred in the axillary, subclavian, and renal veins. Although it is known that the nephrotic syndrome can be caused by renal vein or inferior vena cava thrombosis, it seems more likely that in children at least, the nephrotic syndrome is the primary event, with renal vein thrombosis a secondary complication.

Hypercoagulation may be secondary to increased concentrations of clotting factors or to decreased fibrinolytic activity [98]. Intravascular coagulation is enhanced in the presence of hypovolemia and hemoconcentration. Changes in vascular structure secondary to hyperlipidemia might also promote thrombosis [70]. Work by Bang and associates [5] provided evidence that hypercoagulability in the nephrotic syndrome may be due in part to urinary loss of specific plasma proteins needed to inhibit platelet aggression. Thomson and colleagues [98] demonstrated significant increases in the activities of coagulation factors V and VIII and increases in the concentrations of fibrinogen, plasminogen, and alpha-2-macroglobulins. They also found a significant reduction in antiplasmin activity and alpha-1-antitrypsin activity. Some of these changes favor thrombosis and some favor fibrinolysis. The thrombotic tendency in the nephrotic syndrome may therefore be due to a greater impact on factors favoring thrombosis. It appears that these changes may take place passively as a result of increased protein synthesis and the urinary loss of low-molecular-weight proteins and may not be due to primary changes in the coagulation or fibrinolytic systems.

The possible value of anticoagulant therapy in the treatment of these complications has not been adequately assessed. At present, such therapy cannot be recommended.

INFECTIONS

An increased susceptibility to infection is common in children with nephrotic syndrome in relapse. Before effective antibiotics were available, most deaths in children with the nephrotic syndrome were due to infections, most frequently pneumonitis; bronchitis also occurred, but less commonly.

Septicemia and peritonitis in a child with generalized edema with ascites is a dramatic event. Although it is not seen commonly at present, it still occurs and must be recognized and treated promptly if preventable deaths are to be avoided. The usual history is of a mild respiratory infection followed by the sudden onset of high fever. Abdominal pain and localizing signs or symptoms are often lacking. In some children who survived repeated attacks of pneumococcal peritonitis in the past, the ascitic fluid was found to be sterile, although many leukocytes were present, and blood cultures were positive.

Rarely seen at present, an erysipeloid eruption on the skin of the abdomen or thighs used to be a common occurrence. The borders of the lesion were well demarcated, but less raised than in erysipelas, and no organisms could be cultured from the lesions, which were thought to represent a hypersensitivity reaction to repeated pneumococcal infections.

In a retrospective, 5-year review, Wilfert and Katz [105] enumerated sites of infections and the organisms cultured from these sites. Septicemia, peritonitis, cellulitis, pneumonitis, bronchitis, urinary tract infections, and septic arthritis were seen. Pneumococci were apparently the causative organisms in some of the cases of peritonitis and septicemia, and gram-negative organisms, including *Escherichia coli, Pseudomonas,* and *Serratia* often were implicated. There were no cases of staphylococcal sepsis.

Causes proposed to explain the increased susceptibility to infection include (1) low immunoglobulin levels, (2) decreased resistance because of edema, (3) generalized protein deficiency, (4) decreased bactericidal activity of leukocytes [18], and (5) immunosuppressive therapy [89].

It is recommended that prophylactic antibiotics not be used routinely in children with the nephrotic syndrome. However, prompt recognition and vigorous treatment of intercurrent infections continue to be crucially important, using antibiotic coverage for both gram-positive and gram-negative organisms in severe infections until the organism is identified [105].

IMPAIRED GROWTH

It has long been known that growth in stature diminishes markedly and may cease in children with an uncontrolled nephrotic syndrome [44]. There appears, however, to be no residual growth impairment in those who recover [7], and most children show catch-up growth and resumption of their previous rate along the growth curve after long-term remission [83].

A major cause of growth retardation in patients with the nephrotic syndrome not given corticosteroids was undoubtedly protein-calorie malnutrition. In such patients, malnutrition secondary to poor appetite, protein loss in the urine, and malabsorption due to edema of the gastrointestinal tract was a constant feature.

Today, the major cause of growth impairment in children with the nephrotic syndrome is corticosteroid therapy. Long-term, high-dose corticosteroid therapy delays bone maturation and arrests linear growth [29, 56], especially when dosage exceeds 5 mg/m²/day [106]. There is no deficiency of endogenous production of growth hormone or of its secretion during corticosteroid therapy [69]. It is known, however, that corticosteroids antagonize the effects of endogenous and exogenous growth hormone at the peripheral tissue level through an effect on somatomedins [68, 81]. In addition to the other causes of growth retardation, emotional deprivation and chronic anxiety may play a role [19]. At present, the best way to prevent growth impairment is to avoid unnecessarily prolonged courses of therapy with large doses of corticosteroids, to provide adequate intake of calories and proteins, and to lessen psychological stresses insofar as possible.

Course and Prognosis

The natural history, response to treatment, and prognosis in children with the nephrotic syndrome are determined by the form of primary or secondary glomerular disease present. These are discussed in the appropriate chapters.

The course and prognosis cannot be predicted from the severity of the manifestations of the nephrotic syndrome at the onset. In fact, there appears to be an inverse relationship between the two variables, in that untreated patients with MCNS who have the best prognosis have, in general, more severe proteinuria, hypoalbuminemia, hypercholesterolemia, and edema than those with other glomerular diseases, in whom the onset tends to be more insidious and the manifestations less severe. As shown in Table 52-7, the relatively good prognosis in patients with MCNS sets this disease apart from the other glomerular diseases associated with the nephrotic syndrome, among which the prognosis varies. Thus, during a period of 1 to 18 years after onset, Habib and Kleinknecht [37] found that 71 percent of patients with MCNS were in remission, contrasted with 24, 43, and 7.5 percent respectively of patients with

Table 52-7. Status of 346 Patients with Primary Nephrotic Syndrome

Diagnosis	Period of Follow-up (years)	Number of Patients	Remission (%)	In Chronic Renal Failure or Dead (%)
MCNS	1–18	209	71	7
FSGS	1–18	47	24	38
MGN	1–9	37	43	8
MPGN	1–10	53	7.5	41.5

Source: R. Habib and C. Kleinknecht The Primary Nephrotic Syndrome of Childhood. Classification and Clinicopathologic Study of 406 Cases. In S. C. Sommers (ed.), *Pathology Annual.* New York: Appleton-Century-Crofts, 1971.

FSGS, MGN, and MPGN. The worst prognosis was in patients with FSGS and MPGN, among whom 38 and 41.5 percent were in chronic renal failure or had died. The prognosis for patients with MGN was intermediate, and it appears to be better for younger than for older children [99]. The prognosis for patients with the two major forms of secondary nephrotic syndrome in children, diffuse proliferative lupus nephritis and severe anaphylactoid purpura nephritis is, in general, also poor (Chaps. 58, 61).

References

1. Addis, T. *Glomerular Nephritis.* New York: Macmillan, 1949.
2. Allison, A. C., Hendrickse, R. G., Edington, G. M., Houba, V., de Petris, S., and Adeniyi, A. Immune complexes in the nephrotic syndrome of African children. *Lancet* 2:1232, 1969.
3. Arneil, G. C. Management of the Nephrotic Syndrome in the Child. In E. Lieberman (ed.), *Clinical Pediatric Nephrology.* Philadelphia and Toronto: Lippincott, 1976. Chap. 9, p. 146.
4. Arneil, G. C., Dewhurst, C. J., Houston, I. B., and Winberg, J. Disorders of the Urogenital System. In J. O. Forfar and G. C. Arneil (eds.), *Textbook of Pediatrics.* Edinburgh and London: Churchill Livingstone, 1973. Chap. 17, p. 1020.
5. Bang, N. U., Trygstad, C. W., Schroeder, J. E., Heindenreich, R. O., and Csiscko, B. M. Enhanced platelet function in glomerular renal disease. *J. Lab. Clin. Med.* 81:651, 1973.
6. Bar-Khayim, Y., Teplitz, C., Garella, S., and Chazan, J. A. Trimethadione (Tridione) induced nephrotic syndrome. *Am. J. Med.* 54:272, 1973.
7. Barness, L. S., Mool, G. H., and Janeway, C. A. Nephrotic syndrome I. Natural history of the disease. *Pediatrics* 5:486, 1950.
8. Barnett, H. L. The Natural and Treatment History of Glomerular Diseases in Children—what Can We Learn from International Cooperative Studies? A report of the International Study of Kidney Disease in Children. In S. Giovannetti, V. Bonomini, and G. D'Amico (eds.), *Proceedings of the Sixth Interna-*

tional Congress of Nephrology. Basel: Karger, 1976. Pp. 470–485.

9. Barnett, H. L., Forman, C. W., and Lauson, H. D. The Nephrotic Syndrome in Children. In S. J. Levine (ed.), *Advances in Pediatrics.* Chicago: Year Book, 1952. Vol. 5.

10. Barnett, H. L., Simons, D. J., and Willis, R. E., Jr. Nephrotic syndrome occurring during Tridione therapy. *Am. J. Med.* 4:760, 1948.

11. Barr, J. H., Cole, H. N., Driver, J. R., Deleas, R., Miller, M., and Strauss, L. G. Acute syphilitic nephrosis successfully treated with penicillin. *J.A.M.A.* 131:741, 1946.

12. Baxter, J. H., Goodman, H. C., and Allen, J. C. Effects of infusions of serum albumin on serum lipids and lipoproteins in nephrosis. *J. Clin. Invest.* 40:490, 1961.

13. Baxter, J. H., Goodman, H. C., and Havel, R. J. Serum lipid and lipoprotein alterations in nephrosis. *J. Clin. Invest.* 39:455, 1960.

14. Becker, E. L. Saliva Proteins in Adults with the Nephrotic Syndrome. In *Renal Metabolism and Epidemiology of Some Renal Diseases.* Proceedings of the 15th Annual Conference on the Kidney. New York: National Kidney Foundation, Inc., 1972. Vol. 1, p. 207.

15. Blahd, W. M., Fields, M., and Goldman, R. The turnover rate of serum albumin in the nephrotic syndrome as determined by I^{131} labelled albumin. *J. Lab. Clin. Med.* 46:747, 1955.

16. Blau, E. B., and Haas, J. E. Glomerular sialic acid and proteinuria in human renal disease. *Lab. Invest.* 28:477, 1973.

17. Cameron, J. S. Nephrotic syndrome. *Br. Med. J.* 4:350, 1970.

18. Chandra, R. K., and Seth, V. Reduced bactericidal capacity of polymorphonuclear leucocytes in nephrotic syndrome and effect of steroid therapy. *Experientia* 28:1354, 1972.

19. Chantler, C., and Holliday, M. A. Growth in children with renal disease with particular reference to the effects of calorie malnutrition: A review. *Clin. Nephrol.* 1:230, 1973.

20. Chinard, F. P., Lauson, H. D., Eder, H. A., Greif, R. L., and Hiller, A. A study of the mechanism of proteinuria in patients with the nephrotic syndrome. *J. Clin. Invest.* 33:621, 1954.

21. Chopra, J. S., Mallick, N. P., and Stone, M. C. Hyperlipoproteinaemias in nephrotic syndrome. *Lancet* 1:317, 1971.

22. Churg, J., Habib, R., and White, R. H. R. Pathology of the nephrotic syndrome in children. A report for the International Study of Kidney Disease in Children. *Lancet* 1:1299, 1970.

23. Clapp, J. R., and Robinson, R. R. Distal sites of action of diuretic drugs in the dog nephron. *Am. J. Physiol.* 215:228, 1968.

24. Combes, B., Stastny, P., Shorey, J., Eigenbrodt, E. H., Barera, A., Hull, A. R., and Carter, N. Glomerulonephritis with deposition of Australia antigen-antibody complexes in glomerular basement membrane. *Lancet* 2:234, 1971.

25. Davison, A. M., Lambie, A. T., Verth, A. H., and Cash, J. D. Salt-poor albumin in the management of nephrotic syndrome. *Br. Med. J.* 1:481, 1974.

26. Edelmann, C. M., Jr. The Idiopathic Nephrotic Syndrome of Childhood. In H. L. Barnett (ed.), *Pediatrics* (15th ed.). New York: Appleton-Century-Crofts, 1972. Chap. 22, p. 1499.

27. Epstein, A. A. Concerning the causations of edema in chronic parenchymatous nephritis: Method for its alleviation. *Am. J. Med. Sci.* 154:638, 1917.

28. Farquhar, M. G., and Palade, G. E. Glomerular permeability II. Ferritin transfer across the glomerular capillary wall in nephrotic rats. *J. Exp. Med.* 114:699, 1961.

29. Friedman, M., and Strang, L. B. Effect of long-term corticosteroids and corticotrophin on the growth of children. *Lancet* 2:569, 1966.

30. Gamble, C. N., and Reardan, J. B. Immunopathogenesis of syphilitic glomerulonephritis. *N. Engl. J. Med.* 292:449, 1975.

31. Gitlin, D., and Janeway, C. A. An immunochemical study of the albumins of serum, urine, ascitic fluid, and edema fluid in the nephrotic syndrome. *J. Clin. Invest.* 31:223, 1952.

32. Gitlin, D., Janeway, C. A., and Farr, L. E. Studies on the metabolism of plasma proteins in the nephrotic syndrome. *J. Clin. Invest.* 35:44, 1956.

33. Grausz, H., Lieberman, R., and Earley, L. Effect of plasma albumin on sodium reabsorption in patients with nephrotic syndrome. *Kidney Int.* 1:47, 1972.

34. Greenman, L., Weigand, F. A., and Danowski, T. S. Therapy of the nephrotic syndrome. *Am. J. Dis. Child.* 89:169, 1955.

35. Greifer, I. Personal communication, 1976.

36. Habib, R. The Nephrotic Syndrome. In P. Royer, R. Habib, H. Mathieu, and M. Broyer (eds.), *Pediatric Nephrology.* Philadelphia: Saunders, 1974. Part III, p. 258.

37. Habib, R., and Kleinknecht, C. The Primary Nephrotic Syndrome of Childhood. Classification and Clinicopathologic Study of 406 Cases. In S. C. Sommers (ed.), *Pathology Annual.* New York: Appleton-Century-Crofts, 1971. P. 165.

38. Hangen, H. N. Tridione nephropathy. *Acta Med. Scand.* 159:375, 1975.

39. Hendrickse, R. G., Glasgow, E. F., Adeniyi, A., White, R. H. R., Edington, G. M., and Houba, V. Quartan malaria nephrotic syndrome. *Lancet* 1:1143, 1972.

40. Heymann, W., Horwood, S., Isaacs, E. W., and Cuppage, F. Decreased elasticity of auricular cartilage in the nephrotic syndrome of children. *J. Pediatr.* 62:74, 1963.

41. Hooft, C., van Acker, K., and Deneve, V. Clinical and histological course of the nephrotic syndrome during trimethadione (neoabsentol) therapy. *Helv. Paediatr. Acta* 17:329, 1962.

42. International Study of Kidney Disease in Children. The nephrotic syndrome in children. Prediction of histopathology from clinical and laboratory characteristics at the time of diagnosis. *Kidney Int.* 13:43, 1978.

43. James, J. A. Ethacrynic acid in edematous states in children. *J. Pediatr.* 71:881, 1967.

44. James, J. A. Nephrotic Syndrome. In J. A. James (ed.), *Renal Disease in Childhood.* St. Louis: Mosby, 1968.

45. James, J., Gordillo, G., and Metcoff, J. Effects of infusion of hyperoncotic dextran in children with the nephrotic syndrome. *J. Clin. Invest.* 33:1346, 1954.

46. Kaitz, A. L. Albumin metabolism in nephrotic adults. *J. Lab. Clin. Med.* 53:186, 1959.

47. Katz, J., Bonorris, G., and Sellers, A. L. Albumin metabolism in aminonucleoside nephrotic rats. *J. Lab. Clin. Med.* 62:910, 1963.

48. Kendall, A. G., Lobmann, R. C., and Dossetor, J. B. Nephrotic syndrome—a hypercoagulable state. *Arch. Intern. Med.* 127:1021, 1971.

49. Kibukamusake, J. W. Malaria prophylaxis and immunosuppressant therapy in management of nephrotic syndrome associated with quartan malaria. *Arch. Dis. Child.* 43:598, 1968.

50. Kleit, S. A., Hamburger, R. J., Mertz, B. L., and Fisch, C. Diuretic therapy—current status. *Am. Heart J.* 79:700, 1970.

51. Kluthe, R., Hagemann, V., and Klein, N. The turnover of α2 macroglobulins in the nephrotic syndrome. *Vox Sang.* 12:308, 1967.

52. Knieser, M. R., Jenis, E. H., Lowenthal, D. T., Bancroft, W. H., Burns, W., and Shalhoub, R. Pathogenesis of renal diseases associated with viral hepatitis. *Arch. Pathol.* 97:193, 1974.

53. Kohler, P. F., Cronin, R. E., Hammond, W. S., Olin, D., and Carr, R. I. Chronic membranous glomerulonephritis caused by hepatitis B antigen-antibody immune complexes. *Ann. Intern. Med.* 81:448, 1974.

54. Korsch, B., and Barnett, H. L. The physician, the family, and the child with nephrosis. *J. Pediatr.* 58:707, 1961.

55. Krebs, R. A., and Burrant, M. V. Nephrotic syndrome in association with varicella. *J.A.M.A.* 222:325, 1972.

56. Lam, C. N., and Arneil, G. C. Long-term dwarfing effect of corticosteroid treatment for childhood nephrosis. *Arch. Dis. Child.* 43:589, 1968.

57. Lee, R. E., Vernier, R. L., and Ulstrom, R. A. The nephrotic syndrome as a complication of perchlorate treatment of thyrotoxicosis. *N. Engl. J. Med.* 264:1221, 1961.

58. Leiter, L. Nephrosis. *Medicine (Baltimore)* 10:135, 1931.

59. Lieberman, E., Heuser, E., Gilchrist, G. S., Donnell, G. N., and Landing, B. H. Thrombosis, nephrosis, and corticosteroid therapy. *J. Pediatr.* 73:320, 1968.

60. Loeb, R. F., Atchley, D. W., Richards, D. W., Benedict, D. M., and Driscoll, M. E. On the mechanism of nephrotic syndrome. *J. Clin. Invest.* 11:621, 1932.

61. Luetscher, J. A., Hall, A. D., and Kremer, V. L. Treatment of nephrosis with concentrated human serum albumin. I. Effects on the proteins of body fluids. *J. Clin. Invest.* 28:700, 1949.

62. Luetscher, J. A., Jr., and Johnson, B. B. Chromatographic separation of the sodium retaining corticoids from the urine of children with nephrosis, compared with observations on normal children. *J. Clin. Invest.* 33:276, 1954.

63. Makker, S. P., and Heymann, W. The idiopathic nephrotic syndrome of childhood. *Am. J. Dis. Child.* 127:830, 1974.

64. McGovern, V. J. Persistent nephrotic syndrome: A renal biopsy study. *Aust. Ann. Med.,* 13:306, 1964.

65. McKenzie, I. F. C., and Nestel, P. J. Studies on the turnover of triglyceride and esterified cholesterol in subjects with the nephrotic syndrome. *J. Clin. Invest.* 47:1685, 1968.

66. Mellison, A. W., and Rennie, J. B. Treatment of renal edema with dextran. *Br. Med. J.* 1:893, 1954.

67. Michael, A. F., Blau, E., and Vernier, R. L. Glomerular polyanion alteration in aminonucleoside nephrosis. *Lab. Invest.* 23:649, 1970.

68. Morris, H., Jorgensen, J., Elrick, H., Goldsmith, R., and Subryan, V. Metabolic effects of human growth hormone in corticosteroid-treated children. *J. Clin. Invest.* 47:436, 1968.

69. Morris, H. G., Jorgensen, J. R., and Jenkins, A. Plasma growth hormone concentration in corticosteroid-treated children. *J. Clin. Invest.* 47:427, 1968.

70. Mukherjee, A. P., Toh, B. H., Chan, G. E. L., Lau, K. S., and White, J. C. Vascular complications in the nephrotic syndrome. *Br. Med. J.* 4:273, 1970.

71. Muller, F. Morbus Brightti. *Verh. Dtsch. Pathol. Ges.* 9:64, 1905.

72. Munk, F. Klinische Diagnostik der degenerativen Nierenerkrankungen *Zt. Klin. Med.* 78:1, 1913.

73. Munk, F. Die Nephrosen. *Med. Klin.* 12:1019, 1916.

74. Muth, R. G. Diuretic properties of furosemide in renal disease. *Ann. Intern. Med.* 69:249, 1968.

75. Nabarro, J. D. N., and Rosenheim, N. L. Nephrotic syndrome complicating tridione (Troxidone) therapy. *Lancet* 1:1091, 1952.

76. Newmark, S. R., Anderson, C. F., Donadio, J. V., and Ellefson, R. D. Lipoprotein profiles in adult nephrotics. *Mayo Clin. Proc.* 50:359, 1975.

77. Northway, J. D., and West, C. D. Successful therapy of trimethadione nephrosis with prednisone and cyclophosphamide. *J. Pediatr.* 71:259, 1967.

78. Pierson, M., Lascombes, G., and Vert, P. Syndrome néphrotique par traitment a l'epidione. *Arch. Fr. Pediatr.* 16:1389, 1959.

79. Pollner, P. Nephrotic syndrome associated with congenital syphilis. *J.A.M.A.* 198:263, 1966.

80. Robson, A. M., Giangiacomo, J., Kienstra, R., Naqvi, S. T., and Ingelfinger, J. R. Normal glomerular permeability and its modification by minimal change nephrotic syndrome. *J. Clin. Invest.* 54:1190, 1974.

81. Root, W., Bongiovanni, A. M., and Eberlein, W. R. Studies of the secretion and metabolic effects of human growth hormone in children with glucocorticoid-induced growth retardation. *J. Pediatr.* 75:826, 1969.

82. Rosenblum, J., Sonnenschein, H., and Minsky, A. A. Trimethadione (Tridione) nephrosis. *Am. J. Dis. Child.* 97:790, 1959.

83. Royer, P., Mathieu, H., and Habib, R. Aspects particuliers du syndrome néphrotique de l'enfant. *Pathol. Biol. (Paris)* 10:687, 1962.

84. Royer, P., Mathieu, H. R., and Vermiel, G. Le Syndrome Néphrotique de L'Enfant. In H. Masson (ed.), *Les Syndromes Néphrotiques.* Report of 34th French Congress of Medicine, Paris: Flammarion Press, 1963. Vol. I., p. 265.

85. Rubin, M. I. Nephrotic Syndrome. In M. I. Rubin (ed.), *Pediatric Nephrology.* Baltimore: Williams & Wilkins, 1975. Chap. 19, p. 454.

86. Rytand, D. A. Fatal anuria, the nephrotic syndrome and glomerular nephritis as sequels of the dermatitis of poison oak. *Am. J. Med.* 5:548, 1948.

87. Rytand, D. A. Onset of the nephrotic syndrome during a reaction to bee sting. *Stanford Med. Bull.* 13:224, 1955.

88. Scheinman, J. I., and Stiehm, R. Fibrinolytic studies in the nephrotic syndrome. *Pediatrics* 5:206, 1971.

89. Schreiner, G. E. The Nephrotic Syndrome. In M. B. Strauss and L. G. Welt (eds.), *Diseases of the Kidney* (2nd ed.) Boston: Little, Brown, 1971.

90. Schreiner, G. E., and Bloomer, H. A. The effect of chlorothiazide on edema, cirrhosis, nephrosis, congestive heart failure, and chronic renal insufficiency. *N. Engl. J. Med.* 257:1016, 1957.

91. Shafrir, E., and Brenner, T. Lipoprotein Synthesis in Hypoproteinemia of Experimental Nephrotic Syndrome and Plasmaphoresis. In R. Branchi, G. Mariani, and A. S. McFarlane (eds.), *Plasma Protein Turnover*. Baltimore: University Park Press, 1976. Chapter 3.

92. Smith, H. W. *The Kidney: Structure and Function in Health and Disease.* New York: Oxford University Press, 1951.

93. Soothill, J. F., and Hendrickse, R. G. Some immunological studies of the nephrotic syndrome of Nigerian children. *Lancet* 1:629, 1967.

94. Starling, E. H. The Arris and Gale Lectures on the physiological factors involved in the causation of dropsy. *Lancet* 1:1331, 1896.

95. Starling, E. H. On the absorption of fluids from the connective tissue spaces. *J. Physiol. (Lond.)* 19: 312, 1896.

96. Sterzel, R. B., Krause, P. H., Zobl, H., and Kuhn, K. Acute syphilitic nephrosis: A transient glomerular immunopathy. *Clin. Nephrol.* 2:164, 1974.

97. Talamo, R. C., and Crawford, J. L. Trimethadione nephrosis treated with cortisone and nitrogen mustard. *N. Engl. J. Med.* 269:15, 1963.

98. Thomson, C., Forbes, C. D., Prentice, C. R. M., and Kennedy, A. C. Changes in blood coagulation and fibrinolysis in the nephrotic syndrome. *Q. J. Med.* 43:399, 1974.

99. Trainin, E. B., Boichis, H., Spitzer, A., and Greifer, I. Idiopathic membranous nephropathy. *N.Y. State J. Med.* 76:357, 1976.

100. Volhard, F., and Fahr, T. *Die Brightsche Nierenkrankheit.* Berlin: Springer Verlag, 1914.

101. Weech, A. A. Dietary protein and regeneration of serum albumin. *Bull. Johns Hopkins Hosp.* 70:157, 1942.

102. Westberg, N. G., and Michael, A. F. Human glomerular basement membrane. Preparation and composition. *Biochemistry* 9:3837, 1970.

103. White, J. C. Nephrosis occurring during trimethadione therapy. Report of a case. *J.A.M.A.* 139:376, 1949.

104. White, R. H. R., Glasgow, E. F., and Mills, R. J. Clinicopathologic study of nephrotic syndrome in childhood. *Lancet* 1:1353, 1970.

105. Wilfert, C. M., and Katz, S. L. Etiology of bacterial sepsis in nephrotic children. *Pediatrics* 42: 841, 1968.

106. Wilson, C. J., Kaye, J., Belzer, F. O., Kountz, S. L., and Potter, D. E. Growth following renal transplantation: Daily vs. alternate day steroid therapy. *Pediatric Res.* 6:415, 1972.

107. Wolff, H. P., Kruck, F., Lommer, D., and Schieffer, H. Role of aldosterone in edema formation. *Ann. N.Y. Acad. Sci.* 139:285, 1966.

108. Wren, J. C., and Nutt, R. L. Nephrotic syndrome occurring during paramethadione therapy: Report of case with clinical remission. *J.A.M.A.* 153:918, 1953.

109. Zelazko, M., and Feldman, G. Behavior of the complement system in the nephropathy of congenital syphilis. *J. Pediatr.* 88:359, 1976.

53. Minimal Change Nephrotic Syndrome

Henry L. Barnett, Morris Schoeneman, Jay Bernstein, and Chester M. Edelmann, Jr.

The term *minimal change nephrotic syndrome* (MCNS) defines the form of primary nephrotic syndrome characterized histopathologically by the absence of major structural changes [21]. There may be minor degrees of glomerular abnormality, and diffuse fusion of the epithelial foot processes is usually present. By the generally accepted definition [3, 4, 25, 37, 38, 76, 84], heavy proteinuria and hypoalbuminemia are present at some time in the course of every patient with MCNS. In contrast, they may never be present in some patients with other morphologically defined primary and secondary glomerular diseases that are commonly associated with the nephrotic syndrome (Chap. 52).

Demographic Characteristics

It is difficult to determine the demographic characteristics of children with MCNS, especially the incidence and prevalence. In addition to the usual problems encountered with nonreportable chronic illnesses, the primary nephrotic syndrome creates the problem of differentiating statistics for children with MCNS from those for children with other glomerular abnormalities.

Incidence and Prevalence

Estimates of the annual incidence of the nephrotic syndrome associated with all forms of primary glomerular disease range from 2 to 7 per 100,000 children under 10 years of age [74]. Assuming that the duration of the clinical disease is between 2 and 5 years, the prevalence can be calculated to be between 4 and 35 per 100,000.

Rates observed in Erie County, New York, between 1946 and 1961 [77, 85] are probably the most accurate, since they are based on a survey of a total population rather than of a hospital population. For the 16-year period studied, an overall annual incidence of 2.0 and a cumulative prevalence of 15.7 per 100,000 were found for children under 16 years of age. About four-fifths of children with primary nephrotic syndrome have MCNS (see Table 52-2). Applying this proportion to the rates reported for Erie County yields an incidence and prevalence of MCNS in children under 16 years of age of about 1.6 and 13 per 100,000 respectively.

Geographic Distribution
Minimal change nephrotic syndrome occurs in children in countries throughout the world, but there are no data on geographic variation. As discussed elsewhere (Chap. 52), there is considerable geographic variation in the proportion of all children with primary nephrotic syndrome who have MCNS. Values in the clinics participating in the International Study of Kidney Disease in Children (ISKDC)* ranged from 68 percent at the Hospital of the Albert Einstein College of Medicine in New York to 89 percent at the Royal Hospital for Sick Children in Glasgow [44].

Ethnicity
The data are insufficient for assessing whether or not there are differences in demographic characteristics among children of different ethnic groups. The impression that the primary nephrotic syndrome is less frequent in nonwhite than in white children in the United States has not been borne out by the scanty data reported [74, 77].

Socioeconomic Status
There is some suggestion from the study in Erie County, New York [77, 85], that the incidence of the primary nephrotic syndrome in children is greater in the lower socioeconomic groups. However, no apparent association was found in the ISKDC between histopathologic categories and

* The ISKDC is a multicenter study in which clinical surveys and therapeutic trials (including several in children with MCNS) have been conducted since 1967 in 19 clinics in Europe, North America, Israel, and Japan [6].

socioeconomic status as reflected by the father's occupation [44].

Genetics
It seems certain that familial cases of the primary nephrotic syndrome occur more frequently than can be accounted for by chance. From a European survey of familial cases reported by White and associates [64, 93], it can be inferred that the frequency of familial cases of MCNS is also greater than expected. They found that the primary nephrotic syndrome, excluding the Finnish type of congenital nephrosis, which is clearly an autosomal recessive disease, was familial in about 3.5 percent of patients. About one-half of the patients with familial primary nephrotic syndrome had MCNS, in contrast to about four-fifths in all children with the primary nephrotic syndrome. Of the 209 patients with MCNS reported by Habib and Kleinknecht [38], 7 (3.3 percent) had siblings with the nephrotic syndrome, as did 9 of 393 patients (2.3 percent) in the ISKDC [44]. The separate roles of genetic and environmental determinants in the familial nephrotic syndrome remain to be differentiated.

The male-female ratio in the familial cases of MCNS reported by White and associates [64, 93] was 1.7 : 1, similar to, though somewhat lower than, the nonfamilial cases. Familial nephrosis was confined almost exclusively to siblings, with only one documented instance of involvement of more than one generation. The degree of concordance in regard to type of glomerular disease was so high that if MCNS is present in a first affected child, it will almost certainly be present in a sibling subsequently affected.

Norio [66] has analyzed reported data on the occurrence of the primary nephrotic syndrome in twins. He found a relatively large number of monozygotic twins, all concordant, but no definite dizygotic pairs. If similar environmental factors were the main reason that the twins were concordantly affected, the number of affected dizygotic pairs should be twice that of monozygotic pairs, the expected ratio of dizygotic to monozygotic pairs being about 2 : 1. This discrepancy argues against an independent environmental cause and suggests a genetic one. However, if the mechanism of inheritance were simple, the number of familial nontwin relationships relative to the number of twin pairs found would be greater. Norio therefore suggests that the genetic pattern must be polygenic, affecting several siblings only infrequently and monozygotic twins always. Fanconi [28] observed that the onset in siblings often occurs homeochronously.

Etiology

The cause of MCNS remains unknown. An association with preceding streptococcal infection has not been proved temporally, bacteriologically, or serologically. In most children, MCNS develops without evidence of preceding illness, drug ingestion, or exposure to sensitizing agents [9].

An immunologic basis for MCNS has been suggested on the basis of several lines of evidence. Perhaps the most persuasive argument is found in the minority of patients with seasonal relapses that seem to be precipitated by contact with allergens [47]. Although a controlled study has never been done, Thomson et al. [86] have shown that a history of atopy is more common in children with corticosteroid-responsive nephrotic syndrome than in matched control subjects. Strong support for this hypothesis comes from the success of therapeutic agents such as corticosteroids, cyclophosphamide, and nitrogen mustard, which are thought to have antiinflammatory and immunosuppressive actions. Their induction of a remission in MCNS is very difficult to explain on a nonimmunologic basis. The evidence provided by experimental studies [31, 40, 59, 83] also supports the idea of an immunologic basis for MCNS (Chaps. 3, 6).

Immunologic studies of renal biopsy material have, with few exceptions [32, 75], produced negative results [24, 55, 62], and serum complement levels have been normal [92]. These observations argue against the involvement of antigen-antibody complexes and the activation of the complement system in the pathogenesis of MCNS. Ngu et al. [65] also found normal levels of total complement and C3, but they demonstrated an elevation in immunoconglutinin titers. Although the ultimate significance of this finding is unknown, elevations of immunoconglutinin titers presumably reflect ongoing antigen-antibody reactions mediated by the humoral system. Valdez and coworkers [89] demonstrated that an antigen can induce glomerulonephritis in laboratory animals in the absence of demonstrable immune complex deposition in the glomeruli. These observations make tenable the concept that the renal lesion of MCNS could be an immune complex–mediated disease in which the complexes somehow modify the normal glomerular permeability without being deposited in the glomeruli. Thus, the evidence for primary involvement of the humoral immune system is suggestive but contradictory.

There are now data suggesting involvement of the cell-mediated immune system in the pathogenesis of this syndrome. Mallick and associates [58], using a modified leukocyte migration-inhibition test, produced evidence of cell-mediated immunity against renal antigens in 8 of 8 adults with corticosteroid-sensitive MCNS, in most patients with diffuse or focal glomerular lesions, and in one-half with membranous or membranoproliferative changes. Considering the evidence from a different viewpoint, Shalhoub [81] suggested, on the basis of clinical observations, that MCNS may be a systemic disorder of cell-mediated immunity in which episodic or sustained domination of the immune system by a clone of abnormal T cells results in the production of a circulating chemical mediator that is toxic to an immunologically innocent basement membrane. This toxin augments basement membrane permeability to protein, culminating in the nephrotic syndrome. Lagrue and associates [53] support this argument with an in vitro study showing that cultured lymphocytes from patients with MCNS release a factor that has an inflammatory effect and enhances vascular permeability in guinea pig skin.

Giangiacomo and colleagues [33] measured serum immunoglobulins in 37 children with MCNS and compared them with levels in 36 children with nephrotic syndrome secondary to chronic glomerulonephritis. Serum IgG and IgA levels were reduced below normal in both groups of patients. However, serum IgM levels, which were normal in the group with chronic glomerulonephritis, were twice normal before, during, and after remission in patients with MCNS. Low levels of IgG and high levels of IgM suggest that the primary defect in MCNS could consist of a deficiency in the T cell function that mediates conversion of IgM synthesis to IgG synthesis [23].

These isolated bits of experimental and clinical data do not yield a comprehensive explanation of the etiology of MCNS. However, they should stimulate further investigation into the involvement of the cell-mediated system of immunity in the pathogenesis of this disorder.

Clinical and Laboratory Features at Time of Diagnosis

The characteristics of MCNS and the effects of treatment discussed in this and the following section are based on observations made in three separate studies of large numbers of children in whom a histopathologic diagnosis of MCNS was made by renal biopsy. Most of the data are from the *prospective* study of 398 *unselected* and previously *untreated* children observed between 1967 and

1974 in the ISKDC [44]. The second study is that reported by Habib and Kleinknecht [38] on 209 children referred between 1957 and 1967 to the Unité de Recherches sur les Maladies du Métabolisme chez L'enfant in the Hôpital des Enfants-Malades in Paris. The third study is that of White et al. [94] of 66 *unselected* and 45 *referred* patients seen at Guy's Hospital, London, and the Children's Hospital, Birmingham, between 1962 and 1965 (see Table 52-2).

HISTORY

Present History

The first manifestation is usually edema; less often, it is the chance finding of proteinuria [38]. The interval between awareness of the manifestation and the time of diagnosis was less than 2 months in about three-quarters of the patients with MCNS in the ISKDC; it was 4 months or more in less than 10 percent [44]. This interval tends to be longer in children with other glomerular disease, reflecting a more insidious onset. About one-third to one-half of the patients had preceding infections [38, 44]. Less than 10 percent had either an immunization or an allergic reaction prior to the onset [38, 44].

Past History

Less than 20 percent of patients in the ISKDC [44] had a history of classic allergic manifestations. There was a family history of kidney disease or hypertension in about one-third, including 2.3 percent of patients who had a sibling with the nephrotic syndrome, as described under Genetics.

CLINICAL FINDINGS

Age and Sex Distribution

The age at onset in 209 patients whose cases were reported by Habib and Kleinknecht [38] and in 111 reported by White et al. [94] was before the fourth year in 41 and 53 percent respectively. The distribution by age and sex at the time of diagnosis in 398 children with MCNS in the ISKDC is shown in Fig. 53-1. These patients were among a total of 514 with all forms of primary nephrotic syndrome; they ranged in age from 6 months to 16 years [44]. Almost 60 percent of the children with MCNS were from 2 to less than 6 years of age; 12.3 percent were less than 2 years of age; 7.8 percent were from 10 to less than 15 years of age; none was 15 or 16.

The ratios of males to females in the three series ranged from 2.0 : 1 to 2.6 : 1 [38, 44, 94]. It can be seen in Fig. 53-1 that the ratio of males to females in the ISKDC varied with age, but the differences were not significant.

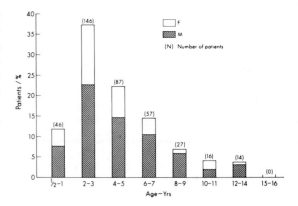

Figure 53-1. Relative frequencies of males and females with MCNS at different ages. (From International Study of Kidney Disease in Children. The nephrotic syndrome in children. Prediction of histopathology from clinical and laboratory characteristics at the time of diagnosis. Kidney Int. 13:43, 1978.)

The age of onset and sex of patients with MCNS beyond the age of 16 years deserve comment [8, 18]. It is of historical interest that until Leiter's 1931 paper, little mention was made of the fact that "nephrosis" was preponderantly a disease of young children. Data on the age of apparent onset in patients with MCNS up to 90 years of age are shown in Fig. 53-2. It would appear that clinical differences between children and adults with the nephrotic syndrome of all forms may be due in large part to differences in the distribution of types of glomerular disease, especially MCNS [39, 63]. However, the fact that the male-

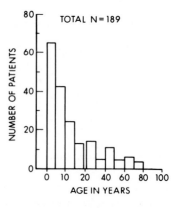

Figure 53-2. Age of onset in MCNS. (From J. S. Cameron et al. Observations on the "Minimal Change" Lesion: Adult Onset Patients and Results of Cyclophosphamide Treatment in Children. In P. Kincaid-Smith, T. H. Mathew, and E. L. Becker [eds.], Glomerulonephritis. New York: Wiley, 1973. Part I, p. 211.)

female ratio in adults with MCNS has been reported to be between 0.9 : 1 and 1.2 : 1 [18], in
contrast to a ratio of over 2 : 1 in children, suggests that there are other determinants. The
change in sex ratio apparently occurs during adolescence, although neither the ISKDC data [44]
nor those reported by Heymann and coworkers
[42] indicate precisely when.

Symptoms
Symptoms are discussed in detail elsewhere
(Chap. 52). The major symptom and often the
only one is *edema*. It is usually the first symptom
to be noted [38] and may become extensive. However, massive edema and the accompanying symptoms are now seen in patients with MCNS only
when treatment is delayed at the onset or when
patients do not respond to corticosteroid therapy.
With current methods of treatment, the clinical
manifestations are due more often to the effects of
corticosteroids than to the disease (see Treatment).

It has been generally believed that children
with MCNS rarely have *hypertension* and that its
presence provides strong evidence of other glomerular disease. It is true that hypertension is less
common in MCNS than in other glomerular diseases, but it is important to know that among 347
children with MCNS observed in the ISKDC
[44], the proportions of children with systolic
and diastolic blood pressures above the 98th percentile for their ages at times of diagnosis were
20.2 and 13.0 percent respectively. Hypertension
was present in 6 and 9 percent, respectively, of patients whose cases were reported by Habib and
Kleinknecht [38] and by White et al. [94]. Data
concerning persistence of hypertension in patients
with MCNS are not available.

LABORATORY FINDINGS
In addition to massive proteinuria and hypoalbuminemia, which define the nephrotic syndrome,
other laboratory findings are important in evaluating a child at the time of diagnosis. The *pathogenesis* of each of these biochemical abnormalities
is discussed elsewhere, as indicated by the cross
references.

Proteinuria
Proteinuria (Chap. 15), is the single most diagnostic clinical laboratory finding in patients with
MCNS. The rate of excretion generally considered
diagnostic is about 1 gm or more per 24 hr; values
of 50 mg/kg/24 hr [38] and 40 mg/hr/m² [1]
have been used to standardize for body size. Children with MCNS in the ISKDC [44] were dis-

tributed almost equally into three groups with
rates of excretion of 40 to 99 mg/hr/m², 100 to
199 mg/hr/m², and equal to or greater than 200
mg/hr/m². Dipstick readings at these rates of excretion are consistently 4 plus.

A highly selective type of proteinuria has been
considered to be characteristic of patients with
MCNS. However, using the method of Cameron
and Blandford [17], highly selective proteinuria
was found in the three series described in only 43
[94], 53 [44], and 75 [38] percent respectively
of patients with MCNS; the proteinuria was
poorly selective (index equal to or greater than
0.2) in 31 of 204 (15.2 percent) patients in
the ISKDC [44] and in 1 of 16 cases reported by
Habib and Kleinknecht [38]. By the method of
Joachim and associates [46], White et al. [94]
found that 47 of 48 patients with MCNS had
highly selective proteinuria. They also found a
high correlation between protein selectivity and
response to corticosteroid therapy. Protein selectivity is discussed further in Chap. 15.

Hypoalbuminemia
Levels of serum albumin used generally to define
the nephrotic syndrome are 2.5 [44, 94] or 3.0
[38] gm or less per deciliter. Severe hypoalbuminemia, with concentrations below 1 gm per
deciliter, occurs in approximately one-fourth [44]
to one-third [38] of patients with MCNS; in
about one-half [38] to two-thirds [44] the concentration is between 1 and 2 gm. (See also
Chap. 52.)

Serum Cholesterol and Total Lipids
An elevation of serum cholesterol and total lipids
(Chap. 52) is almost a constant finding in patients with MCNS, and hyperlipidemia is included
in some of the definitions of nephrosis or idiopathic nephrotic syndrome [78]. The serum
cholesterol exceeded 400 mg per deciliter in approximately two-thirds of patients in the ISKDC;
it was within the normal range in only about 5
percent [44]. Total lipids were increased to values
as high as 4.5 gm per deciliter in 94 percent of
patients whose cases were reported by Habib and
Kleinknecht [38].

Serum Creatinine
The impression is widely held that rates of glomerular filtration in children with MCNS are
within normal limits, and this is generally true.
However, with concentrations of serum creatinine,
corrected for age and sex, used as an estimate of
glomerular filtration rate [79, 80] (see also Chap.
9), one-third of the children in the ISKDC [44]

had values above the 84th percentile (one SD) and one-fourth, above the 98th percentile (two SD) at the time of diagnosis.

White and coworkers [94] found elevated blood urea values before treatment in about 20 percent of children with MCNS. They attributed this evidence of a decrease in glomerular filtration rate to hypovolemia and found that elevated values of blood urea returned to normal following diureses in these children. The results of extensive physiologic studies [10, 67] support this interpretation. Nevertheless, it should be emphasized that evidence of reduced glomerular filtration rate at the time of diagnosis of the nephrotic syndrome cannot be interpreted to mean that the child does not have MCNS. Decreased glomerular filtration rate at the time of diagnosis in children with other glomerular diseases may more often represent a less reversible abnormality.

Hematuria

The absence of hematuria (Chap. 16) is usually considered to be one of the most useful laboratory aids in differentiating between children with MCNS and those with other primary glomerular diseases. However, with rates of urinary excretion of red blood cells greater than 100,000 red cells/hr/m² used as measures of hematuria (Chap. 9), almost *one-fourth of patients with MCNS in the ISKDC [44] had hematuria at the time of diagnosis.* This proportion, taken together with the fact that patients with MCNS represent over four-fifths of all patients with the nephrotic syndrome, accounts for the important finding shown in Fig. 53-3 *that almost 60 percent of patients with the*

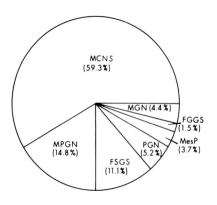

Figure 53-3. Distribution of patients with hematuria by histopathologic diagnosis. For definition of abbreviations see Chap. 52. (From International Study of Kidney Disease in Children. Natural history of the nephrotic syndrome in children. Prediction of histopathology from clinical and laboratory characteristics at the time of diagnosis. Kidney Int. *13:43, 1978.)*

primary nephrotic syndrome who have hematuria at the time of diagnosis have MCNS [44].

Hematuria was present in 13 and 29.1 percent respectively of the patients of White et al. [94] and Habib and Kleinknecht [38]. In the latter series, gross hematuria was exceptional (present in 1.4 percent). Microscopic hematuria, when present, was usually transitory, but was intermittent or persistent in one-third of the patients.

Other Laboratory Findings

Total serum protein is less than 4 gm per deciliter in about one-third of patients [38, 44]. *Serum C3* may very rarely (in 1 percent) be moderately and temporarily reduced [44, 94].

From these clinical and laboratory features of children with MCNS, the typical patient can be described as a boy between 2 and 5 years of age, with edema, massive proteinuria, hypoalbuminemia, and hypercholesterolemia. His blood pressure and serum creatinine are *usually* within normal limits, and hematuria is *usually* absent. The data also show, however, that a clinically significant number of children have, at the time of diagnosis of MCNS, clinical and laboratory findings that are different than those in the usual case. Thus, over one-fourth of children are over 5 years of age, one-third are girls, about one-fifth have hypertension, one-fourth have a reduced glomerular filtration rate (elevated serum creatinine), and between one-fifth and one-fourth have hematuria.

Histopathologic Features

The designation *minimal change* (MC) is used in a histopathologic sense to signify normal or only minimally altered glomerular structure [21]. The emphasis on glomerular morphology stems from the concept that the nephrotic syndrome is primarily a glomerular disease and that tubular, vascular, and interstitial changes are secondary. The histopathologic evaluation of glomeruli involves several crucial judgments, particularly concerning the degrees of mesangial cellularity, mesangial sclerosis, and basement membrane thickening. These judgments are important because the category minimal change permits mild degrees of mesangial hypercellularity, mesangial thickening, and capillary-wall thickening. The inclusion in this category of these histologic variations, which might be regarded as extensions of normal histologic findings, is based on clinicopathologic correlations. Mild thickening of the mesangial stalks and of the capillary walls and basement membranes, for example, carries no implication for corticosteroid unresponsiveness or for an unfavorable prognosis. The significance of mesangial hypercellularity, however, is not entirely settled, since several studies have produced contradictory results. In one investigation, mild mesangial hypercellularity has been reported to be associated with a less-than-favorable response to corticosteroid therapy [45], but in others it has, like the other histologic variations mentioned, been associated with the expected good response [21, 38]. The issue therefore remains in doubt, but additional, carefully controlled data may provide the answer. It must be noted that morphometric studies have shown significantly increased mesangial hypercellularity in MCNS, indicating that the structural abnormality is always present to a greater or lesser degree. More severe hypercellularity would be characterized as proliferative glomerulonephritis, the boundary between it and minimal change being a matter of judgment.

Tubular abnormalities seen in MCNS include protein droplets, lipid accumulation, focal calcification, and disruption by extruded casts. Lipid droplets are small and infrequent early in the course of the disease, the time at which most biopsy sections are taken; massive intratubular accumulation of lipid, described previously in tissue from patients with long-standing active disease, accounts for the earlier designation *lipoid nephrosis*. The tubules may be small and lined by flattened epithelium; occasional tubules are atrophic, with thickened basement membranes. Interstitial and vascular lesions include mild fibrosis, focal mononuclear cell infiltration, and arteriolar hyalinization. Tubular and stromal abnormalities have not been associated with an altered pattern of initial corticosteroid responsiveness in MCNS.

Even when the general glomerular morphology corresponds to minimal change nephrotic syndrome, the presence of focal segmental sclerosis and hyalinosis portends a statistically poor response to corticosteroid therapy and an ultimately poor prognosis. These alterations in their early stages involve only a portion of the glomerular tuft, and their presence even in a single glomerulus is of diagnostic significance. Such cases are no longer categorized as minimal change nephrotic syndrome, but as examples of focal segmental glomerulosclerosis. The presence in renal biopsy specimens of a few totally obsolete glomeruli in children or in adults carries no implication for either treatment or prognosis.

Despite the lack of obvious histologic abnormalities in MCNS, electron microscopy has shown, as in all types of the nephrotic syndrome, swelling and fusion of the foot processes of glomerular epithelial cells [70]. Experimental studies have demonstrated the association of foot-process fusion with proteinuria. The severity of fusion in clinical material is, however, variable and frequently incomplete and unevenly distributed (Fig. 53-4). The degree of fusion and the severity of proteinuria therefore seem to be only partially correlated, and it must be noted that fusion is commonly seen in biopsy sections from nonproteinuric patients, perhaps as an artifact of the biopsy procedure. Current concepts, based on experimental data, hold these changes to be secondary to proteinuria, but the changes in the foot processes have also been interpreted as reflections of a primary epithelial abnormality in which cellular maintenance of the basement membrane is impaired.

Electron-microscopic studies in MCNS have also shown variable thickening of the basement membrane, which is frequently wrinkled or corrugated at its mesangial reflection. Mesangial thickening by increased amounts of extracellular matrix is also seen in long-standing nephrotic syndrome and may be indistinguishable from the early changes of segmental sclerosis.

Differential Diagnosis

The nephrotic syndrome is a clinical state that is defined arbitrarily, and consequently its diagnosis is unequivocal. Important differential diagnoses do have to be made, however, between the several primary and secondary glomerular diseases in which the nephrotic syndrome occurs. This subject is discussed extensively in Chap. 52, in which a formula derived from a multivariate analysis is presented and applied to the differential diagnosis of the primary nephrotic syndromes. It is emphasized there that *if the presence of MCNS in a child with the nephrotic syndrome could be predicted accurately, a renal biopsy would not be recommended at time of diagnosis.*

The occurrence of frequent relapses in a child thought to have MCNS is not considered an indication for biopsy, since frequent relapses are seen rarely, if ever, in children with other glomerular diseases. However, a biopsy is indicated in a child with clinical manifestations of MCNS who fails to respond to an initial intensive course of corticosteroids, since most initial nonresponders have some other glomerular disease (see Chap. 52).

Treatment

The *general treatment* of patients with MCNS must include recommendations about diet and activity, control of edema, and psychological support of patients and their families. These measures are discussed elsewhere (Chap. 52), together with treatment of the important complications of

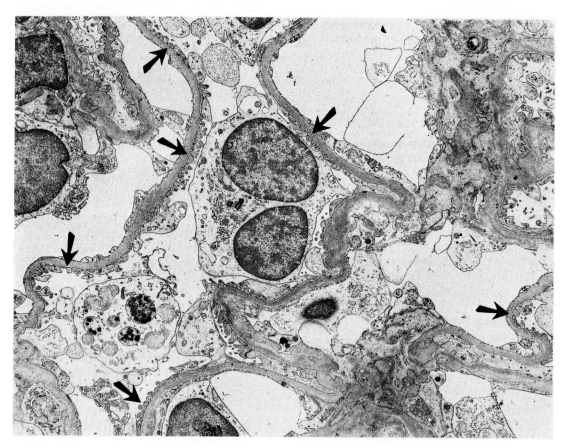

Figure 53-4. Minimal change nephrotic syndrome in a 17-year-old with a 2-year history of disease. The 24-hr excretion of protein was 4.8 gm. She had no diminution of renal function, and her creatinine clearance was 133 ml per minute. Electron microscopy shows swelling of glomerular podocytes with only partial obliteration of foot processes. The foot processes in many areas are swollen (arrows), but fusion is both irregular and incomplete. (×5,440.)

the nephrotic syndrome, including infections, growth retardation, and hypercoagulability.

Specific treatment refers to the use of therapeutic agents that are believed to have a beneficial effect on the underlying glomerular disease. It was shown for the first time in 1950 that two classes of immunosuppressive agents may exert such effects. Farnsworth [29] reported both clinical and biochemical improvement in patients treated with ACTH. Similar results were reported by Luetscher and Deming [56] for cortisone and by Chasis and colleagues [19] for nitrogen mustard. The initial improvement was followed in most patients by recurrences of the signs and symptoms of the disease. Lange, in 1951 [54], and Kramer et al., in 1952 [51], were the first authors to suggest that the initial improvement could be prolonged by continuing treatment in the nonedematous child.

Since 1952, many different regimens with several immunosuppressive agents have been suggested, and these have been reviewed extensively

[15, 16, 35, 91]. The discussion here will be concerned with certain basic principles of specific therapy that have emerged from those studies, and regimens that have had extensive clinical use or are currently being tested in controlled therapeutic trials will be described.

The following general principles of specific treatment are generally accepted at present:

1. Specific treatment should be given as soon as the diagnosis of MCNS is made [41].
2. The initial treatment should be with an intensive course of a corticosteroid.
3. Prednisone appears to be the agent used most commonly, and there is no firm evidence for greater effectiveness of any other agent, including ACTH, which has the disadvantage of requiring parenteral administration.
4. Some form of less intensive "maintenance" treatment with corticosteroids should be given for not less than 1 or 2 months to children

whose edema and proteinuria disappear during initial treatment.

5. The urine should be tested frequently, and treatment with corticosteroids should be reinstituted promptly if proteinuria recurs and persists.

6. Cytotoxic agents should not be used either initially or in patients with recurrences that respond readily to corticosteroids. They should be reserved for patients in whom serious side effects of corticosteroids develop or for those who fail to respond, remain edematous, and are at risk of serious complications (especially, severe infections) from the treatment or the disease.

RECOMMENDED REGIMENS

In this section and in the one following, the terminology used to describe patients' responses to corticosteroids corresponds to that used in the ISKDC [44] (Table 53-1). The definitions of nonrelapsers, late responders, and continuing nonresponders in the following discussions are based on a follow-up period of 10 months from the beginning of corticosteroid treatment.

Initial Treatment

Initial treatment in the ISKDC [7, 44] has been with daily prednisone for 4 weeks followed by in-

Table 53-1. Terminology Used to Describe Response of Patients with MCNS to Treatment with Prednisone

Initial responder   Response[a] during 8 weeks of initial treatment

Nonrelapser   A responder who has no relapses[b]

Infrequent relapser   A responder who relapses but who has less than two relapses within 6 months of the initial response

Frequent relapser   A responder who has two relapses within 6 months of the initial response

Subsequent nonresponder   A responder who fails to respond during treatment of a relapse

Initial nonresponder   No response during 8 weeks of initial treatment

Late responder   Initial nonresponder who responds at some time following the initial 8 weeks of treatment

Continuing nonresponder   Initial nonresponder who does not respond to subsequent or continuing treatment

[a] Protein-free urine (4 mg or less per hour per square meter; negative or trace dipstick) on at least 3 consecutive days within 7 days.

[b] Protein-positive urine (more than 4 mg per hour per square meter; 1+ or greater on dipstick) on at least 3 consecutive examinations on 3 separate days within 7 days.

Table 53-2. Recommended Dosages of Agents Used in the Treatment of Patients with MCNS

Prednisone [44]

Daily: 60 mg/m^2/day in 3 divided doses

Intermittent: 40 mg/m^2/day in three divided doses given on 3 consecutive days out of 7

Alternate-day: 35 mg/m^2 in a single dose given every other day [13].

Cyclophosphamide [60]

2–3 mg/kg/day for no longer than 8 weeks and given with intermittent corticosteroids

Chlorambucil [35, 36]

Starting dosage of 0.1 to 0.2 mg/kg/day in divided doses given with alternate-day corticosteroids; chlorambucil dosage increased weekly until WBC falls, then discontinued abruptly; prednisone continued until WBC stabilized above 5,000, then is gradually discontinued.

Nitrogen Mustard [30, 91]

0.1 mg/kg/day for 4 consecutive days; prednisone, 60 mg/m^2/day for 5 days before and 2 weeks after nitrogen mustard; prednisone then decreased by 20 mg/m^2/week

termittent treatment for 4 weeks (Table 53-2). If a response occurs during the 4 weeks of intermittent treatment, it is continued for 4 weeks from the time of the response.

About 93 percent of patients with MCNS in the ISKDC [44] responded during the initial treatment, with approximately 90 percent doing so during the first 4 weeks of daily treatment (Fig. 53-5). There was little, if any, evidence of

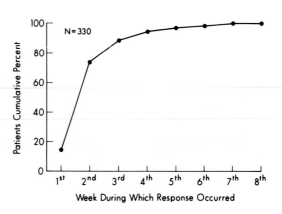

Figure 53-5. Time of response of patients with MCNS to initial treatment with prednisone. (From International Study of Kidney Disease in Children. The nephrotic syndrome in children. Prediction of histopathology from clinical and laboratory characteristics at the time of diagnosis. Kidney Int. *13:43, 1978.)*

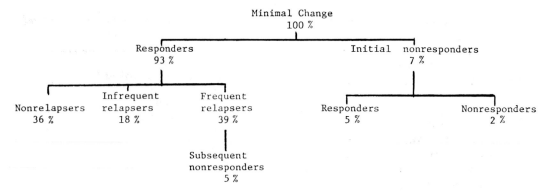

Figure 53-6. Response at 10 months of patients with MCNS treated initially with prednisone. About half of the subsequent nonresponders become nonresponders during a first relapse within 6 months of their initial response. They were therefore potential relapsers rather than actual frequent relapsers. (From International Study of Kidney Disease in Children. The nephrotic syndrome in children. Prediction of histopathology from clinical and laboratory characteristics at the time of diagnosis. Kidney Int. 13:43, 1978.)

harmful corticosteroid toxicity with this regimen, which appears, therefore, to be satisfactory. However, as shown in Fig. 53-6, within 6 months of the initial response, 39 percent of the responders in the ISKDC became frequent relapsers, and of these, 5 percent became subsequent nonresponders [7]. Repeated treatment of these patients with prednisone subsequently places many of them at risk of serious corticosteroid toxicity. Thus, the requirement for improved initial treatment is not so much to increase the proportion of responders or to decrease initial corticosteroid toxicity, but rather to reduce the proportion of patients who become frequent relapsers and subsequent nonresponders. We know no way at present of accomplishing this goal. More intensive initial treatment with prednisone or the use of a cytotoxic agent initially might be considered. More than one-half of the responders have no relapses or relapse infrequently, however, and they would be exposed unnecessarily to the potentially toxic effects of these more intensive regimens.

As shown in Table 53-3, a large proportion of patients who had their first relapse within 6 months of the initial response became frequent relapsers within 6 months of the initial response, and over 90 percent of frequent relapsers had subsequent relapses. These data permit identification early in the course of treatment of a group of patients among whom a very high proportion will become frequent relapsers. This high-risk group might benefit from more intensive initial treatment with corticosteroids or from the use of other agents, but until more effective initial treatment of MCNS is demonstrated by an adequate clinical trial, *we continue to recommend the treatment described at the beginning of the section.*

Treatment of Relapses in Infrequent Relapsers

About 20 [44] to 30 percent [38] of patients who respond to initial treatment are infrequent relapsers. Relapses in these patients are treated with daily prednisone until they respond, and with intermittent therapy thereafter for 4 weeks. If the relapse is recognized and treated within a few days after proteinuria reappears, recurrence of edema is usually prevented, and since most of these patients respond within the first 2 weeks of daily treatment, corticosteroid toxicity is minimal or absent. In this group, therefore, *the prednisone treatment described is considered to be relatively satisfactory and is recommended.*

Treatment of Nonresponders

In the series of White et al. [94] and in the ISKDC [44], 2 and 7 percent of patients repec-

Table 53-3. Proportion of 266 Responders Who Become Frequent Relapsers in Relation to Time of Initial Response

Interval After Initial Response	First (N)	Relapses Within 6 Months			
		Second (Frequent Relapsers)		Subsequent Relapsers Among Frequent Relapsers	
		Number	Percent	Number	Percent
1–3	120	103	85.8	95	92.2
3–6	51	19	37.3	17	89.4
Total	171	122	71.3	112	91.8

Source: International Study of Kidney Disease in Children. To be published.

tively were *initial nonresponders* in contrast with 39 percent in Habib and Kleinknecht's series [38]. These discrepant results cannot be readily explained. There is an unsubstantiated clinical impression that patients who receive intensive initial treatment with corticosteroids may respond more consistently than those treated less intensively. Patients treated initially elsewhere and referred subsequently to a pediatric nephrology center are less certain to have received intensive initial corticosteroid therapy than are unselected patients in a systematic study. Differences in the proportion of initial responders among unselected and referred patients may be related, at least in part, to these differences in initial treatment.

About 60 percent of initial nonresponders have partial remissions with disappearance of the nephrotic syndrome but persistence of proteinuria [38, 44]. Although only 5 of 41 such patients (12.2 percent) in Habib and Kleinknecht's [38] series responded later, 9 of 10 (90 percent) in the ISKDC [44] responded over periods ranging from 1 week to 4 months. The role of the treatment in these late responders becomes increasingly uncertain as the period lengthens; however, *we recommend that intermittent or alternate-day treatment be continued,* at least in initial nonresponders who have only persistent proteinuria.

In about 40 percent of initial nonresponders, edema and its accompanying symptoms persist despite corticosteroid and antibiotic therapy [38, 44]; these present difficult therapeutic problems. Among 29 such patients whose cases were reported by Habib and Kleinknecht [38], only 1 eventually had a remission. However, 3 of 6 in the ISKDC [44] responded over periods of 2 to 8 months.

Other forms of treatment may need to be considered, especially if the patients begin to have serious infections, such as peritonitis, or complications of treatment. In a randomized trial by the ISKDC [43] the proportion of all initial nonresponders who responded subsequently was not different in those who received cyclophosphamide (5 of 7) than in those who received prednisone alone (4 of 7); however, the time of response was significantly shortened in the former (a mean of 38.4 days versus a mean of 95.5 days). It is therefore recommended, that in early nonresponders with MCNS who are considered to be at risk of serious complications, cyclophosphamide or some other cytotoxic agent be considered. It has been reported recently [30] that *nitrogen mustard* may provide an effective treatment with minimal toxicity in these patients.

The presence of active infection, often unrec-ognized, appears to be responsible for failure to respond in some patients. Diagnosis and treatment of these infections may result in response.

Treatment of Subsequent Nonresponders

Subsequent nonresponders appear to be primarily, if not exclusively, patients with MCNS. Of 10 such patients whose cases were reported by Tranin and his associates [87], 8 became nonresponders during a relapse that occurred within 6 months of their initial response, and this occurred in 15 patients in the ISKDC [44]. Thus, these patients were either actual or potential frequent relapsers. It appears that most subsequent nonresponders are either actual or potential frequent relapsers and that nonresponders among infrequent relapsers are probably very rare.

The problems of treatment of subsequent nonresponders are similar to those of initial nonresponders, although those who previously have had frequent relapses are more likely to have serious toxic corticosteroid reactions and to be candidates for treatment with cytotoxic agents.

Treatment of Frequent Relapsers

Between 40 and 50 percent of responders with MCNS become frequent relapsers (Table 53-4). Preventing or minimizing frequent relapses is at present the most pressing unsolved therapeutic need in children with MCNS.

A therapeutic trial of more intensive prednisone treatment for a relapse occurring within 2 to 6 months of the initial response is being conducted by the ISKDC [44], since these patients are at such high risk of becoming frequent relapsers. The results of this trial are not yet known.

Most attempts to treat frequent relapsers more effectively have utilized cytotoxic agents, including azathioprine [1], cyclophosphamide [11, 12, 20, 43, 60, 69, 88] chlorambucil [35, 36], and nitrogen mustard [90]. A critical review of these studies, only a few of which have been ade-

Table 53-4. Frequent Relapsers Among Responders with MCNS

Series	Number of Responders	Frequent Relapsers Number	Percent
Habib [38]	111	55	50.0
White et al. [94]	93	41	44.1
ISKDC [44]	287	120*	41.8

* Includes 15 subsequent nonresponders who were actual or potential frequent relapsers.

quately controlled [1, 11, 12, 20, 35, 36, 43, 60], provided the recommendations that follow.

Prednisone. Maintenance with prednisone is very ineffective in preventing subsequent relapses in patients who have become frequent relapsers. In two reports, one using intermittent prednisone for 180 days [43] and the other alternate-day [20] prednisone for 4 months, the relapse rates were 88.5 and 90.9 respectively, and the relapses per patient per year over periods of approximately 2 years averaged 3.6 and 2.5 respectively. In a controlled trial comparing alternate and intermittent prednisone in frequent relapsers, the multicenter Central European Group [13] found significantly fewer relapses during a 6-month period of treatment in patients given alternate day prednisone (0.75 relapses per patient) than in those given intermittent steroids (1.96 relapses per patient). However, relapse rates during the 6-month period following withdrawal of corticosteroids were almost identical in the two groups (2.80 and 2.83 relapses per patient) and similar to those during the 2-year follow-up in the other studies reported [20, 43].

Continued daily treatment with prednisone is unsatisfactory and exposes the patients to serious corticosteroid toxicity.

Azathioprine. From a controlled clinical trial conducted by the ISKDC [1], it was concluded that azathioprine should not be given to frequent relapsers with MCNS, since its advantages over prednisone, if any, do not warrant exposing children with MCNS to the potential toxicity of azathioprine.

Cyclophosphamide. There is now firm evidence from many studies, some of which were well controlled [11, 12, 20, 43, 60, 69, 88], that cyclophosphamide is effective both in reducing the proportion of frequent relapsers who continue to relapse and in increasing the interval between relapses in patients in whom they do occur. Thus, in two well-controlled trials [20, 43] the proportion of patients who relapsed during a period of almost 2 years after treatment with cyclophosphamide was less than 50 percent compared with about 90 percent in control patients given only prednisone. The relapses per patient per year were reduced from an average of about 3 to between 1 and 2.

In addition to its greater effectiveness, the lowering or absence of corticosteroid toxicity gives cyclophosphamide a great advantage over prednisone in the treatment of frequent relapsers. Cyclophosphamide cannot, however, be considered a completely effective treatment for frequent relapsers. First, almost one-half the patients treated

continue to have relapses even though the interval between them is lengthened in most [20, 43]. Second—and more important—there are a number of side effects, some of which are not readily controlled or assessed. The major short-term side effects are leukopenia, alopecia, hemorrhagic cystitis, anorexia, abdominal pain, nausea, and vomiting. A study of the effect of dosage on toxicity [60] showed that with a daily dosage of 2.5 mg per kilogram for 90 days, severe alopecia did not occur, and the gastrointestinal and genitourinary complaints were almost eliminated, *especially when the drug was given with a meal followed by a large intake of fluid.* However, lymphopenia (1,000 or less lymphocytes per cubic millimeter) was still common with this regimen, and serious leukopenia (2,000 or less leukocytes per cubic millimeter) was not eliminated.

The most disturbing toxic effect of cyclophosphamide, however, especially in young patients with a good long-term prognosis, is the effect on gonadal function. It is now well established that diminished spermatogenesis and menstrual disturbances occur in adult patients receiving prolonged cyclophosphamide therapy [26, 27, 52, 71]. It has been shown also that cyclophosphamide may affect gonadal function in prepubertal boys, [2, 34, 72], although the relationship between dosage and degree of gonadal toxicity has not been defined. The results of several studies suggest that daily dosages of 2 to 3 mg per kilogram for no more than 8 weeks in prepubertal boys may not damage the germinal epithelium, and even longer periods of treatment may be safe for prepubertal girls [27, 68]. Caution should be used in accepting these dose relationships, however, since oligospermia has been reported in 2 prepubertal boys treated with 2 to 3 mg/kg/day for only 2-week and 8-week intervals [68]. It has been suggested that for further investigation of this problem, testing for luteinizing hormone releasing factor may provide a means of identifying the patient who has sustained testicular injury and may require testicular biopsy [48]. The long-term effects of cyclophosphamide on ovulation and on female fertility also need to be clarified.

It is difficult at present to make a firm recommendation about treating frequent relapsers with cyclophosphamide. If the degree of corticosteroid toxicity is not considered dangerous to the patient, it is probably wise to continue treating relapsers with prednisone as described under Treatment of Relapses in Infrequent Relapsers. If the degree of corticosteroid toxicity is believed to be unacceptable, some form of cytotoxic therapy should be considered. The elimination or significant reversal of corticosteroid-induced growth retardation, obesity, and psychological impairment by a single course of treatment with a cytotoxic agent has persuaded many clinicians to use it without waiting for more serious side reactions from corticosteroids, such as osteoporosis and impending vertebral collapse. On the other hand, inducing permanent azoospermia in a boy with a good ultimate prognosis is a serious matter. The factors involved should be discussed thoroughly with parents and older children, who will have to decide whether to accept or reject the physician's recommendation.

Chlorambucil. Chlorambucil has been reported by Gruppe and his associates [36] to be completely effective in preventing subsequent relapses over periods from 18 to 30 months in a randomized controlled trial in 21 children with either corticosteroid-dependent or frequently relapsing nephrotic syndrome, presumably MCNS. Although they observed minimal complications, Kleinknecht and coworkers [49], from their experience in treating 250 children with various nephropathies over a period of 10 years, reported severe long-term adverse effects, including testicular injury in prepubertal boys. They also observed acute leukemia in 2 children, renal carcinoma in 1, and 4 children who died of viral infections. On the basis of their experience, and until other patients have been followed longer, chlorambucil cannot be recommended in these patients.

Nitrogen Mustard. The beneficial effects of nitrogen mustard (mechlorethamine NH-2), were reported first by Chasis and coworkers [19]. In 1958, West [90] reported that in children with pure lipoid nephrosis (probably MCNS), the addition of nitrogen mustard at the end of a course of corticotropin, or of corticosteroid followed by corticotropin, resulted in remissions of greater duration than those observed after hormone therapy alone. Although there are no recent reports of the use of nitrogen mustard in frequent relapsers, its apparent effectiveness reported in nonresponders [30] suggests that it might be more effective and less toxic than cyclophosphamide in the treatment of frequent relapsers.

Prognosis

Before effective antibiotic treatment was available, about two-thirds of all children with the nephrotic syndrome died; with effective antimicrobial therapy, about two-thirds survived. Since the widespread use of corticosteroids, the survival rate has increased to about 75 percent [5, 14, 22, 61, 73]. These findings are from reports of children in whom the diagnosis of the nephrotic syndrome was made before a renal biopsy enabled diagnosis of the underlying glomerular diseases. The survival rate of approximately 75 percent with the use of both antibiotics and corticosteroids is similar to the proportion of children with the nephrotic syndrome who have MCNS, and it is likely that most of the deaths during this period were in children with other glomerular diseases. The duration of active disease among those who recovered was between 2 and 3 years on the average [6, 61].

It appears now that patients with MCNS rarely progress to chronic renal failure, at least during the first 10 years of their disease (Table 53-5). Among 95 patients followed for 4 to 7 years at Guy's Hospital in London and at the Children's Hospital in Birmingham, there were 4 deaths (4.2 percent), only 1 of which was due to renal insufficiency (1.1 percent); the other 3 were due to complications of treatment or intercurrent infections [94]. Among 209 patients followed by Habib and Kleinknecht [38] for 1 to 10 years, there were 14 deaths (6.7 percent); only 3 were due to chronic renal insufficiency (1.4 percent), and they occurred after 5, 6, and 8 years. The other 11 deaths were secondary to intercurrent complications, including 2 each to thrombosis of the pulmonary arteries, diarrhea with malnutrition and severe metabolic disorders, acute adrenal failure, and unknown causes, and 1 each due to measles pneumonia, van Bogaert encephalitis, and pneumococcal meningitis.

Among 399 patients observed prospectively in the ISKDC for periods of 3 to 10 years [44], there were 9 deaths (2.3 percent), 1 of which was due to renal insufficiency (0.3 percent); 6 were due to intercurrent infection, 1 to cerebral sinus thrombosis, and 1 to congestive heart failure occurring as a complication of therapy. The death due to renal insufficiency was in a child who had MCNS on the initial biopsy, who was a nonre-

Table 53-5. Deaths in Children with MCNS

		Deaths			
	Number of	Total		Renal	
Series	Patients	N	%	N	%
Habib and Kleinknecht [38]	209	14	6.7	3	1.4
White et al. [94]	95	4	4.2	1	1.1
ISKDC [44]	399	9	2.3	1	0.3
Total	613	27	4.4	5	0.8

Table 53-6. Course of MCNS Between 1 and 15 Years After Onset

Series	Number of Patients	Follow-up (years)	Complete Remission						Persistent Proteinuria or Active Disease		Deaths	
			Treatment Withdrawn		With Treatment		Total					
			No.	%	No.	%	No.	%	No.	%	No.	%
Habib and Kleinknecht [38]	209[a]	1–10	130[b]	62.2[b]	18	8.6	148	70.8	47	22.5	14	6.7
Siegel and Associates [82]	51[c]	5–15	25	49[d]	13	25.5	38	74.5	9	17.6	4	7.8

[a] Histopathologic diagnosis of MCNS.
[b] Of these 130, 80 (61.5%) were in complete remission for more than 2 years.
[c] Patients with relapsing course, probably MCNS.
[d] All in complete remission for more than 2 consecutive years.

sponder, and who at autopsy was found to be one of the two children in the series of 399 who had an initial histologic diagnosis of MCNS and was later shown to have FSGS (see Chap. 55).

Although the proportion of children with MCNS in whom progressive renal failure develops is less than 1 percent, it needs to be emphasized that over 4 percent of patients treated in nephrology centers in these three studies died [38, 44, 94], and that most of the deaths were preventable. Early recognition and prompt treatment of potentially fatal intercurrent infections and of iatrogenic complications, should nearly eliminate mortality in this disease.

The status of patients during the first 8 months with current treatment has been described (Recommended Regimens). The status from 1 to 15 years after the onset in two series in which patients were known [38] or thought very likely [82] to have MCNS is shown in Table 53-6. Neither of these series was prospective, and it is possible that results may be somewhat better in patients treated systematically with intensive corticosteroid therapy at the onset of their disease (see Treatment of Nonresponders). Follow-up of patients in the ISKDC [44] will provide such data. It appears, however, that between 1 and 15 years after onset, roughly three-fourths of patients with MCNS will be in remission, about 20 percent will continue to have active disease, about 4 percent will have died of nonrenal causes, and about 1 percent will have died of renal failure or require chronic hemodialysis or transplantation (Table 53-6).

There are several other reports on the status of patients with the nephrotic syndrome during this period of 1 to 15 years after the onset [39, 57, 63]. Although patients with MCNS cannot be identified as such in these reports, the results appear to be similar to those described here.

The more distant prognosis of children with MCNS is difficult to assess [22, 50]. Kohn and Obrinsky [50] reported observations made over a period of 26 years on 57 children with "lipid nephrosis." Data on the course of the disease in most of these children, including a mortality of 63 percent, are no longer pertinent, since 33 were treated before antibiotics were introduced, none received corticosteroids, and the nature of their glomerular disease was not known. The course of 12 patients followed 10 to 26 years however, is of interest. With the exception of 1 patient with progressive renal disease, all these patients were leading normal lives. Of the remaining 11, 7 had albuminuria and 2 had hypertension. From the case histories and summaries given for the 12 patients, it seems likely that they all had MCNS. From these admittedly scanty data and from the experience of many physicians who have followed individual patients for periods of 25 years or longer, there seems to be little question that complete and lasting recovery of patients with MCNS occurs. However, until data on long-term follow-up of patients with histologically proved MCNS treated by current methods are available, predictions about the distant prognosis are tenuous.

References

1. Abramowicz, M., Barnett, H. L., Edelmann, C. M., Jr., Griefer, I., Kobayashi, O., Arneil, G. C., Barron, B. A., Gordillo, G., Hallman, N., and Tiddens, H. A. Controlled trial of azathioprine in children with ne-

phrotic syndrome. A report of the International Study of Kidney Disease in Children. *Lancet*, 2:959, 1970.

2. Arneil, G. C. Cyclophosphamide and the pubertal testis. *Lancet* 2:1259, 1972.

3. Arneil, G. C. Management of the Nephrotic Syndrome in the Child. In E. Lieberman, (ed.), *Clinical Pediatric Nephrology*. Philadelphia and Toronto: Lippincott, 1976. Chap. 9, p. 146.

4. Arneil, G. C., Dewhurst, C. J., Houston, I. B., and Winberg, J. Disorders of the Urogenital System. In J. O. Forfar and G. C. Arneil (eds.), *Textbook of Pediatrics*. Edinburgh and London: Churchill Livingstone, 1973.

5. Arneil, G. C., and Lam, C. N. Long-term assessment of steroid therapy in childhood nephrosis. *Lancet*, 2:819, 1966.

6. Barnett, H. L. Nephrosis in children. *Mo. Med.* 56:772, 1956.

7. Barnett, H. L. The Natural and Treatment History of Glomerular Diseases in Children—What Can We Learn from International Cooperative Studies? A report of the International Study of Kidney Disease in Children. In *Proceedings of the Sixth International Congress of Nephrology*. Basel: Karger, 1976. Pp. 470–485.

8. Barnett, H. L., and Eder, H. A. The nephrotic syndrome. *J. Chronic Dis.* 5:108, 1957.

9. Barnett, H. L., Forman, C. W., and Lauson, H. D. The Nephrotic Syndrome in Children. In S. Z. Levine (ed.), *Advances in Pediatrics*. Chicago: Year Book, 1952. Vol. 5.

10. Barnett, H. L., Forman, C. W., McNamara, H., McCrory, W., Rapport, M., Michie, A. J., and Barbero, G. The effect of adrenocorticotrophic hormone on children with the nephrotic syndrome. II. Physiologic observations on discrete kidney functions and plasma volume. *J. Clin. Invest.* 20:227, 1951.

11. Barratt, T. M., Osofsky, S. G., Bercowsky, A., Soothill, J. F., and Kay, R. Cyclophosphamide treatment in steroid-sensitive nephrotic syndrome of childhood. *Lancet* 1:55, 1975.

12. Barratt, T. M., and Soothill, J. F. Controlled trial of cyclophosphamide in steroid-sensitive relapsing nephrotic syndrome of childhood. *Lancet* 2:479, 1970.

13. Brodehl, J. Unpublished data, personal communication, 1977.

14. Brown, R. B., Burke, E. C., and Stickler, G. B. Studies in nephrotic syndrome. I. Survival of 135 children with nephrotic syndrome treated with adrenal steroids. *Mayo Clin. Proc.* 40:384, 1965.

15. Cameron, J. S. Immunosuppressant agents in the treatment of glomerulonephritis: Part I. Corticosteroid drugs. *J. R. Coll. Physicians (London)* 5:282, 1971.

16. Cameron, J. S. Immunosuppressant agents in the treatment of glomerulonephritis: Part II. Cytotoxic drugs. *J. R. Coll. Physicians (London)* 5:301, 1971.

17. Cameron, J. S., and Blandford, G. The simple assessment of selectivity in heavy proteinuria. *Lancet*, 2:242, 1966.

18. Cameron, J. S., Turner, D. R., Ogg, C. S., Sharpstone, P., and Brown, C. B. The nephrotic syndrome in adults with minimal change glomerular lesions. *Q. J. Med.* 171:461, 1974.

19. Chasis, H., Goldring, W., and Baldwin, D. S. The effect of nitrogen mustard on renal manifestations of human glomerulo-nephritis. *J. Clin. Invest.* 29:804, 1950.

20. Chiu, J., McLain, P. N., and Drummond, K. N. A controlled prospective study of cyclophosphamide in relapsing, corticosteroid-responsive, minimal-lesion nephrotic syndrome in childhood. *J. Pediatr.* 82:607, 1973.

21. Churg, J., Habib, R., and White, R. H. R. Pathology of the nephrotic syndrome in children. A report for the International Study of Kidney Disease in Children. *Lancet* 1:1299, 1970.

22. Cornfeld, D., and Schwartz, M. W. Nephrosis: A long-term study of children treated with corticosteroids. *J. Pediatr.* 68:507, 1966.

23. Davie, J. M., and Paul, W. E. Role of T lymphocytes in the humoral immune response. *J. Immunol.* 113:89, 1974.

24. Drummond, K. N., Michael, A. F., Good, R. A., and Vernier, R. L. The nephrotic syndrome: Immunologic, clinical and pathologic correlations. *J. Clin. Invest.* 45:620, 1966.

25. Edelmann, C. M., Jr. The Idiopathic Nephrotic Syndrome of Childhood. In H. L. Barnett (ed.), *Pediatrics* (15th ed). New York: Appleton-Century-Crofts, 1972. Chap. 22, p. 1499.

26. Etteldorf, J. N., West, C. D., Pitcock, J. A., and Williams, D. L. Gonadal function, testicular histology, and meiosis following cyclophosphamide therapy in patients with the nephrotic syndrome. *J. Pediatr.* 88:206, 1976.

27. Fairley, K. F., Barrie, J. V., and Johnson, W. Sterility and testicular atrophy related to cyclophosphamide therapy. *Lancet* 1:568, 1972.

28. Fanconi, G., Konsmine, C., and Frischknecht, W. Die konstitutionelle Bereitschaft Zum Nephrosesyndrom. *Helv. Paediatr. Acta* 6:199, 1951.

29. Farnsworth, E. B. Studies on Influence of Adrenocorticotrophin in Acute Nephritis, in Simple Nephrosis, and in Nephrosis with Azotemia. In J. R. Mote (ed.), *Proceedings of the First Clinical ACTH Conference*. Philadelphia: Blakiston, 1950.

30. Fine, B. P., Munoz, A. R., Uy, C. S., and Ty, A. Nitrogen mustard therapy in children with nephrotic syndrome unresponsive to corticosteroid therapy. *J. Pediatr.* 89:1014, 1976.

31. Fouts, P. J., Corcoran, A. C., and Page, I. H. Observations on the clinical and functional course of nephrotoxic nephritis in dogs. *Am. J. Med. Sci.* 201:313, 1941.

32. Gerber, M. A., and Paronetto, F. IgE in glomeruli of patients with nephrotic syndrome. *Lancet* 1:1097, 1971.

33. Giangiacomo, J., Cleary, T. G., Cole, B. R., Hoffsten, P., and Robson, A. M. Serum immunoglobulins in the nephrotic syndrome. *N. Engl. J. Med.* 294:8, 1975.

34. Greifer, I., and Barnett, H. L. International workshop on risk-benefit assessment of cyclophosphamide in renal disease. *Kidney Int.* 2:352, 1972.

35. Grupe, W. E. Chlorambucil in steroid-dependent nephrotic syndrome. *J. Pediatr.* 82:598, 1973.

36. Grupe, W. E., Makker, S. P., and Ingelfinger, J. R. Chlorambucil treatment of frequently relapsing nephrotic syndrome. *N. Engl. J. Med.* 295:746, 1976.

37. Habib, R. The Nephrotic Syndrome. In P. Royer, R. Habib, H. Mathieu, and M. Broyer (eds.), *Pediatric Nephrology*. Philadelphia: Saunders, 1974. Part III, p. 258.

38. Habib, R., and Kleinknecht, C. The Primary Nephrotic Syndrome of Childhood. Classification and

Clinicopathologic Study of 406 Cases. In S. C. Sommers (ed.), *Pathology Annual*. New York: Appleton-Century-Crofts, 1971.

39. Hayslett, J. P., Kashgarian, M., Bensch, K. G., Spargo, B. H., Freedman, L. R., and Epstein, F. H. Clinicopathologic correlations in the nephrotic syndrome due to primary renal disease. *Medicine (Baltimore)* 52:93, 1973.

40. Heymann, W., Hackel, D. B., Harwood, S., Wilson, S. G., and Hunter, J. E. Production of nephrotic syndrome in rats by Freund's adjuvants *Exp. Biol. Med.* 100:660, 1959.

41. Heymann, W., and Hunter, J. L. Importance of early treatment of the nephrotic syndrome. *J.A.M.A.* 175:563, 1961.

42. Heymann, W., Makker, S. P., and Post, R. S. The preponderance of males in the idiopathic nephrotic syndrome of childhood. *Pediatrics* 50:814, 1972.

43. International Study of Kidney Disease in Children. Prospective, controlled trial of cyclophosphamide therapy in children with the nephrotic syndromes. *Lancet* 1:423, 1974.

44. International Study of Kidney Disease in Children. The nephrotic syndrome in children. Prediction of histopathology from clinical and laboratory characteristics at the time of diagnosis. *Kidney Int.* 13:43, 1978.

45. Jao, W., Lewy, P., Norris, S. H., Pollak, V. E., and Pirani, C. L. Lipoid Nephrosis: A Reassessment. In P. Kincaid-Smith, T. H. Mathew, and E. L. Becker (eds.), *Glomerulonephritis*. New York: Wiley, 1973. Part I, p. 183.

46. Joachim, G. R., Cameron, J. S., Schwartz, M., and Becker, E. L. Selectivity of protein excretion in patients with the nephrotic syndrome. *J. Clin. Invest.* 43:2332, 1964.

47. Kark, R. M., Pirani, C. L., Pollak, V. E., Muercke, R. C., and Blainey, J. D. The nephrotic syndrome in adults: A common disorder with many causes. *Ann. Intern. Med.* 49:751, 1958.

48. Kirkland, R. T., Bongiovanni, A. M., Cornfeld, D., McCormick, J. B., Parks, J. S., and Tenore, A. Gonadotropin responses to luteinizing releasing factor in boys treated with cyclophosphamide for nephrotic syndrome. *J. Pediatr.* 89:941, 1976.

49. Kleinknecht, D., Guesvy, P., Lenoir, G., and Broyer, M. High-cost benefit of chlorambucil in frequently relapsing nephrosis (letter to editor). *N. Engl. J. Med.* 296:48, 1977.

50. Kohn, J. L., and Obrinsky, W. Lipid nephrosis in children. Observations over a period of 26 years. *Am. J. Dis. Child.* 84:587, 1952.

51. Kramer, B., Goldman, H., and Cason, L. The treatment of the non-edematous nephrotic child with ACTH. *J. Pediatr.* 41:792, 1952.

52. Kumar, R., Biggart, J. D., and McEvoy, J. Cyclophosphamide and reproductive function. *Lancet* 1:1212, 1972.

53. Lagrue, G., Xheneumont, S., Branellec, A., and Weil, B. Lymphokines and nephrotic syndrome. *Lancet* 1:271, 1975.

54. Lange, K. Experimental Nephritis. In J. Metcoff (ed.), *Proceedings of the Third Annual Conference on the Nephrotic Syndrome*. New York: National Nephrosis Foundation Inc., 1951. Vol. 3, p. 16.

55. Lewis, E. J., and Kallen, R. J. Glomerular localisation of IgE in lipoid nephrosis. *Lancet* 1:1395, 1973.

56. Luetscher, J. A., Jr., and Deming, Q. B. Treatment

of nephrosis with cortisone. *J. Clin. Invest.* 29:1576, 1950.

57. Makker, S. P., and Heymann, W. The idiopathic nephrotic syndrome of childhood. *Am. J. Dis. Child.* 127:830, 1974.

58. Mallick, N. P., McFarlane, H., Taylor, G., Williams, R. J., Orr, W., and Williams, G. Cell-mediated immunity in nephrotic syndrome. *Lancet* 1:507, 1972.

59. Masugi, M. Uber die Experimentelle Glomerulonephritis durch das spezifische Antinierenserum. *Beitr. Pathol. Anat. Allg. Pathol.* 92:429, 1934.

60. McCrory, W. W., Shibuya, M., Lu, W.-H., and Lewy, J. E. Therapeutic and toxic effects observed with different dosage programs of cyclophosphamide in treatment of steroid-responsive, but frequently relapsing nephrotic syndrome. *J. Pediatr.* 82:614, 1973.

61. McDonald, J., Murphy, A. V., and Arneil, G. C. Long-term assessment of cyclophosphamide therapy for nephrosis in children. *Lancet* 2:980, 1974.

62. Michael, A. F., McLean, R. H., Roy, L. P., Westberg, N. G., and Vernier, R. L. Immunologic aspects of the nephrotic syndrome. *Kidney Int.* 3:105, 1973.

63. Miller, R. B., Harrington, J. T., Ramos, C. P., Relman, A. S., and Schwartz, W. B. Long-term results of steroid therapy in adults with idiopathic nephrotic syndrome. *Am. J. Med.* 46:919, 1969.

64. Moncrieff, M. W., White, R. H. R., Glasgow, E. F., Winterborn, M. H., Cameron, J. S., and Ogg, C. S. The familial nephrotic syndrome: II. A clinicopathological study. *Clin. Nephrol.* 1:220, 1973.

65. Ngu, J. L., Barratt, T. M., and Soothill, J. F. Immunoconglutinin and complement changes in steroid sensitive relapsing nephrotic syndrome of children. *Clin. Exp. Immunol.* 6:109, 1970.

66. Norio, R. The nephrotic syndrome and heredity. *Hum. Hered.* 19:113, 1969.

67. Oliver, W. J., and Owings, C. L. Sodium excretion in the nephrotic syndrome. Relation to serum albumin concentration, glomerular filtration rate, and aldosterone excretion rate. *Am. J. Dis. Child.* 113:352, 1967.

68. Pennisi, A. J., Grushkin, C. M., and Lieberman, E. Gonadal function in children with nephrosis treated with cyclophosphamide. *Am. J. Dis. Child.* 129:315, 1975.

69. Pennisi, A. J., Grushkin, C. M., and Lieberman, E. Cyclophosphamide in the treatment of idiopathic nephrotic syndrome. *Pediatrics* 57:948, 1976.

70. Powell, H. R. Relationship between proteinuria and epithelial cell changes in minimal lesion glomerulopathy. *Nephron* 16:310, 1976.

71. Qureshi, M. S. A., Goldsmith, H. J., and Pennington, J. H. Cyclophosphamide therapy and sterility. *Lancet* 2:1290, 1972.

72. Rapola, J., Koskimies, O., and Huttunen, N. P. Cyclophosphamide and the pubertal testis. *Lancet* 1:98, 1973.

73. Riley, C. M., and Scaglione, P. R. Current management of nephrosis. *Pediatrics* 23:561, 1959.

74. Rothenberg, M. B., and Heymann, W. The incidence of the nephrotic syndrome in children. *Pediatrics* 19:446, 1957.

75. Roy, L. P., Westberg, N. G., and Michael, A. F. Nephrotic syndrome—no evidence for a role for IgE. *Clin. Exp. Immunol.* 13:553, 1973.

76. Rubin, M. I. Nephrotic Syndrome. In M. I. Rubin (ed.), *Pediatric Nephrology*. Baltimore: Williams & Wilkins, 1975. Chap. 19, p. 454.

77. Schlesinger, E. R., Sultz, H. A., Misher, W. E., and

Feldman, J. G. The nephrotic syndrome. Its incidence and implications for the community. *Am. J. Dis. Child.* 116:623, 1968.

78. Schreiner, G. E. The Nephrotic Syndrome. In M. B. Strauss and L. G. Welt (eds.), *Diseases of the Kidney* (2nd ed.). Boston: Little, Brown, 1971.

79. Schwartz, G. J., Haycock, G. B., Edelmann, C. M., Jr., and Spitzer, A. A simple estimate of glomerular filtration rate in children derived from body length and plasma creatinine. *Pediatrics* 58:259, 1976.

80. Schwartz, G. J., Haycock, G. B., and Spitzer, A. Plasma creatinine and urea concentration in children: Normal values for age and sex. *J. Pediatr.* 88:828, 1976.

81. Shalhoub, R. J. Pathogenesis of lipoid nephrosis: A disorder of T-cell function. *Lancet* 2:556, 1974.

82. Siegel, N. J., Goldberg, B., Krassner, L. S., and Hayslett, J. P. Long-term follow-up of children with steroid-responsive nephrotic syndrome. *J. Pediatr.* 81:251, 1972.

83. Smadel, J. E., and Farr, L. E. Experimental nephritis in rats induced by injection of anti-kidney serum. II. Clinical and functional studies. *J. Exp. Med.* 65:527, 1937.

84. Smith, H. W. *The Kidney: Structure and Function in Health and Disease.* New York: Oxford University Press, 1951.

85. Sultz, H. A., Schlesinger, E. R., Misher, W. E., and Feldman, J. G. *Long-Term Childhood Illness.* Pittsburgh: University of Pittsburgh Press, 1972.

86. Thomson, P. D., Stokes, C. R., Barratt, T. M., Turner, M. W., and Soothill, J. F. HLA antigens and atopic features in steroid-responsive nephrotic syndrome of childhood. *Lancet* 2:765, 1976.

87. Tranin, E. B., Boichis, H., Spitzer, A., Edelmann, C. M., Jr., and Greifer, I. Late nonresponsiveness to steroids in children with the nephrotic syndrome. *J. Pediatr.* 87:519, 1975.

88. Tsao, Y. C., and Yeung, C. H. Paired trial of cyclophosphamide and prednisone in children with nephrosis. *Arch. Dis. Child.* 46:327, 1971.

89. Valdez, A. J., Germuth, F. G., and Rodriguez, E. Fatal immune complex glomerulonephritis without deposits. *Fed. Proc.* 34:878, 1975.

90. West, C. D. Use of combined hormone and mechlorethamine (nitrogen mustard) therapy in lipoid nephrosis. *Am. J. Dis. Child.* 95:498, 1958.

91. West, C. D. Alkylating Agents in the Treatment of Nephrotic Syndrome. In P. Kincaid-Smith, T. H. Mathew, and E. L. Becker (eds.), *Glomerulonephritis.* New York: Wiley, 1973. Part I, p. 199.

92. West, C. D., Northway, J. D., and Davis, N. C. Serum levels of β_1C globulin, a complement component, in nephritis, lipoid nephrosis, and other conditions. *J. Clin. Invest.* 32:1507, 1964.

93. White, R. H. R. The familial nephrotic syndrome. I.A. European survey. *Clin. Nephrol.* 1:215, 1973.

94. White, R. H. R., Glasgow, E. F., and Mills, R. J. Clinicopathologic study of nephrotic syndrome in childhood. *Lancet* 1:1353, 1970.

54. Congenital Nephrotic Syndrome

Niilo Hallman
and Juhani Rapola

Definition and Classification

Nephrotic syndrome is a common condition of childhood that rarely presents before the age of 1 year. In several large series, only a small proportion of the children were under 1 year of age. *Congenital nephrotic syndrome* (CN) clinically is similar to childhood nephrotic syndrome, but it is present at birth. The appearance of the signs of the fully developed syndrome, including proteinuria, hypoproteinemia, and edema, may, however, be delayed for some days or even for a few months after birth. Because it is often difficult to decide whether the disease is truly congenital or whether it develops later, many authors include all nephrotic patients presenting during the first year of life in the category of CN. Several series and case reports of the nephrotic syndrome occurring in infancy thus represent heterogeneous populations of diseases. We shall try to separate from this group of infantile nephrotics those that are truly congenital.

Nephrotic syndrome presenting after birth or during the first months of life is either idiopathic or secondary to some known causative factor (Table 54-1). In this discussion, we are dealing only with the congenital nephrotic syndrome, principally of Finnish type (CNF). Some of the exogenous factors listed in Table 54-1 are well established as causes of the nephrotic syndrome in infants, but the causal relationships in the rare cases of CN that are associated with renal vein thrombosis or many of the infectious diseases require further clarification. The CN caused by syphilis provides a unique example of an immune complex type of glomerulonephritis in the newborn [4, 6, 36]. It is the most important of the CNs of known cause for two reasons: first, in a population with a high incidence of syphilis, most

Research presented in this chapter has been supported by the Sigrid Jusélius Foundation and Foundation of Pediatric Research, Helsinki, Finland.

Table 54-1. Etiologic Classification of Infantile Nephrotic Syndrome

---

Idiopathic
  Congenital nephrotic syndrome of Finnish type (CNF) [15]
  Other types of congenital and infantile nephrotic syndrome [3, 11, 14, 37]
Secondary
  Infections: syphilis, toxoplasmosis, cytomegalic inclusion disease, other [5, 8, 26, 34, 37]
  Heavy metal (mercurial) poisoning [37]
  Renal venous thrombosis [1]
  Renal tumor [39]
  Other

---

patients with CN belong to this group [26]; and second, highly effective specific treatment for it is available, which is not the case for most other types of the CN.

Congenital Nephrotic Syndrome, Finnish Type

GENETICS AND EPIDEMIOLOGY

The Finnish type of congenital nephrotic syndrome is inherited as an autosomal recessive disease [27, 28]. Reports of typical cases in various ethnic groups and races have been published all over the world. The incidence of the disease, however, is highest in Finland, particularly in certain areas where population isolates were formed in the past. The CNF gene frequency for the whole country has been calculated to be 1 : 200. The incidence of the disease in Finland is 10 to 12.5 per 10^5 live births.

Habib and Bois [11] have collected the largest series of carefully analyzed patients with different types of infantile nephrotic syndrome. Their 37 cases included 11 of typical CNF, a ratio that may indicate the relative incidence of CNF in infantile nephrosis outside Finland.

The pathogenesis of CNF is not known, but the most likely hypothesis is that it is the result of an inborn error of metabolism that leads to a faulty structure of glomerular basal lamina. As a result, abnormally large amounts of plasma protein can cross the glomerular barrier.

The heterozygotes for CNF gene are healthy, and we have not been able to confirm the observation that they excrete more basement membrane–like products into the urine than do control subjects [20, 22]. The disease is often diagnosed at birth, and there are no sex differences. No exogenous factors precipitating the disease have been found.

CLINICAL MANIFESTATIONS

Several nonspecific but almost constant pathologic features are found in the obstetric and perinatal histories of the patients. The placenta is always larger than normal [14, 18]; in our series it averaged 40 percent of the birth weight of the child and only exceptionally less than 25 percent. The large placenta is the most important early sign of the disease. The course of the pregnancy is usually normal, but almost 90 percent of the children are born about 4 weeks before term. Consequently, the birth weight in most children is less than 3,000 gm.

Signs of fetal asphyxia (meconium-stained amniotic fluid and a low Apgar score) are found in three-quarters of the patients. During the first days of life, paleness, marmorization of the skin, and breathing difficulties are very common. It is evident that some of these children die during the neonatal period without CNF having been diagnosed. High perinatal mortality has been recorded in some families having affected children. As a further evidence of intrauterine anoxia and birth asphyxia, high hemoglobin values, erythroblasts, and increased amounts of reticulocytes have been found in the newborn patients. Later, the children consistently are anemic.

The newborn baby typically has a small, low-bridged nose and wide sutures of the skull, without increased intracranial pressure. These are probably the result of retarded bone formation. The feet are often in a talipes calcaneus position, apparently owing to the muscular weakness.

The main signs of nephrosis, edema, abdominal distention, or both, are present at birth in 25 percent of children [18]. They appear in an additional 25 percent during the first week of life. In our patients the edema has always been found by the end of the first 3 months. It is often extensive at about 2 weeks, with the simultaneous presence of ascites. Even in the absence of edema the laboratory findings indicate the changes of the nephrotic syndrome. In our patients, proteinuria has been detected consistently in the first urine sample studied, usually right after birth. The protein fractions of amniotic fluid and urine have been found to be identical, indicating intrauterine proteinuria [24]. Further evidence of this has been obtained by a recent observation on a therapeutically aborted 20-week fetus who showed a highly increased amount of protein in the bladder urine. Later, the CNF patients have a characteristic appearance. In addition to the edematous legs, the abdomen is distended by ascitic fluid, and the peripheral veins on the abdomen are clearly visible. The patients do not thrive and remain in very poor general condition. The weight and height hardly increase. The face remains infantile, and bone age is severely retarded. The teeth develop slowly, with abnormal enamel.

Motor development is very poor. The patients are bedridden; none of them has ever learned to sit without support or reached any further milestone of normal infantile motor development. Mental development, too, is retarded. Some patients apparently learn to recognize their mother, but none has ever learned to speak. The general retardation of development may be due, however, to the extremely severe somatic disease and lack of protein rather than to some inherent abnormality in the central nervous system.

The patients are very susceptible to infections, pneumonia and gastroenteritis being the most common. During gastroenteritic periods the edema often disappears. In general, the edema is less prominent in older infants than at the beginning of the clinical disease. The older infants are dystrophic, with extensively distended abdomens.

In our experience the disease is consistently fatal. The increased mortality is already present during the perinatal period; only about 25 percent of the patients reach the age of 1 year, and 3 percent live up to the age of 2 years; our record is 3 years and 10 months (Fig. 54-1). The immediate cause of death often is infection, but in many cases the actual mechanism of death has remained unclear [18]. None of the patients has died in uremia.

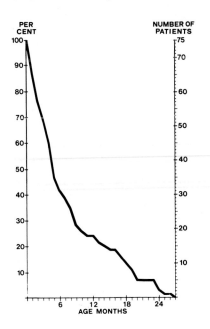

Figure 54-1. Survival curve of 75 CNF patients from 1965–1973 [19].

CLINICAL PATHOLOGIC FEATURES
The laboratory findings in CNF do not differ from those of nephrotic syndrome in general. The amount of protein in the urine is usually very large, varying from 4 to 13 gm per liter, usually increasing with the age of the patient [13]. Proteinuria is, in general, highly selective, but in some patients low selectivity, as judged by the ratio of orosomucoid (mw 44,100) to IgG (mw 160,000), has been found [21]. Microscopic hematuria and a slightly increased number of urinary leukocytes are common. Slight generalized aminoaciduria and glucosuria are also frequent findings, due to renal tubular atrophy. Renal insufficiency is not a feature of the disease, but in patients surviving the longest, blood urea nitrogen shows a tendency to increase.

The total amount of serum protein is always low; mean values are 3.0 to 3.5 gm per deciliter. The protein profile in the cord blood is typical of the nephrotic syndrome. The albumin is always low, and the alpha globulin fraction is high, owing to the large amount of alpha-2-macroglobulin. The IgG fraction of gamma globulin is low, whereas IgM is high, especially in the long-lasting cases. The protein content of ascitic fluid is variable and may be as high as 1 gm per deciliter. Serum cholesterol and total lipids are increased in the newborn and increase further during the course of the disease. In interpreting the cholesterol values, one has to remember the low values of healthy infants. Levels of serum electrolytes, particularly potassium and calcium, are low. The ionized fraction of calcium, however, is normal.

RENAL PATHOLOGIC FEATURES
Gross Examination
At autopsy, the kidneys of CNF patients appear pale, smooth surfaced, and slightly softer and larger than in control children of a corresponding age. The mean kidney weight, relative to body weight, is almost twice that of control children [31].

Light Microscopy
Pathologic changes are limited to the cortex, and the medulla appears spared. Rare findings of medullary lesions in autopsied patients can always be attributed to secondary causes, such as thrombosis or pyelonephritis.

The most characteristic lesion of the CNF kidney is the dilatation of the tubules. Although this lesion is very common, it cannot be considered as a sine qua non for the diagnosis of the CNF, as it sometimes is presented in the literature [12]. On the other hand, all infantile nephropathies with cystic tubular dilatations [29] do not belong to the same etiopathogenetic group. In patients in whom dilatation is minimal, the abnormality typically is found in the tubules of the deep cortex (Fig. 54-2). They seem to spread radially from the deep to the outer cortex, and the proximal tubules are primarily involved. In the full-blown disease, the whole cortex appears cystic, and distal tubules are also involved (Fig. 54-3). In the early phase of tubular dilatation the epithelium is tall and edematous, and the apical parts of the cells appear rounded. Ghostlike cell particles are common in the lumen. Along with the increase of the size of the cysts, the epithelium becomes flat and atrophic. The epithelial atrophy is progressive with age, as evidenced on repeated biopsies. The cystic tubular dilatation reaches a maximal inner diameter of about 0.5 mm.

The microdissection studies of CNF kidneys in our laboratory [30] and elsewhere [7, 9, 37] have confirmed the tubular alterations seen in the his-

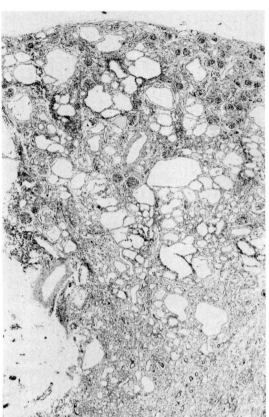

Figure 54-3. Renal cortex of an 8-month-old CNF patient. Note that several microcysts involve the whole cortex. Atrophic epithelium can be seen. (H&E, ×60.)

tologic sections. Paatela [30] reported that the proximal tubules are primarily involved, showing wide dilatation and irregularities in shape and size. In some cases, small saclike dilatations were also detected in the distal tubule, whereas the loop of Henle was normal.

The glomeruli display progressive changes. In young patients the abnormalities are very subtle, but three basic types of altered glomeruli are present in varying proportions. Glomeruli that resemble the immature glomerulus, with small shrunken capillary tufts, covered by a continuous layer of visceral epithelial cells, and surrounded by a cystic urinary space, are most frequent in the youngest age group. They differ from the normally developing glomeruli of the premature newborn by their larger size, owing to the cystic urinary space, and by their presence deeper in the cortex.

Mesangial cell proliferation is a typical feature of mature glomeruli (Fig. 54-4). It is relatively mild in some patients, but comparison with age-matched control subjects showed significantly in-

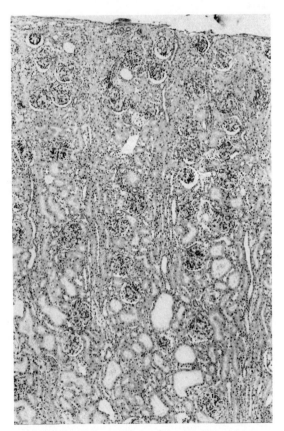

Figure 54-2. Renal cortex of a 3-month-old CNF patient. Ectatic tubuli with relatively high epithelium are seen mainly deep in the cortex. (H&E, ×110.)

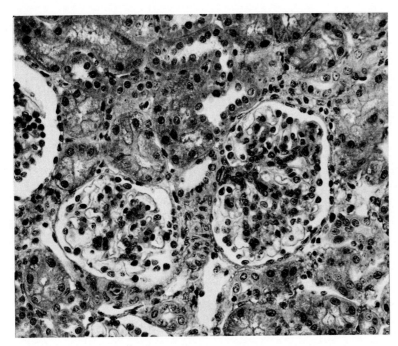

Figure 54-4. Two glomeruli showing mesangial cell proliferation, but open peripheral capillaries. (H&E, ×250.)

creased mesangial cellularity in all age groups [31]. The mesangial hypercellularity is accompanied by an increase of PAS-positive and silver-positive mesangial matrix, but it does not lead to the narrowing of the peripheral capillaries; on the contrary, the capillaries often are very wide, almost ectatic. Periglomerular, concentric, onion-like fibrosis leading to the complete obstruction and finally hyalinization of the glomerulus becomes evident in the latter part of the first year (Fig. 54-5). In the rare patients who live longer than 1.5 years, up to one-half the glomeruli may be totally hyalinized.

Like the tubular and glomerular changes, the amount of interstitial tissue and the number of inflammatory cells show progression with age. In infants under 6 months of age the changes are either absent or minimal and focal. By the age of 1 year, the changes are always present and later become very marked. The inflammatory cells are mainly lymphocytes and plasma cells. Polymorphonuclear leukocytes are usually rare, and histiocytes are not very prominent. In the oldest patients, true lymphoid follicles with germinal centers are formed. At this stage, glomerular hyalinization, tubular atrophy, and interstitial scarring with inflammatory cells are very similar to any type of end-stage nephritis.

From the individual pathologic changes of the

CNF at different stages, the following general pattern emerges. In patients up to 2 to 3 months of age the histologic picture may be near normal. One has to look carefully for tubular dilatation near the medullary border. Immature-looking glomeruli may occur in excess, but the mesangial hypercellularity is sometimes very slight. The classic picture of the CNF kidney consists in microcystic tubular dilatation and glomerular mesangial hypercellularity. It may be present at any age, but most often is encountered in patients several months of age. Finally, advanced glomerular sclerosis and chronic interstitial inflammation with scarring is typical in patients approaching the age of 2 years.

In our experience with CNF we have not observed the glomerular lesions associated with the corticosteroid-resistant forms of nephrosis seen in older children, such as membranous glomerulonephropathy, membranoproliferative glomerulonephritis, focal sclerosis, or fibroepithelial crescents of Bowman's capsule (see Chap. 52).

Immunofluorescence Studies

Contrary to the early reports of positive findings for gamma globulin and complement fractions in the CNF [23–25], more recent studies have proved negative [2, 10, 17, 32]. We have recently studied 11 biopsy specimens from CNF patients

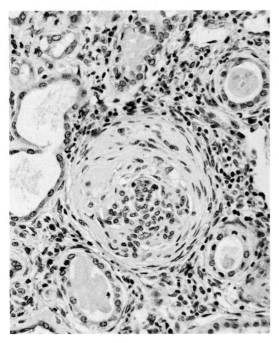

Figure 54-5. Peripheral onion skin–like fibrosis leading to the obstruction of a glomerulus. (H&E, ×250.)

for the presence of IgG, IgM, IgA, and C3 complement, with negative results.

Electron-microscopic Studies

By electron microscopy, visceral epithelial cells in well-spared mature glomeruli show swollen cytoplasm with numerous clear vesicles. The foot processes are usually fused, and the basal membrane is covered by a thin layer of epithelial cytoplasm. Microvillous projections of the epithelial cells are often abundant. The basal membrane is usually thin; endothelial cells are usually normal. Mesangial hypercellularity is conspicuous, and the cells are embedded in a matrix composed of convoluted pieces of basement membrane–like material. Dense deposits that are typically associated with the basal membrane or mesangium in the immune complex type of glomerulonephritis have not been encountered. Except for the mesangial changes, the fine structure of glomeruli in CNF is thus essentially the same as in minimal change nephrosis.

In partially sclerosed glomeruli the capillary lumina become narrowed through the wrinkling and the collapse of the basal membranes and through the hyperplasia of the endothelial and mesangial cells. Occasional fibrin deposits are also present in the capillaries and mesangium of the sclerosed glomeruli.

In the early phase of the proximal tubular dila-

tation the tubular cells are tall and contain more and larger dark cytosomes than do normal tubules. Large cytoplasmic fragments appear to lie free in the lumen of the tubules. This hyperplastic phase is gradually followed by atrophy of the cells. Their cytoplasm is diminished, and microvilli are irregular and finally almost disappear. The scanty cytoplasm contains numerous residual dense bodies. The change from initial hypertrophy to final atrophy is probably the result of the heavy protein load on the absorptive cells, ending in functional and structural exhaustion.

TREATMENT

Treatment of the Finnish type of congenital nephrotic syndrome is symptomatic. The response to cortisone therapy is very poor. The same is true of the response to cyclophosphamide and other antimetabolites. Kidney transplantation can be tried if the child attains sufficient size. Before transplantation, both kidneys have to be removed and peritoneal dialysis performed in order to normalize blood chemistry, including proteins and lipids. If this is not done, the risk of thrombosis is great. So far, all our attempts have failed, but all the patients have weighed less than 5 kg at the time of operation. However, Hoyer et al. [16] have published one report of a patient with CNF, in whom successful transplantation was performed at the age of 5 years.

Examination of amniotic fluid early in pregnancy has shown elevated concentration of alpha fetoprotein [35]. With this method it is now possible to detect affected fetuses and to terminate the pregnancy before 20 weeks gestation.

Other Types of Congenital and Infantile Idiopathic Nephrotic Syndrome

These diseases are rare in infants. They vary in the age at which the clinical manifestations appear and in the course of the disease, the clinical and renal pathologic features, and prognosis. Some cases have proved to be familial, but in others this has not been shown [28].

A specific type of infantile nephrotic syndrome, which in young infants may be confused with CNF, deserves a short description. Habib and Bois [11] described 6 cases and named the entity *diffuse mesangial sclerosis* (DMS) on the basis of the characteristic histologic lesions. We have personal experience with 1 similar case, and it is very likely that other cases published under different titles also belong to this category [33, 38]. Abnormalities in the gestation, birth weight, or placenta have not been recorded in DMS. The involvement of siblings in two of five families in the series of Habib and Bois [11] is compatible with recessive inheritance. The time of onset of proteinuria and edema ranges from the first week of life to as late as the eleventh month, but the cases with early onset are those easily confused with the CNF. After a variable period, during which the nephrotic syndrome is the primary clinical feature, uremia develops, and the patients die in renal insufficiency. Therapy has been ineffective. The age at death has varied from 10 to 36 months.

On histologic examination the glomeruli are seen to be affected in a uniform manner. The capillary tuft appears somewhat contracted and is often lined with a layer of epithelial cells. Consequently, the urinary space often appears wider than normal. The capillaries are obstructed, and patent capillaries are difficult to find. The main cause of the glomerular obsolescence seems to be a diffuse increase of mesangial PAS-positive and silver-positive fibrils protruding into the capillaries. The number of glomerular cells is not increased, although the contraction of the tuft may give this impression. The tubules are atrophic and often show dilatation. Hyaline casts in the tubules are frequent. Marked interstitial fibrosis with some inflammatory cells is an additional feature.

Based on the histologic classification of the infantile nephrotic syndrome, Habib and Bois [11] found 17 patients who showed either minimal glomerular lesions or focal glomerular sclerosis. These changes were by all histologic criteria similar to those of corresponding nephrotic patients of older ages. Three additional patients with typical membranous nephropathy associated with the onset of the nephrotic syndrome in the latter part of the first year were presented. It is thus possible that, rarely, the same types of glomerular disease that are responsible for the nephrotic syndrome in older children may present in infancy.

The clinical and morphologic variations in the remaining cases of the infantile nephrotic syndrome are so great that classification is not feasible. A later onset and a milder course compared with CNF and DMS have frequently been reported [13]. Corticosteroid therapy may sometimes be effective in these patients.

References

1. Alexander, F., and Campbell, A. B. Congenital nephrotic syndrome and renal vein thrombosis in infancy. *J. Clin. Pathol.* 24:27, 1971.
2. Bach, C., Schaeffer, P., Tixier, J.-L., and Bach, J. F. Une observation de syndrome néphrotique congénital. Etude immunologique. *Ann. Pediatr.* 16:756, 1969.
3. Bouton, J. M., and Coulter, J. B. S. The nephrotic syndrome of infancy. *Acta Paediatr. Scand.* 63:769, 1974.
4. Braunstein, G. D., Lewis, E. J., Galvanek, E. G., Hamilton, A., and Bell, W. R. The nephrotic syndrome associated with secondary syphilis: An immune deposit disease. *Am. J. Med.* 48:643, 1970.
5. DeLuca, G., Delendi, N., and D'Andrea, S. Un raro caso di nefrosi congenita e malattia da inclusioni citomegaliche. *Nota I. Minerva Pediatr.* 16:1164, 1964.
6. Falls, W. F., Ford, K. L., Aschworth, C. T., and Carter, N. W. The nephrotic syndrome in secondary syphilis. *Ann. Intern. Med.* 63:1047, 1965.
7. Fetterman, G. H., and Feldman, J. D. Congenital anomalies of renal tubules in a case of "infantile nephrosis." *Am. J. Dis. Child.* 100:319, 1960.
8. Flatz, G. Nephrotisches Syndrom und Pyknocytose bei einem jungen Säugling. *Monatsschr. Kinderheilkd.* 112:102, 1964.
9. Giles, H. McC., Pugh, R. C. B., Darmady, E. M., Stranack, F., and Woolf, L. I. The nephrotic syndrome in early infancy: A report of three cases. *Arch. Dis. Child.* 32:167, 1957.
10. Griswold, W., and McIntosh, R. M. Immunological studies in congenital nephrosis. *J. Med. Genet.* 9:245, 1972.
11. Habib, R., and Bois, E. Hétérogénéité des syndromes néphrotiques à debut précoce du nourrisson (syndrome néphrotique "infantile"). *Helv. Paediatr. Acta* 28:91, 1973.
12. Habib, R., and Kleinknecht, C. The Primary Nephrotic Syndrome of Childhood. Classification and Clinicopathologic Study of 406 Cases. In S. C. Sommers (ed.), *Pathology Annual.* New York: Appleton-Century-Crofts, 1971. Pp. 417–474.
13. Hallman, N., Hjelt, L., and Ahvenainen, K. Nephrotic syndrome in newborn and young infants. *Ann. Paediatr. Fenn.* 2, 227, 1956.
14. Hallman, N., Norio, R., Kouvalainen, K., Vilska, J., and Kojo, N. Das kongenitale Syndrom. *Ergeb. Inn. Med. Kinderheilkd.* 30:3, 1970.
15. Hallman, N., Norio, R., and Rapola, J. Congenital nephrotic syndrome. *Nephron* 11:101, 1973.
16. Hoyer, J. R., Kjellstrand, C. M., Simmons, R. L., Najarian, J. S., Mauer, S. M., Buselmeier, T. J., Michael, A. F., and Vernier, R. L. Successful renal transplantation in 3 children with congenital nephrotic syndrome. *Lancet* 1:1410, 1973.
17. Hoyer, J. R., Michael, A. F., Jr., Good, R. A., and Vernier, R. L. The nephrotic syndrome of infancy: Clinical, morphologic, and immunologic studies of four infants. *Pediatrics* 40:233, 1967.
18. Huttunen, N. P. Congenital nephrotic syndrome of Finnish type: Study of 75 patients. *Arch. Dis. Child.* 51:344, 1976.
19. Huttunen, N. P. Unpublished data, 1975.
20. Huttunen, N. P., Hallman, N., and Rapola, J. Glomerular basement membrane antigens in congenital and acquired nephrotic syndrome in childhood. *Nephron* 16:401, 1976.
21. Huttunen, N. P., Savilahti, E., and Rapola, J. Selectivity of proteinuria in congenital nephrotic syndrome of Finnish type. *Kidney Int.* 8:255, 1976.
22. Kniker, T. W., and Sweeney, M. J. Increased urinary basement membrane—like products (BMP) in infants with congenital nephrosis (CN) and their healthy relatives. *Clin. Res.* 20:115, 1972.
23. Kobayashi, N. An immunohistochemical study on

renal biopsies in children. *Arch. Dis. Child.* 41:477, 1966.

24. Kouvalainen, K.   Immunological features in the congenital nephrotic syndrome. A clinical and experimental study. *Ann. Paediatr. Fenn.* [Suppl. 22] 9:1, 1963.

25. Lange, K., Wachstein, M., Wasserman, E., Alptekin, F., and Slobody, L. B.   The congenital nephrotic syndrome. *Am. J. Dis. Child.* 105:338, 1963.

26. McDonald, R., Wiggelinkhuizen, J., and Kaschula, R. O. C.   The nephrotic syndrome in very young infants. *Am. J. Dis. Child.* 122:507, 1971.

27. Norio, R.   Heredity in the congenital nephrotic syndrome: A genetic study of 57 Finnish families with a review of reported cases. *Ann. Paediatr. Fenn.* [Suppl. 27] 12:1, 1966.

28. Norio, R.   The nephrotic syndrome and heredity. *Hum. Hered.* 19:113, 1969.

29. Oliver, T.   Microcystic renal disease and its relation to "infantile nephrosis." *Am. J. Dis. Child.* 100:312, 1960.

30. Paatela, M.   Renal microdissection in infants with special reference to the congenital nephrotic syndrome. *Ann. Paediatr. Fenn.* [Suppl. 21], 9:1, 1963.

31. Rapola, J., Huttunen, N. P., and Savilahti, E.   Unpublished data, 1975.

32. Rapola, J., and Savilahti, E.   Immunofluorescent and morphological studies in congenital nephrotic syndrome. *Acta paediatr. Scand.* 60:253, 1971.

33. Rossenbeck, H. G., Margraf, O., and Hofmann, D.   Über das infantile nephrotische Syndrom bei kongenitalen Glomerulonephritis. *Dtsch. Med. Wochenschr.* 91:348, 1966.

34. Scully, J. P., and Yamazaki, J. N.   Congenital syphilitic nephrosis successfully treated with penicillin. *Am. J. Dis. Child.* 77:652, 1949.

35. Seppälä, M., Aula, P., Rapola, J., Karjalainen, O., Huttunen, N.-P., and Ruoslahti, E.   Congenital nephrotic syndrome: Prenatal diagnosis and genetic counseling by estimation of amniotic-fluid and maternal serum alpha-fetoprotein. *Lancet* 2:123, 1976.

36. Wiggelinkhuizen, J., Kaschula, R. O. C., Uys, C. J., Kuijten, R. H., and Dale, J.   Congenital syphilis and glomerulonephritis with evidence for immune pathogenesis. *Arch. Dis. Child.* 48:375, 1973.

37. Worthen, H. G., Vernier, R. L., and Good, R. A.   Infantile nephrosis. Clinical, biochemical and morphologic studies of the syndrome. *Am. J. Dis. Child.* 98:731, 1959.

38. Zeithofer, J., and Zweymüller, E.   Congenitales Nephrosesyndrom. *Pathol. Anat.* 130:226, 1964.

39. Zunin, C., and Soave, F.   Association of nephrotic syndrome and nephroblastoma in siblings. *Ann. Paediatr. (Basel)* 203:29, 1964.

55. Focal Segmental Glomerulosclerosis

Martin A. Nash

Focal segmental glomerulosclerosis (FSGS) is a lesion characterized on light microscopy by sclerosis of only a portion of the affected glomerulus, with the remainder of the glomerulus being normal or showing mild mesangial hypercellularity (Fig. 55-1). It should not be confused with focal global glomerulosclerosis, which is characterized by total sclerosis of all affected glomeruli (Fig. 55-2). The latter lesions may be seen normally in kidneys during the first year of life, a finding termed *congenital glomerulosclerosis* [5, 6]. Usually not associated with tubular atrophy, these obsolescent glomeruli probably represent errors in nephrogenesis. They generally constitute less than 1 percent of the glomeruli present [5].

In some patients with the nephrotic syndrome, renal biopsy reveals a much higher frequency of glomeruli with global glomerulosclerosis than that seen in congenital glomerulosclerosis; in these patients, glomerular sclerosis is associated with tubular atrophy. We have been unable to differentiate this group of patients from children with minimal lesion disease, either by clinical findings at onset or by prognosis [24]. All responded to corticosteroid therapy, although they had frequent relapses. Glomerular filtration rates have remained normal.

Focal global glomerulosclerosis with extensive tubular atrophy may be seen in the advanced stage of focal segmental glomerulosclerosis. If sufficient numbers of glomeruli are present on the renal biopsy specimen, both segmental and global lesions usually can be seen.

Thus, the finding on renal biopsy of totally sclerotic glomeruli associated with tubular atrophy may be difficult to interpret. This lesion in a child with the nephrotic syndrome *unresponsive* to corticosteroid therapy should suggest the possibility of a missed focal segmental lesion with its attendant guarded prognosis. The presence of global sclerosis in a child with the nephrotic syndrome *responsive* to corticosteroids would suggest the presence of minimal lesion disease and an excellent prognosis.

History and Significance of Focal Segmental Glomerulosclerosis

Focal segmental glomerulosclerosis is found in renal biopsy sections from about 10 percent of

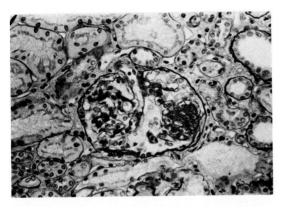

Figure 55-1. Focal segmental sclerosis. (×320.) (From M. A. Nash, I. Greifer, H. Olbing, J. Bernstein, B. Bennett, and A. Spitzer. The significance of focal sclerotic lesions of glomeruli in children. J. Pediatr. 88:806, 1976.)

children with the nephrotic syndrome and in about 40 percent of those who continue to have proteinuria after 8 weeks of corticosteroid therapy. In addition, this lesion may be seen in children with proteinuria without the nephrotic syndrome. Focal segmental sclerosis was described by Rich [25] in 1957 from autopsies of 20 children with the nephrotic syndrome. The lesion was reported as initially affecting juxtamedullary glomeruli, which contained segmental areas of hyaline sclerosis. The changes gradually involved the entire glomerulus and eventually spread to cortical glomeruli (Fig. 55-3). This evolution was associated with renal failure and death. The significance of Rich's observations was not appreciated for several years, when investigators using renal biopsies were able to associate FSGS

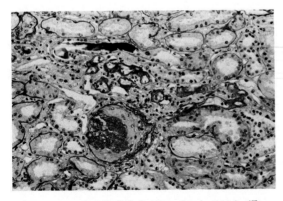

Figure 55-2. Focal global sclerosis. (×200.) (From M. A. Nash, I. Greifer, H. Olbing, J. Bernstein, B. Bennett, and A. Spitzer. The significance of focal sclerotic lesions of glomeruli in children. J. Pediatr. 88:806, 1976.)

with corticosteroid-resistant nephrotic syndrome and progressive renal disease [3, 9, 12, 30]. The results of subsequent surveys of patients with this lesion have been in general agreement that the presence of FSGS on renal biopsy distinguishes a group of patients at high risk for the development of renal insufficiency, although the frequency of such deterioration varies among these series. Habib and Gubler [10] described two clinical groups, one with persistent nephrotic syndrome (60 percent) and a high incidence of functional deterioration and a second with a remitting nephrotic syndrome (40 percent) and no functional deterioration. McGovern and Lauer [21] believed the course to be "inexorably progressive," leading to renal insufficiency, while Kincaid-Smith [17] stated that the prognosis is not bad. Nash et al. [24] described almost invariable histologic deterioration in serial biopsy specimens despite the early maintenance of normal renal function. Thus, while the lesion appears to be morphologically distinctive, its clinical significance has not been completely ascertained.

Pathologic Features

On light microscopy [3, 8, 14, 15, 24] the affected segment appears as a dense nodule in sections stained with periodic acid–Schiff or trichrome. The diagnosis rests on the demonstration of a single lesion, regardless of the glomerular count. Collapsed capillaries appear to be obliterated by increased mesangial matrix. There also may be a mild or moderate increase in the number of mesangial cells, but this is not a constant feature; hypocellularity of the affected area is seen more frequently. Entrapped endothelial cells and foam cells are also visible. Hyaline deposits are often present within the involved areas [14], appearing as globules of brightly acidophilic material. Sclerotic segments often adhere to Bowman's capsule, with a localized proliferation of epithelial cells. Grishman and Churg [7] have emphasized focal proliferation of the visceral epithelial cells over the sclerotic segment. Tubular atrophy, apparently involving the tubule of the same nephron, and interstitial fibrosis are often present.

Several glomerular alterations have been described in electron microscopic studies (Fig. 55-4) [7, 8, 14, 15, 24, 26]. Abnormalities similar to those of minimal change nephrotic syndrome can be identified in all glomeruli, not only in those shown by light microscopy to be sclerotic. The abnormalities include capillary basement membrane wrinkling and segmental thickening, subendothelial accumulation of filamentous material, and epithelial cell hyperplasia. The sclerotic areas

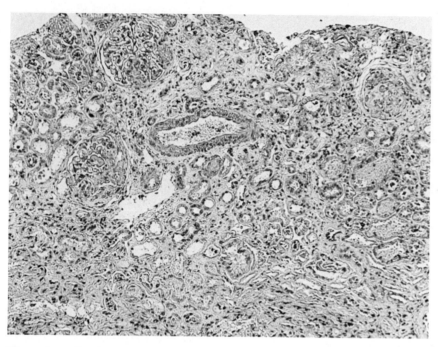

Figure 55-3. Focal segmental sclerosis, advanced lesion. Both segmental sclerosis and global sclerosis are present, with extensive tubular atrophy and interstitial fibrosis. (×94.) (Courtesy of Dr. Jacob Churg, Mount Sinai Hospital, New York.)

contain degenerating mesangial and endothelial cells that accumulate lipid, bands of mesangial matrix, clumps of hyaline and lipid material, and deposits of electron-dense granular material. Immunofluorescence microscopy has revealed frequent granular or globular deposits of IgM associated with complement [11, 14, 15, 21, 24a].

It may be difficult to distinguish this lesion from the resolving phase of focal proliferative glomerulonephritis (Chap. 46), as seen, for example, in Schönlein-Henoch purpura. In this condition, glomerular segments severely affected during the acute stage may heal with scar formation. Helpful distinguishing features may be the proliferation of visceral epithelial cells in focal segmental sclerosis, indicating an active lesion [2, 7]. The healing phase of focal proliferative disease is rarely associated with the nephrotic syndrome, and immunofluorescence microscopy in this condition is more likely to reveal diffuse mesangial immunoglobulin deposition than the focal pattern seen in focal segmental sclerosis [1, 8, 24a]. Despite these features, the distinction is often difficult. Including patients with these healing lesions with those with progressive sclerosing lesions accounts in part for the differences in prognosis reported in the literature.

Clinical Features

The best-recognized clinical picture associated with FSGS is that of the nephrotic syndrome, and in most, but not all, series of patients this is the most frequent kind of presentation as well. However, Kincaid-Smith [17] has stated that the vast majority of her patients with this lesion do not have the nephrotic syndrome. She attributed this difference to the fact that all patients in her clinic with asymptomatic proteinuria undergo renal biopsy. Other estimates have varied from 0 to 60 percent of patients without the nephrotic syndrome at time of initial presentation [1, 10, 14–16, 21, 24, 24a, 27, 29, 31]. The second most frequent form of presentation is that of asymptomatic proteinuria, with or without hematuria. The initial finding of isolated macroscopic hematuria has also been described, as have recurrent episodes of gross hematuria [31]. There is no striking sex difference, although most series have a slight preponderance of males. Clinical onset may be at any age of life.

Treatment and Prognosis

The response to treatment with corticosteroids in patients with FSGS and the nephrotic syndrome has not been encouraging. While some patients have

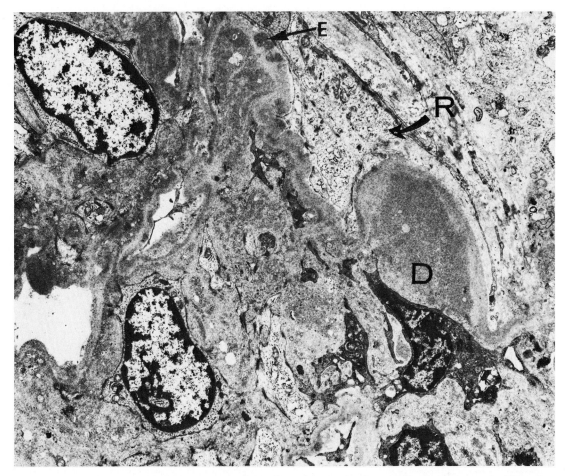

Figure 55-4. Electron micrograph of area of glomerular sclerosis showing capillary collapse and obliteration. Granular, electron-dense subendothelial (D) and apparently intramembranous (E) deposits are present. The lamina densa has a corrugated appearance around the collapsed segment. Note the small crescent formed by epithelial proliferation and the adhesion (R) between the glomerular tuft and the capsule. (×5,800.) (Courtesy of Dr. Jay Bernstein, William Beaumont Hospital, Royal Oak, Michigan.)

been described as having a "partial remission"— meaning an improvement in the degree of edema or a decrease in the quantity of proteinuria—it is not clear that this represents improvement in the underlying disease process. Most patients with FSGS are unresponsive to corticosteroid therapy, when response is defined as disappearance of proteinuria. While it is generally believed that disappearance of proteinuria reflects histologic resolution or improvement, Saint-Hillier et al. [27] described progression of the disease histologically despite a full remission of proteinuria. The response to cytotoxic therapy has been equally unrewarding. A controlled trial to determine the efficacy of cyclophosphamide in focal segmental sclerosis is in progress under the auspices of the International Study of Kidney Disease in Chil-

dren. Histologic deterioration has been nearly invariable in our experience, regardless of the type of therapy and despite the early maintenance of normal renal function [24]. In general, the lesion of FSGS in a child with corticosteroid-nonresponsive nephrotic syndrome portends a grave prognosis. It is unlikely that progression of the disease will be halted by cytotoxic therapy, although sufficient data are not available to determine whether or not such therapy might decrease the rate of progression.

The natural history of this lesion in patients without the nephrotic syndrome is less clear. The frequency with which isolated proteinuria, with or without hematuria, is associated with FSGS varies from one reported series to another, being as high as 65 percent in one [27]. The higher frequencies reported have been attributed to the practice in some clinics of performing biopsies on all patients with asymptomatic proteinuria [17]. The prognosis in children with asymptomatic proteinuria associated with hematuria and FSGS on biopsy does not appear to be different from that in children with the same lesion who have the nephrotic syndrome. The progression to renal failure in these patients has been well documented [10, 14, 21, 24, 27], but it perhaps occurs less rapidly than in patients with the nephrotic syndrome [27]. Risk factors signaling a poor prognosis appear to be hematuria and hypertension [10, 27]. The only patient in our own series who did not show histologic deterioration on serial biopsies was a child who had proteinuria that was not associated with hematuria or hypertension [24]. This finding is in agreement with the experience of other investigators [27], although renal failure has been observed even in patients without hematuria or hypertension [10].

Patients whose clinical presentation is isolated hematuria—either persistent microscopic or recurrent gross hematuria—yet whose renal biopsy reveals FSGS may have a different prognosis; their lesion may represent a separate pathogenetic process characterized by mesangial proliferation, either focal or diffuse and with or without the glomerular deposition of IgA. There are insufficient data to comment on the natural history of these lesions, but the general opinion is that they represent a relatively benign process. We have observed 2 patients thought to represent pure mesangial proliferation on initial biopsy, but who on serial biopsies showed FSGS that was associated with functional deterioration. However, careful sectioning of the initial biopsy material revealed the presence of focal segmental lesions that had been missed. Other investigators have noted an association between mesangial proliferation and FSGS [10, 24a]. Sufficient information is not available to enable a clear statement regarding this relationship, since it is always possible that a focal sclerotic lesion has been missed. Nonetheless, we would regard the presence of pure mesangial proliferation in a child with a nephrotic syndrome unresponsive to corticosteroids as a danger signal, suggesting the possibility of progressive disease, perhaps a prelude to focal segmental glomerulosclerosis.

There appears to be an unusually large number of heroin addicts among young adult patients with FSGS [7, 19]. The unfortunate encroachment of the drug problem on the younger age group makes this relationship of potential importance to those treating pediatric patients.

We have noted the early appearance of glomer-ulotubular imbalance in several patients with FSGS and the nephrotic syndrome. The apparent imbalance appeared as glycosuria and bicarbonaturia at levels of glomerular filtration rate that were either normal or slightly decreased, but not to the level at which such imbalance is expected (less than 20 ml/min/1.73 m^2). Although this observation has not been investigated thoroughly, others have noted similar aberrations of proximal tubular function in patients with this lesion [22, 23].

The recurrence of FSGS in renal transplants [13, 27, 29] suggests that the disorder is systemic rather than local [4]. Supporting this idea is the observation that serum from patients with FSGS infused into the renal arteries of rats produced more epithelial cell swelling, greater decrease in glomerular polyanion content, and more proteinuria than serum from normal patients or those with minimal change nephrotic syndrome [32]. However, the development of this lesion in transplanted kidneys has been described as well in several patients whose original disease was not FSGS [20]. The possibility is suggested that this may represent a form of graft rejection. In addition, this glomerular lesion has been found associated with vesicoureteral reflux both in original kidneys and renal transplants [18, 20]. Thus, recurrence of the original disease is not the only mechanism whereby FSGS can appear in renal transplants.

Pathogenesis

The pathogenesis of FSGS remains controversial. It is possible that this lesion is a later development in some patients with minimal lesion nephrotic syndrome and represents one possible course for some of these patients [12, 28]. Additionally, such a development might be an adverse effect of the prolonged administration of corticosteroids. The experience of most investigators, however, does not support either of these suggested relationships; the lesion has been identified frequently in patients who have never received corticosteroid therapy. Analysis of clinical features at the time of presentation of the disease enables the separation, at the time of onset, of this group of patients from those with minimal lesion disease [14–16, 24, 31], suggesting that FSGS is a separate process. The focal distribution of the lesion and concentration of lesions in the juxtamedullary nephrons make it difficult to resolve this question completely. The finding of minimal lesions on initial biopsy, with the later appearance of FSGS on serial biopsies, is probably a reflection of this unequal distribution and focal nature, but this supposition is difficult to prove. The occurrence of hematuria, hypertension, and lack of response to corticosteroid therapy (disappearance of proteinuria) in a child whose biopsy suggests minimal lesion disease should alert one to the strong possibility of FSGS missed by the biopsy needle. Thus, most investigators view minimal lesion disease and focal segmental sclerosis as separate processes.

The evidence for an immunologic pathogenesis is sparse. Immunoglobulin deposition within glomeruli is not striking and appears in no characteristic pattern. The lack of response to corticosteroids and cytotoxic agents does not support an immune mechanism. Grishman and Churg [7] have suggested primary podocyte injury and degeneration, perhaps on a nephrotoxic basis, in some patients, particularly heroin addicts. An experimental model of FSGS produced by repeated injections of aminonucleoside in rats also has indicated that such epithelial cell injury may be the primary event that leads to proteinuria and development of sclerotic lesions [29a].

It would seem probable that FSGS is a lesion of heterogeneous pathogenesis and represents a stage in the course of several pathologic processes. The associated clinical prognosis is related more to the dynamic pathologic process than to the presence of this particular lesion. At least in the setting of the nephrotic syndrome or of persistent proteinuria and hematuria, the process is one of progressive functional and histologic deterioration. In mesangial proliferation unassociated with the nephrotic syndrome, one is less certain of the prognosis, and the same is true for its occurrence in pyelonephritis, reflux nephropathy, and following transplantation when the original disease was one other than FSGS. In some patients a similar lesion appears during the recovery phase of focal proliferative nephritis, and in these children it carries a favorable prognosis.

References

1. Cameron, J. S., Ogg, D. R., Turner, D. R., and Weller, R. O. Focal Glomerulosclerosis. In P. Kincaid-Smith, T. H. Mathew, and E. L. Becker (eds.), *Glomerulonephritis*. New York: Wiley, 1973. P. 249.
2. Churg, J., and Grishman, E. Nephrotic Syndrome of Focal Glomerular Sclerosis. In E. L. Becker (ed.), *Cornell Seminars in Nephrology*. New York: Wiley, 1973. P. 35.
3. Churg, J., Habib, R., and White, R. H. R. Pathology of the nephrotic syndrome in children. *Lancet* 1: 1299, 1970.
4. Editorial. Focal glomerulosclerosis. *Lancet* 2:367, 1972.
5. Emery, J. L., and MacDonald, M. S. Involuting and scarred glomeruli in the kidneys of infants. *Am. J. Pathol.* 36:713, 1960.
6. Friedman, H. H., Grayzel, D. M., and Lederer, M. Kidney lesions in stillborn and newborn infants:

"Congenital glomerulosclerosis." *Am. J. Pathol.* 18: 699, 1942.
7. Grishman, E., and Churg, J. Focal glomerular sclerosis in nephrotic patients: An electron microscopic study of glomerular podocytes. *Kidney Int.* 7:111, 1975.
8. Habib, R. Focal glomerular sclerosis. *Kidney Int.* 4: 355, 1973.
9. Habib, R., and Gubler, M. C. Les lésions glomérulaires focales des syndromes néphrotiques idiopathiques de l'enfant: A propos de 49 observations. *Nephron* 8:382, 1971.
10. Habib, R., and Gubler, M. Focal Sclerosing Glomerulonephritis. In P. Kincaid-Smith, T. H. Mathew, and E. L. Becker (eds.), *Glomerulonephritis*. New York: Wiley, 1973. P. 263.
11. Habib, R., and Kleinknecht, C. The Primary Nephrotic Syndrome of Childhood: Classification and Clinicopathologic Study of 406 Cases. In S. C. Sommers (ed.), *Pathology Annual*. New York: Appleton-Century-Crofts, 1971. P. 417.
12. Hayslett, J. P., Krassner, L. S., Klaus, G., Bensch, M. D., Kashgarian, M., and Epstein, F. H. Progression of lipoid nephrosis to renal insufficiency. *N. Engl. J. Med.* 281:181, 1969.
13. Hoyer, J. R., Vernier, R. L., Najarian, J. S., Raij, L., Simmons, R. L., and Michael, A. F. Recurrence of idiopathic nephrotic syndrome after renal transplantation. *Lancet* 2:343, 1972.
14. Hyman, L. R., and Burkholder, P. M. Focal sclerosing glomerulonephropathy with segmental hyalinosis: A clinicopathologic analysis. *Lab. Invest.* 28:533, 1973.
15. Hyman, L. R., and Burkholder, P. M. Focal sclerosing glomerulonephropathy with hyalinosis: A clinical and pathologic analysis of the disease in children. *J. Pediatr.* 84:217, 1974.
16. Jenis, E. H., Teichman, S., Briggs, W. A., Sandler, P., Hollerman, C. E., Calcagno, P. L., Knieser, M. R., Jensen, G. E., and Valeski, J. E. Focal segmental glomerulosclerosis. *Am. J. Med.* 57:695, 1974.
17. Kincaid-Smith, P. Discussion. In P. Kincaid-Smith, T. H. Mathew, and E. L. Becker (eds.), *Glomerulonephritis*. New York: Wiley, 1973. P. 280.
18. Kincaid-Smith, P. Glomerular lesions in atrophic pyelonephritis and reflux nephropathy. *Kidney Int.* 8:S81, 1975.
19. Matalon, R., Katz, L., Gallo, G., Waldo, E., Cabaluna, C., and Eisinger, R. P. Glomerular sclerosis in adults and nephrotic syndrome. *Ann. Intern. Med.* 80:488, 1974.
20. Mathew, T. H., Mathews, D. C., Hobbs, J. B., and Kincaid-Smith, P. Glomerular lesions after renal transplantation. *Am. J. Med.* 59:177, 1975.
21. McGovern, V. J., and Lauer, C. S. Focal Sclerosing Glomerulonephritis. In P. Kincaid-Smith, T. H. Mathew, and E. L. Becker (eds.), *Glomerulonephritis*. New York: Wiley, 1973. P. 223.
22. McVicar, M. I., Exeni, R., and Susin, M. Renal glycosuria, an early sign of focal segmental glomerulosclerosis. *Pediatr. Res.* 9:376, 1975.
23. Nagi, A. H., Alexander, F., and Lannigan, R. Light and electron microscopical studies of focal glomerular sclerosis. *J. Clin. Pathol.* 24:846, 1971.
24. Nash, M. A., Greifer, I., Olbing, H., Bernstein, J., Bennett, B., and Spitzer, A. The significance of focal sclerotic lesions of glomeruli in children. *J. Pediatr.* 88:806, 1976.
24a. Newman, W. J., Tisher, C. C., McCoy, R. C.,

Gunnels, J. C., Krueger, R. P., Clapp, J. R., and Robinson, R. R. Focal glomerular sclerosis: Contrasting clinical patterns in children and adults. *Medicine* 55:67, 1976.

25. Rich, A. R. A hitherto undescribed vulnerability of the juxtamedullary glomeruli in lipoid nephrosis. *Bull. Johns Hopkins Hosp.* 100:173, 1957.

26. Rumpelt, H. J., and Thoenes, W. Fokal-sklerosierende Glomerulopathie (Glomerulonephritis)—ein diffuser Prozess. *Klin. Wochenschr.* 50:1143, 1972.

27. Saint-Hillier, Y., Morel-Magroder, L., Woodrow, D., and Richet, G. Focal and Segmental Hyalinosis. In J. Hamburger, J. Crosnier, and M. H. Maxwell (eds.), *Advances in Nephrology*. Chicago: Year Book, 1975. Vol. 5, p. 67.

28. Sigel, N. J., Hayslett, J. P., Spargo, B. H., and Kashgarian, M. Focal sclerotic lesions in steroid sensitive nephrotic syndrome. *Pediatr. Res.* 7:290, 1973.

29. Velosa, J. A., Donadio, J. V., Jr., and Holley, K. E. Focal sclerosing glomerulonephropathy: A clinicopathologic study. *Mayo Clin. Proc.* 50:121, 1975.

29a. Velosa, J. A., Glasser, R. J., Nevins, T. E., and Michael, A. F. Focal glomerular sclerosis: An experimental model. *Proceedings of the American Society of Nephrology, Ninth Annual Meeting.* Washington, D.C., 1976. P. 66.

30. White, R. H. R., and Glasgow, E. F. Focal glomerulosclerosis—a progressive lesion associated with steroid-resistant nephrotic syndrome. *Arch. Dis. Child.* 46:877, 1971.

31. White, R. H. R., Glasgow, E. F., and Mills, R. J. Focal Glomerulosclerosis in Childhood. In P. Kincaid-Smith, T. H. Mathew, and E. L. Becker (eds.), *Glomerulonephritis.* New York: Wiley, 1973. P. 231.

32. Zimmerman, S. W., and Moorthy, A. V. Renal pathophysiologic effects of serum from nephrotics: Studies in the rat. *Proceedings of the American Society of Nephrology, Ninth Annual Meeting,* Washington, D.C., 1976. P. 66.

Section Three. Renal Abnormalities in Systemic Disease

56. Hemolytic-Uremic Syndrome

Carlos A. Gianantonio

The hemolytic-uremic syndrome is characterized by the abrupt onset of hemolytic anemia and rapidly progressive renal failure. It may be associated with signs of central nervous system injury, gastrointestinal bleeding, and additional hematologic abnormalities, including red cell fragmentation, thrombocytopenia, and evidence of intravascular coagulation [17, 19].

The hemolytic-uremic syndrome is predominantly a disease of infancy, although it does occur in older children and adults [10]. An expanded view of the hemolytic-uremic syndrome must include some of its late consequences, such as neurologic sequelae, hypertension, and chronic renal failure.

History
In 1955, Gasser et al. [17] published the first communication about the association of acute hemolytic anemia and bilateral renal cortical necrosis in infants. This report clarified several previous ones on the combination of anemia with distorted red blood cells and apparently unrelated conditions, such as burns, thrombocytopenia, malignancy, uremia, and "nephritis."

Brain and colleagues [7] contributed to the understanding of the pathogenesis of the erythrocyte abnormalities, attributing it to the extensive compromise of the endothelium of the vascular tree. A new and important definition was achieved when the concept "microangiopathic hemolytic anemia" was established.

It is true, however, that the concept of "hemolytic uremic syndrome" as a clear-cut entity [22] developed slowly, since it was confused with other conditions [75], or it was assumed that the hemolytic anemia was related to acute renal failure [50] or to "nephritis" [46]. There also was concern about the possibility of curable versus lethal forms of the syndrome [30], and even of a localized renal microangiopathy, as distinct from a generalized vascular disease. Several later reports [19, 49, 51, 66, 76] brought clarity to the clinical and pathologic aspects of the hemolytic-uremic syndrome.

In more recent years, the participation of intravascular coagulation in the pathogenesis of the hemolytic-uremic syndrome has been established [36, 74]. The importance of the early management of acute renal failure on the immediate prognosis has been recognized [21], the late consequences of the hemolytic-uremic syndrome are now known [20], and suggestive evidence of a viral etiology is accumulating [70, 87].

Epidemiology

During the past 10 years there has been a progressive increase in the number of reported cases of hemolytic-uremic syndrome in many countries, including Argentina [21], Australia [71], Belgium [57], Chile [83], Czechoslovakia [73], England [58], France [31, 53], Germany [86], Italy [89], Mexico [27, 65], South Africa [44], Uruguay [69], and the United States [48]. In the Children's Hospital of Buenos Aires, 32 patients with the hemolytic-uremic syndrome were admitted from 1957 to 1961; 130 were admitted from 1962 to 1966; and 776 were admitted from 1967 to 1974. It is likely that the increase in the number of patients in pediatric hospitals around the world is due to a growing awareness of the syndrome rather than to a real increment in incidence. In our hospital, and probably in many others, several autopsied cases of typical hemolytic-uremic syndrome were described several years before it was defined clinically.

In many series the patients are admitted in small "epidemics," although clustering is not absolute. At the present time we treat patients year round. Nevertheless, two or three times a year there is a marked rise in the number of infants with hemolytic-uremic syndrome admitted to the wards. These peaks are erratic and do not follow a seasonal distribution.

There are some reports on the simultaneous occurrence of the hemolytic-uremic syndrome in related and in nonrelated adopted siblings [9, 37a]. Moreover, in a prospective familial epidemiologic survey, Tune et al. [79] have found evidence of the hemolytic-uremic syndrome in 3 siblings of 13 index patients.

Although in Argentina most of the patients come from the large cities, they also are found in rural areas. An interesting aspect of our experience is the high socioeconomic status of the families of infants with the hemolytic-uremic syndrome: 67 percent were middle class families, 11 percent upper class, and only 22 percent belonged to the lowest level. As a group, these families significantly exceeded the socioeconomic level of a matched group of patients admitted for other reasons.

The hemolytic-uremic syndrome is basically a disease of late infancy. Our patients had an average age of 12.4 months, with a range of 2 months to 8 years, a distribution similar to that of other observers [44, 66]. The incidence is similar in both sexes, and it does not appear to have a racial predilection.

Etiology

The etiology of the hemolytic-uremic syndrome remains unknown. Initial research, directed chiefly toward a possible bacterial or toxic course, was unrewarding [22]. The occasional finding of gram-negative bacterial pathogens in the stools of some patients is not sufficient evidence for a causal relationship, since acute infectious diarrhea may be complicated by gram-negative sepsis, in which intravascular coagulation, hemolysis, and, occasionally, acute renal tubular necrosis may be part of the clinical picture. Not only are all the bacterial cultures negative, but also, endotoxin is not detectable in the blood of infants with the hemolytic-uremic syndrome during the acute stage [39]. Evidence of preceding streptococcal infections (either by history or serology) is missing.

In Buenos Aires, a viral agent, provisionally called Portillo virus, of the Tacaribe group (an arenavirus), was isolated from the blood in 8 patients during the acute phase [60, 87]. In 36 of 55 patients, complement-fixing antibodies against an antigen prepared with the initial isolate were demonstrated during convalescence. Recently, arenavirus antigens were detected by immunofluorescence in kidney specimens of patients with the hemolytic-uremic syndrome [45].

The similarities between the hemolytic-uremic syndrome and some experimental and natural viral infections in which intravascular coagulation is a prominent finding [55, 56], together with the "epidemic" presentation of the cases in many countries [22, 79], have prompted many investigations. Serologic evidence of group A coxsackievirus infection was found, not only in some patients, but also in their contacts [25, 70]. Other authors have reported occasional evidence of viral infections, such as Asian influenza, echovirus 29, and respiratory syncytial virus. A rickettsialike agent has been isolated in 2 unrelated patients [61]. Several reports refer to the occasional relationship of the hemolytic-uremic syndrome to previous vaccination with live attenuated virus (measles, mumps, smallpox, poliomyelitis). This association is very likely a chance occurrence. Finally, there are excellent reports with completely negative findings [44].

With the exception of Argentina, where a specific viral agent may be involved, it is not possible at the present time to identify a single cause for the hemolytic-uremic syndrome. It is possible, however, that in most instances it may be precipitated by a viral infection, the specific type differing from one geographical area to another. These viruses may act either singly or in combination with other viruses or bacteria to precipitate the pathogenetic mechanisms of the hemolytic-uremic syndrome.

Pathogenesis

Most of the pathogenetic processes involved in the hemolytic-uremic syndrome are unknown. The mechanism responsible [4] must explain not only the renal component of the syndrome but also the widespread vascular compromise, the anemia, and the abnormalities of coagulation.

An immunologic mechanism has been proposed in the pathogenesis of the renal injury. However, the histologic pattern of the acute lesions does not resemble any immune-mediated pattern of glomerular injury. Only endothelial damage and capillary thrombosis are found, and immunofluorescence studies do not reveal substances other than fibrin [3, 18, 32]. The same findings are present in the other compromised vascular areas. Furthermore, in our experience, the levels of complement in serum are normal, although they have been found depressed by others [40]. Persistent intravascular C3 activation in 3 adult patients was reported by Kourilsky and coworkers [44a]. Finally, the hemolytic-uremic syndrome has been described in immunodeficient patients [14].

A widespread disturbance of the coagulation mechanism is present in the hemolytic-uremic syndrome, pointing to an initial and usually a single episode of acute intravascular coagulation [42]. The likelihood of initially diffuse, intravascular coagulation is supported by the presence of thrombocytopenia, the abnormality lasting longest after acute defibrination, and by the increase in fibrinogen and in other factors, especially factor VIII, that are thought to represent a rebound phenomenon after intravascular consumption [13, 63, 74, 82]. This sequence is neatly demonstrated in the few patients with recurrent bouts of intravascular coagulation, related either to the persistence of the etiologic agent or to an added inciting stimulus, such as complicating bacterial infection [74, 88]. It is only in these patients that vascular thromboses of different ages are found at autopsy.

It is attractive to link the extensive vascular thromboses of the hemolytic-uremic syndrome with those of the experimental generalized Shwartzman phenomenon, a supposition supported by its occurrence in young persons, the evidence of preceding "infectious" disease, the sudden onset, and the predominant involvement of the kidney [11, 35].

It should be noted that to produce the Shwartzman phenomenon, the initial and the inciting infections may be either of an identical or of a different nature, and that the second is not necessary if the reticuloendothelial system has been previously blocked. The vascular endothelium is modified by the first injection, so that after the second, extensive intravascular coagulation takes place, with fibrin deposits in the lumens and in the subendothelial spaces; the latter event is followed by ischemic necrosis of the tissues involved in the process. The kidney is the chief target organ, and bilateral cortical necrosis often follows.

The microvascular lesions observed in the hemolytic-uremic syndrome may be secondary to acute intravascular coagulation. A more likely explanation, however, may be found in a primary alteration of the vascular endothelia, due to the action of a vasculotropic virus or other agent, with secondary activation of the coagulation mechanism. It is also possible that the glomerular endothelial damage may impair the capacity of such cells for fibrinolytic activation, thus contributing to the persistence of locally deposited fibrin.

The intravascular deposition of fibrin, either primary or secondary, has outstanding importance in the pathogenesis of the hemolytic-uremic syndrome, not only in the acute phase, but also in the consequent postischemic renal and cerebral scarring; this may be true also for the late glomerulosclerosis.

Bleeding is observed as a consequence of diffuse intravascular coagulation [72]; it is prominent in the hemolytic-uremic syndrome, especially as a consequence of the extensive necrosis of the colonic mucosa.

Brain and colleagues [7] brought together under the term *microangiopathic hemolytic anemia* a group of apparently unrelated anemias with fragmented erythrocytes, suggesting that hemolysis might be a consequence of pathologic changes in small vessels. The altered intima and the partially occluding thrombi subject the erythrocytes of patients with the hemolytic-uremic syndrome to mechanical stress, followed by partial or total alteration of erythrocyte morphology and a marked decrease in their life span [16]. The high blood flow per unit of kidney mass explains the severity of anemia in the hemolytic-uremic syndrome in which the renal vascular tree is specifically damaged. Once fibrin is removed and the most severely damaged vessels are completely occluded, hemolysis stops. Bilateral nephrectomy in infants with severe arterial hypertension during the acute phase of the hemolytic-uremic syndrome completely corrects their anemia, pointing again to the grinding action that the kidney exerts on the red cells in this syndrome [8].

The pathogenesis of the late renal lesions has not been established. In patients in whom recovery is complete, only minimal cicatricial and resolving sequelae are found 2 to 3 years after the beginning of the disease [18]. Massive scarring, of ischemic origin, is found in patients in whom chronic renal failure developed soon after the diuretic period of the acute phase. In an important group of children, a very prolonged reparative process apparently is still taking place several years after the initial renal insult. In the patients with chronic active glomerulonephritis, the pathogenesis of the glomerular damage remains speculative. Serum complement levels are normal, and immunopathologic studies do not suggest an immune mechanism. It is possible that intravascular clotting, with fibrin deposition in the glomerular capillaries, may be followed, as it is in experimental animals, by proliferative and sclerotic glomerular changes.

Clinical Picture

In the most common clinical situation, several of the following symptoms develop in a previously well infant over a period of several days: mild fever, coryza, vomiting, diarrhea, and abdominal pain. Then, suddenly, the patient is struck by a severe illness, characterized by extreme pallor, irritability, restlessness, stupor and convulsions, cardiac failure, edema, arterial hypertension, gastrointestinal bleeding, and oliguria or anuria. Acute renal failure persists for 1 to 3 weeks and is followed by slow improvement of the anemia and renal function. In some infants, neurologic or renal sequelae are incompatible with full clinical recovery. In others, there is slowly progressive renal disease, that leads to uremia several years later.

PRODROMAL PHASE

The manifestations of the prodromal phase are usually mild; because the symptoms are not alarming, less than 5 percent of the patients are admitted to the hospital during this period. The general picture is that of a nonspecific infectious disease, with fever, malaise, irritability, vomiting, and slight diarrhea.

Fever is moderate (37.5 to 38.5°C) and is accompanied by pharyngitis and coryza in one-third of the patients. Vomiting is the most troublesome manifestation during this phase; it is profuse, persistent, and composed of ingested food and gastric juice, occasionally tinged with fresh or partially digested blood. Diarrhea is a nearly con-

stant occurrence, although it is not severe enough to cause dehydration and usually subsides in 24 to 72 hr. The stools are mucous and watery, with clumps or filaments of coagulated blood. Colicky abdominal pain, sometimes severe, is present in most of the patients.

This prodromal phase evolves 1 to 7 days and is followed, with or without a free interval of 1 to 5 days, by the manifestations of the acute stage.

ACUTE PHASE

In nearly every instance, the severity of the illness is only discovered during the first hours of the acute phase. This phase is initiated by oliguria, striking pallor, and, in some patients, convulsions. Unless the physician is familiar with the syndrome, serious and immediate consequences may result from delay in the management of the multiple derangements of this phase. Before 1956, most of these infants in our hospital died shortly after admission, and the most common diagnoses were encephalitis, meningitis, poisoning, fulminant sepsis, cryptogenic cardiac failure, myocarditis, intestinal intussusception, hemolytic crisis, acute angiitis, and acute renal failure. Although Argentinian pediatricians are now well aware of the condition, the very low incidence of the hemolytic-uremic syndrome still reported in some countries may represent misdiagnoses.

Most of the recent interest in the hemolytic-uremic syndrome has been concentrated on the acute phase [15, 31, 34, 48] because of the high fatality rates that existed before effective procedures were available for the management of acute renal failure in infants.

Hemolytic anemia

Hemolytic anemia is one of the hallmarks of the hemolytic-uremic syndrome. As a rule, anemia is severe from onset (admission blood hemoglobin levels are from 2 to 12 gm per deciliter), constituting a medical emergency in some patients. Pallor is extreme, but jaundice of any degree is absent [19]. In many infants, anemia, together with hypervolemia and electrolyte disturbances, causes congestive heart failure [47].

During the first 2 weeks of the illness, anemia may be aggravated by a hemolytic crisis, during which the blood hemoglobin concentration may fall 3 to 5 gm per deciliter in a few hours. These bouts of hemolysis decrease slowly in number and clinical severity and disappear after the second week.

The intensity of anemia does not correlate with the degree of renal and central nervous system involement. Moreover, in some patients, acute hemolytic anemia is the only relevant clinical finding.

Acute Renal Failure

The renal injury is established abruptly and simultaneously with the anemia and the other manifestations of the acute phase. In some infants the renal manifestations are minimal, with a transient decrease in urinary volume, abnormal urinary findings, and slight depression of renal function. Cases of this type, in which the patients have so-called laboratory hemolytic-uremic syndrome, may occur more frequently than has been recognized. However, of patients admitted to hospitals, acute renal failure is present in over 90 percent. As a rule it is severe because of the high catabolic rate and intercurrent complications; prolonged oliguria persists for an average of 2 weeks. In a few patients, oliguria lasts only 2 to 3 days, while in others, it may be present for as long as 8 weeks; it lasts more than 2 weeks (mean 25 days) in one-third of the patients [19]. Half the patients have anuria of more than 4 days' duration (mean 10 days, range 4 to 47 days) [19].

In some infants, one or both kidneys are enlarged, firm and easily palpable. All the complications of acute renal insufficiency are found, including hypervolemic cardiac failure, hyperkalemia, metabolic acidosis, hyperuricemia [39a], and pulmonary and generalized edema. These complications are more common when the local pediatrician is not aware of the initial manifestations of the hemolytic-uremic syndrome and there is a delay in diagnosis. Furthermore, most of the fatalities are due to these complications, which can be minimized by early diagnosis and comprehensive management.

Bilateral renal cortical necrosis develops in some infants who never have a diuresis or put out only minute amounts of urine and usually die after weeks of dialytic treatment.

The diuretic phase is never abrupt. The most common occurrence is a stepwise increase in the urinary volume that requires several days before homeostasis is achieved. In the usual case, convalescence is prolonged, with a slow return to good general health and normal renal function.

Arterial hypertension is found in one-third of the patients. In some it is related to sodium and water retention; in the remainder, it persists after overhydration is corrected. In these infants it may markedly complicate the clinical course, with left ventricular failure, hypertensive encephalopathy, and signs of hypertensive vascular damage to the kidneys and other organs. In addition to hypervolemia and arterial hypertension, cardiac failure may be precipitated by anemia, metabolic derangements, and myocardial ischemia, due to thrombotic compromise of the coronary vasculature.

Hemorrhagic diathesis

Hemorrhagic signs are present in nearly every patient; bloody stools and blood-tinged vomitus may be present during the prodromal phase. It is during the acute stage, however, that the gastrointestinal blood loss attains clinical relevance [2, 19]. Melena is found in 60 percent of the patients and hematemesis in 20 percent.

The association of pallor, intermittent crying, vomiting, rectal blood loss, and abdominal tenderness may confuse the unaware physician and suggest an abdominal emergency, such as intestinal intussusception. If this unfortunate error results in surgical intervention, multiple intramural and subserosal extravasations of blood will be found in the colon and terminal ileum.

With the exception of an occasional subdural hematoma and hemorrhages into the retina of some infants, no other obvious sites of bleeding are observed. Petechiae are rare, and ecchymoses are never seen. However, in one-third of the patients, several slightly raised dermal hematomas, 1 to 3 mm in diameter, are scattered over the trunk, face, and root of the limbs.

Neurologic Involvement

Nearly all patients manifest signs of involvement of the central nervous system during the initial days of the oliguric period [19, 59]. In about half the patients, these signs are mild, consisting of somnolence, irritability, myoclonic jerks, tremor, and slight ataxia.

In other patients, however, the problems are much more severe, and include generalized convulsions, either single or recurrent, self-limited or prolonged, and life-threatening; they are accompanied by alterations in the level of consciousness and focal neurologic signs. Deep and prolonged coma is not uncommon and may be associated with respiratory depression and death.

Decerebrate rigidity, muscular hypotonia or hypertonia, increased deep tendon reflexes, transient hemiparesis, nystagmus, and pupillary abnormalities are found in many of these severely compromised infants. Retinal hemorrhages are observed in one-third. There is no strict correlation between the degree of neurologic involvement and either the severity of renal impairment or the intensity of the anemia.

The great majority of patients recover completely after days or weeks, without obvious sequelae. Nonetheless, some infants die as a result of the insult to the central nervous system, and a small group with disabling sequelae remains.

CHRONIC RENAL DISEASE

In the average patient, recovery of sufficient renal function to sustain life is attained rapidly after the diuretic phase. A moderate to marked restriction in the capacity to handle sodium loads persists, however, for many weeks. In some of these infants, sodium retention, edema, hypervolemia, arterial hypertension, and cardiac failure may reappear during the first months after discharge if a low-sodium formula is not given.

A small group of patients (1 to 3 percent), all of whom had oliguria or anuria for more than 3 weeks during the acute stage, does not return to normal level of renal function; during the first 3 years of follow-up they die in chronic renal failure or require dialysis or renal transplantation. Another distressing group of children have persistent urinary abnormalities, intermittent arterial hypertension, and slowly deteriorating renal function, leading to terminal uremia 5 to 13 years after onset [20].

The overall incidence of chronic renal disease varies from 9.5 to 40 percent [20, 80], depending on the initial severity and the length of time intervening before follow-up. However, progression to end-stage renal insufficiency during the school years and adolescence is probably restricted to about 15 percent of patients.

NEUROLOGIC SEQUELAE

Variable manifestations of permanent neurologic impairment are encountered in some patients. The spectrum is wide, ranging from behavioral and learning difficulties to severe mental retardation and quadriparesis or hemiparesis. Convulsive episodes, either akinetic, myoclonic, jacksonian, or grand mal, are present in some children, either singly or in combination with motor, intellectual, or sensory handicaps. It should be noted that, as a rule, there is a marked tendency to initial improvement, and many neurologic symptoms present at the end of the acute phase will subside during the ensuing months.

Laboratory Findings

ANEMIA

Of the diminished erythrocyte population, 5 to 50 percent is morphologically abnormal. The finding of fragmented, distorted, triangular, helmetlike erythrocytes, and burr erythrocytes, together with very small spherocytes, ghost cells, eggshell cells, and other bizarre forms, is constant and very striking. The proportion of damaged erythrocytes increases during hemolytic crises, and they persist, in decreasing proportions, for an average of 70 days [22]. The reticulocyte number is increased (mean 7.8 percent, range 2.6 to 20 percent). The serum bilirubin levels are moderately elevated (mean 1.88 mg per deciliter, range 1.06 to 3.5 mg per deciliter) during the hemolytic crises. The high plasma hemoglobin levels, hemoglobinuria, and depressed haptoglobin levels are indicative of the intravascular nature of the hemolysis [21, 77]. The life span of transfused erythrocytes is markedly shortened during the first 2 weeks of the hemolytic-uremic syndrome [16, 41, 62]. Leukocytosis (mean leukocyte count 17,000 per square millimeter, range 4,600 to 62,000 per square millimeter), with an increase in the percentage of neutrophils, is found during the same period.

Marked erythroblastic and moderate myeloid hyperplasia, together with abundant but immature megakaryocytes, are found in the bone marrow. The findings of a Coombs test, erythrocyte enzyme assays (glucose 6-phosphate dehydrogenase, pyruvate kinase) and the hemoglobin structure are normal [37].

PLATELETS AND COAGULATION FACTORS

Thrombocytopenia is present on initial examination in about 90 percent of the patients, with a mean platelet count of 75,000 per cubic millimeter and a range of 16,000 to 175,000 per cubic millimeter. In the remainder, platelet counts are either normal or elevated, suggesting a rebound phenomenon after an undetected initial fall [74]. Thrombocytopenia persists for 7 to 15 days and is followed by a progressive increase in the platelet count, very often to the level of thrombocytosis. However, in some patients with extremely severe clinical involvement, recovery from thrombocytopenia is irregular, transient, or absent until death [74, 88]. Platelet survival is normal [41, 62].

Quick's prothrombin time is prolonged in half the cases and is related to decreases in factors II, VII, VIII, IX, and X. Partial thromboplastin time with kaolin is shorter than normal during the first 3 weeks in most patients. These infants have simultaneously elevated levels of factor VIII and, to a lesser extent, of factors IX and XI. Plasma fibrinogen concentrations are elevated in half the patients, while fibrin degradation products may be demonstrated in about one-third.

If the patients are studied very early, i.e., during the first hours of the initial phase, thrombocytopenia, together with low fibrinogen, depressed levels of factors VIII, IX, and XI, and increased fibrinogen degradation products, may be documented. Secondary drops in fibrinogen and factors VIII, IX, and XI are found in the few patients with late thrombocytopenia and clinical deterioration during the initial weeks of the acute phase of the hemolytic-uremic syndrome.

These observations suggest that intravascular coagulation is present in every patient, but as a very transient, initial phenomenon. Since most of the infants are seen a few days after onset, the most frequent finding is a rebound in the coagulation factors, signaled by high levels of fibrinogen and factors VIII, IX, and XI.

Although there are communications describing persistent and slow deposition of fibrin during the acute phase [88], it is generally held that a single, initial bout of intravascular coagulation heralds the clinical catastrophic events, and that it does not usually recur [62, 74]. This observation has obvious implications with regard to treatment.

KIDNEY FUNCTION AND URINARY ABNORMALITIES

Metabolic acidosis, hyperkalemia of varying degrees of severity, and high levels of blood urea (mean 326 mg per deciliter, range 46 to 696 mg per deciliter) are present on admission in all patients. There is a rapid increment in the concentration of blood urea (46 mg/dl/day in one series) during the first week of oliguria in nondialyzed patients [21].

Gross hematuria is present in only 10 percent of the patients, while microscopic hematuria is found in every case, together with hyaline, granular, and epithelial casts and leukocytes. Nonselective proteinuria (2 to 10.0 gm per liter) is a constant finding during the acute phase, decreasing slowly thereafter. Hemoglobinuria is present in patients with severe hemolysis. Serum immunoglobulins and concentrations of C3 are normal during the acute and late phases of the hemolytic-uremic syndrome.

In patients with a favorable late prognosis, the urinary sediment returns to normal in 6 months, and the proteinuria subsides in 1 year. Glomerular filtration rates reach normal values about the same time, from 6 to 12 months after the onset of the disease. The group of patients with massive parenchymal necrosis and renal scarring show critically low glomerular filtration rates immediately after the diuretic phase and run a downhill course during the following months. There is a third heterogeneous group, composed of children with decreased but stable renal function; some of these patients subsequently have progressive improvement in their glomerular filtration rates, whereas other patients show slow, relentless deterioration of kidney function, accompanied by persistent proteinuria and, commonly, arterial hypertension.

RADIOLOGIC AND ELECTROCARDIOGRAPIC FINDINGS

During the acute phase, radiographs of the abdomen show a moderate increase in the size of the kidneys. In patients with severe renal scarring, a marked reduction of renal size, with eventual linear deposits of calcium in the cortical areas, can be demonstrated.

During the oliguric period, the ECG may reflect either high output cardiac failure of the overhydrated infant or metabolic abnormalities such as hyperkalemia or hypocalcemia. In some infants the ECG tracings are suggestive of myocardial ischemia; these abnormalities persist for weeks after the acute phase of the disease.

Pathologic Features
ACUTE PHASE

The basic lesion consists of damage to the microvasculature of the kidney, and eventually of other organs, by an extensive thrombotic process. There is no conclusive pathologic evidence favoring either primary vascular damage or thrombosis as the initial step in the development of thrombotic microangiopathy [3, 21, 29, 81, 85]. Part of the difficulty encountered in the interpretation of the initial pathologic findings arises from the fact that specimens are not usually obtained during the first week.

The former controversy about the possibility of two different forms of the hemolytic-uremic syndrome, one with the microthrombosis limited to the renal vascular tree and the other with simultaneous involvement of other organs, has been resolved. The disease covers a wide spectrum of clinical abnormalities that are expressions of varying degrees of involvement by the thrombotic process in different vascular areas. The kidney is always maximally involved, but, in most cases, identical lesions can be found in other organs.

The early renal abnormalities belong to three pathologic categories:

1. Occluding fibrin thrombi (Fig. 56-1) and linear deposits of fibrin on the endothelial surface of the glomerular capillaries involve a variable proportion of the glomeruli in a focal fashion. In biopsy material obtained in mild cases, thrombosis is segmental and focal. However, in the most grave forms, with prolonged oliguria, more than 75 percent of the glomeruli are damaged. The basal membrane is normal, and there are neither in-

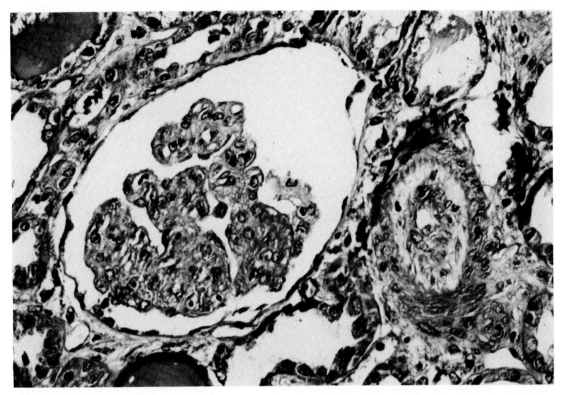

Figure 56-1. Renal biopsy section from a 10-month-old boy with the hemolytic-uremic syndrome. The interlobular artery on the right shows striking intimal thickening, with only a small lumen remaining. The glomerulus is normocellular, but the capillary walls are markedly thickened. (Trichrome, ×50.)

flammatory changes nor endothelial or mesangial proliferation. Extensions of the glomerular thrombi may be found in the adjacent part of the afferent arterioles.

2. The vascular lesions are concentrated in the preglomerular and interlobular arteries (Fig. 56-1). Most often, they consist of subendothelial edema, with or without foci or fibrinoid necrosis and thrombotic occlusion of their lumens. There is no perivascular cellular infiltration. The coalescence of areas of ischemic necrosis leads to massive or partial bilateral renal cortical necrosis (Fig. 56-2).

3. Foci of hemorrhagic necrosis, not related to thrombosis of the adjacent vasa recta, are frequently observed in the outer medulla, with occasional extension to the pyramids.

The following findings, with a patchy distribution, are not considered specific: degeneration and necrosis of the convoluted tubules, hemorrhagic necrosis of isolated glomeruli, and occasional epithelial crescents.

If the kidneys are studied after the second week of the disease, the following abnormalities are apparent:

1. Marked centrilobular thickening, due mainly to an increase in the mesangial matrix, with only slight focal mesangial proliferation.

2. Thickening of the capillary walls due to irregular hyalinization, duplication of the basement membrane, or pale subendothelial deposits.

3. Varying degrees of glomerular scarring, with some glomeruli reduced to sclerotic nodules.

Well-established, bilateral renal cortical necrosis is found in infants who die after several weeks of oliguria or anuria.

There is an inverse correlation between the duration of the disease and the extent of glomerular capillary thrombi; they have nearly disappeared after 30 days.

Hypertensive vascular changes that may be extremely severe and widespread are present in some patients. Other findings, of secondary importance, include tubular atrophy, interstitial fibrosis and infiltration with mononuclear cells, and deposits of calcium and hemosiderin.

Immunofluorescence studies performed on kidney specimens obtained during the acute phase of the hemolytic-uremic syndrome have confirmed the presence of fibrin in the capillary lumens and

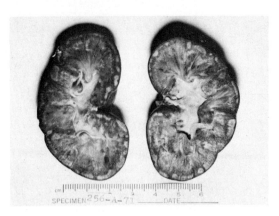

Figure 56-2. Kidney from a 6-month-old infant who died 7 days after onset of oliguria showing bilateral renal cortical necrosis.

walls and in the walls of the small and medium-sized arteries. With few exceptions [54], search for deposits of immunoglobulins and complement components has produced negative results [18, 21, 32].

Electron-microscopic studies [29, 54] have confirmed the findings on light-microscopy, with the important addition that hypertrophy and increased phagocytic activity in glomerular endothelial cells were better demonstrated. Abundant platelets in the foci of thrombosis, and irregular deposits in the lamina densa of the basement membranes, also have been described [12].

A meticulous scrutiny reveals small-vessel thrombosis in other organs; these may be severe and extensive. The colonic wall is most intensely affected, followed by the pancreas (islets of Langerhans), myocardium, central nervous system, adrenals, skin, and lungs. Seen microscopically, the lesions in the colon consist, in addition to the thromboses, of large areas of hemorrhage and necrosis with mucosal ulceration, more intense in the cecum and the ascending colon. Microscopic foci of necrosis are found in the myocardium, while in the brain the predominant changes are edema and gross and microscopic hemorrhages, with small-vessel thrombosis, fibrin deposits in the choroid plexuses, and minute areas of spongiosis.

LATE PHASE

The pathologic findings of the late phase belong in three main categories [21]. In the first group of patients, only renal scarring is present, with generalized and segmental hyalinization of the glomeruli, capsular adhesions, fibrous crescents, tubular atrophy, and marked interstitial fibrosis. Often, these lesions are grouped, conforming to small healed infarcts. The remaining glomeruli are normal or have minimal focal mesangial proliferation. These sequelae may be minimal in children with normal renal function, or they may be widespread in those who die in early uremia or live with low but stable glomerular filtration rates.

In the second group, scarring of variable severity is also present, but it is accompanied by mesangial proliferation, either segmental or generalized, in the nonscarred glomeruli. This lesion may progress over the years and eventuate in an end-stage kidney. Hypertensive vascular changes also may be observed.

The third group comprises the children with advanced nephrosclerosis and severe hypertensive changes. Some of these children reflect the end result of severe kidney scarring, while others may be instances of the terminal stage of diffuse mesangial proliferation.

Diagnosis

The diagnosis of hemolytic-uremic syndrome depends on the pediatrician's awareness of this entity. In the average case, the syndrome is so dramatic and clear-cut that there is little difficulty in making a correct and early diagnosis. Since the incidence varies considerably, it is essential to keep physicians informed about the presence of the hemolytic-uremic syndrome in their area. The initial suspicion arises when a well baby, 6 to 14 months old, becomes ill with cramping and blood-streaked diarrhea and persistent vomiting. Confirmation comes when, suddenly, intense pallor or a generalized convulsion ushers in the acute phase of the syndrome. A history of a recent decrease in the quantity of urine or a change in its color to reddish brown coincides with an unexplained increase in weight. At this time, urinalysis shows heavy proteinuria, red cells, and granular casts; the BUN is markedly elevated, and a blood smear confirms the diagnosis, revealing the abnormal erythrocytes and the scant platelets.

Acute glomerular damage due to other causes is uncommon during infancy. Acute tubular necrosis of toxic or ischemic origin or renal vein thrombosis should be considered in the differential diagnosis. Also to be considered are acute poststreptococcal glomerulonephritis, Schönlein-Henoch nephritis, lupus nephritis, and thrombotic thrombocytopenic purpura [1, 26, 52].

If the diagnosis is delayed, the complications of acute renal insufficiency, including cardiac failure, hyperkalemia, metabolic acidosis, and massive edema, may become dramatically apparent. Difficult diagnostic problems may be posed by patients in whom one symptom is predominant, such as extreme anemia, grave neurologic manifestations, or profuse rectal bleeding.

The anemia may be erroneously ascribed to blood loss through the gastrointestinal tract. Other causes of hemolysis, such as erythrocyte enzymatic defects, abnormal hemoglobins, congenital microspherocytosis, immunohemolytic anemias, poisoning, bacterial sepsis, or malignancy, may have to be ruled out. The erythrocyte fragmentation syndrome may be observed also in thrombotic thrombocytopenic purpura, cavernous hemangioma, renal transplant rejection, metastatic tumor, gram-negative sepsis, congenital heart disease, and surgical repair of valvular and other cardiac defects.

The neurologic symptoms may suggest the diagnosis of viral or bacterial infection of the central nervous system, acute metabolic brain dysfunction, poisoning, or trauma.

Treatment

Since the cause is unknown, the treatment of the hemolytic-uremic syndrome is symptomatic. Of prime importance is intense management of acute renal failure. In our initial experience (1957), the mortality was about 50 percent; however, since the introduction of early and iterative peritoneal dialysis, with the simultaneous provision of an adequate caloric and protein intake, mortality during the acute stage has dropped to about 6 percent [21].

Hyperkalemia, extreme acidosis, hypervolemia, and other life-threatening complications can be either prevented or effectively treated through conservative measures or dialysis.

Adequate measures to prevent hospital-acquired infections are essential. Anemia often requires repeated transfusions of packed red blood cells. The neurologic manifestations of the hemolytic-uremic syndrome deserve special attention because they contribute heavily to the mortality. Status epilepticus, deep coma, and respiratory depression require the usual treatment for these states, together with peritoneal dialysis.

There is an ample literature on anticoagulation with heparin [5, 6, 23, 24, 36, 38, 42a, 43, 68, 78a, 80] with favorable results in the experience of some investigators, but with poor or no results in the majority of recent studies. In the only controlled study in which supportive therapy and peritoneal dialysis were contrasted with similar management plus heparin, no advantage of anticoagulant therapy was observed [84]. Many of the reports are difficult to evaluate, since mild to moderate cases have been included, and the progress made in conservative and dialytic management of infants was not taken into account. Therefore, the improved prognosis ascribed to heparin therapy may simply be the result of better care. At the present time, most centers no longer use heparin, because the very early occurrence of intravascular coagulation precludes its administration at the time it could be effective. Treatment usually begins, after the process of coagulation has already ended. Heparin may have a place in the management of recurrent bouts of intravascular coagulation. The value that heparin treatment may have in the prevention of chronic renal disease is unknown.

Several investigators have reported the results of streptokinase therapy in the hemolytic-uremic syndrome [28, 64, 78], suggesting that it improves early mortality. Obviously, the removal of fibrin is a more rational approach than anticoagulation, but the effectiveness, as well as the limitations and dangers, of such therapy are not well established. Theoretically, its value, if any, may be related more to the late sequelae (hypertension and reduced renal function) than to early mortality. Powell and Ekert [67] reported that treatment with streptokinase, aspirin, and dipyridamole [67] did not improve the results obtained with heparin. However, chronic renal disease did not occur in any of the surviving patients. Arensen and August [1a] reported good results with aspirin and dipyridamole. Anticoagulant and fibrinolytic treatment of the hemolytic-uremic syndrome is considered further in Chap. 70.

There are no reports on medical treatment of the chronic glomerular disease that develops in some children, aside from symptomatic management of uremia. Patients with end-stage renal disease as a consequence of the hemolytic-uremic syndrome are good candidates for renal transplantation [8].

Prognosis

The immediate prognosis is dependent on the severity of acute renal failure and the extent of injury to the central nervous system (Table 56-1). Mortality approaches zero in patients with mild disease, while it rises to 25 percent in those with more than 25 days of oliguria. Anuria of more than 4 days' duration is also a sign of poor prognosis, since it often coincides with extensive renal cortical necrosis. Factors of prime importance to the prognosis are the quality of care offered to these infants and the experience of the physician in the management of acute renal failure in early life. Recurrent episodes of the hemolytic-uremic syndrome have been reported rarely [13a].

Chronic renal insufficiency can be expected to follow the initial phase in 3 to 4 percent of pa-

Table 56-1. Clinical Grading of Severity

Severity	Oliguria (days)	Anuria (days)	CNS Symptoms	Arterial Hypertension	Bleeding Diathesis	Anemia
Mild	<7	–	0 to +	0 to +	0 to +	+ to + + +
Moderate	7–14	<7	0 to + + +	0 to + +	0 to + +	+ to + + +
Severe	>14	>7	+ + to + + +	+ to + + +	+ + to + + +	+ to + + +

0 to + + + = intensity and duration of sign

tients. They belong to the severe group and present massive scarring of the kidneys. Late renal failure, with terminal uremia during childhood or early adolescence, develops in about 15 percent of patients. Most of them had either severe or moderately severe disease, but chronic glomerular disease may develop even in a few patients with the mild form of hemolytic-uremic syndrome.

An accurate prognosis must be based on the serial study of renal function and on biopsy specimens. However, undue concern about patients with normal blood pressure, normal and stable renal function, and absence of proteinuria after the first year of follow-up is not warranted, and it may pose an unjustified emotional burden on the parents.

Renal transplantation has been reported to be successful, despite recurrence of the hemolytic-uremic syndrome [36a].

References

1. Adelson, E., Heitzman, E. J., and Fennesey, J. F. Thrombohemolytic thrombocytopenic purpura. *A.M.A. Arch. Intern. Med.* 94:42, 1954.
1a. Arensen, E. B., Jr., and August, C. S. Preliminary report: Treatment of the hemolytic-uremic syndrome with aspirin and dipyridamole. *J. Pediatr.* 86:957, 1975.
2. Berman, W., Jr. The hemolytic-uremic syndrome. Initial clinical presentation mimicking ulcerative colitis. *J. Pediatr.* 81:275, 1972.
3. Bouissou, H., Familiades, J., Fabre, J., Regnier, C., and Hamousin-Metregiste, B. La glomerulo-nécrose, lesion initiale de la nécrose corticale symetrique des reins. *Sem. Hop. (Ann. Pediatr.)* 39:282, 1963.
4. Brain, M. C., Baker, L. R. I., McBride, J. A., and Rubenberg, M. L. Heparin therapy in hemolytic-uremic syndrome. *Q. J. Med.* 36:608, 1967.
5. Brain, M. C. The haemolytic-uremic syndrome. *Semin. Hematol.* 6:162, 1969.
6. Brain, M. C., Baker, L. R. I., McBride, J. A., Rubenberg, M. L., and Dacie, J. U. Treatment of patients with microangiopathic hemolytic anemia with heparin. *Br. J. Haematol.* 15:603, 1968.
7. Brain, M. C., Dacie, J. U., and Hourihane, D. O'B. Microangiopathic haemolytic anemia: The possible role of vascular lesions in pathogenesis. *Br. J. Haematol* 8:358, 1962.
8. Cerilli, G. J., Nelsen, C., and Dorfmann, L. Renal

homotransplantation in infants and children with the hemolytic-uremic syndrome. *Surgery* 71:66, 1972.
9. Corrigan, J. J., Abilgaard, C. F., Vanderheiden, J. F., and Schulman, I. Quantitative aspects of blood coagulation in the generalized Shwartzman reaction. *Pediatr. Res.* 1:39, 1967.
10. Craig, J., and Gitlin, D. The nature of hyaline thrombi in thrombotic thrombocytopenic purpura. *Am. J. Pathol.* 33:251, 1957.
11. Chan, J. C. M., Eleff, M. G., and Campbell, R. A. The hemolytic-uremic syndrome in nonrelated adopted siblings. *J. Pediatr.* 75:1050, 1969.
12. Churg, J., Loffler, D., Paronetto, F., Rorat, E., and Barnett, R. N. Hemolytic uremic syndrome as a cause of postpartum renal failure. *Am. J. Obstet. Gynecol.* 108:253, 1970.
13. Desmit, E. M., and En Hart, H. C. L. Behandeling van het hemolytisch-uramisch Syndrom. *Ned. Tijdschr. Geneeskd.* 110:355, 1966.
13a. Drukker, A., Winterborn, M., Bennett, B., Churg, J., Spitzer, A., and Greifer, I. Recurrent hemolytic-uremic syndrome: A case report. *Clin. Nephrol.* 4:48, 1975.
14. Dubilier, L. D., Chadwick, J. A., and Leddy, J. P. Thymic alymphoplasia associated with the hemolytic-uremic syndrome. *J. Pediatr.* 73:714, 1968.
15. European Society for Pediatric Nephrology. Prospective survey of the hemolytic-uremic syndrome. Second International Symposium of Pediatric Nephrology, Paris, 1971, pp. 149–150.
16. Fleisher, D. S., McElfresh, A. E., and Arey, J. B. The hemolytic-uremic syndrome in children (abstract 56). Seventy-Second Annual Meeting of the American Pediatric Society, Atlantic City, N.J., 1962, p. 65.
17. Gasser, C. von, Gautier, E., Steck, A., Siebermann, R. E., and Oechslin, R. Hämolytisch-urämische syndrome. Bilaterale Nierenrindennekrosen bei akuten erworbenen hämolytischen Anämien. *Schweiz. Med. Wochenschr.* 85:905, 1955.
18. Gervais, M., Richardson, J. B., Chiu, J., and Drummond, K. N. Inmunofluorescent and histologic findings in the hemolytic uremic syndrome. *Pediatrics* 47:352, 1971.
19. Gianantonio, C. A., Vitacco, M., and Mendilaharzu, F. The hemolytic-uremic syndrome. In *Proceedings of the Third International Congress of Nephrology.* New York: Karger, 1967. Vol. 3, pp. 24–36.
20. Gianantonio, C. A., Vitacco, M., Mendilaharzu, F., and Gallo, G. E. The hemolytic uremic syndrome. Renal status of 76 patients at long-term follow-up. *J. Pediatr.* 72:757, 1968.
21. Gianantonio, C. A., Vitacco, M., Mendilaharzu, F., Gallo, G. E., and Sojo, E. T. The hemolytic-uremic syndrome. *Nephron* 11:174, 1973.
22. Gianantonio, C. A., Vitacco, M., Mendilaharzu, F.,

Rutty, A., and Mendilaharzu, J. The hemolytic-uremic syndrome. *J. Pediatr.* 64:478, 1964.

23. Gilchrist, G., and Lieberman, E. Haemolytic uremic syndrome and heparin therapy. *Lancet* 2:1069, 1969.

24. Gilchrist, G. S., Lieberman, E., Ekert, H., Fine, R. N., and Grushkin, C. Heparin therapy in the Haemolytic-uraemic syndrome. *Lancet* 1:1123, 1969.

25. Glasgow, L. A., and Balduzzi, P. Isolation of Coxsackie virus group A, type 4, from a patient with hemolytic-uremic syndrome. *N. Engl. J. Med.* 273:754, 1965.

26. Goldenfarb, P. B., and Finch, S. C. Thrombotic thrombocytopenic purpura. *J.A.M.A.* 226:644, 1973.

27. Gordillo, G. Personal communication, 1977.

28. Guillin, M. C., Boyer, C., Beaufils, F., and Lejeune, C. Traitement par la streptokinase dans deux cas de syndrome hémolytique et urémique. *Arch. Fr. Pediatr.* 30:401, 1973.

29. Habib, R., Courtecuisse, V., Leclerc, F., Mathieu, H., and Royer, P. Etude anatomopathologique de 35 observations de syndrome hémolytique et urémique de l'enfant. *Arch. Fr. Pediatr.* 26:391, 1969.

30. Habib, R., Leclerc, F., Mathieu, H., and Royer, P. Comparaison clinique et anatomo-pathologique entre les formes mortelles et curables du syndrome hémolitique et urémique. *Arch. Fr. Pediatr.* 26:417, 1969.

31. Habib, R., Mathieu, H., and Royer, P. Le syndrome hémolitique et urémique de l'enfant. *Nephron.* 4:139, 1967.

32. Hadley, W., and Rosenan, W. Study of human renal disease by immunofluorescent methods. *Arch. Pathol.* 83:342, 1967.

33. Hagge, W. W., Holley, K. E., Burke, E. C., and Stickler, G. B. Hemolytic uremic syndrome in two siblings. *N. Engl. J. Med.* 277:138, 1967.

34. Hammond, D., and Lieberman, E. The hemolytic uremic syndrome. *Arch. Intern. Med.* 126:816, 1970.

35. Hitzig, W. H. Phenomene de Sanarelli-Shwartzman lors de syndrome par manque d'anticorps. *Med. et Hyg.* 21:1106, 1963.

36. Hitzig, W. H. Therapie mit antikoagulantien in der pädiatric. *Helv. Pediatr. Acta* 19:213, 1964.

36a. Howard, E. J., Mauer, S. M., Miller, K., Simmons, R. L., and Najarian, J. S. Biopsy proven recurrence of hemolytic uremic syndrome early after kidney transplantation with a favorable outcome. *Kidney Int.* 10:544, 1976.

37. Javett, S. N., and Senior, B. Syndrome of hemolysis, thrombocytopenia and nephropathy in infancy. *Pediatrics* 29:209, 1962.

37a. Kaplan, B. S., Chesney, R. W., and Drummond, K. N. Hemolytic-uremic syndrome in families. *N. Engl. J. Med.* 292:1090, 1975.

38. Kaplan, B. S., Katz, J., Krawitz, S., and Lurie, A. An analysis of the results of therapy in 67 cases of the hemolytic-uremic syndrome. *J. Pediatr.* 78:420, 1971.

39. Kaplan, B. S., and Koornhof, H. J. Haemolytic-uraemic syndrome. Failure to demonstrate circulating endotoxin. *Lancet* 12:1424, 1969.

39a. Kaplan, B. S., and Thomson, P. D. Hyperuricemia in the hemolytic-uremic syndrome. *Am. J. Dis. Child.* 130:854, 1976.

40. Kaplan, B. S., Thomson, P. D., and MacNab, G. M. Serum-complement levels in hemolytic-uremic syndrome. *Lancet* 2:1505, 1973.

41. Katz, J., Krawitz, S., Sacks, P., Levin, S. E., Thomson, P., Levin, J., and Metz, J. Platelet, erythrocyte and fibrinogen kinetics in the hemolytic-uremic syndrome of infancy. *J. Pediatr.* 83:739, 1973.

42. Katz, J., Lurie, A., Kaplan, B. S., Krawitz, S., and Metz, J. Coagulation findings in the hemolytic uremic syndrome of infancy. Similarity to hyperacute renal allograft rejection. *J. Pediatr.* 78:426, 1971.

42a. Khanh, B. J., Bhatena, D., Vazquez, M. T., and Luke, R. G. Role of heparin therapy in the outcome of adult hemolytic uremic syndrome. *Nephron* 16:292, 1976.

43. Kibel, M. A., and Barnard, P. J. Treatment of acute haemolytic-uraemic syndrome with heparin. *Lancet* 2:259, 1964.

44. Kibel, M. A., and Barnard, P. J. The haemolytic-uraemic syndrome: A survey in South Africa. *S. Afr. Med. J.* 42:692, 1968.

44a. Kourilsky, O., Vandewalle, A., Smith, M. D., Stühlinger, W., Verroust, P. J., Gonzalo, A., Neuilly, G., Kanfer, A., Sraer, J. D., and Morel-Maroger, L. Persistent intravascular C3 activation after bilateral nephrectomy in patients with thrombotic microangiopathy. *Clin. Nephrol.* 6:437, 1976.

45. Laguens, R. P., Cossio, P. M., Patin, D. J., Maiztegui, J. L., Voyer, L. E., Segal, A., and Arana, R. M. Presencia de antígenos de arenavirus y partículas de tipo viral en riñones de enfermos con sindrome urémico hemolítico (SUH) de la ciudad de Buenos Aires. *Medicina* 35:611, 1975.

46. Lamvik, J. O. Acute glomerulonephritis with hemolytic anemia in infants. *Pediatrics* 29:224, 1962.

47. Leikin, S. L. Hematological aspects of renal disease. *Pediatr. Clin. North Am.* 11:667, 1964.

48. Lieberman, E. Hemolytic uremic syndrome. *J. Pediatr.* 80:1, 1972.

49. Lieberman, E., Heuser, E., Donnell, G. N., Landing, B. H., and Hammond, G. D. Hemolytic-uremic syndrome. *N. Engl. J. Med.* 275:227, 1966.

50. Lock, S. P., and Dormandy, K. M. Red-cell fragmentation syndrome. A condition of multiple aetiology? *Lancet* 1:1020, 1961.

51. Loeb, H., Batman, J., Dustin, P., and Nameche, J. Néphropathie avec anemie hémolytique et purpura thrombocytopenique. *Acta Paediatr. Belg.* 13:111, 1959.

52. MacWhinney, J. B., Packer, J. T., Miller, G., and Greendyke, R. M. Thrombotic thrombocytopenic purpura in childhood. *Blood* 19:181, 1962.

53. Mathieu, H., Leclerc, F., Habib, R., and Royer, P. Etude clinique et biologique de 37 observations de syndrome hémolitique et urémique. *Arch. Fr. Pediatr.* 26:369, 1969.

54. McCoy, R. C., Abramowsky, C. R., and Krueger, R. The hemolytic-uremic syndrome with positive immunofluorescence studies. *J. Pediatr.* 85:170, 1974.

55. McKay, D. G., and Margaretten, W. Disseminated intravascular coagulation in virus diseases. *Arch. Intern. Med.* 120:129, 1967.

56. McKay, D. G., Phillips, L. L., Kaplan, H., and Henson, J. B. Chronic intravascular coagulation in Aleutian disease of mink. *Am. J. Pathol.* 50:899, 1967.

57. McKay, D. G., and Shapiro, S. S. Alterations in the blood coagulation system induced by bacterial endotoxin. *J. Exp. Med.* 107:353, 1958.

58. McLean, M. M., Hilton Jones, C., and Sutherland, D. A. Haemolytic-uraemic syndrome. *Arch. Dis. Child.* 41:76, 1966.

59. Meadow, R.   Central nervous system involvement in the hemolytic uraemic syndrome. *Dev. Med. Child Neurol.* 13:812, 1971.

60. Mettler, N. E., Gianantonio, C. A., and Parodi, A. Aislamiento del agente causal del sindrome urémico-hemolítico. *Medicina* 23:139, 1963.

61. Mettler, N. E.   Isolation of a microtatobiote from patients with hemolytic-uremic syndrome and thrombotic thrombocytopenic purpura and from mites in the United States. *N. Engl. J. Med.* 281:1023, 1969.

62. Metz, J.   Observations on the mechanisms of the haematological changes in the haemolytic uraemic syndrome of infancy. *Br. J. Haematol.* [Suppl.] 23: 53, 1972.

63. Monnens, L., and Schretlen, E.   Intravascular coagulation in an infant with the hemolytic-uremic syndrome. *Acta Paediatr. Uppsala* 56:430, 1967.

64. Monnens, L., Kleynen, F., Van Munster, P., Schretlen, E., and Bonnerma, A.   Coagulation studies and streptokinase therapy in the haemolytic uraemic syndrome. *Helv. Paediatr. Acta* 27:45, 1972.

65. Mota Hernandez, F., and Gordillo Paniagua, G. Microangiopatia trombótica renal. *Bol. Med. Hosp. Infant. (Mexico)* 21:691, 1964.

66. Piel, C.   Hemolytic uremic syndrome. *Pediatr. Clin. North Am.* 13:295, 1966.

67. Powell, H. R., and Ekert, H.   Streptokinase and anti-thrombotic therapy in the hemolytic-uremic syndrome. *J. Pediatr.* 84:345, 1974.

68. Proesmans, W., and Eeckels, R.   Heparin and the hemolytic uremic syndrome. *J. Pediatr.* 85:142, 1974.

69. Ramon-Guerra, A. V.   Sindrome hemolítico-urémico. *Arch. Pediatr. Urug.* 36:26, 1965.

70. Ray, C. G., Tucker, V. L., Harris, D. J., Cuppage, F. E., and Chin, T. D. Y.   Enteroviruses associated with the hemolytic uremic syndrome. *Pediatrics* 46: 377, 1970.

71. Robertson, S. E. J.   Hemolytic anemia associated with acute glomerulonephritis in infancy. *Med. J. Aust.* 2:686, 1957.

72. Rodriguez Erdmann, F.   Bleeding due to increased intravascular coagulation. *N. Engl. J. Med.* 273:1370, 1965.

73. Sajičk, M., and Pelikan, L.   Haemolytic-uremic syndrome. *Cesk. Pediatr.* 14:504, 1959.

74. Sanchez Avalos, J., Vitacco, M., Molinas, F., Peñalver, J., and Gianantonio, C. A.   Coagulation studies in the hemolytic uremic syndrome. *J. Pediatr.* 76:538, 1970.

75. Shumway, C. N., Jr., and Miller, G.   An unusual syndrome of hemolytic anemia, thrombocytopenic purpura and renal disease. *Blood* 12:1045, 1957.

76. Shumway, C., and Terplan, K.   Hemolytic anemia, thrombocytopenia, and renal disease in childhood. The hemolytic-uremic syndrome. *Pediatr. Clin. North Am.* 11:577, 1964.

77. Skinton, N. K., Galpine, J. F., Kendall, A. C., and Williams, H. P.   Haemolytic anemia in acute renal disease. *Arch. Dis. Child.* 39:455, 1964.

78. Stuart, J., Winterborn, M. H., White, R. H. R., and Flinn, R. M.   Thrombolytic therapy in the haemolytic-uraemic syndrome. *Br. Med. J.* 3:217, 1974.

78a. Thomson, P. D., and Kaplan, B. S.   The treatment of the hemolytic-uremic syndrome (HUS). *Pediatr. Res.* 9:380, 1975.

79. Tune, B. M., Groshong, E., Plumer, L. B., and Mendoza, S. A.   The hemolytic uremic syndrome in siblings: A prospective survey. *J. Pediatr.* 85:682, 1974.

80. Tune, B. M., Leavitt, T. J., and Gribble, T. J.   The hemolytic uremic syndrome in California: A review of 28 non-heparinized cases with long-term follow-up. *J. Pediatr.* 82:304, 1973.

81. Umlas, J., and Kaiser, J.   Thrombohemolytic thrombocytopenic purpura. *Am. J. Med.* 49:723, 1970.

82. Uttley, W. S.   Serum levels of fibrin/fibrinogen degradation products in the haemolytic-uremic syndrome. *Arch. Dis. Child.* 45:587, 1970.

83. Vildosola, S. M. J., Bravo, R. I., and Emparanza, S. E.   Sindrome hemolítico-urémico en la infancia. *Pediatria (Napoli)* 5:292, 1962.

84. Vitacco, M., Sanchez Avalos, J., and Gianantonio, C. A.   Heparin therapy in the hemolytic-uremic syndrome. *J. Pediatr.* 83:271, 1973.

85. Vitsky, B., Suzuki, Y., Strauss, L., and Churg, J. The hemolytic-uremic syndrome. *Am. J. Pathol.* 57: 627, 1969.

85a. Wardle, E. N.   Radio-fibrinogen catabolism and fibrin products for the assessment of renal disease. *Nephron* 18:193, 1977.

86. Wehinger, H., and Künzer, W.   Hämolytisch-urämische syndrom. *Klin. Wochenschr.* 47:445, 1969.

87. World Health Organization.   Arboviruses and Human Disease. W.H.O. Technical Report Series. No. 369. Geneva, 1967, p. 83.

88. Willoughby, M. L. N., Murphy, A. V., McMorris, S., and Jewell, F. G.   Coagulation studies in haemolytic uraemic syndrome. *Arch. Dis. Child.* 47:766, 1972.

89. Zanesco, L.   Sindrome emolitica thrombocitopenica con nefropatia. *Minerva Pediatr.* 15:1317, 1963.

57. Pulmonary Hemorrhage and Glomerulonephritis (Goodpasture's Syndrome)

Edmund J. Lewis

The syndrome of pulmonary alveolar hemorrhage and progressive glomerulonephritis is a distinct entity that often has an acute onset of frightening severity. The original description was made in the course of Goodpasture's detailed analysis of the etiology and pathology of pulmonary lesions found in patients dying during the 1918 "swine influenza" pandemic [32]. One patient in this series was an 18-year-old male who had an apparently typical influenzal illness. After a brief hospitalization, the patient continued to complain of a cough and weight loss. He died 1 month later with hemoptysis. At postmortem examination gross pulmonary hemorrhage, proliferative glomerulonephritis, and vascular lesions in the intestine and spleen were described. The findings in this patient attracted little attention, and the significance of Goodpasture's description remained obscure for decades. The concurrence of hemorrhagic lung disease and glomerulonephritis was once again described in 1955 by Parkin et al. [61]. Stanton and Tange were aware of Goodpasture's description and recommended the currently accepted eponymic designation [8, 73]. Synonyms include pulmonary hemorrhage with glomerulonephritis, lung purpura with nephritis, hemorrhagic pulmonary-renal syndrome, pulmonary hemosiderosis with glomerulonephritis, and hemorrhagic and interstitial pneumonitis with nephritis.

In 1967 a major advance in the understanding of the role of the humoral immune response in the pathogenesis of glomerulonephritis was achieved when Lerner et al. observed that patients with Goodpasture's syndrome had deposits of anti–glomerular basement membrane antibodies (anti-GBM) in their glomeruli [44]. This first insight into the pathogenesis of the glomerular lesion of Goodpasture's syndrome provided an immunologic test that relieved much of the diagnostic confusion surrounding this condition. The presence of anti-GBM antibody deposits on the renal glomeruli effectively differentiates patients with Goodpasture's syndrome from those with other diseases that also cause coexistent renal and pulmonary disease, such as systemic lupus erythematosus, polyarteritis nodosa, Wegener's granulomatosis, disseminated intravascular coagulation, essential cryoglobulinemia, and other forms of glomerulonephritis associated with pulmonary edema or pulmonary infarction. Patients with pulmonary hemorrhage and immunologically mediated glomerular disease associated with immune complex deposits therefore do not fall within the diagnostic rubric of Goodpasture's syndrome.

The diagnosis of Goodpasture's syndrome rests upon the demonstration of (1) glomerulonephritis, (2) pulmonary alveolar hemorrhage, and (3) evidence of the glomerular deposition of anti-GBM antibodies. Many reports antedate the use of immunologic techniques to confirm the presence of anti-GBM antibodies, and therefore literature on the subject of the pulmonary hemorrhage-glomerulonephritis syndromes must be interpreted with caution.

Clinical Features

The syndrome has been reported in patients ranging in age from 16 to 60 years, with a mean age of onset in the twenties. There is clearly a predisposition in males, the prevalence ratio in various series ranging from 3 : 1 to 10 : 1 [7, 40, 64, 79]. The majority of patients present with pulmonary symptoms. A cough and scanty hemoptysis may be accompanied by dyspnea. However, while hemoptysis is often scanty and intermittent, it can also be massive, life-threatening, or fatal. The radiologic findings reveal diffuse, powdery, and nodular opacifications of the air spaces characteristic of alveolar consolidation. The nodular infiltrates are usually bilateral and tend to become confluent in the hilar areas. The functional effect of extensive alveolar hemorrhage is to cause the lung to become noncompliant; hence pulmonary function tests reveal evidence of restricted ventilation during periods of active hemorrhage. There is often impaired respiratory gas exchange with arterial hypoxemia. In addition, a respiratory alkalosis occurs due to a dysjunction of alveolar ventilation and perfusion characteristics and hyperpnea. Prussian-blue staining of sputum cytology may reveal iron-laden macrophages (siderophages).

The alveolar hemorrhages may be extensive despite little or no hemoptysis early in the course of the disease. As a result of the quantity of blood lost in the parenchyma of the lung, a profound iron-deficient, microcytic-hypochromic anemia is a striking feature of the illness [7, 64]. Several radioisotopic techniques have been employed as investigative techniques to document active pulmonary hemorrhage in these patients. Benoit et al. utilized a radioiron ferrokinetic technique in order to measure pulmonary sequestration of red blood cells [7]. Ewan et al. showed that the pulmonary uptake of radioactive carbon monoxide (^{15}CO) was increased and the clearance rate of ^{15}CO from the lungs was decreased as the result of the sequestered hemoglobin within the alveoli [27b]. Neither of these radioisotopic techniques are generally available in the clinic, however, and evidence of massive pulmonary hemorrhage usually rests upon the clinical documentation of hemoptysis, iron-deficiency anemia, and siderophages in the sputum.

The loss of blood into pulmonary alveoli during periods of active disease causes a markedly shortened radiochromium (^{59}Cr) labeled red cell half-life. This finding is due to pulmonary sequestration and is often mistaken for, and must be differentiated from, a shortened red cell life span due to a hemolytic process.

Evidence of pulmonary disease usually precedes

or is noted concomitant with clinical abnormalities [7, 40, 79]. Goodpasture's syndrome can also present as mild to severe glomerulonephritis, with the development of clinical pulmonary abnormalities later in the course of the disease [79]. Proteinuria, while often lacking early in the course of the disease, becomes manifest at some stage in virtually every patient and may be so profound as to cause the nephrotic syndrome [9]. Microscopic hematuria with red blood cell casts is also noted as the disease progresses. Severe hematuria may cause the patient to note a darkened color of the urine; however, gross hematuria is rare.

Clinical manifestations other than those attributable to the effects of severe renal or pulmonary disease are uncommon. The older literature contains numerous cases in which arthritis, arthralgias, or myalgias were clinical problems; however, these complaints were noted almost exclusively in patients with pathologic evidence of arteritis. It is likely that many of these older cases represented polyarteritis nodosa with pulmonary hemorrhage and glomerulonephritis [40].

Abnormalities of the optic fundi have been noted in as many as 11 percent of patients with Goodpasture's syndrome [38, 64]. These changes generally have been attributed to acute or severe hypertension, although one report suggests that retinal detachment may not be merely secondary to changes in the blood pressure of uremic patients. Studies of the choroid of two patients revealed the deposition of anti–basement membrane antibodies along Bruch's membrane analogous to the immune phenomenon in lung and kidney [38]. As there is evidence in an experimental model that immunization with choroid plexus can cause the development of anti-GBM antibodies, this latter clinical phenomenon may indeed be a specific finding [54].

Etiology and Pathogenesis

In view of the circumstances of Goodpasture's original description, it is relevant to consider the possibility of an infectious etiology. The report of occasional "mini-epidemics" of Goodpasture's syndrome is compatible with this possibility [62]. Nondescript viral-like illnesses and upper respiratory infections have been noted to precede the onset of the syndrome in a significant proportion of patients; however, the diagnosis of a specific antecedent infection is rare. Wilson and Dixon reported a review of 32 patients in whom the complaint of sore throat or respiratory infection was noted in 44 percent and a flulike syndrome in 17 percent [79]. Wilson and Smith described a

patient with Goodpasture's syndrome and anti-GBM antibodies whose serum influenza A2 titers rose during the disease, while other viral titers remained normal [80]. The role that influenza viral infection may have played in the latter patient's clinical problems was only inferential. Etiologic and epidemiologic factors other than viral illness have also been considered. An exposure to petroleum products appeared to be a common risk factor in one series; however, the significance of this report remains speculative [3].

The infectious and toxic etiologic factors hypothesized to be capable of triggering Goodpasture's syndrome have failed to explain the reason for the development of anti-GBM antibodies. The proposed mechanisms that may be capable of initiating the development of anti-GBM antibodies are reviewed in Chaps. 3, 48. The pathogenetic role of anti-GBM antibodies in the glomerular lesion appears established. Because of the in vitro cross-reactivity of antibodies eluted from glomeruli with alveolar and glomerular basement membrane antigens, a unitary explanation has been developed to explain the pathogenetic process in both lung and kidney. Deposits of immunoglobulin have been observed in alveolar septa, and anti-GBM antibody has been eluted from affected lung parenchyma [5, 43, 50, 56]. Immunoglobulins eluted from both lung and kidney have been shown to have similar or identical activity against tissue antigens, with a broader specificity than anti-GBM antibodies obtained from those patients with rapidly progressive glomerulonephritis who have no pulmonary lesions [56a]. Despite this in vitro evidence, however, investigators have been unable to reproduce the pulmonary lesion in vivo using antibody of human origin. The inability to induce alveolar lesions in squirrel monkeys by the intravenous injection of anti-GBM antibodies may be due to the preferential in vivo fixation of the antibody to glomeruli [56a]. Although pulmonary and renal lesions have been produced in experimental animals using heterologous antiserum against alveolar basement membrane antigens [56b], the search for additional mechanisms of pulmonary damage in these patients continues, since the disruption of the functional continuity of the alveolar wall is presently unexplained.

Pathology

Pulmonary Findings

Histologic examination of the alveoli in Goodpasture's syndrome reveals large amounts of red cells and iron-laden macrophages in alveolar spaces. The alveolar septa usually appear normal or congested. It is unusual to find necrosis or inflammation of the alveolar wall, although this has been described [79]. Bronchial arterioles are usually normal, although vasculitis has been described in a number of cases. Immunofluorescence microscopy has been performed in several cases, and the results have been variable [5, 43, 50, 56, 67, 74]. Immunoglobulin G has been found in a linear and segmental linear pattern within the alveolar wall in some cases [5, 43, 50, 56, 74, 75], with negative results for IgG and C3 being found in others [24, 67]. Donald et al. described fragmentation of the alveolar basement membrane, gaps between endothelial cells, and platelet occlusion of capillaries [23]. A broad experience in the electron microscopy of the lung in Goodpasture's syndrome has not yet been accrued.

Renal Findings

Light microscopy of the established renal lesion is identical to that described for rapidly progressive glomerulonephritis (Chap. 48). Early glomerular involvement is characteristically focal and segmental with necrosis of the tuft. However, more advanced lesions are characterized by diffuse proliferation in the glomerular tuft and abundant crescent formation. When the lesion of the glomerular tuft is advanced, multinucleated giant cells can be found. Accumulation of periglomerular lymphoid cells is often a striking histologic feature.

Because hemoptysis may antedate clinical renal disease by months, a renal biopsy may be performed at a relatively early stage of the glomerular lesion. At this stage glomerular histology may be normal, although immunofluorescence microscopy and electron microscopy are abnormal, as described below [19, 23, 52].

Linear deposition of IgG is noted along the glomerular basement membrane in the typical pattern for anti-GBM antibodies [24, 44, 79]. Immunoglobulin M may be present in a linear or segmental linear pattern. Other immunoglobulins are usually absent. Complement components have been found quite variably. Component C3 has been absent in up to 20 percent of specimens [79]; when present, it may be distributed in a linear fashion or in an interrupted, segmental linear pattern. Fibrin is found in the glomerular crescents.

As noted in Chap. 48, there are no consistent lesions associated with anti-GBM antibody-induced injury. Gaps or defects in the continuity in the GBM may be noted. Dense osmiophilic changes in the basement membranes have been described in Goodpasture's syndrome [63]. Expansion of the lamina rara interna to form an electron-lucent subendothelial zone has been noted in some cases.

Differentiation of Goodpasture's Syndrome from Other Entities with Pulmonary Hemorrhage

The differential diagnosis of Goodpasture's syndrome is summarized in Table 57-1.

Idiopathic Pulmonary Hemosiderosis

Idiopathic pulmonary hemosiderosis (IPH) is seen primarily in the pediatric age group, usually in patients less than 7 years old [71]. It can occur, however, in young adults. There is no sex predilection. The differential diagnosis between IPH and Goodpasture's syndrome can be extremely difficult, insofar as pulmonary hemorrhage usually precedes the glomerulonephritis [19, 23, 52, 79]. There are now several reports of patients presenting with pulmonary hemorrhage with an apparent diagnosis of pulmonary hemosiderosis; these patients had linear deposition of IgG along the glomerular basement membrane despite normal renal function and normal glomerular histology [19, 23, 52]. Presumably these patients represent the earliest stage of the glomerulitis of Goodpasture's syndrome.

There has been little agreement regarding a characteristic alveolar histologic lesion in the lungs of patients with IPH [23, 31, 37, 71]. Several studies have shown ultrastructurally normal lung. Abnormalities that have been noted include fragmentation of elastic fibers, fracture of the capillary membrane, and duplication of the structure of the capillary basement membrane. Fibrils, presumably collagen, have been described within the basement membrane. Immunoglobulin deposition has not been noted.

Laboratory tests other than the demonstration of serum anti-GBM activity in Goodpasture's syndrome are not of differential diagnostic value. Cold agglutinins have been described in IPH [70], and the titer was reported in one instance to vary with disease activity [71]. Iron deficiency anemia may occur. These patients can hemorrhage as much as 11 percent of their total blood volume into the lung in a single day [35].

There is therefore little to differentiate between IPH and Goodpasture's syndrome in their earliest stages. Anti–glomerular basement membrane antibodies diagnostic of Goodpasture's syndrome may be consistently or intermittently undetectable in the circulation. While immunofluorescent microscopy for alveolar immunoglobulin deposits has been reported to be positive in Goodpasture's syndrome, negative findings have been noted in some patients, and focal immunoglobulin deposits have been described in others [5, 43, 50, 56, 67]. Therefore, while the finding of immunoglobulins

Table 57-1. Differential Diagnosis of Goodpasture's Syndrome

Goodpasture's & Other Entities	Age Predilection	Serum Anti-GBM	Serum Anti-DNA	Cold Agglutinins	Cryoglobulins	Serum Complement	Immunofluorescence	
							Lung	Kidney
Goodpasture's syndrome	3rd decade	+	−	−	±	Normal	Focal linear IgG in alveolar walls	Linear IgG along GBM
Idiopathic pulmonary hemosiderosis	1st decade	−	−	+	−	Normal	Negative	Negative
Immune complex glomerulonephritis and pulmonary hemorrhage	None	−	−	+	±	Low or normal	Unknown	Granular IgG
Systemic lupus erythematosus	2nd–3rd decade	−	+	+	+	Low	Granular IgG in alveolar walls	Mesangial and granular IgG
Disseminated intravascular coagulation	None	−	−	−	−	Normal	Unknown	Fibrin in capillaries
Essential mixed cryoglobulinemia	None	−	−	−	+	Low	Negative in one case	Granular[b] IgG, IgM
Polyarteritis nodosa	4th decade	±[a]	−	−	±	Normal	Unknown	Variable, often negative

Note: + = common manifestation; ± = unusual manifestations; − = usually negative; GBM = glomerular basement membrane.
[a] Low titer, low affinity antibodies [49].
[b] IgG-IgM deposits have been described in the reports of essential cryoglobulinemia although there was no immunoglobulin deposit in the one reported patient with cryoglobulins associated with pulmonary hemorrhage and glomerulonephritis [51].

on the alveolar basement membrane speaks strongly in favor of Goodpasture's syndrome, negative findings are not helpful.

The diagnostic procedure that differentiates best between IPH and Goodpasture's syndrome is the renal biopsy. The finding of linear IgG along the GBM, possibly with histologic features of necrotizing or proliferative glomerulonephritis, establishes the diagnosis of Goodpasture's syndrome. Renal biopsy may be indicated, therefore, in a patient without clinical evidence of renal disease. The establishment of the diagnosis of Goodpasture's syndrome at the earliest stages of the disease can be important in the light of reports of effective therapeutic programs, particularly with respect to plasmapheresis in conjunction with immunosuppressive therapy [46, 47, 66].

Pulmonary Hemorrhage and Glomerulonephritis with Immune Complex Disease
A number of patients with clinically demonstrable pulmonary hemorrhage and glomerulonephritis have had no evidence of anti-GBM antibodies [4,

16, 17a, 45, 51]. Several cases have been reported in which the pathogenesis of the glomerular lesion appeared to be due to immune complex deposition [45, 51]. The concept that acute immune complex deposition could be responsible for acute alveolar damage as well as glomerulonephritis was established in experimental serum sickness by Gregory and Rich in 1946 [34]. Brentjens et al. confirmed that immune complexes may deposit within the alveolar capillary wall [11]. It is likely that an analogous lesion occurs in certain clinical situations [27a, 33].

There appears to be a variant of systemic lupus erythematosus that falls into this group of immune complex diseases. Immune complex-associated glomerulonephritis and pulmonary hemorrhage in these patients is associated with antinuclear antibodies, although anti-DNA antibodies may not be detectable in serum. Cold agglutinins and cryoglobulins have also been noted. The immunohistology of the glomeruli reveals granular deposits suggesting immune complex-mediated systemic disease [45, 60].

One patient has been reported with essential cryoglobulinemia and a similar clinical constellation [51]. While the presence of cryoglobulins in serum was demonstrated and presumed to represent immune complexes, no immunoglobulins were demonstrated in lung or kidney. The immunopathogenesis of the organ lesions was unexplained.

Systemic Lupus Erythematosus
The presentation of systemic lupus erythematosus (SLE) as pulmonary hemorrhage and glomerulonephritis is relatively rare, but it has been described in several patients [13, 27a, 33]. Since the usual skin and joint manifestations can be absent in these patients, the diagnosis on clinical grounds alone may be difficult. Typical serologic abnormalities of SLE usually are present. Lupus cell preparations, antinuclear antibodies, anti-DNA antibodies, and serum complement levels may all help in the differentiation of these syndromes. Cold agglutinins have been noted in SLE [78], but the significance of cold agglutinins in the pulmonary hemorrhage syndromes of idiopathic pulmonary hemosiderosis and SLE is not known. The reason for the genesis of this autoantibody in these disorders similarly is unclear. Anti-GBM antibodies have not been among the autoimmune antibodies described in the serum of patients with SLE, and so their presence provides a differential serologic feature.

Renal biopsy in SLE may reveal glomerular abnormalities on light microscopy similar to those noted in Goodpasture's syndrome. However, electron microscopy in SLE often reveals mesangial and subendothelial electron-dense deposits as well as endothelial cell tubuloreticular inclusions that are often referred to as myxovirus-like particles. The fluorescence microscopic examination in lupus may demonstrate immunoglobulin deposits in peripheral capillary loops or mesangium or both. It should be noted that in rare instances, biopsy specimens from SLE patients have had linear immunofluorescence of IgG without C3 along the basement membrane. In these latter cases there is no evidence that this deposit has anti-GBM antibody activity [42].

Biopsy of the lung in patients with SLE who have had pulmonary hemorrhage has revealed deposits of granules of IgG along the alveolar capillary wall [33], and electron microscopy of the lung may show electron-dense deposits [27a]. Some of the deposits have the organized "fingerprint" pattern, associated with DNA–anti-DNA aggregates, which has also been described in the renal deposits in this disease [27a].

Disseminated Intravascular Coagulation
A pulmonary hemorrhage syndrome has been described in disseminated intravascular coagulation [17b, 57]. As these patients may also have renal microvascular involvement by the coagulopathy, they can present a pulmonary-renal syndrome requiring differentiation. The primary diseases underlying intravascular coagulation in the reported patients have generally been neoplastic [57]. Clinically these patients have had dyspnea, chest pain, and a pleural friction rub accompanying the hemoptysis, and the entity may be confused with pulmonary infarction. Pulmonary hemorrhage was reported to be the cause of death in four of five patients with this manifestation of neoplasia-related disseminated intravascular coagulation [57].

Vasculitis Associated with Pulmonary Hemorrhage and Glomerulonephritis
Respiratory manifestations can precede other systemic manifestations of polyarteritis nodosa and can be associated with glomerulonephritis as well [12, 14–16, 25, 65]. Rose and Spencer [65] reported 32 patients with respiratory symptoms, 13 of whom had hemoptysis. Two of the 13 patients with hemoptysis died of massive hemorrhages. Reports in the literature that preceded the identification of anti-GBM antibodies often described vasculitis as a histologic feature of the pulmonary hemorrhage–glomerulonephritis ("Goodpasture's") syndrome. Undoubtedly many of these cases represented instances of polyarteritis nodosa [18, 40]. In addition to the lung and renal manifestations, joint and muscle symptoms were prominent in these patients [16, 40]. While low-affinity anti-GBM antibodies have been reported to be present in polyarteritis nodosa [49], linear glomerular deposits have not been described. The renal histologic lesions in polyarteritis nodosa present the same spectrum as in Goodpasture's syndrome, varying from a focal, segmental glomerulitis to a diffuse, crescentic, proliferative lesion. There are many similarities between anti-GBM antibody–mediated glomerulonephritis and polyarteritis nodosa (Chap. 48). Glomerular immunoglobulin deposits, when present in polyarteritis nodosa, are often segmental and granular. Florid histologic glomerular lesions may have negative immunofluorescence results.

Other forms of vasculitis also enter into the differential diagnosis. Hypersensitivity angiitis may be confused with Goodpasture's syndrome, as pulmonary hemorrhage and rapidly progressive glomerulonephritis can occur. Sulfonamide hypersensitivity has been suspected as the cause in one case of hypersensitivity angiitis [29]. Wegener's granulomatosis usually presents with upper and lower respiratory symptomatology [28], and while frank pulmonary hemorrhage is not characteristic of the syndrome, hemoptysis can occur and can be accompanied by typical x-ray findings of alveolar hemorrhage [30, 39]. Biopsy of nasal sinus or pulmonary tissue may be diagnostic in Wegener's syndrome. The renal lesion of Wegener's syndrome is a segmental or diffuse necrotizing glomerulonephritis [28]. Glomerular immunoglobulin deposition is focal, segmental, and readily differentiated from the pattern of anti-GBM–mediated disease.

Schönlein-Henoch purpura has rarely been reported to cause pulmonary hemorrhage [81]. The major vasculitic manifestations of this syndrome are in the kidney, skin, joints, and intestine. While the differential diagnosis between Goodpasture's syndrome and instances of vasculitis can be difficult, differentiation from classic Schönlein-Henoch purpura should present little problem.

Clinical Course and Therapy

Although Goodpasture's syndrome has the well-deserved reputation of being an acute and fulminant disease that leads to pulmonary or renal failure within months after onset, a broad spectrum of clinical courses actually has been described. Reports of apparent response to therapy [20, 22, 36, 46, 68], prolonged survival [2, 20, 52, 53, 72, 75], and spontaneous remission [72] all emphasize the unpredictability of the natural history of Goodpasture's syndrome in a given patient.

The classically described course begins with either pulmonary symptomatology or the simultaneous onset of pulmonary and renal disease [64]. In their summary of 32 cases, Wilson and Dixon describe a pulmonary onset in about one-third of the patients and simultaneous onset of pulmonary and renal disease in an equal number of cases [79]. In those patients with a pulmonary onset of disease, clinical evidence of renal disease usually became manifest in less than 3 months; however in unusual cases this was delayed for a year or more [79]. The renal lesion often progressed rapidly, and the mean time to the requirement of maintenance dialysis was $3\frac{1}{2}$ months (range, <1 to 14 months). When death was caused by respiratory failure due to massive pulmonary hemorrhage, it occurred within 4 months of the initial symptoms [79]. When the initial clinical manifestations were renal, pulmonary symptoms were generally manifest within a 3-month period.

Despite the overall poor prognosis of Goodpasture's syndrome, there is considerable variability in the course in a given patient, and it is thus difficult to evaluate the effect of therapy. Corticosteroids have been widely used, and many uncontrolled therapeutic observations have been reported. The pulmonary hemorrhages appear to be improved in patients receiving steroids [22, 79]. In some instances the apparent cessation of pulmonary hemorrhage with high-dose steroid therapy has been reported to be dramatic [4, 22]. There is little to suggest that the course of the glomerular lesion is altered by steroids [79]. Immunosuppressive drugs, including azathioprine [68, 79], 6-mercaptopurine [68, 79], cyclophosphamide [79], and nitrogen mustard [20], have been reported to be of benefit in individual cases; however, there are many documented failures of the use of these agents [79]. Anticoagulants, while possibly of value in the therapy of extracapillary glomerulonephritis [59, 76, 77] (see Chap. 48), are usually considered a danger to patients with active pulmonary hemorrhage.

One contemporary approach to therapy has been the use of plasmapheresis in conjunction with steroid and alkylating agent therapy [46, 47, 66]. Plasma exchanges have been reported to decrease serum anti-GBM titers and promote concomitant improvement in the clinical picture, particularly with regard to the lung disease [47]. This combination of the physical removal of antibody with a drug-induced suppression of antibody synthesis may achieve decreased anti-GBM–mediated injury in patients with Goodpasture's syndrome. In addition to this specific immune suppressive mechanism, the removal of mediators of tissue damage such as complement components and coagulation proteins may also be involved in the response to plasmapheresis. While the mechanism of the reported effectiveness of the procedure remains unclear, the ease of the procedure, and the reported beneficial effects all make plasmapheresis an attractive form of therapy. Further experience by more investigators, hopefully using controlled trials, will undoubtedly provide valuable information on this subject.

Spontaneous remission is rare, but it has been noted in several patients with Goodpasture's syndrome. Characteristically these patients have had a mild pulmonary onset of disease with very little renal involvement [2, 20, 68, 79]. Recovery has been reported to follow severe renal damage and anuria in a patient diagnosed prior to the use of immune diagnostic techniques [58].

Bilateral nephrectomy has been associated with a prompt, dramatic cessation of massive pulmonary hemorrhage in some patients [48, 69, 70, 79]. While the explanation of this phenomenon is not clear, the numerous reports of this effect of nephrectomy often makes the procedure a serious consideration when life-threatening hemorrhage and pulmonary insufficiency are present. It should be noted, however, that numerous patients have undergone bilateral nephrectomy with no apparent benefits [26, 79]. The judgment of whether and when to consider bilateral nephrectomy in a given patient is therefore complicated and difficult. It is recommended only when other therapeutic measures, including plasmapheresis and a steroid-immunosuppression regimen, have failed to alter the progression of the disease and there is life-threatening pulmonary hemorrhage.

Patients with established renal failure have been treated by hemodialysis and transplantation [21]. While the recurrent deposition of anti-GBM antibody in the allograft with consequent severe glomerulonephritis has been reported [6], good transplant results have been achieved in several patients [79]. Transplantation carried out several months after the initiation of hemodialysis, at a time when serum anti-GBM levels are undetectable, appears to afford the greatest opportunity for the avoidance of recurrent glomerulonephritis. Allograft biopsies in the latter group of patients have been reported to be negative [79]. Allografts in some patients with anti-GBM–mediated rapidly progressive glomerulonephritis (not Goodpasture's syndrome) have also been reported to show little or no evidence of recurrent glomerulonephritis, despite the deposition of anti-GBM [21]. The latter response may be explained by a low titer of antibody, or conversely, it is possible that less pathogenic antibodies may form at a later stage of disease. In view of the reported effective results, renal transplantation in the appropriate circumstances is an acceptable therapy in patients whose renal failure is due to Goodpasture's syndrome.

References

1. Agodoa, L. C. Y., Striker, G. E., George, C. R. P., Glassock, R., and Quadracci, L. J. The appearance of nonlinear deposits of immunoglobulins in Goodpasture's syndrome. *Am. J. Med.* 61:407, 1976.
2. Azen, E. A., and Clatanoff, D. V. Prolonged survival of Goodpasture's syndrome. *Arch. Intern. Med.* 114:453, 1964.
3. Beirne, G. J., and Brennan, J. T. Glomerulonephritis associated with hydrocarbon solvents: Mediated by antiglomerular basement membrane antibody. *Arch. Environ. Health* 25:365, 1972.
4. Beirne, G. J., Kopp, W. L., and Zimmerman, S. W. Goodpasture's syndrome: Dissociation from antibodies to glomerular basement membrane. *Arch. Intern. Med.* 132:261, 1973.
5. Beirne, G. J., Octaviano, G. N., Kopp, W. L., and Burns, R. O. Immunohistology of the lung in Goodpasture's syndrome. *Ann. Intern. Med.* 69:1207, 1968.
6. Beliel, O. M., Coburn, J. W., Shinaberger, J. H., and Glassock, R. J. Recurrent glomerulonephritis due to anti-glomerular basement membrane antibodies in two successive allografts. *Clin. Nephrol.* 1:377, 1973.
7. Benoit, F. L., Rulon, D. B., Theil, G. B., Doolan, P. D., and Watten, R. H. Goodpasture's syndrome: A clinicopathologic entity. *Ann. Intern. Med.* 37:424, 1964.
8. Bialestock, D., and Tange, J. D. Acute necrotizing glomerulonephritis: The clinical features and pathology in nine cases. *Australas. Ann. Med.* 8:281, 1959.
9. Bloom, V. R., Wayne, D. J., and Wrong, O. L. Lung purpura and nephritis (Goodpasture's syndrome) complicated by the nephrotic syndrome. *Ann. Intern. Med.* 63:750, 1965.
10. Brannan, H. M., McCaughey, W. T. E., and Good, C. A. Roentgenographic appearance of pulmonary hemorrhage associated with glomerulonephritis. *Ann. J. Roentgenol.* 90:83, 1963.
11. Brentjens, J. R., O'Connell, D. W., Pawlowski, I. B., Hsu, K. C., and Andres, G. A. Experimental immune complex disease of the lung: The pathogenesis of a laboratory model resembling certain human interstitial lung diseases. *J. Exp. Med.* 140:105, 1974.
12. Brewer, A. J., Kennedy, R. L. J., and Edwards, J. E. Recurrent pulmonary hemorrhage with hemosiderosis: So-called idiopathic pulmonary hemosiderosis. *Am. J. Roentgenol.* 76:98, 1976.
13. Byrd, R. B., and Trunk, G. Systemic lupus erythematosus presenting as pulmonary hemosiderosis. *Chest* 64:128, 1973.
14. Clinicopathologic Conference: A variant of periarteritis nodosa. *Bull. N. Engl. Med. Center* 15:161, 1953.
15. Clinicopathologic Conference, Barnes Hospital. Joint pains, anemia, neuropathy, fever, convulsions and blindness. *Am. J. Med.* 18:335, 1955.
16. Clinicopathologic Conference, Barnes Hospital. Unclassified pulmonary-renal syndrome. *Am. J. Med.* 45:933, 1958.
17a. Clinicopathologic Conference, Barnes Hospital. Proliferative glomerulonephritis and pulmonary hemorrhage. *Am. J. Med.* 55:199, 1973.
17b. Clinicopathologic Conference, Barnes Hospital. Pulmonary hemorrhage and renal failure. *Am. J. Med.* 60:397, 1976.
18. Clinicopathological Conference, Hammersmith Hospital. Polyarteritis or glomerulonephritis? *Postgrad. Med.* 30:35, 1954.
19. Clinicopathological Conference, Massachusetts General Hospital. Hemoptysis and severe dyspnea in a 19-year-old woman. *N. Engl. J. Med.* 294:944, 1976.
20. Couser, W. G. Goodpasture's syndrome: A response to nitrogen mustard. *Am. J. Med. Sci.* 268:175, 1974.
21. Couser, W. G., Wallace, A., Monaco, A. P., and Lewis, E. J. Successful renal transplantation in patients with circulating antibody to glomerular basement membrane: Report of 2 cases. *Clin. Nephrol.* 1:381, 1973.
22. de Torrente, A., Popovitzer, M. M., Guggenheim, S. J., and Schrier, R. W. Serious pulmonary hemorrhage, glomerulonephritis, and massive steroid therapy. *Ann. Intern. Med.* 83:218, 1975.
23. Donald, K. J., Edwards, R. L., and McEvoy, J. D. S. Alveolar capillary basement membrane lesions in

Goodpasture's syndrome and idiopathic pulmonary hemosiderosis. *Am. J. Med.* 59:642, 1975.

24. Duncan, D. A., Drummond, K. N., Michael, A. F., and Vernier, R. L. Pulmonary hemorrhage and glomerulonephritis: Report of six cases and study of the renal lesion by the fluorescent antibody technique and electron microscopy. *Ann. Intern. Med.* 62:920, 1965.

25. Edwards, J. E., Parkin, T. W., and Burchell, H. B. Recurrent hemoptysis and necrotizing pulmonary alveolitis in a patient with acute glomerulonephritis and periarteritis nodosa. *Mayo Clin. Proc.* 29:193, 1954.

26. Eisinger, A. J. Goodpasture's syndrome: Failure of nephrectomy to cure pulmonary hemorrhage. *Am. J. Med.* 55:565, 1973.

27a. Elliott, M. L., and Kuhn, C. Idiopathic pulmonary hemosiderosis: Ultrastructural abnormalities in the capillary walls. *Am. Rev. Resp. Dis.* 102:895, 1970.

27b. Ewan, P. W., Jones, H. A., Rhodes, C. G., and Hughes, J. M. B. Detection of intrapulmonary hemorrhage in Goodpasture's syndrome. *N. Engl. J. Med.* 295:1391, 1976.

28. Fauci, A. S., and Wolff, S. M. Wegener's granulomatosis: Studies in eighteen patients and a review of the literature. *Medicine (Baltimore)* 52:535, 1973.

29. French, A. J. Hypersensitivity in pathogenesis of histopathologic changes associated with sulfonamide chemotherapy. *Am. J. Pathol.* 22:679, 1946.

30. Felson, B. *Chest Roentgenology* (rev. ed.). Philadelphia: Saunders, 1973. P. 303.

31. Gonzalez-Crussi, F., Hull, M. T., and Grosfeld, J. L. Idiopathic pulmonary hemosiderosis: Evidence of capillary basement membrane abnormality. *Am. Rev. Resp. Dis.* 114:689, 1976.

32. Goodpasture, E. W. The significance of certain pulmonary lesions in relation to the etiology of influenza. *Am. J. Med. Sci.* 158:863, 1919.

33. Gould, D. B., and Soriano, R. Z. Acute alveolar hemorrhage in lupus erythematosus. *Ann. Intern. Med.* 83:836, 1975.

34. Gregory, J. E., and Rich, A. R. The experimental production of anaphylactic pulmonary lesions with the basic characteristics of rheumatic pneumonitis. *Bull. Johns Hopkins Hosp.* 78:1, 1946.

35. Hamilton, H. E., Sheets, R. F., and Evans, T. C. Erythrocyte destruction in the lungs as the major cause for anemia in primary pulmonary hemosiderosis. *Proc. Cent. Soc. Clin. Res.* 33:44, 1960.

36. Hayslett, J. P., Berte, J. B., and Kashgarian, M. Successful treatment of renal failure in Goodpasture's syndrome. *Arch. Intern. Med.* 127:953, 1971.

37. Irwin, R. S., Cotrell, T. S., Hsu, K. C., Griswold, W. R., and Thomas, H. M., III. Idiopathic pulmonary hemosiderosis: An electron microscopic and immunofluorescent study. *Chest* 65:41, 1974.

38. Jampol, L. M., Lahav, M., Albert, D. M., and Craft, J.. Ocular clinical findings and basement membrane changes in Goodpasture's syndrome. *Am. J. Ophthalmol.* 79:452, 1975.

39. Johnson, J. R., and McGovern, V. J. Goodpasture's syndrome and Wegener's granulomatosis. *Australas. Ann. Med.* 11:250, 1962.

40. Jordan, W. P., Jr. Hemorrhagic pulmonary-renal syndrome. *N.C. Med. J.* 25:386, 1964.

41. Knight, V., Badger, T. L., Schulz, E., and Suskind, G. Recurrent pulmonary disease in a child: Clinicopathologic conference at the National Institutes of Health. *Ann. Intern. Med.* 53:556, 1960.

42. Koffler, D., Agnello, V., Carr, I., and Kunkel, H. G. Variable patterns of immunoglobulin and complement deposition in the kidneys of patients with systemic lupus erythematosus. *Am. J. Pathol.* 56:305, 1969.

43. Koffler, D., Sandson, J., Carr, I., and Kunkel, H. G. Immunologic studies concerning the pulmonary lesions in Goodpasture's syndrome. *Am. J. Pathol.* 54: 293, 1969.

44. Lerner, R., Glassock, R. J., and Dixon, F. J. The role of anti-glomerular basement membrane antibody in the pathogenesis of human glomerulonephritis. *J. Exp. Med.* 126:989, 1967.

45. Lewis, E. J., Schur, P. H., Busch, G. J., Galvanek, E., and Merrill, J. P. Immunopathologic features of a patient with glomerulonephritis and pulmonary hemorrhage. *Am. J. Med.* 54:507, 1973.

46. Lockwood, C. M., Boulton-Jones, J. M., Lowenthal, R. M., Simpson, I. J., Peters, D. K., and Wilson, C. B. Recovery from Goodpasture's syndrome after immunosuppressive treatment and plasmapheresis. *Br. Med. J.* 1:252, 1975.

47. Lockwood, C. M., Rees, A. J., Pearson, T. A., Evans, D. J., Peters, D. K., and Wilson, C. B. Immunosuppression and plasma exchange in the treatment of Goodpasture's syndrome. *Lancet* 1:711, 1976.

48. Maddock, R. K., Stevens, L. E., Reetsma, K., and Bloomer, H. A. Goodpasture's syndrome: Cessation of pulmonary hemorrhage after bilateral nephrectomy. *Ann. Intern. Med.* 67:1258, 1967.

49. Mahieu, P., Dardenne, M., and Bach, J. F. Detection of humoral and cell-mediated immunity to kidney basement membranes in human renal diseases. *Am. J. Med.* 53:185, 1972.

50. Markowitz, A. S., Battifora, H. A., Schwartz, F., and Aseron, C. Immunological aspects of Goodpasture's syndrome. *Clin. Exp. Immunol.* 3:585, 1968.

51. Martinez, J. S., and Kohler, P. F. Variant "Goodpasture's syndrome"? The need for immunologic criteria in rapidly progressive glomerulonephritis and hemorrhagic pneumonitis. *Ann. Intern. Med.* 75:67, 1971.

52. Mathew, T. H., Hobbs, J. B., Kalnoski, S., Sutherland, P. W., and Kincaid-Smith, P. Goodpasture's syndrome: Normal renal diagnostic findings. *Ann. Intern. Med.* 82:215, 1975.

53. McCall, C. B., Ham, T. R., and Hatch, F. E. Nonfatal pulmonary hemorrhage and glomerulonephritis. *Am. Rev. Resp. Dis.* 91:424, 1965.

54. McIntosh, R. W., Koss, M. N., Chernack, W. B., Griswold, W. R., Copack, P. B., and Weil, R. Experimental pulmonary disease and autoimmune nephritis in the rabbit produced by homologous and heterologous choroid plexus. *Proc. Soc. Exp. Biol. Med.* 147:216, 1974.

55. McPhaul, J. J., Jr., and Dixon, F. J. The presence of anti-glomerular basement membrane antibodies in peripheral blood. *J. Immunol.* 103:1168, 1969.

56a. McPhaul, J. J., Jr., and Dixon, F. J. Characterization of human anti-glomerular basement membrane antibodies eluted from glomerulonephritic kidneys. *J. Clin. Invest.* 49:308, 1970.

56b. Mercola, K. E., and Hagadorn, J. E. Complement dependant acute immunologic lung injury in an experimental model resembling Goodpasture's syndrome. *Exp. Mol. Pathol.* 19:230, 1973.

57. Minna, J. D., Robboy, S. J., and Colman, R. W. *Disseminated Intravascular Coagulation in Man.* Springfield, Ill.: Thomas, 1974. Pp. 78–85.

58. Munro, J. F., Geddes, A. M., and Lamb, W. L. Goodpasture's syndrome: Survival after acute renal failure. *Br. Med. J.* 4:95, 1967.

59. Naish, P., Penn, G. B., Evans, D. J., and Peters, D. K. The effect of defibrination in nephrotoxic serum nephritis in rabbits. *Clin. Sci.* 42:643, 1972.

60. O'Donohue, W. J., Jr. Idiopathic pulmonary hemosiderosis with manifestations of multiple connective tissue immune disorders: Treatment with cyclophosphamide. *Am. Rev. Resp. Dis.* 109:473, 1974.

61. Parkin, T. W., Rusted, I. E., Burchell, H. B., and Edwards, J. E. Hemorrhagic and interstitial pneumonitis with nephritis. *Am. J. Med.* 18:220, 1975.

62. Perez, G. O., Bjornsson, S., Roso, A. H., Amato, J., and Rothfield, N. A miniepidemic of Goodpasture's syndrome: Clinical and immunological studies. *Nephron* 13:161, 1974.

63. Poskitt, T. R. Immunologic and electron microscopic studies in Goodpasture's syndrome. *Am. J. Med.* 49:250, 1970.

64. Proskey, A. J., Weatherbee, L., Easterling, R. E., Greene, J. A., and Weller, J. M. Goodpasture's syndrome: A report of five cases and review of the literature. *Am. J. Med.* 48:162, 1970.

65. Rose, G. A., and Spencer, H. Polyarteritis nodosa. *Q. J. Med.* 26:43, 1957.

66. Rossen, R. D., Duffy, J., McCredie, K. B., Reisberg, M. A., Sharp, J. T., Herd, E. M., Eknoyan, G., and Suki, W. N. Treatment of Goodpasture's syndrome with cyclophosphamide, prednisone and plasma exchange transfusions. *Clin. Exp. Immunol.* 24:218, 1976.

67. Scheer, R. L., and Grossman, M. A. Immune aspects of the glomerulonephritis associated with pulmonary hemorrhage. *Ann. Intern. Med.* 60:1009, 1964.

68. Seaton, A., Meland, J. M., and Lapp, N. L. Remission of Goodpasture's syndrome: Report of two patients treated by immunosuppression and review of the literature. *Thorax* 26:683, 1971.

69. Shires, D. L., Pfaff, W. W., DeQuesada, A., Miller, G. H., and Cade, J. R. Pulmonary hemorrhage and glomerulonephritis: Treatment of two cases by bilateral nephrectomy and renal transplantation. *Arch. Surg.* 97:699, 1968.

70. Siegel, R. R. The basis of pulmonary disease resolution after nephrectomy in Goodpasture's syndrome. *Am. J. Med. Sci.* 259:201, 1970.

71. Soergel, K. H., and Sommers, S. C. Idiopathic pulmonary hemosiderosis and related syndromes. *Am. J. Med.* 32:499, 1962.

72. Solberg, C. O. Glomerulonephritis with lung purpura (Goodpasture's syndrome). *Acta Med. Scand.* 186:401, 1969.

73. Stanton, M. C., and Tange, J. D. Goodpasture's syndrome (pulmonary hemorrhage associated with glomerulonephritis). *Australas. Ann. Med.* 7:132, 1958.

74. Sturgill, B. C., and Westerwelt, F. B. Immunofluorescence studies in a case of Goodpasture's syndrome. *J.A.M.A.* 194:914, 1965.

75. Teichman, S., Briggs, W. A., Knieser, M. R., and Enquist, R. W. Goodpasture's syndrome: Two cases with contrasting early course and management. *Am. Rev. Resp. Dis.* 113:223, 1976.

76. Thomson, N. M., Moran, J., Simpson, I. J., and Peters, D. K. Defibrination with ancrod in nephrotoxic nephritis in rabbits. *Kidney Int.* 10:343, 1976.

77. Vassalli, P., and McCluskey, R. T. The pathogenic role of the coagulation process in rabbit Masugi nephritis. *Am. J. Pathol.* 45:653, 1964.

78. Videbaek, A. Auto-immune haemolytic anaemia in systemic lupus erythematosus. *Acta Med. Scand.* 171:187, 1962.

79. Wilson, C. B., and Dixon, F. J. Anti-glomerular basement membrane antibody-induced glomerulonephritis. *Kidney Int.* 3:74, 1973.

80. Wilson, C. B., and Smith, R. C. Goodpasture's syndrome associated with influenza A$_2$ virus infection. *Ann. Intern. Med.* 76:91, 1972.

81. Zollinger, H. U., and Hegglin, R. Die idiopathische Lungen—Haemosiderose als pulmonale form der purpura Schönlein-Henoch. *Schwiez. Med. Wochenschr.* 88:439, 1958.

58. Systemic Lupus Erythematosus

Alfred J. Fish, Robert L. Vernier, and Alfred F. Michael

Systemic lupus erythematosus (SLE) is a generalized disease of unknown etiology that affects persons of all ages with progressive involvement of the skin, joints, kidneys, central nervous system, and pulmonary and cardiovascular systems. The basic lesion appears to be a diffuse vasculitis, probably mediated by soluble antigen-antibody complexes and the complement system. The course, consequences, and complications of this disorder are greatly attenuated by corticosteroid and immunosuppressive therapy.

Historical Aspects

The earliest descriptions of SLE deal with the cutaneous manifestations of the disease; the term *lupus,* derived from the Latin, meaning "wolf," was used by Paracelsus and others in the sixteenth century to characterize the erythematous, ulcer-

Supported by grants from American Heart Association, Minnesota Arthritis Foundation, Minnesota Heart Association, and the U.S. Public Health Service (AI-10704) (HL 06314) (AM 05671).

ating facial lesions that "bite, destroy and eat away" the skin tissues [186]. Physicians later described the progressive cutaneous lesions, often in a butterfly distribution on the face, but unfortunately did not differentiate this lesion clinically from cutaneous tuberculosis. In the twentieth century the observation of multiple organ system involvement in SLE was first appreciated by Osler and others, who noted arthritic, pulmonary, and central nervous system disease; Osler speculated that vascular involvement was present in involved tissues. In 1923, Libman and Sachs [116] described a form of verrucous endocarditis that was histologically distinct from rheumatic endocarditis. Subsequent observers described glomerular wire-loop lesions [13], associated hematologic abnormalities with thrombocytopenia [118], and cytoid bodies in the retina [124] and adopted the term *diffuse collagen disease* [97].

Discovery of the LE cell by Hargraves in 1948 [83] provided both a way to differentiate SLE from rheumatoid arthritis and an approach to the autoimmune features of the disease. Within recent years, the association of drug-induced SLE, the autoimmune features of Coombs-positive hemolytic anemia, and a false-positive test for syphilis were appreciated. With development of the immunofluorescent technique by Coons and Kaplan, the observations of immunoglobulin and complement deposition in glomeruli and antinuclear antibody formation in SLE were established. During the past two decades these findings have led to the concept of SLE as a state of tissue injury that is mediated by antigen-antibody complexes.

Etiology and Pathogenesis

Considerable evidence has accumulated supporting the concept of an immune pathogenesis of the vascular and renal injury in SLE. Depression of serum complement is present in most cases. It was discovered by Freedman and colleagues [58] that immunoglobulin and complement are deposited in the glomeruli [107, 142]. It has been shown that electron-dense deposits in the subendothelial space, within the glomerular basement membrane, and in the subepithelial space are a prominent feature of the ultrastructural alteration in this disease. The immune deposits observed by fluorescence and electron microscopy are the hallmark of glomerular injury by soluble immune complexes [53, 198a] (see Chap. 3). Presumably, immune complexes of antigen and antibody form in the circulation, bind complement, cause lowering of serum complement levels, and localize in the glomeruli. The characteristics of the deposited im-

munoglobulin [100] and complement components of the classic and alternative pathways [125, 131, 165, 197], as well as the nature of the immunopathologic changes, are discussed subsequently. Immunoglobulins eluted from glomeruli have antinuclear activity [57, 104] and are deposited in the glomerulus as immune complexes with DNA [102].

Antibodies against a large number of nuclear and cytoplasmic antigens are present in the sera of patients with SLE. Antibody to native or double-stranded DNA (nDNA) has been shown to correlate well with the degree of activity and is widely used both diagnostically and to regulate therapy. When tissue sections are examined by immunofluoresence after incubation with the patients' sera and staining for IgG, the antibody produces a peripheral or rim nuclear pattern [161]. The antibodies also may be detected by a variety of other immunologic methods, such as the Farr-type assay that employs radiolabeled DNA [150, 201]; the latter has been used to examine patients with childhood SLE [149]. Earlier studies by Gewurz et al. [60] demonstrated the anticomplementary nature of SLE sera; this test has provided evidence for circulating immune complexes in SLE. Similarly, Agnello and coworkers [1] have shown the presence of C1q precipitins in the sera of patients with SLE. Studies by Tan et al. [189] revealed that elevated levels of circulating DNA may be detected in the serum of certain patients during the acute phase of SLE, indicating soluble immune complexes in antigen excess. Combining the sensitive Farr radioimmunoassay and exposure of SLE sera to DNase, Harbeck et al. [82] demonstrated a significant increase in DNA binding after enzyme digestion, indicating the presence of in vivo bound DNA and anti-DNA. These studies provided strong supportive evidence of circulating immune complexes in SLE that correlate well with the extent of renal injury.

Involvement of the central nervous system in SLE occasionally may result in elevated cerebrospinal fluid pressure, increased protein, and pleocytosis, depending on the proximity of the area of nervous system damage to the cerebrospinal fluid (CSF). Increased decay of C4 in CSF in vitro has been shown in some patients [76, 143]. Keeffe and coworkers [96] have demonstrated antibody to DNA, and DNA–anti-DNA complexes in the CSF. These findings may relate to the observation by Atkins et al. [12] of immune complex deposition in the choroid plexus in 2 patients with SLE.

Antibodies to other nuclear constituents have been observed in SLE, including denatured or single stranded DNA (SSDNA), deoxyribonucleoprotein (DNP), RNA, ribonucleoprotein (RNP) (extractable nuclear antigen [ENA]), and Sm antigen (carbohydrate-protein antigen). Various investigators have examined the presence of antibody to these antigens [141, 163] and their relationship to renal injury. In a review of the current information in this area, Koffler [99] speculated on the possible bacterial or viral origin of these polynucleotide antigens, but suggested that they probably are endogenous. Studies of glomeruli obtained at autopsy, using acidic buffers or DNase, have revealed anti-nDNA [102, 104] and anti-RNP [101] antibodies. Similarly, nDNA, SSDNA, but not RNP, antigens have been detected within glomerular deposits [8, 101]. These studies further support the concept of immune complex glomerular injury, although the elution studies have not always correlated well with the presence of circulating antibodies to these antigens. The discrepancies may reflect the possibility that various immunoreactants may be deposited secondarily in damaged glomeruli of end-stage SLE nephropathy and thus may not always relate directly to the primary immune processes.

There have been numerous recent observations by electron microscopy of virallike particles in the glomerular endothelium in patients with SLE. These virallike inclusions are dense, tubular, or filamentous structures that have the morphologic appearance of myxoviruses or paramyxoviruses [69, 89, 95, 140, 191]; they may be found also in other tissues [56, 59, 69, 98, 166]. These structures have been observed also in a large number of other collagen and renal diseases, although in much lower frequency [44, 69, 90, 148]. Of great interest are the reports of C-type RNA virus infection in SLE patients [115a, 126a, 140b, 145a]. It also has been noted that antibody titers to a variety of viral agents are elevated in SLE; this observation may reflect a hyperactive immunologic state [86]. The nature, origin [15], and significance of viruses relative to the pathogenesis of SLE must await further investigation.

Recent attention has been drawn to various aspects of cellular immunity in SLE. Lymphocyte stimulation by nuclear, nonnuclear, bacterial, and fungal antigens and various mitogens has yielded remarkably variable results; in some instances, impaired cellular reactivity [78, 87, 184] and in others, heightened or normal responses [55, 67, 168] have been found. The percentage of bone marrow–derived (B cell) and thymus-derived (T cell) lymphocytes also has been examined. By using different techniques to study each cell type, it was initially reported that increased numbers of immunoglobulin-bearing B lymphocytes and de-

creased T cells were present [129, 198]. Based on more recent studies, Winchester and associates [199, 199a, 200], and others [128a] have attributed these observations to binding of cold-reactive, antilymphocyte antibodies to T cells, which resulted in anomalously high numbers of immunoglobulin-bearing lymphocyte (B cell) counts. These investigators showed that the elevated levels of B cells could be reduced to normal numbers by incubating SLE lymphocytes in tissue culture, thus presumably washing off the cold-reactive antibody.

Specific infectious or exogenous etiologic agents have not been identified, except for drugs such as isoniazid, sulfonamides, phenytoin sodium, chlorpromazine, trimethadione, alpha methyldopa, nitrofurantoin, hydralazine and procainamide [2, 114, 187]. The role of drugs in the induction of SLE has been reviewed extensively [41]; the underlying mechanism is not known. Tan [187] has shown reactivity of antibody to a hydralazine-soluble nucleoprotein complex in the serum of a patient with SLE induced by hydralazine. A relationship may exist between patients who are slow acetylators (action of hepatic acetyltransferase) and the incidence of hydralazine-induced SLE [144].

Extensive studies of drug-induced SLE have been reported by Alarcón-Segovia with respect to anticonvulsants [4], isoniazid [3, 4], and hydralazine [5]. Jacobs [91] has described anticonvulsant-induced SLE in children. Beernink and Miller [16] found that the course of drug-induced SLE in childhood is relatively benign. Their patients had systemic symptoms—fever, rashes, and arthritis—but no evdience of renal, pulmonary, cardiac, or central nervous system involvement. The children had normal serum complement levels, although anti-DNA, anti-DNP, and anti-ENA antibodies were present. Progressive improvement usually occurred after the offending drugs were discontinued. Only low-dose corticosteroid therapy was required.

Familial and Genetic Factors
There is direct evidence of familial and genetic factors operating in the pathogenesis of SLE. Studies of sera from relatives of SLE patients have shown an increased incidence of biologic false-positive reactions for syphilis, elevated titers of rheumatoid factor, and positive Coombs' tests. Studies by Pollak [154], Fennell et al. [50] and Peterson et al. [145] have demonstrated an increased incidence of antinuclear antibodies in family members of patients with SLE. A significantly increased incidence of SLE in siblings dur-

ing childhood has been reported by Peterson et al. [145] and others [32, 70, 80, 126, 152]; SLE in 4 of 12 children in one family was reported by Brunjes and associates [21], and there have been multiple reports of SLE in identical twins. Systemic or discoid SLE in one parent of a child with SLE also has been sporadically observed [32].

There have been reports of a high incidence of certain HL-A histocompatibility antigens in patients with SLE. Associations based on population studies utilizing HL-A1 [66], HL-A8 [66, 75], HL-A5 [177], HL-A3 [11], and W15 [75, 196] are somewhat conflicting. Nies et al. [139] have observed a statistically significant incidence of HL-A5 only in black American patients with SLE. Extensive experimental observations have been made of the SLE-like disorder that develops spontaneously in certain genetic strains of mice, such as the NZB/NZW F1 hybrids [108, 120, 185] and other strains [190].

An increased incidence of SLE has been observed in patients with rare inherited deficiencies of serum complement components [7]. Homozygous autosomal recessive modes of inheritance for C1r, C1s, C2, and C4 deficiencies [33, 84, 134, 147] occur in families and may be associated with SLE in certain persons, suggesting the possibility that genetic factors may be involved.

Epidemiology
INCIDENCE
The occurrence rate and incidence of SLE in childhood appear to be 4 to 10 percent that of adults [70]. Definitive data on the incidence in the general population are not available, although several reports suggest that the apparent increasing frequency in recent years represents greater clinical awareness and more sensitive diagnostic procedures. Larsen [111] has observed an average incidence of 6.5 cases per 100,000 in Norway; Kurland et al. [105] have reported 48 cases per 100,000 in southeastern Minnesota; Siegel and Lee [173] have found 16 cases per 100,000 in New York City. Fessel [51] has examined the incidence of SLE in the general population of California and found 50 cases per 100,000, including 140 cases per 100,000 in women aged 15 to 64 years and 400 cases per 100,000 in black women.

DISTRIBUTION
Sixty percent of cases of SLE occur between the ages of 15 and 40 years [42]. The younger population, within the first two decades of life, thus accounts for approximately 20 to 25 percent of the total. The majority of reports of SLE in children [32, 80, 91, 126, 145, 195a] indicate a peak

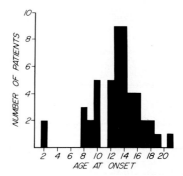

Figure 58-1. Frequency curve for age of onset in 49 patients at the University of Minnesota. The mean age of onset is 12.97 years. (From A. J. Fish et al. Am. J. Med. 62:99, 1977.)

incidence between the ages of 10 and 14, during the prepubertal and adolescent periods (Fig. 58-1); approximately one-third are between the ages of 5 and 10 years. Only a few congenital and infantile cases have been reported [52, 138].

As in adults, the majority of children with SLE are girls, with the incidence of female patients varying from 80 percent [126] to 90 to 95 percent [80, 145]. Only two childhood series contained a lower incidence of female children with SLE [195a, 203]. The age of onset of the male children in each series seems to be more broadly distributed, without the striking peak at puberty.

There is little evidence of a seasonal predilection for the onset of SLE, although Cook [32] noted a peak incidence of rash and possibly onset of SLE in the spring. Geographic or socioeconomic factors do not appear to play a role.

Clinical Manifestations
Systemic lupus erythematosus is a systemic illness in childhood, and most patients present with a wide and variable spectrum of symptoms. Initial complaints, which may have been present for several weeks to 2 or 3 months, are nonspecific and include fever, malaise, irritability, anorexia, and weight loss. Rarely, a child may have a history of several years' duration before the diagnosis is made, with failure to thrive, arthritis, or a low-grade illness. The most common presenting symptoms in childhood are fever, skin rash, arthralgia, and arthritis in reported series (Table 58-1) [32, 52, 70, 80, 91, 140a, 145, 195a, 203].

CUTANEOUS LESIONS
The majority of children exhibit an erythematous rash over the face in a butterfly distribution, involving the bridge of the nose and malar areas. As the lesions progress, vesicular and bullous changes

Table 58-1. Clinical Signs and Symptoms of Systemic Lupus Erythematosus

Sign or Symptom	Minnesota 1958–1974 (49 patients) (%)	Reported Pediatric Cases* (241 patients) (%)
Fever	63	86
Arthritis	57	82
Rash	78	79
Weight loss	31	42
Cardiovascular	31	46
Hypertension	15	29
Splenomegaly or lymphadenopathy	31	38
Central nervous system	29	28

* See references 32, 52, 70, 80, 91, 127, 145, 195a, 202.

occur, leading to focal areas of necrosis of epidermal and subcutaneous tissues. The initial erythematous rash may spread to involve the remainder of the face, scalp, neck, upper chest, and arms. Macular and petechial lesions involving the hands, fingertips, and feet with periungual inflammation and secondarily infected paronychiae are frequently observed early in the course of the disease [32]. Histologic examination of the variety of papular, hemorrhagic, and urticarial lesions usually reveals diffuse inflammation and vasculitis [145]. Exposed areas of the body, particularly the fingers and lower extremities, often exhibit a diffuse dusky suffusion and increased vascularity, with mottling that resembles livedo reticularis [34, 145]; the latter, which is thought to be due to cutaneous angiitis, often remains after corticosteroid therapy has been initiated and gradually disappears when a sustained remission has been attained. The cutaneous manifestations of SLE are photosensitive and exacerbate on exposure to sunlight. In some instances, cutaneous photosensitivity has preceded the onset of SLE [153]. Exacerbation of the systemic manifestations of SLE on exposure to sunlight is frequently observed in patients previously in remission on corticosteroid therapy.

By placing a drop of microscopy immersion oil over the finger or toenails, the capillaries of the nail beds can be examined using a dissecting microscope. In SLE the vessels demonstrate increased tortuosity and dilatation and small hemorrhages [22, 145].

JOINT SYMPTOMS
Musculoarticular abnormalities are present in most patients [48, 52, 145]. Adult patients [106, 175] frequently (22 to 35 percent) have deforming arthritic changes similar to those of rheumatoid arthritis, with destruction of joint surface cartilage and ankylosis. Although rarely, findings indistinguishable from juvenile rheumatoid arthritis have been reported in children with SLE [160], arthralgia, myalgia, and an acute arthritic process, with periarticular joint swelling and effusions, are most frequently observed [32, 80, 140a, 145].

MUCOUS MEMBRANES
Involvement of the mucous membranes of the oral cavity and lips by punctate hemorrhagic or ulcerating lesions has been observed. Perforation of the nasal septum has also been reported in SLE [6, 194].

RENAL DISEASE
On the basis of morphologic studies, involvement of the kidney in SLE occurs with a frequency of about 40 [48] to 80 percent [52]. Symptomatic renal findings, however, are manifest only in 6 percent of patients [48]. Clinical symptoms and signs of renal disease in SLE may not be present at the onset of the disease, but may develop later as the disease progresses. Hypertension has been reported in 50 [32] and 15 percent [52] of patients. Without adequate therapy, progressive renal disease ensues, often associated with nephrotic syndrome, uremia, and death due to renal insufficiency.

CARDIOPULMONARY DISORDERS
The incidence of cardiac involvement in childhood SLE varies from 10 [32] to 25 percent [91]. Pericarditis and pericardial effusions are encountered and frequently are asymptomatic; occasionally, large effusions are associated with pulsus paradoxus and tamponade. In some series, generalized cardiomegaly has been reported in up to 50 percent of children [32]. These findings are probably the result of myocarditis in the acute stage of SLE and may lead to congestive heart failure. Endocarditis leading to valvular insufficiency has been seen in a smaller percentage of children, with involvement of the mitral and aortic valves. Recent reports by Bernard and associates [19] and others have shown that perforation of the valve cusps may occur. Libman-Sachs verrucous endocarditis of the mitral valve, which can be diagnosed only at autopsy, has been seen in children with SLE [32, 145].

Pulmonary and pleural involvement is frequently noted in all series in childhood [32, 80, 91, 203]. Bilateral or unilateral pleuritic chest pain has been reported as a presenting symptom in over 50 percent of cases in adults [10, 42] and children [91]. Areas of hemorrhage and pulmonary arteriolar vasculitis also have been observed [74]. Recent reports [42, 65, 88] have described marked alterations in the results of pulmonary function tests in adults, including reduction in vital capacity, maximal expiratory flow rate, and carbon monoxide diffusion capacity, even in the absence of clinical or radiologic manifestations of lung disease. One childhood case of primary pulmonary hypertension, with cor pulmonale and severe cyanosis, was reported by Zetterström and Berglund [203]; we have recently seen a patient with similar clinical presentation and established the presence of recurrent pulmonary emboli from extensive thrombosis of the inferior vena cava and pelvic veins.

NERVOUS SYSTEM

Disorders of the nervous system in SLE have been observed in all reported series and reviewed extensively by Johnson and Richardson [92]. Involvement of the nervous system reportedly occurs in from 20 to 75 percent of children [64] and adults [48, 92], with similar clinical manifestations. All portions of the nervous system have been involved, probably by the same mechanism of injury, namely, a form of angiitis that results in edema, hemorrhage, necrosis, and infarction of nerve tissue [169]. Seizure disorders have been observed in all childhood series [32, 80, 91, 145, 203] and appear to involve 25 to 40 percent of patients. Lesions of the cranial nerves occur, most frequently related to extraocular movements [92]. Myelitis and peripheral motor (wrist and footdrop) and sensory neuropathies have been reported in children [64, 80, 91]. Disorders of movement [52, 145, 174], which often resemble childhood Sydenham's chorea, have been described, and when seen with other clinical findings of fever, malaise, and arthritis, may lead to the misdiagnosis of acute rheumatic fever. It has been reported that abnormal brain scans were found in a majority of patients with central nervous system symptoms [17]. A wide spectrum of neuropsychiatric disorders has been reported [145, 203], and such disorders were a prominent feature of central nervous system involvement in our series [52].

Ocular and eyeground changes in SLE reflect changes in intracranial pressure and injury to the nervous system. Papilledema, exudates, hemorrhages, and cytoid bodies have been reported [27, 124].

Clinical Course

In the majority of children with SLE, there is involvement of multiple organ systems; without corticosteroid therapy, the disease process is progressive and leads inevitably to death. In a series of adult patients the cumulative 5-year survival rate was only 5 percent in patients not treated with corticosteroids [43]. The progressive deterioration of patients relates primarily to ongoing renal and central nervous system involvement [43, 48]. Infrequently in adults, and rarely in children, the course may be more indolent and nonprogressive; typical symptomatology includes fatigue, mild skin eruptions, and arthralgia or more severe arthritis that resembles rheumatoid arthritis. These patients have no clinical evidence of systemic organ involvement and minimal or no renal disease. Such patients have a good prognosis and require only moderate doses of corticosteroid therapy, but they must be carefully followed at regular intervals.

The clinical course and prognosis in SLE have been highly correlated with the nature of the renal lesion (Fig. 58-2). Whereas patients with normal kidneys, mesangial nephritis, and focal proliferative nephritis have a good prognosis, a much lower survival rate has been observed in patients with diffuse proliferative nephritis [14, 28, 48, 157, 159]. Pollak and coworkers [158] first described the beneficial effect of high-dose corticosteroid therapy in the latter group of patients. It has been shown that patients with membranous glomerulopathy and focal proliferative nephritis have a much higher survival rate than that of patients with other histologic lesions [26, 28, 159], although this experience is not uniformly reported [14, 181]. Hagge et al. [77] demonstrated an improved survival rate in children with SLE and clinical evidence of renal disease who were treated intensively with corticosteroids, as compared with a 100 percent mortality in a comparable group of children treated with only low doses. These workers emphasized that children with drug-induced SLE, and the rare childhood cases in which rheumatoid arthritic changes with no renal involvement occur, could be managed successfully with low-dose corticosteroid therapy.

The clinical course of SLE in children has become more complex as survival has been extended by newer and more successful modes of therapy [195a]. Children now regularly survive to adulthood, but the clinical course may be punctuated by recurrent exacerbations and a host of complications relating both to the basic disease process and to therapy itself. As mortality and the frequency

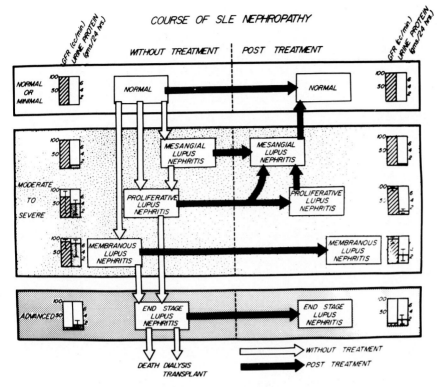

Figure 58-2. The clinical course of SLE nephropathy. On the right side the course with adequate treatment is depicted with black arrows; on the left the course without therapy is shown with white arrows. Proliferative lupus nephritis includes both the focal and diffuse forms of this entity.

of complications decrease through more skillful application of effective therapy, the prognosis in this lifelong disease undoubtedly will improve.

Complications

The complications of SLE leading to death have changed over the last three decades as modifications in management have evolved. Dubois et al. [43] have observed a changing pattern in the complications leading to death (Table 58-2). Among adult patients there has been a declining rate of death from central nervous system involvement and renal failure, but an increase in fatal infections and malignancies. The incidence of renal failure leading to death has decreased, due to more effective management of lupus nephropathy and the availability of chronic dialysis and transplantation for treatment of end-stage renal disease. Cardiovascular complications such as hypertension may be worsened by corticosteroid therapy. Recurrent venous thrombosis and multiple pulmonary emboli have been observed in some series [24, 52]. Increased mortality late in the course of SLE has been attributed to the increased frequency of myocardial infarction [193a].

Additional complications encountered in the course of SLE are related in part to corticosteroid therapy. Severe life-threatening infections are a major problem. Bacterial infections with multiple abscesses, septicemia, meningitis, pneumonitis, and endocarditis were observed in 25 percent of our series of 49 patients [52]. Constant careful surveillance for infections due to opportunistic pathogens, such as *Candida, Aspergilla, Cryptococcus,* cytomegalovirus, and *Pneumocystis carinii,* is essential. We have observed a very high incidence (45 percent) of herpes zoster infection; some patients have experienced multiple herpes zoster infections, but in all instances the infection was managed successfully without serious complications.

Other complications resulting from corticosteroid therapy include peptic ulcer of the upper gastrointestinal tract and acute pancreatitis. In addition, we have observed a high incidence of avascular necrosis of bone [18, 52], both occult and symptomatic, with an overall incidence of 31 percent. The major long-term complication involving the central nervous system relates to behavioral and emotional difficulties. Although major aberra-

Table 58-2. Complications Leading to Death in Systemic Lupus Erythematosus

Years	Percentage of Patients			
	CNS	Uremia	Infection	Malignancy
1950–1956 (precorticosteroid)	26	26	16	2
1956–1962 (low-dose corticosteroids)	11	36	12	2
1963–1973 (high-dose corticosteroids, dialysis, diuretics)	8	14	19	6.5

Source: Dubois and coworkers [43].

tions of behavior with psychotic episodes can be caused by both SLE itself or by corticosteroids, there seems to be a high incidence of low-grade emotional disturbance in these patients. Cade and coworkers [24] have observed a high incidence of behavioral disorders when compared either with that in other patients receiving long-term corticosteroid therapy or with that in SLE patients treated with azathioprine alone or azathioprine and heparin. This observation may suggest an unusual predilection of SLE patients to emotional instability, which is accentuated in some manner by corticosteroid therapy.

A small percentage of patients have a relentless, progressive course that responds neither to high-dose corticosteroids nor to immunosuppressive therapy. These patients have continuing renal damage, with a "malignant," progressive, systemic process in which serum anti-DNA titers are persistently elevated and serum complement values cannot be normalized, despite high doses of corticosteroids. Such patients frequently succumb either to renal failure or sepsis.

Clinical Pathologic Features

There are strong correlations between the form and extent of pathologic involvement of the kidney in SLE and the clinical and laboratory findings of renal disease [155]. Proteinuria, with erythrocytes, leukocytes, and casts in the urine, is observed regularly in diffuse proliferative and membranous nephritis. These abnormalities often are absent, and renal function may be normal, in patients with normal glomeruli, mesangial nephritis, or focal proliferative nephritis. The most marked impairment in renal function is present in patients with diffuse proliferative nephritis.

Many hematologic abnormalities are present in SLE [48, 126]. Hemolytic anemia is frequently

encountered and is usually of the Coombs'-positive type. Leukopenia in the range of 3,000 to 4,500 cells per cubic millimeter is commonly seen, associated with an increase in segmented neutrophils and a relative lymphopenia [199a]. Thrombocytopenia is present in 8 to 20 percent of patients. The majority of patients have an elevated erythrocyte sedimentation rate. Positive LE clot tests are most easily detected in the acute phase of SLE at the onset of the disease [39]; it is frequently difficult to correlate the state of clinical activity with the presence of positive LE clot tests [122, 132].

Changes in serum proteins are observed; elevations of serum immunoglobulin levels are often found, and marked hypergammaglobulinemia may be present occasionally. The presence of immunoglobulin light chains in the serum and urine has been reported by Epstein and coworkers [46, 47, 176] to correlate well with the degree of SLE activity. Cryoglobulins are found in a high percentage of patients and have been shown to be complexes of IgG, IgM, rheumatoid factor, and C1q [79, 178]. Depression of serum hemolytic complement activity and C3 (β_1C globulin) are regularly found [110]. The activity of SLE and lupus nephropathy correlates well with levels of serum complement (see Chap. 3) [20, 68, 103, 110, 115, 133, 167]. Return of serum complement levels to normal usually occurs after about 1 month of corticosteroid therapy, but may fluctuate below normal in association with exacerbations of the disease.

Numerous autoantibodies have been found in SLE, including antibodies to a wide variety of nuclear antigens, of which anti-DNA and anti-DNP are the most common. The latter are most easily detected by overlaying dilutions of the patient's serum on frozen sections of mouse liver; various staining patterns, corresponding to different antinuclear antibodies [161], are observed. More recently, a Farr-type assay for anti-DNA antibody has been employed and has been shown to correlate well with the degree of clinical and renal activity [117a, 146, 149, 150]. Rheumatoid factor is encountered in about 50 percent of children with SLE [81]. Approximately 15 percent have a biologically false-positive test for syphilis, which apparently represents an autoantibody to cardiolipin antigens [202].

A variety of disorders of coagulation has been described. It is widely recognized that a circulating anticoagulant ("lupus inhibitor") is found in the sera of about 9 percent of patients with SLE [49]. Prolonged activated (kaolin) partial thromboplastin times and occasionally factor II (prothrombin) deficiency are noted. It is believed that the lupus anticoagulant interferes with the interaction of prothrombin activator with prothrombin and may be mediated by antilipoidal antibodies [20a, 49, 195]. This autoantibody may react with platelet lipids to produce thrombocytopenia and may have activity to cardiolipin, thus producing the biologically false-positive Wasserman reaction that is seen in these patients. Abnormal platelet aggregation studies with collagen and epinephrine have been reported in SLE patients with circulating lupus anticoagulant [162]. The presence of lupus anticoagulant with or without abnormal platelet function has been associated with vascular thrombosis [24, 195]. Specific factor inhibitors (lupus inhibitor inactivators) against factors VIII, IX, X, XI [112, 113] may be differentiated from lupus anticoagulant and are associated with increasing bleeding tendency. Unlike the lack of effect upon lupus anticoagulant, steroid therapy is effective in eliminating lupus inhibitor inactivators as evidenced by return of the PTT to normal.

Increased fibrin split products are regularly found in the serum and urine of patients with SLE [94]. Marchesi et al. [123] failed to establish a relationship between the level of urinary fibrin split products and the degree of renal injury or other measures of SLE activity.

Histopathologic Findings

Major contributions to the understanding and description of SLE nephropathy have been made by Muehrcke, Pollak, and coworkers [136, 158, 159], Baldwin and coworkers [14, 164], and Méry and coworkers [128]. The availability of percutaneous renal biopsy has allowed investigators to follow the natural history of SLE nephropathy and the pathologic alterations associated with therapy. Since it appears that the clinical course and prognosis of SLE nephropathy depend to a large extent on the nature of the glomerular lesions, it is essential that a uniform classification be used to permit evaluation and comparison of data by different investigators. The classification described here is a modification of the scheme used by Baldwin and coworkers [14] and is basically similar to that of Pollak and coworkers [158, 159] (Table 58-3).

The overall incidence of histologic renal involvement in SLE varies from 70 to 88 percent, although a lower incidence may be detected clinically [52, 128, 136, 157, 204]. Because of the variable course in childhood, uncertainties regarding the nature and response to therapy, and the lifelong course of this disorder, it has been our policy to perform a renal biopsy in all childhood patients when first seen [52].

Table 58-3. Classification of Lupus Nephropathy

Normal
Mesangial lupus nephritis
Proliferative lupus nephritis
Focal proliferative lupus nephritis
Diffuse proliferative lupus nephritis
Membranous lupus nephritis

MESANGIAL LUPUS NEPHRITIS

We have adopted the term *mesangial lupus nephritis* to describe a range of mild proliferative changes in the glomerular mesangium [52]. This lesion in its least extensive form corresponds to the "minimal glomerular involvement" of Pollak and Pirani [156] or to the "equivocal glomerular lesions" described by Cheatum and coworkers [28] and consists of focal and segmental proliferation of mesangial cells and mild increases in mesangial matrix (Fig. 58-3*A*). This term also describes glomerular lesions with more diffuse proliferation of mesangial cells that corresponds to the "mesangial glomerulitis" lesion of Cheatum [28] and the "mesangial lesion" defined by Ginzler and colleagues [62]. Mesangial lupus nephritis is closely related to the term *lupus glomerulitis* previously used by Pollak et al. [158] and may show minimal amounts of fibrinoid deposition, but no polymorphonuclear leukocyte infiltration, necrosis, or karyorrhexis.

Occasionally, biopsy specimens may contain glomeruli that appear completely normal by light microscopy, yet show finely granular deposits of immunoglobulin and complement components in the mesangial areas [85a, 100, 135]; subendothelial and subepithelial deposits usually are not present (Fig. 58-3*B*). Mesangial proliferation, increases in mesangial matrix, and dense deposits in the mesangium typically are seen by electron microscopy of such specimens.

PROLIFERATIVE LUPUS NEPHRITIS

Proliferative lupus nephritis, as defined by Baldwin and coworkers [14], is focal and segmental when only some glomeruli are involved (focal proliferative lupus nephritis) or diffuse when all or nearly all (more than 90 percent) are altered (diffuse proliferative lupus nephritis). The changes in the focal form generally are less extensive and less severe than those seen in the diffuse lesion. In proliferative nephritis, marked hypercellularity of endothelial and mesangial cells is present that may vary in degree from one glomerular lobule to another. Glomerular basement membrane thickening, with "wire-loop" lesions, polymorphonuclear leukocyte infiltration, fibri-

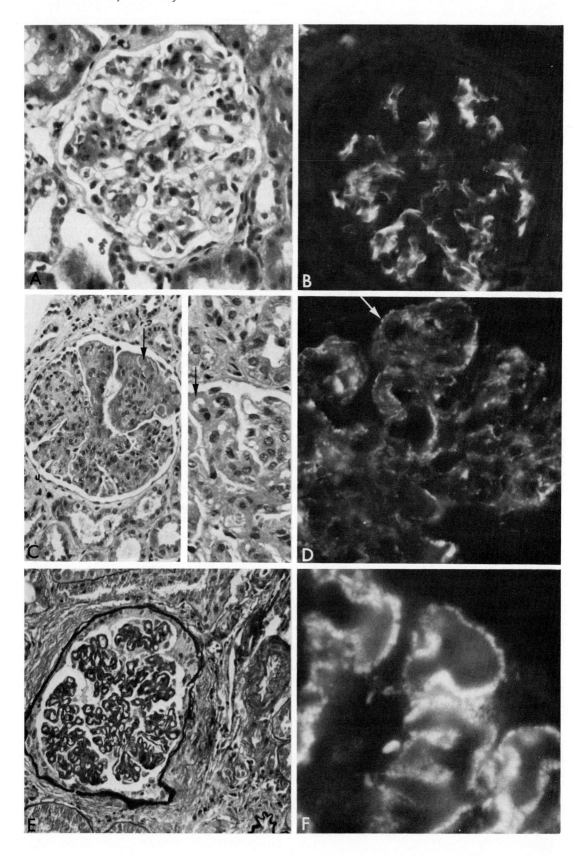

noid deposition, capillary thrombi, glomerular necrosis, fragmentation of polymorphonuclear leukocytes, karyorrhexis, hematoxyphil bodies, glomerular crescents, and sclerotic glomeruli, are the usual component lesions (Fig. 58-3C). Tubular damage, interstitial edema, and lymphocytic infiltration commonly are present. Larger vessel-wall abnormalities, with inflammation and necrosis, may be observed. Except for hematoxyphil bodies, none of the glomerular changes observed is thought to be solely pathognomonic for SLE.

By immunofluorescence microscopy, proliferative lupus nephritis is associated with numerous fine granular deposits in the glomerular mesangium that extend throughout the subendothelial space and follow the capillary loops (Fig. 58-3D). These deposits may be very extensive (Fig. 58-4A–C), with nodular aggregates of immunoglobulin and complement within the glomerular basement membrane and in subepithelial loci. There are electron-dense deposits in the mesangium, subendothelial space (Fig. 58-4D), glomerular basement membrane, and in a subepithelial location [31, 45, 73]. The deposits in the subendothelial space may be extensive, corresponding to the aggregates of immunoprotein detected by fluorescence microscopy (Fig. 58-4C) and representing the components of the wire-loop lesion observed by light microscopy; some electron-dense deposits have a unique organized ("fingerprint") appearance [72].

MEMBRANOUS LUPUS NEPHRITIS
Glomerular changes in membranous lupus nephritis feature a diffuse, generalized thickening of the glomerular basement membranes, without evidence of a cellular proliferative reaction. There are no areas of necrosis, karyorrhexis, crescent formation, or polymorphonuclear leukocyte infiltration (see Fig. 58-3E). By immunofluorescence microscopy, diffuse, discrete immune deposits are present within the glomerular basement membrane. Remarkably uniform deposits of immunoglobulins and complement, which vary from fine

deposits to larger immunoprotein aggregates, project toward the epithelial side of the glomerular basement membrane (see Fig. 58-3F). By electron microscopy, regular electron-dense osmiophilic deposits are noted on the epithelial surface of the glomerular basement membrane, lying between "spikes" of basement membrane material. The latter projections result in a "toothcomb" appearance of the outer, epithelial aspect of the glomerular basement membrane. No deposits are found in the mesangium or subendothelial space. The lesions in membranous nephritis in SLE, by light, immunofluorescence, and electron microscopy, are identical to those of idiopathic membranous nephropathy.

Extensive immunofluorescence studies have shown that IgG and IgM are the predominant immunoglobulins found in the lesions [100, 127, 131, 182]; in addition, a large proportion of patients has deposits of IgA. Elution studies have demonstrated that the deposited immunoglobulins have antinuclear antibody activity [101, 104]. In general, the sites of immunoprotein deposition within the glomerulus correspond to the areas of abnormality seen by light microscopy. That is, in mesangial lupus nephritis, deposits are found within the mesangium; in proliferative lupus nephritis, deposition is within the subendothelial space and the glomerular basement membrane; while in the membranous lesion, deposits are found only within the basement membrane. Dujovne and coworkers [45] have shown that only the subendothelial deposits of immunoprotein contain albumin and transferrin and have suggested that an insudative process is involved in the pathogenesis of these lesions. It has been shown that immunoproteins may be deposited also in glomeruli that are normal when seen by light microscopy, possibly representing the earliest stage of glomerular injury in SLE nephropathy [52, 100]. Remission of glomerular injury during therapy is associated with the disappearance of immune deposits, as observed by immunofluorescence and electron microscopy.

Figure 58-3. A. Photomicrograph showing mesangial nephritis. Proliferation of mesangial cells and increased mesangial matrix is evident. (H&E, ×400.) B. Fluorescent micrograph showing mesangial nephritis. Deposition of IgG can be seen in the mesangium. (×300.) C. Photomicrograph showing diffuse proliferative nephritis with glomerular enlargement, lobulation, endothelial proliferation, necrosis, and hyaline thrombi (arrow). (H&E, ×225.) Higher magnification insert illustrates thickened glomeruli "wire" loops (arrow). (H&E, ×1,100.) D. Fluorescent micrograph showing diffuse proliferative nephritis. IgG in a fine granular distribution is seen in the subendothelial space and mesangium. (×900.) E. Photomicrograph showing membranous nephritis with diffuse thickening of the glomerular basement membrane and absent cellular proliferation. (PAS, ×260.) F. Fluorescent micrograph showing nephritis with diffuse thickening and deposition of IgG within the glomerular basement membrane. (×1,200.) (Figure 58-3 was kindly prepared and provided by Dr. Robert McLean, University of Connecticut, Hartford.)

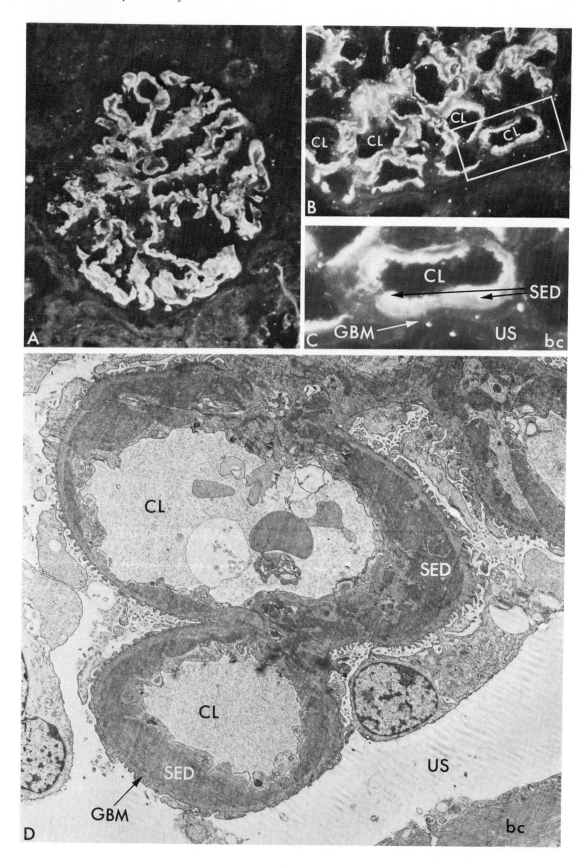

Pollak and coworkers [158, 159] have classified glomerular lesions in SLE into two forms, "active" or "inactive," both to differentiate patients with proliferative nephritis from those with other forms of renal injury in SLE (mesangial lupus nephritis and membranous lupus nephritis) and to quantify the extent of ongoing active glomerular injury. The active lesion is characterized by glomerular cell proliferation, necrosis, crescents, wire-loop lesions, and interstitial infiltrates with edema. The "activity" of SLE glomerular lesions has been evaluated semiquantitatively [151] and used by several investigators [14, 20, 36, 157] to provide a guide to corticosteroid therapy, high doses being recommended for the patients with glomerular lesions of high activity. In the management of our patients with SLE, we have directed therapy toward maximal and optimal suppression of autoimmune phenomena and varied the intensity of treatment with the degree of glomerular injury and with the clinical progress, as evaluated by glomerular filtration rate and urinary excretion of protein [52].

Immunopathologic study of normal and involved skin in SLE has revealed granular deposition of immunoglobulin and complement along the basal membrane at the dermal-epidermal junction [23, 93, 188]. By electron microscopy, dense deposits similar to those found in SLE nephropathy are evident [71]. Immunoglobulin eluted from involved skin has been shown to have antinuclear antibody activity. Rothfield and associates [165] have reported the deposition of properdin in these areas. Gilliam and coworkers [61] reported an overall incidence of positive immunofluorescence in clinically uninvolved skin in 55 percent of SLE patients; 81 percent of patients with more severe proliferative glomerular lesions had positive skin immunofluorescence, as compared with 23 percent of patients with mild renal injury. Such interesting observations may be explained by either qualitative or quantitative variables in host antigen-antibody complex formation.

Differential Diagnosis

Preliminary criteria to characterize patients with SLE have been proposed by the American Rheumatism Association of the Arthritis Foundation [30]. The presence of four or more of the following fourteen items has been used to diagnose SLE and to differentiate between rheumatoid arthritis and other collagen diseases: (1) facial erythema, (2) discoid lupus, (3) Raynaud's phenomenon, (4) alopecia, (5) photosensitivity, (6) oral or nasopharyngeal ulceration, (7) arthritis without deformity, (8) LE cells, (9) false-positive biologic syphilis test, (10) proteinuria, (11) cellular casts, (12) pleuritis or pericarditis, (13) psychosis or convulsions, (14) hemolytic anemia or leukopenia or thrombocytopenia. These criteria have been shown to be satisfactory for establishing the diagnosis of SLE [29], although it has been suggested that low serum complement [117] and the presence of elevated titers of antinuclear antibody [192, 201a] should be included. In childhood, it is usually not difficult to differentiate SLE from juvenile rheumatoid arthritis. Other collagen diseases, such as acute rheumatic fever, periarteritis nodosa, anaphylactoid purpura, thrombotic thrombocytopenic purpura, mixed connective tissue disease, scleroderma, dermatomyositis, and serum sickness, should be considered in the differential diagnosis, in addition to lupoid hepatitis and other forms of glomerulonephritis.

In the acute phase of rheumatic fever, differentiation from SLE may be difficult. Fever, arthritis, elevated erythrocyte sedimentation rate, valvular heart disease, and chorea may be present in both conditions. However, erythema marginatum, subcutaneous nodules, the absence of significant renal involvement and antinuclear antibodies, and a normal serum complement characterize acute rheumatic fever.

Although LE clot tests become positive in a significant number of adults with deforming rheumatoid arthritis of long duration, this circumstance is seldom found in childhood. Occasionally, a child with SLE may have arthritic joint changes that are very similar to those of rheumatoid arthritis; the correct diagnosis is usually established by the presence of anti-nDNA antibodies, low serum complement, and evidence of renal disease. However, evidence of involvement of other organ systems in rheumatoid arthritis, such as hepatospleno-

Figure 58-4. A. Fluorescent micrograph showing diffuse proliferative nephritis with extensive deposition of C1q adjacent to the glomerular basement membrane and within the mesangium. (×375.) B. Fluorescent micrograph of same biopsy section showing mesangial and subendothelial deposition of IgG in most glomerular capillaries (CL). (×525.) C. Fluorescent micrograph of boxed area from B showing subendothelial deposits (SED) of IgG beneath the glomerular basement membrane (GBM). CL = capillary lumen; US = urinary space; bc = Bowman's capsule. (×1,250.) D. Electron micrograph showing diffuse proliferative nephritis. Extensive deposition of electron-dense subendothelial deposits (SED) is seen in two glomerular capillaries (CL); bc = Bowman's capsule; GBM = glomerular basement membrane; US = urinary space. (×6,300.)

megaly, lymphadenopathy, and restrictive lung disease, may make differentiation from SLE more difficult. Since complement levels are usually normal or high in rheumatoid arthritis and other multiple-system diseases, complement determinations have become a critical laboratory diagnostic procedure.

The arthritic changes in dermatomyositis may be indistinguishable from SLE. The predominance of muscle pain and weakness are a major feature of dermatomyositis; the distinctive features of the skin rash include the heliotrope discoloration of the eyelids and the atrophic extensor joint skin surfaces. The absence of renal disease or other systemic involvement in dermatomyositis, the negative serologic studies for SLE, and the presence of elevated serum levels of muscle enzymes aid in establishing the correct diagnosis.

Rarely, an "overlap syndrome" occurs in scleroderma (progressive systemic sclerosis), to the extent that patients with this disease may have skin changes very similar to SLE. Such cases may be differentiated by the absence of pleuritis, pericarditis, fever, arthritis, glomerulonephritis, hemolytic anemia, and hypocomplementemia. These two conditions may share features such as Raynaud's phenomenon, finger ulceration, hyperglobulinemia, and antinuclear antibodies. Although renal disease occurs in scleroderma, the predominant lesion involves the renal vasculature (intimal proliferation) and interstitium, with fibrosis and periglomerular scarring out of proportion to the glomerular involvement. The overlap syndrome of scleroderma and SLE has been successfully treated with corticosteroids.

Sharp and colleagues [171] have described a new disorder called *mixed connective tissue disease,* in which arthritis, arthralgia, hand swelling, Raynaud's phenomenon, myositis, lymphadenopathy, fever, hepatosplenomegaly, and hyperglobulinemia are present. Renal disease occurs only rarely, and these cases can be differentiated from SLE by the absence of hypocomplementemia and the detection of antinuclear antibody to extractable nuclear antigens; the latter has been shown by hemagglutination assay to be present in extremely high titer and to be directed specifically to ribonucleoprotein. It is believed that patients with this disorder benefit from corticosteroid therapy. Very few cases have been recognized in children.

Treatment

The beneficial effects of corticosteroid therapy in childhood SLE have been observed by many investigators [32, 80, 145]. Control of systemic signs and symptoms, such as malaise, fever, and arthritis, usually is achieved rapidly following initiation of therapy and may even be accomplished using low corticosteroid doses. The systemic manifestations of SLE involving the central nervous system and cardiovascular and pulmonary systems also have been shown to respond well to corticosteroid therapy.

Numerous reports in the early literature suggested that therapy with high doses of prednisone (60 mg/m^2/day) produced a remission of SLE, but as the dose was reduced to avoid corticosteroid side effects, exacerbation often occurred. Since progressive renal involvement is inevitably fatal and has accounted for half of the reported mortality in SLE in children [59a, 126, 145], therapy should be directed to the control of the renal disease. Pollak and colleagues [156, 158] first showed in adult patients that high-dose corticosteroid therapy in diffuse lupus nephritis was superior to low-dose therapy, and that significant improvement in survival resulted from this approach (Fig. 58-5). This was shown by Hagge et al. in children [77]. Many investigators [14, 20, 48, 126, 159, 181] believe that if the kidneys are normal, or show evidence only of mesangial lupus nephritis, focal proliferative lupus nephritis, or membranous lupus nephritis, progressive glomerular injury is not likely to occur; in such cases they recommend treatment with low doses of corticosteroids. This concept is still in dispute, however, since several workers [62, 203a] have documented progression of mesangial lupus nephritis and focal proliferative lupus nephritis to diffuse proliferative disease in serologically active patients. We share this view and thus have recommended that doses of corticosteroids, with or without immunosuppressive therapy, be sufficient to maintain normal concentrations of complement in serum and negative anti-DNA titers, as well as normal levels of creatinine clearance and rates of excretion of protein in the urine [52, 62].

During the first 4 to 5 weeks of treatment, it is recommended that 60 mg of prednisone per square meter be given daily in three divided doses (maximum dose of 100 mg) [54]. Levels of complement in serum usually rise to normal or near-normal levels within a few weeks, and the anti-DNA antibody titers become negative. Prednisone therapy is then gradually reduced to 60 mg per square meter given as a single morning dose (maximum dose of 100 mg) on alternate days. The usual side effects of corticosteroids are evident in these patients, but alternate-day, single-dose therapy is associated with minimal incidence of the more serious complications, such as severe infections, osteoporosis, avascular necrosis, carbo-

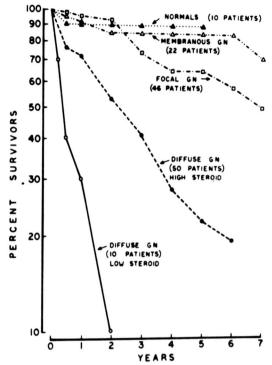

Figure 58-5. Survival curves by Pollak and coworkers using the life table technique. Survival in SLE patients with diffuse and focal proliferative lupus nephritis, membranous lupus nephritis, and normal kidneys is shown. (From V. E. Pollak et al. The Clinical Course of Lupus Nephritis: Relationship to the Renal Histologic Findings. In P. Kincaid-Smith, T. H. Mathew, and E. L. Becker [eds.], Proceedings of International Symposium on Glomerulonephritis. New York: Wiley, 1973.)

hydrate intolerance, and psychosis. Serum complement and anti-DNA levels are closely monitored over the next 1 to 2 years, and the dose of alternate-day corticosteroid therapy is slowly reduced to maintenance levels of 20 to 30 mg per square meter.

This form of corticosteroid therapy has been shown to be beneficial in lupus nephropathy, resulting in significant improvement in renal function and in the pathology of the glomerular lesions, as well as in decreased mortality [14, 48, 109, 121, 137, 157, 159]. In the large majority of patients treated appropriately at the onset of the disease, it should be possible to reverse the renal injury completely. Patients seen later in the course of SLE, sometimes initially having received inadequate doses of corticosteroids, often have irreversible injury, with glomerular scarring and sclerosis. When patients are treated with a high-dose regimen, the severity of the renal process may stabilize, with varying degrees of impairment of renal func-

tion, and they may subsequently experience a nonprogressive course.

While it seems appropriate to treat patients exhibiting minimal renal involvement with corticosteroid therapy alone, it has become apparent that the addition of immunosuppressive agents to the therapeutic regimen of patients with significant nephropathy may provide additional benefit [193]. Several investigators have described their experiences with combined prednisone and azathioprine. Interpretation of these studies is difficult, since the circumstances, dose, duration of therapy, and other conditions vary widely, and the results of very few well-controlled trials are available. Hayslett et al. [85] and Shelp et al. [172] have reported improvements in the clinical and histologic manifestations of lupus nephropathy. Sztejnbok and coworkers [183] showed decreased mortality and morbidity, fewer exacerbations, and improved renal function in patients receiving azathioprine and prednisone when compared with controls on prednisone alone. Drinkard and coworkers [38] followed 20 adults who were initially treated with corticosteroids alone and then placed on azathioprine because of deteriorating renal status. Although clinical improvement was observed, no significant histologic improvement in kidney lesions was evident. Cade and coworkers [24] have reported on the management of a group of patients with diffuse lupus glomerulonephritis in whom superior results were obtained using azathioprine (alone or in combination with prednisone or heparin) when compared with those of prednisone alone. Maher and Schreiner [122] were unable to show significant clinical improvement in adult patients with the addition of azathioprine therapy when prolonged corticosteroid administration alone had been unsuccessful. Donadio and coworkers [36] reported no additional benefit from the use of azathioprine and prednisone compared with that of corticosteroids alone in the initial 6-month course of SLE in 16 adult patients. A 3-year follow-up failed to reveal any difference in the two groups with regard to the nature and frequency of exacerbations. The two groups, however, were not strictly comparable, since the combined therapy group did not receive azathioprine for the entire 3-year study period [37]. Similarly Hahn et al. [78a] report no additional benefit of azathioprine. Ginzler et al. [63] reported the results of a controlled study in adult patients that indicated a more favorable clinical course with fewer exacerbations and hospitalizations in patients receiving azathioprine and prednisone compared with those receiving corticosteroids alone. In a childhood series of SLE,

Walravens and Chase [195a] did not find that immunosuppressive therapy enhanced survival.

Our experience in the management of SLE in children with significant nephropathy [52] supports the value of combined therapy. The addition of azathioprine in a dose of 2 mg/kg/day to the standard corticosteroid program previously outlined, either at the onset of therapy (in the most severe cases) or at a later time (in patients with poor serologic or clinical control), appears to be of value. We believe that this approach results in improved salvage of renal function, fewer exacerbations on alternate-day corticosteroid therapy, less toxicity (especially from corticosteroids), better patient acceptance, and improved survival. Patients receiving azathioprine should have white blood cell counts every 1 to 2 weeks; if leukopenia is present (less than 5,000 leukocytes per cubic millimeter), the drug should be discontinued until the white cell count returns to normal.

The long-term management of SLE involves careful monitoring of renal function, urinary excretion of protein, serum complement, and anti-DNA titers. In patients who are stable for 2 or 3 years, azathioprine is gradually tapered and discontinued, and they are maintained on low-dose, alternate-day prednisone alone [170]. The majority of children experience several exacerbations of SLE within the first 5 years of the disease, ranging from laboratory evidence of activity, with low serum complement levels and elevated anti-DNA titers alone, to complete clinical recrudescence of symptoms, with rash, fever, arthritis, and changes in urinary sediment and renal function. Although renal injury with increasing proteinuria or loss of renal function is seldom encountered in the closely observed patient, a repeat kidney biopsy should be performed if this occurs. Exacerbations are treated as described, that is, with azathioprine and daily prednisone, until remission is achieved, and then corticosteroid therapy is maintained, using the alternate-day regimen.

The combined use of prednisone and azathioprine therapy in our patients during the past 17 years has provided a 10-year survival in 86 percent of a group of 49 children, which is more favorable than that reported in any other series of patients with SLE [52]. We have observed improvement or stabilization of renal disease in all except 4 patients, 2 of whom could not be relied on to take their medications. There were no deaths due to progressive renal insufficiency; the main cause of death was infection (septicemia, bacterial endocarditis, systemic candidiasis, and Pneumocystis carinii pneumonia). Other side effects and complications included osteoporosis, avascular ne-crosis of bone, hypertension, gastrointestinal tract ulceration, leukopenia, a high incidence of herpes zoster infection (27 percent), and growth retardation. We have observed only 2 patients who have had a "malignant," inexorably progressive downhill course with renal damage; these patients demonstrated persistent hypocomplementemia and elevated anti-DNA titers in spite of maximum prednisone and azathioprine therapy. Pneumocystis carinii pneumonia developed in both these patients, and 1 died; the other patient was treated successfully with pentamidine and finally achieved sustained remission of SLE following the addition of cyclophosphamide.

The mechanisms of action of corticosteroid and azathioprine therapy are unknown, but the beneficial effects are believed to be derived from changes in the size, nature, and site of glomerular localization of immune complexes and in the antiinflammatory and antiphlogistic properties of these drugs [130].

Other immunosuppressive drugs, including alkylating agents and antimetabolites, have been used to a lesser extent than azathioprine; these experiences have been reviewed and summarized by Dillard and associates [35]. Combined therapy with prednisone and cyclophosphamide has been described by Cameron et al. [25, 26], Donadio et al. [35a], and Steinberg et al. [9, 179, 180], who suggested some beneficial effect from the latter drug, especially at high (neutropenic) doses. Decker et al. [33a] subsequently have reported no benefit of cyclophosphamide or azathioprine. However, the recent demonstration of the gonadal toxicity of cyclophosphamide raises serious questions as to its value in a chronic process such as SLE. Dillard and associates [35] reported the results of a single course of nitrogen mustard at the onset of SLE, along with high-dose prednisone therapy, and found little additional benefit compared with that of corticosteroids alone. Epstein and Grausz [47] reported a 73 percent 5-year survival in 67 adult patients treated with prednisone and chlorambucil. Ginzler et al. [61a] did not observe additional benefit using triple therapy of prednisone, azathioprine, and cyclophosphamide compared to prednisone and azathioprine alone.

Careful attention to all aspects of patient care in SLE contributes in a major way to the overall success and survival. The avoidance of direct exposure to sunlight is highly recommended; various sunscreen preparations are available for topical use that reduce the risk of exacerbation of SLE. Topical application of corticosteroids is helpful in providing a better cosmetic appearance, but should not be used unless serologic remission with corticosteroid therapy has been attained. Restriction of activity and bed rest have no specific value. The use of antimalarials in the management of childhood SLE has been described in the older literature [80, 91, 126] and is carefully reviewed by Dubois [40]. It is doubtful that there is any indication for this form of therapy in children.

Prognosis

The prognosis of SLE has improved dramatically during the past three decades. The data of Dubois et al. [43] have shown clearly that prior to corticosteroid therapy, survival did not exceed 5 years. Today, with a large armamentarium of therapeutic modalities, survival at 5 years has been extended to nearly 70 percent in some series of adults. Although it has been suggested that SLE in childhood is more severe and has a worse prognosis than in adults [126], it seems likely that the outlook in SLE is independent of age. Our observations in children have documented a 10-year survival of 86 percent [52].

Considerable attention has been focused on the relationship of the type of renal injury to the prognosis. Pollak et al. [157–159], Baldwin et al. [14], and Estes and Christian [48] have shown that patients with diffuse proliferative lupus nephritis have a poorer prognosis (45 percent 5-year survival) compared with that of patients having normal kidneys, mesangial lupus nephritis, focal proliferative lupus nephritis, or membranous lupus nephritis. It is possible that an improved prognosis in the diffuse proliferative group will be attained by earlier referral and more aggressive therapy [35, 52].

It now appears that the major mortality in SLE is from nonrenal causes. Mackay [119] has aptly characterized the current status of this disease:

. . . modern treatment has transformed SLE from an acute severe, to a chronic attenuated disease. The florid febrile lupus erythematosus of former years is, of course, still seen, but most transiently so, by reason of precise serological diagnostic procedures and effective suppressive therapy. Hence, today we are more concerned with long-term disabling effects and less familiar clinical manifestations resulting from slowly ebbing and partially or intermittently suppressed autoimmune reactions.

Mackay's evaluation underscores both the current status of SLE and the enormity and magnitude of the problems facing physicians engaged in the care of these patients. It is our feeling that if the prognosis of this disease is to continue to improve, highly coordinated, consistent, and aggressive care in large centers is essential.

References

1. Agnello, V., Winchester, R. J., and Kunkel, H. G. Precipitin reactions of the C1q component of complement with aggregated gamma-globulin and immune complexes in gel diffusion. *Immunology* 19: 909, 1970.
2. Alarcón-Segovia, D. Drug induced lupus syndromes. *Mayo Clin. Proc.* 44:664, 1969.
3. Alarcón-Segovia, D., Fishbein, E., and Betancourt, V. M. Antibodies to nucleoprotein and to hydrazide-altered soluble nucleoprotein in tuberculous patients receiving isoniazid. *Clin. Exp. Immunol.* 5: 429, 1969.
4. Alarcón-Segovia, D., Fishbein, E., Reyes, P. A., Dies, H., and Shwadsky, S. Antinuclear antibodies in patients on anticonvulsant therapy. *Clin. Exp. Immunol.* 12:39, 1972.
5. Alarcón-Segovia, D., Wakim, K. G., Worthington, J. W., and Ward, L. E. Clinical and experimental studies on the hydralazine syndrome and its relationship to systemic lupus erythematosus. *Medicine (Baltimore)* 46:1, 1967.
6. Alcala, H., and Alarcón-Segovia, D. Ulceration and perforation of the nasal septum in systemic lupus erythematosus. *N. Engl. J. Med.* 281:722, 1969.
7. Alper, C. A., and Rosen, F. S. The Role of Complement in Vivo as Revealed by Genetic Defects. In L. Brent and J. Holborow (eds.), *Progress in Immunology II, Proceedings of the Second International Congress of Immunology.* Amsterdam: North-Holland Publishing Co., 1974. Pp. 201–208.
8. Andres, G. A., Accinni, L., Beiser, S. M., Christian, C. L., Cinotti, G. A., Erlanger, B. F., Hsu, K. C., and Seegal, B. C. Localization of fluorescein-labeled antinucleoside antibodies in glomeruli of patients with active systemic lupus erythematosus nephritis. *J. Clin. Invest.* 49:2106, 1970.
9. Aptekar, R. G., Steinberg, A. D., and Decker, J. L. Complications of cytotoxic agents in systemic lupus erythematosus (SLE) and rheumatoid arthritis (RA) (abstract). *Arthritis Rheum.* 16:533, 1973.
10. Armas-Cruz, R., Harnecker, J., Ducach, G., Jalil, J., and Gonzalez, F. Clinical diagnosis of systemic lupus erythematosus. *Am. J. Med.* 25:409, 1958.
11. Arnett, F. C., Bias, W. B., and Shulman, L. E. HL-A antigens in systemic lupus erythematosus (SLE). *Arthritis Rheum.* 15:428, 1972.
12. Atkins, C. J., Kondon, J. J., Jr., Quismorio, F. P., and Friou, G. J. The choroid plexus in systemic lupus erythematosus. *Ann. Intern. Med.* 76:65, 1972.
13. Baehr, G., Klemperer, P., and Schifrin, A. A diffuse disease of the peripheral circulation (usually associated with lupus erythematosus and endocarditis). *Trans. Assoc. Am. Physicians* 50:139, 1935.
14. Baldwin, D. S., Lowenstein, J., Rothfield, N. F., Gallo, G., and McCluskey, R. T. The clinical course of the proliferative and membranous forms of lupus nephritis. *Ann. Intern. Med.* 73:929, 1970.
15. Baringer, J., and Swoveland, P. Tubular aggregates in endoplasmic reticulum: Evidence against their viral nature. *J. Ultrastruct. Res.* 41:270, 1972.
16. Beernink, D. H., and Miller, J. J. Anticonvulsant-induced antinuclear antibodies and lupus-like disease in children. *J. Pediatr.* 82:113, 1973.
17. Bennahum, A., Messner, P., and Shoop, J. D. Brain scan findings in central nervous system in-

volvement by lupus erythematosus. *Ann. Intern. Med.* 81:763, 1974.

18. Bergstein, J. M., Wiens, C., Fish, A. J., Vernier, R. L., and Michael, A. F. Avascular necrosis of bone in systemic lupus erythematosus. *J. Pediatr.* 85:31, 1974.

19. Bernard, G. C., Lange, R. L., and Hensley, G. T. Aortic disease with valvular insufficiency as the principal manifestation of systemic lupus erythematosus. *Ann. Intern. Med.* 71:81, 1969.

20. Boelaert, J., Morel-Maroger, L., and Méry, J. P. Renal Insufficiency in Lupus Nephritis. In J. Hamburger, J. Crosnier, and M. H. Maxwell (eds.), *Advances in Nephrology*. Chicago: Year Book, 1974. Pp. 249–289.

20a. Boxer, M., Ellman, L., and Carvalho, A. The lupus anticoagulant. *Arthritis Rheum.* 19:1244, 1976.

21. Brunjes, S., Zikeik, K., and Julian, R. Familial systemic lupus erythematosus. A review of the literature with a report of ten additional cases in four families. *Am. J. Med.* 30:529, 1961.

22. Buchanan, I. S., and Humpston, D. J. Nail-fold capillaries in connective tissue disorders. *Lancet* 1:845, 1968.

23. Burnham, T. K., Fine, G., and Neblett, T. R. Immunofluorescent "band" test for lupus erythematosus: II. Employing skin lesions. *Arch. Dermatol.* 102:42, 1970.

24. Cade, R., Spooner, G., Schlein, E., Pickering, M., DeQuesada, A., Holcomb, A., Juncos, L., Richard, G., Shires, D., Levin, D., Hackett, R., Free, J., Hunt, R., and Fregly, M. Comparison of azathioprine, prednisone and heparin alone or combined in treating lupus nephritis. *Nephron* 10:37, 1973.

25. Cameron, J. S., Boulton-Jones, M., Robinson, R., and Ogg, C. Treatment of lupus nephritis with cyclophosphamide. *Lancet* 2:846, 1970.

26. Cameron, J. S., and Jones, M. B. Lupus Nephritis: Long-Term Follow-up. In P. Kincaid-Smith, T. H. Mathew, and E. L. Becker (eds.), *Proceedings International Symposium on Glomerulonephritis*. New York: Wiley, 1972. Pp. 1187–1191.

27. Carlow, T. J., and Glaser, J. S. Pseudotumor cerebri syndrome in systemic lupus erythematosus. *J.A.M.A.* 228:197, 1974.

28. Cheatum, D. E., Hurd, E. R., Strunk, S. W., and Ziff, M. Renal histology and clinical course of systemic lupus erythematosus. *Arthritis Rheum.* 16:670, 1973.

29. Cohen, A. S., and Canoso, J. J. Criteria for the classification of systemic lupus erythematosus—status 1972. *Arthritis Rheum.* 15:540, 1972.

30. Cohen, A. S., Reynolds, W. E., Franklin, E. C., Kulka, J. P., Ropes, M. W., Shulman, L. E., and Wallace, S. L. Preliminary criteria for the classification of systemic lupus erythematosus. *Bull. Rheum. Dis.* 21:643, 1971.

31. Comerford, F. R., and Cohen, A. S. The nephropathy of systemic lupus erythematosus. *Medicine (Baltimore)* 46:425, 1967.

32. Cook, C. D., Wedgwood, R. J. P., Craig, J. M., Hartmann, J. R., and Janeway, C. A. Systemic lupus erythematosus. Description of 37 cases in children and a discussion of endocrine therapy in 32 of the cases. *Pediatrics* 26:570, 1960.

33. Day, N. K., Geiger, H., McLean, R., Michael, A., and Good, R. A. C2 deficiency. Development of lupus erythematosus. *J. Clin. Invest.* 52:1601, 1973.

33a. Decker, J. L., Klippel, J. H., Plotz, P. H., and Steinberg, A. D. Cyclophosphamide or azathioprine in lupus glomerulonephritis. *Ann. Intern. Med.* 83:606, 1975.

34. Desser, K. B., Sartiano, G. P., and Cooper, J. L. Lupus livedo and cutaneous infarction. *Angiology* 20:261, 1969.

35. Dillard, M. G., Dujovne, I., Pollak, V. E., and Pirani, C. L. The effect of treatment with prednisone and nitrogen mustard on the renal lesions and life span of patients with lupus glomerulonephritis. *Nephron* 10:273, 1973.

35a. Donadio, J. V., Holley, K. E., Ferguson, R. H., and Ilstrup, D. M. Progressive lupus glomerulonephritis. Treatment with prednisone and combined prednisone and cyclophosphamide. *Mayo Clin. Proc.* 51:484, 1976.

36. Donadio, J. V., Jr., Holley, K. E., Wagoner, R. D., Richard, D., Ferguson, R. H., Richard, H., McDuffie, F. C., and Frederic, C. Treatment of lupus nephritis with prednisone and azathioprine. *Ann. Intern. Med.* 77:829, 1972.

37. Donadio, J. V., Jr., Holley, K. E., Wagoner, R. D., Richard, D., Ferguson, R. H., Richard, H., McDuffie, F. C., and Frederic, C. Further observations on the treatment of lupus nephritis with prednisone and combined prednisone and azathioprine. *Arthritis Rheum.* 17:573, 1974.

38. Drinkard, J. P., Stanley, T. M., Dornfield, L., Austin, C., Barnett, E. V., Pearson, C. M., Vernier, R. L., Adams, D. A., Latta, H., and Gonick, H. C. Azathioprine and prednisone in the treatment of adults with lupus nephritis. Clinical histological and immunological changes with therapy. *Medicine (Baltimore)* 49:411, 1970.

39. Dubois, E. L. Effect of L.E. cell test on clinical picture of systemic lupus erythematosus. *Ann. Intern. Med.* 38:1265, 1953.

40. Dubois, E. L. Management of Discoid and Systemic Lupus Erythematosus. In E. Dubois (ed.), *Lupus Erythematosus* (2nd ed.). Los Angeles: University of Southern California Press, 1974. P. 537.

41. Dubois, E. L. The Clinical Picture of Systemic Lupus Erythematosus. In E. Dubois (ed.), *Lupus Erythematosus* (2nd ed.). Los Angeles: University of Southern California Press, 1974. P. 385.

42. Dubois, E. L. The Clinical Picture of Systemic Lupus Erythematosus. In E. Dubois (ed.), *Lupus Erythematosus* (2nd ed.). Los Angeles: University of Southern California Press, 1974. P. 232.

43. Dubois, E. L., Wierzchowiecki, M., Cox, M. B., and Weiner, J. M. Duration and death in systemic lupus erythematosus. An analysis of 249 cases. *J.A.M.A.* 227:1399, 1402, 1974.

44. Duffy, J. L. Myxovirus-like particles in lipoid nephrosis. *N. Engl. J. Med.* 281:562, 1969.

45. Dujovne, I., Pollak, V. E., Pirani, C. L., and Dillard, M. G. The distribution and character of glomerular deposits in systemic lupus erythematosus. *Kidney Int.* 2:33, 1972.

46. Epstein, W. Immunologic events preceding clinical exacerbation of systemic lupus erythematosus. *Am. J. Med.* 54:631, 1973.

47. Epstein, W. V., and Grausz, H. Favorable outcome in diffuse proliferative glomerulonephritis of systemic lupus erythematosus. *Arthritis Rheum.* 17:129, 1974.

48. Estes, D., and Christian, C. L. The natural history

of systemic lupus erythematosus by prospective analysis. *Medicine (Baltimore)* 50:85, 1971.

49. Feinstein, D. I., and Rapaport, S. I.   Acquired Inhibitors of Blood Coagulation. In T. H. Spaet (ed.), *Progressive Hemostasis and Thrombosis*. New York: Grune & Stratton, 1972. Vol. 1, pp. 75–95.

50. Fennell, R. H., Jr., Maclachlan, M. J., and Rodnan, G. P.   Occurrence of antinuclear factors in sera of relatives of patients with systemic rheumatic disease (abstract). *Arthritis Rheum.* 5:296, 1962.

51. Fessel, W. J.   Systemic lupus erythematosus in the community. *Arch. Intern. Med.* 134:1027, 1974.

52. Fish, A. J., Blau, E. B., Westberg, N. G., Burke, B. A., Vernier, R. L., and Michael, A. F.   SLE within the first two decades of life. *Am. J. Med.* 62:99, 1977.

53. Fish, A. J., Michael, A. F., and Good, R. A.   Pathogenesis of Glomerulonephritis. In M. B. Strauss and L. G. Welt (eds.), *Diseases of the Kidney* (2nd ed.). Boston: Little, Brown, 1971. Pp. 373–403.

54. Fish, A. J., Vernier, R. L., and Michael, A. F.   Glomerular Disorders. In H. F. Conn (ed.), *Current Therapy* (1976 ed.). Philadelphia: Saunders, 1976. P. 519.

55. Foad, B. S. I., Khuller, S., Freimer, E. H., Kirsner, A. B., and Sheon, R. P.   Cell-mediated immunity in systemic lupus erythematosus: Alterations with advancing age. *J. Lab. Clin. Med.* 85:132, 1975.

56. Fraire, A. E., Smith, M. N., Greenberg, S. D., Weg, J. G., and Sharp, J. T.   Tubular structures in pulmonary endothelial cells in systemic lupus erythematosus. *Am. J. Clin. Pathol.* 56:244, 1971.

57. Freedman, P., and Markowitz, A. S.   Isolation of antibody-like gamma-globulin from lupus glomeruli. *Br. Med. J.* 1:1175, 1962.

58. Freedman, P., Peters, J. H., and Kark, R. M.   Localization of gamma-globulin in the diseased kidney. *Arch. Intern. Med.* 105:524, 1960.

59. Garancis, J. C., Komorowski, R. A., Bernhard, G. C., and Staumfjord, J. V.   Significance of cytoplasmic microtubules in lupus nephritis. *Am. J. Pathol.* 64:1, 1971.

59a. Garin, E. H., Donnelly, W. H., Fennell, R. S., and Richard, G. A.   Nephritis in systemic lupus erythematosus in children. *J. Pediatr.* 89:366, 1976.

60. Gewurz, H., Pickering, R. J., Mergenhagen, S. E., and Good, R. A.   The complement profile in systemic lupus erythematosus, acute glomerulonephritis. *Int. Arch. Allergy* 34:557, 1968.

61. Gilliam, J. N., Cheatum, D. E., Hurd, E. R., Stastny, P., and Ziff, M.   Immunoglobulin in clinically uninvolved skin in systemic lupus erythematosus. Association with renal disease. *J. Clin. Invest.* 53:1434, 1974.

61a. Ginzler, E., Diamond, H., Guttadauria, M., and Kaplan, D.   Prednisone and azathioprine compared to prednisone plus low-dose azathioprine and cyclophosphamide in the treatment of diffuse lupus nephritis. *Arthritis Rheum.* 19:693, 1976.

62. Ginzler, E. M., Nicastri, A. D., Chen, C. K., Friedman, E. A., Diamond, H. S., and Kaplan, D.   Progression of mesangial and focal to diffuse lupus nephritis. *N. Engl. J. Med.* 291:693, 1974.

63. Ginzler, E., Sharon, E., Diamond, H., and Kaplan, D.   Long-term maintenance therapy with azathioprine in systemic lupus erythematosus. *Arthritis Rheum.* 18:27, 1975.

64. Gold, A. P., and Yahr, M. D.   Childhood lupus

erythematosus. *Trans. Am. Neurol. Assoc.* 85:96, 1960.

65. Gold, W. M., and Jennings, D. B.   Pulmonary function in patients with systemic lupus erythematosus. *Am. Rev. Resp. Dis.* 93:556, 1966.

66. Goldberg, M. A., Arnett, F. C., and Bias, W. B.   Histocompatibility (HL-A) antigens in systemic lupus erythematosus. Thirty-seventh Annual Meeting of the American Rheumatism Association, Sect. Arthritis Foundation, Los Angeles, California, June 6–9, 1973.

67. Goldman, J. A., Litwin, A., Adams, L. E., Krueger, R. C., and Hess, E. V.   Cellular immunity to nuclear antigens in systemic lupus erythematosus. *J. Clin. Invest.* 51:2669, 1972.

68. Gotoff, S. P., Issacs, E. W., Muehrcke, R. C., and Smith, R. D.   Serum β_1C-globulin in glomerulonephritis and systemic lupus erythematosus. *Ann. Intern. Med.* 71:327, 1969.

69. Grausz, H., Earley, L. E., Stephens, B. G., Lee, J. C., and Hopper, J., Jr.   Diagnostic import of virus-like particles in the glomerular endothelium of patients with systemic lupus erythematosus. *N. Engl. J. Med.* 283:506, 1970.

70. Gribetz, D., and Henley, W. L.   Systemic lupus erythematosus in childhood. *Mt. Sinai Hosp. J.* 26:289, 1959.

71. Grishman, E., and Churg, J.   Ultrastructure of dermal lesions in systemic lupus erythematosus. *Lab. Invest.* 22:189, 1970.

72. Grishman, E., Porush, J. G., Lee, S. L., and Churg, J.   Renal biopsies in lupus nephritis. *Nephron* 10:25, 1973.

73. Grishman, E., Porush, J. G., Rosen, S. M., and Churg, J.   Lupus nephritis with organized deposits in the kidneys. *Lab. Invest.* 16:717, 1967.

74. Gross, M., Esterly, J. R., and Earle, R. H.   Pulmonary alterations in systemic lupus erythematosus. *Am. Rev. Resp. Dis.* 105:572, 1972.

75. Grumet, F. C., Coukell, A., Bodmer, J. G., Bodmer, W. F., and McDevitt, H. O.   Histocompatibility (HL-A) antigens associated with systemic lupus erythematosus. *N. Engl. J. Med.* 285:193, 1971.

76. Hadler, N. M., Gerwin, R. D., Frank, M. M., Whitaker, J. N., Baker, M., and Decker, J. L.   The fourth component of complement in the cerebrospinal fluid in systemic lupus erythematosus. *Arthritis Rheum.* 16:507, 1973.

77. Hagge, W. W., Burke, E. C., and Stickler, G. B.   Treatment of systemic lupus erythematosus complicated by nephritis in children. *Pediatrics* 40:822, 1967.

78. Hahn, B. H., Bagby, M. K., and Osterland, C. K.   Abnormalities of delayed hypersensitivity in systemic lupus erythematosus. *Am. J. Med.* 55:25, 1973.

78a. Hahn, B. H., Kantor, O. S., and Osterland, C. K.   Azathioprine plus prednisone compared with prednisone alone in the treatment of systemic lupus erythematosus. *Ann. Intern. Med.* 83:597, 1975.

79. Hanauer, L. B., and Christian, C. L.   Studies of cryoproteins in SLE. *J. Clin. Invest.* 46:400, 1967.

80. Hanson, V., and Kornreich, H.   Systemic rheumatic disorders ("collagen disease") in childhood. Lupus erythematosus, anaphylactoid purpura, dermatomyositis, and scleroderma. *Bull. Rheum. Dis.* Parts I and II, 17:435, 1967.

81. Hanson, V., Kornreich, H. K., and Drexler, E.

Rheumatoid factor in children with lupus erythematosus. *Am. J. Dis. Child.* 112:28, 1966.

82. Harbeck, R. J., Bardana, E. J., Kohler, P. F., and Carr, R. I. DNA: Anti-DNA complexes. Their detection in systemic lupus erythematosus sera. *J. Clin. Invest.* 52:789, 1973.

83. Hargraves, M. M., Richmond, H., and Morton, R. Presentation of two bone marrow elements, the "tart" cell and "L.E." cell. *Proc. Staff. Meet. Mayo Clin.* 23:25, 1948.

84. Hauptmann, G., Grosshans, E., Heid, R., Mayer, S., and Basset, A. Lupus erythemateux aigu avec déficit complet de la fraction C4 du complement. *Nouv. Presse Med.* 3:881, 1974.

85. Hayslett, J. P., Kashgarian, M., Cook, C. D., and Spargo, B. H. The effect of azathioprine on lupus glomerulonephritis. *Medicine (Baltimore)* 51:393, 1972.

85a. Hollcraft, R. M., Dubois, E. L., Lundberg, G. D., Chandor, S. B., Gilbert, S. B., Quismorio, F. P., Barbour, B. H., and Friou, G. J. Renal damage in systemic lupus erythematosus with normal renal function. *J. Rheumatol.* 3:251, 1976.

86. Hollinger, R., Sharp, J. T., Lidsky, M. D., and Rawls, W. E. Antibodies to viral antigens in systemic lupus erythematosus. *Arthritis Rheum.* 14:1, 1971.

87. Horwitz, D. A. Impaired delayed hypersensitivity in systemic lupus erythematosus. *Arthritis Rheum.* 15:353, 1972.

88. Huang, C. T., and Lyons, H. A. Comparison of pulmonary function in patients with systemic lupus erythematosus, scleroderma and rheumatoid arthritis. *Am. Rev. Resp. Dis.* 93:865, 1966.

89. Hurd, E. R., Eigenbrodt, E., Worthen, H., Strunk, S. S., and Ziff, M. Glomerular cytoplasmic tubular structures in renal biopsies of patients with systemic lupus erythematosus and other diseases. *Arthritis Rheum.* 14:539, 1971.

90. Hurd, E. R., Eigenbrodt, E., Ziff, M., and Strunk, S. W. Cytoplasmic tubular structures in kidney biopsies in systemic lupus erythematosus. *Arthritis Rheum.* 12:541, 1969.

91. Jacobs, C. Systemic lupus erythematosus in childhood. *Pediatrics* 32:257, 1963.

92. Johnson, R. T., and Richardson, E. P. The neurological manifestations of systemic lupus erythematosus. *Medicine (Baltimore)* 47:337, 1968.

93. Kalsbeek, G. L., and Cormane, R. H. "Bound" complement in the skin of patients with chronic discoid lupus erythematosus and systemic lupus erythematosus. *Lancet* 2:178, 1964.

94. Kanyerezi, B. R., Lwanga, S. K., and Bloch, K. J. Fibrinogen degradation products in serum and urine of patients with systemic lupus erythematosus. *Arthritis Rheum.* 14:267, 1971.

95. Kawano, K., Miller, L., and Kimmelstiel, P. Virus-like structures in lupus erythematosus. *N. Engl. J. Med.* 281:1228, 1969.

96. Keeffe, E. B., Bardana, E. J., Jr., Harbeck, R. J., Pirofsky, B., and Carr, R. I. Lupus meningitis. *Ann. Intern. Med.* 80:58, 1974.

97. Klemperer, P., Pollack, A. D., and Baehr, G. Pathology of disseminated lupus erythematosus. *Arch. Pathol.* 32:569, 1941.

98. Klippel, J. H., Grimley, P. M., Decker, J. L., and Michelitch, H. J. Lymphocyte tubuloreticular structures in lupus erythematosus. Correlation with disease activity. *Ann. Intern. Med.* 81:355, 1974.

99. Koffler, D. Immunopathogenesis of systemic lupus erythematosus. *Ann. Rev. Med.* 25:149, 1974.

100. Koffler, D., Agnello, V., Carr, R. I., and Kunkel, H. G. Variable patterns of immunoglobulin and complement deposition in the kidneys of patients with systemic lupus erythematosus. *Am. J. Pathol.* 56:305, 1969.

101. Koffler, D., Agnello, V., and Kunkel, H. G. Polynucleotide immune complexes in serum and glomeruli of patients with systemic lupus erythematosus. *Am. J. Pathol.* 74:109, 1974.

102. Koffler, D., Schur, P. H., and Kunkel, H. G. Immunological studies concerning the nephritis of systemic lupus erythematosus. *J. Exp. Med.* 126:607, 1967.

103. Kohler, P. F., and ten Bensel, R. Serial complement alterations in acute erythematosus. *Clin. Exp. Immunol.* 4:191, 1969.

104. Krishnan, C., and Kaplan, M. H. Immunopathologic studies of systemic lupus erythematosus. II. Antinuclear reaction of γ-globulin eluted from homogenates and isolated glomeruli of kidneys from patients with lupus nephritis. *J. Clin. Invest.* 46:569, 1967.

105. Kurland, L. T., Hauser, W. A., Ferguson, R. H., and Holley, K. E. Epidemiologic features of diffuse connective tissue disorders in Rochester, Minnesota, 1951 through 1967 with special reference to systemic lupus erythematosus. *Mayo Clin. Proc.* 44:649, 1969.

106. Labowitz, R., and Schumacher, H. R. Articular manifestations of systemic lupus erythematosus. *Ann. Intern. Med.* 74:911, 1971.

107. Lachmann, P. J., Müller-Eberhard, H. J., Kunkel, H. G., and Paronetto, F. The localization of *in vitro* bound complement in tissue sections. *J. Exp. Med.* 115:63, 1962.

108. Lambert, P. H., and Dixon, F. J. Pathogenesis of the glomerulonephritis of NZB/W mice. *J. Exp. Med.* 127:507, 1968.

109. Lange, K., Ores, R., Strauss, W., and Wachstein, M. Steroid therapy of systemic lupus erythematosus based on immunologic considerations. *Arthritis Rheum.* 8:244, 1965.

110. Lange, K., Wasserman, E., and Slobody, L. B. Significance of serum complement levels for diagnosis and prognosis of acute and subacute glomerulonephritis and lupus erythematosus disseminatus. *Ann. Intern. Med.* 53:636, 1960.

111. Larsen, R. A. I. A proband material from central eastern Norway in family studies in systemic lupus erythematosus (SLE). *Acta Med. Scand. [Suppl.]* 543:11, 1972.

112. Lechner, K. A new type of coagulation inhibitor. *Thromb. Diath. Haemorrh.* 21:482, 1969.

113. Lee, S. L., and Miotti, A. B. Disorders of hemostatic function in patients with systemic lupus erythematosus. *Semin. Arthritis Rheum.* 4:241, 1975.

114. Lee, S. L., Rivero, I., and Siegel, M. Activation of systemic lupus erythematosus by drugs. *Arch. Intern. Med.* 117:620, 1966.

115. Lewis, E. J., Carpenter, C. B., and Schur, P. H. Serum complement levels in human glomerulonephritis. *Ann. Intern. Med.* 75:555, 1971.

115a. Lewis, R. M., Tannenberg, W., Smith, C., and

Schwartz, R. S. C-type viruses in systemic lupus erythematosus. *Nature* 252:78, 1974.

116. Libman, E., and Sachs, B. A hitherto undescribed form of valvular and mural endocarditis. *Arch. Intern. Med.* 33:701, 1924.

117. Lie, T. H., and Rothfield, N. F. An evaluation of the preliminary criteria for the diagnosis of systemic lupus erythematosus. *Arthritis Rheum.* 15:532, 1972.

117a. Lightfoot, R. W., Jr., and Hughes, G. R. V. Significance of persisting serologic abnormalities in SLE. *Arthritis Rheum.* 19:837, 1976.

118. Lyon, J. M. Acute lupus erythematosus. *Am. J. Dis. Child.* 45:572, 1933.

119. Mackay, I. R. Chronic Lupus Erythematosus. Observations on Long-Term Survivors of "Suppressive" Therapy of Lupus Nephritis with Prednisolone. In P. Kincaid-Smith, T. H. Mathew, and E. L. Becker (eds.), *Proceedings International Symposium on Glomerulonephritis.* New York: Wiley, 1972. Pp. 1211–1217.

120. Mackay, I. R. Autoimmune Aspects of Systemic Lupus Erythematosus and the Forbidden Clone Hypothesis: A Revision. In E. Dubois (ed.), *Lupus Erythematosus* (2nd ed.). Los Angeles: University of California Press, 1974. Pp. 142–152.

121. Mackay, I. R., Chan, D., and Robson, G. Prednisolone treatment of lupus nephritis: Effect of high doses on course of disease, renal function, histological lesions and immunological reactions. *Aust. Ann. Med.* 2:123, 1970.

122. Maher, J. F., and Schreiner, G. E. Treatment of lupus nephritis with azathioprine. *Arch. Intern. Med.* 125:293, 1970.

123. Marchesi, S. L., Aptekar, R. G., Steinberg, A. D., Gralnick, H. R., and Decker, J. L. Urinary fibrin split products in lupus nephritis. Correlation with other parameters of renal disease. *Arthritis Rheum.* 17:158, 1974.

124. Maumenee, A. E. Retinal lesions in lupus erythematosus. *Am. J. Ophthalmol.* 23:971, 1940.

125. McLean, R. H., and Michael, A. F. Activation of the Complement System in Renal Conditions in Animals and Man. In L. Brent and J. Holborow (eds.), *Progress in Immunology II.* Amsterdam: North-Holland Publishing Co., 1974. Vol. 5, pp. 69–79.

126. Meislin, A. G., and Rothfield, N. Systemic lupus erythematosus in childhood. *Pediatrics* 42:37, 1968.

126a. Mellors, R. C., and Mellors, J. W. Antigen related to mammalian type-C RNA viral p30 proteins is located in renal glomeruli in human systemic lupus erythematosus. *Proc. Natl. Acad. Sci. U.S.A.* 73:233, 1976.

127. Méry, J. P., Morel-Maroger, L., and Boelaert, J. Glomerulonephritis in SLE. *N. Engl. J. Med.* 292:480, 1975.

128. Méry, J. P., Morel-Maroger, L., Boelaert, J., and Richet, G. Clinical and anatomical evaluation of diffuse and focal glomerulonephritis in the course of SLE. *J. Urol. Nephrol. (Paris)* 79:321, 1973.

128a. Messner, R. P., Kennedy, M. S., and Jelinek, J. G. Antilymphocyte antibodies in systemic lupus erythematosus. *Arthritis Rheum.* 18:201, 1975.

129. Messner, R. P., Lindstrom, F. D., and Williams, R. C., Jr. Peripheral blood lymphocyte cell surface markers during the course of systemic lupus erythematosus. *J. Clin. Invest.* 52:3046, 1973.

130. Michael, A. F., Vernier, R. L., Drummond, K. N.,

Levitt, J. I., Herdman, R. C., Fish, A. J., and Good, R. A. Immunosuppressive therapy of chronic renal disease. *N. Engl. J. Med.* 276:817, 1967.

131. Michael, A. F., and McLean, R. H. Evidence for Activation of the Alternate Pathway in Glomerulonephritis. In J. Hamburger, J. Crosnier, and M. H. Maxwell (eds.), *Advances in Nephrology.* Chicago: Year Book, 1974. Vol. 4.

132. Miescher, P. A., Rothfield, N., and Miescher, A. Immunologic Phenomena in Patients with Systemic Lupus Erythematosus. In E. Dubois (ed.), *Lupus Erythematosus* (2nd ed.). Los Angeles: University of Southern California Press, 1974. Pp. 153–163.

133. Miyasato, F., Pollak, V. E., and Barcelo, R. Serum $\beta_1 C$ ($\beta_1 C$) globulin levels in systemic erythematosus: Their relationship to clinical and histologic findings. *Arthritis Rheum.* 9:308, 1966.

134. Moncada, B., Day, N. B. K., Good, R. A., and Windhorst, D. B. Lupus erythematosus-like syndrome with a familial defect of complement. *N. Engl. J. Med.* 286:689, 1972.

135. Morel-Maroger, L., Méry, J. P., Delrieu, F., and Richet, G. Etude immuno-histochimique de 29 biopsies rénales faites au cours du lupus érythémateux disséminé. *J. Urol. Nephrol. (Paris)* 77:367, 1970.

136. Muehrcke, R. C., Kark, R. M., Pirani, C. L., and Pollak, V. E. Lupus nephritis: A clinical and pathologic study based on renal biopsies. *Medicine (Baltimore)* 36:1, 1957.

137. Nanra, R. S., and Kincaid-Smith, P. Lupus Nephritis: Clinical Course in Relation to Treatment. In P. Kincaid-Smith, T. H. Mathew, and E. L. Becker (eds.), *Proceedings International Symposium on Glomerulonephritis.* New York: Wiley, 1972. Pp. 1193–1210.

138. Nice, C. M. Congenital disseminated lupus erythematosus. *Am. J. Roentgenol.* 88:585, 1962.

139. Nies, K. M., Brown, J. C., Dubois, E. L., Quismorio, F. P., Friou, G. J., and Terasaki, P. I. Histocompatibility (HL-A) antigens and lymphocytotoxic antibodies in systemic lupus erythematosus (SLE). *Arthritis Rheum.* 17:397, 1974.

140. Norton, W. L. Endothelial inclusions in active lesions of systemic lupus erythematosus. *J. Lab. Clin. Med.* 74:369, 1969.

140a. Okawa, K. I., Wada, H., and Kobayashi, O. Systemic lupus erythematosus in children. *Acta Med. Biol.* 23:149, 1976.

140b. Panem, S., Ordonez, N. G., Kirstein, W. H., Katz, A. I., and Spargo, B. H. C-type virus expression in systemic lupus erythematosus. *N. Engl. J. Med.* 295:470, 1976.

141. Parker, M. D. Ribonucleoprotein antibodies: Frequency and clinical significance in systemic lupus erythematosus, scleroderma, and mixed connective tissue disease. *J. Lab. Clin. Med.* 82:769, 1973.

142. Paronetto, F., and Koffler, D. Immunofluorescent localization of immunoglobulins, complement, and fibrinogen in human diseases. I. Systemic lupus erythematosus. *J. Clin. Invest.* 44:1657, 1965.

143. Petz, L. D., Sharp, G. C., Cooper, N. R., and Irvin, W. D. Serum and cerebral spinal fluid complement and serum autoantibodies in systemic lupus erythematosus. *Medicine (Baltimore)* 50:259, 1971.

144. Perry, H., Tan, E. M., Carmody, S., and Sakamoto, A. Relationship of acetyl transferase activity to

antinuclear antibodies and toxic symptoms in hypertensive patients treated with hydralazine. *J. Lab. Clin. Med.* 76:114, 1970.

145. Peterson, R. D. A., Vernier, R. L., and Good, R. A. Lupus erythematosus. *Pediatr. Clin. North Am.* 10: 941, 1963.

145a. Phillips, P. E. The virus hypothesis in systemic lupus erythematosus. *Ann. Intern. Med.* 83:709, 1975.

146. Pick, A. I., Levo, Y., and Weiss, C. The value of antiDNA antibody titers in the early diagnosis, treatment and follow-up of systemic lupus erythematosus. *Isr. J. Med. Sci.* 10:725, 1974.

147. Pickering, R. J., Michael, A. F., Herdman, R. C., Good, R. A., and Gewurz, H. The complement system in chronic glomerulonephritis: Three newly associated aberrations. *J. Pediatr.* 78:30, 1971.

148. Pincus, T., Blacklow, N. R., Grimley, P. M., and Bellanti, J. A. Glomerular microtubules of systemic lupus erythematosus. *Lancet* 2:1058, 1970.

149. Pincus, T., Hughes, G. R. V., Pincus, D., Tina, L. U., and Belanti, J. A. Antibodies to DNA in childhood systemic lupus erythematosus. *J. Pediatr.* 78:981, 1971.

150. Pincus, T., Schur, P. H., Rose, J. A., Decker, J. L., and Talal, N. Measurement of serum DNA-binding activity in systemic lupus erythematosus. *N. Engl. J. Med.* 281:701, 1969.

151. Pirani, C. L., Pollak, V. E., and Schwartz, F. D. The reproducibility of semiquantitative analyses of renal histology. *Nephron* 1:230, 1964.

152. Pirofsky, B., and Shearn, M. A. The familial occurrence of disseminated lupus erythematosus. *N.Y. State J. Med.* 53:3022, 1953.

153. Pollak, B. H., Steven, M. B., and Shulman, L. E. Photosensitivity in lupus erythematosus, abstract. *Arthritis Rheum.* 9:533, 1966.

154. Pollak, V. E. Antinuclear antibodies in families of patients with systemic lupus erythematosus. *N. Engl. J. Med.* 271:165, 1964.

155. Pollak, V. E., and Pirani, C. L. Renal histologic findings in systemic lupus erythematosus. *Mayo Clin. Proc.* 44:630, 1969.

156. Pollak, V. E., and Pirani, C. L. Pathology of the Kidney in Systemic Lupus Erythematosus: Serial Renal Biopsy Studies and the Effects of Therapy on Kidney Lesions. In E. Dubois (ed.), *Lupus Erythematosus* (2nd ed.). Los Angeles: University of Southern California Press, 1974. Pp. 72–89.

157. Pollak, V. E., Pirani, C. L., Dujovne, I., and Dillard, M. G. The Clinical Course of Lupus Nephritis: Relationship to the Renal Histologic Findings. In P. Kincaid-Smith, T. H. Mathew, and E. L. Becker (eds.), *Proceedings International Symposium on Glomerulonephritis*. New York: Wiley, 1972. Pp. 1167–1181.

158. Pollak, V. E., Pirani, C. L., and Kark, R. M. Effect of large doses of prednisone on the renal lesions and life span of patients with lupus glomerulonephritis. *J. Lab. Clin. Med.* 57:495, 1961.

159. Pollak, V. E., Pirani, C. L., and Schwartz, F. D. The natural history of the renal manifestations of systemic lupus erythematosus. *J. Lab. Clin. Med.* 63: 537, 1964.

160. Prachuabmoh, C., and Stickler, G. B. Rheumatoid arthritis with positive LE clot test in children. *Clin. Pediatr.* 8:695, 1969.

161. Quismorio, F. P., and Friou, G. J. Immunologic

Phenomena in Patients with Systemic Lupus Erythematosus. In E. Dubois (ed.), *Lupus Erythematosus* (2nd ed.). Los Angeles: University of Southern California Press, 1974. P. 164.

162. Regan, M. G., Lackner, H., and Karpatkin, S. Platelet function and coagulation profile in lupus erythematosus. *Ann. Intern. Med.* 81:462, 1974.

163. Reichlin, M., and Mattioli, M. Correlation of a precipitin reaction to an RNA protein antigen and a low prevalence of nephritis in patients with systemic lupus erythematosus. *N. Engl. J. Med.* 286:908, 1972.

164. Rothfield, N. F., McCluskey, R. T., and Baldwin, D. S. Renal disease in systemic lupus erythematosus. *N. Engl. J. Med.* 269:537, 1963.

165. Rothfield, N., Ross, A. H., Minta, J. O., and Lepow, I. H. Glomerular and dermal deposition of properdin in systemic lupus erythematosus. *N. Engl. J. Med.* 287:681, 1972.

166. Schaff, Z., Barry, D. W., and Grimley, P. M. Cytochemistry of tubuloreticular structures in lymphocytes from patients with systemic lupus erythematosus and in cultured human lymphoid cells. *Lab. Invest.* 29:577, 1973.

167. Schur, P. H., and Sandson, J. Immunologic factors and clinical activity in systemic lupus erythematosus. *N. Engl. J. Med.* 278:533, 1968.

168. Senyk, G., Hadley, W. K., Attias, M. R., and Talal, N. Cellular immunity in systemic lupus erythematosus. *Arthritis Rheum.* 17:553, 1974.

169. Sergent, J. S., Lockshin, M. D., Klempner, M. S., and Lipsky, B. A. Central nervous system disease in systemic lupus erythematosus. Therapy and prognosis. *Am. J. Med.* 58:644, 1975.

170. Sharon, E., Kaplan, D., and Diamond, H. S. Exacerbation of systemic erythematosus after withdrawal of azathioprine therapy. *N. Engl. J. Med.* 288:122, 1973.

171. Sharp, G. C., Irvin, W. S., Tan, E. M., Gould, R. G., and Holman, H. R. Mixed connective tissue disease—an apparently distinct rheumatic disease syndrome associated with a specific antibody to an extractable nuclear antigen (ENA). *Am. J. Med.* 52: 148, 1972.

172. Shelp, W. D., Bloodworth, J. M. B., Jr., and Rieselbach, R. E. Effect of azathioprine on renal histology and function in lupus nephritis. *Arch. Intern. Med.* 128:566, 1971.

173. Siegel, M., and Lee, S. L. The epidemiology of systemic lupus erythematosus. *Semin. Arthritis Rheum.* 3:1, 1973.

174. Silber, S. J., Gikas, P. W., and McDonald, F. D. Active lupus glomerulitis and hematoxylin bodies with normal urinalysis. *J. Urol.* 106:812, 1971.

175. Silver, M., and Steinbrocker, O. The musculoskeletal manifestations of systemic lupus erythematosus. *J.A.M.A.* 176:1001, 1961.

176. Spriggs, B., and Epstein, W. V. Clinical and laboratory correlates of L-chain proteinuria in systemic lupus erythematosus. *J. Rheumatol.* 1:3, 287, 1974.

177. Stastny, P. The distribution of HL-A antigens in black patients with systemic lupus erythematosus (SLE). *Arthritis Rheum.* 15:455, 1972.

178. Stastny, P., and Ziff, M. Cold-insoluble complexes and complement levels in SLE. *N. Engl. J. Med.* 280:1376, 1969.

179. Steinberg, A. D., and Decker, J. L. A double-blind controlled trial comparing cyclophosphamide, azathi-

oprine and placebo in the treatment of lupus glomerulonephritis. *Arthritis Rheum.* 17:923, 1974.

180. Steinberg, A. D., Kaltreider, H. B., Staples, P. J., Goetzl, E. J., Talal, N., and Decker, J. L. Cyclophosphamide in lupus nephritis: A controlled trial. *Ann. Intern. Med.* 75:165, 1971.

181. Striker, G. E., Kelly, M. R., Quadracci, L. J., and Scribner, B. H. The Course of Lupus Nephritis: A Clinical-Pathological Correlation of Fifty Patients. In P. Kincaid-Smith, T. H. Mathew, and E. L. Becker (eds.), *Proceedings International Symposium on Glomerulonephritis.* New York: Wiley, 1972. Pp. 1141–1166.

182. Svec, K. H., Blair, J. D., and Kaplan, M. H. Immunopathologic studies of systemic lupus erythematosus (SLE) I. Tissue-bound immunoglobulins in relation to serum antinuclear immunoglobulins in systemic lupus and in chronic liver disease with LE cell factor. *J. Clin. Invest.* 46:558, 1967.

183. Sztejnbok, M., Stewart, A., Diamond, H., and Kaplan, D. Azathioprine in the treatment of systemic lupus erythematosus. A controlled study. *Arthritis Rheum.* 14:639, 1971.

184. Talal, N. Immunologic and viral factors in the pathogenesis of systemic lupus erythematosus. *Arthritis Rheum.* 13:887, 1970.

185. Talal, N., and Steinberg, A. D. The pathogenesis of autoimmunity in New Zealand black mice. *Curr. Top. Microbiol. Immunol.* 64:79, 1974.

186. Talbott, J. H. Historical Background of Discoid and Systemic Lupus Erythematosus. In E. Dubois (ed.), *Lupus Erythematosus* (2nd ed.). Los Angeles: University of Southern California Press, 1974. P. 1.

187. Tan, E. M. Drug-induced autoimmune disease. *Fed. Proc.* 33:1894, 1974.

188. Tan, E. M., and Kunkel, H. G. An immunofluorescent study of the skin lesions in systemic lupus erythematosus. *Arthritis Rheum.* 9:37, 1966.

189. Tan, E. M., Schur, P. H., Carr, R. I., and Kunkel, H. G. Deoxyribonucleic acid (DNA) and antibodies to DNA in the serum of patients with systemic lupus erythematosus. *J. Clin. Invest.* 45:1732, 1966.

190. Teague, P. O., Yunis, E. J., Rodey, G. E., Fish, A. J., Stutman, O., and Good, R. A. Autoimmune phenomena and renal disease in inbred mice: Role of thymectomy aging and involution of immunologic capacity. *Lab. Invest.* 22:121, 1970.

191. Tisher, C. C., Kelso, H. B., Robinson, R. R., Gunells, J. C., and Burkholder, P. M. Intraendothelial inclusion in kidneys of patients with systemic lupus erythematosus. *Ann. Intern. Med.* 75:537, 1971.

192. Trimble, R. B., Townes, A. S., Robinson, H., Kaplan, S. B., Chandler, R. W., Hanissian, A. S., and Masi, A. T. Preliminary criteria for the classification of systemic lupus erythematosus (SLE). *Arthritis Rheum.* 17:184, 1974.

193. Urizar, R. E., Tinglof, B., McIntosch, R., Litman, N., Barnett, E., Wilkerson, J., Smith, F., Jr., and Vernier, R. L. Immunosuppressive therapy of proliferative glomerulonephritis in children. *Am. J. Dis. Child.* 118:411, 1969.

193a. Urowitz, M. B., Bookman, A. A. M., Koehler, B. E., Gordon, D. A., Smythe, H. A., and Ogryzlo, M. A. The bimodal mortality pattern of systemic lupus erythematosus. *Am. J. Med.* 60:221, 1976.

194. Vachtenheim, J., and Grossmann, J. Perforation of the nasal septum in systemic lupus erythematosus. *Br. Med. J.* 2:98, 1969.

195. Veltkamp, J. J., Kerkhoven, P., and Loeliger, E. A. Circulating anticoagulant in disseminated lupus erythematosus. *Haemostasis* 2:253, 1974.

195a. Walravens, P. A., and Chase, H. P. The prognosis of childhood systemic lupus erythematosus. *Am. J. Dis. Child.* 130:929, 1976.

196. Waters, H., Konrad, P., and Walford, R. L. The distribution of HL-A histocompatibility factor and genes in patients with systemic lupus erythematosus. *Tissue Antigens* 1:68, 1971.

197. Westberg, N. G., Naff, G., Boyer, J., and Michael, A. F. Glomerular deposition of properdin in acute and chronic glomerulonephritis with hypocomplementemia. *J. Clin. Invest.* 50:642, 1971.

198. Williams, R. C., Jr., DeBoard, J. R., Mellbye, O. J., Messner, R. P., and Lindstrom, F. D. Studies of T- and B-lymphocytes in patients with connective tissue diseases. *J. Clin. Invest.* 52:283, 1973.

198a. Wilson, C. B., and Dixon, F. J. The Renal Response to Immunologic Injury. In B. M. Brenner and F. C. Rector, Jr. (eds.), *The Kidney.* Philadelphia: Saunders, 1976. P. 838.

199. Winchester, R. J., Winfield, J. B., Siegal, F., Wernet, P., Bentwich, Z., and Kunkel, H. G. Analyses of lymphocytes from patients with rheumatoid arthritis and systemic lupus. *J. Clin. Invest.* 54:1082, 1974.

199a. Winfield, J. B., Winchester, R. J., and Kunkel, H. G. Association of cold-reactive antilymphocyte antibodies with lymphopenia in systemic lupus erythematosus. *Arthritis Rheum.* 18:587, 1975.

200. Winfield, J. B., Winchester, R. J., Wernet, P., and Fu, S. M. Nature of cold-reactive antibodies to lymphocyte surface determinants in systemic lupus erythematosus. *Arthritis Rheum.* 18:1, 1975.

201. Wold, R. T., Young, F. E., Tan, E. M., and Farr, R. S. Deoxyribonucleic acid antibody: A method to detect its primary interaction with deoxyribonucleic acid. *Science* 161:806, 1968.

201a. Wolf, L., Sheahan, M., McCormick, J., Michel, B., and Moskowitz, W. Classification criteria for systemic lupus erythematosus. Frequency in normal patients. *J.A.M.A.* 236:1497, 1976.

202. Zellman, H. E. Incidence of positive serologic tests for syphilis in the collagen diseases. *Am. J. Syph.* 36:163, 1952.

203. Zetterström, R., and Berglund, G. Systemic lupus erythematosus in childhood. *Acta Pediatr. Scand.* 45:189, 1956.

203a. Zimmerman, S. W., Jenkins, P. G., Shelp, W. D., Bloodworth, J. M. B., and Burkholder, P. M. Progression from minimal or focal to diffuse proliferative lupus nephritis. *J. Lab. Invest.* 32:665, 1975.

204. Zweiman, B., Kornblum, J., Cornog, J., and Hildreth, E. A. The prognosis of lupus nephritis: The role of clinical-pathologic correlations. *Ann. Intern. Med.* 69:441, 1968.

59. Renal Manifestations in Connective Tissue Disease

*Jack S. Resnick
and Alfred F. Michael*

Connective-tissue or collagen-vascular diseases are a group of chronic disorders that affect many body systems, including the kidney. The common feature in these diseases appears to be progressive damage to the vasculature throughout the body, resulting in clinical manifestations in the skin, joints, muscles, gastrointestinal tract, kidneys, lungs, heart, and serosal membranes. This chapter will discuss the renal involvement in four common connective tissue diseases: (1) juvenile rheumatoid arthritis (JRA), (2) scleroderma, or progressive systemic sclerosis (PSS), (3) dermatomyositis, and (4) mixed connective tissue disease (MCTD). Systemic lupus erythematosus, anaphylactoid purpura, polyvasculitides, and metabolic diseases are discussed elsewhere. Because of the overlapping clinical features found in these diseases, special emphasis is placed on the characteristic clinical and laboratory findings that help to differentiate and correctly classify them.

Juvenile Rheumatoid Arthritis

Juvenile rheumatoid arthritis, which is a chronic disease of childhood of unknown etiology, is often progressive and crippling. It is essential to rule out other systemic diseases that share many of the articular or extraarticular features of JRA, such as systemic lupus erythematosus or MCTD, since the risk of renal involvement in these diseases is significantly higher; renal involvement in JRA has been documented infrequently.

In studies of the prognosis in children with JRA and in adults whose arthritis began in childhood, 643 cases with 31 deaths were analyzed [2, 8, 24, 27, 39, 48]. Of these deaths, 6 were caused by amyloidosis; 4 of these 6 had chronic renal failure. Amyloidosis was detected as early as 1 to 2 years after the onset of JRA, although in the majority of patients it occurred after many years of active disease. We have seen a death due to amyloidosis with renal failure in a girl who had severe JRA for 15 years (Fig. 59-1). No mention is made of clinical renal disease unassociated with amyloidosis in these reports, except that "febrile proteinuria" was noted in one study [8].

Antilla [3] reviewed the world literature on JRA with kidney involvement, including renal findings in 165 children studied prospectively. Re-

nal biopsies were performed on every third patient, with or without clinical renal involvement, and were evaluated by light microscopy. Proteinuria without nephrotic syndrome was noted at some time in 42.5 percent of the patients; however, this persisted in only 2.4 percent. One-half the patients with proteinuria had received gold therapy. Addis counts revealed that 23.0 percent had hematuria, which was persistent or recurrent in only 4 percent and was associated with either amyloidosis, gold therapy, or (in 1 patient) coagulopathy.

Pyuria was noted in 25.5 percent, of whom almost one-half had a urinary tract infection. Pyuria was not associated with analgesic use. Renal function studies showed a decreased creatinine clearance in 10 percent and a decreased maximal concentrating ability in 31.4 percent; however, no association with therapy or biopsy abnormalities was noted. Hypertension was present in 31 percent and was seen more frequently in patients with a decreased creatinine clearance. It was not associated with drug therapy (including corticosteroids).

Amyloidosis involving the kidney was present in 1 of the 3 patients who died and was found in one renal biopsy specimen. The lesions were mild in both cases and were not observed in glomeruli. Glomerular changes were seen in 28 percent (17 patients). They included the following: focal glomerulonephritis (mostly mesangial proliferation) in 22 percent (13 patients); glomerular basement membrane thickening in 6.7 percent (4 patients); and isolated interstitial nephritis in 3.4 percent (2 patients). Unfortunately, fluorescence or electron microscopy was not performed. Abnormalities on renal biopsy were more frequent in patients with extraarticular manifestations when the duration of disease was longer than 5 years and also were correlated with prior treatment with gold. Although changes on renal biopsy were noted in 38.4 percent of patients, these findings did not correlate with functional abnormalities and did not lead to significant clinical renal disease. Many of the abnormalities were due to treatment with gold and were reversible.

Studies in adults have confirmed the concept of rheumatoid arthritis as a systemic disease with many extraarticular features [19, 26, 61], includ-

Aided by grants AI10704 and HL06314 from the National Institutes of Health.

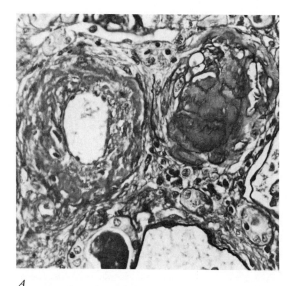

A

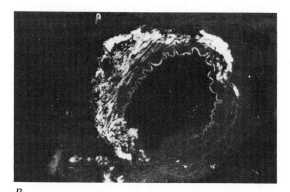

B

Figure 59-1. A. Kidney of a patient with JRA of 15 years' duration. There is extensive involvement of the glomerulus with amyloid, so that only remnants remain. Severe infiltration of an interlobular artery with amyloid can be seen. (PAS, ×350.) B. Thioflafin-T stain of artery from same specimen showing extensive amyloid infiltration of media and adventitia. (×175.)

ing nodules, pulmonary fibrosis, vasculitis, cutaneous ulceration, lymphadenopathy, neuropathy, splenomegaly, episcleritis, pericarditis, and serious bacterial infections. Laboratory findings have included the presence of rheumatoid factors (both 19S and 7S) in high titer and low values for serum complement (CH50, C4, and C2), indicating activation of the classic complement pathway. The presence of soluble immune complexes in serum has also been noted. The association of vasculitis with IgG, rheumatoid factor (IgM), and low-molecular-weight (7S) IgM in a group of patients with rheumatoid arthritis suggests a role for these

factors in the development of vasculitis [58]. Supporting evidence has been the finding of immune deposits (IgM and C3) in cutaneous vessels of seropositive rheumatoid patients [11]. A careful study of cryoglobulinemia in adult patients with rheumatoid arthritis has demonstrated consistent cryoglobulinemia (IgG and IgM) in all patients with rheumatoid vasculitis (neuropathy, dermal vasculitis, or nodules) associated with higher rheumatoid factor (antiglobulin) activity and lower C3 levels than found in patients with uncomplicated rheumatoid arthritis. Rheumatoid factor activity was detected in the cryoglobulins and resided in the 19S IgM fraction only. Immunosuppressive therapy resulted in improvement of clinical disease and a decrease in cryoglobulins, thus implicating circulating immune complexes in the pathogenesis of vascular injury [59].

Antilla [3] also noted a higher incidence of extraarticular findings in patients with renal biopsy changes, especially in those with hypergammaglobulinemia, cryoglobulinemia, and positive antinuclear antibodies. The occurrence of antinuclear antibodies in JRA is common (occurs in 24 percent); however, they are usually in low titer, and rarely, if ever, is anti-DNA antibody detectable [48]. This is in contrast to patients with SLE, in whom high titers of anti-DNA antibodies are found. In an autopsy study of adults with rheumatoid arthritis, Pollack and coworkers [40] found a mild glomerulitis characterized by endothelial cell hyperplasia in 6 of 16 patients. We have seen a 1-year-old girl with severe JRA and extraarticular disease in whom hematuria and decreased creatinine clearance unassociated with gold treatment developed, and whose renal biopsy showed focal glomerulitis (mesangial) and fluorescent deposits of IgM and C3 in the mesangium (Fig. 59-2).

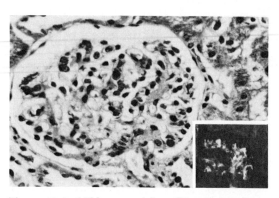

Figure 59-2. Mild mesangial proliferation and segmental increase of mesangial matrix in a child with JRA (H&E, ×445.) Inset shows granular deposits of IgM in the mesangium. (×150.)

Therefore, despite the frequency of renal histologic abnormalities found in JRA, the majority of these findings are clinically and functionally insignificant and often are related to prior gold therapy or are secondary to circulating immune complexes. Vasculitis may also be observed in some patients with severe rheumatoid arthritis and may be related to circulating immune complexes and cryoglobulins. The frequent finding of generalized and renal amyloidosis as a cause of renal failure in patients with chronic JRA should be emphasized, although no specific treatment is available (see Chap. 63).

Scleroderma (Progressive Systemic Sclerosis)

Scleroderma is a rare disease of unknown cause. The clinical spectrum, including extracutaneous involvement, has been well defined in children [13, 21]. The clinical features include cutaneous sclerosis, with typical, waxy, nonpliable skin of the fingers, and variable progression to involve the trunk and face, hyperpigmentation and depigmentation, subcutaneous calcifications, characteristic Raynaud's phenomenon, arthralgias, muscle weakness, dyspnea and, commonly, dysphagia. Renal abnormalities are not seen initially, although in one report, 2 of the 4 deaths were due to the rapid onset of renal failure [1]. Heart disease (myocardial fibrosis or pericardial involvement) and pulmonary disease (fibrosis) are uncommon in children with progressive systemic sclerosis (PSS), although they occur frequently in adults. A poor prognostic sign, noted late in the course, is the onset of severe vasospasm, leading to digital gangrene [21].

Routine laboratory findings are nondiagnostic, although rheumatoid factors and antinuclear antibodies have been positive in about one-third of the patients. Specific antibodies to DNA have been reported in children with PSS [20], although studies in adults have shown predominantly (or characteristically) fluorescent nucleolar antibodies (large nuclear speckling) in the majority of patients [46, 47]. These antibodies have been shown to be directed specifically against the uracil base of single-stranded RNA and not related to the high-titered antiribonucleoprotein (RNP) antibody found in MCTD [1]. The role of these antibodies in the pathogenesis of PSS is unknown, although their presence is useful in confirming the diagnosis.

The major value in defining the type of antinuclear antibody is to rule out SLE, dermatomyositis, or MCTD. Nevertheless, there are patients who defy classification, as exemplified by one child in whom features of SLE developed 4 years after the onset of PSS and who died of central nervous system involvement [13]. We have seen a patient with features of both PSS and dermatomyositis, with deposition of IgM at the dermal-epidermal junction, IgM antinuclear antibody (diffuse pattern), and a favorable response to corticosteroid therapy.

Special diagnostic procedures that are helpful in confirming the diagnosis of PSS include digital plethysmography, demonstration of digital tuft resorption, esophageal radiograms, pulmonary diffusion studies, and skin biopsies.

In a study carried out by Cannon et al. [9], in adults with PSS, renal involvement occurred in about 45 percent of patients, usually within 3 years of onset of the disease and was established by proteinuria (36 percent), hypertension (24 percent), or azotemia (19 percent); the mortality in those with renal involvement was 60 percent. In a series of 358 patients reported by Medsger and Masi [34], renal involvement noted at the onset in 17 patients was uniformly fatal within 1 year. Among patients dying with PSS, renal involvement was the cause of death in almost one-half [9]. The clinical manifestations of renal involvement rarely have included severe proteinuria or nephrotic syndrome [9]. The hypertensive patterns seen have been either malignant hypertension or mild chronic hypertension with superimposed abrupt renal failure. However, in the report of Cannon and associates [9], one-fourth of the patients with azotemia never had hypertension, and the azotemia was often precipitated by infection or dehydration.

Renal histologic abnormalities in patients with PSS have been well described. They affect predominantly the interlobular and small arcuate vessels and often spare the larger vessels. The vascular changes consist of a loose, mucinous intimal thickening of the interlobular arteries (Fig. 59-3A), similar to that seen in malignant hypertension, and fibrinoid necrosis of smaller arteries and afferent arterioles [9, 22]. Variable glomerular changes are seen, including mesangial hypercellularity, thickening of glomerular capillary walls, and ischemic or infarcted segments. Immunofluorescence microscopy has demonstrated fibrinogen and antihemophilic factor in the intima of affected interlobular arteries (Fig. 59-3B) [25], and immunoglobulins, especially IgM, in vascular lesions [33]. Other studies [32] have shown, in addition, rheumatoid factor (antiglobulin) in the vascular deposits and antinuclear (speckled and antinucleolar) antibody from renal eluates. These findings suggest a role for antinuclear antibodies and rheumatoid factors (immune complexes) in the renal vascular lesions of PSS [32]. A role for the renin-angiotensin system in the development

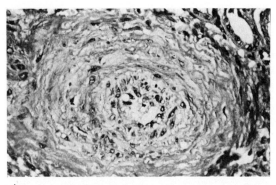

A

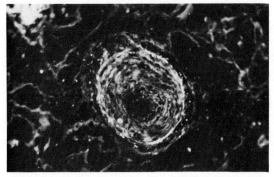

B

Figure 59-3. A. Interlobular artery showing loose, mucinous intimal thickening and collagenous thickening of adventitia in an adult with PSS (H&E, ×280.) B. Deposition of fibrin-fibrinogen in intima of interlobular artery from same specimen. (×415.)

of vascular damage also has been suggested because of the marked elevations of plasma renin activity in patients with scleroderma and azotemia [9, 29]. An increase in collagen synthesis by fibroblasts from skin [31] and increased reducible collagen cross-links [23] lend support to previous theories of defects in the quantity or quality of collagen synthesis in this disease. Whatever the etiology of PSS, renal involvement is common, augurs a poor prognosis, and is a frequent cause of death.

Therapy of renal involvement in PSS has been unsuccessful. However, reports of successful renal transplantation in 3 patients with renal failure and PSS have been encouraging [9, 29, 45]. In addition, following transplantation, all 3 patients have had cessation of or improvement in Raynaud's phenomenon and cutaneous involvement, which possibly may be a consequence of the immunosuppressive drugs used to prevent transplant rejection (corticosteroids and azathioprine). Confirmation of these clinical observations is required.

Dermatomyositis

Dermatomyositis (polymyositis) of childhood is an inflammatory disease of unknown cause that characteristically involves muscle, skin, and blood vessels. The distinctive clinical features that separate this disease from other forms of myositis and myopathies in childhood include the following: erythematous skin lesions over the extensor surfaces of joints (elbows, knees, knuckles, cuticles, and occasionally the neck); a facial erythematous rash, often in a "butterfly" distribution, with a violaceous discoloration of the eyelids; and the insidious development of muscle weakness, occasionally with pain and induration, which is most marked in the proximal, large muscles (deltoids and hip and thigh muscles). To the unfamiliar observer, the skin eruptions and associated symptoms may resemble SLE. However, the characteristic skin lesions over the knuckles (erythema and telangiectasia of underlying small vessels and atrophy with scaling and depigmentation of the overlying epidermis) are diagnostic of dermatomyositis. Other diseases that must be differentiated from dermatomyositis include polyvasculitis involving skin and muscle (periarteritis, allergic angiitis, anaphylactoid purpura), PSS with myositis, rheumatoid arthritis with myositis, primary cryoglobulinemia, and MCTD [54].

The multisystem involvement seen in dermatomyositis may in addition lead to intermittent low-grade fever, fatigue, anorexia, dysphagia, abdominal pain, and arthralgias with or without arthritis. Inflammatory vascular involvement may also be seen in the gastrointestinal tract, subcutaneous tissue, and small nerves [5]. Less commonly noted are involvement of the cardiac musculature, conduction defects and arrhythmias [50, 55], and interstitial lung disease characterized by inflammation and fibrosis without vascular inflammatory changes [4, 18, 37, 51].

The primary pathologic alteration in dermatomyositis is a vasculitis of small vessels within the skeletal muscle, skin, gastrointestinal tract, cardiac musculature, peripheral nerves, and subcutaneous tissues. The vessels show proliferative and infiltrative lesions of the intima and, in later stages, occlusion by fibrin thrombi and subsequent infarction [5]. Electron-microscopic studies have revealed major changes in the endothelial cells of capillaries, arterioles, and veins, with varying degrees of endothelial cell degeneration. It is likely that the microthrombi found in the vessels of some patients are a consequence of endothelial damage. Three pathologic changes have been demonstrated: (1) separation of the endothelial cell junction, (2) necrosis of endothelium with subsequent retraction and cell loss, and (3) endothelial hyperplasia [4]. A widely quoted study has shown immunofluorescent deposits of IgG, IgM, and C3 in blood vessels of skeletal muscle in the majority of children with dermatomyositis, implicating an immune complex vasculitis as the mechanism of muscle injury [60]. We have been unable to confirm this observation in 6 children; muscle biopsies were completely negative for immunoglobulins, complement components, and fibrinogen or properdin in vessels and muscle [44].

A great deal of evidence exists implicating a cell-mediated (lymphocyte or lymphotoxin myotoxicity) immunologic reaction against skeletal muscle by lymphocytes in patients with dermatomyositis and indicating that this abnormality improves after treatment with immunosuppressive agents, correlating with clinical improvement [14, 15]. It has been suggested that a humoral (B cell) deficiency state may exist in dermatomyositis, predisposing to development of a cell-mediated (T cell) inflammatory response [16]. An interesting case of a patient with hereditary deficiency of complement (C2) and typical dermatomyositis has been reported, raising the possibility of complement-dependent immunodeficiency states predisposing to the development of vasculitis diseases such as SLE, anaphylactoid purpura, and dermatomyositis [30]. There has also been a recent description of an antibody to a calf thymus extract antigen that appears to be specific for patients with dermatomyositis [43] and may explain the occasional occurrence of weak antinuclear antibodies found in some patients. Antibody to DNA, however, is not present.

A suggestion of a causal relationship between dermatomyositis and infection with *Toxoplasma gondii* has been reported, although attempts at isolation of the organism and therapy directed toward this infection have been unsuccessful [28]. A virus etiology of dermatomyositis has also been suggested in numerous reports, and prominent tubular aggregates in vascular endothelium have been seen. However, evidence that these represent virus particles is lacking [4].

Renal manifestations in dermatomyositis are uncommon and usually of little clinical significance, but there are reports of a sclerosing glomerulonephritis in a 7-year-old girl with proteinuria and microscopic hematuria [7], a 9-year-old boy with nephrotic syndrome associated with membranoproliferative glomerulonephritis, which resolved completely both clinically and histologically following therapy with corticosteroids and chlorambucil [17], and an adult with nephrotic syndrome and focal glomerulosclerosis that was resistant to therapy with corticosteroids [36].

In well over a hundred cases of dermatomyositis in children [10, 12, 21, 35, 56], signs or symptoms of renal disease were noted in only 3 patients. Two .of these patients had hematuria associated with immobilization, hypercalciuria, and microscopic calcium deposits in the kidney [5, 12], and renal vasculitis and nephritis developed in another patient after corticosteroid therapy was stopped, which was probably due to polyvasculitis mimicking dermatomyositis [56]. The renal histologic findings in 8 children examined at autopsy were normal except for calcium deposition [5].

An exception to the infrequent occurrence of renal involvement in dermatomyositis is found in the paper by Bitnum et al. [6], in which 3 of 13 patients had proteinuria without nephrotic syndrome or renal insufficiency. Renal biopsies in 6 patients demonstrated abnormalities in 5: mild to moderate glomerular hypercellularity, capillary wall thickening, glomerular adhesions, and "hyperplastic changes" in the walls of small blood vessels. One specimen showed diffuse glomerular hyalinization and interstitial nephritis at autopsy after a duration of 9 years. This patient had persistent pyuria, although no mention is made of urinary tract infection or administration of drugs other than corticosteroids. We have seen a 6-year-old child with dermatomyositis and isolated proteinuria (200 mg per day) that disappeared completely after a week of corticosteroid therapy. Additionally, a 10-year-old boy developed typical dermatomyositis one month after the onset of classical poststreptococcal glomerulonephritis.

Since significant renal involvement, either clinical or histological, appears to be rare in children with dermatomyositis, when it occurs, it should suggest the possibility of another diagnosis, such as SLE, vasculitis, or MCTD.

Mixed Connective Tissue Disease

Mixed connective tissue disease is a discrete clinical and laboratory entity that has recently been described [52, 54] and is characterized by overlapping features of SLE, PSS, dermatomyositis (polymyositis), and rheumatoid arthritis. Its clinical features include polyarthralgias or polyarthritis, Raynaud's phenomenon, decreased esophageal motility, decreased pulmonary diffusion, inflammatory polymyositis, and, less frequently, skin rash, sclerodermatous skin features, lymphadenopathy, fever, serositis, hepatosplenomegaly, parotitis, and thyroiditis. Renal disease is uncommon in MCTD, being reported in only 10 percent of patients. One-half the deaths, however, are due to renal failure [52, 53].

Laboratory findings reflect multisystem involvement, with anemia and leukopenia, elevated erythrocyte sedimentation rate, muscle enzymes, and serum immunoglobulins, positive rheumatoid factor, and a characteristic high-titer fluorescent antinuclear antibody showing a speckled pattern on tissue targets (Fig. 59-4). This antibody has been studied by hemagglutination methods and is directed against a saline extractable nuclear antigen (ENA) in a very high titer (up to $1 : 10^7$). The antigen is susceptible to enzymatic treatment with ribonuclease (RNase) (elimination or reduction of titer) while being only partially reduced by treatment with trypsin. This antibody contrasts with a similarly speckled antinuclear antibody seen in SLE that is unaffected by RNase treatment but is susceptible to trypsin digestion. The antibody of MCTD has specificity for the RNP fraction, whereas the antibody seen in SLE reacts with a nuclear component termed *Sm* antigen. These differences have been useful in differentiating these two diseases, which have different morbidities, mortalities, and responses to therapy [52, 53].

The pathogenesis of MCTD is unknown. The overlapping features of SLE, scleroderma, and dermatomyositis, however, suggest a vasculitislike disease. Muscle biopsies have revealed lymphocytic infiltration, and renal biopsies have disclosed a variety of pathologic findings: membranoproliferative changes, membranous nephropathy, mesangial hypercellularity, glomerulitis with focal basement membrane thickening, arterial changes similar to scleroderma, and hypertensive vasculopathy [52, 53]. A group of patients similar to those with MCTD, described as a subgroup of SLE, have antibodies to soluble nuclear RNP antigen, a low frequency of anti-DNA antibodies, and a paucity of renal disease [42]. Of 21 such patients, 3 had renal disease that consisted of diffuse proliferative glomerulonephritis with interstitial nephritis and renal failure, or focal glomerulonephritis with normal renal function. Parker [38] has emphasized that patients with the clinical picture of MCTD and antibody to RNP but not other nuclear antigens have no renal disease. In contrast, patients with antibody to RNP and other nuclear antigens (DNA and others) had a high incidence of nephritis (8 of 15), and all met the criteria for the diagnosis of SLE.

An early report of a case of MCTD in a young woman with proteinuria described a renal biopsy showing proliferative glomerulonephritis and fluorescent deposits of immunoglobulins and complement along the glomerular basement membranes [57]. A recent report in a young woman with MCTD without clinical renal involvement described a renal biopsy with focal mesangial proliferation and vascular sclerosis; immunofluorescence microscopy showed granular mesangial and capillary-loop deposits of IgG, IgM, and C3, and electron microscopy showed dense mesangial deposits [41].

The pathogenesis of MCTD thus is presumably that of an immune complex disease affecting blood vessels in a variety of target organs, including the kidney. Cryoglobulins, decreased complement levels, and anti-DNA antibodies are found infrequently, and their presence may suggest the diagnosis of SLE with overlapping features. High-titer rheumatoid factor is often found (in 62 percent), and glomerular deposits of immunoglobulins (IgM and IgG) have been found in patients with renal disease. Rheumatoid factor (IgM) may be involved in the formation of soluble immune complexes that damage the kidney; however, proof for this is lacking. No instances of circulating immune complexes in the sera of patients with MCTD have been reported.

Mixed connective tissue disease has been reported infrequently in children, although a 13-year-old was included in the original series of Sharp and colleagues [54]. A case reported in a 9-year-old girl included the typical symptoms, together with absent serum and salivary IgA [49]. No clinical renal disease was noted. We have observed a 9-year-old girl with a 4-year history of Raynaud's phenomenon, dysphagia, parotitis, fevers, arthritis and arthralgias, and growth retardation, without clinical evidence of renal disease. A renal biopsy revealed normal findings by both light and fluorescence microscopy. Mixed connec-

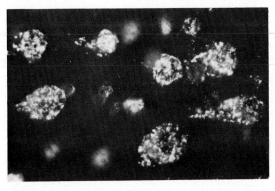

Figure 59-4. Speckled antinuclear antibody pattern in a child with MCTD. (Indirect fluorescence on mouse liver nuclei.) ($\times$675.)

tive tissue disease has been seen in a 14-year-old girl with hematuria, proteinuria, and renal insufficiency; the kidney biopsy revealed necrotizing glomerulonephritis with crescents and immune deposits of IgM, IgG, and C3 (personal communication, Dr. E. Blau).

Baldassare et al. [3a] have reported 5 children with MCTD, 2 of whom had renal involvement consisting of membranous glomerulonephropathy and focal mesangial glomerulonephritis, with deposits of IgG, IgM, and C3 in the mesangium and subepithelial deposits detected by electron microscopy. A report by Singsen et al. [54a] described 14 children with MCTD. They noted the frequent findings of thrombocytopenia (6 of 14 patients), cardiac involvement (9 of 14 patients), and renal involvement (7 of 14 patients). Only five of the patients had clinical evidence of renal disease (proteinuria or abnormal renal function) and 2 patients had histologic evidence of renal disease at autopsy. Renal pathology included interstitial nephritis, proliferative glomerulonephritis with glomerular basement membrane thickening, and membranous glomerulonephropathy. One patient had an initial renal biopsy showing mild glomerulitis that progressed 5 years later to a severe, proliferative glomerulonephritis with IgG deposition on capillary walls. Corticosteroid therapy alone or with immunosuppressive therapy appeared to be beneficial in the patients with severe renal disease.

Mixed connective tissue disease in children may be a more common disease than previously realized. Because of the broad spectrum of clinical findings, the likelihood of erroneous diagnoses (scleroderma, JRA, SLE, and dermatomyositis) is high. It is important to make the correct diagnosis, since MCTD appears to be particularly responsive to therapy with corticosteroids, especially if used early in the course of the disease. The recent observations of a high frequency of renal involvement in children with MCTD should be emphasized, since aggressive therapy, including immunosuppressive agents, may be required to prevent progressive renal damage.

References

1. Alarcon-Segova, D., Fishbein, E., Garcia-Ortigoza, E., and Estrada-Parra, S. Uracil-specific anti-R.N.A. antibodies in scleroderma. *Lancet* 1:363, 1975.
2. Ansell, B. M., and Bywaters, E. G. L. Rheumatoid arthritis (Still's disease). *Pediatr. Clin. North Am.* 10:921, 1963.
3. Antilla, R. Renal involvement in juvenile rheumatoid arthritis. A clinical and histopathological study. *Acta Paediatr. Scand.* [Suppl. 227]61:1, 1972.
3a. Baldassare, A., Weiss, T., Auclair, R., and Zuckner, J. Mixed connective tissue disease (M.C.T.D.) in children. (Abstract) *Arthritis Rheum.* 19:788, 1976.
4. Banker, B. Q. Dermatomyositis of childhood. Ultrastructural alterations of muscle and intra muscular blood vessels. *J. Neuropathol. Exp. Neurol.* 34:46, 1975.
5. Banker, B. Q., and Victor, M. Dermatomyositis (systemic angiopathy) of childhood. *Medicine (Baltimore)* 45:261, 1966.
6. Bitnum, S., Daeschner, C. W., Travis, L. B., Dodge, W. F., and Hopps, H. C. Dermatomyositis. *J. Pediatr.* 64:101, 1964.
7. Bradley, J. E., Drake, M. E., and Mack, H. P. Dermatomyositis with nephritis in a Negro girl. *Am. J. Dis. Child.* 81:403, 1951.
8. Calabro, J. J., and Marchesano, J. M. The early natural history of juvenile rheumatoid arthritis. A 10 year follow-up of 100 cases. *Med. Clin. North Am.* 52:567, 1968.
9. Cannon, P. J., Hassar, M., Case, D. B., Casarella, W. J., Sommers, S. C., and LeRoy, C. The relationship of hypertension and renal failure in scleroderma (progressive systemic sclerosis) to structural and functional abnormalities of the renal cortical circulation. *Medicine (Baltimore)* 55:1, 1974.
10. Carlisle, J. W., and Good, R. A. Dermatomyositis in childhood. Report of studies on 7 cases and a review of literature. *J. Lancet* 79:266, 1959.
11. Conn, D. L., Schroeter, A. L., and McDuffie, F. C. Cutaneous vessel immune deposits in rheumatoid arthritis. *Arthritis Rheum.* 19:15, 1976.
12. Cook, C. D., Rosen, F. S., and Banker, B. Q. Dermatomyositis and focal scleroderma. *Pediatr. Clin. North Am.* 10:979, 1963.
13. Dabich, L., Sullivan, D. B., and Cassidy, J. T. Scleroderma in the child. *J. Pediatr.* 85:770, 1974.
14. Dawkins, R. L. Experimental autoallergic myositis, polymyositis and myesthenia gravis. Autoimmune muscle disease associated with immunodeficiency and neoplasia. *Clin. Exp. Immunol.* 21:185, 1975.
15. Dawkins, R. L., and Mastaglia, F. L. Cell mediated cytotoxicity to muscle in polymyositis. *N. Engl. J. Med.* 288:434, 1973.
16. Dawkins, R. L., and Zilka, P. J. Polymyositis and myesthenia gravis. Immunodeficiency disorders involving skeletal muscle. *Lancet* 1:200, 1975.
17. Debauchez, C., Beissiere, M., and Etienne, M. Syndrome néphrotique associé à une dermatomyosite. *Ann. Pediatr.* 20:153, 1973.
18. Duncan, P. E., Griffin, J. P., Garcia, A., and Kaplan, S. B. Fibrosing alveolitis in polymyositis. *Am. J. Med.* 57:621, 1974.
19. Gordon, D. A., Stein, J. L., and Broder, I. The extra-articular features of rheumatoid arthritis. A systematic analysis of 127 cases. *Am. J. Med.* 54:445, 1973.
20. Hanson, V., Drexler, E., and Kornreich, H. DNA antibodies in childhood scleroderma. *Arthritis Rheum.* 13:798, 1970.
21. Hanson, V., and Kornreich, H. Systemic rheumatic disorders ("collagen disease") in childhood; lupus erythematosus, anaphylactoid purpura, dermatomyositis, and scleroderma. *Bull. Rheum. Dis.* 17:441, 1967.
22. Heptinstall, R. H. *Pathology of the Kidney.* Boston: Little, Brown, 1974. P. 698.
23. Herbert, C. M., Jayson, M. I. V., Lindberg, K. A., and Bailey, A. J. Biosynthesis and maturation of skin collagen in scleroderma, and effect of D-penicillamine. *Lancet* 1:187, 1974.

24. Hill, R. H., Herstein, A., and Walters, K. Juvenile rheumatoid arthritis: Follow-up into adulthood—medical, sexual and social status. *Can. Med. Assoc. J.* 114:790, 1976.

25. Hoyer, J. R., Michael, A. F., and Hoyer, L. W. Immunofluorescent localization of antihemophiliac factor antigen and fibrinogen in human renal diseases. *J. Clin. Invest.* 53:1375, 1974.

26. Hunder, G. G., and McDuffie, F. C. Hypocomplementemia in rheumatoid arthritis. *Am. J. Med.* 54:461, 1973.

27. Jeremy, R., Schaller, J., Arkless, R., Wedgewood, R. J., and Healey, L. A. Juvenile rheumatoid arthritis persisting into adulthood. *Am. J. Med.* 45:419, 1968.

28. Kagen, L. J., Kimball, A. C., and Christian, G. L. Serologic evidence of toxoplasmosis among patients with polymyositis. *Am. J. Med.* 56:186, 1974.

29. Keane, W. F., Danielson, B., and Raij, L. Successful renal transplantation in progressive systemic sclerosis. *Ann. Intern. Med.* 85:199, 1976.

30. Leddy, J. P., Griggs, R. C., Klemperer, M. R., and Frank, M. M. Hereditary complement (C2) deficiency with dermatomyositis. *Am. J. Med.* 58:83, 1975.

31. LeRoy, E. C. Increased collagen synthesis by scleroderma skin fibroblasts in vitro. *J. Clin. Invest.* 54:880, 1974.

32. McCoy, R. C., Tisher, C. C., Pepe, P. F., and Cleveland, L. A. The kidney in progressive systemic sclerosis; immunohistochemical and antibody elution studies. *Lab. Invest.* 35:124, 1976.

33. McGiven, A. R., deBoer, W. G. R. M., and Barnett, A. J. Renal immune deposits in scleroderma. *Pathology* 3:145, 1971.

34. Medsger, T. A., Jr., and Masi, A. T. Survival with scleroderma. II. A life table analysis of clinical and demographic factors in 358 male U.S. veteran patients. *J. Chron. Dis.* 26:647, 1973.

35. Miller, J. J. Late progression in dermatomyositis in childhood. *J. Pediatr.* 83:543, 1973.

36. Moutsopoulos, H., and Fye, K. H. Lipoid nephrosis and focal glomerulosclerosis in a patient with polymyositis. *Lancet* 1:1039, 1975.

37. Park, S., and Nyhan, W. L. Fatal pulmonary involvement in dermatomyositis. *Am. J. Dis. Child.* 129:723, 1975.

38. Parker, M. D. Ribonucleoprotein antibodies; frequency and clinical significance in systemic lupus erythematosus, scleroderma and mixed connective tissue disease. *J. Lab. Clin. Med.* 82:769, 1973.

39. Pazirandeh, M., Mackenzie, A. H., and Scherbel, A. L. The natural course of juvenile rheumatoid arthritis. *Cleve. Clin. Q.* 36:109, 1969.

40. Pollack, V. E., Pirani, C. I., Steck, I. E., and Kark, R. M. The kidney in rheumatoid arthritis: Studies by renal biopsy. *Arthritis Rheum.* 5:1, 1962.

41. Rao, K. V., Berkseth, R. O., Crosson, J. T., Raij, L., and Shapiro, F. L. Immune-complex nephritis in mixed connective tissue disease. *Ann. Intern. Med.* 84:174, 1976.

42. Reichlin, M., and Mattioli, M. Correlation of a precipitin reaction to an RNA protein antigen and a low prevalence of nephritis in patients with systemic lupus erythematosus. *N. Engl. J. Med.* 286:908, 1972.

43. Reichlin, M., and Mattioli, M. Description of a serological reaction characteristic of polymyositis. *Clin. Immunol. Immunopathol.* 5:12, 1976.

44. Resnick, J. S., and Michael, A. F. Unpublished observations.

45. Richardson, J. A. Hemodialysis and kidney transplantation for renal failure from scleroderma. *Arthritis Rheum.* 16:265, 1973.

46. Ritchie, R. F. Antinucleolar antibodies. Their frequency and diagnostic association. *N. Engl. J. Med.* 282:1174, 1970.

47. Rothfield, N. F., and Rodman, G. P. Serum antinuclear antibodies in progressive systemic sclerosis (scleroderma). *Arthritis Rheum.* 11:607, 1968.

48. Rudnicki, R. D., Ruderman, M., Scull, E., Goldenberg, A., and Rothfield, N. Clinical features and serologic abnormalities in juvenile rheumatoid arthritis. *Arthritis Rheum.* 17:1007, 1974.

49. Sanders, D. Y., Huntley, C. C., and Sharp, G. C. Mixed connective tissue disease in a child. *J. Pediatr.* 83:642, 1973.

50. Schaumburg, H. H., Nielson, S. L., and Yunchak, P. M. Heart block in polymyositis. *N. Engl. J. Med.* 284:480, 1971.

51. Schwarz, M. I., Matthay, R. A., Sahn, S. A., Stanford, R. E., Marmorstein, B. L., and Scheinhorn, D. J. Interstitial lung disease in polymyositis and dermatomyositis. Analysis of six cases and review of the literature. *Medicine (Baltimore)* 55:89, 1976.

52. Sharp, G. C. Mixed connective tissue disease. *Bull. Rheum. Dis.* 25:828, 1975.

53. Sharp, G. C., Irvin, W. S., May, C. M., Holman, H. R., McDuffie, F. C., Hess, E. V., and Schmid, F. R. Association of antibodies to ribonucleoprotein and Sm antigens with mixed connective tissue disease, systemic lupus erythematosus and other rheumatic diseases. *N. Engl. J. Med.* 295:1149, 1976.

54. Sharp, G. C., Irvin, W. S., Tan, E. M., Gould, R. G., and Holman, H. R. Mixed connective tissue disease. An apparently distinct rheumatic disease syndrome associated with a specific antibody to an extractable nuclear antigen (ENA). *Am. J. Med.* 52:148, 1972.

54a. Singsen, B. H., Bernstein, B. H., Kornreich, H. K., King, K. K., Hanson, V., and Tan, E. M. Mixed connective tissue disease in childhood: A clinical and serologic survey. *J. Pediatr.* 90:893, 1977.

55. Singsen, B., Goldreyen, B., Stanton, R., and Hanson, V. Childhood polymyositis with cardiac conduction defects. *Am. J. Dis. Child.* 130:72, 1976.

56. Sullivan, D. B., Cassidy, J. T., Petty, R. E, and Burt, A. Prognosis in childhood dermatomyositis. *J. Pediatr.* 80:555, 1972.

57. Tan, E. M., Northway, J. D., and Pinnas, J. L. The clinical significance of antinuclear antibodies. *Postgrad. Med.* 54:143, 1973.

58. Theofilopoulos, A. N., Burtonboy, G., LoSpalluto, J. J., and Ziff, M. IgG rheumatoid factor and low molecular weight IgM. An association with vasculitis. *Arthritis Rheum.* 17:272, 1974.

59. Weisman, M., and Zvaifler, N. Cryoglobulinemia in rheumatoid arthritis: Significance in serum of patients with rheumatoid vasculitis. *J. Clin. Invest.* 56:725, 1975.

60. Whitaker, J. N., and Engel, W. K. Vascular deposits of immunoglobulin and complement in idiopathic inflammatory myopathy. *N. Engl. J. Med.* 286:333, 1972.

61. Zubler, R. H., Nydegger, U., Perrin, L. H., Fehr, K.,

McCormick, J., Lambert, P. H., and Miescher, P. A. Circulating and intra-articular immune complexes in patients with rheumatoid arthritis. Correlation of

125I-C1q binding activity with clinical and biological features of the disease. *J. Clin. Invest.* 57:1308, 1976.

60. Sickle Cell Nephropathy

José Strauss and Rawle M. McIntosh

Sickle cell nephropathy is one of the nephrologist's most challenging therapeutic problems; it also has promising potential for studying basic mechanisms of renal disease.

Genetic and Biochemical Aspects

Sickle cell disease is the consequence of inheriting abnormal hemoglobin S rather than normal adult hemoglobin A or A_2. Hemoglobin S is one of several mutant hemoglobin genes. It is produced by relatively simple changes in the DNA structure: the shifting of a single base pair or peptide unit, with a valine replacing a glutamic acid of hemoglobin A [17, 89]. The consequences are far reaching: valine is hydrophobic; glutamic acid is hydrophilic [72]. Mechanical problems, increased red blood cell fragility and hemolysis, vascular occlusion, and poor oxygen transport and delivery occur, as well as elevation of the concentration of 2,3-diphosphoglycerate (DPG) [50, 73], a phosphate compound that normally is part of the hemoglobin molecule. The increase in 2,3-DPG leads to a decrease in the oxygen transport capacity of hemoglobin; however, release of available oxygen to the tissues is facilitated [30, 50, 81].

Hemoglobin S is easily polymerized during deoxygenation, increasing its internal viscosity and leading to the formation of a gel that causes the irregular, sickled red blood cell shape and lack of the flexibility needed for free circulation. The rigidity, rather than the sickle shape of the cell, seems to cause the mechanical problems [73].

Polymerization of the hemoglobin requires certain conditions, the best known being low oxygen, hyperosmolality [92], and an increased level of prostaglandin E_2 (PGE_2) [58]. Since these conditions exist in the medulla of the kidney, sickling is expected there. The functions of the medulla, especially concentration of the urine, are affected

in sickle cell disease; medullary necrosis, focal scarring, and interstitial fibrosis may develop [4, 41, 85].

Inheritance of hemoglobin S occurs in simple mendelian fashion [89, 100]. Heterozygous persons (genotype SA) have sickle cell trait; homozygous individuals (genotype SS) have sickle cell disease. Studies suggest that the presence of this abnormal hemoglobin is protective against the malarial parasite *Plasmodium falciparum,* which infects red blood cells and alters their biochemical composition. Heterozygous persons are relatively immune to this parasite; normal persons (AA) are highly susceptible [15, 17].

Because phenotypic frequencies (p.f.) of hemoglobin S are high among African populations (p.f. 10 to 40 percent) [15, 17] and among blacks in the United States (p.f. 6 to 14 percent) [77], some consider it to be a "race marker." However, the same mutant gene—or at least one with similar action—is present in Greeks, Turks, and other populations around the Mediterranean (p.f. < 10 percent) and in parts of South Asia (p.f. 5 to 30 percent). The distribution of the trait is throughout these areas and also in populations that have emigrated from these areas into South America and the Caribbean Islands. The trait is not found in northern Europe, most of Asia, Australia, or among the aboriginal populations of North or South America [15, 17]. Thus, the common denominator seems not to be race but an environmental condition: the tropical *P. falciparum* parasite, which is highly destructive to human life. Heterozygote inheritance of hemoglobin S seems to have a selective advantage in these areas, and some consider its persistence in the gene pool to be an example of genetic adaptation, or balanced polymorphism. Since movement of peoples from one area to another and "crossbreeding" are now common occurrences, we can expect to see an in-

Supported in part by grants from the Division of Children's Medical Services, State of Florida, The Miami Dolphins Wives Charity Organization through the Kidney Foundation of Dade County, Inc., and Abbott Laboratories.

creasing number of patients with this abnormal hemoglobin and its resultant complications [15, 17].

History of Renal Involvement

Although sickle cell disease has been identified in Africa for centuries [64, 65], Herrick [54] gave the first published description of renal involvement in 1910. He reported "peculiarly elongated and sickle-shaped" red blood cells in a West Indies student with anemia, white blood cells and casts in the urine, slightly increased urinary output, and low urinary specific gravity. In 1923, Sydenstricker et al. [121] described renal morphologic changes at autopsy in a child with sickle cell disease, noting prominent glomeruli distended with blood, and necrosis and pigmentation of tubules. In 1948, Abel and Brown [1] reported hematuria in SS patients. In 1949, Pauling and coworkers [89] conclusively defined the genetic basis of the disease, as postulated by Emmel [35] in 1917.

Interest increased in renal involvement in sickle cell disease, including renal structural, vascular, and functional changes, as well as clinical manifestations. Infarction of the renal medulla was reported by Goodwin et al. [41] in 1950 as one of the causes of the hematuria in SS patients. McCrory et al. [71] in 1953 and Keitel et al. [60] in 1956 reported clinical and physiologic studies of hyposthenuria. Berman and Schreiner [12] in 1958 postulated a casual relationship between glomerular involvement and the nephrotic syndrome in these patients. McCoy [70] in 1969 and Antonovych [6] in 1972 reported the occurrence of membranoproliferative glomerulonephritis, which we have confirmed [86, 87, 115], providing the first description of glomerular damage due to an autologous immune complex disease in an SS patient [113, 114]. Ho Ping Kong and Alleyne [56] in 1971, Goosens et al. [42] in 1972, and Oster et al. [83] in 1976 described a renal tubular defect that appears in many SS patients and limits their ability to secrete hydrogen ions. In 1974, Friedman et al. [39] reported on chronic dialysis in SS patients with end-stage renal disease.

The general impression has been that the renal disease associated with sickle cell disease is mild, usually transient, and most often only functional. However, the experience of several groups in the last few years has demonstrated that it can be organic, progressive, and severe. The belief that renal problems develop only in older SS patients, not in children, as a result of their hematologic problem has been shattered. Reevaluation of the nephritis of sickle cell disease and the renal complications of the trait require consideration of structural and physiologic alterations as a basis for recognition and understanding of clinical manifestations and therapeutic possibilities.

Physiologic Alterations

Several renal functional alterations have been observed in patients with sickle cell disease and sickle cell trait. A urinary concentrating defect has been recognized and well studied over the past several years. More recently, a defect in hydrogen ion production and progressive deterioration of renal ability to maintain other aspects of metabolic homeostasis adequately have been observed.

CONCENTRATING DEFECT

The renal concentrating defect is constant in sickle cell anemia, and, although of lesser degree, it is also frequent in sickle cell trait [4, 23, 52, 70, 103, 104, 109–111, 129, 130]. The inability to concentrate urine appropriately has been the most consistent renal functional derangement of sickle cell disease, and it is regarded as typical [52, 60, 66, 70, 71, 102, 109, 110, 126, 128]. This defect has also been observed in SC patients [129, 130]. In very young children, early in the disease, the defect is reversible by multiple transfusions with normal erythrocytes [60, 110]. This reversibility is lost progressively with age and is almost negligible in patients after age 15 years.

Patients with sickle cell disease are known to dilute urine normally [4, 52, 60, 70, 109, 111]. Radel et al. [96] concluded that SS patients in crisis have a narrow range of solute concentration in the urine, with limited diluting as well as concentrating capacity. Studies by Hatch and associates [52] suggest that the ability to reabsorb sodium in the loop of Henle and distal tubule is intact.

Several explanations have been given for the defect in urinary concentration in patients with sickle cell anemia. A decrease in medullary blood flow [129, 130], possibly due to local sickling because of high osmolality [92], or a reduced number of vasa recta and their branches [109] has been suggested. The renal medulla is also relatively anoxemic as a result of countercurrent exchange. Other possible explanations include decreased oxygen transport resulting from increased levels of 2,3-DPG; osmotic diuresis of juxtamedullary nephrons [124]; medullary ischemic necrosis [14]; enhanced lymph flow with decreased osmotic gradient [19]; and the presence of PGE_2 in the medulla [58, 95, 101]. The defect may be related to an inability to maintain a high concentration of solute in the medullary interstitium [4].

The decreased urinary concentration is not a severe threat to life. The obligatory volume to excrete the usual solute load amounts to about 2,000 ml per day in the adult sickle cell patient as compared with 600 ml in the normal person. This amount, however, is not unusual even in normal subjects [4]. Nevertheless, fluid deprivation or excessive fluid loss will cause dehydration and an increase in plasma osmolality more rapidly in SS patients than in normal persons. This is reminiscent of patients with diabetes insipidus and is an important clinical consideration.

URINARY ACIDIFICATION DEFECT
Following the administration of ammonium chloride, patients with sickle cell disease did not achieve as low a urinary pH as control subjects, and their rate of excretion of titratable acid and total hydrogen ion was lower [4, 42, 55, 56, 83]. Excretion of ammonia and total hydrogen ion was also lower in patients with sickle cell trait [4, 82]. In contrast, patients with a similar degree of anemia secondary to iron deficiency were found to have a reduction in ammonia excretion, although the minimal urine pH was the same as that of control subjects [4]. Alleyne et al. [4] found that patients with SS disease could lower their pH to the same level as controls when given sodium sulfate while avidly retaining sodium. These investigators also found no difference between SS and control patients in bicarbonate handling. They concluded that patients with sickle cell anemia have a mild form of distal renal tubular acidosis and suggested that this defect may be related to a disturbance of the medullary vasculature, resulting in organic destruction of cells.

Studies have shown that the greatest defect in acidification appears to occur in patients with the most severe concentrating abnormalities [42]. Recently, Oster and coworkers found that 40 percent of patients with sickle cell disease excreted abnormally low amounts of hydrogen ion after ammonium chloride administration [83]. They also found that the Pco_2 plasma-urine gradient was abnormally high after administration of sodium bicarbonate, suggesting a decrease in carbonic anhydrase activity and a consequent reduction in carbon dioxide conversion to H_2CO_3.

OTHER FUNCTIONAL ALTERATIONS
Higher-than-normal rates of glomerular filtration, effective renal plasma flow, and maximal tubular excretion of paraaminohippuric acid have been reported in children with sickle cell disease [36, 37, 123]. These values appear to decrease gradually until 30 to 50 years of age, when they reach critically low levels. Decreased creatinine clearances have been observed in children with sickle cell disease [18, 87, 114]; this may be associated with glomerular abnormalities. On the other hand, patients have been observed who had severe glomerular morphologic alterations and normal or elevated creatinine clearance [87, 123].

Gross and Godel [46] found that blood volume was higher in children with sickle cell disease than in control subjects when related to body weight, but the same when related to height. In SS patients, presumably without severe renal disease, there was a retarded bone age and a progressive increase in growth impairment when compared with a normal population [80]. The effect of overt renal impairment on these variables remains to be determined.

Structural Alterations
GROSS FINDINGS
The kidneys of patients with sickle cell disease are of nearly normal size [4], except in the event of cortical scarring and atrophy. Small, yellowish-white, shallow infarcts are sometimes present on the capsular surface and may occasionally be extensive, resembling cortical necrosis. In kidneys removed for hematuria, hemorrhages are found in the cortex, medulla, and under the pelvic mucosa [3, 76]. Medullary or papillary necrosis has been observed [3, 51]. Caliectasis was found by radiographic examination in 59 percent of 17 patients with sickle cell disease [69], and it has been suggested from autopsy studies in 3 patients that caliectasis is indicative of pyelonephritis. Renal vein thrombosis has been found in some patients [116].

MICROSCOPIC FINDINGS
The most constant histopathologic change is dilatation of the glomerular capillaries and of the interstitial vascular plexus. The glomerular capillaries are filled with red cells showing the characteristic sickled form in formalin-fixed tissue. Glomerular enlargement and congestion, mainly in the juxtamedullary glomeruli [14, 16], are more severe in children than in older patients, in whom glomerular scarring and fibrosis develop [123]. Bernstein and Whitten [14] examined kidneys from children 1 to 15 years of age and found that the congestion of the glomeruli became increasingly severe in the older children, and ischemic glomeruli began to appear in the two oldest. Glomerular fibrosis was present in the oldest patient, and focal fibrosis was seen in others. These changes may be very mild in the absence of

clinical manifestations of renal disease. Small cortical infarcts of varying ages [61], hemosiderin deposits in the epithelium of the proximal convoluted tubules [14], and focal tubular necrosis also have been described. Medullary changes include edema progressing to focal scarring and interstitial fibrosis.

Until recent years, information on the glomerular involvement in patients with overt renal disease, such as the nephrotic syndrome, has been limited. Berman and Schreiner [12] studied a series of patients in whom the nephrotic syndrome was associated with sickle cell disease and hypothesized a causal relationship. Subsequently, additional instances of this association were reported [8, 38, 75, 116, 120]. In a study that included electron-microscopic examination of the kidneys of 3 patients with sickle cell disease, McCoy [70] demonstrated a membranoproliferative glomerulonephritis with circumferential mesangial extension into the capillary loops. Similar findings were reported by Antonovych [6] and Elfenbein et al. [32]. Duplication of the glomerular basement membranes [6, 7, 32, 93], mesangial proliferation, iron-containing deposits in glomerular epithelial cells [70], and glomerular sclerosis have been observed. The histologic findings in other patients with nephrotic syndrome have been those of minimal change disease [8].

We have reported the findings of histologic, ultrastructural, and immunohistologic studies in 7 patients with sickle cell disease [86, 87]. Proteinuria was present in all patients. The nephrotic syndrome, hypertension, hematuria, and renal insufficiency were found in 4 of the 7 patients. All patients had membranoproliferative glomerulonephritis of varying severity; glomerular basement membrane splitting, electron-dense deposits in the glomerulus, interstitial fibrosis, tubular atrophy, and hemosiderin deposits were frequent (Figs. 60-1, 60-2). Immunoglobulin, complement components (in the classic complement pathway), and renal tubular epithelial antigen were distributed in a granular pattern along the glomerular basement membranes of all patients studied. Cryoprecipitable immune complexes of

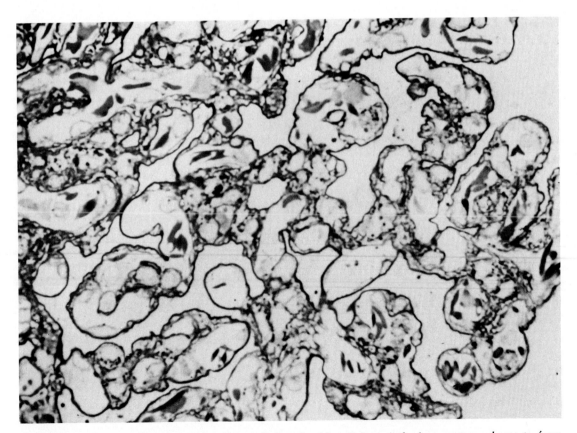

Figure 60-1. The glomerular capillary wall is thickened with splitting of the basement membrane to form double contours. The mesangium is thickened, and the pattern resembles that of membranoproliferative glomerulonephritis. (Jones silver methenamine stain, approximately ×800.)

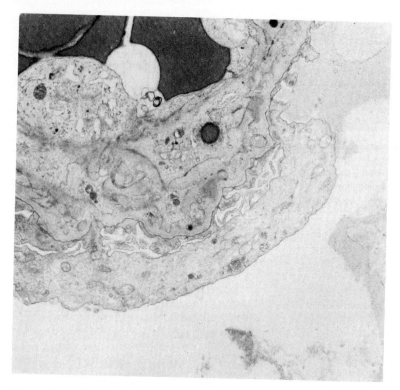

Figure 60-2. Electron micrograph showing mesangial interposition and duplication of basement membrane in the peripheral capillary wall. Granular electron-dense subendothelial deposits can be identified. There is partial fusion of epithelial foot processes. (Approximately ×12,000.)

renal tubular epithelial antigen and antibody to renal tubular epithelial antigen were detected in the circulation of some patients. There was no serologic evidence of activation of the alternate complement pathway [113]. We have seen 2 patients, 1 with proliferative glomerulonephritis associated with sickle cell anemia and 1 with sickle trait and mild morphologic aberrations, who had similar immunohistologic deposits of IgG, complement components, and renal tubular epithelial antigen [84].

PATHOGENESIS OF GLOMERULAR DISEASE
Whether or not there is a causal relationship between sickle cell disease and the nephrotic syndrome is a matter of controversy. The association may be fortuitous, and some patients have had incidental lipoid nephrosis [108], poststreptococcal glomerulonephritis [119], or other renal diseases. Fortuitous renal disease, however, does not account for the great majority of patients with nephrotic syndrome, although minimal change disease may occur with greater-than-usual frequency in patients with sickle cell disease.

Sickle cell disease may produce glomerular lesions through multiple pathogenic mechanisms.

Sickling of erythrocytes within glomerular and postglomerular capillaries may result in stasis and anoxemia. Renal vein thrombosis does occur in sickle cell disease [53, 116], but it cannot account for the glomerular pathologic changes.

Renal involvement has also been attributed to the toxic effect of the extensive deposition of iron in these patients' kidneys [70]. However, in patients with sickle cell disease, there is no correlation between the severity of these deposits, which are minimal in glomeruli, and the presence of renal disease. The patient in our study who presented the most extensive hemosiderin deposition has been followed for 6 years without any deterioration in his renal status [87]. Furthermore, experimental glomerular lesions produced by iron overload [27, 33, 34] do not resemble those encountered in our study. In addition, the glomerular involvement in hemochromatosis is related to the development of diabetes and not to the degree of iron content.

Phagocytosis of fragmented sickled erythrocytes by mesangial cells and subsequent stimulation of these cells has been considered an important factor by Antonovych [6] and Elfenbein et al. [32]. The finding of electron-dense deposits in 4 of our 7 patients and the localization of IgG and C3 in the glomeruli of all 4 patients investigated by immunofluorescence suggest the presence of immune deposits [87]. It has been proposed that there is an alternate complement pathway defect in sickle cell disease [21, 59].

The increased incidence of bacterial infections [10, 127] and exposure to exogenous antigens from multiple blood transfusions suggest that sickle cell patients may have an immune complex glomerulonephritis related to antigens from microbial agents or blood products. The association of streptococcal and other bacterial infections, and of hepatitis B antigenemia with immune complex glomerulonephritis, is well documented [24, 47, 63, 78, 97].

The splenic dysfunction [40, 90] and abnormalities of the reticuloendothelial system, as well as the impaired immunity observed in patients with sickle cell disease [59, 98, 105, 106, 127], may render them more susceptible to persistent progressive glomerulonephritis, as encountered with low antibody producers in the persistent progressive experimental serum sickness model of Dixon et al. [29]. Furthermore, reduced clearance of immune complexes by a defective reticuloendothelial system may facilitate localization of the complexes in the kidney. Local factors, such as impacted red cell masses in the capillary loops or mesangial proliferation, also may influence glomerular perfusion or filtration and facilitate deposition and localization of the immune complexes.

The findings of granular deposits of IgG and complement components in association with renal tubular epithelial antigen in 4 of our sickle cell anemia patients with membranoproliferative glomerulonephritis, as well as in 2 patients with proliferative glomerulonephritis, suggest an autologous immune complex nephropathy caused by deposition of complexes of renal tubular epithelial antigen and antibody to this antigen. Furthermore, the detection of cryoprecipitable immune complexes of this antigen and its antibody in the sera of some of these patients, and demonstration in 1 patient that the glomerular bound antibody was directed against this antigen, support the concept of an autologous immune complex pathogenesis [114]. We have suggested that in some patients with sickle cell disease, ischemic tubular damage may lead to release of renal tubular epithelial antigen, with autosensitization and an autologous immune complex nephritis.

Clinical Manifestations

The manifestations of renal disease in patients with sickle cell disease or trait may or may not occur at the same time as other manifestations of the basic hematologic problem. However, our focus here is on the clinical picture related to the kidney.

Hematuria

Sickle cell crises may present with hematuria. Factors such as hypoxia, acidosis, hypertonicity, and stasis have been described as favoring crises and hematuria [44, 45]. Hematuria at times may be only microscopic [104]. Gross hematuria has been associated with sickle cell disease [1, 41, 67, 68, 107, 123] and, less frequently, with the trait [11, 41]; it usually is unilateral and most often from the left kidney [41]. The radiologic findings associated with hematuria may lead to the diagnosis of renal cancer [1]; a thorough urologic evaluation may be necessary [20].

Hyposthenuria

The inability to concentrate the urine up to normal levels under conditions of proper stimulation has been described repeatedly [4, 104]. It also is found in SA patients [123] and, like other conditions with defective concentrating ability, can be the cause of enuresis [79] or of dehydration. In both SS and SA patients it may be present at young ages. In SS patients it is accompanied by a diluting defect in some [123] but not in others [52]; in SA patients the diluting mechanism seems to be intact [4, 123].

Hyposthenuria appears to be a chronic and stable problem, unrelated to any acute or organic development. It is found during as well as between sickle cell crises and, in general, before any evidence of renal disease appears. Some patients with sickle cell disease have tubular and interstitial changes that probably contribute to the concentrating defect [11, 123]. Hyposthenuria is correctable in young children by the administration of blood [4, 60, 110].

Nephrotic Syndrome

The nephrotic syndrome can occur in patients with sickle cell disease [12]. Membranoproliferative glomerulonephritis [86, 87], minimal change disease [8], and other lesions have been reported in these patients. They may have normal or even subnormal levels of serum cholesterol [70, 120, 123]. There seems to be a correlation between partial remission of the nephrotic syndrome (as evidenced by diuresis) and sickle cell crises, and between relapses and flank pain (thrombotic episodes?) [120]. Proteinuria has been described, sometimes with [94] and sometimes without renal vein thrombosis, as an isolated finding in SS patients [99, 123].

Sickle Cell Crises

Four types of sickle cell crises have been described [90]: aplastic, hyperhemolytic, acute splenic sequestration, and vaso-occlusive. Their significance in respect to the nephropathy is still unclear, but they cannot be dismissed entirely [45, 84, 112, 122].

Acidosis

As an isolated manifestation of renal disease, acidosis seems to appear only under extreme conditions. Acidemia has not been detected between or even during crises, even though up to 40 percent of patients studied show deficient production of H^+ [4, 55, 82, 83]. Acidemia is present as a manifestation of end-stage renal disease, as in severe kidney damage due to other causes [87, 114]. Although painful crises have been induced by administration of acidifying agents [44], the association between acidosis and painful crises is not always present [4].

An acid pH induces sickling in vitro [4]. A similar change in blood pH following ammonium chloride administration failed to induce sickling in vivo [83]; it was concluded from these studies that the acidosis and sickling that may be present during a crisis do not represent cause and effect. Whether or not an acid pH may induce sickling in the presence of hyperosmolality remains to be evaluated.

Pyelonephritis

Bacteriuria seems to occur more frequently in black pregnant women with sickle cell trait than in comparable control subjects [85, 88, 125]. Pyelonephritis seems to be more frequent in SS [104] and SA [5] patients than in control subjects, but a final statement on the matter will require further agreement among nephrologists and pathologists as to what is meant by this diagnosis [48].

Chronic Renal Failure

Until rather recently it was accepted that renal failure does not occur in sickle cell anemia, at least in young patients [4, 36, 49]. Although true in general, as stated previously, there have been exceptions [18, 87, 114], and it may be found more often as awareness of the possibility increases and if an intensive search for these patients is launched. Improved patient care seems to allow patients to survive longer and to manifest the whole picture of chronic renal failure and end-stage renal disease. Although renal failure has been reported even during childhood [87, 114], it is expected that there will be increasing

numbers of older SS patients with chronic renal failure [4] as survival improves.

Chronic renal failure has been reported in patients with sickle cell trait [84, 122], some reports indicating that SA patients may die in end-stage renal disease [14, 70, 87, 114, 123]. Unlike other investigators [123], we do not believe that the manifestations of progressive renal disease are related to the number or severity of sickle cell crises [87].

Hypertension

Elevation of arterial blood pressure, a constant finding in most types of nephropathies that have reached the end stage, has not been emphasized in sickle cell nephropathy. According to the authors of exhaustive reviews [4, 16, 104, 123], hypertension does not seem to be much of a problem in adult SS patients prior to or during the period of hemodialysis [39]. Three children at the University of Miami had severe hypertension requiring treatment [87, 114], which in one included bilateral nephrectomy. It is not yet clear whether or not severe hypertension unresponsive to therapy is more common in SS children than in those with other nephropathies with comparable renal damage. The mechanism of the hypertension has not been elucidated and requires further study.

Growth and Bone Age

Children with sickle cell disease are known to have delayed bone age and stunted growth [80]. The degree of growth reduction correlates well with the number and severity of the crises. Once renal disease and failure ensue, assessment of the cause of growth alterations becomes a complex problem. It is difficult to determine which changes are due to the hemoglobinopathy and which to the nephropathy. It seems that they can be independent, since 2 patients seen by one of the authors at the University of Miami have grown normally, although they ultimately reached end-stage renal disease.

Enuresis

Enuresis in the SA and SS pediatric population seems related primarily to the decreased capacity to concentrate the urine [2, 4, 60, 71, 130] and to the reversal or absence of diurnal rhythm in urine flow and solute excretion [2, 4]. Low environmental temperature aggravates this problem and may induce a crisis [4, 28].

Treatment

General management of sickle cell crises and specific measures for renal complications can be recommended. Further studies are needed, however, to clarify the exact role played by each treatment modality.

GENERAL MEASURES

Necessary prophylactic therapeutic measures include early detection [91, 117], avoidance of dehydration, acidosis, hyperosmolality, hypoxia, ischemia, infection, and extreme anemia.

Dehydration, Acidosis, and Hyperosmolality

Administration of adequate amounts of fluids will prevent or correct dehydration due to excessive output of dilute urine. The criteria usually followed in fluid-electrolyte derangements should be used, with volumes and composition tailored to the patient's needs [97]. Whether or not systemic acidosis or hyperosmolality induces sickling is yet to be determined [4, 83]. Nonetheless, based on laboratory evidence [92] and on the general principles of good medical practice, these derangements should be avoided if possible, or corrected if they develop.

Urea, alkali, and invert sugar administered IV all have been found to be equally effective in relieving painful, febrile, vaso-occlusive crises [25]. Citrate-containing fluids have either corrected or decreased both hematuria and sickle cell crises [9, 62]. In agreement with the concept that these benefits may be due mainly to the administration of fluid, Alleyne et al. [4] conclude regarding sodium bicarbonate that ". . . clinical experience has not shown that there is any consistent benefit from this therapy."

Hypoxia, Ischemia, and Anemia

The problem of ischemia and the subsequent hypoxia is intimately related to the sickling process, degree of anemia, and alterations in macrocirculation and microcirculation. Anemia may protect sickle cell disease patients by decreasing blood viscosity and thus facilitating blood flow [45, 73, 112]. Even in normal experimental animals, decreasing the blood hematocrit to a critical level of 19 percent increases the surface Po_2 of the kidney and other organs, with a concomitant increase in cardiac output and presumably of the microcirculation [74, 112]. Accordingly, in treating the acute problems of these patients, the goal is to restore their hematocrits only to a level about 50 percent of normal and to provide adequate circulating fluid volume. This concept needs further experimental and clinical evaluation.

Anticoagulants, phenothiazines, and plasma expanders have been used in patients with circulatory problems. Among the latter, dextran has

seemed useful [90]. In this regard, blood replacement solutions may offer a desirable alternative to the use of blood under acute conditions of hypovolemic shock or of ischemic episodes [112]. Two solutions seem to offer attractive possibilities: a cell-free hemoglobin solution [118] and fluorocarbons [22]. Determination of their usefulness and safety in patients requires further testing.

Recently, efforts have been made to modify the abnormal polymerization of hemoglobin S to prevent gel formation and sickling. Urea and cyanate have been used for this purpose. Urea in vitro seems to block the SS hemoglobin binding sites and interrupt its hydrophobic change; clinical trials have yielded questionable results [25].

Cyanate in vitro and in vivo carbamylates in the N-terminal amino group of alpha and beta hemoglobin chains, blocking intermolecular bindings, shifting the hemoglobin oxygen dissociation to the left (thus increasing its affinity for oxygen), and increasing the survival time of sickle cells [50, 73]. Despite all these benefits, tissue oxygenation is not increased and may even be decreased. Cyanate currently is under clinical testing in several centers in the United States, but ". . . in view of the human toxicity already demonstrated, such clinical trials are probably not justified" [50].

Acute and Chronic Splenic Dysfunction, and Hemolytic, Aplastic, and Vaso-occlusive Crises. If anemia becomes extreme, packed or sedimented red blood cells should be administered; fresh blood may be needed [90]. The possible future need of a renal transplant suggests the use of buffy coat–free washed or frozen red blood cells whenever possible; this would seem especially indicated in patients with autologous renal disease [114].

Aplastic crises [90] may complicate immunosuppressive management in an SS patient with a renal transplant. To our knowledge, transplantation has been attempted in one patient with this condition (R. Fine, personal communication).

SPECIFIC MEASURES FOR RENAL COMPLICATIONS

In addition to the general measures that have been described, renal complications require specific treatment.

Hematuria

Modified exchange transfusion, hydration with distilled water and urinary alkalinization [62], and epsilon aminocaproic acid and epinephrine during selective renal angiography [57] have been proposed as treatments for either gross or microscopic hematuria. Gross hematuria frequently has been treated with unilateral nephrectomy, but the rate of recurrence in the remaining kidney has been high enough to suggest that conservative management may be a better approach [104].

Hyposthenuria
Besides prophylactic or therapeutic fluid intake, little need be done for the concentrating defect. Electrolyte losses should be evaluated and the intake modified accordingly. No specific recommendations have been made regarding protein or electrolyte ingestion. The use of diuretics, generally accepted in diabetes insipidus, has not been reported in SS or SA patients, probably because of its potential dangers.

Nephrotic Syndrome
The general therapeutic approach to the nephrotic syndrome secondary to systemic diseases has been followed in sickle cell disease patients. The problem is compounded by the tendency to severe infections and thrombosis. Extreme care should be exercised if the use of corticosteroids, diuretics, or immunosuppressant agents is considered necessary.

Corticosteroids seem to help in controlling the SS nephrotic syndrome [8, 120], though it is usually regarded as a corticosteroid-resistant type [11]. In general, this mode of therapy does not have many supporters [13, 123] and may be hazardous [26]. One patient was reported to have had convulsions and hemiplegia during corticosteroid therapy and the induced diuresis [120].

Sickle Cell Crises, Acidosis, and Pyelonephritis
Sickle cell crises, acidosis, and pyelonephritis seem properly handled by following general measures. Pyelonephritis, if properly diagnosed, is a serious development under any circumstances. It may need more aggressive treatment in patients with sickle cell disease or trait than in AA patients.

Glomerulopathies
Glomerulopathies seem to be due either to stasis and occlusion of glomerular capillaries or to deposition of RTE (renal tubular epithelium) –anti-RTE complexes. With stasis, general measures to ensure proper hydration and microcirculation are indicated. In autologous antigen-antibody nephropathy the problem is in getting to the factors responsible for the transformation of renal tubular epithelial protein into an antigenically active substance. Again, general measures may be sufficient as soon as a crisis develops. Various immunologic maneuvers may be indicated once a suitable experimental model is found or developed

and its efficacy properly tested. As previously stated, corticosteroids or immunosuppressant drugs seem not to be useful modes of therapy.

End-Stage Renal Disease
A patient with sickle cell disease in whom end-stage renal disease develops poses special problems [39, 43]. The degree of involvement of other organs must be a factor in deciding the course of treatment. The tendency for these patients to develop obstruction of small and large vessels and for severe infections to develop are also factors to be weighed. If the medical and family decision is to proceed with dialysis, preference should be given to a subcutaneous access to the circulation in the form of a fistula or a bovine graft. In many pediatric nephrology centers, admission to a dialysis program is limited to those acceptable for renal transplantation. If this approach is followed, a special decision will have to be made in terms of the risk to live, related donors, their eligibility in the presence of an autologous renal disease, and the chances for a successful transplantation.

Hypertension
Because of the tendency toward dehydration and thrombosis in sickle cell anemia, administration of diuretics for hypertension requires greater care than in AA patients. Antihypertensives used include the whole spectrum available; no drugs have been found to be especially harmful or beneficial to the SS or SA patient. Sound principles of pathophysiology should be applied, as in the treatment of all types of hypertension [31] (Chap. 32).

References
1. Abel, M. S., and Brown, C. R. Sickle cell disease with severe hematuria simulating renal neoplasm. *J.A.M.A.* 136:624, 1948.
2. Addae, S. K., and Konotey-Ahulu, F. I. D. Lack of diurnal variations in sodium, potassium and osmolar excretion in the sickle cell patient. *Afr. J. Med. Sci.* 2:349, 1971.
3. Akinkugbe, O. O. Renal papillary necrosis in sickle cell haemoglobinopathy. *Br. Med. J.* 3:283, 1967.
4. Alleyne, G. A. O., Statius Van Eps, L. W., Addae, S. K., Nicholson, G. D., and Schouten, H. The kidney in sickle cell anemia. *Kidney Int.* 7:371, 1975.
5. Amin, U. F., and Ragbeer, M. M. S. The prevalence of pyelonephritis among sicklers and non-sicklers in an autopsy population. *West Indian Med. J.* 21:166, 1972.
6. Antonovych, T. T. Ultrastructural changes in glomeruli of patients with sickle cell disease and the nephrotic syndrome (abstract). *Abs. Am. Soc. Nephrol.,* 1972, p. 3.
7. Arakawa, M., and Kimmelstiel, P. Circumferential mesangial interposition. *Lab. Invest.* 21:276, 1969.

8. Barnett, H. L., and Bernstein, J. Clinical pathological conference. *J. Pediatr.* 73:936, 1968.

9. Barreras, L., and Diggs, L. W. Bicarbonates, pH and percentage of sickled cells in venous blood of patients in sickle cell crisis. *Am. J. Med. Sci.* 247:710, 1964.

10. Barrett-Connor, E. Bacterial infection and sickle cell anemia. *Medicine (Baltimore)* 50:97, 1971.

11. Berman, L. B. Sickle cell nephropathy. *J.A.M.A.* 228:1279, 1974.

12. Berman, L. B., and Schreiner, G. E. Clinical and histologic spectrum of the nephrotic syndrome. *Am. J. Med.* 24:249, 1958.

13. Berman, L. B., and Tublin, I. The nephropathies of sickle-cell disease. *A.M.A. Arch. Intern. Med.* 103:602, 1959.

14. Bernstein, J., and Whitten, C. F. A histologic appraisal of the kidney in sickle cell anemia. *Arch. Pathol.* 70:407, 1960.

15. Birdsell, J. B. *Human Evolution.* Chicago: Rand McNally, 1972.

16. Buckalew, V. M., Jr., and Someren, A. Renal manifestations of sickle cell disease. *Arch. Intern. Med.* 133:660, 1974.

17. Buettner-Janusch, J. *Origins of Man.* New York: Wiley, 1966.

18. Calcagno, P. L., McLavy, J., and Kelley, T. Glomerular filtration rate in children with sickle cell disease. *Pediatrics* 5:127, 1950.

19. Carone, F. A. Patho-Physiology of Renal Concentrating Defects. In F. W. Sunderman and F. W. Sunderman, Jr. (eds.), *Laboratory Diagnosis of Kidney Diseases.* St. Louis: W. H. Green, 1970. P. 54.

20. Carrion, H., Machiz, S., and Politano V. Sickle cell disease and transitional cell carcinoma of the renal pelvis: A case report. *J. Urol.* 109:569, 1973.

21. Casper, J., Koethe, S., and Rodey, G. Evidence for an alternate complement pathway defect other than C3 proactivator (C3PA) deficiency in sickle cell disease (SCD) (abstract). *J. Clin. Invest.* 53:15a, 1974.

22. Clark, L. C., Jr., Kaplan, S., and Becattini, F. The physiology of synthetic blood. *J. Thorac. Cardiovasc. Surg.* 60:757, 1970.

23. Cochran, R. T. Hyposthenuria in sickle cell states. *Arch. Intern. Med.* 112:222, 1963.

24. Combes, B., Stastny, P., Shorey, J., Eigenbrodt, E. H., Barrera, A., Hull, A. R., and Carter, N. W. Glomerulonephritis with desposition of Australia antigen-antibody complexes in glomerular basement membrane. *Lancet* 2:234, 1971.

25. Cooperative Urea Trials Group. Clinical trials of therapy for sickle cell vaso-occlusive crises. *J.A.M.A.* 228:1120, 1974.

26. Cosgriff, S. W., Diefenbach, A. F., and Vogt, W. Hypercoagulability of the blood associated with ACTH and cortisone therapy. *Am. J. Med.* 9:752, 1950.

27. Dachs, S., and Churg, J. Iron nephropathy (abstract). *Fed. Proc.* 24:619, 1965.

28. Diggs, L. W. Sickle cell crisis. *Am. J. Clin. Pathol.* 44:1, 1965.

29. Dixon, F. J., Feldman, J. D., and Vazquez, J. A. Experimental glomerulonephritis. The pathogenesis of a laboratory model resembling the spectrum of human glomerulonephritis. *J. Exp. Med.* 113:899, 1961.

30. Duc, G. Assessment of hypoxia in the newborn. Suggestions for a practical approach. *Pediatrics* 48:469, 1971.

31. Dustan, H. P., and Tarazi, R. C. Hemodynamics of Hypertension in Adolescence. In J. Strauss (ed.), *Pediatric Nephrology: Epidemiology, Evaluation and Therapy.* New York: Stratton Intercontinental, 1976. Vol. 2, p. 385.

32. Elfenbein, I. B., Patchefsky, A., Schwartz, W., and Weinstein, A. G. Pathology of the glomerulus in sickle cell anemia with and without nephrotic syndrome. *Am. J. Pathol.* 77:357, 1974.

33. Ellis, J. T. Glomerular lesions and the nephrotic syndrome in rabbits given saccharated iron oxide intravenously with special reference to the part played by intracapillary precipitates in the pathogenesis of the lesions. *J. Exp. Med.* 103:127, 1956.

34. Ellis, J. T. Glomerular lesions in rabbits with experimentally induced proteinuria as disclosed by electron microscopy (abstract). *Am. J. Pathol.* 34:559, 1958.

35. Emmel, V. E. A study of the erythrocytes in a case of severe anemia with elongated and sickle-shaped red blood corpuscles. *Arch. Intern. Med.* 20:586, 1917.

36. Etteldorf, J. N., Smith, J. D., Tuttle, A. H., and Diggs, L. W. Renal hemodynamic studies in adults with sickle cell anemia. *Am. J. Med.* 18:243, 1955.

37. Etteldorf, J. N., Tuttle, A. H., and Clayton, G. W. Renal function studies in pediatrics. Renal hemodynamics in children with sickle cell anemia. *Am. J. Dis. Child.* 83:185, 1952.

38. Evans, P. V., and Symmes, A. T. Bone marrow infarction with fat embolism and nephrosis in sickle cell disease. *J. Indiana State Med. Assoc.* 50:1101, 1957.

39. Friedman, E. A., Sreepada, T. K., Sprung, C. L., Smith, A., Manis, T., Bellevue, R., Butt, K. M. H., Levere, R. D., and Holden, D. M. Uremia in sickle-cell anemia treated by maintenance hemodialysis. *N. Engl. J. Med.* 291:431, 1974.

40. Gavrilis, P., Rothenberg, S. P., and Guy, R. Correlation of low serum IgM levels with absence of functional splenic tissue in sickle cell disease syndromes. *Am. J. Med.* 57:542, 1974.

41. Goodwin, W. E., Alston, E. F., and Semans, J. H. Hematuria and sickle cell disease: Unexplained, gross unilateral, renal hematuria in Negroes, coincident with the blood sickling trait. *J. Urol.* 63:79, 1950.

42. Goosens, J. P., Statius Van Eps, L. W., Schouten, H., and Giterson, A. L. Incomplete renal tubular acidosis in sickle cell disease. *Clin. Chim. Acta* 41:149, 1972.

43. Gordillo-Paniagua, G. Supportive Therapy of Chronic Uremia. In J. Strauss (ed.), *Pediatric Nephrology: Current Concepts in Diagnosis and Management.* New York: Stratton Intercontinental, 1974. Vol. 1, p. 409.

44. Greenberg, M. S., and Kass, E. H. Studies on the destruction of red blood cells. XIII. Observations on the role of pH in the pathogenesis and treatment of painful crisis in sickle-cell disease. *Arch. Intern. Med.* 101:355, 1958.

45. Greenberg, M. S., Kass, E. H., and Castle, W. B. Studies on the destruction of red blood cells. XII. Factors influencing the role of S hemoglobin in the

pathologic physiology of sickle cell anemia and related disorders. *J. Clin. Invest.* 36:833, 1957.

46. Gross, S., and Godel, J. C. Comparative studies of height and weight as blood volume reference standard in normal children and children with sickle cell anemia. *Am. J. Clin. Pathol.* 55:662, 1971.

47. Gyorkey, F., Min, K. W., and Gyorkey, P. Renal changes in hepatitis-associated antigenemia with hematuria: Immunofluorescent and electronmicroscopic study (abstract). *Am. J. Pathol.* 66:59a, 1972.

48. Habib, R. Discussion. In J. Strauss (ed.), *Pediatric Nephrology: Current Concepts in Diagnosis and Management.* New York: Stratton Intercontinental, 1974. Vol. 1, p. 351.

49. Hamburger, J. (ed.). *Nephrology.* Philadelphia: Saunders, 1968. Vol. 2, p. 926.

50. Harkness, D. R., and Roth, S. Clinical evaluation of cyanate in sickle cell anemia. *Prog. Hematol.* 9: 157, 1975.

51. Harrow, B. R., Sloane, J. A., and Liebman, N. C. Roentgenologic demonstration of renal papillary necrosis in sickle-cell trait. *N. Engl. J. Med.* 268: 969, 1963.

52. Hatch, F. E., Culbertson, J. W., and Diggs, L. W. Nature of the renal concentrating defect in sickle cell disease. *J. Clin. Invest.* 46:336, 1967.

53. Heptinstall, R. H. *Pathology of the Kidney* (2nd ed.). Boston: Little, Brown, 1974. P. 1152.

54. Herrick, J. B. Peculiar elongated and sickle-shape red blood corpuscles in a case of severe anemia. *Arch. Intern. Med.* 6:517, 1910.

55. Ho Ping Kong, H., and Alleyne, G. A. O. Defect in urinary acidification in adults with sickle-cell anaemia. *Lancet* 2:954, 1968.

56. Ho Ping Kong, H., and Alleyne, G. A. O. Studies on acid excretion in adults with sickle cell anaemia. *Clin. Sci.* 41:505, 1971.

57. Hoffman, R. B., and Zucker, M. O. Epinephrine infusion in a patient with sickle cell trait. *Calif. Med.* 118:49, 50, 1973.

58. Johnson, M., Rabinowitz, I., Willis, A. L., and Wolf, P. L. Detection of prostaglandin induction of erythrocyte sickling. *Clin. Chem.* 19:23, 1973.

59. Johnston, R. B., Jr., Newman, S. L., and Struth, A. G. An abnormality of the alternate pathway of complement activation in sickle-cell disease. *N. Engl. J. Med.* 288:803, 1973.

60. Keitel, H. G., Thompson, D., and Itano, H. A. Hyposthenuria in sickle cell anemia: A reversible renal defect. *J. Clin. Invest.* 35:998, 1956.

61. Kimmelstiel, P. Vascular occlusion and ischemic infarction in sickle cell disease. *Am. J. Med. Sci.* 216:11, 1948.

62. Knochel, J. P. Hematuria in sickle cell trait: The effect of intravenous administration of distilled water, urinary alkalinization, and diuresis. *Arch. Intern. Med.* 123:160, 1969.

63. Kohler, P. F., Cronin, R. E., Hammond, W. S., Olin, D., and Carr, R. I. Chronic membranous glomerulonephritis caused by hepatitis B antigen-antibody immune complexes. *Ann. Intern. Med.* 81: 448, 1974.

64. Konotey-Ahulu, F. I. D. Hereditary qualitative and quantitative erythrocyte defects in Ghana: A historical and geographical survey. *Ghana Med. J.* 7:118, 1968.

65. Lebby, R. Case of absence of the spleen. *South. J. Med. Pharmacol.* 1:481, 1846.

66. Levitt, M. F., Hauser, A. D., Levy, M. S., and Polimeros, D. The renal concentrating defect in sickle cell disease. *Am. J. Med.* 29:611, 1960.

67. Lucas, W. M., and Bullock, W. H. Hematuria in sickle cell disease. *J. Urol.* 83:733, 1960.

68. Mahurkar, S. D., Dunea, G., and Bush, I. M. Hematuria in sickle C disease: Precipitation by acidosis and correction by dialysis. *J. Urol.* 110:443, 1973.

69. Margulies, S. I., and Minkin, S. D. Sickle cell disease: The roentgenologic manifestations of urinary tract abnormalities in adults. *Am. J. Roentgenol. Radium Ther. Nucl. Med.* 107:702, 1969.

70. McCoy, R. C. Ultrastructural alterations in the kidney of patients with sickle cell disease and the nephrotic syndrome. *Lab. Invest.* 21:85, 1969.

71. McCrory, W. W., Goren, N., and Gornfeld, D. Demonstration of impairment of urinary concentration ability of "Pitressin-resistance," in children with sickle-cell anemia (abstract). *Am. J. Dis. Child.* 86: 512, 1953.

72. Meessen, H., and Litton, M. A. Morphology of the kidney in morbus caeruleus. *A.M.A. Arch. Pathol.* 56:480, 1953.

73. Messer, M. S. Discussion. Sickle cell disease medical staff conference, University of California, San Francisco. *Calif. Med.* 118:48, 1973.

74. Messmer, K., Görnandt, L., Sinagowitz, E., Sunder-Plassmann, L., Jesch, F., and Kessler, M. Local Oxygen Tension in Tissue of Different Organs During Limited Normovolemic Hemodilution. In J. Ditzel and D. H. Lewis (eds.), *Seventh European Conference on Microcirculation. Part II: Clinical Aspects of Microcirculation.* Basel: Karger, 1973. P. 327.

75. Miller, R. E., Hartley, M. W., Clark, E. C., and Lupton, C. H., Jr. Sickle cell nephropathy. *Ala. J. Med. Sci.* 1:233, 1964.

76. Mostofi, F. K., Vorder Bruegge, C. F., and Diggs, L. W. Lesions in kidneys removed for unilateral hematuria in sickle-cell disease. *A.M.A. Arch. Pathol.* 63:336, 1957.

77. Motulsky, A. G. Frequency of sickling disorders in U.S. blacks. *N. Engl. J. Med.* 288:31, 1973.

78. Myers, B. D., Griffel, B., Naveh, D., Jankielowitz, T., and Klajman, A. Membrano-proliferative glomerulonephritis associated with persistent viral hepatitis. *Am. J. Clin. Pathol.* 60:222, 1973.

79. Noll, J. B., Newman, A. J., and Gross, S. Enuresis and nocturia in sickle cell disease. *J. Pediatr.* 70: 965, 1967.

80. Olambiwonnu, N. O., Penny, R., and Frasier, S. B. Sexual maturation in subjects with sickle cell anemia: Studies of serum gonadotropin concentration, height, weight, and skeletal age. *J. Pediatr.* 87:459, 1975.

81. Oski, F. A., and Delivoria-Papadopoulos, M. The red cell, 2-3, diphosphoglycerate and tissue oxygen release. *J. Pediatr.* 77:941, 1970.

82. Oster, J. R., Lee, S. M., Lespier, L. E., Pellegrini, E. L., and Vaamonde, C. A. Renal acidification in sickle-cell trait (HbAS) (abstract). *Arch. Intern. Med.* 136:30, 1976.

83. Oster, J. R., Lespier, L. E., Lee, S. M., Pellegrini, E. L., and Vaamonde, C. A. Renal acidification in sickle-cell disease. *J. Lab. Clin. Med.* 88:389, 1976.

84. Ozawa, T., Mass, M. F., Guggenheim, S., Strauss, J., and McIntosh, R. M. Autologous immune complex nephritis associated with sickle cell trait: Diagnosis

of the hemoglobinopathy following isolation of immune complexes, renal morphologic studies and immunohistological demonstration of glomerular bound autologous antigen and immunoglobulins. *Br. Med. J.* 1:369, 1976.

85. Papper, S. *Clinical Nephrology.* Boston: Little, Brown, 1971. Pp. 379–381.

86. Pardo, V., Kramer, H., Levi, D., and Strauss, J. Glomerular changes in patients with sickle cell disease and the nephrotic syndrome (abstract). *Am. J. Pathol.* 70:4a, 1973.

87. Pardo, V., Strauss, J., Kramer, H., Ozawa, T., and McIntosh, R. M. Nephropathy associated with sickle cell anemia: An autologous immune complex nephritis. II. Clinicopathologic studies in seven patients. *Am. J. Med.* 59:650, 1975.

88. Pathak, U. N., Tang, K., Williams, L. L., and Stuart, K. L. Bacteriuria of pregnancy: Results of treatment. *J. Infect. Dis.* 120:91, 1969.

89. Pauling, L., Itano, H. A., Singer, S. J., and Wells, I. C. Sickle cell anemia, a molecular disease. *Science* 110:543, 1949.

90. Pearson, H. A., and Diamond, L. K. The critically ill child: Sickle cell disease crises and their management. *Pediatrics* 48:629, 1971.

91. Pearson, H. A., and O'Brien, R. T. Sickle cell testing programs. *J. Pediatr.* 81:1201, 1972.

92. Perillie, P. E., and Epstein, F. H. Sickling phenomenon produced by hypertonic solutions: A possible explanation for the hyposthenuria of sicklemia. *J. Clin. Invest.* 42:570, 1963.

93. Pitcock, J. A., Muirhead, E. E., Hatch, F. E., Johnson, J. G., and Kelly, B. J. Early renal changes in sickle cell anemia. *Arch. Pathol.* 90:403, 1970.

94. Pollak, V. E., Pirani, C. L., Seskind, C., and Griffel, B. Bilateral renal vein thrombosis: Clinical and electron microscopic studies of a case with complete recovery after anticoagulant therapy. *Ann. Intern. Med.* 65:1056, 1966.

95. Rabinowitz, I. N., Wolf, P. L., Shikuma, N., and Berman, S. Prostaglandin E_2 effects on oxygen carriage by intact sickle cell erythrocytes (abstract). *Am. J. Pathol.* 74:92a, 1974.

96. Radel, E., Kochen, J., and Finberg, L. Hyponatremia in sickle crisis—a defect in renal diluting capacity (abstract). *Pediatr. Res.* 8:460, 1974.

97. Rammelkamp, C. H. Microbiologic aspects of glomerulonephritis. *J. Chronic Dis.* 5:28, 1957.

98. Rosen, F. S. Sickle-cell disease and the properdin system. *N. Engl. J. Med.* 288:845, 1973.

99. Rosenmann, E., Pollak, V. E., and Pirani, C. Renal vein thrombosis in the adult. A clinical and pathologic study based on renal biopsies. *Medicine (Baltimore)* 47:269, 1968.

100. Rucknagel, D. L. The genetics of sickle cell anemia and related syndromes. *Arch. Intern. Med.* 133:595, 1974.

101. Salyer, D. C., and Salyer, W. R. Sickle cell disease and the kidney: A hypothesis (letter to the editor). *Arch. Intern. Med.* 134:181, 1974.

102. Saxena, U. H., Scott, R. B., and Ferguson, A. D. Studies in sickle cell anemia. XXV. Observations on fluid intake and output. *J. Pediatr.* 69:220, 1966.

103. Schlitt, L., and Keitel, H. G. Pathogenesis of hyposthenuria in persons with sickle cell anemia of the sickle cell trait. *Pediatrics* 26:249, 1960.

104. Schlitt, L. E., and Keitel, H. G. Renal manifestations of sickle cell disease: A review. *Am. J. Med. Sci.* 239:773, 1960.

105. Schwartz, A. D., and Pearson, H. A. Impaired antibody response to intravenous immunizations in sickle cell anemia. *Pediatr. Res.* 6:145, 1972.

106. Shulman, S. T., Bartlett, J., Clyde, W. A., and Ayoub, E. M. The usual severity of mycoplasmal pneumonia in children with sickle-cell disease. *N. Engl. J. Med.* 287:164, 1972.

107. Sperber, A., and Tessler, A. N. Gross hematuria in white man with sickling disorder. *J. Urol.* 111:528, 1974.

108. Squire, J. R., Blainey, J. D., and Hardwicke, J. The nephrotic syndrome. *Br. Med. Bull.* 13:43, 1957.

109. Statius Van Eps, L. W., Pinedo-Veels, C., De Vries, C. H., and De Konig, J. Nature of the concentrating defect in sickle-cell nephropathy: Microradioangiographic studies. *Lancet* 1:450, 1970.

110. Statius Van Eps, L. W., Schouten, H., La Porte-Wijsman, L. W., and Struyker Boudier, A. M. The influence of red blood cell transfusions on the hyposthenuria and renal hemodynamics of sickle cell anemia. *Clin. Chim. Acta* 17:449, 1967.

111. Statius Van Eps, L. W., Schouten, H., Ter Harr Romeny-Wachter, C. C. H., and La Porte-Wijsman, L. W. The relation between age and renal concentrating capacity in sickle cell disease and hemoglobin C disease. *Clin. Chim. Acta* 27:501, 1970.

112. Strauss, J., Baker, R., Kessler, M., and McIntosh, R. M. Renal Hemodynamics and Oxygenation. In J. Strauss (ed.), *Pediatric Nephrology: Epidemiology, Evaluation and Therapy.* New York: Stratton Intercontinental, 1976. Vol. 2, p. 205.

113. Strauss, J., Koss, M., Griswold, W., Chernack, W., Pardo, V., and McIntosh, R. M. Cryoprecipitable immune complexes, nephropathology, and sickle-cell disease (letter to the editor). *Ann. Intern. Med.* 81:114, 1974.

114. Strauss, J., Pardo, V., Koss, M. N., Griswold, W., and McIntosh, R. M. Nephropathy associated with sickle cell anemia. An autologous immune complex nephritis. I. Studies on nature of the glomerular-bound antibody and antigen identification in a patient with sickle cell disease and immune deposit glomerulonephritis. *Am. J. Med.* 58:382, 1975.

115. Strauss, J., Pardo, V., Kramer, H., Koss, M. N., Griswold, W. R., and McIntosh, R. M. Sickle cell nephropathy and autologous immune-complex nephritis. *Abs. Am. Soc. Nephrol.,* 1973, p. 101.

116. Strom, T., Muehrcke, R. C., and Smith, R. D. Sickle cell anemia with the nephrotic syndrome and renal vein obstruction. *Arch. Intern. Med.* 129:104, 1972.

117. Stuart, J., Schwartz, F. C. M., Little, A. J., and Raine, D. N. Screening for abnormal hemoglobins: A pilot study. *Br. Med. J.* 4:284, 1973.

118. Sunder-Plassmann, L., Jesch, F., Seifert, J., Grohmann, W., and Messmer, K. The hemodynamic and hemorrheological effects of stroma-free hemoglobin solution. Preliminary report. *Bibl. Anat.* 11:104, 1973.

119. Susamano, S., and Lewy, J. E. Sickle cell disease and acute glomerulonephritis. *Am. J. Dis. Child.* 118:615, 1969.

120. Sweeney, M. J., Dobbins, W. T., and Etteldorf, J. N. Renal disease with elements of the nephrotic

syndrome associated with sickle cell anemia: A report of 2 cases. *J. Pediatr.* 60:42, 1962.

121. Sydenstricker, V. P., Mulherin, W. A., and Houseal, R. W. Sickle cell anemia. Report of two cases in children, with necropsy in one case. *Am. J. Dis. Child.* 26:132, 1923.

122. Tellem, M., Rubenstone, A. I., and Frumin, A. M. Renal failure and other unusual manifestations in sickle-cell trait. *A.M.A. Arch. Pathol.* 63:508, 1957.

123. Walker, B. R., Alexander, F., Birdsall, T. R., and Warren, R. L. Glomerular lesions in sickle cell nephropathy. *J.A.M.A.* 215:437, 1971.

124. Welt, L. G., and Lyle, C. B., Jr. The Kidney in Sickle Cell Anemia. In M. B. Strauss and L. G. Welt (eds.), *Diseases of the Kidney* (2nd ed.). Boston: Little, Brown, 1971. Vol. 2, pp. 1207–1213.

125. Whalley, P. J., Martin, F. G., and Pritchard, J. A. Sickle cell trait and urinary tract infections during pregnancy. *J.A.M.A.* 189:903, 1964.

126. Whitten, C. F., and Younes, A. A. A comparative study of renal concentrating ability in children with sickle cell anemia and in normal children. *J. Lab. Clin. Med.* 55:400, 1960.

127. Winkelstein, J. A., and Drachman, R. H. Deficiency in pneumococcal serum opsonizing activity in sickle-cell disease. *N. Engl. J. Med.* 279:459, 1968.

128. Wirz, H., Hargitay, B., and Kuhn, W. Lokalisation des Konzentrierungsprozesses in der Niere durch direkte Kryoskopie. *Helv. Physiol. Acta* 9: 196, 1951.

129. Zarafonetis, C. J. D., McMaster, J. D., Molthan, L., and Steiger, W. A. Apparent renal defect in sicklemic individuals. *Am. J. Med. Sci.* 232:76, 1956.

130. Zarafonetis, C. J. D., Steiger, W. A., Molthan, L., McMaster, J., and Colville, V. F. Renal defects associated with sickle cell trait and sickle cell disease (abstract). *J. Lab. Clin. Med.* 44:959, 1954.

61. Schönlein-Henoch Syndrome

Roy Meadow

"Another boy, five years old, was seized with pains and swellings in various parts, and the penis in particular was so distended, though not discoloured, that he could hardly make water. He had sometimes pains in his belly, with vomiting, and at the time some streaks of blood were perceived in his stools, *and the urine was tinged with blood.* When the pain attacked his leg, he was unable to walk; and presently the skin of his leg was all over full of bloody points. After a truce of three or four days the swelling returned, and the bloody dots, as before" (Heberden, 1801 [18]).

The association of characteristic skin, joint, and gastrointestinal symptoms has been recognized in children for more than 100 years. In the early case reports, urine abnormalities were sometimes reported [18] or suspected [44]. Schönlein [38] named the association of purpura and joint pains "peliosis rheumatica," purpura rheumatica, and reported "frequent precipitates in the urine." Henoch [19] drew attention to the gastrointestinal manifestations of purpura rheumatica and 30 years later pointed out that the kidney was sometimes involved [20].

The syndrome itself is usually clearly identifiable in childhood, even though it is called variously Henoch-Schönlein syndrome, Schönlein-Henoch syndrome (by those who believe in the rights of historical precedence), purpura rheumatica, anaphylactoid purpura, and allergic purpura.

In the last 50 years it has become increasingly clear that the main mortality of Schönlein-Henoch syndrome results from glomerulonephritis.

Schönlein-Henoch syndrome represents an important cause of nephritis in childhood and also a potentially serious one. Habib and Levy [16] reported that in France it represents 15 percent of glomerular nephropathies in children. Experience in other western countries is similar. It represents an even higher proportion of the glomerular nephropathies leading to end-stage renal failure in children of school age in Europe.

The illness of Schönlein-Henoch syndrome is preceded, 1 to 3 weeks earlier, by an upper respiratory tract infection in as many as two-thirds of the affected children [3].

There have been reports implicating many different organisms, ranging from hemolytic streptococci [9] and *Mycoplasma pneumoniae* [29] to varicella [34a]. However, no specific microorganism has been implicated consistently. Moreover, careful controlled studies in large numbers of affected children do not support a causal relationship between group A streptococci and the syndrome [4]. Specific food allergens have been identified as the stimulus for the syndrome in a number of children [2], and in others, drugs have been incriminated [1, 17]. It has also occurred 1 to 2 weeks after smallpox vaccination [24, 28], after insect bites [6], and on exposure to cold

[37]. While the syndrome may follow different identifiable causes, the manifestations do not appear to vary according to the cause, and in most cases there is no identifiable cause. Thus, the syndrome is a common end result of a process that can originate from different causes.

Analysis of many different surveys shows that the incidence in males is higher than in females by a factor of between 1.15 and 2. The incidence of associated nephritis follows this male preponderance. Although 50 percent of patients are under the age of 5 years, the syndrome is rarely identified under the age of 6 months [3]. Severe renal manifestations tend to occur in children over the age of 5 [33].

It is rare for other members of the family to be affected. In a series of 131 patients with the syndrome, only 1 had an affected sibling [3]. Of another 88 children with Schönlein-Henoch nephritis, 1 had a sister who had similar nephritis 9 years earlier [33]. There is a report of the syndrome occurring in three members of a family [30].

Systemic Manifestations
SKIN
The characteristic rash is purpuric and is symmetrically distributed over the extensor surfaces of the lower legs and arms and over the sides of the buttocks (Figs. 61-1, 61-2). It is nearly always present in the area of the lateral malleolus and at times is present only there (Fig. 61-3). Pressure areas, for example, beneath a waist band, are commonly affected, and a few spots may be present on the penis. It usually begins as a red maculopapular rash that then becomes purpuric and eventually takes on a fawn color as it fades. The patches of purpura may be tiny or very large. Sometimes the rash does not have a purpuric stage. It does not itch. In children under 5 years of age, the illness may start with a generalized urticarial rash, which later may become purpuric. Edema of the scalp and face and of the dorsa of the hands and feet is common. Subcutaneous bleeding may occur anywhere. It is often seen in the scrotum (mimicking torsion of the testicle), eyelids, and conjunctiva.

JOINTS
Pain, with or without swelling and tenderness, affects predominantly the ankles and knees. Other joints of the hands and feet may be affected. There is periarticular edema that is of short duration. There is no residual damage to the joints.

GASTROINTESTINAL TRACT
Colicky abdominal pain is common and may be severe enough to mimic an acute abdominal emergency. Vomiting and diarrhea are also common and may be accompanied by hematemesis and melena. The alimentary problems can be most severe.

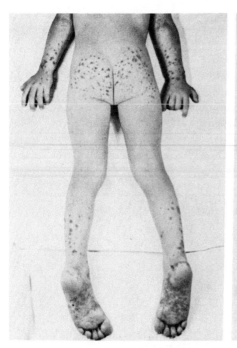
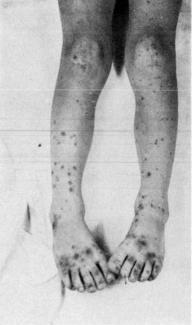

Figure 61-1. The symmetrical distribution of the purpuric spots.

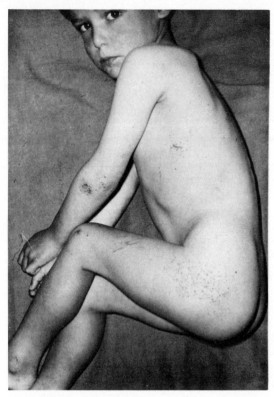

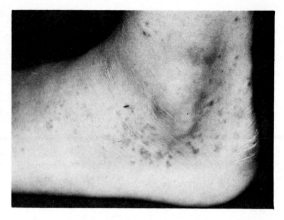

Figure 61-3. Lateral view of the ankle showing the commonest site for the rash of Schönlein-Henoch syndrome (in mild cases, it may be the only site).

Figure 61-2. Purpuric spots most marked on the extensor aspects of the elbow, knee, and ankle and on the side of the buttock.

Intussusception is a rare complication; paralytic ileus or severe alimentary symptoms requiring parenteral fluids are more common.

OTHER EXTRARENAL MANIFESTATIONS
A large variety of different problems may occur. Nosebleeds may be severe; bleeding into the calf may occur, simulating a deep vein thrombosis. Convulsions, encephalopathy, facial palsy, and chorea occasionally occur. The liver may be enlarged. The peripheral blood shows a normal hemoglobin and platelet count and no clotting defect. The white cell count and the erythrocyte sedimentation rate may be moderately raised.

RENAL MANIFESTATIONS
Incidence of Renal Involvement
The proportion of patients reported to have renal involvement varies between 20 and 100 percent [3, 21, 27, 31, 32, 35, 36, 39]. Part of this variation can be accounted for by the different criteria used to define "renal involvement," as well as by the different methods used to detect microscopic hematuria. Urinary abnormalities may be transient, and unless repeated checks are made, they

may be missed. Study of the surveys referred to suggests that 20 to 30 percent of children have macroscopic hematuria, while 30 to 70 percent have albuminuria, or microscopic hematuria, or both, persisting for more than a week. However, raised red cell excretion rates in urine have been found in all children with the syndrome [33], and an abnormal renal histologic picture has been reported in children with Schönlein-Henoch syndrome who had normal urine on routine testing [12].

Renal Presentation
Just as the skin, joint, and gut symptoms may occur in any order and at any time over a period of several days or weeks, so too may the kidney manifestations occur at any time. In general, the first urinary abnormality is noticed after other symptoms, but hematuria occasionally may be the initial feature. In 80 percent of children with a urinary abnormality, the first abnormality is detected within 4 weeks of onset of the illness. In most of the remainder, the urine abnormality develops within the next 8 weeks, and a small minority are found to have urinary abnormalities several months later [22, 23].

The nonrenal manifestations of the illness fluctuate over a period of days or weeks before disappearing. Recurrences are common and appear to be particularly so in those in whom severe renal damage develops. My colleagues and I [33] found that 25 percent of 88 children with Schönlein-Henoch nephritis had had a late relapse of the syndrome 2 months or more after the initial episode. The relapses may occur at the time of an upper respiratory tract infection [9].

It has been found in most investigations that severe alimentary system involvement is particularly likely to be associated with renal involvement [33], though this association was not found in a study done in Montreal [22]. There is agreement, however, that even with the mildest skin, joint, or gut symptoms, renal involvement may occur. Apparently, Henoch realized this for he wrote, "I must advise, in the presence of purpura no matter what its manifestations, to not omit an examination of the urine, since I have observed nephritis in apparently simple cases" [32].

The commonest urinary abnormalities are albuminuria and microscopic hematuria. A smaller number of patients have macroscopic hematuria. Acute nephritic syndrome occurs in the more severe cases and may lead to a nephrotic syndrome or to renal insufficiency. Both of these may develop independently and insidiously, but they are much more likely to develop in the child who has had an acute nephritic stage in the illness. In a series of 34 children with Schönlein-Henoch nephrotic syndrome reported by Marchal et al. [31], there were only 8 who did not have an acute nephritic syndrome [33]. There is one report of severe hypertension occurring in a child without urinary abnormality [7].

Certain features of the syndrome may lead to a mistaken diagnosis of renal involvement: (1) edema not associated with hypoalbuminemia and (2) hypoalbuminemia provoked by excess loss from the gut. Facial and scalp edema is a common feature of the rash, particularly in children under the age of 4. Peripheral edema of the dorsum of the hands and feet is common at all ages and, according to Willan [44], was particularly common 170 years ago in the legs of "delicate young women who live luxuriously, but use very little exercise." Hypoalbuminemia provoked by excess protein loss from the gut is more likely in those with severe gastrointestinal manifestations [25].

Blood and Urine Findings
The peripheral blood count may show a neutrophil leukocytosis at onset. The erythrocyte sedimentation rate is variable and may be elevated. Platelet count, bleeding time, and clotting time are normal (the purpura is of vascular, not thrombocytopenic origin). Serum C3 complement level is normal. In the cases of 3 patients reported by Evans et al. [8], total hemolytic complement and the serum concentrations of the components of the classic pathway (C1q and C4) and the alternate pathway proteins (glycine rich β-glycoprotein and properdin) were in the normal range. Elevated titers for ASO, anti-DNase B, or anti-NADase are present in a third of children, but the titers do

not differ significantly from those of matched normal control subjects [4]. Serum IgG, IgM, and IgD are normal. Of 20 children with Schönlein-Henoch purpura observed by Trygstad and Stiehm [41], 10 had significant elevations of serum IgA globulin.

When there is appreciable proteinuria, measurement of differential renal clearance of plasma proteins usually shows poorly or moderately selective proteinuria. The few patients with highly selective proteinuria tend to have mild renal lesions [33]. In common with other types of hematuria originating from the kidneys, red cell and granular casts are present in the urine.

Significant cryoglobulinemia has been found in children with recent Schönlein-Henoch purpura and also in those with current glomerular disease resulting from previous Schönlein-Henoch syndrome. Analysis of the cryoglobulins showed IgA and properdin, suggesting activation of complement via the alternative pathway, but isolated cryoglobulins capable of splitting C3 in vitro did so via the classical pathway. Because of this and the occasional finding of hypocomplementemia in a minority of patients, it has been suggested that complement may participate in the tissue damage of Schönlein-Henoch purpura [9a]. Circulating immune complexes of IgA have been detected in children with Schönlein-Henoch purpura [28a].

Morphology
The focal nature of Schönlein-Henoch nephritis has been emphasized rightly in the past. More recent studies of children have tended to stress that it is mainly a focal variation imposed on a diffuse glomerulonephritis of varying severity [15, 33]. The appearance on light microscopy varies from an insignificant to a major abnormality. The mildest cases show merely minimal changes, with most of the glomeruli optically normal; a minority show small areas of mesangial thickening with or without minor foci of hypercellularity. Tubules and interstitium are normal. The most common appearance is of a focal and segmental glomerulonephritis (Fig. 61-4). Focal proliferation is present in many glomeruli, with minor adhesions or small crescents involving a segment of the glomerulus. Biopsies performed 6 months or more after onset may show lobular scars. Minor degrees of tubular atrophy, or interstitial inflammation, or both may be present. The more severe cases show this focal glomerulonephritis superimposed on a diffuse proliferative glomerulonephritis. The appearance, together with lobular stalk thickening, is similar to that seen in late poststreptococcal nephritis [23], but there is more focal and segmen-

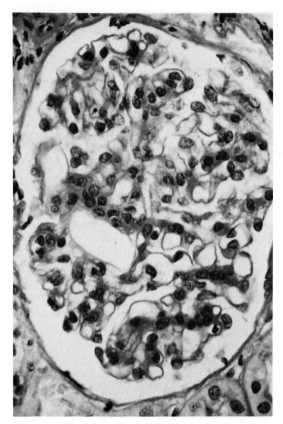

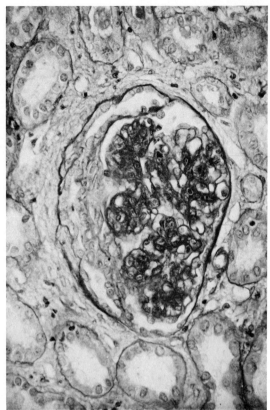

Figure 61-4. Biopsy specimen from an 11-year-old girl. The glomerulus shows mild diffuse mesangial proliferation with segmental variation. Marked focal variation was seen in the specimen, some glomeruli being almost normal. (PAS, ×160.)

Figure 61-5. Biopsy specimen from a 9-year-old boy. The specimen showed diffuse proliferative glomerulonephritis, and there were crescents in 40 percent of the glomeruli seen here. (PAS, ×100.)

tal variation. Epithelial cell crescents are common. The most severe cases are associated with a severe diffuse proliferative picture. There may be polymorphonuclear infiltration, with interstitial inflammation and tubular atrophy. Most glomeruli contain crescents (Fig. 61-5), and late biopsies show glomerular sclerosis. A typical membranoproliferative appearance is occasionally seen in Schönlein-Henoch syndrome.

Immunofluorescent Appearance. Most glomeruli show granular deposits of IgA, IgG, C3 globulin, and fibrin on immunofluorescence microscopy. These are in the mesangium and also occasionally spread along the basement membrane in severe cases [17a] (Fig. 61-6). They may be found as long as 5 years after onset [16]. The mesangial IgA deposits are particularly characteristic of Schönlein-Henoch nephritis. Evans et al. [8] found properdin to be deposited with IgA in the glomerular mesangium. Since they could not detect C1q, they suggested that the glomerular injury is mediated by the properdin system. Al-

though glomerular lesions on light microscopy tend to have marked focal variation, immunofluorescence generally shows diffuse involvement [14, 28b].

Electron-microscopic Appearance. Various ultrastructural changes have been described [5, 10, 15, 33, 42]. These range from open capillary loops with slightly thickened basement membranes and fusion of foot processes to almost totally sclerosed glomeruli with the loops occluded by basement-membrane type of material. The mesangial areas in less severely affected glomeruli contain increased amounts of mesangial matrix. Subendothelial aggregations of varying size and electron density may give a wrinkled or scalloped appearance to the basement membrane. Occasionally, larger aggregations of electron-dense material may be seen between the lamina densa and endothelium, similar to those seen in long-standing renal disease and diabetic nephropathy. The aggregations may be seen within 8 weeks of onset. Deposited material is most common in the mesangium alone, but may also be subendothelial and

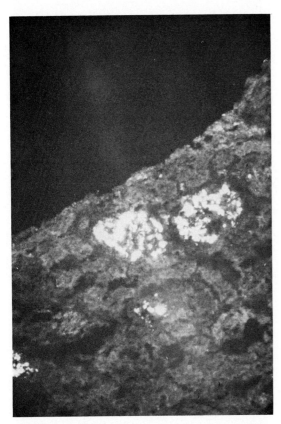

Figure 61-6. Biopsy specimen from an 8-year-old boy. Granular fluorescence is apparent in the mesangium and also involves the capillary walls of the glomeruli. (Anti-IgA antiserum stain, ×20.)

subepithelial. Those with both subendothelial and subepithelial deposits tend to have a severe diffuse proliferative appearance on light microscopy with many crescents [17a].

Differential Diagnosis

Any child with purpura should have a platelet count and simple screening tests for a bleeding disorder. When the results of these studies are normal in the presence of the characteristic skin, joint, and gut abnormalities, diagnosis of Schönlein-Henoch syndrome is relatively easy. Somewhat similar findings may occur in meningococcal septicemia, but fever is usually more marked and the pupuric rash much more generally distributed.

The collagen diseases, particularly polyarteritis nodosa, may present an identical clinical picture. Other systemic manifestations are more likely with a collagen disease, but these also may occur in severe Schönlein-Henoch syndrome. Lung manifestations are very rare in Schönlein-Henoch syndrome.

Confusion sometimes arises when the illness

continues for many months, with recurrence of purpura and other symptoms. A long, progressive course does increase the possibility of a collagen disease such as polyarteritis, but a long course does not necessarily mean a progressive collagen disease and a bad prognosis. One boy had severe Schönlein-Henoch syndrome with renal involvement and recurrent purpura, alimentary, and joint symptoms for 3 years, yet eventually recovered completely [33].

Diagnosis is more difficult when one or two components of the syndrome occur late or not at all. It is particularly difficult if, for instance, the alimentary symptoms or joint symptoms precede the rash by a lengthy period. In the former instance the appearance is that of an acute abdominal emergency, and laparotomy may be needed to exclude appendicitis. When the joint symptoms are the initial presentation, rheumatic fever (acute rheumatism) or rheumatoid arthritis may have to be considered.

Course and Clinicopathologic Correlations

To obtain an unbiased picture of the natural history of Schönlein-Henoch syndrome, one must study the data on children from unselected populations [3, 13, 21, 27, 31, 36, 39], rather than from those in whom severe renal problems predominate. From the former, it is clear that the mortality from renal causes for children with Schönlein-Henoch syndrome is 1 to 5 percent. Of those who have a urinary abnormality in the first month of illness, 50 percent will have abnormal urine 3 months later. Between 10 to 20 percent still will have abnormal urine 2 years after onset. In addition, 2 to 5 percent of children who had no urinary abnormality in the first month will have abnormal urine 2 years later. The detailed follow-up studies from several large departments of pediatric nephrology allow interpretation and prediction of the meaning of abnormal urinary and renal findings [6a, 15, 22, 28b, 33, 40].

The course can be related to the renal presentation. In general, those with microscopic hematuria alone are completely normal 2 years later. Their urine, blood pressure, and renal function are all normal. They are developing healthily and they remain well. Of the large group of children who have appreciable proteinuria and hematuria at onset, 75 percent are also normal 2 years later, though a few subsequently reveal abnormality. Those who have an acute nephritic syndrome at onset do worst, particularly if a nephrotic syndrome also develops. Of those with previous acute nephritic and nephrotic syndrome, 40 percent will have normal renal function and normal urine 2 years later, 20 percent will have minor urinary abnormalities, and the rest will have either severe proteinuria, hypertension, or renal insufficiency.

The longest follow-up study (mean follow-up 10 years from onset of disease) shows that progressive deterioration occurring 2 or more years after onset of disease, although uncommon, does occur in a small minority of children [6a]. Poor outcome was most commonly associated with a clinical presentation of acute nephritis with a nephrotic syndrome and a high proportion of crescents in the first renal biopsy specimen. However, neither the clinical presentation nor the renal morphology was a clear discriminant of outcome; for example, half the children with acute nephritic syndrome and nephrotic syndrome were fully recovered 10 years later, and 15 percent of those who had merely proteinuria and hematuria nevertheless had severe renal insufficiency 10 years later (Fig. 61-7).

The renal morphology is roughly correlated with the severity of clinical presentation and is of definite value as a predictor of outcome. In a disease with such focal variation within the kidney, it is important to evaluate specimens containing at least 20 glomeruli. Children with minimal changes or mild focal segmental glomerulonephri-

tis are usually completely normal 2 years later and remain so; a minority have minor abnormalities of urine. Of those with focal segmental changes superimposed on a diffuse glomerulonephritis, 75 percent have normal or only mildly abnormal urine; the other 25 percent have more active renal disease. Those with marked diffuse proliferation and crescents have a worse prognosis in that more than half will have persistent severe proteinuria, hypertension, or renal insufficiency 2 years later. Nevertheless, there will be some in these groups who will be either normal or have mild proteinuria or microscopic hematuria. It is a remarkable fact that a kidney showing severe proliferative glomerulonephritis, and with the majority of glomeruli containing crescents, may recover to allow normal renal function and normal urine many years later. When biopsies are repeated in children 1 to 2 years after onset, the majority show considerable healing. A "worse" appearance on a repeat biopsy may be seen in 10 percent [34].

Complete apparent recovery is more common in children under the age of 5 than in older children. The rather exceptional finding of highly selective proteinuria appears to be evidence of a good prognosis.

Treatment

There is no evidence from adequately controlled studies that any specific treatment affects the course of either Schönlein-Henoch syndrome or the associated nephritis. There are many anecdotal reports of diminution of gastrointestinal symptoms with corticosteroid therapy [3]. Corticosteroids have also been given for the renal disease; analysis of retrospective data does not show a definite benefit [33]. Immunosuppressive drugs have been used, including azathioprine [11, 22, 33], cyclophosphamide [33, 40, 43], and combinations of corticosteroids, cyclophosphamide, dipyridamole, and oral anticoagulants [26].

Although many spectacular recoveries have been documented, it is not possible to demonstrate convincingly any favorable effect of corticosteroids, cytotoxic drugs, or anticoagulants used singly or in combination. As with most other forms of glomerulonephritis, carefully controlled therapeutic trials are needed. In view of the natural history of the condition, the use of potentially dangerous drugs can be justified only for those with a severe renal presentation and a marked abnormality on biopsy or for rapidly progressive nephritis. Therefore, therapy of Schönlein-Henoch nephritis is symptomatic. Patients with mild and moderate disease require no particular therapy.

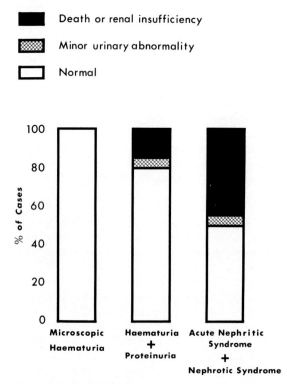

Figure 61-7. The relationship between presentation at onset and clinical state 10 years later.

Bed rest has not been shown to alter the course of the illness. More severe disease will require dietary measures for treatment of nephrotic syndrome or renal insufficiency and sometimes hypotensive drugs.

Energetic symptomatic therapy is worthwhile because of the considerable potential for recovery from Schönlein-Henoch nephritis. Relapses of the syndrome and of the nephritis sometimes occur at the time of an upper respiratory infection. Therefore, some clinicians, particularly those who have seen severe relapses associated with streptococcal pharyngitis, give a daily prophylactic dose of oral penicillin for 1 year.

References

1. Ackroyd, M. B. Allergic purpura, including purpura due to foods, drugs and infections. *Am. J. Med.* 14: 605, 1953.
2. Alexander, H. L., and Eyermann, C. H. Food allergy in Henoch's purpura. *Arch. Derm. Syph.* 16:322, 1927.
3. Allen, D. M., Diamond, L. K., and Howell, D. A. Anaphylactoid purpura in children (Schönlein-Henoch syndrome) *Am. J. Dis. Child.* 99:833, 1960.
4. Ayoub, E. M., and Hoyer, J. Anaphylactoid purpura: Streptococcal antibody titers and β_{1c}-globulin levels. *J. Pediatr.* 75:193, 1969.
5. Ben-Bassat, M., and Stark, N. Diffuse ultrastructural glomerular alterations in apparent 'focal' Schönlein-Henoch nephritis. *Pathol. Microbiol. (Basel)* 38: 278, 1972.
6. Burke, D. M., and Jellinek, J. L. Nearly fatal case of Schoenlein-Henoch syndrome following insect bite. *Am. J. Dis. Child.* 88:772, 1954.
6a. Counahan, R., Winterborn, M. H., Meadow, S. R., Heaton, J., Cameron, J. S., White, R. H. R., Bluett, N. H., Swetschin, H., and Chantler, C. The prognosis of Schönlein-Henoch nephritis. *Br. Med. J.* 2: 11, 1977.
7. DuBois, D. R. Severe hypertension in Schönlein-Henoch purpura without hematuria. *J. Pediatr.* 75: 731, 1969.
8. Evans, D. J., Williams, G. D., Peters, D. K., Sissons, J. G. P., Boulton-Jones, J. M., Ogg, C. S., Cameron, J. S., and Haffrand, B. I. Glomerular deposition of properdin in Henoch-Schönlein syndrome and idiopathic focal nephritis. *Br. Med. J.* 3:326, 1973.
9. Gairdner, D. The Schönlein-Henoch syndrome (anaphylactoid purpura) *Q. J. Med.* 17:95, 1948.
9a. Garcia-Fuentes, M., Chantler, C., and Williams, D. G. Cryoglobulinaemia in Henoch-Schönlein purpura. *Br. Med. J.* 2:163, 1977.
10. Glasgow, E. F. Renal changes in Henoch-Schönlein purpura. *Arch. Dis. Child.* 45:151, 1970.
11. Goldbloom, R. B., and Drummond, K. N. Anaphylactoid purpura with massive gastrointestinal hemorrhage and glomerulonephritis. *Am. J. Dis. Child.* 116:97, 1968.
12. Greifer, I., Bernstein, J., Kikkawa, Y., and Edelmann, C. M., Jr. Histologic evidence of nephritis in patients with Henoch-Schönlein syndrome without clinical evidence of renal disease. *Proc. Am. Soc. Nephrol.* 1966.
13. Haahr, J., Thomsen, K., and Sparrenohn, S. Renal involvement in Henoch-Schönlein purpura. *Br. Med. J.* 4:405, 1974.
14. Habib, R. Discussion. In P. Kincaid-Smith, T. H. Mathew, and E. L. Becker (eds.), *Glomerulonephritis II.* New York: Wiley, 1973. P. 1137.
15. Habib, R., and Levy, M. Les nephropathies du purpura rhumatoide chez l'enfant. Etude clinique et anatomique de 60 observations. *Arch. Pediatr.* 29:305, 1972.
16. Habib, R., and Levy, M. Anaphylactoid purpura nephritis. *Clin. Pediatr. (Phila.)* 12:445, 1973.
17. Handa, S. P. The Schönlein-Henoch syndrome: Glomerulonephritis following erythromycin. *South. Med. J.* 65:917, 1972.
17a. Heaton, J. M., Turner, D. R., and Cameron, J. S. Localization of glomerular "deposits" in Henoch-Schönlein nephritis. *Histopathology* 1:93, 1977.
18. Heberden, W. *Commentarii di Marlbaun. Historia et Curatione.* London: T. Payne, 1801. Chap. 78.
19. Henoch, E. Verhandlungen ärztlicher Gesellschaffen. *Berl. Klin. Wochenschr.* 5:517, 1868.
20. Henoch, E. Neunter Abschnitt III. Die hämorrhagische Diathese—Purpura, 847. *Vorlesungen über Kinderkrankheiten.* Berlin: Hirschwald. 1895.
21. Hughes, L. A., and Wenyl, J. C. Anaphylactoid purpura nephritis in children. *Clin. Pediatr. (Phila.)* 8:594, 1969.
22. Hurley, R. M., and Drummond, K. N. Anaphylactoid purpura nephritis: Clinicopathological correlations. *J. Pediatr.* 81:904, 1972.
23. Jennings, R. B., and Earle, D. P. Post-streptococcal glomerulonephritis: Histopathologic and clinical studies of the acute, subsiding acute and early chronic latent phases. *J. Clin. Invest.* 40:1525, 1961.
24. Jimenez, E. L., and Darrington, H. J. 1968. Vaccination and Henoch-Schoenlein purpura. *N. Engl. J. Med.* 279:1771, 1968.
25. Jones, N. F., Creamer, B., and Gimlette, T. M. D. Hypoproteinaemia in anaphylactoid purpura. *Br. Med. J.* 2:1166, 1966.
26. Kalowski, S., and Kincaid-Smith, P. Glomerulonephritis in Henoch-Schönlein Syndrome. In P. Kincaid-Smith, T. H. Mathew, and E. L. Becker (eds.), *Glomerulonephritis.* New York: Wiley, 1973. P. 1123.
27. Koskimies, O., Rapola, J., Sanilakt, E., and Vilska, J. Renal involvement in Schönlein-Henoch purpura. *Acta Paediatr. Scand.* 63:357, 1974.
28. Lane, J. M. Vaccination and Henoch-Schoenlein purpura (concluded). *N. Engl. J. Med.* 280:781, 1969.
28a. Levinsky, R. J., Barratt, T. M., and Soothill, J. F. Circulating immune complexes in disease (abstract). *Arch. Dis. Child.* 52:808, 1977.
28b. Levy, M., Broyer, M., Arsan, A., Levy-Bentolila, D., and Habib, R. Glomérulonephrites du purpura rhumatoide chez l'enfant. Histoire naturelle et étude immunopathologique. In *Actualités Néphrologiques de l'Hôpital Necker.* Paris: Flammarion Medecine-Sciences, 1976.
29. Liew, S. W., and Kessel, I. Mycoplasmal pneumonia preceding Henoch-Schönlein purpura. *Arch. Dis. Child.* 49:912, 1974.
30. Lofters, W. S., Pineo, G. F., Luke, K. H., and Yaworsky, R. G. Henoch-Schönlein purpura occurring in three members of a family. *Can. Med. Assoc. J.* 109:46, 1973.

31. Marchal, A., Bost, M., Dieterlen, M., Rossignol, A.-M., Gout, J.-P., and Beaudoing, A. Syndrome de Schoenlein-Henoch de l'enfant. *Ann. Pediatr.* 21: 379, 1974.

32. Marx, K. Henoch purpura revisited. *Am. J. Dis. Child.* 128:74, 1974.

33. Meadow, S. R., Glasgow, E. F., White, R. H. R., Moncrieff, M. W., Cameron, J. S., and Ogg, C. S. Schönlein-Henoch nephritis. *Q. J. Med.* 41:241, 1972.

34. Meadow, S. R., Glasgow, E. F., White, R. H. R., Moncrieff, M. W., Cameron, J. S., and Ogg, C. S. Schönlein-Henoch Nephritis. In P. Kincaid-Smith, T. H. Mathew, and E. L. Becker (eds.), *Glomerulonephritis II.* New York: Wiley, 1973. P. 1089.

34a. Pedersen, F. K., and Petersen, E. A. Varicella followed by glomerulonephritis. *Acta Paediatr. Scand.* 64:886, 1975.

35. Philpott, M. G. The Schoenlein-Henoch syndrome in childhood with particular reference to the occurrence of nephritis. *Arch. Dis. Child.* 27:480, 1952.

36. Potanin, N. V. Klinicka Charakteristika Postizeni Ledvin Pri Chorobe Schönleinove-Henochove u deti. *Cesk. Pediatr.* 25:147, 1970.

37. Rogers, P. W., Bunn, S. M., Kurtyman, M. C., and White, M. C. Schonlein-Henoch syndrome associated with exposure to cold. *Arch. Intern. Med.* 128: 782, 1971.

38. Schonlein, J. L. *Allgemeine und Specielle Pathologie und Therapie.* Wurzburg: Etlinger, 1832. P. 41.

39. Sterkey, G., and Thilen, A. A study on the onset and prognosis of acute vascular purpura (the Schönlein-Henoch syndrome) in children. *Acta Pediatr. (Ups.)* 49:217, 1960.

40. Striker, G. E., Quadracci, L. J., Larter, W., Hichman, R. O., Kelly, M. R., and Schaller, J. The Nephritis of Henoch-Schönlein Purpura. In P. Kincaid-Smith, T. H. Mathew, and E. L. Becker (eds.), *Glomerulonephritis II.* New York: Wiley, 1973. P. 1105.

41. Trygstad, C. W., and Stiehm, E. R. Elevated serum IgA globulin in anaphylactoid purpura. *Pediatrics* 47: 1023, 1971.

42. Urizar, R. E., Michael, A., Sisson, S., and Vernier, R. L. Anaphylactoid purpura—immunofluorescent and electron microscopic studies of the glomerular lesions. *Lab. Invest.* 19:437, 1968.

43. White, R. H., Cameron, J. S., and Traunce, J. R. Immunosuppressive therapy in steroid-resistant proliferative glomerulonephritis accompanied by the nephrotic syndrome. *Br. Med. J.* 2:853, 1966.

44. Willan, R. *Cutaneous Disease.* London: J. Johnson, 1808.

62. Polyarteritis Nodosa (Periarteritis Nodosa)

Roy Meadow

Polyarteritis nodosa is a disease of arteries and, less commonly, of veins. It may occur in all or any parts of the body, and thus its clinical manifestations are protean. It is extremely rare in childhood.

The literature on polyarteritis nodosa (PAN) is confusing because of some lack of agreement about its definition, particularly in publications during the first half of this century. Reviewing the literature, Zeek [33] traced the development of knowledge from the early work of Kusmaul and Maier [15]. She suggested first that the genetic term *necrotizing angiitis* should be applied to the group of vascular lesions, both arterial and venous, that in the fully developed stage consist of fibrinoid necrosis and inflammatory reaction involving all three coats of the vessel wall. Second, she pointed out that five groups of conditions were being included in the polyarteritis syndrome: hypersensitivity angiitis, allergic granulomatous angiitis, rheumatic arteritis, periarteritis nodosa, and temporal arteritis. The studies of Davson et al. [6], Churg and Strauss [4], Rose and Spencer [24], and others have helped to clarify the situation further. In general, rheumatic granulomatous angiitis may be considered a variety of polyarteritis with lung involvement that at times amounts to Wegener's granulomatosis.

From a pediatric standpoint, two varieties predominate: (1) an infantile form, generally confined to children below the age of 1 year, in which heart lesions predominate and cause early death, and (2) the adult form, with or without lung involvement.

Incidence

Earlier reports suggested that between 10 and 15 percent of cases of PAN occurred in childhood [5, 18, 25]. This does not fit in with current experience in Britain or North America. It may be that some of the earlier reports included children with rheumatic fever and other conditions. Alternatively, the disease might have become more rare. Inquiry at three English centers for pediatric nephrology in Birmingham, Leeds, and Manchester, which serve a combined total population of about 18 million, revealed that in the 5-year period 1970–1975, two infants with PAN had been seen, together with two older children with possible PAN. It is certain that PAN with significant renal complications is extremely rare in English children. This is what might be expected in a disease that is rare in adults and has a peak incidence at the age of 60 to 70 years.

Cause and Relationship to Schönlein-Henoch Syndrome

The cause of PAN is unknown. There have been many suggestions that it represents some form of hypersensitivity to microorganisms or to drugs, but no consistent association has emerged. Au-SH antigen is found with an unexpectedly high frequency in the serum [28].

In adults there is sometimes confusion between Schönlein-Henoch syndrome and PAN. There are reports of adults initially diagnosed as having Schönlein-Henoch syndrome who later are proved to have PAN. I have seen the same occurrence in older teenagers, but never in younger children. The age distribution of the two conditions is intriguing: PAN occurs in young infants, hardly ever in childhood, and in adults. Schönlein-Henoch syndrome does not occur in early infancy, occurs in childhood, and is rare in adults. Whether or not the two conditions represent different responses to similar agents remains to be seen. Regardless of any similarities, the end results are vastly different, for PAN carries a poor prognosis.

Adult Form

WITHOUT LUNG INVOLVEMENT

Clinical Features

The syndrome of PAN is twice as common in males as in females. A preceding or present respiratory infection is found in 50 percent of patients. Usually, there is weight loss, fever, and a variety of symptoms, dependent on the systems involved. Compared with adults, children tend to have a higher incidence of convulsions, skin eruptions and purpura, peripheral gangrene, arthritis, and lymphadenopathy [18, 25, 30]. Generally, the erythrocyte sedimentation rate is elevated, and mild anemia and a neutrophil leukocytosis are present. There may be a moderate eosinophilia. The serum globulin tends to be increased and the albumin reduced.

Renal Features

Renal abnormality is present in 80 percent [23] and is the cause of death in most of these patients. The presentation may vary from microscopic hematuria and symptomless proteinuria to acute nephritic syndrome or renal insufficiency of acute or gradual onset. Rarely, nephrotic syndrome has been reported [7]. Hypertension may occur and, when developing during the illness, is usually preceded by urinary abnormalities [23]. Once started, it is usually progressive. It has been suggested that hypertension is a sign of advanced or healed (scarred) lesions [24].

There are two main types of pathologic changes, renal polyarteritis and glomerulonephritis. Renal polyarteritis is found in about 75 percent of those with renal involvement [10, 20, 23]. The destructive inflammatory necrotizing process begins in the vessels of the cortex. It starts in the media and subsequently involves the adventitia and intima. Thrombi and aneurysms may occur and lead to cortical infarcts. At first, the lesions may be associated merely with mild urinary abnormalities, but cortical infarcts may cause sudden renal failure and death [27].

Glomerulonephritis is present in 44 percent of those with renal involvement. One-third of those with glomerulonephritis have marked renal polyarteritis. Rose [23] listed the characteristics as capillary microthrombi, focal fibrinoid necrosis, polymorphonuclear infiltration, and capsular infiltration with crescent formation. However, a variety of changes are possible. Benitez et al. [1] found pure membranous changes in 1 patient. Tubular changes are nonspecific and inconsistent. Immunofluorescence usually is positive for fibrin only. The focal nature of early PAN creates difficulties both in diagnosis and in study of kidney tissue. It is generally recognized that a large piece of medium-sized artery may be needed for the clinical diagnosis. Renal polyarteritis may be similarly patchy.

Treatment

Corticosteroids have been widely used in the treatment of PAN. It is uncertain whether or not they alter the course of the renal disease. However, there are some intriguing anecdotal reports. For example, a 16-year-old with severe hypertension and multiple aneurysms on renal arteriography was found to have an improved arteriogram after corticosteroid therapy [17]. Cytotoxic drugs and anticoagulants have been used and sometimes appear to bring about improvement [14].

WITH LUNG INVOLVEMENT

One-third of persons with histologically proved PAN have major lung involvement, including such features as pulmonary symptoms, nodular and caseous lesions in the lungs, and granulomatous lesions in the upper respiratory tract and ears. This group comprises a number of subgroups, including Wegener's granulomatosis, the Löffler syndrome, allergic granulomatosis, and allergic angiitis. The pulmonary features may precede involvement of other systems by many years. Renal involvement may occur just as in PAN without lung involvement, but it is less likely to dominate the clinical picture.

Polyarteritis nodosa with lung involvement is extremely rare in childhood. However, 13 cases of allergic granulomatosis and allergic angiitis reviewed by Churg and Strauss [4] included 2 children. Churg and Strauss found diffuse or focal interstitial nephritis with a predominance of eosinophilic infiltration of the capillary walls, with necrosis of cells and fragmentation of nuclei. Focal segmental lesions were present in a minority of glomeruli and were usually seen as a terminal fibrosis of the affected segment, with complete obliteration of the involved loop with capsular adhesions. Afferent and efferent arterioles were involved in the same process.

Wegener's Granulomatosis

Wegener's granulomatosis is applied to a fairly well defined group with the triad of respiratory tract involvement, vasculitis, and glomerulonephritis. By Wegener's [31] definition all have glomerulonephritis. There are isolated reports of its occurrence in childhood [21a]. Raised serum IgA and C3 complement has been found in adults [26].

Morphologically, the kidneys show a focal and segmental glomerulonephritis of varying severity. Immunofluorescence studies show a variety of deposits ranging from fibrin alone to immunoglobulins and C3. Subepithelial deposits have been seen on electron microscopy; they are composed of dense material consistent with antibody-antigen complexes [8, 19].

Before the advent of cytotoxic therapy, death from renal disease usually occurred within 6 months of onset. Cytotoxic drugs have altered this dramatically. Although the rarity of the condition has not allowed controlled trials, there is very little doubt from comparative case reports that cytotoxic drugs are effective and sometimes curative in Wegener's granulomatosis. Further, it is not merely the local granulomas in the upper respiratory tract that regress; other systemic manifestations, including the glomerulonephritis, improve or go into total remission [16, 21, 29]. Cyclophosphamide and azathioprine have been most widely used, but all cytotoxic drugs appear to be effective. At times, they have been combined with corticosteroids and heparin in the treatment of the nephritis [11, 32]. It appears that although lengthy courses may be needed, treatment can be stopped once cure seems to have been achieved [16].

Infantile Polyarteritis

Polyarteritis is more common in the first year of life than in any other year of childhood. The infantile form of the disease is characteristic and is confined to the early months of life [22]. The infant presents with an upper respiratory tract infection that persists. There is prolonged or intermittent fever, rashes, conjunctivitis, cardiomegaly, and heart failure. Hematuria and proteinuria are common, and there may be hypertension [2, 22]. Serum IgE has been found elevated in 2 infants [13]. The course is rapidly fatal, most infants dying of heart failure within a few weeks [12, 22].

Diagnosis is possible in life, but more often is made at autopsy. The kidneys may show arterial lesions and infarcts. However, the coronary artery involvement is the most significant lesion in polyarteritis of infancy; it is this that kills the infants and makes the renal lesions somewhat irrelevant.

Mucocutaneous Lymph Node Syndrome

Mucocutaneous lymph node syndrome is an acute illness affecting infants and young children. It is widespread in Japan and occurs in Hawaii, but is seldom reported elsewhere. It is characterized by fever, a scarlet-fever type of rash, sore lips, red oral mucosa, conjunctivitis, and cervical lymphadenopathy. There may be mild proteinuria and leukocytosis. The cause is unknown. Most infants recover completely within 2 weeks. However, 1 to 2 percent of infants die suddenly during the illness, and autopsy reveals myocardial infarction secondary to coronary thromboarteritis. The autopsy findings are indistinguishable from those of infantile polyarteritis [9, 16a].

References

1. Benitez, L., Mathews, M., and Mallory, G. K.   Platelet thrombosis with polyarteritis nodosa. *A.M.A. Arch. Pathol.* 77:117, 1964.
2. Benyo, R. B., and Perrin, E. V.   Periarteritis nodosa in infancy. *Am. J. Dis. Child.* 116:539, 1968.
3. Carrington, C. B., and Liebow, A. A.   Limited forms of angiitis and granulomatosis of Wegener's. *Am. J. Med.* 41:497, 1966.
4. Churg, J., and Strauss, L.   Allergic granulomatosis, allergic angiitis, and periarteritis nodosa. *Am. J. Pathol.* 27:277, 1951.
5. Coe, M., Reisman, H. A., and DeHoff, J.   Periarteritis nodosa in a nine-year-old child. *J. Pediatr.* 18:793, 1941.
6. Davson, J., Ball, J., and Platt, R.   The kidney in periarteritis nodosa. *Q. J. Med.* 17:175, 1948.
7. DeWardener, H. E.   *The Kidney.* London: Churchill, 1957.
8. Fauci, A. S., and Wolff, S. M.   Wegener's granulomatosis: Studies in eighteen patients and a review of the literature. *Medicine (Baltimore)* 52:535, 1973.
9. Fetterman, G. H., and Hashida, Y.   Mucocutaneous

lymph node syndrome (MLNS): A disease widespread in Japan which demands our attention. *Pediatrics* 54:269, 1974.

10. Fujimaki, S., Oonish, Y., and Urano, T. Nature of collagen disease, particularly of systemic lupus erythematosus (SLE), with special reference to renal lesion. *Acta Med. Biol. Niigata* 11:57, 1963.

11. Fuller, T., Olsen, N., Block, A., and Cade, J. Wegener's granulomatosis. Treatment with heparin in addition to azathioprine and corticosteroids. *Nephron* 9:225, 1972.

12. Gotz, E. G. Panarteriitis nodosa der Koronargefässe bei einem neuneinhalb Monate alten Kind. *Klin. Paediatr.* 184:288, 1972.

13. Kraus, H. F., Clausen, C. R., and Ray, C. G. Elevated immunoglobulin E in infantile polyarteritis nodosa. *J. Pediatr.* 84:841, 1974.

14. Kühner, U., Ackerman, R., and Frohmuller, H. Zur Diagnose und Therapie einer Panarteriites im Kindesalter. *Klin. Paediatr.* 184:399, 1972.

15. Kusmaul, A., and Maier, R. Ueber eine bisher nicht beschriebene eigenthümliche Arterienerkrankung (Periarteritis nodosa), die mit Morbus Brightii und rapid forschreitender allgemeiner Muskellähmung einhergeht. *Dtsch. Arch. Klin. Med.* 1:484, 1866.

16. Lancet. Annotation. Wegener's granulomatosis, *Lancet* 2:519, 1972.

16a. Landing, B. H., and Larson, E. J. Are infantile periarteritis nodosa with coronary artery involvement and fatal mucocutaneous lymph node syndrome the same? *Pediatrics* 59:651, 1977.

17. McLain, L. G., Bookstein, J. J., and Kelsch, R. C. Polyarteritis nodosa diagnosed by renal arteriography. *J. Pediatr.* 80:1032, 1972.

18. Miller, H. G., and Daley, R. Clinical aspects of polyarteritis nodosa. *Q. J. Med.* 15:255, 1946.

19. Norton, W. L., Suki, W., and Strunk, S. Combined corticosteroid and azathioprine therapy. *Arch. Intern. Med.* 121:554, 1968.

20. Patalano, V. J., and Sommers, S. C. Biopsy diagnosis of periarteritis nodosa. *A.M.A. Arch. Pathol.* 72:1, 1961.

21. Pickering, J. G. Wegener's granuloma treated with azathioprine. *Proc. R. Soc. Med.* 65:592, 1972.

21a. Roback, S. A., Herdman, R. C., Hoyer, J., and Good, R. A. Wegener's granulomatosis in a child. *Am. J. Dis. Child.* 118:608, 1969.

22. Roberts, F. B., and Fetterman, G. N. Polyarteritis nodosa in infancy. *J. Pediatr.* 63:519, 1963.

23. Rose, G. A. The natural history of polyarteritis. *Br. Med. J.* 2:1148, 1957.

24. Rose, G. A., and Spencer, H. Polyarteritis nodosa. *Q. J. Med.* 26:43, 1957.

25. Rothstein, J. L., and Welt, S. Periarteritis nodosa in infancy and in childhood. *Am. J. Dis. Child.* 45:1277, 1933.

26. Shillitoe, E. J., Lehner, T., Lessof, M. H., and Harrison, D. F. N. Immunological features of Wegener's granulomatosis. *Lancet* 1:281, 1974.

27. Taylor, A. W., and Jacoby, N. M. Acute polyarteritis nodosa in children. *Lancet* 1:792, 1949.

28. Trepo, C. G., Thivolet, J., and Prince, A. M. Australia antigen and polyarteritis nodosa. *Am. J. Dis. Child.* 123:390, 1972.

29. Trethowan, J. D., McEnedy, M. B., and King, R. C. Treatment of Wegener's granulomatosis. *Lancet* 1:318, 1973.

30. Vining, C. W. A case of periarteritis nodosa with subcutaneous lesions and recovery. *Arch. Dis. Child.* 13:31, 1938.

31. Wegener, F. Über generalisierte, septische Gefässerkrankungen. *Verh. Dtsch. Ges. Pathol.* 29:202, 1936.

32. Whitaker, A. N., Emmerson, B. T., Bunce, I. H., Nicoll, P., and Sands, J. M. Reversal of renal failure in Wegener's granulomatosis by heparin. *Am. J. Med. Sci.* 265:399, 1973.

33. Zeek, P. M. Periarteritis nodosa: A critical review. *Am. J. Clin. Pathol.* 22:777, 1952.

63. Renal Involvement in Amyloidosis

Eugene B. Trainin

Classification

Amyloidosis is a disorder characterized by the deposition in various organs of the body of a proteinaceous material, amyloid, an inert substance that elicits no inflammatory reaction and produces disease by compressing and replacing normal tissue. The disease occurs in a "primary" form and in association with a number of diseases, the most common of which are (1) chronic infections and inflammatory conditions, such as tuberculosis, osteomyelitis, endocarditis, bronchiectasis, ulcerative colitis, regional ileitis, and rheumatoid arthritis; (2) heredofamilial conditions, such as familial Mediterranean fever (FMF); and (3) multiple myeloma. There have been attempts to classify amyloidosis on the basis of either the distribution of organ involvement or the pattern of amyloid deposition in blood vessels [15]. Amyloidosis in chronic inflammatory diseases and FMF is said to have a "parenchymal" distribution, involving mainly the liver, spleen, kidneys, and adrenals. In multiple myeloma and in primary amyloidosis it is said to have a "mesenchymal" distribution, involving mainly smooth and striated muscle and connective tissue [15]. This classification has not been particularly useful, however, since there is much overlapping among the various conditions [11, 15]. In inflammatory disease and FMF, amyloid is said to be deposited along reticulin fibers in vascular intima, in contrast to its deposition along collagen fibers in vascular adventitia in multiple myeloma and primary disease [34]. This also has not been a useful classification, since in many cases it is difficult to differentiate these two patterns [15]. A more useful and potentially meaningful classification can be based on recently acquired knowledge concerning the chemical composition of amyloid in different conditions, as discussed in the next section.

Chemistry and Pathogenesis

Amyloid deposits are composed of fibrillar subunits, which are responsible for the histologic properties by which amyloid is identified (see later) [26]. These fibrils are insoluble under physiologic conditions and are resistant to proteolysis, features that account, in part, for the body's difficulty in eliminating amyloid deposits [31]. It is now possible, however, to solubilize and purify the major protein constituents of amyloid fibrils [29] and to determine their composition and sequence of amino acids [30]. Such studies have revealed that, although amyloid, whatever its type, has identical structural and histologic characteristics, [15] amyloid fibrils are derived from two separate sources. In some cases the major protein constituent is of immunoglobulin origin [26]. This protein is derived most commonly from the variable region of either kappa or lambda light chains, although it may also consist of either intact light chains or combinations of intact and fragmented light chains [31]. The amino acid sequence of these polypeptide chains appears to be homogeneous and unique in each individual; antibodies made against fibrils from one patient will not react with those from another [26]. In other cases the major constituent of amyloid fibrils appears to be unique, with an amino acid composition that differs from that of all other known proteins [20, 44, 45]. The protein has been variously designated as "amyloid A" [59] or "amyloid of unknown origin" [31]. Slight differences reported by various workers in the structure of this protein suggest that amyloid A, like amyloid of immunoglobulin origin, is ultimately derived from a larger precursor protein [31].

The mechanisms by which amyloid deposits are formed have not yet been completely elucidated, but recent studies suggest a reasonable hypothesis. By utilizing Bence Jones proteins as precursors and incubating these light chains with pepsin at pH 3.5 and 37°C, Glenner and his associates [27] have been able to create fibrils in vitro with all the characteristic physical properties of amyloid fibrils seen in vivo [27]. Since these conditions are comparable to an intralysosomal environment, it was con-

cluded that amyloid fibrils may be formed following uptake and subsequent intralysosomal proteolysis of circulating light chains by phagocytic cells [28]. The polypeptide fragments formed, because of their intrinsic physical properties, then aggregate into fibrils, which are extruded into the surrounding extracellular space [28]. In support of this hypothesis, the intralysosomal presence of amyloid fibrils [26] has been demonstrated by electron microscopy, and deposits are frequently found to be in proximity to phagocytic cells [31]. Such a mechanism, however, does not account for the formation of fibrils composed of intact light chains. In such cases it has been suggested that there may be some defect in lysosomal function, resulting in incomplete light-chain digestion and in consequent amyloid formation [31].

Similar studies of the formation of amyloid A fibrils have not been done because the nature of the precursor protein is unknown. However, a large protein called amyloid A–related serum component (SAA) that is antigenically similar to amyloid A has been found to be present in low titers in sera from normal subjects and in high titers in sera from patients with several diseases, including amyloidosis [59]. It is conceivable that amyloid A is derived from this protein, although the mechanisms are unknown. However, all amyloid fibrils, independent of origin and composition, have the same physico-optical properties; it is therefore reasonable to conclude that the mechanisms of formation of the various fibrils are similar.

The twofold origin of amyloid fibrils has a clinical counterpart in the observation that the immunoglobulin variety has been found, with rare exceptions, in patients with either "primary" amyloidosis or various plasma cell dyscrasias; amyloid A has been found in patients with chronic inflammatory disease and FMF [31]. This clinicopathologic correlation has important implications for the pathogenesis of amyloidosis. Since amyloid fibrils of predominantly immunoglobulin origin develop in patients with both plasma-cell dyscrasias and primary amyloidosis, patients with the latter may also have an abnormality in immunoglobulin metabolism. In fact, Isobe and Osserman [37] found that all 50 of their patients with primary amyloidosis had M-proteins in their serum, or Bence Jones proteinuria, or both. On the other hand, Rosenthal and Franklin [59] have shown that many patients with chronic inflammatory disease produce SAA in high titers. This may also be true in patients with FMF, but has not been tested; however, one might anticipate similar findings, since FMF is a chronic inflammatory disease. Rosenthal and Franklin [59] also found high SAA titers in patients with several acute inflammatory conditions. Thus, it was hypothesized that SAA may actually be an acute phase reactant that normally is cleared rapidly from the plasma, but, when produced in large amounts or for a prolonged time, may somehow result in amyloid fibril formation [59].

Renal Pathologic Features
GROSS APPEARANCE
The kidneys in amyloidosis are pale and firm. They are usually enlarged, with as much as a two-fold increase in weight. Treating the cut surface with Lugol's iodine results in a mahogany-brown coloration of amyloid deposits, and the glomeruli appear as small brown dots. The kidneys may on occasion be scarred and contracted, especially when there is significant intrarenal vascular involvement [15].

MICROSCOPIC APPEARANCE
Light-Microscopic Findings
The *glomeruli* commonly are all affected, but the severity of involvement is variable and often segmental. The earliest findings are small, eosinophilic nodules that are located within the mesangium [35]. As the disease progresses, these nodules enlarge and obstruct capillary lumina (Fig. 63-1). Eventually, the nodules coalesce, and the entire tuft may be replaced by masses of amyloid. Glomerular obsolescence, sclerosis, and tubular atrophy in advanced disease are probably also secondary to vascular involvement.

Interstitial deposition of amyloid, particularly in the inner medulla, is occasionally severe. When present, these amyloid deposits are usually seen in relationship to the basement membranes of loops of Henle and collecting tubules [35]. The degree of intrarenal vascular involvement varies considerably from one patient to another, lacking correlation with the severity of glomerular disease [35]. There is amyloid infiltration of the media and adventitia of the interlobular arteries and arterioles [35]. Thrombosis of the smaller tributaries of the renal vein occurs occasionally, and may spread to involve the main renal vein [6]. The basis for this complication, which is not rare, is uncertain, but it does not appear to be secondary to amyloid deposition in the walls of the veins [33].

Electron-Microscopic Findings
Electron-microscopic examination is an extremely reliable way to diagnose amyloidosis (Fig. 63-2). It reveals that amyloid is essentially fibrillar, despite its apparent hyaline appearance on light microscopy. The fibrils are about 80 to 100 Å in diameter, up to 1 μ in length, and randomly arranged

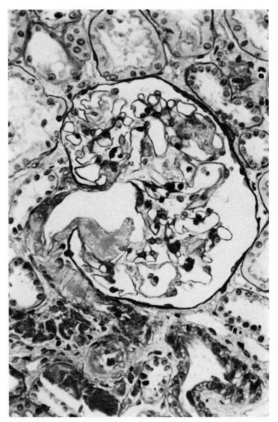

Figure 63-1. Photomicrograph of glomerulus showing deposition of fluffy, lightly eosinophilic material expanding the mesangium and extending about loops. Similar material is present in areas of the interstitium and about blood vessels. The Congo red stain was positive for amyloid. (PAS, ×250.) (Courtesy of Dr. B. Bennet, Albert Einstein College of Medicine.)

[35]. There will often be a periodicity of 55 Å within the fibrils. Deposits are seen in the mesangium, where fibrils lie within the mesangial matrix [35]. Apparently by extension, deposits also involve the glomerular capillary walls, lying along the endothelial side of the basement membrane. Mesangial involvement is one of the earliest findings in amyloidosis and may be present despite negative findings on light microscopy. It is noteworthy because of the known phagocytic properties of mesangial cells and the proposed importance of phagocytosis in the pathogenesis of amyloidosis.

Immunofluorescence Findings
Complement (C3) and immunoglobulin are occasionally demonstrable, [41, 70, 71] by immunofluorescence microscopy, but the results are inconsistent and appear not to have value in the diagnosis or evaluation of the disease.

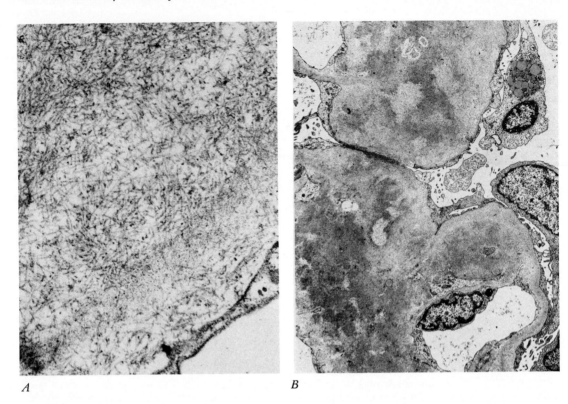

A   *B*

Figure 63-2. A. *Electron microscopy reveals expansion of the mesangium by an accumulation of acellular, fibrillary material that has a periodicity of 50 Å. (×60,000.)* B. *The material is somewhat variable in electron density and extends partially around the peripheral capillary walls. (×4,800.) (Courtesy of Dr. B. Bennet, Albert Einstein College of Medicine.)*

Staining Characteristics

Amyloid exhibits certain tinctorial histologic features that facilitate its identification. Amyloid characteristically gives a metachromatic reaction on staining with crystal violet or by the standard toluidine method. It takes up the fluor, thioflavin T, which is a very sensitive but nonspecific technique. Other dyes and staining methods are available. The most specific reaction is thought to be the green birefringence of Congo red–treated sections under polarized light [15, 35, 40]. The Congo red stain may be too pale in the thin (3- to 4-μ) sections customarily cut for renal biopsies, and thicker sections (6 to 7 μ) are necessary.

Clinical Features

Amyloidosis in children is a relatively rare disease and has been described almost exclusively in association with three conditions: (1) chronic infection, notably tuberculosis and osteomyelitis, (2) FMF, and (3) juvenile rheumatoid arthritis (JRA) [65]. With the advent of modern antimicrobial drugs, however, infection has been all but eliminated as a cause of amyloidosis. Amyloidosis occurs in certain ethnic groups [64] (mainly Sephardic Jews and Armenians) in association with FMF, a condition that is rarely seen in the United States and Europe. Thus, in the Western world, amyloidosis in children is seen now almost exclusively among patients with JRA.

The incidence of amyloidosis among children with JRA is low, ranging in reported series from about 1 to 4 percent [3, 19, 31, 46, 61, 63]. Its frequency is in sharp contrast to that in adults with rheumatoid arthritis, in whom amyloidosis develops with a frequency of 5 to 12 percent in prospective studies [4, 12, 47, 54] and 15 to 60 percent in retrospective studies [23, 51, 67]. The stated incidence in children may, however, be low, since amyloidosis can be present subclinically for many years [4, 5, 15, 67]. Despite the low incidence of amyloidosis in children with JRA, it must be realized that the 10-year survival rate of these patients is less than 50 percent [68], and that amyloidosis accounts for about 25 percent of all deaths in children with JRA [2].

The average duration of JRA before the clinical detection of amyloidosis is about 5 years, but has ranged from as little as 9 months [53] to as long as 23 years [63]. In general, there is little, if any, correlation between the severity of JRA and the development of amyloidosis [63]. The sexes are affected about equally, but because JRA is more common in females [60], it is possible that in males with JRA there may actually be a greater tendency toward the development of amyloidosis.

Amyloidosis in JRA involves many organs, but most commonly affects the liver, spleen [55], adrenals, and kidneys. The liver and spleen are palpable in about 50 percent of cases [63], but significant dysfunction of these organs is rare. Adrenal involvement is also rarely clinically evident. Significant renal disease is the major complication, and death in amyloidosis is almost always due to renal failure.

The clinical presentation of renal amyloidosis is nonspecific, and there are no features that establish the diagnosis beyond the level of clinical suspicion [69]. Proteinuria, almost always present [65], may in some cases be mild and go undetected and in others be severe enough to result in the nephrotic syndrome. There is often not a very good correlation between the degree of proteinuria and the severity of glomerular involvement as seen on histologic examination [25]. One unusual feature is that patients often continue to excrete large amounts of protein, even when little renal function is left [11, 69]. The proteinuria is usually nonselective, and a variety of plasma proteins may appear in the urine [25]. Renal vein thrombosis is not an infrequent occurrence, presenting either as a sudden increase in proteinuria or as acute renal failure [6]. Abnormalities of the urinary sediment are only occasionally present.

Radiography usually reveals the kidneys to be enlarged [56], although, as previously mentioned, significant renovascular involvement results in shrunken kidneys [15]. An additional radiographic finding in children with FMF is narrowing and shortening of the ureter, interpreted as being due to diffuse amyloid infiltration in the ureteral submucosa [56].

The incidence of hypertension in renal amyloidosis is controversial. Some authors claim it to be unusual [8], found only in patients with advanced renal insufficiency, and then even less frequently than in patients with renal failure due to other causes [8]. Others [35, 69] claim that hypertension is common, and that the low incidence figures in other series is due to the inclusion of many patients debilitated by their primary disease, such as

tuberculosis. Other factors, however, might tend to make hypertension infrequent in renal amyloidosis. First, there may be extensive amyloid deposits in the medulla, resulting in the salt and water wasting that is often observed clinically [2, 8]. Second, there is often extensive amyloid deposition in the adrenals; although gross adrenal insufficiency is rare, there is evidence that patients may have subclinical disease, as determined by impaired responsiveness to ACTH [10]. In any case, when hypertension occurs, it often heralds rapid deterioration with accelerated renal failure; vigorous control of blood pressure may prolong life in affected patients [69].

Diagnosis

The diagnosis of amyloidosis at one time was based on the finding that, following IV injection, affected patients retain about 80 percent or more of Congo red dye, while normal subjects retain about 40 percent or less [15]. The sensitivity of the test, however, depends on the amount of amyloid present in the body [18, 35], and there is a high incidence of false-negative results [18, 21, 52]. Other problems include occasional false-positive results and hypersensitivity reactions [15].

The clinical suggestion of amyloidosis must be confirmed by the histologic demonstration of amyloid in biopsy sections. A site that is accessible and allows for reliable examination is the rectum [15, 21, 52]; in two reports, the diagnostic accuracy of rectal biopsy has been 85 and 96 percent [21, 52]. The specimen must contain submucosa, since amyloid deposits are often found localized around blood vessels. Gingival biopsy has been advocated as a reliable test [14], but despite its ease and safety, it appears not to be as reliable as rectal biopsy [13, 35]. Other sites recently reported to yield as good or better results than the rectum are the spleen and adipose tissue obtained from the abdominal wall [72]; these reports await confirmation.

A renal biopsy is necessary for establishing the presence of amyloid in the kidney. It has been stated that amyloid-laden tissue may bleed profusely [15], and this complication on occasion has necessitated a nephrectomy [65]. Rectal biopsy may result in severe bleeding, but adequate hemostasis is more readily achieved in this method than in renal biopsy.

It is of great interest that amyloid fibrils have recently been found by electron microscopy to be present in the urinary sediment [17]. Although the sensitivity of this finding has not yet been established, it would be most helpful if renal amyloidosis could be detected by this method, obviating the need for renal biopsy.

Treatment

There is no specific therapy for any of the clinical varieties of amyloidosis. However, recent advances in our understanding of the composition of amyloid have provided a theoretical basis for a rational approach to treatment. As mentioned, "primary" amyloidosis appears to be associated usually with occult plasma cell dyscrasias; it is logical, therefore, to assume that chemotherapy might be helpful in diminishing plasmacytic proliferation and hence production of amyloid. Indeed, there have been several reports [7, 16, 38] on the use of melphalan (L-phenylalanine mustard, commonly used in patients with multiple myeloma) in the treatment of primary amyloidosis. Although the results are inconclusive [7], some patients appear to have benefited from this therapy [16, 38]. In one report of a patient whose glomerular filtration rate had fallen from 84 to 14 ml per minute in only 4 months, renal function stabilized following initiation of melphalan therapy and had improved slightly 4 years later [38].

Treatment of amyloidosis associated with chronic inflammatory conditions and FMF is somewhat more complicated. In patients with amyloidosis secondary to chronic suppurative conditions, it is clear that clinical remission may follow treatment of the primary disorder if renal function has not yet deteriorated [48, 69]. However, amyloidosis in children is now nearly always secondary to JRA and FMF, conditions for which no curative treatment exists. Nevertheless, one might expect that immunosuppression could be of some benefit in some cases, since fibrils from some patients, although composed mainly of amyloid A, also contain significant amounts of immunoglobulin-derived protein [36, 44]. In addition, these forms of amyloidosis apparently are characterized by overproduction of amyloid A percursor, and, although it is unclear which cell produces this protein, it is possible that its synthesis could be suppressed by nonspecific cytotoxic therapy. In one report of 10 children with JRA and amyloidosis treated with chlorambucil, 3 showed improvement, as determined by a decrease in proteinuria [1]. Another report suggests that chloroquine and methotrexate might be of benefit [52].

As previously discussed, it has been proposed that circulating precursor proteins are taken up by phagocytic cells, where they undergo proteolysis, the fragments being extruded into the extracellular compartment [26, 31]. Thus, one way to interfere with amyloid formation would be to interrupt these cellular processes. A drug that might be useful in this regard is colchicine, whose main mechanism of action appears to be the prevention of aggregation of microtubules, a mechanism necessary for lysosomal degranulation and enzyme release [49, 74]. Colchicine has been shown in an experimental model to decrease significantly or to block completely the formation of amyloid [24, 39, 62]. Although the drug has not been used for this purpose clinically, it has been reported to decrease the number and severity of inflammatory episodes in patients with FMF [73]. It will be of great interest to see whether or not the incidence and severity of amyloidosis can also be diminished with this treatment.

Corticosteroids have been tried in the treatment of all types of amyloidosis, but have been found to be ineffective [22, 50, 63, 65]. There is some controversy as to whether or not they actually enhance amyloid formation [9, 42, 43, 57, 66].

For patients who reach end-stage renal failure, there remains room for cautious optimism. The 1975 ACS/NIH renal transplant registry [58] reports that of 21 patients with amyloidosis who received a renal transplant, only 1 had shown evidence of recurrence; 11 had well-functioning grafts, and 5 had had functioning kidneys for more than 3 years. These data must be tempered by the fact that if amyloidosis is still active, it may ultimately affect other organs, such as the heart. However, in a child with JRA, there is a good chance that a long-term remission of the arthritis eventually will occur and, with it, the stimulus for further production of amyloid.

References

1. Ansell, B. M., Eghtedari, A., and Bywaters, E. G. L. Chlorambucil in the management of juvenile chronic polyarthritis complicated by amyloidosis. *Ann. Rheum. Dis.* 30:331, 1971.
2. Antilla, R. Renal involvement in children and adult patients with rheumatoid arthritis. *Acta Paediatr. Scand.* [Suppl.] 227:3, 1972.
3. Antilla, R., and Laaksonen, A. L. Renal disease in juvenile rheumatoid arthritis. *Acta Rheum. Scand.* 15:99, 1969.
4. Arapkis, G., and Tribe, C. R. Amyloidosis in rheumatoid arthritis investigated by means of rectal biopsy. *Ann. Rheum. Dis.* 22:256, 1963.
5. Armstrong, J. A fatal case of Still's disease complicated by amyloidosis. *Br. Med. J.* 11:1261, 1951.
6. Barclay, G. P. T., Cameron, H. M., and Loughridge, L. W. Amyloid disease and renal vein thrombosis. *Q. J. Med.* 29:137, 1960.
7. Barth, W. F., Willerson, J. T., Waldmann, T. A., and Decker, J. L. Primary amyloidosis. Clinical, immunochemical and immunoglobulin metabolism studies in fifteen patients. *Am. J. Med.* 47:259, 1969.
8. Bentwich, Z., Rosenmann, E., and Eliakim, M.

Prevalence of hypertension in renal amyloidosis. Correlation with chemical and histological parameters. *Am. J. Med. Sci.* 262:93, 1971.

9. Bestetti, A., Pirani, C. L., and Catchpole, H. R. Studies on experimental amyloidosis. *Arthritis Rheum.* 1:274, 1958.

10. Beter, O. S., Tuma, S., Barzilai, D., Peleg, I., and Chaimovitz, C. Diminished Adrenocortical Function Reserve in Patients with Familial Mediterranean Fever and Renal Amyloidosis. In *Frontiers of Internal Medicine, 1974.* Twelfth International Congress of Internal Medicine. Basel: Karger, 1975. Pp. 339–342.

11. Brandt, K., Carthcart, E. S., and Cohen, A. S. A clinical analysis of the course and prognosis of forty-two patients with amyloidosis. *Am. J. Med.* 44:955, 1968.

12. Brun, C., Olsen, T. S., Raaschou, F., and Sorensen, A. W. S. Renal biopsy in rheumatoid arthritis. *Nephron* 2:65, 1965.

13. Calkins, E., and Cohen, A. S. Diagnosis of amyloidosis. *Bull. Rheum. Dis.* 10:215, 1960.

14. Clinicopathological conference. *N. Engl. J. Med.* 294:831, 1976.

15. Cohen, A. S. Amyloidosis. *N. Engl. J. Med.* 277:522, 574, 628, 1967.

16. Cohen, H. J., Lessin, L. S., Hallal, J., and Burkholder, P. Resolution of primary amyloidosis during chemotherapy. Studies in a patient with nephrotic syndrome. *Ann. Intern. Med.* 82:646, 1975.

17. Derosena, R., Koss, M. N., and Pirani, C. L. Demonstration of amyloid fibrils in urinary sediment. *N. Engl. J. Med.* 293:1131, 1975.

18. Editorial. Diagnosis of amyloidosis. *Br. Med. J.* 4:1090, 1966.

19. Edstrom, G. Rheumatoid arthritis and Still's disease in children. A survey of 161 cases. *Arthritis Rheum.* 1:497, 1958.

20. Ein, D., Kimura, S., Terry, W. D., Magnotta, J., and Glenner, G. G. Amino acid sequence of an amyloid fibril protein of unknown origin. *J. Biol. Chem.* 247:5653, 1972.

21. Gafni, J., and Sohar, E. Rectal biopsy for the diagnosis of amyloidosis. *Am. J. Med. Sci.* 102:332, 1960.

22. Gardner, D. L. Amyloidosis in rheumatoid arthritis treated with hormones. *Ann. Rheum. Dis.* 21:298, 1962.

23. Gedda, P. O. On amyloidosis and other causes of death in rheumatoid arthritis. *Acta Med. Scand.* 150:443, 1955.

24. Gillespie, E. Colchicine binding in tissue slices. Decrease by calcium and biphasic effect of adenosine 3'5' monophosphate. *J. Cell Biol.* 50:544, 1971.

25. Glassock, R. J., and Bennett, C. M. The Glomerulopathies. In B. M. Brenner and F. C. Rector, Jr. (eds.), *The Kidney.* Philadelphia: Saunders, 1976: Pp. 941–1078.

26. Glenner, G. G. The Nature and Pathogenesis of Systemic Amyloidosis. In J. Hamburger, J. Crosnier, and M. H. Maxwell (eds.), *Advances in Nephrology.* Chicago: Year Book, 1974. Vol. 4, pp. 291–300.

27. Glenner, G. G., Ein, D., Eanes, E. D., Bladen, H. A., Terry, W. D., and Page, D. L. The creation of "amyloid" fibrils from Bence Jones proteins in vitro. *Science* 171:712, 1971.

28. Glenner, G. G., Ein, D., and Terry, W. D. The immunoglobulin origin of amyloid. *Am. J. Med.* 52:141, 1972.

29. Glenner, G. G., Harada, M., and Isersky, C. The purification of amyloid fibril proteins. *Prep. Biochem.* 2:39, 1972.

30. Glenner, G. G., Terry, W. D., Harada, M., Isersky, C., and Page, D. L. Amyloid fibril proteins: Proof of homology with immunoglobulin light chains by sequence analysis. *Science* 171:1150, 1971.

31. Glenner, G. G., Terry, W. D., and Isersky, C. Amyloidosis: Its nature and pathogenesis. *Semin. Hematol.* 10:65, 1973.

32. Goel, K. M., and Shanks, R. A. Follow-up study of 100 cases of juvenile rheumatoid arthritis. *Ann. Rheum. Dis.* 33:25, 1974.

33. Harrison, C. V., Milne, M. D., and Steiner, R. E. Clinical aspects of renal vein thrombosis. *Q. J. Med.* 25:285, 1956.

34. Heller, H., Missmahl, H.-P., Sohar, E., and Gafni, J. Amyloidosis: Its differentation into perirecticulin and pericollagen types. *J. Pathol. Bacteriol.* 88:15, 1964.

35. Heptinstall, R. M. *Pathology of the Kidney.* Boston: Little, Brown, 1974. Pp. 737–753.

36. Isersky, C., Ein, D., Page, D. L., Harada, M., and Glenner, G. G. Immunochemical cross-reactions of human amyloid proteins with immunoglobulin light polypeptide chains. *J. Immunol.* 108:486, 1972.

37. Isobe, T., and Osserman, E. F. Patterns of amyloidosis and their association with plasma-cell dyscrasia, monoclonal immunoglobulins and Bence Jones proteins. *N. Engl. J. Med.* 290:473, 1974.

38. Jones, N. F., Hilton, P. J., Tighe, J. R., and Hobbs, J. R. Treatment of "primary" amyloidosis with melphalan. *Lancet* 1:616, 1972.

39. Kedar, I., Ravid, M., Sohar, E., and Gafni, J. Colchicine inhibition of casein-induced amyloidosis in mice. *Isr. J. Med. Sci.* 10:787, 1974.

40. Kyle, R. A., and Bayrd, E. D. Amyloidosis: Review of 236 cases. *Medicine (Baltimore)* 54:271, 1975.

41. Lachmann, P. J., Muller-Eberhard, H. J., Kunkel, H. G., and Paronetto, F. The localization of in vivo bound complement in tissue sections. *J. Exp. Med.* 115:63, 1962.

42. Latvalahti, J. The effect of ACTH and cortisone on experimental amyloid degeneration. *Acta Path. Microbiol. Scand.* [Suppl.] 93:81, 1952.

43. Laufer, A., Tal, C., and Kolander, N. Experimental amyloidosis and the effect of cortisone treatment. *Pathol. Microbiol.* 31:85, 1968.

44. Levin, M., Franklin, E. C., Frangione, B., and Pras, M. The amino acid sequence of a major non-immunoglobulin component of some amyloid fibrils. *J. Clin. Invest.* 51:2773, 1972.

45. Levin, M., Pras, M., and Franklin, E. C. Immunologic studies of the major non-immunoglobulin protein of amyloid. *J. Exp. Med.* 138:373, 1973.

46. Lindbjerg, I. F. Juvenile rheumatoid arthritis. A follow-up of 75 cases. *Arch. Dis. Child.* 39:576, 1964.

47. Linder, M., and Wolf, E. Incidence of amyloidosis in rheumatoid arthritis. *Scand. J. Rheumatol.* 1:109, 1972.

48. Lowenstein, J., and Gallo, G. Remission of the nephrotic syndrome in renal amyloidosis. *N. Engl. J. Med.* 282:128, 1970.

49. Malawista, S. E. Colchicine: A common mechanism for its anti-inflammatory and anti-mitotic effects. *Arthritis Rheum.* 11:191, 1968.

50. Maxwell, M. H., Adams, D. A., and Goldman, R.

Corticosteroid therapy of amyloid nephrotic syndrome. *Ann. Intern. Med.* 60:539, 1964.

51. Missen, G. A. K., and Taylor, J. D. Amyloidosis in rheumatoid arthritis. *J. Pathol. Bacteriol.* 71:179, 1956.

52. Missmahl, H.-P. Follow-up Studies for a 30 Year Period on Patients with Amyloidosis; Diagnostic Methods; Treatment. In E. Mandema, L. Ruinen, J. H. Scholten, and A. S. Cohen (eds.), *Amyloidosis.* Amsterdam: Excerpta Medica, 1968. Pp. 429–435.

53. Moschowitz, E. The clinical aspects of amyloidosis. *Ann. Intern. Med.* 10:73, 1936–1937.

54. Ozdemir, A. I., Wright, J. R., and Calkins, E. Influence of rheumatoid arthritis on amyloidosis of aging. *N. Engl. J. Med.* 285:534, 1971.

55. Pasternack, A. Fine-needle aspiration biopsy of spleen in diagnosis of generalized amyloidosis. *Br. Med. J.* 2:20, 1974.

56. Pirnar, T., and Coruh, M. Radiological findings in renal amyloidosis of children. *Pediatr. Radiol.* 1:172, 1973.

57. Polliack, A., Laufer, A., George, R., and Fields, M. The effect of cortisone on the formation and resorption of experimental amyloid. *Br. J. Exp. Pathol.* 54:6, 1973.

58. Renal transplantation in congenital and metabolic diseases. A report from the ACS/NIH renal transplant registry. *J.A.M.A.* 323:148, 1975.

59. Rosenthal, C. J., and Franklin, E. C. Variation with age and disease of an amyloid A protein—related serum component. *J. Clin. Invest.* 55:746, 1975.

60. Schaller, J., and Wedgwood, R. J. Juvenile rheumatoid arthritis. A review. *Pediatrics* 50:940, 1972.

61. Schlesinger, B. E., Forsyth, C. C., White, R. H. R., Smellie, J. M., and Stroud, C. E. Observations on the clinical course and treatment of 100 cases of Still's disease. *Arch. Dis. Child.* 36:65, 1960.

62. Shirahama, T., and Cohen, A. S. Blockage of amyloid induction by colchicine in an animal model. *J. Exp. Med.* 140:1102, 1974.

63. Smith, M. E., Ansell, B. M., and Bywaters, E. G. L.

Mortality and prognosis related to the amyloidosis of Still's disease. *Ann. Rheum. Dis.* 27:137, 1968.

64. Sohar, E., Gafni, J., Pras, M., and Heller, H. Familial Mediterranean fever. A survey of 470 cases and review of the literature. *Am. J. Med.* 43:227, 1967.

65. Strauss, R. G., Schubert, W. K., and McAdams, A. J. Amyloidosis in childhood. *J. Pediatr.* 74:272, 1969.

66. Teilum, G. Cortisone-ascorbic acid interaction and the pathogenesis of amyloidosis. Mechanism of action of cortisone on mesenchymal tissue. *Ann. Rheum. Dis.* 11:119, 1952.

67. Teilum, G., and Lindahl, A. Frequency and significance of amyloid changes in rheumatoid arthritis. *Acta Med. Scand.* 149:449, 1954.

68. Trainin, E., Greifer, I., and Spitzer, A. Amyloidosis in juvenile rheumatoid arthritis. *N.Y. State J. Med.,* in press.

69. Triger, D. R., and Joekes, A. M. Renal amyloidosis: A fourteen-year follow-up. *Q. J. Med.* 42:15, 1973.

70. Vazquez, J. J., and Dixon, F. J. Immunohistochemical analysis of amyloidosis by the fluorescence technique. *J. Exp. Med.* 104:727, 1956.

71. Verroust, P., Mery, J.-P., Morel-Maroger, L., Clauvel, J.-P., and Richet, G. Glomerular Lesions in Monoclonal Gammopathies and Mixed Essential Cryoglobulinemias IgG-IgM. In J. Hamburger, J. Crosnier, and M. H. Maxwell (eds.), *Advances in Nephrology.* Chicago: Year Book, 1971. Vol. 1, pp. 161–194.

72. Westermark, P., and Stenkvist, B. A new method for the diagnosis of systemic amyloidosis. *Ann. Intern. Med.* 132:522, 1973.

73. Zemer, D., Revach, M., Pras, M., Modan, B., Schor, S., Sohar, E., and Gafni, J. A controlled trial of colchicine in preventing attacks of familial Mediterranean fever. *N. Engl. J. Med.* 291:932, 1974.

74. Zurier, R. B., Hoffstein, S., and Weissmann, G. Mechanisms of lysosomal enzyme release from human leukocytes. I. Effect of cyclic nucleotides and colchicine. *J. Cell Biol.* 58:27, 1973.

64. Renal Disease in Juvenile Diabetes

Harvey C. Knowles, Jr.

Renal disease is the most serious hazard eventually faced by the young diabetic patient. Whereas the patient with the diagnosis of diabetes made at an older age is more prone to large-vessel disease, the young diabetic is at risk of small-vessel disease of the kidneys and eyes. It is the purpose of this chapter to describe the renal lesions observed in juvenile diabetes and to discuss their development, course, and prognosis. Recent reviews have covered the general problem of renal disease in diabetes in a more extensive fashion [2, 29].

Renal Lesions

The renal lesions usually seen in long-term diabetes are diabetic glomerulosclerosis (DGS) and arteriolar nephrosclerosis. Data on the frequency of pyelonephritis are not available, though there may be an increased incidence of chronic urinary tract infection in diabetics beyond that associated with long-term debilitating disease. Medullary necrosis is very uncommon in children, but does occur occasionally in the patient with long-standing juvenile diabetes. Finally, there is no evidence at present to support an unusual incidence of glomerulonephritis or other nephropathies in diabetes. For the purpose of this presentation, the term *diabetic renal disease* will include DGS, arteriolar nephrosclerosis, and chronic pyelonephritis.

The intercapillary nodular glomerular lesions described by Kimmelstiel are generally held to be specific for diabetes. In 1936, Kimmelstiel and Wilson [17] described nodular renal glomerular lesions in several patients with hypertension and nephrosis. The next step was the description of thickened glomerular basement membranes by Bell [4] in 1942. Finally, some 20 years later, Kimmelstiel [16] emphasized thickening of the mesangial stalk, a possible precursor of the thickened peripheral capillary walls. Thus, a diffuse increase in mesangial matrix and glomerular capillary basement membranes and intercapillary nodules of basement membrane materials constitute the major components of DGS. Nodules appear to develop late in the course of DGS and are preceded by the diffuse thickening of the glomerular stalks and capillary walls [10]. The lesions progress to obliterative hyalinization of glomeruli and subsequent nephron atrophy.

Bell [4] has emphasized that in contrast to nondiabetic arteriolosclerosis, which is usually associated with benign hypertension, efferent as well as afferent arterioles are involved in the kidney of a diabetic patient. The hyaline thickening of arterioles is characteristically attended by the mural deposition of lipid and plasma proteins, forming the so-called insudative lesion of diabetic arteriopathy [30]. Additional insudative deposits of fibrinlike material in glomerular capillaries form the "fibrin-cap" lesions and, in Bowman's capsule, the "hyaline-droplet" lesion, both frequently observed with advanced DGS. These four glomerular lesions, nodular and diffuse sclerosis, fibrin cap, and capsular droplet, are collectively referred to as renal diabetic microangiopathy, whereas the arteriole lesion is categorized as an arteriopathy. Of particular importance is the fact that it is only the nodular glomerulosclerosis that is pathognomonic of diabetes mellitus, whereas the other lesions including the arteriole may occur without diabetes. The nodular lesions follow the development of diffuse glomerulosclerosis, and therefore diffuse glomerulosclerosis is always present whenever there is typical nodular glomerulosclerosis. Finally, although the nodular lesion is the most characteristic, it is the diffuse sclerosis that is of the greatest clinical significance, since it correlates best with renal symptomatology.

Idiopathic membranous nephropathy has been reported to occur in the juvenile diabetic patient

[34]. This author has observed one instance of it in his juvenile diabetic population.

Urinary Tract Disorders

Urinary tract infections can pose serious problems in the juvenile diabetic patient, especially after long duration of the disease. Asymptomatic infection in the young patient, however, is unusual. In a group of 170 girls and boys at a summer camp, Etzwiler [9] found only 1 patient with significant infection. In contrast, this writer has observed recurrent urinary tract infection in about 10 percent of 175 juvenile diabetic patients over 16 years of age and followed for 10 years or more. Infection occurred predominantly in females. Although there is still debate as to the incidence of pyelonephritis in older juvenile diabetic patients, this writer has observed chronic pyelonephritis, according to the criteria of Kimmelstiel et al. [15], in about one quarter of such patients coming to autopsy. Using the same criteria, Halverstadt et al. [11] found chronic pyelonephritis on renal biopsy in about 10 percent of juvenile diabetic patients. Organisms found on urine culture are similar to those found in nondiabetic controls, with gram-negative organisms predominating.

Other urinary tract disorders seen in juvenile diabetes include neuropathy of the bladder and its consequences, medullary necrosis and fungal infections. Neuropathy of the bladder is rare before age 20. Its association with urinary stasis often results in infection and may predispose to pyelonephritis. Medullary necrosis also is unusual in young diabetic patients [1]. It may cause extreme toxicity; in contrast, necrotic tissue may break off and be seen by intravenous pyelogram to lie free in the renal pelvis in a patient without symptoms. Fungal infections are common in the diabetic patient, and symptoms of cystitis may accompany candidal vulvovaginitis. Fungal invasion of the kidney has been reported in a juvenile diabetic patient [33].

The Development of Diabetic Glomerulosclerosis

The mechanisms of development of DGS are not understood. Although the lesion may appear in older diabetic patients at any age, it is much more common in the juvenile patient. As with many other aspects of diabetes, the development of DGS may be related to a combination of genetic and acquired factors. The studies by Pyke and Tattersall [28] in identical twins with diabetes suggest a significant contribution from heredity in the development of microangiopathy, at least insofar as retinopathy is concerned. In their observations, retinopathy occurred particularly when there was a strong family history of diabetes, and malignant retinopathy tended to be concordant. This suggests that microangiopathy might be related to the degree of diabetic penetrance. Studies of a similar nature dealing with familial aggregation of DGS are needed to evaluate the influence of heredity.

It is not known what acquired factors may be responsible for the development of DGS. Many hold to the view that insulin insufficiency and poor control are important [23]. Bloodworth [5] reported nodular lesions in male dogs made diabetic with alloxan, and the studies by Spiro [32] of glomerular changes in alloxan-treated, diabetic rats indicate hyperactivity of glucosyltransferase in the presence of insulin insufficiency, leading to increased polysaccharide formation [32]. More recently, the findings of the ingenious experiments of Mauer et al. [24] with islet cell transplantation in rats support a role for pancreatic deficiency in the development of DGS. Also, there are sporadic case reports of DGS in patients with chronic pancreatitis and diabetes, a situation in which hereditary factors presumably are absent [19]. There also have been reports of DGS with hemochromatosis. These clinical observations and the animal studies support the view that insulin insufficiency is a major factor. However, studies intending to show a positive correlation between vascular disease and poor diabetic control have not met the criteria for adequately controlled clinical trials [13], and the applicability of the animal models to human diabetes remains to be determined.

The present means of treatment do not allow for acquisition of complete chemical control in the young insulin-dependent diabetic patient, and insulin deficiency could be at fault. In regard to grossly inadequate control, Engleson [8] has suggested that this may predispose to DGS. In a group of 40 diabetic juveniles less than 20 years of age at the time of diagnosis and with a duration of diabetes of 10 or more years, proteinuria and azotemia developed in 87 percent. The degree of control in these patients was considered unsatisfactory in that urinary glucose averaged 120 gm per day, and blood sugar concentrations fluctuated, with an average of 348 mg per deciliter.

Other approaches to elucidate the development of DGS have dealt with circulating lipids, decreased rates of fibrinolysis, and immunologic mediators, all without satisfactory results. The one factor that appears to be related clearly to the development of DGS is duration of the disease. In this regard, two points are of note: First, it is unusual for proteinuria to appear before 10 years of known duration of diabetes, and the risk seems to decrease after 30 years. Second, the development of DGS proceeds in a more orderly fashion when the duration of diabetes is measured from puberty [6, 21]; the presence of diabetes prior to this time does not seem to be influential. It may be that microangiopathy has its onset at puberty, the time at which it has been proposed that atherosclerosis starts.

Studies of the biochemistry of the glomerular basement membrane have permitted investigations of the abnormalities in diabetic nephropathy [26]. The morphologic observation of increased basement membrane material has been confirmed by chemical analysis. Glomerular basement membranes from diabetic kidneys show an increase in hydroxylysine and a reciprocal decrease in lysine content. An increase in the number of glucosylgalactose disaccharide units also has been observed. This has suggested to Spiro [32] that there is increased hydroxylation of lysine residues, with subsequent glycosylation of newly formed attachment sites, which might account for the altered character of the basement membrane. Smaller differences have been observed in glycine, hydroxyproline, tyrosine, and valine contents. The contents of other amino acid and sugar components have not differed from those in normal subjects.

The Prevalence of Diabetic Renal Disease

The reported prevalence of diabetic renal disease in populations of juvenile diabetic patients has varied considerably. In a review published in 1965, this author listed published prevalence figures, based on proteinuria, in groups in which the diagnosis of diabetes had been made before 20 years of age and with known duration of diabetes of 10 or more years [21]. The frequencies ranged from 4 to 100 percent. However, these figures referred only to survivors who came in for evaluation. Although published 20 years ago, the extensive long-term observations of White [35] are probably the most revealing. In 1956, she reported on 1,072 surviving juvenile diabetic patients. By the thirty-fifth to thirty-ninth years of disease, 63 percent had proteinuria and 70 percent had hypertension (Table 64-1). Recently, White and her colleagues presented data on the course of 73 juvenile diabetic patients with disease of 40 or more years' duration [27]; 42 percent of these patients had evidence of renal disease.

The prevalence of diabetic renal disease by histologic diagnosis in juvenile diabetes is not known, since most studies have included patients of all ages, and those with onset at a young age have not always been separated. If patients dying before age 50 are assumed, for the most part, to have long-

Table 64-1. Incidence of Proteinuria and Hypertension at Known Duration of Juvenile Diabetes

Duration (Years)	Albumin (%)	Hypertension (%)
0–9	2	1
15–19	18	15
25–29	39	44
35–39	63	70

Source: P. White, *Diabetes* 5:445, 1956.

standing diabetes, the observations of Bell [4] would indicate that DGS and arteriolar nephrosclerosis occurred in 21 and 43 percent of patients respectively coming to autopsy.

The Signs and Symptoms of Diabetic Glomerulosclerosis

The signs and symptoms of DGS vary from proteinuria, to the nephrotic syndrome, to a progressive course leading to renal failure and death. The features of nephrosis in diabetes differs somewhat from those of the idiopathic nephrotic syndrome; the degree of proteinuria is less, and the concentration of albumin in serum is higher. Hypertension is common and may appear shortly after proteinuria is first noted. Whether or not early hypertension accelerates the course of arteriolosclerosis remains to be determined.

Two aspects of laboratory evaluation warrant comment. First, Albustix may miss minimal degrees of proteinuria; radioimmunoassay, which can detect very low concentrations of protein, may some day be of value in earlier detection of DGS [14]. Second, a normal glomerular filtration rate does not necessarily indicate unimpaired renal function, since an increased rate may be found in juvenile diabetes [7], attributed to enlarged kidneys [12]. Thus, a normal level of glomerular filtration rate may represent a decrease from a previously much higher value.

The Natural History of Diabetic Renal Disease

The appearance of symptoms of DGS before puberty is extremely unlikely. Balodimos et al. [3] reported the case of a 9-year-old boy with diabetes of 8 years' duration who died in diabetic acidosis. At autopsy, thick glomerular membranes and mesangial thickening believed compatible with DGS were observed. The authors reviewed previous reports of glomerulosclerosis in childhood diabetes and advised caution in acceptance of the diagnosis on the basis of the casual appearance of thickening of the glomerular capillary wall seen

on light microscopy. The methods developed by Østerby-Hansen and Lundbaek [26] offer an approach to objective quantitative membrane measurement, which may detect abnormal glomeruli even before proteinuria appears [26]. The present author, in his own prospective studies of juvenile diabetic patients whose disease was diagnosed in childhood, has not seen proteinuria before the ninth year of known diabetes. On the other hand, lesions believed to be those of DGS have been reported in the presence of normal or only minimal glucose intolerance [25].

Attempts have been made to plot the course of diabetic renal disease over time. Wilson et al. [36] reported 13 fatal cases in which the patients' mean age at diagnosis of diabetes was 14.2 years. The average time at which proteinuria appeared was 13.9 years from onset, followed by edema in 3 years and death from renal disease 2 years later, in the nineteenth year of disease. These observations refer only to fatal cases, however, and were collected retrospectively. Deckert and Poulsen [6] observed a mortality of 80 percent after 10 years of proteinuria. In the experience of the present author, the cumulative rate of proteinuria at 15 and 25 years' duration of diabetes in patients followed prospectively was 12 and 38 percent respectively [20]. When proteinuria appeared, the cumulative azotemia and death rates were 57 and 48 percent at 5 years and 81 and 77 percent at 10 years (Table 64-2). Of 25 patients observed with azotemia, 23 died within 3 years, and 2 had survived over 3 years at the time the data were assembled. This author has observed that proteinuria can exist for 10 years or more without appearance of azotemia, and that proteinuria may remit, possibly to recur later. In essence, although proteinuria may exist for years, survival after establishment of azotemia is usually less than 2 years. Hypertension is present in almost all cases and usually appears before the serum urea nitrogen rises. Malignant hypertension is unusual, occurring only once in 45 cases of diabetic renal disease in this author's experience.

Table 64-2. Mortality in Juvenile Diabetic Patients with Proteinuria

Year of Proteinuria	Azotemia (%)	Death (%)
1	2	0
3	43	17
5	57	48
8	68	77
10	81	77
12	81	88

Treatment of Diabetic Renal Disease

Until recently, the management of diabetic renal disease has been mainly supportive, directed toward treatment of hypertension, the nephrotic syndrome, and renal insufficiency.

Treatment of sodium retention is similar to that used in other forms of renal disease. The use of potent diuretics, such as furosemide, permits dietary intake of sodium to be only moderately restricted, so that food does not become unpalatable. This is particularly important for the younger patient, in whom a balanced food intake is especially necessary.

Dietary manipulation for renal failure is complicated by the requirement that there be an even intake of food throughout the day to aid in good diabetic management [22]. Carbohydrate ingestion should be neither low nor excessive, in view of certain aspects of insulin and glucose metabolism peculiar to renal insufficiency. As renal failure progresses, insulin sensitivity develops, so that small doses of insulin suffice for diabetic control; hypoglycemia may develop suddenly. The mechanism of the marked insulin sensitivity is unknown, but it seems as if uremia causes a decrease in gluconeogenesis and thus increases sensitivity to small doses of insulin. The author often has seen patients whose insulin requirement decreased to a range of 6 to 10 units daily, with symptoms of insulin in excess if the range was exceeded. Insulin sensitivity may make diabetic control difficult to attain, particularly when renal failure causes anorexia and vomiting.

Two other complications compounding the treatment of diabetic renal disease have been neuropathy and infection. Atony of the bladder may lead to an irregular voiding pattern and incomplete bladder emptying, making it difficult to judge diabetic control, as well as predisposing to cystitis. Urinary tract infection may be extremely difficult to eradicate, and fungal infection already prevalent in the diabetic patient may be increased when renal disease develops. Management of bladder hypotonia is difficult. Manual pressure to enforce emptying and urocholine to increase contraction are recommended, but have little effect.

In patients with neuropathy, gastroparesis and diabetic diarrhea add to the problem of maintaining good nutrition. The antihypertensive drugs may accentuate orthostatic hypotension.

Until recently, diabetic renal disease often has been rapidly progressive, with death within 2 years of the appearance of azotemia. Although treatment that prevents or slows the progression of diabetic nephropathy is still not available, in the past few years, programs of long-term dialysis and transplantation for the diabetic patient have been mounted [18, 31]. Survival has been lengthened, and the discomforts of immunosuppressive therapy have been considerably less than those endured prior to transplantation. It is likely that more programs in diabetic renal transplantation will be instituted.

References

1. Abdulhayoglu, S., and Marble, A. Necrotizing renal papillitis (papillary necrosis) in diabetes mellitus. *Am. J. Med. Sci.* 248:623, 1964.
2. Balodimos, M. C. Diabetic Nephropathy. In A. Marble, P. White, R. F. Bradley, and L. P. Krall (eds.), *Joslin's Diabetes Mellitus* (11th ed.). Philadelphia: Lea & Febiger, 1971.
3. Balodimos, M. C., Legg, M. A., and Bradley, R. F. Diabetic glomerulosclerosis in children. *Diabetes* 20: 622, 1971.
4. Bell, E. T. Renal vascular disease in diabetes mellitus. *Diabetes* 2:376, 1953.
5. Bloodworth, J. M. B., Jr., and Engerman, R. L. Diabetic microangiopathy in the experimentally diabetic dog and its prevention by careful control with insulin (abstract). *Diabetes* 22:290, 1973.
6. Deckert, T., and Poulsen, J. E. Prognosis for juvenile diabetics with late diabetic manifestations. *Acta Med. Scand.* 183:351, 1968.
7. Ditzel, J., and Schwartz, M. Abnormally increased glomerular filtration rate in short-term insulin-treated diabetic subjects. *Diabetes* 16:264, 1967.
8. Engleson, G. *Studies in Diabetes Mellitus.* Lund: Berlingska Boktryckeriet, 1954.
9. Etzwiler, D. D. Incidence of urinary-tract infections among juvenile diabetes. *J.A.M.A.* 191:93, 1965.
10. Gellman, D. D., Pirani, C. L., Soothill, J. F., Muehrcke, R. C., and Kark, R. M. Diabetic nephropathy: A clinical and pathologic study based on renal biopsies. *Medicine (Baltimore)* 38–39:321, 1959–1960.
11. Halverstadt, D. B., Leadbetter, G. W., and Field, R. A. Pyelonephritis in the diabetic. *J.A.M.A.* 195: 827, 1966.
12. Kahn, C. B., Raman, P. G., and Zic, Z. Kidney size in diabetes mellitus. *Diabetes* 23:788, 1974.
13. Kaplan, M. H., and Feinstein, A. R. A critique of methods in reported studies of long-term vascular complications in patients with diabetes mellitus. *Diabetes* 22:160, 1973.
14. Keen, H., and Chlouverakis, C. Urinary albumin excretion and diabetes mellitus. *Lancet* 2:1155, 1964.
15. Kimmelstiel, P., Kim, O. J., Beres, J. A., and Wellmann, K. Chronic pyelonephritis. *Am. J. Med.* 30: 589, 1961.
16. Kimmelstiel, P., Osawa, G., and Beres, J. Glomerular basement membrane in diabetics. *Am. J. Clin. Pathol.* 45:21, 1966.
17. Kimmelstiel, P., and Wilson, C. Intercapillary lesions in the glomeruli of the kidney. *Am. J. Pathol.* 12:83, 1936.
18. Kjellstrand, C. M., Shideman, J. R., Simmons, R. L., Buselmeier, T. J., Von Hartitzsch, B., Goetz F. C., and Najarian, J. S. Renal transplantation in insulin dependent diabetic patients. *Kidney Int.* 6:515, 1974.
19. Knowles, H. C., Jr. Pancreatic diabetes and vascular disease. *Diabetes* 13:315, 1964.

20. Knowles, H. C., Jr. Long-term juvenile diabetes treated with unmeasured diet. *Trans. Assoc. Am. Physicians* 84:95, 1971.
21. Knowles, H. C., Jr., Guest, G. M., Lampe, J., Kessler, M., and Skillman, T. G. The course of juvenile diabetes treated with unmeasured diet. *Diabetes* 14:239, 1965.
22. Kurtzman, N. A., and Pillay, V. K. G. Renal reabsorption of glucose in health and disease. *Arch. Intern. Med.* 131:901, 1973.
23. Marble, A. Angiopathy in diabetes: An unsolved problem. *Diabetes* 16:825, 1967.
24. Mauer, S. M., Sutherland, D. E. R., Steffes, M. W., Leonard, R. J., and Najarian, J. S., Michael, A. F., and Brown, D. M. Pancreatic islet transplantation. Effects on the glomerular lesions of experimental diabetes in the rat. *Diabetes* 23:748, 1974.
25. Nash, D. A., Jr., Rogers, P. W., Langlinais, P. C., and Bunn, S. M., Jr. Diabetic glomerulosclerosis without glucose intolerance. *Am. J. Med.* 59:191, 1975.
26. Østerby-Hansen, R., and Lundbaek, K. The Basement Membrane Morphology in Diabetes Mellitus. In M. Ellenberg and H. Rifkin (eds.), *Diabetes Mellitus: Theory and Practice.* New York: McGraw-Hill, 1970.
27. Paz-Guevara, A. T., Hsu, T. H., and White, P. Juvenile diabetes mellitus after forty years. *Diabetes* 23:357, 1974.
28. Pyke, D. A., and Tattersall, R. B. Diabetic retinopathy in identical twins. *Diabetes* 22:613, 1973.
29. Rifkin, H., and Berkman, J. Diabetes and the Kidney. In M. Ellenberg and H. Rifkin (eds.), *Diabetes Mellitus: Theory and Practice.* New York: McGraw-Hill, 1970.
30. Salinas-Madrigal, L., Pirani, C. L., and Pollak, V. E. Glomerular and vascular "insudative" lesions of diabetic nephropathy: Electron microscopic observations. *Am. J. Pathol.* 59:369, 1970.
31. Shapiro, F. L., Leonard, A., and Comty, C. M. Mortality, morbidity and rehabilitation results in regularly dialyzed diabetics. *Kidney Int.* [Suppl. 1] 6:5–8, 1974.
32. Spiro, R. G. Biochemistry of the renal glomerular basement membrane and its alterations in diabetes mellitus. *N. Engl. J. Med.* 288:1337, 1973.
33. Tennant, F. S., Remmers, A. R., Jr., and Perry, J. E. Primary renal candidiasis. *Arch. Intern. Med.* 122:435, 1968.
34. Urizar, R. E., Schwartz, A., Top, F., Jr., and Vernier, R. L. The nephrotic syndrome in children with diabetes mellitus of recent onset. *N. Engl. J. Med.* 281:173, 1969.
35. White, P. Natural course and prognosis of juvenile diabetes. *Diabetes* 5:445, 1956.
36. Wilson, J. L., Root, H. F., and Marble, A. Diabetic nephropathy. A clinical syndrome. *N. Engl. J. Med.* 245:513, 1951.

65. Effects of Extrarenal Neoplasms on the Kidney

A. Vishnu Moorthy, Stephen W. Zimmerman, and Peter M. Burkholder

Some nonrenal malignant tumors are capable of altering renal function. Such pathophysiologic effects may result from direct invasion of the kidneys, their vasculature or collecting system; from ectopic production of hormones; or from an immunologic response of the patient to tumor antigen. In addition, extrarenal tumors may affect the kidney by causing disturbances in the metabolism of uric acid, calcium, potassium, sodium, and water. These secondary effects, generated by remote tumors, may create unpleasant and unnecessary morbidity in a patient already jeopardized by a tumor. Some effects of nonrenal tumors are of great intrinsic interest in that they may provide insight into the pathogenesis of certain renal diseases, such as the idiopathic nephrotic syndrome or immune complex disease; sometimes they are the first sign of an occult or recurrent neoplasm [56].

The possible disturbances in renal function and electrolyte metabolism that may occur in malignancy are listed in Table 65-1.

Direct Invasion of the Kidney, Renal Vasculature, and Ureters

The kidneys are a relatively uncommon site for metastatic tumors. Lymphomas and leukemias have a much higher incidence of invasion of the kidney than do carcinomas; rarely, renal involvement may be the only obvious site of a lymphoma [70, 104, 109]. However, metastases may occur from carcinoma of the other kidney, lung, uterus, breast, or other organs [1].

Richmond et al. [176] have reported lymphomatous infiltration of the kidneys in 33.5 percent of patients with lymphoma, 13 percent in Hodgkin's disease, 63 percent in lymphosarcoma with marrow involvement or 38.5 percent in lymphosarcoma without marrow involvement, and 46 per-

This study was supported by the National Kidney Foundation, the Kidney Foundation of Wisconsin, and Research Grant AM05582 from the National Institutes of Health, Bethesda, Maryland.

Table 65-1. Pathophysiologic Effects of Nonrenal Tumors on the Kidney

Direct invasion of the kidney, renal blood vessels, and ureters by the tumor

Disturbanecs in the metabolism of sodium, water, potassium, calcium, and uric acid

Membranous glomerulonephropathy

Minimal change nephrotic syndrome

Amyloidosis of the kidney

Myeloma kidney

Renal complications of cancer chemotherapeutic agents

Miscellaneous renal complications of malignancy

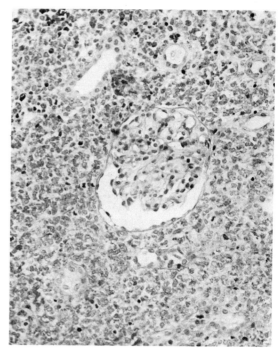

Figure 65-1. Diffuse lymphocytic infiltration of the renal cortex in a 12-year-old girl with acute lymphatic leukemia. (×150.)

cent in reticulum cell sarcoma. Infiltration of the kidneys can be unilateral, but bilateral involvement is more common [176]. Leukemic [105, 129a, 137, 152, 195a, 237] and lymphomatous infiltrates are most commonly in the form of multiple nodules, but diffuse infiltration (Fig. 65-1) and large or small single nodules also occur. Occasionally, infiltration will be detected only on microscopic examination [176]. Invasion of the kidneys from adjacent retroperitoneal tumors occurs but is not common [237].

Despite the frequency of leukemic and lymphomatous infiltration of the kidneys, renal involvement is usually not recognized antemortem. In one study, renal parenchymal infiltration was recognized antemortem in only 14 percent of 142 patients; it was responsible for death in only a few patients [176].

Azotemia, proteinuria, and an abnormal urinary sediment are uncommon manifestations of parenchymal infiltration, although renal failure can occur. Radiation therapy has been reported to be of benefit [2, 6, 100, 138, 198, 246]. Early diagnosis is rarely made, since the roentgenographic findings are nonspecific [18, 126]. Bilateral enlargement of the kidneys with regular renal outlines has been described in diffuse leukemia or lymphomatous involvement [3, 77, 125a, 154, 176, 198]. Single or multiple cortical lesions lead to localized bulges in the renal outline as well as calyceal and pelvic distortion [176, 198], and the radiographic findings may mimic those of polycystic kidneys.

Involvement of retroperitoneal lymph nodes is frequent in patients with lymphoma [96], and displacement and obstruction of a ureter may be the first clue to the diagnosis of the tumor [13, 23, 45, 104, 132, 202]. Occult neoplasm has been observed to cause the syndrome of retroperitonal fibrosis [121]. Ureteral compression by tumors can result in unilateral or bilateral obstruction and hydronephrosis, leading to urinary stasis and subsequent infection and pyelonephritis [132, 176]. Treatment with radiation or chemotherapy may relieve the ureteral block, and renal function may return even if obstruction had been present for several weeks [104, 202]. These measures should usually precede surgical intervention to relieve obstruction from radiosensitive or chemosensitive tumors. When undertaken in conjunction with radiation treatment of radiosensitive tumors, dialytic support for renal failure due to bilateral ureteral obstruction is a reasonable alternative to surgical urinary drainage.

Hypertension can result from the mechanical effects of a tumor as well as from the more common and better known hormonal mechanisms of tumors elaborating excessive amounts of aldosterone or catecholamines. Since the early report of Blatt and Page [20] describing constriction of a renal artery by a massive retroperitoneal lymphosarcoma, other cases of hypertension resulting from constriction of renal arteries by tumors have been reported [86, 87, 99, 114, 181, 188, 216, 238]. The majority of these tumors have been pheochromocytomas, but leiomyosarcoma, papillary carcinoma of the renal pelvis, ganglioneuromas, and lymph node metastases from carcinoma of lung and colon also have been reported [238]. Response of the blood pressure to surgical removal of the offending tumor usually has been gratifying. Elevated renin levels noted on occasion [238] and response to removal of the tumor or kidney suggest that the mechanisms involved in the pathogenesis of the hypertension are similar to those in renal artery stenosis resulting from atherosclerosis or fibromuscular hyperplasia [190].

A second but rare cause of hypertension related to a tumor is unilateral ureteral or pelvic obstruction and hydronephrosis [104]. The pathogenesis of hypertension seen in patients with unilateral hydronephrosis is not entirely clear, since there are reports of patients with both elevated [14] and normal [160] renal vein renin levels on the involved side. Vander and Miller [230] have reported elevation in renal vein renin activity as a consequence of acute ureteral obstruction in dogs. It seems likely that the renin-angiotensin system is involved in the pathogenesis of the increased blood pressure in this situation, but the stimulus for increased release of renin remains conjectural. If surgical correction of the obstruction is performed early, the blood pressure responds satisfactorily.

Renal vein thrombosis can result from direct invasion by a tumor [85]; when bilateral, it can result in a rapid decline of renal function. Lee et al. [117] have reported a 6 percent incidence of renal vein thrombosis in patients with a malignant tumor.

Disturbances in Sodium and Water Metabolism

Vomiting and diarrhea, with consequent loss of significant amounts of fluid from the gastrointestinal tract, may occur in patients with malignant tumors. Tumors of the stomach, pancreas, and colon can result in obstruction of the bowel and loss of gastrointestinal secretions. Massive diarrhea, which may occur in association with villous adenoma of the colon, pancreatic adenoma, and the Zollinger-Ellison syndrome, as well as the carcinoid syndrome, may result in significant depletion of sodium. In addition, a deficit of sodium may be observed in patients with vomiting and polyuria associated with the hypercalcemia of cancer or as a result of malabsorption in intestines involved with amyloidosis or infiltration by lymphomas.

Sodium retention, with consequent edema, hypertension, and hypokalemia, is known to occur in adrenocortical adenoma or carcinoma, adrenal hyperplasia secondary to pituitary tumors, and after prednisone therapy for cancer [53].

Interference with the ability of kidneys to concentrate urine in patients with malignant tumors may be due to a variety of mechanisms. Diabetes insipidus due to inadequate production of antidi-uretic hormone (ADH) can result from cranio-pharyngioma, chromophobe adenoma, and other primary tumors of the pituitary gland, as well as from metastatic tumors or leukemic infiltrates in the pituitary [217].

Nephrogenic diabetes insipidus also is observed in patients with malignant tumors [182] as a consequence of hypokalemia or hypercalcemia [35, 59, 131]. Nephrogenic diabetes insipidus observed in patients with amyloidosis or multiple myeloma may be a consequence of amyloid deposits around the medullary collecting ducts [34].

Defects in urinary concentration have been noted after relief of ureteral obstruction by a tumor. The mechanism of this "postobstructive diuresis" is not clearly defined.

Schwartz et al. [195] described the syndrome of inappropriate ADH secretion in 2 patients with bronchogenic carcinoma. This condition has been described mostly in oat cell carcinoma of the lung and also in other malignant tumors arising in the duodenum, pancreas, colon, ovary, and nasopharynx and in Hodgkin's disease [62, 119, 211]. ADH-like activity has been shown by bioassay and by radioimmunoassay of tumor extracts [38, 229]. Furthermore, hyponatremia with hyperosmolar urine has been reported in 11 patients with acute myeloid leukemia [141].

Disturbances in Potassium Metabolism

Depression of serum potassium below 3 mEq per liter can occur with a variety of neoplasms. The following are examples of the association between malignant disease and hypokalemia: villous adenoma and adenocarcinoma of the rectum with abundant liquid stools rich in potassium [186]; pancreatic adenoma with Zollinger-Ellison syndrome and gastric hypersecretion; primary hyperaldosteronism; Cushing's syndrome secondary to ectopic production of ACTH by tumor [11, 65a]; myelomonocytic leukemia with lysozymuria [147]; hypernephroma with renal potassium wasting [61]; the Fanconi syndrome in multiple myeloma [16]; and renal tubular acidosis of the distal type in Hodgkin's disease [67].

Hypokalemia in the presence of normal serum and urinary lysozyme concentrations has also been noted in patients with acute myeloid leukemia [140a, 156a]. Prolonged hypokalemia can impair the kidney's ability to concentrate urine and result in polyuria resistant to vasopressin [76, 130, 174] (see Chap. 82).

Disturbances in Calcium Metabolism

Hypercalcemia with subsequent renal injury in patients with malignant tumors can be due to a variety of mechanisms. The most common is direct involvement of bone by the malignant process, as seen in lymphoproliferative diseases, including leukemia [17, 101, 134], lymphomas [104, 146], and multiple myeloma, as well as in carcinomas. The majority of patients with leukemia have acute or subacute leukemia, which is of the lymphocytic variety in as many as 90 percent [110, 213]. Hypercalcemia has been noted in reticulum cell sarcoma [201], chronic lymphocytic leukemia [17], and chronic myeloid leukemia [17]. Tumors of the parathyroid gland, both adenoma and adenocarcinoma, can cause hypercalcemia by release of excessive parathormone. Nonparathyroid malignant tumors may also release parathormonelike substances, with resulting hypercalcemia [205], as noted in carcinoma of the lung, kidney, ovary, and colon [166, 193], in reticulum cell sarcoma [201], and in acute leukemia of different cell types, such as myeloblastic [249a], lymphatic [98b], and undifferentiated [151a] variety. In some instances, hypercalcemia may result from prostaglandins produced by tumors [224]. Brereton et al. [25] have shown the usefulness of indomethacin in lowering serum calcium in a patient with renal cell adenocarcinoma and hypercalcemia. It has been shown that supernatant fluid from cultures of lymphoid cells derived from patients with myeloma, Burkitt's lymphoma, and malignant lymphoma has bone-reabsorbing activity [149]. Treatment of hypercalcemia [74, 219] and its effects on the kidney are discussed in Chap. 74.

Acid-Base Disturbances in Malignancies

Metabolic acidosis, especially lactic acidosis in patients with malignant tumors, may be the consequence of poor tissue perfusion or rapid proliferation of tumor cells [63, 168, 233]. Field et al. [63] have described elevated lactate levels ranging between 12 to 42 mEq per liter in 11 cases of acute leukemia, in the absence of tissue hypoperfusion. Lactic acidosis has also been described in lymphosarcoma [217] and in Burkitt's lymphoma [21]. The elevation of blood lactate could be due either to overproduction of lactic acid by tumor cells [21] or to an increased number of cells producing lactic acid at a normal rate [233]. Rarely, lactic acidosis may be chronic [184, 233]. Besides supportive and alkali therapy, chemotherapy of the tumor results in improvement of the acidosis.

Metabolic acidosis with concomitant renal failure due to uric acid nephropathy or direct renal involvement can be seen in patients with malignant tumors. Renal tubular acidosis, of either the proximal or the distal tubular variety, has also been noted in the absence of renal failure. Proximal re-

nal tubular acidosis, often as a part of the Fanconi syndrome, with renal glycosuria, aminoaciduria, and phosphaturia, has been associated with multiple myeloma [55, 58, 203, 206], leukemia [142], certain carcinomas [57, 183, 239], and amyloidosis. Distal renal tubular acidosis has been observed in some patients with Hodgkin's disease and hyperglobulinemia [145]. Proximal tubular dysfunction in patients with myeloma is thought to be due to the injurious effect of myeloma protein on renal tubules and their transport mechanisms. Peculiar cytoplasmic inclusion bodies in proximal tubular cells have been noted by electron microscopy in such patients [43]. The pathogenesis of distal renal tubular dysfunction in this situation is unclear, but immunologic mechanisms may be involved [145]. Metabolic alkalosis occurring in the setting of malignant tumors is often secondary to vomiting and extracellular fluid volume depletion. Profound potassium depletion due to any cause can also lead to metabolic alkalosis.

Hyperuricemia and Uric Acid Nephropathy

Uric acid is the ultimate end product of purine catabolism in human beings, since they do not possess the enzyme uricase. In diseases involving increased turnover of cells, such as in various blood dyscrasias, the precipitation of both uric acid and monosodium urate, both of which are sparingly soluble, is of considerable pathogenic importance [12, 75, 102, 107, 129, 177, 194, 212]. Since Virchow's initial observation in 1851 that hyperuricemia and uricosuria can complicate the course of leukemia [222], renal insufficiency with associated hyperuricemia in patients with leukemia has been noted by several observers [73, 78, 111, 112, 137, 167]. In recent years, with the advent of more effective chemotherapy and x-ray therapy for malignant tumors, the incidence of hyperuricemia has increased. Hyperuricemia occasionally may be a problem even before the diagnosis of leukemia is established [5, 102, 232]. Hyperuricemia with hyperuricosuria has been noted in malignant lymphoma [172] and in disseminated neoplasms, associated more often with anaplastic tumors than with well-differentiated tumors [45a, 228]. Although the turnover of nucleic acids is greatly increased in all malignant tumors, uric acid nephropathy with subsequent renal failure usually is a problem only in patients with lymphoma and leukemia. (The effects of hyperuricemia on the kidney are discussed in Chap. 73).

Malignancy and Membranous Glomerulonephropathy

The association between solid tumors of various organs and membranous glomerulonephropathy

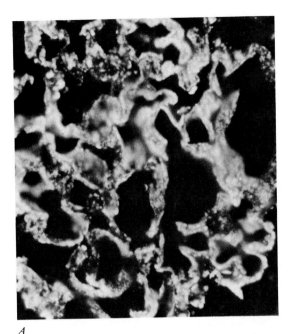

A

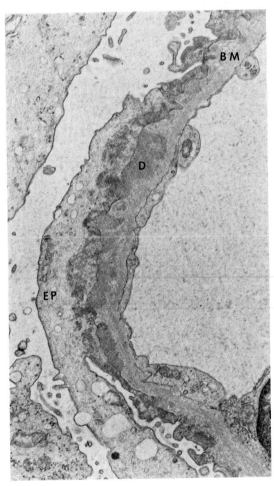

B

has been reported in a number of patients [55a, 66, 103, 117, 185]. This phenomenon is generally observed in older patients and is uncommon in children. However, a brief review is appropriate, since this association illustrates an important pathogenic relationship between malignant neoplasms and renal glomerular disease.

Recent advances in nephrology, such as examination of renal biopsy specimens by electron microscopy and immunofluorescence histochemistry, have led to inferences regarding the immunopathogenesis of so-called immune complex, autoimmune anti–glomerular basement membrane, and alternate C3 pathway activation glomerular diseases [30].

While the most common mechanism of immunologically mediated renal glomerular diseases involves deposition of immune complexes along the glomerular capillary walls, in most instances the antigen(s) responsible for initiation of this process has (have) not been identified. In membranous glomerulonephropathy, one variety of immune complex disease, a few exogenous antigens, such as drugs (gold [204], penicillamine [98]), or microbial agents (malarial parasite [88], hepatitis-associated antigen [39]) have been implicated. One consequence of neoplastic disease—and of carcinoma in particular—is development of antibodies against tumor antigens that have been demonstrated to be deposited in glomerular capillary walls and result in membranous glomerulonephropathy with or without the nephrotic syndrome [185].

About 80 percent of more than 40 patients reported to have carcinoma-associated glomerular disease had membranous glomerulonephropathy; the other patients had mixed membranous and proliferative lesions [9, 33, 42, 44, 47, 68, 71, 90, 92, 118, 123, 125, 178, 241, 250]. The subepithelial electron-dense deposits and granular pattern of glomerulus-localized immunoglobulin and complement observed in membranous glomerulonephropathy associated with malignant tumors are indistinguishable from any other form of membranous glomerulonephropathy (Fig. 65-2A, B).

Figure 65-2. A. Immunofluorescence micrograph showing diffuse granular deposition of IgG along glomerular capillary walls. (×450.) B. Subepithelial electron-dense deposits typical of membranous glomerulonephropathy. From a patient with colonic carcinoma and membranous glomerulonephropathy. (BM = basement membrane; D = deposit; EN = endothelial cell; EP = epithelial cell.) (×13,500.) (A and B from W. G. Couser et al., Am. J. Med. 57: 962, 1974.)

Carcinoma of the lung and colon have been the most common tumors implicated, with 16 and 5 cases respectively; other malignant tumors have included tumors of the stomach, thyroid, gallbladder, kidney, ovary, breast, carotid body, ovarian dermoid, melanoma, basal cell carcinoma of the skin, and squamous cell carcinoma of the cervix. Significant glomerular disease in early childhood (0 to 6 years of age) has been observed with embryonal neoplasm. Thirteen such cases have been associated with Wilms' tumors (nephroblastoma) and a single instance with gonadoblastoma [55a]. Immune complex mediated glomerulonephropathy was probable in one patient [12a], but the pathology in other patients is unknown. Glomerular deposits of immunoglobulins have been seen at autopsy in patients with cancer who had no clinical symptoms of renal involvement [220, 221]. This finding is not without precedent, since glomerular deposition of immunoglobulins without symptoms of renal disease has been observed in some patients with systemic lupus erythematosus [54]. Why nephritic syndrome develops in only a few patients with glomerular deposition of immune complexes is unclear. The determining factors may be the physical properties of the antigen-antibody complexes and the rate at which they are deposited.

Carcinoembryonic antigen has been identified in the glomerular deposits of a patient with carcinoma of the colon [42], and other tumor specific antigens have been found in glomeruli of patients with bronchogenic carcinoma, carcinoma of the colon [44], malignant myeloma [241], and renal cell carcinoma [159]. In addition, immunoglobulins eluted from glomeruli of a patient with bronchogenic carcinoma have been noted to react specifically with tumor antigen extracted from the primary carcinoma [118]. Carcinoembryonic antigen, however, was not present in the glomerular deposits of a patient with membranous glomerulonephropathy and polypoid adenocarcinoma of the colon [242]. In some instances, antibody may be directed against DNA released from large necrotic tumors [90]. Although an increased incidence of β-hemolytic streptococcal infection has been noted in patients with neoplastic disease [89], antecedent streptococcal infection has not been found in patients with concurrent malignancy and glomerular disease.

The association between membranous glomerulonephropathy and malignant tumors is very impressive. Because in more than 50 percent of the patients reported the renal lesion is evident before an associated tumor is discovered, Fichman and Bethune [60] and Hopper [92] have urged

that investigation for hidden malignancy be undertaken in adult patients with membranous glomerulonephropathy. Reports of rapid remission of heavy proteinuria after excision of the malignant tumor support the causal relationship between carcinoma and glomerular disease [41, 125, 175]. Revol et al. [175] described gynecomastia, hypertrophic pulmonary osteoarthropathy, and heavy proteinuria in a patient with bronchial carcinoma. Proteinuria disappeared completely within 2 weeks of resection of the carcinoma, returned 6 months postoperatively when metastases became apparent, and finally disappeared during treatment with cyclophosphamide. Proteinuria ceased 3 weeks after excision of a gastric adenocarcinoma in a patient whose case was reported by Cantrell [33], and neither the carcinoma nor the proteinuria had recurred 10 years later. Unfortunately, renal tissue was not examined in either of these 2 patients. In a case described by Couser and coworkers [44], resection of a carcinoma of the colon resulted in return of levels of carcinoembryonic antigen to normal and resolution of glomerular ultrastructural lesions.

There is considerable evidence from studies in animal models supporting a causal association between malignant tumors and glomerular injury [169]. Membranous glomerulonephropathy developed within 10 days in rats with a Walker 256 adenocarcinoma transplantation. Chronic antigenemia with antibody production in near equivalence has been noted in these animals. Glomerulonephritis has been reported also in mice and cats with leukemia [4, 161] and in dogs with several different types of neoplasms [151]. Immune complex glomerulonephritis, with granular deposits of immunoglobulin and complement along glomerular capillary walls, has been noted in a strain of mice that demonstrate a lupuslike syndrome with antinuclear antibodies, chronic murine leukemia virus (MuLV) infection, circulating MuLV–antiviral antibody complexes, and lymphoma [93].

Minimal Glomerular Change Disease with Nephrotic Syndrome (MCNS) in Patients with Malignant Tumors

The occurrence of the nephrotic syndrome in patients with Hodgkin's disease without amyloidosis or vena cava or renal vein occlusion has been appreciated since the 1940s [40, 180]. No statistical studies are available, however, that would establish a significant pathogenetic relationship rather than a fortuitous concurrence of Hodgkin's disease and nephrotic syndrome.

The cases of 45 patients with Hodgkin's disease and the nephrotic syndrome have been reported

[19, 37, 40, 45a, 65, 69, 82–84, 95, 97, 103a, 104, 106, 115, 120, 124, 135, 139, 144, 162, 164, 168, 180, 185, 199, 200, 208, 223, 249], and we have recently reviewed reports on 35 of these patients [144]. Renal biopsy specimens were examined by light microscopy in 13 of 15 of these patients and were interpreted as showing minimal change nephrotic syndrome (MCNS). One renal biopsy specimen, originally interpreted as membranous glomerulonephropathy, was later reexamined and diagnosed as MCNS [200]. Proliferative glomerulonephritis and minimal cellular proliferation with minimal basement membrane thickening were seen in the renal biopsies from 2 remaining patients.

In only 23 patients with Hodgkin's disease and nephrotic syndrome has a renal biopsy specimen been studied by light and immunofluorescence and/or electron microscopy. Of these patients, 17 had MCNS [37, 69, 83, 95, 115, 164, 200, 249]. Light-microscopic examination did not reveal any thickening of the capillary walls or increase in cellularity of glomeruli. Immunofluorescence microscopy revealed negative findings for immunoglobulins and complement, and electron microscopy revealed only extensive effacement of foot processes of glomerular capillary epithelial cells (Fig. 65-

3). Clinically, these patients had heavy proteinuria, generalized edema with hypoalbuminemia, and elevated serum cholesterol. The clinical and pathologic findings in these patients were very similar to those of patients with idiopathic minimal change disease. Glomerular filtration rate, as measured by creatinine clearance, was normal, and serum complement was not decreased [144]. In those patients whose urinary proteins were examined qualitatively, selective proteinuria similar to that observed in MCNS was noted [83, 143].

Membranous glomerulonephropathy with epimembranous electron-dense deposits was described in 2 patients [84, 185], one of whom had early (stage 1) membranous glomerulonephropathy [185]. No information was provided with regard to glomerular immunofluorescence in these patients. One patient had proliferative glomerulonephritis with crescents demonstrated in an initial renal biopsy [65]. In a later renal biopsy, membranous glomerulonephropathy was found, with granular IgG and C3 by immunofluorescence microscopy and epimembranous electron-dense deposits. This patient was said to have had a preceding group A streptococcal pharyngitis. Renal biopsy in another patient showed focal prolifera-

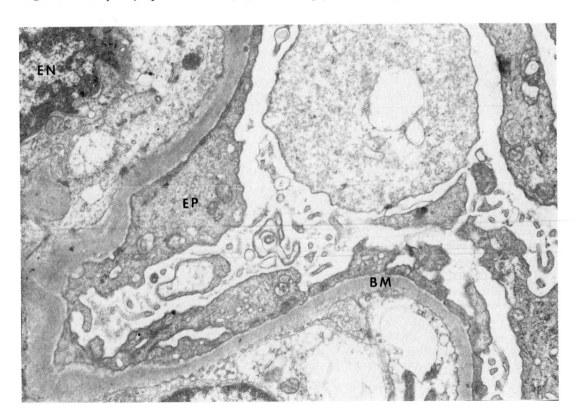

Figure 65-3. Minimal glomerular change disease in a 26-year-old woman with Hodgkin's disease and nephrotic syndrome. (BM = basement membrane; EN = endothelial cell; EP = epithelial cell.) (×11,200.)

tive glomerulonephritis with immunoglobulins G, M, and A and complement in the glomeruli and subendothelial electron-dense deposits [120]. Membranoproliferative glomerulonephritis with intramembranous and subendothelial electron-dense deposits was responsible for proteinuria in one patient with Hodgkin's disease [221a]. A patient with the nephrotic syndrome described by Yum and colleagues [249] had the Sjögren syndrome as well as Hodgkin's disease and nephrotic syndrome. Renal biopsy in this patient revealed an increase in mesangial cellularity, with immunoglobulins G and M and complement and subendothelial electron-dense deposits. Another patient's biopsy specimen had IgG and C3 in glomeruli, with only subendothelial electron-dense deposits [199]. Membranous glomerulonephropathy seems to be rare in patients with Hodgkin's disease who have the nephrotic syndrome, in contrast to those who have carcinoma and the nephrotic syndrome.

The course of nephrotic syndrome usually has paralleled the course of the disease in patients with Hodgkin's disease [144], although the stage of disease has varied from stage IA to stage IVB. Of 20 patients, 13 have had the mixed cellularity type of Hodgkin's disease [115, 144, 249]. Whereas the usual incidence of this type among patients with Hodgkin's disease is only 33 percent [153], it is curious that over 60 percent of patients with Hodgkin's disease and nephrotic syndrome have this type. It is not clear whether or not the immunologic status of these patients is different from patients with other types of Hodgkin's disease. Remissions of the nephrotic syndrome have followed surgical excision, irradiation of tumor tissue, or chemotherapy with prednisone or alkylating agents [144]. A spontaneous remission of the nephrotic syndrome was noted in 1 patient. Disappearance of proteinuria in response to therapy has been rapid [144, 200]. Recurrence of Hodgkin's disease seems often to be associated with relapse of the nephrotic syndrome, sometimes repeatedly [165]. Nephrotic syndrome initially resistant to prednisone in some patients has subsequently responded more satisfactorily to cyclophosphamide [95]. Minimal change nephrotic syndrome also has been reported in patients with mesenteric angiofollicular lymph node hyperplasia (lymphoid hamartoma) and chronic lymphatic leukemia [94, 103a]. Removal of the abdominal tumor or chemotherapy, resulted in remission of the nephrotic syndrome.

No satisfactory explanation has been made to account for the association between Hodgkin's disease and MCNS. The etiology of both these conditions is of course still unknown. Several observations suggest that MCNS may be a consequence of altered T lymphocyte function [59a, 197, 125b]. An abnormality in cell-mediated immunity is suggested by the following: the therapeutic response of patients with MCNS to prednisone, or cyclophosphamide, or both; remission of the nephrotic syndrome during measles virus infection, which suppresses cell-mediated immunity; increased susceptibility of these patients to pneumococcal peritonitis; high IgM levels in the serum with depressed IgG and IgA; and the inhibitory effect of plasma from patients on the blastogenic response of lymphocytes in vitro [95a, 143]. Although the immunology of Hodgkin's disease is complicated and as yet incompletely understood, it may be that the anergy observed in many Hodgkin's disease patients may actually be a consequence of hyperactivity of suppressor T lymphocytes [227]. The serum of patients with a variety of lymphoproliferative disorders, including Hodgkin's disease, has been shown to inhibit chemotactic activity [236]. The serum of 1 patient with Hodgkin's disease and MCNS had inhibitory activity against migration of guinea pig peritoneal macrophages [144]. Sherman et al. [200] have noted a diminished mitogenic response in lymphocytes incubated in the serum of these patients [200].

It is quite possible that some lymphoid tumors may produce substances toxic to, or capable of altering, metabolic properties of glomerular visceral epithelial cells. The ultimate barrier to protein in the glomerular capillaries resides not in the basement membrane itself but probably in the "zipper-like" slit diaphragm extending between the foot processes of the epithelial cells [179]. An alteration in effective maintenance by glomerular epithelial cells of this complex slit diaphragm and probably of the capillary basement membrane as well could represent the origin of proteinuria.

Although the glomerular lesion in patients with Hodgkin's disease and the nephrotic syndrome is most often similar to MCNS, with no or only minimal glomerular immunoglobulin deposition, immunofluorescence microscopy reveals significant glomerular deposition of immune complexes in the glomeruli of some patients. In 1 patient described by Hyman et al. [95] the initial diagnosis by renal biopsy was MCNS; progression to focal proliferative and sclerosing glomerulonephritis was observed on a repeat renal biopsy and in an autopsy specimen 2 years later. The findings of immunofluorescence and electron-microscopic studies were negative in the initial biopsy, but a later biopsy and autopsy material revealed immunoglobulin and complement components as well as subendothelial electron-dense deposits and viruslike particles in the glomeruli.

In patients with or without nephrotic syndrome and Burkitt's lymphoma [95], chronic lymphatic leukemia [26, 27, 32, 49, 80, 196], lymphosarcoma [69], or reticulum cell sarcoma [148], immune complex deposition has been evident in glomeruli on renal biopsy. Association of the Ebstein-Barr (EB) virus with Burkitt's lymphoma is reasonably well established [79], and the patient described by Hyman et al. [95] had a gradual elevation of serum antibody titer to EB virus. It was not possible to identify EB virus by immunohistochemical techniques in the kidney of that patient, but this may have been due to its absence or, alternatively, to unavailability of viral antigenic sites. The occurrence of glomerular lesions in patients with infectious mononucleosis, also caused by EB virus, has been noted [226]. The possible role of immune complexes involving virus particles or viral antigens in the pathogenesis of glomerulonephritis is increasingly appreciated. Eluates from kidney biopsy material from 20 patients with immune complex glomerulonephritis had demonstrable antibody reactivity with measles virus in 7 cases and with EB virus in 6 cases [247]. Mammalian type-C RNA virus–related antigen has been demonstrated in glomeruli of patients with the nephritis of systemic lupus erythematosus [136]. Vianna and Greenwald [231] have postulated that Hodgkin's disease may be due to a virus of low virulence. Such a virus might give rise to slow and persistent generation of immune complexes that become trapped in the glomerular basement membrane. However, an opportunistic virus infection, resulting from the partial immunoincompetence in some of these patients, may represent another possible explanation for glomerular injury in lymphomatous disease.

Renal Amyloidosis in Patients with Malignant Tumors

Systemic amyloidosis with renal involvement was noted in patients with lymphomas as early as 1856 [244]. The incidence of amyloidosis complicating malignant tumors is variable [10, 36, 113]. Of 52 patients with Hodgkin's disease studied by Steinberg [214], 11 percent were found to have amyloidosis, while autopsy series from the Mayo Clinic revealed positive amyloid cases in only 3 percent of patients with Hodgkin's disease [235, 245]. Lymphoma usually precedes the development of amyloidosis by several months to years; occasionally, both conditions have been diagnosed simultaneously. There is often amyloid involvement of other organs, such as the liver, spleen,

adrenal glands, intestinal mucosa, and skin. Development of amyloidosis as a complication of lymphoma is often masked by lack of distinguishing clinical features apart from proteinuria. Development of proteinuria and renal dysfunction in patients with lymphoma as a consequence of amyloidosis often is a poor prognostic sign; death usually occurs within a year.

Renal amyloidosis occurs in 6 to 15 percent of patients with multiple myeloma [10, 24, 31, 113, 156]. Other lymphomas and carcinomas are less frequently associated with renal amyloidosis [10, 24, 113]. The pathogenesis of amyloidosis is unclear at present. Amyloid fibrils in patients with multiple myeloma are composed in part of light chains, and such amyloid is referred to as "amyloid of immunoglobulin origin." Amyloid fibrils of patients with so-called secondary amyloidosis unrelated to myeloma appear not to involve immunoglobulin G peptide chains, and this condition is referred to as "amyloid of unknown origin" [15, 72]. Whereas casein-induced amyloidosis in mice is related to an associated T lymphocyte deficiency preventable by thymosin therapy, nitrogen mustard therapy of lymphoma has been suggested as one of the factors favoring the development of amyloidosis [210, 225].

Renal Involvement in Multiple Myeloma

Renal involvement with or without renal failure is a frequent and usually ominous manifestation of multiple myeloma [50, 52, 133, 189, 192, 234]. Multiple myeloma is rare in childhood [89a]; however, a discussion of the several ways in which the kidney may become involved in patients with multiple myeloma contributes to our understanding of the diverse mechanisms by which renal function is affected. Hyperuricemia, hypercalcemia, plasma hyperviscosity, amyloidosis, plasma cell infiltration, urinary tract obstruction, and pyelonephritis are some of the means by which renal functions are altered in patients with multiple myeloma [71a, 133, 189, 209]. However, mechanical obstruction due to precipitation of Bence Jones protein within the renal tubule has been postulated as the major cause of renal failure [29, 156]. Myeloma proteins may also exert a toxic effect directly on the renal tubules, resulting in the Fanconi syndrome, with renal tubular acidosis, glycosuria, phosphaturia, aminoaciduria, and vasopressin-resistant polyuria [43, 58, 171]. Renal failure usually develops insidiously and progresses slowly over a period of several months to years. In the majority of these patients, sudden deterioration of renal function has been attributed to dehydration, reactions to intravenous pyelography, or to both [28, 163, 234]. Radiographic contrast material has been shown to cause precipitation of Bence Jones proteins in vitro [116]. This, along with the common practice of restricting fluid intake prior to intravenous pyelography, may increase the risk of renal impairment in patients with multiple myeloma [52].

Occasionally, the nephrotic syndrome may be the presenting feature of patients with multiple myeloma. The renal lesion in these patients is most often amyloidosis.

Renal Complications of Cancer Therapy

A consequence of earlier diagnosis of malignancy is more extensive use of cancer chemotherapy, thus increasing the potential for adverse effects of these agents on renal function. Some of these effects are transient and of little concern, whereas others are of great clinical significance. Release of substances such as uric acid and potassium from tumor cells as a consequence of therapy may lead to severe hyperuricemia and hyperkalemia. Hyperkalemia, noted within 48 hours of the institution of chemotherapy in 5 of 22 patients with Burkitt's lymphoma, was fatal in 2 patients, suggesting that this acute complication is not an unusual or innocuous sequel of chemotherapy in this disease [7]. The response of Burkitt's lymphoma to chemotherapy is frequently gratifying, and long-term remissions may be achieved in a substantial percentage of cases, but renal function and serum electrolytes should be monitored closely during treatment [8]. Fatal hyperkalemia has developed in a patient with acute lymphatic leukemia within 12 hr of starting chemotherapy [59b].

While conventional doses of cyclophosphamide do not have a significant effect on renal function, larger doses (50 mg per kilogram) impair water excretion, leading to weight gain, hyponatremia, and unusually highly concentrated urine [51]. These effects could be a greater problem in patients who have a preexisting, tumor-related syndrome of inappropriate ADH secretion [150]. This syndrome may develop in a manner similar to hyponatremia induced by chlorpropamide [240]. Also a direct effect of a metabolite of cyclophosphamide on the distal renal tubule has been noted [51]. Hyponatremia has been reported to occur more frequently in association with therapeutic doses of vincristine [46, 64, 81, 207].

Hypocalcemia with hyperphosphatemia has been observed in patients with acute lymphatic leukemia [251], Burkitt's lymphoma [25b], and chronic leukemia [98a]. This occurs usually in the severely ill patient, after chemotherapy, and may

be present for variable periods of time ($\frac{1}{2}$ hour to 25 days) despite treatment. The phosphorus load comes primarily from the lymphoblasts, which have four times the amount of organic and inorganic phosphorus than mature lymphocytes, and the hypocalcemia may be secondary to the hyperphosphatemia. Other factors contributing to the development of hypocalcemia in these patients include administration of blood and platelets containing citrate, hypoproteinemia, monilial infection associated with hypoparathyroidism [98a], and drugs such as busulphan, and L-asparaginase. In rabbits L-asparaginase has been noted to have a direct toxic effect on the chief cells of the parathyroid glands [248].

Patients with leukemia and lymphoma with or without chemotherapy are generally prone to life-threatening infections requiring the use of potent antibiotics, including gentamicin, kanamycin, polymyxin B, and cephaloridine. The potential of these agents for causing renal toxicity and injury is well known.

Despite the frequent use of radiation therapy in the management of malignant tumors, the incidence of radiation nephritis is waning because of the increased awareness of the need to shield the kidneys [218]. If the kidneys are not well protected, acute or chronic radiation nephritis can result [22, 48, 127, 128, 187, 191] (Chap. 77).

Miscellaneous Renal Complications Due to Malignancy

There are several additional pathogenetic mechanisms by which impairment of renal function may occur in patients with malignant tumors. Patients with monocytic and myelomonocytic leukemia have been noted to excrete large quantities of lysozyme in the urine, associated with significant hypokalemia [158]. These patients show renal tubular dysfunction, with hyperkaliuria, glycosuria, and "tubular" proteinuria [147, 173]. Lysozyme is an enzyme of molecular weight 14,000 to 15,000 originating from granulocytes and macrophages. "Lysozyme nephropathy" could result from increased renal excretion of this enzyme and subsequent damage to proximal tubular epithelial cells [157]. Accumulation of cytoplasmic droplets and distortion of mitochondria and nuclei have been noted in the proximal tubular cells of patients with lysozymuria [243] and of animals such as the Wistar/Furth rats with Shay chloroleukemia and lysozymuria [108]. Whether or not hypergammaglobulinemia, also noted in these patients, contributes additionally to renal injury is unclear [173]. Significant proteinuria with azotemia was noted in 50 percent of patients with myelomonocytic leukemia and lysozymuria studied by Pruzanski and Platts [173].

In patients with pancreatic adenocarcinoma, thrombophlebitis migrans may be an important clinical problem. Rarely, this process may involve renal arterioles, veins, or both, resulting in renal cortical necrosis and renal failure [122]. Acute renal failure due to renal cortical necrosis secondary to disseminated intravascular coagulation has been noted in many patients with carcinoma [155, 215] and in patients with myeloma, particularly during chemotherapy [170]. Renal tubular obstruction by mucoproteins similar to that due to Bence Jones proteins in "myeloma kidney" has been reported in patients with pancreatic carcinoma [91, 140]. Protein obtained from the urine of this patient was immunologically identical to protein extracted from the tumor and to that found in his ascitic fluid and serum.

References

1. Abeshouse, B. S., and Goldstein, A. E. Metastatic malignant tumors of the kidney. A review of the literature and report of 23 cases. *Urol. Cutan. Rev.* 45:163, 1941.
2. Aledort, L. M., Hodges, M., and Brown, J. A. Irreversible renal failure due to malignant lymphoma. *Ann. Intern. Med.* 65:117, 1966.
3. Allen, D. H., Berg, O. C., and Rosenblatt, W. Lymphosarcoma of the kidney: A case report and description of roentgen findings. *Radiology* 55:731, 1950.
4. Anderson, L. J., and Jarret, W. F. Membranous glomerulonephritis associated with leukemia in cats. *Res. Vet. Sci.* 12:179, 1971.
5. Appleyard, W. J. Hyperuricemia and renal failure preceding the onset of acute lymphoblastic leukemia. *Proc. R. Soc. Med.* 64:728, 1971.
6. Armstrong, D., and Myers, W. P. L. Renal failure incident to reticulum cell sarcoma of the kidneys: Response to radiotherapy. *Ann. Intern. Med.* 65:109, 1966.
7. Arseneau, J. C., Bagley, C. L., Anderson, T., and Canellos, G. P. Hyperkalemia, a sequel to the chemotherapy of Burkitt's lymphoma. *Lancet* 1:10, 1973.
8. Arseneau, J. C., Canellos, G. P., DeVira, V. T., and Sherins, R. J. Recently recognized complications of cancer chemotherapy. *Ann. N.Y. Acad. Sci.* 230:481, 1974.
9. Asamer, H., Stühlinger, W., and Dittrich, P. Paraneoplastic nephrotic syndrome. *Dtsch. Med. Wochenschr.* 99:573, 1974.
10. Azzopardi, J. G., and Lehner, J. Systemic amyloidosis and malignant disease. *J. Clin. Pathol.* 19:539, 1966.
11. Bagshawe, K. D. Hypokalemia, carcinoma and Cushing's syndrome. *Lancet* 2:284, 1960.
12. Band, P. R., Silverberg, D. S., Ulan, R. A., Wensel, R. M., Banerjee, T. K., and Little, A. S. Xanthine nephropathy in a patient with lymphosarcoma treated with allopurinol. *N. Engl. J. Med.* 283:365, 1970.
12a. Barakat, A. Y., Papadopoulous, Z. L., Chandra, R. S., and Hollerman, C. E. Pseudohermaphroditism, nephron disorder and Wilms' tumor: A unifying concept. *Pediatrics* 54:366, 1974.
13. Bell, J. C., Heublein, G. W., and Hammer, H. J. The roentgen examination of the urinary tract: With special reference to methods of examination and findings in individuals with testicular tumors. *Am. J. Roentgenol.* 53:527, 1945.
14. Belman, A. B., Kropp, K. A., and Simon, N. M. Renal-pressin hypertension secondary to unilateral hydronephrosis. *N. Engl. J. Med.* 278:1133, 1968.
15. Benditt, E. P., and Erikson, N. Chemical classes of amyloid substance. *Am. J. Pathol.* 65:231, 1971.
16. Ben-Ishay, D., Dreyfuss, F., and Ullman, T. D. Fanconi syndrome with hypouricemia in an adult. *Am. J. Med.* 31:793, 1961.
17. Benvenisti, D. S., Sherwood, L. M., and Heinemann, H. O. Hypercalcemic crisis in acute leukemia. *Am. J. Med.* 46:976, 1969.
18. Besse, B. E., Lieberman, J. E., and Lusted, L. B. Kidney size in leukemia. *Am. J. Roentgenol.* 80:611, 1968.
19. Bichel, J., and Jensen, K. B. Nephrotic syndrome and Hodgkin's disease. *Lancet* 2:1425, 1971.
20. Blatt, E., and Page, I. H. Hypertension and constriction of renal arteries in man: Report of a case. *Ann. Intern. Med.* 12:1690, 1939.
21. Block, J. B., Bronson, W. R., and Bell, W. R. Metabolic abnormalities of lactic acid in Burkitt-type lymphoma with malignant effusions. *Ann. Intern. Med.* 65:101, 1966.
22. Bloomfield, D. K., Schneider, D. H., and Vertes, V. Renin and angiotensin: II: Studies in malignant hypertension after X-irradiation for seminoma. *Ann. Intern. Med.* 68:146, 1968.
23. Boyd, H. L. Lymphomatous involvement of the genitourinary tract. *N.Y. State J. Med.* 52:197, 1952.
24. Brandt, K., Cathcart, E. S., and Cohen, A. A clinical analysis of the course and prognosis of 42 patients with amyloidosis. *Am. J. Med.* 44:955, 1968.
24a. Brereton, H. D., Anderson, T., Johnson, R. A., and Schein, P. Hyperphosphatemia and hypocalcemia in Burkitt lymphoma. *Arch. Intern. Med.* 135:307, 1975.
25. Brereton, H. D., Halushka, P. V., Alexander, R. W., Mason, D. M., Kaiser, H. R., and DeVita, V. T., Jr. Indomethacin responsive hypercalcemia in a patient with renal-cell adenocarcinoma. *N. Engl. J. Med.* 291:83, 1974.
26. British Medical Journal. Clinicopathology conference. A case of chronic lymphatic leukemia. 1:546, 1970.
27. Brodovsky, H. S., Samuels, M. L., Migliore, P. J., and Howe, C. D. Chronic lymphatic leukemia, Hodgkins disease and the nephrotic syndrome. *Arch. Intern. Med.* 12:71, 1968.
28. Brown, M., and Battle, J. D. The effect of urography on renal function in patients with multiple myeloma. *Can. Med. Assoc. J.* 91:788, 1964.
29. Brownell, E. G. Multiple myeloma, review of 61 proved cases. *Arch. Intern. Med.* 95:699, 1955.
30. Burkholder, P. M. *Atlas of Human Glomerular*

Pathology. Hagerstown, Md.: Hoeber Med. Div., Harper & Row, 1974.

31. Calkins, E., and Cohen, A. S. Diagnosis of amyloidosis and malignant disease. *J. Clin. Pathol.* 19: 539, 1966.

32. Cameron, S., and Ogg, C. S. Nephrotic syndrome in chronic lymphatic leukemia. *Br. Med. J.* 4:164, 1974.

33. Cantrell, E. G. Nephrotic syndrome cured by removal of gastric Ca. *Br. Med. J.* 1:739, 1969.

34. Carone, F. A., and Epstein, F. H. Nephrogenic diabetes insipidus caused by amyloid disease. *Am. J. Med.* 28:539, 1960.

35. Carone, F. A., Epstein, F. H., Beck, D., and Leviten, H. The effects upon the kidney of transient hypercalcemia induced by parathyroid extract. *Am. J. Pathol.* 36:77, 1960.

36. Case records of the Massachusetts General Hospital. *N. Engl. J. Med.* 284:95, 1971.

37. Case records of the Massachusetts General Hospital. *N. Engl. J. Med.* 289:1241, 1973.

38. Claxton, C. P., Jr., McPherson, H. T., Sealy, W. C., and Young, W. G., Jr. Hyponatremia from inappropriate antidiuretic hormone elaboration in carcinoma of the lung. *J. Thorac. Cardiovasc. Surg.* 52: 331, 1966.

39. Combes, B., Stastny, P., Shorey, J., Eigenbrodt, E. H., Barera, A., Hull, A. R., and Carter, N. Glomerulonephritis with deposition of Australia antigen-antibody complexes in glomerular basement membrane. *Lancet* 2:234, 1971.

40. Cornic, H. J. Une forme nouvelle de la maladie de Hodgkin. La granulomatose maligne à type de néphrose lipoïdique. Thèse 547. Faculté de Médecine de Paris, 1939.

41. Cosby, R., Yamauchi, H., Lee, J. C., and Hopper, J. Tumor related renal lesions—reversal following tumor excision (abstract). *Clin. Res.* 12:136A, 1974.

42. Costanza, M. E., Pinn, V., Schwartz, R. S., and Nathanson, L. Carcinoembryonic antigen-antibody complexes in a patient with colonic carcinoma and nephrotic syndrome *N. Engl. J. Med.* 289:520, 1973.

43. Costanza, D. J., and Smoller, M. Multiple myeloma with the Fanconi syndrome. *Am. J. Med.* 34: 125, 1963.

44. Couser, W. G., Wagonfeld, J. B., Spargo, B. H., and Lewis, E. J. Glomerular deposition of tumor antigen in membranous nephropathy associated with colonic carcinoma. *Am. J. Med.* 57:962, 1974.

45. Cowen, R. L. Lymphodenomatous ureteral obstruction. Structure of the ureter from Hodgkins disease; report of first case. *Urol. Cutan. Rev.* 53:521, 1949.

45a. Crittenden, D. R., and Ackerman, G. L. Hyperuricemic acute renal failure in disseminated carcinoma. *Arch. Intern. Med.* 137:97, 1977.

45b. Crowley, J. P. Personal communication, 1977.

46. Cutting, H. O. Inappropriate secretion of antidiuretic hormone secondary to vincristine therapy. *Am. J. Med.* 51:269, 1971.

47. DaCosta, C. R., Dupont, E., Hamers, R., Hooghe, R., Dupuis, F., and Potvliege, R. Nephrotic syndrome in bronchogenic carcinoma: Report of 2 cases with immunochemical studies. *Clin. Nephrol.* 2:245, 1974.

48. Danforth, D. N., and Javadpour, N. Total unilateral renal destruction caused by irradiation for Hodgkins disease. *Urology* 5:790, 1975.

49. Dathan, J. R. E., Heyworth, M. F., and MacIver,

A. G. Nephrotic syndrome in chronic lymphatic leukemia. *Br. Med. J.* 4:655, 1974.

50. Dawson, A. A., and Ogstrom, D. Factors influencing the prognosis in myelamatosis. *Postgrad. Med. J.* 47:635, 1971.

51. DeFronzo, R. A., Colvin, O. M., Braihe, H., Robertson, G. L., and Davis, P. J. Cyclophosphamide and the kidney. *Cancer* 33:483, 1974.

52. DeFronzo, R. A., Humphrey, R. L., Wright, J. R., and Cooke, C. R. Acute renal failure in multiple myeloma. *Medicine (Baltimore)* 54:209, 1975.

53. De Wardener, H. E. Control of sodium reabsorption. *Br. Med. J.* 3:611, 1969.

54. Dillard, M. G., Tillman, R. L., and Sampson, C. C. Lupus nephritis: Correlations between clinical course and presence of electron dense deposits. *Lab. Invest.* 32:261, 1975.

55. Dragsted, P. J., and Hjorth, N. The association of Fanconi syndrome and malignant disease. *Dan. Med. Bull.* 3:177, 1956.

55a. Eagen, J. W., and Lewis, E. J. Glomerulopathies of neoplasia. *Kidney Int.* 11:297, 1977.

56. Editorial. Non-renal neoplasms and the kidney. *Lancet* 1:24, 1975.

57. Editorial. Renal tubular syndromes, immunological disorders and cancer. *Ann. Intern. Med.* 67:213, 1967.

58. Engle, R. L., and Wallis, L. A. Multiple myeloma and the adult Fanconi syndrome. *Am. J. Med.* 22:5, 1957.

59. Epstein, F. H. Calcium and the kidney. *Am. J. Med.* 45:700, 1968.

59a. Eyres, K. E., Mallick, N. P., and Taylor, G. Evidence for cell mediated immunity to renal antigens in minimal change nephrotic syndrome. *Lancet* 1: 1158, 1976.

59b. Fennelly, J. J., Smyth, H., and Muldowney, F. P. Extreme hyperkalemia due to rapid lysis of leukemic cells. *Lancet* 1:27, 1974.

60. Fichman, M., and Bethune, J. Effect of neoplasms on renal electrolyte function. *Ann. N.Y. Acad. Sci.* 230:448, 1974.

61. Fichman, M. P., Crane, M. G., and Bethune, J. E. Hypokalemia with normal blood pressure aldosterone and renin levels secondary to a renal or adrenal tumor. *Am. J. Med.* 48:509, 1970.

62. Fichman, M. P., and Telfer, N. Unusual hypotonic syndromes. *Clin. Res.* 19:195, 1971.

63. Field, M., Block, J. B., Levin, R., and Rall, D. P. Significance of blood lactate elevations among patients with acute leukemia and other neoplastic proliferative disorders. *Am. J. Med.* 40:528, 1966.

64. Fine, R. N., Clarke, R. R., and Shore, N. A. Hyponatremia and vincristine therapy—syndrome possibly resulting from inappropriate anti diuretic hormone secretion. *Am. J. Dis. Child.* 112:256, 1966.

65. Froom, D. W., Franklin, W. A., Hano, J. E., and Potter, E. V. Immune deposits in Hodgkin's disease with nephrotic syndrome. *Arch. Pathol.* 94: 547, 1972.

65a. Gabrilove, J. L., Nicolis, G. L., and Kirschner, P. A. Cushing's syndrome in association with carcinoid tumor. *Ann. Surg.* 169:240, 1969.

66. Gault, M. H., Kaplan, B. S., Chirito, E., Klassen, J., and Knaack, J. Glomerulopathy associated with neoplasia (abstract). *Am. Soc. Nephrol.* 1973, p. 39.

67. Geary, C. G., Platts, M. M., and Stewart, A. K.

Hypokalemia of unknown etiology complicating Hodgkins disease. *Br. Med. J.* 2:507, 1966.

68. Germuth, F. H., Jr., and Rodriguez, E. *Immunopathology of the Renal Glomerulus.* Boston: Little, Brown, 1973.

69. Ghosh (Banerji), L., and Muehrcke, R. The nephrotic syndrome: A prodrome to lymphoma. *Ann. Intern. Med.* 72:379, 1970.

70. Gibson, T. E. Lymphosarcoma of kidney. *J. Urol.* 60:838, 1948.

71. Glassock, R. J., and Bennet, C. M. The Glomerulopathies. In B. M. Brenner and F. C. Rector (eds.), *The Kidney.* Philadelphia: Saunders, 1976.

71a. Glassock, R. J., Friedler, R. M., and Massry, S. G. Kidney and Electrolyte Disturbances in Neoplastic Diseases. In S. G. Massry (ed.), *Contributions to Nephrology.* Basel: Karger, 1977. Vol. 7.

72. Glenner, G. G., Terry, W. D., and Isersky, C. Amyloidosis: Its nature and pathogenesis. *Semin. Haematol.* 10:65, 1973.

73. Gold, L. G., and Fritz, B. D. Hyperuricemia associated with the treatment of acute leukemia. *Ann. Intern. Med.* 47:428, 1957.

74. Goldstein, R. S. Treatment of hypercalcemia. *Med. Clin. North Am.* 56:951, 1972.

75. Gonic, H., Rubins, M. E., Gleason, I. O., and Sommers, S. C. The renal lesion in gout. *Ann. Intern. Med.* 62:667, 1965.

76. Gottschalk, C. W., Mylie, M. L., Jones, N. F., and Winters, R. W. Osmolality of renal fluid in potassium depleted rodents. *Clin. Sci.* 29:249, 1965.

77. Gowdy, J. F., and Neuhauser, E. B. D. The roentgen diagnosis of diffuse leukemic infiltration of the kidneys in children. *Am. J. Roentgenol.* 60:13, 1948.

78. Greenbaum, D., and Stone, H. Dangers of uric acid excretion during treatment of leukemia and lymphosarcoma. *Lancet* 1:73, 1959.

79. Guneven, P., Klein, G., Henle, G., Henle, W., and Clifford, P. Epstein-Barr virus in Burkitt's lymphoma and nasopharyngeal carcinoma. *Nature* 228:1053, 1970.

80. Gupta, R. K. Immunohistochemical study of glomerular lesions in retroperitoneal lymphomas. *Am. J. Pathol.* 71:427, 1973.

81. Haggard, M. E., Fernbach, D. J., Molcomb, T. M., Sutow, W. W., Viette, T. J., and Windmiller, J. Vincristine in acute leukemia of childhood. *Cancer* 22:438, 1968.

82. Hamburger, J., Richet, G., Crosnier, J., Funck-Brentano, J. L., Antoine, B., Ducrot, H., Mery, J. P., and de Montera, H. *Nephrology.* Philadelphia: Saunders, 1968. Vol. 1, p. 226.

83. Hansen, H. E., Skov, P. E., Askjaer, S. A., and Albertson, K. Hodgkin's disease associated with nephrotic syndrome without kidney lesion. *Acta Med. Scand.* 191:307, 1972.

84. Hardin, J. G., Jr., Coker, A. S., and Blanton, J. H. Medical grand rounds. *South. Med. J.* 62:1111, 1969.

85. Harrison, C. V., Milne, M. D., and Steener, R. E. Clinical aspects of renal vein thrombosis. *Q. J. Med.* 25:285, 1956.

86. Harrison, J. H., Gardner, F. H., and Dammin, G. J. A note on pheochromocytoma and renal hypertension. *J. Urol.* 79:173, 1958.

87. Heberer, G., Engelking, R., and Eigler, F. W. Diagnostische und therapeutische Besonderheiten bei einigen Hochdruckkranken mit Nierenarterienstenosen. *Dtsch. Med. Wochenschr.* 92:581, 1957.

88. Hendricks, R. G., Glasgow, E. F., Adeniyi, A., White, R. H. R., Edington, G. M., and Houba, V. Quartan malarial nephrotic syndrome. *Lancet* 1:1143, 1972.

89. Henkel, J. S., Armstrong, D., Blevins, A., and Moody, M. D. Group A—hemolytic streptococcus bacteremia in a cancer hospital. *J.A.M.A.* 211:983, 1970.

89a. Hewell, G. M., and Alexanian, R. Multiple myeloma in young persons. *Ann. Intern. Med.* 84:441, 1976.'

90. Higgins, M. R., Randall, R. E., and Still, W. J. S. Nephrotic syndrome with oat cell carcinoma. *Br. Med. J.* 3:450, 1974.

91. Hobbs, J. R., Evans, D. J., and Wrong, O. M. Renal tubular obstruction by mucoproteins from adenocarcinoma of pancreas. *Br. Med. J.* 2:87, 1974.

92. Hopper, J., Jr. Tumor related renal lesions. *Ann. Intern. Med.* 81:550, 1974.

93. Howie, J., and Helyer, B. Immunology and pathology of NZB mice. *Adv. Immunol.* 9:215, 1968.

94. Humphreys, S. R., Holley, K. E., Smith, L. H., and McIlrath, D. C. Mesenteric angiofollicular lymph node hyperplasia (lymphoid hamartoma) with nephrotic syndrome. *Mayo Clinic Proc.* 60:317, 1975.

95. Hyman, L. R., Burkholder, P. M., Joo, P. A., and Segar, W. E. Malignant lymphoma and nephrotic syndrome. *J. Pediatr.* 82:207, 1973.

95a. Iitaka, K., and West, C. D. Response of lymphocytes from patients with idiopathic nephrotic syndrome to phytomitogens (abstract). *Am. Soc. Nephrol.* 1976. P. 59A.

96. Jackson, H., Jr., and Parker, F., Jr. *Hodgkin's Disease and Allied Disorders.* New York: Oxford University Press, 1947.

97. Jackson, R. H., and Oo, M. Nephrotic syndrome with Hodgkin's disease. *Lancet* 2:821, 1971.

98. Jaffe, I. A., Treser, G., Suzuki, Y., and Ehrenreich, T. Nephropathy induced by D-penicillamine. *Ann. Intern. Med.* 69:549, 1968.

98a. Jaffe, N., Paed, D., Kim, B. S., and Vawter, G. F. Hypocalcemia—a complication of childhood leukemia. *Cancer* 29:392, 1972.

98b. Jayaraman, J., and David, R. Hypercalcemia as a presenting manifestation of leukemia: Evidence of excessive PTH secretion. *J. Pediatr.* 90:609, 1977.

99. Jennings, R. C., Shaikh, V. A. R., and Allen, W. M. C. Renal ischemia due to thrombosis of renal artery resulting from metastasis from primary carcinoma of the bronchus. *Br. Med. J.* 2:1053, 1964.

100. Jones, G. W., Odel, H. M., and Popp, W. C. Lymphoblastoma with signs of renal involvement improved by roentgen therapy. II. *Mayo Clin. Proc.* 24:264, 1949.

101. Jordan, G. W. Serum calcium and phosphorus abnormalities in leukemia. *Am. J. Med.* 41:381, 1966.

102. Kanwar, Y. S., and Manaligod, J. R. Leukemic urate nephropathy. *Arch. Pathol.* 99:467, 1975.

103. Kaplan, B. S., Klassen, J., and Gault, M. H. Glomerular injury in patients with neoplasia. *Annu. Rev. Med.* 27:117, 1976.

103a. Kerkhoven, P., Briner, J., and Blumberg, A. Nephrotisches syndrom als erstmanifestation maligner lymphome. *Schweiz. Med. Wochenschr.* 103:1706, 1973.

104. Kiely, J. M., Wagoner, R. D., and Holley, K. E. Renal complications of lymphoma. *Ann. Intern. Med.* 71:1159, 1969.

105. Kirshbaum, J. D., and Preuss, F. S. Leukemia: Clinical and pathologic study of 123 fatal cases in series of 14,400 necropsies. *Arch. Intern. Med.* 71: 777, 1943.

106. Kiy, Y. Sindrome nefrotica associada a doenca de Hodgkins. *Rev. Hosp. Clin. Fac. Med. Sao Paulo* 22:186, 1967.

107. Kjellstrand, C. M., Campbell, D. C., II, Von Hartitzsch, B., and Buselmeier, T. J. Hyperuricemic acute renal failure. *Arch. Intern. Med.* 133:349, 1974.

108. Klockars, M., Azar, M. A., Hermida, R., Isobe, T., Hsu, C. C. S., Ansari, H., and Osserman, E. F. The relationship of lysozyme to the nephropathy in chloroleukemic rats and the effects of lysozyme loading on normal rat kidneys. *Cancer Res.* 34:47, 1974.

109. Knoepp, L. F. Lymphosarcoma of kidney. *Surgery* 39:510, 1956.

110. Knisley, R. E. Hypercalcemia associated with leukemia. *Arch. Intern. Med.* 118:14, 1966.

111. Krahoff, I. H., and Murphy, M. L. Hyperuricemia in neoplastic disease in children: Prevention with allopurinol, a xanthine oxidase inhibitor. *Pediatrics* 41:52, 1968.

112. Kritzler, R. A. Anuria complicating the treatment of leukemia. *Am. J. Med.* 25:532, 1958.

113. Kyle, R. A., and Bayrd, E. D. Amyloidosis: Review of 236 cases. *Medicine (Baltimore)* 54:271, 1975.

114. Lampe, W. T. Renovascular hypertension. A review of reversible causes due to extrinsic pressure on the renal artery and report of three unusual cases. *Angiology* 16:677, 1965.

115. Larson, L. S., and Fritz, R. D. Nephrotic syndrome in association with Hodgkin's disease. *Wis. Med. J.* 75:S14, 1976.

116. Lasser, E. C., Lang, J. H., and Zawadzki, Z. A. Contrast media. Myeloma protein precipitates in urography. *J.A.M.A.* 198:273, 1966.

117. Lee, J. C., Yamauchi, H., and Hopper, J., Jr. The association of cancer and the nephrotic syndrome. *Ann. Intern. Med.* 64:41, 1966.

118. Lewis, M. G., Loughridge, L. W., and Phillips, T. M. Immunological studies in nephrotic syndrome associated with extrarenal malignant disease. *Lancet* 2:134, 1971.

119. Linton, A. L., and Hutton, I. Hyponatremia and bronchial carcinoma: Therapy with nitrogen mustard. *Br. Med. J.* 2:277, 1965.

120. Lokich, J. J., Galvenek, E. G., and Moloney, W. C. Nephrosis of Hodgkin's disease. *Arch. Intern. Med.* 132:597, 1973.

121. Longley, J. R., Bush, J., and Brunsting, C. D. Occult neoplasm causing syndrome of retroperitoneal fibrosis. *Calif. Med.* 103:279, 1965.

122. Lorge, R. E., and Richards, P. Carcinoma of the pancreas and acute renal failure. *Br. Med. J.* 1:24, 1976.

123. Loughridge, L. W., and Lewis, M. G. Nephrotic syndrome in malignant disease of non-renal origin. *Lancet* 1:256, 1971.

124. Lowry, W. S., Munzenrider, J. E., and Lynch, G. A. Nephrotic syndrome in Hodgkin's disease. *Lancet* 1:1127, 1971.

125. Lumeng, J., and Moran, J. F. Carotid body tumor associated with mild membranous glomerulonephritis. *Ann. Intern. Med.* 54:1266, 1966.

125a. Lundberg, W. B., Cadman, E. D., Finch, S. C., and Capizzi, R. L. Renal failure secondary to leukemic infiltration of the kidneys. *Am. J. Med.* 62:636, 1977.

126. Lusted, L. B., Besse, B. E., and Fritz, R. The intravenous urogram in acute leukemia. *Am. J. Roentgenol.* 80:608, 1958.

127. Luxton, R. W. Radiation nephritis: A long term study of 54 patients. *Lancet* 2:1221, 1961.

128. Luxton, R. W., and Kunkler, P. B. Radiation nephritis. *Acta Radiol [Ther.] (Stockh.)* 2:169, 1964.

129. Maher, J. F., Rath, C. E., and Schreiner, G. E. Hyperuricemia complicating leukemia. Treatment with allopurinol and dialysis. *Arch. Intern. Med.* 123:198, 1969.

129a. Mallick, N. P. The pathogenesis of minimal change nephropathy. *Clin. Nephrol.* 7:87, 1977.

130. Manitus, A., Levitin, H., Beck, D., and Epstein, F. H. On the mechanism of impairment of renal concentrating ability in potassium deficiency. *J. Clin. Invest.* 39:684, 1960.

131. Maromo, F., and Edelman, I. S. Effects of calcium and prostaglandin E on vasopressin activation of renal adenyl cyclase. *J. Clin. Invest.* 50:1613, 1971.

132. Martinez-Maldonado, M., and Ramirez De Arellano, G. A. Renal involvement in malignant lymphomas: A survey of 49 cases. *J. Urol.* 95:485, 1966.

133. Martinez-Maldonado, M., Yium, J., Suki, W. N., and Ekonyan, G. Renal complications of multiple myeloma pathophysiology and some aspects of clinical management. *J. Chronic Dis.* 24:221, 1971.

134. McKee, L. C., Jr. Hypercalcemia in leukemia. *South. Med. J.* 67:1976, 1974.

135. Mehta, S. R., Kumar, K. K., and Gupta, M. L. Hodgkin's disease with nephrotic syndrome and erythema multiforma. *J. Indian Med. Assoc.* 48:279, 1967.

136. Mellors, R. C., and Mellors, J. W. Mammalian type c RNA virus–related antigen in human systemic lupus erythematosus. *Fed. Proc. 60th Ann. Meeting Abstr.* 35:574, 1976.

137. Merrill, D., and Jackson, H., Jr. The renal complications of leukemia. *N. Engl. J. Med.* 228:271, 1943.

138. Meyer, L. M. Pathology of the genitourinary tract in leukemia. *Urol. Cutan. Rev.* 45:693, 1941.

139. Miller, D. G. The association of immune disease and malignant lymphoma. *Ann. Intern. Med.* 66: 507, 1967.

140. Min, K.-W., Cain, G. D., Györkey, P., and Györkey, F. Myeloma-like lesions of the kidney: Occurrence in a case of acinic cell adenocarcinoma of the pancreas. *Arch. Intern. Med.* 136:1299, 1976.

140a. Mir, M. A., Brabin, B., Tang, O. T., Leyland, M. J., and Delamore, I. W. Hypokalemia in acute myeloid leukemia. *Ann. Intern. Med.* 82:54, 1975.

141. Mir, M. A., and Delamore, I. W. Hyponatremia syndrome in acute myeloid leukemia. *Br. Med. J.* 1: 62, 1974.

142. Mir, M. A., and Delamore, I. W. Hypouricemia and proximal tubular dysfunction in acute myeloid leukemia. *Br. Med. J.* 3:775, 1974.

143. Moorthy, A. V., Zimmerman, S. W., and Burkholder, P. M. Inhibition of lymphocyte blastogenesis by plasma of patients with minimal change nephrotic syndrome. *Lancet* 1:1160, 1976.

144. Moorthy, A. V., Zimmerman, S. W., and Burkholder, P. M. Nephrotic syndrome in Hodgkin's disease: Evidence alternative to immune complex pathogenesis. *Am. J. Med.* 61:471, 1976.

145. Morris, R. C., Jr., and Fudenberg, H. H. Impaired

renal acidification in patients with hypergamma-globulinemia. *Medicine (Baltimore)* 46:57, 1967.

146. Moses, A. M., and Spencer, H. Hypercalcemia in patients with malignant lymphoma. *Ann. Intern. Med.* 59:531, 1963.

147. Muggia, F. M., Heinemann, H. O., Farhangi, M., and Osserman, E. F. Lysozymuria and renal tubular dysfunction in monocytic and myelomonocytic leukemia. *Am. J. Med.* 47:351, 1969.

148. Muggia, F. M., and Ultmann, J. E. Glomerulonephritis or nephrotic syndrome in malignant lymphoma, reticulum-cell type. *Lancet* 1:805, 1971.

149. Mundy, G. R., Luben, R. A., Raisz, L. G., Oppenheim, J. J., and Buell, D. N. Bone-resorbing activity in supernatants from lymphoid cell lines. *N. Engl. J. Med.* 290:857, 1974.

150. Munro, A. M. G., and Crompton, G. K. Inappropriate antidiuretic hormone secretion in oat-cell carcinoma of the bronchus. *Thorax* 27:640, 1972.

151. Murray, M., and Wright, N. G. Morphologic study of canine glomerulonephritis. *Lab. Invest.* 30:213, 1974.

151a. Neiman, R. S., and Li, H. C. Hypercalcemia in undifferentiated leukemia. *Cancer* 30:942, 1972.

152. Norris, H. J., and Weiner, J. The renal lesions in leukemia. *Am. J. Med. Sci.* 241:512, 1961.

153. O'Connor, G. T., Correa, P., Christine, B., Axtell, L., and Myers, M. International symposium on Hodgkin's disease. *NCI Monographs* No. 36L7, 1973.

154. Odel, H. M., and Popp, W. C. Lymphoblastoma with signs of renal involvement improved by roentgen therapy: Report of three cases. *Radiology* 31:687, 1938.

155. O'Meara, R. A., and Jackson, R. D. Cytological observations of carcinoma. *Irish J. Med. Sci.* 391:327, 1958.

156. Ooi, B. S., Pesce, A. J., Pollak, V. E., and Mandalenakis, N. Multiple myeloma with massive proteinuria and terminal renal failure. *Am. J. Med.* 52:538, 1972.

156a. O'Regan, S., Kaplan, B. S., Chesney, R. W., Ayoub, J. I. G., and Drummond, K. N. Hypokalemia: An indicator of poor immediate prognosis in childhood leukemia. *Am. J. Dis. Child.* 130:937, 1976.

157. Osserman, E. F. Lysozymia in Renal and Nonrenal Disease. In Y. Manuel, J. P. Revillard, and H. Betuel (eds.), *Proteins in Normal and Pathological Urine.* Basel: Karger, 1970.

158. Osserman, E. F., and Lawlor, D. P. Serum and urinary lysozyme (muramidase) in monocytic and monomyelocytic leukemia. *J. Exp. Med.* 124:921, 1966.

159. Ozawa, T., Pluss, R., Lacher, J., Boedecker, E., Guggenheim, S., Hammond, W., and McIntosh, R. Endogenous immune complex nephropathy associated with malignancy. I. Studies on the nature and immunopathogenic significance of glomerular bound antigen and antibody, isolation and characterization of tumor specific antigen and antibody and circulating immune complexes. *Q. J. Med.* 44:523, 1975.

160. Palmer, J. M., Zweiman, F. G., and Assaykeen, T. A. Renal hypertension due to hydronephrosis with normal plasma renin activity. *N. Engl. J. Med.* 283:1032, 1970.

161. Pascal, R. R., Koss, M. N., and Kassel, R. L. Glomerulonephritis associated with immune complex deposits and viral particles in spontaneous murine leukemia. An electron microscopic study with immunofluorescence. *Lab. Invest.* 29:159, 1973.

162. Paslawska-Udolf, E. Przypadek nerczycy lipoidowej w przebiegu ziarnicy zlosliwej u dziecka 2-letniego. *Pediatr. Pol.* 42:591, 1967.

163. Perillie, P. B., and Conn, H. O. Acute renal failure after intravenous pyelography in plasma cell myeloma. *J.A.M.A.* 167:2186, 1958.

164. Perlin, E., Powers, J. M., Dickson, L. G., and Moquin, R. B. The nephrotic syndrome in Hodgkin's disease. *Med. Ann. D.C.* 41:354, 1972.

165. Plager, J., and Stutzman, L. Acute nephrotic syndrome as a manifestation of active Hodgkin's disease: Report of 4 cases and review of the literature. *Am. J. Med.* 50:56, 1971.

166. Plimpton, C. H., and Gellhorn, A. Hypercalcemia in malignant disease without evidence of bone destruction. *Am. J. Med.* 21:750, 1956.

167. Pochedly, C. Hyperuricemia in leukemia and lymphoma: III. Clinical and pathophysiology. *N.Y. State J. Med.* 73:1085, 1973.

168. Pochedly, C., Miller, D. R., Sarrafi, G., Defuna, F. G., and Chua, E. B. Lactic acidosis in acute leukemia. *Mt. Sinai. Med. J.* 41:557, 1974.

169. Poskitt, P. K. F., Poskitt, T. R., and Wallace, J. H. Renal deposition of soluble immune complexes in mice bearing B-16 melanoma. *J. Exp. Med.* 140:410, 1974.

170. Preston, F. E., and Milford, W. A. Acute renal failure in myelomatosus from intravascular coagulation. *Br. Med. J.* 1:604, 1972.

171. Preuss, H. G., Weiss, F. R., Iammarino, R. M., Hammock, W. J., and Murdaugh, H. V. Effects on rat kidney slice function in vitro of proteins from the urines of patients with myelomatosus and nephrosis. *Clin. Sci. Mol. Med.* 46:283, 1974.

172. Primikirios, N., Stutzman, L., and Sandberg, A. A. Uric acid excretion in patients with malignant lymphomas. *Blood* 17:701, 1961.

173. Pruzanski, W., and Platts, M. E. Serum and urinary proteins, lysozyme (muramidase), and renal dysfunction in a mono- and myelomonocytic leukemia. *J. Clin. Invest.* 49:1694, 1970.

174. Relman, A. S., and Schwartz, W. B. The kidney in potassium depletion. *Am. J. Med.* 24:764, 1958.

175. Revol, L., Viala, J. J., Revillard, J. P., and Manuel, Y. Proteinurie associée à des manifestation paranéoplasiques au cours d'un cancer bronchique. *Lyon Med.* 212:907, 1964.

176. Richmond, J., Sherman, R. S., Diamond, H. D., and Craver, L. F. Renal lesions associated with malignant lymphomas. *Am. J. Med.* 32:184, 1962.

177. Rieselbach, R. E., Bentzel, C. J., Cotlove, E., Frei, E., III, and Freireich, E. J. Uric acid excretion and renal function in the acute hyperuricemia of leukemia: Pathogenesis and therapy of uric acid nephropathy. *Am. J. Med.* 37:872, 1964.

178. Rizutto, V. J., Mazzara, J. T., and Grace, W. J. Pheochromocytoma with nephrotic syndrome. *Am. J. Cardiol.* 16:432, 1965.

179. Rodewald, R., and Karnovsky, M. J. Porous substructure of the glomerular slit diaphragm in the rat and mouse. *J. Cell. Biol.* 60:423, 1974.

180. Rohmer, P., and Sacrez, R. Un cas de néphrose lipoidique au cours d'une maladie de Hodgkin. *Strasbourg Med.* 108:45, 1948.

181. Rosenheim, M. L., Ross, E. J., Wrong, O. M., Hodson, C. J., Davies, D. R., and Smith, J. F. Unilateral renal ischemia due to compression of renal artery by a pheochromocytoma. *Am. J. Med.* 34:735, 1963.

182. Rosenzweig, A. I., and Kendall, J. W. Diabetes insipidus as a complication of acute leukemia. *Arch. Intern. Med.* 117:397, 1966.

183. Ross, E. J. Hyponatremic syndromes associated with carcinoma of the bronchus. *Q. J. Med.* 32:297, 1963.

184. Rother, J. R., and Porte, D. Chronic lactic acidosis and acute leukemia. *Arch. Intern. Med.* 125:317, 1970.

185. Row, P. G., Cameron, J. S., Turner, D. R., Evans, D. J., White, R. H. R., Ogg, C. S., Chantler, C., and Brown, C. B. Membranous nephropathy: Long term follow up and association with neoplasia. *Q. J. Med.* 44:207, 1975 (new series).

186. Roy, A. D., and Ellis, H. Potassium secreting tumor of the large intestine. *Lancet* 1:759, 1959.

187. Rubenstone, A. I., and Fitch, L. B. Radiation nephritis: A clinicopathological study. *Am. J. Med.* 33:545, 1962.

188. Sato, T., Sakamato, S., Maebashi, M., Suzuki, C., Furuyama, T., Yoshinaya, K., and Sudo, K. Hypertension due to combination of pheochromocytoma and unilateral renal ischemia by tumor compression. *Jap. Heart J.* 8:202, 1967.

189. Scachez, L. M., and Domz, C. A. Renal patterns in myeloma. *Ann. Intern. Med.* 52:44, 1960.

190. Schaffer, A. J., and Marhowitz, M. Hypertension treated by nephrectomy. A report of 4 additional cases and a re-evaluation of prognoses and criteria for operation. *Am. J. Med. Sci.* 227:417, 1954.

191. Schreiner, B. F., and Greendyke, R. M. Radiation nephritis: Report of a fatal case. *Am. J. Med.* 26:146, 1959.

192. Schubert, G. E., Veigel, J., and Lennert, K. Structure and function of the kidney in multiple myeloma. *Virchows Arch. (Pathol. Anat.)* 355:135, 1972.

193. Schultz, A. L., Adatepe, M., Barron, J., and Barron, M. Hypercalcemia in malignancy without bony metastasis. *Minn. Med.* 47:360, 1964.

194. Schumacher, H. R., and Phelps, P. Sequential changes in Shuman polymorphonuclear leukocytes after urate crystal phagocytosis: An electron microscopic study. *Arthritis Rheum.* 14:513, 1971.

195. Schwartz, W. B., Bennett, W., Curelop, S., and Bartter, F. C. A syndrome of renal sodium loss and hyponatremia probably resulting from inappropriate secretion of ADH. *Am. J. Med.* 23:529, 1957.

195a. Schwarze, E. W. Pathoanatomical features of the kidney in myelomonocytic and chronic lymphatic leukemia. *Virchows Arch. [Pathol. Anat.]* 368:243, 1975.

196. Scott, R. B. Chronic lymphatic leukemia. *Lancet* 1:1162, 1957.

197. Shalhoub, R. J. Pathogenesis of lipoid nephrosis: A disorder of T-cell function. *Lancet* 2:556, 1974.

198. Shapiro, J. H., Ramsay, C. G., Jacobson, H. G., Botstein, C. C., and Allen, L. B. Renal involvement in lymphomas and leukemias in adults. *Am. J. Roentgenol. J.* 88:928, 1962.

199. Sharma, H. M., Hurtubise, P. E., and Stevenson, T. D. The nephrotic syndrome in Hodgkin's disease. *Lab. Invest.* 30:404, 1974.

200. Sherman, R. L., Susin, M., Weksler, M. E., and Becker, E. L. Lipoid nephrosis in Hodgkin's disease. *Am. J. Med.* 52:699, 1972.

201. Sherwood, L. M., O'Riordan, J. L. H., Aurbach, G. D., and Potts, J. T., Jr. Production of parathyroid hormone by non-parathyroid tumors. *J. Clin. Endocrinol. Metab.* 27:140, 1967.

202. Shivers, C. H. D., and Axilrod, H. D. Lymphoblastomatous nephropathy. *J. Urol.* 65:380, 1951.

203. Short, I. A., and Smith, V. P. Myelomatosis associated with glycosuria and amino aciduria. *Scott. Med. J.* 4:89, 1959.

204. Silverberg, D. S., Kidd, E. G., and Shmitka, T. K. Gold nephropathy: A clinical and pathologic study. *Arthritis Rheum.* 13:812, 1970.

205. Singer, F. R., Powell, D., Minkin, C., Bethune, J. E., Brickman, A., and Coburn, J. W. Hypercalcemia in reticulum cell sarcoma without hyperparathyroidism or skeletal metastasis. *Ann. Intern. Med.* 78:365, 1973.

206. Sirota, J. H., and Hamerman, D. Renal function studies in an adult subject with the Fanconi syndrome. *Am. J. Med.* 16:138, 1954.

207. Slater, L. M., Warner, R. A., and Serpick, A. A. Vincristine neurotoxicity with hyponatremia. *Cancer* 23:122, 1969.

208. Solsona-Conillera, J. Linfogranulomatosis maligna: Forma monoganglionar y nefrosica. *Med. Clin. (Barcelona)* 20:37, 1953.

209. Somer, T. The viscosity of blood, plasma and serum dys- and para-proteinemias. *Acta. Med. Scand.* 180 [Suppl. 456]:1, 1966.

210. Spain, D. M. Rapid and extensive development of amyloidosis in association with nitrogen mustard therapy: Report of a case. *Am. J. Clin. Pathol.* 26:52, 1956.

211. Spittle, M. F. Inappropriate antidiuretic hormone secretion in Hodgkin's disease. *Postgrad. Med. J.* 42:523, 1966.

212. Steele, T. H., and Rieselbach, R. E. The Renal Handling of Urate and Other Organic Anions. In B. M. Brenner and F. C. Rector, Jr. (eds.), *The Kidney.* Philadelphia: Saunders, 1976. Pp. 442–476.

213. Stein, R. C. Hypercalcemia in leukemia. *J. Pediatr.* 78:861, 1971.

214. Steinberg, C. Lymphogranulomatose und reticuloendotheliose Ergeben. *Allg. Pathol.* 30:1, 1936.

215. Straub, P. W., von Felton, A., and Frick, P. G. Recurrent intravascular coagulation with renal cortical necrosis and recovery. *Ann. Intern. Med.* 64:643, 1966.

216. Straube, K. R., and Hodges, C. V. Pheochromocytoma causing renal hypertension. *Am. J. Roentgenol.* 98:222, 1966.

217. Suki, W. N., and Eknoyan, G. Renal Involvement in Leukemia and Lymphoma. In *The Kidney in Systemic Disease.* New York: Wiley, 1976.

218. Suki, W. N., and Eknoyan, G. Radiation Nephritis. In B. M. Brenner and F. C. Rector, Jr. (eds.), *The Kidney.* Philadelphia: Saunders, 1976.

219. Suki, W. N., Yium, J. J., Von Minden, M., Saller-Hebert, C., Eknoyan, G., and Martinez-Maldonado, M. Acute treatment of hypercalcemia with furosemide. *N. Engl. J. Med.* 283:836, 1970.

220. Sutherland, J. C., Markham, R. V., and Mardiney, M. R. Subclinical immune complexes in the glomeruli of kidneys postmortem. *Am. J. Med.* 57:536, 1974.

221. Sutherland, J. C., Markham, R. V., Jr., Ramsey, H. E., and Mardiney, M. R., Jr. Subclinical immune complex nephritis in patients with Hodgkin's disease. *Cancer Res.* 34:1179, 1974.

221a. Szabo, J., Lustyik, G., Szabo, T., Erdei, I., and Szegedi, G. Glomerulonephritis of immune complex origin associated with Hodgkin's disease. *Acta Med. Acad. Sci. Hung.* 31:187, 1974.

222. Talbott, J. H., and Terplan, K. L. The kidney in gout. *Medicine (Baltimore)* 39:405, 1960.

223. Tapie, J., Laporte, J., and Richalens, J. Syndrome néphrotique au cours de la maladie de Hodgkin-Sternberg. *Presse Med.* 65:287, 1957.

224. Tashjian, A. H., Jr., Voelkel, E. F., Levine, L., and Goldhaber, P. Successful treatment of hypercalcemia by indomethacin in mice bearing a prostaglandin-producing fibrosarcoma. *Prostaglandins* 3:515, 1973.

225. Teilum, G. Studies on pathogenesis of amyloidosis. II. Effect of nitrogen mustard in inducing amyloidosis. *J. Lab. Clin. Med.* 43:367, 1960.

226. Tennant, F. S., Jr. The glomerulonephritis of infectious mononucleosis. *Tex. Rep. Biol. Med.* 26:603, 1968.

227. Twomey, J. J., Laughter, A. H., Farrow, S., and Douglass, C. C. Hodgkin's disease: An immuno-depleting and immunosuppressive disorder. *J. Clin. Invest.* 56:467, 1975.

228. Ultmann, J. E. Hyperuricemia in disseminated neoplastic diseases other than lymphomas and leukemias. *Cancer* 15:122, 1962.

229. Utiger, R. D. Inappropriate antidiuresis and carcinoma of the lung: Detection of argininine vasopressin in tumor extracts by immunoassay. *J. Clin. Endocrinol. Metab.* 26:970, 1966.

230. Vander, A. J., and Miller, R. Control of renin secretion in the anesthetized dog. *Am. J. Physiol.* 207:537, 1964.

231. Vianna, N. J., and Greenwald, P. Nature of Hodgkins disease agent. *Lancet* 1:733, 1971.

232. Vining, C. W., and Thomson, J. G. Gout and aleukemic leukemia in a boy aged five. *Arch. Dis. Child.* 9:277, 1934.

233. Wainer, R. A., Wiernik, P. M., and Thompson, W. L. Metabolic and therapeutic studies of a patient with acute leukemia and severe lactic acidosis of prolonged duration. *Am. J. Med.* 55:255, 1973.

234. Waldenstrom, J. *Diagnosis and Treatment of Multiple Myeloma.* New York: Grune & Stratton, 1970. Pp. 196–203.

235. Wallace, S. L., Feldman, D. J., Berlin, I., Harris, C., and Glass, I. Amyloidosis in Hodgkin's disease. *Am. J. Med.* 8:552, 1950.

236. Ward, P. A., and Barenberg, J. L. Defective regulation of inflammatory mediators in Hodgkin's disease; supernormal levels of chemotactic-factor inactivator. *N. Engl. J. Med.* 290:76, 1974.

237. Watson, E. M., Sauer, H. R., and Sadugor, M. G. Manifestations of the lymphoblastomas in the genitourinary tract. *J. Urol.* 61:626, 1949.

238. Weidmann, P., Siegenthaler, W., Ziegler, W. H.,

Sulser, H., Endres, P., and Werning, C. Hypertension associated with tumors adjacent to renal arteries. *Am. J. Med.* 47:528, 1969.

239. Weinstein, I. B., Irreverre, F., and Watkin, D. M. Lung carcinoma hypouricemia and aminoaciduria. *Am. J. Med.* 39:520, 1965.

240. Weissman, P. N., Shenkman, L., and Gregerman, R. I. Chlorpropamide hyponatremia: Drug induced inappropriate ADH activity. *N. Engl. J. Med.* 284:65, 1970.

241. Weksler, M. E. Nephrotic syndrome in malignant melanoma: Demonstration of melanoma antigen-antibody complexes in the kidney. *Am. Soc. Nephrol. Abstr.* 99, 1974.

242. Whitworth, J. A., Unger, A., and Cameron, J. S. Carcinoembryonic antigen in tumor-associated membranous nephropathy. *Lancet* 2:611, 1975.

243. Wiernik, P. M., and Serpick, A. A. Clinical significance of serum and urinary muramidase activity in leukemia and other hematologic malignancies. *Am. J. Med.* 46:330, 1969.

244. Wilks, S. Cases of lardaceous disease and some allied affections with remarks. *Guys Hospital Rep.* 2:103, 1856.

245. Winawer, S. J., and Feldman, S. M. Amyloid nephrosis in Hodgkin's disease: Presentation of a case and review of the literature. *Arch. Intern. Med.* 104:793, 1959.

246. Wolfsohn, A. W. Uremia due to renal lymphomatosis. *Ann. Intern. Med.* 53:197, 1960.

247. Woodroffe, A. J., and Wilson, C. B. Improved techniques in the identification of antigen and antibody in immune complex glomerulonephritis and the detection of anti–measles virus antibody in eluates from human immune complex glomerulonephritis. *Fed. Proc.* 35:574, 1976.

248. Young, D. M., Olson, H. M., Prieur, D. J., Cooney, D. A., Regan, R. L. Clinicopathological and ultrastructural studies of L-asparaginase induced hypocalcemia in rabbits. *Lab. Invest.* 29:374, 1973.

249. Yum, M. N., Edwards, J. L., and Kleit, S. Glomerular lesions in Hodgkin's disease. *Arch. Pathol.* 99:645, 1975.

249a. Zidar, B. L., Shadduck, R. K., Winkelstein, A., Zeigler, Z., and Hawker, C. D. Acute myeloblastic leukemia and hypercalcemia. A case of probable ectopic parathyroid hormone production. *N. Engl. J. Med.* 295:692, 1976.

250. Zunin, C., and Soave, F. Association of nephrotic syndrome and nephroblastoma in siblings. *Ann. Paediatr. (Basel)* 203:29, 1964.

251. Zusman, J., Brown, D. M., and Nesbit, M. E. Hyperphosphatemia, hyperphosphaturia in acute lymphoblastic leukemia. *N. Engl. J. Med.* 289:1335, 1973.

The occurrence of glomerulonephritis has been recognized in a variety of systemic infections caused by agents such as bacteria, viruses, fungi, rickettsiae, and protozoa (Table 66-1). Although the pathogenesis of this association is not entirely understood, recent studies suggest that the immune response of the host to infectious agents plays a major role, resulting in immune-mediated renal disease.

Bacterial Infections

A number of bacterial infections have been associated with the development of significant glomerulonephritis in human beings (Table 66-1). This review will include a discussion of glomerulonephritis associated with bacterial endocarditis, ventriculoatrial shunt infections, and syphilis.

BACTERIAL ENDOCARDITIS

Renal involvement in bacterial endocarditis was relatively frequent in the preantibiotic era, and it has been associated with various infectious agents such as *Streptococcus viridans* [4], *Staphylococcus aureus* [100], enterococci [63], pneumococci [6], *Hemophilus influenzae* [5], *Neisseria gonorrhoeae* [6], *Bacteroides* [20], and *Brucella suis* [25]. The presence of bacteria in renal lesions of some patients with bacterial endocarditis led Löhlein [65] and Baehr [4] to suggest that these lesions were the direct consequence of bacterial embolization of the kidney, leading to necrosis and infarction. However, most of the subsequent studies failed to demonstrate any organisms in renal lesions, raising questions of their role in the pathogenesis. Williams and Kunkel [110] were the first to propose that the injury was immune-mediated, as evidenced by the presence of circulating rheumatoid factor and hypocomplementemia. Studies utilizing immunofluorescence and electron microscopy revealed the presence of immune proteins and electron-dense deposits, similar to those found in other forms of immune complex glomerulonephritis, such as lupus nephropathy and poststreptococcal glomerulonephritis. Additionally, Levy and Hong [63] were able to elute antibody from the kidney of a patient with nephritis secondary to subacute bacterial endocarditis that reacted specifically with bacteria cultured from the patient's blood. All these findings strongly indicate that these renal lesions are due to immune complexes as a result of host immune response to bacterial antigens.

Hematuria and proteinuria are usually present when there is renal involvement in bacterial endocarditis. Renal function may be impaired, depending on the severity of the renal lesions. Morel-Maroger et al. [71], however, reported the cases of a few patients without overt renal abnormalities in whom renal lesions were found in biopsy material.

Light microscopy shows diffuse or focal proliferative glomerular changes with areas of necrosis [40]. Granular deposits of IgG, IgM, IgA, and C3 are found by immunofluorescence microscopy along glomerular basement membrane (GBM) and in the mesangium [40, 55, 63]. Electron microscopy reveals electron-dense deposits along GBM (subepithelial, intramembranous, or subendothelial) and occasionally in the mesangium [40].

In the majority of patients, specific antibiotic treatment of bacterial endocarditis results in prompt reversal of abnormal renal function and hypocomplementemia, even though an abnormal urinary sediment may persist for several months [40]. Repeat biopsy in these patients shows complete healing of the renal lesions [40].

SHUNT NEPHRITIS

Since the original description in 1965 by Black et al. [14] of the nephrotic syndrome associated with bacteremia following shunt operations for hydrocephalus, this association has been well documented by other investigators [15, 26, 54, 70, 80, 90, 92]. Several lines of evidence point to an immune complex origin of the shunt nephritis:

1. Demonstration of immunoproteins and electron-dense material in diseased glomeruli by immunofluorescence and electron microscopy [26, 92].
2. Decreased levels of complement in serum.
3. Presence of bacterial antigen and antibody in cryoglobulins [92].
4. Fixation of antibody against the infecting bacteria on the diseased glomeruli by immunofluorescence techniques [26, 54].
5. The presence of C1q precipitating material, presumably immune complexes, in the patient's serum [15].

Table 66-1. Infection and Nephritis

Clinical Condition	Renal Pathologic Findings	Infectious Agents	References
Bacterial and rickettsial			
Endocarditis	Proliferative glomerulonephritis	*Streptococcus viridans*	4, 65, 71, 102
		Staphylococcus aureus	40, 100
		Enterococci	63
		Pneumococci	6
		Hemophilus influenzae	5
		Gonococci	6, 102
		Bacteroides	20
		Brucella suis	25
		Coxiella burnetii	24
Infected ventriculo-atrial shunt	Membranoproliferative glomerulonephritis	*Staphylococcus albus*	14, 26, 54, 70, 80, 90, 92
		Corynebacterium bovis	15
		Staphylococcus aureus	90
		Listeria monocytogenes	92
Syphilis, congenital and secondary	Proliferative glomerulonephritis	*Treponema pallidum*	13, 17, 31, 32, 42, 46, 52, 53, 74, 78, 81, 83, 89, 93, 94, 97, 99, 109, 115, 116
Typhoid fever	Mesangioproliferative glomerulonephritis Interstitial nephritis	*Salmonella typhi*	29, 85
Leprosy	Proliferative glomerulonephritis	*Mycobacterium leprae*	51
Tuberculosis	Proliferative glomerulonephritis	*Mycobacterium tuberculosis*	11
Osteomyelitis	Membranoproliferative glomerulonephritis	*Staphylococcus aureus*	16
Abdominal abscess	Membranoproliferative glomerulonephritis Focal proliferative glomerulonephritis Extracapillary glomerulonephritis	*Staphylococcus aureus* *Moraxella alcaligenes* *Pseudomonas aeruginosa* *Escherichia coli* Proteus mirabilis	8
Pneumonia	Membranoproliferative glomerulonephritis	Pneumococci	50
Otitis media with sepsis	Proliferative glomerulonephritis	*Staphylococcus aureus* Pneumococci	67
Viral			
Serum Hepatitis	Proliferative glomerulonephritis Membranous nephropathy Membranoproliferative glomerulonephritis Focal glomerulosclerosis	Hepatitis B virus	19, 22, 27, 28, 60, 61, 72, 91
Infectious mono-nucleosis	Interstitial nephritis	Epstein-Barr virus	2, 18, 23, 38, 64, 76, 95, 96, 98, 101, 113, 117
Goodpasture's syndrome	Proliferative glomerulonephritis	Influenza A2 virus	111
Pharyngitis	Proliferative glomerulonephritis	Echovirus type 9	114
Pneumonia	Not done	Coxsackievirus B4	7
Varicella	Proliferative glomerulonephritis	Varicella virus	62, 68
Guillain-Barré-Strohl syndrome	Membranous nephropathy Proliferative glomerulonephritis	Unknown	9, 82
Smallpox vaccination	Proliferative glomerulonephritis	Vaccinia virus	45
Parasitic and fungal			
Malaria			
Quartan malaria	Quartan nephropathy	*Plasmodium malariae*	1, 3, 34, 43, 44, 56–59, 79, 87, 106, 107, 112
Falciparum malaria	Proliferative glomerulonephritis	*Plasmodium falciparum*	10, 12, 41
Toxoplasmosis	Proliferative glomerulonephritis Interstitial nephritis	*Toxoplasma gondii*	35, 39, 66, 84, 108
Schistosomiasis	Membranoproliferative glomerulonephritis	*Schistosoma mansoni*	30
Filarial loiasis	Membranous nephropathy	*Loa loa*	77
Chronic mucocutaneous candidiasis	Membranoproliferative glomerulonephritis	*Candida albicans*	21

Renal involvement is manifested by hematuria (gross or microscopic), proteinuria, azotemia, and edema [14, 80, 90]. The nephrotic syndrome is a frequent manifestation of shunt nephritis, but it never occurs in nephritis associated with bacterial endocarditis. Rheumatoid factor and cryoglobulin are frequently present in the serum [26, 92]. The serum complement profiles show depressed levels of C1q, C4, C2, C3, C5, C6, and C7 [26, 92] (Fig. 66-1). Serum concentrations of factor B and properdin are only occasionally depressed, indicating predominantly classical pathway activation [26, 92]. Renal pathologic changes are very similar to the findings in idiopathic chronic membranoproliferative glomerulonephritis [26, 92]. There is diffuse involvement of glomeruli, with lobulation, increase in mesangial matrix and cellularity, focal GBM thickening with splitting, and occasional infiltration of polymorphonuclear leukocytes.

Immunofluorescence microscopy demonstrates extensive granular deposition of IgG, IgM, C1q, C3, and C4 in the mesangium and along the GBM, especially of the peripheral capillary loops. Properdin and fibrin may be found in the same location, but in a lesser intensity (Fig. 66-2). Electron microscopy reveals an increase in mesangial matrix and cellularity, with interposition of mesangial cell cytoplasmic processes. True GBM is not thickened. In addition, electron-dense deposits are found in the subendothelial and mesangial areas.

Although antibiotics alone have been successful in the treatment of some patients [15], most patients ultimately require removal of the shunt [14, 26, 80, 90]. Once the bacteriologic cure is achieved, there is usually rapid improvement in renal manifestations, although some patients may have persistent, low-grade proteinuria [26, 90].

SYPHILITIC NEPHROPATHY

Renal involvement in congenital and acquired syphilis has been well documented by many investigators [13, 17, 31, 32, 42, 46, 52, 53, 74, 78, 81, 83, 89, 93, 94, 97, 99, 109, 115, 116]. Thomas and Schur [97] reported the incidence of nephropathy to be 0.3 percent in patients with secondary syphilis. Sartain [83] found an 8 percent incidence in infants with congenital syphilis. The most common renal manifestation in both forms of syphilis is the nephrotic syndrome, with proteinuria, hypoalbuminemia, edema, and hypercholesterolemia. Hematuria, azotemia, and hypertension, although uncommon in the secondary type, are frequently

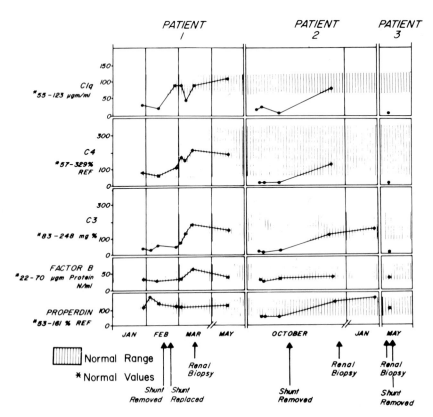

Figure 66-1. Complement levels in 3 patients with shunt nephritis. Note the increase in levels following removal of the shunt in patients 1 and 2. (From R. S. Dobrin et al., Am. J. Med. 59:660, 1975.)

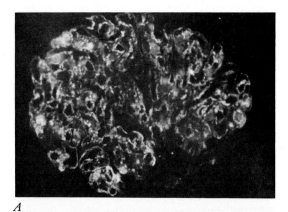

A

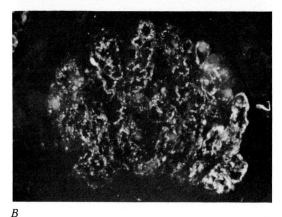

B

Figure 66-2. Immunofluorescence studies on kidney of patient with shunt nephritis demonstrating deposition of C3 (A) and properdin (B).

present in the congenital disease. The levels of serum complement components are usually depressed in congenital syphilitic nephropathy [53, 109, 115]. A recent study of 2 infants with congenital syphilitic nephropathy by Zelazko and Feldman [116] showed depressed serum levels of C1q, C4, C3, and C5, indicating activation of the classical pathway. This differs from patients with secondary syphilitic nephropathy, in whom serum complement is usually normal [13, 17, 32, 89].

The pathologic picture of both congenital and acquired syphilitic nephropathy are very similar. On light microscopy, glomeruli are hypercellular, mainly due to endothelial cell proliferation, as described in secondary syphilis, or visceral epithelial cell proliferation, seen in congenital syphilis; mesangial cell proliferation with an increase in mesangial matrix is also observed. The GBM is thickened, frequently in a segmental distribution. The interstitium shows focal areas of edema, with cellular infiltration, consisting of polymorphonu-

clear leucocytes, plasma cells, and mononuclear cells; the blood vessels are normal [13, 17, 31, 32, 52, 53, 74, 94, 99]. Occasionally, renal tissue may appear to be normal [89]. Immunofluorescence microscopy demonstrates granular deposition of IgG and C3 along the GBM and, to a lesser extent, in the mesangium; IgM also may be detected in the mesangium, whereas IgA usually is not observed [13, 17, 32, 46, 52, 53, 74, 89, 99, 109, 115]. Electron microscopy shows irregular thickening of the GBM, with electron-dense deposits. These deposits are localized in subepithelial areas, less frequently in intramembranous, subendothelial, or mesangial areas. Extensive fusion of epithelial cell foot processes and an increase in mesangial matrix and cellularity may be seen [13, 17, 31, 32, 46, 53, 74, 99, 109, 115].

The presence of immunoproteins and electron-dense deposits in glomeruli suggests an immune complex renal injury. Treponemal antigenic material has been detected in glomeruli of patients with both congenital and secondary syphilitic nephropathy, confirming the role of immune complexes in the pathogenesis of this renal lesion [74, 99]. Antisyphilitic treatment results in prompt alleviation of renal manifestations within 2 to 4 weeks [13, 17, 109, 115]. Although syphilitic nephropathy may remit spontaneously, some patients may require 4 to 18 months to achieve full recovery [32, 42, 46, 89].

Parasitic Diseases: Malarial Nephropathy

Although glomerulonephritis has been demonstrated in several parasitic diseases, this discussion will be limited to malarial nephropathy.

The association between malarial infection and renal disease has long been recognized. Although a causal relationship between them has not been definitely proved, several lines of indirect evidence point to a role for malarial infection as an etiologic agent;

1. A higher incidence of *Plasmodium malariae* infection with the nephrotic syndrome than observed in the rest of the population in Nigeria and Uganda [34, 57].
2. A markedly decreased incidence of renal disease following the eradication of malaria in British Guiana [33].
3. Detection of malarial antigen in glomeruli of patients with the nephrotic syndrome [44, 106].
4. Production of experimental glomerulonephritis resembling human malarial nephropathy in an *Aotus* monkey following infection with human *P. malariae* [103].

In man, malarial nephropathy can be subdivided into acute (transient, reversible) and chronic (progressive) lesions [48].

ACUTE MALARIAL NEPHROPATHY

Acute malarial nephropathy occurs during the course of infection with *P. falciparum* [10, 41, 48, 79]. The clinical manifestations are those of acute glomerulonephritis with or without nephrotic syndrome. The levels of serum complement components are depressed. This is not surprising in view of the findings of Srichaikul et al. [88] that increased clearance of radioactive C1q and reduction of serum C3 were found in 15 of 18 patients during *P. falciparum* infection.

On histologic examination, irregular thickening of the GBM with hyperplasia and hypertrophy of endothelial cells is seen; the mesangial matrix and cellularity are increased. Electron microscopy reveals thickening of the GBM with subendothelial deposits and endothelial and mesangial proliferation. By immunofluorescence microscopy, granular deposition of IgM, IgG, and C3 can be seen along the GBM and within the mesangium.

Immunopathologic and ultrastructural findings support an immunopathogenesis of this renal lesion. Bhamarapravati and colleagues [12] demonstrated the presence of *P. falciparum* antigen in diseased glomeruli and were able to elute immunoglobulins with antimalarial activity from the kidney. Additionally, they detected the C1q-precipitating material in the sera of these patients, further strengthening the evidence for the role of immune complexes in the pathogenesis.

Antimalarial therapy usually results in reversal of renal manifestations within 4 to 6 weeks [12, 41], although Berger et al. [10] reported the cases of 3 patients with persistently abnormal urinalysis 6 to 15 months after treatment.

CHRONIC MALARIAL NEPHROPATHY

Chronic malarial nephropathy (quartan malarial nephropathy) is associated with *P. malariae* infection, which, in contrast to *P. falciparum* nephropathy, tends to be progressive [44, 48, 57, 107, 112]. The clinical manifestations are invariably those related to the nephrotic syndrome. Serum complement is normal. Most of the patients, however, have circulating breakdown products of C3 in sera, indicating in vivo activation of the complement system [87]. Reports of the histologic findings in the renal lesion are conflicting. Hendrickse and coworkers [44] studied 51 children with chronic malarial nephropathy in Nigeria (West Africa). They reported that the basic lesion consisted of segmental thickening of glomer-

ular capillary walls with PAS-positive double-contour appearances. As this lesion progressed, it caused obliteration of the capillary lumen, resulting in segmental sclerosis of the peripheral capillary loops. This sclerosing process also involved the mesangium. The segmental nature of this lesion later became diffuse, leading to total glomerular sclerosis with secondary tubular atrophy and interstitial fibrosis. Cellular proliferation was usually absent. Superficially, this lesion resembled membranous nephropathy or membranoproliferative glomerulonephritis [107]. However, the absence of spikes by PAS–silver methenamine stain and the lack of mesangial proliferation and lobulation, could differentiate the malarial renal lesion from the other two nephropathies. In malarial nephropathy, the capillary wall thickening was always more advanced than the associated mesangial sclerosis, and might even be present without mesangial sclerosis, whereas in focal glomerular sclerosis in other diseases the uninvolved capillary wall was normal. Electron microscopy revealed thickening of the GBM that consisted of an increase in subendothelial basement membrane–like material of varying density. A unique feature was the invariable presence of small lacunae distributed throughout the basement membrane, often containing an island of material similar in density to the basement membrane; the nature of this abnormality is unknown. Subepithelial electron-dense deposits were absent [44, 107]. Immunofluorescence study revealed nodular or granular deposition of IgG, IgM, and C3 along the GBM [3, 44, 106].

On the other hand, Kibukamusoke et al. [56] studied 77 patients with nephrotic syndrome in Uganda (East Africa). By light microscopy, 55 patients had proliferative glomerulonephritis, ranging from minimal to diffuse changes. Nil lesions were found in 3 children and membranous nephropathy in 9 adults. *Plasmodium malariae* parasitemia was found in 29 of 48 patients with proliferative changes and in none with membranous nephropathy.

It is not clear at the present time why there is such a geographic discrepancy in histologic findings. The demonstration of malarial antigen [44, 49, 106] in diseased renal tissue supports the immunopathologic finding that immune complexes may play a role in the pathogenesis. What is not known at present are the factors responsible for the chronicity of *P. malariae* nephropathy. It seems unlikely that chronicity is the result of constant availability of malarial antigen, since antimalarial therapy has proved to be ineffective [34, 43, 57]. The results of treatment with corticosteroid or immunosuppressive agents have also been very disappointing [1, 44, 57, 112]. The uncontrolled study by Hendrickse et al. [44] suggests that corticosteroid therapy may occasionally be beneficial in young patients with mild glomerular change and highly selective proteinuria.

In a study of 115 patients with nephrotic syndrome associated with *P. malariae* infection in Uganda, Wing and colleagues [112] were able to follow 89 patients for at least 2 years, and 26 patients for 5 years or longer. Complete remission with loss of proteinuria occurred in 26 percent, asymptomatic proteinuria in 45 percent, and chronic renal failure in 29 percent. The results of this study clearly emphasize that one has to be cautious in interpreting the results of any therapeutic trial unless it is well controlled.

Viral Infections
SERUM HEPATITIS
Serum hepatitis is frequently associated with arthralgia, arthritis, urticaria, rashes, and angioneurotic edema [69]. In a study of 3 patients with polyarthritis and rash as a prodrome of hepatitis, Onion and coworkers [73] demonstrated the presence of Australia antigen (HBag) and depressed complement levels in both serum and synovial fluid. At the onset of clinically apparent jaundice, the arthritis resolved with return of the serum complement to normal, disappearance of HB antigenemia, and appearance of HB antibody. These clinical manifestations and immunologic events are similar to those seen in experimental serum sickness, in which soluble immune complexes formed in antigen excess cause tissue damage. Circulating immune complexes containing HBag, immunoglobulin, and complement have been detected in patients with serum hepatitis with arthritis, further confirming the role of immune complexes in this disease [104].

In 1970, Gocke et al. [36] reported the cases of 4 patients with HB antigenemia in whom systemic vasculitis, indistinguishable clinically and pathologically from polyarteritis nodosa, developed. These patients manifested polyarthralgia, myalgia, rash, mild hepatic dysfunction, and hypocomplementemia, and subsequently, peripheral neuropathy, hypertension, hematuria, and azotemia developed. Immunofluorescence studies of tissue revealed deposition of HBag, IgM, and C3 in blood-vessel walls. Circulating immune complexes composed of HBag and immunoglobulin also were detected in these patients, suggesting that the immune complex induced vessel injury.

Combes et al. [22] were the first to recognize the association of HB antigenemia and glomerulo-nephritis, when HB antigenemia and nephrotic syndrome developed in a 53-year-old man following blood transfusion. The association of antigenemia and renal disease has been reported in diffuse proliferative glomerulonephritis [19], membranous nephropathy [19, 20, 60, 61], membranoproliferative glomerulonephritis [19, 60, 72, 91], and focal glomerulosclerosis [60]. Clinical, morphologic, ultrastructural, and immunopathologic features in these patients were identical to those observed in patients with these diseases without HB antigenemic features. Immunofluorescence study of the diseased kidneys in patients with HB antigenemia and glomerulonephritis invariably reveals the presence of HBag in a distribution similar to that of immunoglobulins and complement, indicating renal injury mediated by an HB antigen-antibody complex. Additionally, Kohler and associates [61] were able to demonstrate circulating HBag-ab complexes by serum cryoprecipitation in a patient with membranous nephropathy and chronic HB antigemia. Serum complement components were normal in patients with membranous nephropathy [22, 61], whereas they were depressed in patients with membranoproliferative glomerulonephritis [72, 91]. Very little information is available regarding the efficacy of any mode of therapy in these patients. In 1 patient with HB antigenemia whose case was reported by Combes et al. [22], corticosteroid therapy was not successful either in the prevention or treatment of membranous nephropathy.

INFECTIOUS MONONUCLEOSIS
The occurrence of renal involvement in infectious mononucleosis (IM) has been recognized for many years [2, 18, 23, 38, 64, 76, 95, 96, 98, 101, 113, 117]. In a review of renal lesions in this disease, Tennant [96] found an incidence of abnormal urinary findings of 0 to 13 percent in different series. This, however, may not reflect the actual incidence of renal involvement because of either misdiagnosis of IM or erroneous diagnosis of hematuria in instances in which the red color of urine was due to the presence of large amounts of uric acid crystals, urates, or hemoglobin, all known to occur in IM [37, 86]. Rarely, hematuria may be the consequence of thrombocytopenia or due to the concomitant occurrence of poststreptococcal glomerulonephritis. In a study of 200 patients with IM, Hoagland [47] found β-hemolytic streptococcus in 30 percent of throat cultures.

The most consistent renal manifestation of IM is hematuria, frequently macroscopic. It usually appears within the first week of the illness, lasting from a few days to several months [18, 64, 95, 96,

98]. The occurrence of edema, oliguria, azotemia, or diastolic hypertension is uncommon, a distinguishing feature from poststreptococcal glomerulonephritis [96]. Proteinuria is either absent or low grade, though Greenspan [38] reported the case of 1 patient with frank nephrotic syndrome. The level of serum complement is not depressed [96, 113]. The most common renal lesion seen on pathologic examination is interstitial nephritis with mononuclear cell infiltration and foci of tubular necrosis [2, 18, 23, 113, 117]. Glomeruli show normal basement membrane and varying degrees of mesangial proliferation that may be present without any interstitial changes [18, 96, 113]. However, Peters et al. [76] reported thickening of the GBM in 11 of 12 patients with IM, none of whom had any clinical renal disease. Using immunofluorescence techniques, they also demonstrated the presence of specific heterophile reactive antigen in glomeruli, tubular cytoplasm, and vascular intima in these patients [75, 76]. Recently, Wands et al. [105] demonstrated the presence of circulating immune complexes composed of complement, Epstein-Barr antibody, and particles resembling Epstein-Barr virus in a patient with IM complicated by an urticarial rash.

The pathogenesis of renal disease in IM is unknown. Although autoimmune phenomema (positive Coombs' test, antinuclear antibody) have been reported, conclusive evidence of immune complex nephritis is lacking.

References

1. Adeniyi, A., Hendrickse, R. G., and Houba, V. Selectivity of proteinuria and response to prednisolone or immunosuppressive drugs in children with malarial nephrosis. *Lancet* 2:644, 1970.
2. Allen, F. H., and Kellner, A. Infectious mononucleosis. An autopsy report. *Am. J. Pathol.* 23:463, 1947.
3. Allison, A. C., Houba, V., Hendrickse, R. G., De Petris, S., Edington, G. M., and Adeniyi, A. Immune complexes in the nephrotic syndrome of African children. *Lancet* 1:1232, 1969.
4. Baehr, G. Glomerular lesions of subacute bacterial endocarditis. *J. Exp. Med.* 15:330, 1912.
5. Baehr, G. Renal complications of endocarditis. *Trans. Assoc. Am. Physicians* 46:87, 1931.
6. Bain, R. C., Edward, J. E., Scheifley, C. H., and Geraci, J. E. Right-sided bacterial endocarditis and endarteritis. A clinical and pathologic study. *Am. J. Med.* 24:98, 1958.
7. Bayatpour, M., Zbitnew, A., Dempster, G., and Miller, K. R. Role of coxsackievirus B4 in the pathogenesis of acute glomerulonephritis. *Can. Med. Assoc. J.* 109:873, 1973.
8. Beaufils, M., Morel-Maroger, L., Sraer, J.-D., Kanfer, A., Kourilsky, O., and Richet, G. Acute renal failure of glomerular origin during visceral abscesses. *N. Engl. J. Med.* 295:185, 1976.
9. Behan, P. O., Lowenstein, L. M., Stilmant, M., and Sax, D. S. Landry-Guillain-Barré-Strohl syndrome and immune-complex nephritis. *Lancet* 1:850, 1973.
10. Berger, M., Birch, L. M., and Conte, N. F. The nephrotic syndrome secondary to acute glomerulonephritis during falciparum malaria. *Ann. Intern. Med.* 67:1163, 1967.
11. Berman, L. B., Antonovych, T. T., and Duke, J. Glomerular abnormalities in tuberculosis. *Arch. Pathol.* 69:278, 1960.
12. Bhamarapravati, N., Boonpucknavig, S., Boonpucknavig, V., and Yaemboonruang, C. Glomerular changes in acute *plasmodium falciparum* infection. An immunopathologic study. *Arch. Pathol.* 96:289, 1973.
13. Bhorade, M. S., Carag, H. B., Lee, H. J., Potter, E. V., and Dunea, G. Nephropathy of secondary syphilis. A clinical and pathological spectrum. *J.A.M.A.* 216:1159, 1971.
14. Black, J. A., Challacombe, D. N., and Ockenden, B. G. Nephrotic syndrome associated with bacteraemia after shunt operations for hydrocephalus. *Lancet* 2:921, 1965.
15. Bolton, W. K., Sande, M. A., Normansell, D. E., Sturgill, B. C., and Westervelt, F. B. Ventriculojugular shunt nephritis with corynebacterium bovis. Successful therapy with antibiotics. *Am. J. Med.* 59:417, 1975.
16. Boonshaft, B., Maher, J. F., and Schreiner, G. E. Nephrotic syndrome associated with osteomyelitis without secondary amyloidosis. *Arch. Intern. Med.* 125:322, 1970.
17. Braunstein, G. D., Lewis, E. J., Galvanek, E. G., Hamilton, A., and Bell, W. R. The nephrotic syndrome associated with secondary syphilis. An immune deposit disease. *Am. J. Med.* 48:643, 1970.
18. Brun, C., Madsen, S., and Olsen, S. Infectious mononucleosis with hepatic and renal involvement. *Scand. J. Gastroenterol.* 5 [Suppl. 7]:89, 1970.
19. Brzosko, W. J., Krawczynski, K., Nazarewicz, T., Morzycka, M., and Nowoslawski, A. Glomerulonephritis associated with hepatitis-B surface antigen immune complexes in children. *Lancet* 2:7879, 1974.
20. Case records of the Massachusetts General Hospital. *N. Engl. J. Med.* 291:242, 1974.
21. Chesney, R. W., O'Regan, S., Cuyda, H. J., and Drummond, K. N. Candida endocrinopathy syndrome with membranoproliferative glomerulonephritis: Demonstration of glomerular candida antigen. *Clin. Nephrol.* 5:232, 1976.
22. Combes, B., Stastny, P., Shorey, J., Eigenbrodt, E. H., Barrera, A., Hull, A. R., and Carter, N. W. Glomerulonephritis with deposition of Australia antigen-antibody complexes in glomerular basement membrane. *Lancet* 2:234, 1971.
23. Custer, R. P., and Smith, E. B. The pathology of infectious mononucleosis. *Blood* 3:830, 1948.
24. Dathan, J. R. E., and Heyworth, M. F. Glomerulonephritis associated with Coxiella burnetii endocarditis. *Br. Med. J.* 1:376, 1975.
25. DeGowin, E. L., Carter, J. R., and Borts, I. H. A case of infection with brucella suis, causing endocarditis and nephritis; death from rupture of mycotic aneurysm. *Am. Heart J.* 30:77, 1945.
26. Dobrin, R. S., Day, N. K., Quie, P. G., Moore, H. L., Vernier, R. L., Michael, A. F., and Fish, A. J. The role of complement, immunoglobulin and bacterial antigen in coagulase-negative staphylococcal shunt nephritis. *Am. J. Med.* 59:660, 1975.

27. Duffy, J., Lidsky, M. D., Sharp, J. T., Davis, J. S., Person, D. A., Hollinger, F. B., and Min, K.-W. Polyarthritis, polyarteritis and hepatitis B. *Medicine (Baltimore)* 55:19, 1976.

28. Eknoyan, G., Gyorkey, F., Dichoso, C., Martinez-Maldonado, M., Suki, W. N., and Gyorkey, P. Renal morphological and immunological changes associated with acute viral hepatitis. *Kidney Int.* 1: 413, 1972.

29. Faierman, D., Ross, F. A., and Seckler, S. G. Typhoid fever complicated by hepatitis, nephritis and thrombocytopenia. *J.A.M.A.* 221:60, 1972.

30. Falcao, H. A., and Gould, D. B. Immune complex nephropathy in schistosomiasis. *Ann. Intern. Med.* 83:148, 1975.

31. Falls, W. F., Ford, K. L., Ashworth, C. T., and Carter, N. W. The nephrotic syndrome in secondary syphilis. Report of a case with renal biopsy findings. *Ann. Intern. Med.* 63:1047, 1965.

32. Gamble, C. N., and Reardan, J. B. Immunopathogenesis of syphilitic glomerulonephritis. Elution of antitreponemal antibody from glomerular immune-complex deposits. *N. Engl. J. Med.* 292:449, 1975.

33. Giglioli, G. Malaria and renal disease, with special reference to British Guiana. II. The effect of malaria eradication on the incidence of renal disease in British Guiana. *Ann. Trop. Med. Parasitol.* 56: 225, 1962.

34. Gilles, H. M., and Hendrickse, R. G. Nephrosis in Nigerian children. Role of plasmodium malariae, and effect of antimalarial treatment. *Br. Med. J.* 3: 27, 1963.

35. Ginsburg, B. E., Wasserman, J. Huldt, G., and Bergstrand, A. Case of glomerulonephritis associated with acute toxoplasmosis. *Br. Med. J.* 3:664, 1974.

36. Gocke, D. J., Hsu, K., Morgan, C., Mombardieri, S., Lockshin, M., and Christian, C. L. Association between polyarteritis and Australia antigen. *Lancet* 2: 1149, 1970.

37. Green, N., and Goldenberg, H. Acute hemolytic anemia hemoglobulinuria complicating infectious mononucleosis. *Arch. Intern. Med.* 105:108, 1960.

38. Greenspan, G. The nephrotic syndrome complicating infectious mononucleosis. *Calif. Med.* 98:162, 1963.

39. Guingnard, J. P., and Torrado, A. Interstitial nephritis and toxoplasmosis in a 10 year old child. *J. Pediatr.* 85:381, 1974.

40. Gutman, R. A., Striker, G. E., Gililand, B. C., and Cutler, R. E. The immune complex glomerulonephritis of bacterial endocarditis. *Medicine (Baltimore)* 51:1, 1972.

41. Hartenbower, D. L., Kantor, G. L., and Rosen, V. J. Renal failure due to acute glomerulonephritis during falciparum malaria: Case report. *Milit. Med.* 137:74, 1972.

42. Hellier, M. D., Webster, A. D. B., and Risinger, A. J. M. F. Neprotic syndrome: A complication of secondary syphilis. *Br. Med. J.* 4:404, 1971.

43. Hendrickse, R. G., and Gilles, H. M. The nephrotic syndrome and other renal diseases in children in Western Nigeria. *East Afr. Med. J.* 40:186, 1963.

44. Hendrickse, R. G., Glasgow, E. F., Adeniyi, A., White, R. H. R., Edington, G. M., and Houba, V. Quartan malarial nephrotic syndrome. Collaborative clinicopathological study in Nigerian children. *Lancet* 1:1143, 1972.

45. Herbut, P. Diffuse glomerulonephritis following revaccination for smallpox. *Am. J. Pathol.* 20:1011, 1944.

46. Hill, L. L., Singer, D. B., Falletta, J., and Stasney, R. The nephrotic syndrome in congenital syphilis. An immunopathy. *Pediatrics* 49:260, 1972.

47. Hoagland, R. J. *Infectious Mononucleosis.* New York: Grune & Stratton, 1967. P. 65.

48. Houba, V. Immunopathology of nephropathies associated with malaria. *Bull. W.H.O.* 52:199, 1975.

49. Houba, V., Allison, A. C., Adeniyi, A., and Houba, J. E. Immunoglobulin classes and complement in biopsies of Nigerian children with nephrotic syndrome. *Clin. Exp. Immunol.* 8:761, 1971.

50. Hyman, L. R., Jens, E. H., Hill, G. S., Zimmerman, S. W., and Burkholder, P. M. Alternate C3 pathway activation in pneumococcal glomerulonephritis. *Am. J. Med.* 58:810, 1975.

51. Iveson, J. M. I., McDougall, A. C., Leathem, A. J., and Harris, H. J. Lepromatous leprosy presenting with polyarthritis, myositis, and immune-complex glomerulonephritis. *Br. Med. J.* 3:619, 1975.

52. Kaplan, B. S., Wiglesworth, F. W., Marks, M. I., and Drummond, K. N. The glomerulopathy of congenital syphilis—an immune deposit disease. *J. Pediatr.* 81:1154, 1972.

53. Kaschula, R. O. C., Uys, C. J., Kuijten, R. H., Dale, J. R. P., and Wiggelinkhuizen, J. Nephrotic syndrome of congenital syphilis. Biopsy studies in four cases. *Arch. Pathol.* 97:289, 1974.

54. Kaufman, D. B., and McIntosh, R. The pathogenesis of the renal lesion in a patient with streptococcal disease, infected ventriculoatrial shunt cryoglobulinemia and nephritis. *Am. J. Med.* 50:262, 1971.

55. Keslin, M. H., Messner, R. P., and Williams, R. C. Glomerulonephritis with subacute bacterial endocarditis. Immunofluorescent studies. *Arch. Intern. Med.* 132:578, 1973.

56. Kibukamusoke, J. W., and Hutt, M. S. R. Histological features of the nephrotic syndrome associated with quartan malaria. *J. Clin. Pathol.* 20:117, 1967.

57. Kibukamusoke, J. W., Hutt, M. S. R., and Wilks, N. E. The nephrotic syndrome in Uganda and its association with quartan malaria. *Q. J. Med.* 143: 393, 1967.

58. Kibukamusoke, J. W. Malaria prophylaxis and immunosuppressant therapy in management of nephrotic syndrome associated with quartan malaria. *Arch. Dis. Child.* 43:598, 1968.

59. Kibukamusoke, J. W., and Voller, A. Serological studies on nephrotic syndrome of quartan malaria in Uganda. *Br. Med. J.* 1:406, 1970.

60. Knieser, M. P., Jenis, E. H., Lowenthal, D. T., Bancroft, W. H., Burns, H., and Shalboub, R. Pathogenesis of renal disease associated with viral hepatitis. *Arch. Pathol.* 97, 193, 1974.

61. Kohler, P. F., Cronin, R. E., Hammond, W. S., Olin, D., and Carr, R. I. Chronic membranous glomerulonephritis caused by hepatitis B antigen-antibody immune complexes. *Ann. Intern. Med.* 81: 448, 1974.

62. Krebs, R. A., and Burvant, M. U. Nephrotic syndrome in association with varicella. *J.A.M.A.* 222: 325, 1972.

63. Levy, R. L., and Hong, R. The immune nature of

subacute bacterial endocarditis (SBE) nephritis. *Am. J. Med.* 54:645, 1973.

64. Lindsey, D. C., and Chrisman, W. P. Gross hematuria as the presenting symptom of infectious mononucleosis. *J.A.M.A.* 157:1406, 1955.

65. Löhlein, M. Ueber hamorrhagische Nierenaffektionen bei chronischer ulzeroser Endokarditis. (Embolische nichteiterige Herdnephritis). *Med. Klin.* 10:375, 1910.

66. Michael, A. F., Herdman, R. C., Fish, A. J., Pickering, R. J., and Vernier, R. L. Chronic membranoproliferative glomerulonephritis with hypocomplementemia. *Transplant. Proc.* 1:4, 1969.

67. Michael, A. F., Westberg, N. G., Fish, A. J., and Vernier, R. L. Studies on chronic membranoproliferative glomerulonephritis with hypocomplementemia. *J. Exp. Med.* 134:208s, 1971.

68. Minkowitz, S., Wenk, R., Friedman, E., Yucoeoglu, A., and Berkovich, S. Acute glomerulonephritis associated with varicella infection. *Am. J. Med.* 44:489, 1968.

69. Mirick, G. S., and Shank, R. E. An epidemic of serum hepatitis studied under controlled conditions. *Trans. Am. Clin. Climatol. Assoc.* 71:176, 1960.

70. Moncrieff, M. W., Glasgow, E. F., Arthur, L. J. H., and Hargreaves, H. M. Glomerulonephritis associated with *Staphylococcus albus* in a Spitz Holter valve. *Arch. Dis. Child.* 48:69, 1973.

71. Morel-Maroger, L., Sraer, J.-D., Herreman, G., and Godeau, P. Kidney in subacute endocarditis. Pathological and immunofluorescence findings. *Arch. Pathol.* 94:205, 1972.

72. Myers, B. D., Griffel, B., Naveh, D., Jankielowitz, T., and Klajman, A. Membranoproliferative glomerulonephritis associated with persistent viral hepatitis. *Am. J. Clin. Pathol.* 60:222, 1973.

73. Onion, D. K., Crumpacker, C. S., and Gilliland, B. C. Arthritis of hepatitis associated with Australia antigen. *Ann. Intern. Med.* 75:29, 1971.

74. O'Regan, S., de Chadarevian, J.-P., Rishikof, J. R., and Drummond, K. N. Treponemal antigens in congenital and acquired syphilitic nephritis. *Ann. Intern. Med.* 85:325, 1976.

75. Peters, J. H. Heterophile reactive antigen in infectious mononucleosis. *Science* 157:1200, 1967.

76. Peters, J. H., Flume, J., and Fuccillo, D. Nephritis in infectious mononucleosis. *Clin. Res.* 10:254, 1962.

77. Pillay, V. K. G., Kirch, E., and Kurtzman, N. A. Glomerulopathy associated with filarial loiasis. *J.A.M.A.* 225:179, 1973.

78. Pollner, P. Nephrotic syndrome associated with congenital syphilis. *J.A.M.A.* 198:173, 1966.

79. Powell, K. C., and Meadows, R. The nephrotic syndrome in New Guinea. A clinical and histological spectrum. *Aust. N.Z. J. Med.* 4:363, 1971.

80. Rames, L., Wise, B., Goodman, J. R., and Piel, C. F. Renal disease with *staphylococcus albus* bacteremia. A complication in ventriculoatrial shunts. *J.A.M.A.* 212:1671, 1970.

81. Robins, D. E., and Ladd, A. T. Acute syphilitic nephrosis. Case report and review of the literature. *Am. J. Med.* 32:817, 1962.

82. Rodriquez-Iturbe, B., Garcia, R., Rubio, L., Zabala, J., Moros, G., and Torres, R. Acute glomerulonephritis in the Guillain-Barré-Strohl syndrome. Report of nine cases. *Ann. Intern. Med.* 78:391, 1973.

83. Sartain, P. The anemia of congenital syphilis. *South. Med. J.* 58:27, 1965.

84. Shahin, B., Papadopolou, Z. L., and Jenis, E. H. Congenital nephrotic syndrome associated with congenital toxoplasmosis. *J. Pediatr.* 85:366, 1974.

85. Sitprija, V., Pipatanagul, V., Boonpucknavig, V., and Boonpucknavig, S. Glomerulitis in typhoid fever. *Ann. Intern. Med.* 81:210, 1974.

86. Sonkin, N. Unusual causes of color changes in urine. Excessive metabolites in infectious mononucleosis and paprika ingestion are incriminated. *R.I. Med. J.* 52:441, 1969.

87. Soothill, J. F., and Hendrickse, R. G. Some immunological studies of the nephrotic syndrome of Nigerian children. *Lancet* 2:629, 1967.

88. Srichaikul, T., Puwasatien, P., Puwasatien, P., Karnjanajetanee, J., and Bokisch, V. A. Complement changes and disseminated intravascular coagulation in plasmodium falciparum malaria. *Lancet* 1:770, 1975.

89. Sterzel, R. B., Krause, P. H., Zobl, H., and Kuhn, K. Acute syphilitic nephrosis: A transient glomerular immunopathy. *Clin. Nephrol.* 2:164, 1974.

90. Stickler, G. B., Shin, M. H., Burke, E. C., Holley, K. E., Miller, R. H., and Segar, W. E. Diffuse glomerulonephritis associated with infected ventriculoatrial shunt. *N. Engl. J. Med.* 279:1077, 1968.

91. Stratta, P., Camussi, G., Ragni, R., and Vercellone, A. Hepatitis-B antigen-aemia associated with active chronic hepatitis and mesangioproliferative glomerulonephritis. *Lancet* 2:179, 1975.

92. Strife, C. F., McDonald, B. M., Ruley, E. J., McAdams, A. J., and West, C. D. Shunt nephritis: The nature of the serum cryoglobulins and their relation to the complement profile. *J. Pediatr.* 88:403, 1976.

93. Suskind, R., Winkelstein, J. A., and Spear, G. A. Nephrotic syndrome in congenital syphilis. *Arch. Dis. Child.* 48:237, 1973.

94. Taitz, L. S., Isaacson, C., and Stein, H. Acute nephritis associated with congenital syphilis. *Br. Med. J.* 2:152, 1961.

95. Taub, E. A. Renal lesions, gross hematuria, and marrow granulomas in infectious mononucleosis. *J.A.M.A.* 195:1153, 1966.

96. Tennant, F. S. The glomerulonephritis of infectious mononucleosis. *Tex. Rep. Biol. Med.* 26:603, 1968.

97. Thomas, E. W., and Schur, M. Clinical nephropathies in early syphilis. *Arch. Intern. Med.* 78:679, 1946.

98. Thompson, W. T., and Pitt, C. Frank hematuria as a manifestation of infectious mononucleosis. *Ann. Intern. Med.* 33:1274, 1950.

99. Tourville, D. R., Byrd, L. H., Kim, D. U., Zajd, D., Lee, I., Reichman, L. B., and Baskin, S. Treponemal antigen in immunopathogenesis of syphilitic glomerulonephritis. *Am. J. Pathol.* 82:479, 1976.

100. Tu, W. H., Shearn, M. A., and Lee, J. C. Acute diffuse glomerulonephritis in acute staphylococcal endocarditis. *Ann. Intern. Med.* 71:335, 1969.

101. Utian, H. L., Fanaroff, A. A., and Plit, M. Glomerular disease in childhood: A review of 150 consecutive cases. *S. Afr. Med. J.* 38:162, 1964.

102. Villarreal, H., and Sokoloff, L. The occurrence of renal insufficiency in subacute bacterial endocarditis. *Am. J. Med. Sci.* 220:655, 1950.

103. Volle, A., Draper, C. C., Shwe, T., and Hutt, M. S. R. Nephrotic syndrome in monkey infected with human quartan malaria. *Br. Med. J.* 4:208, 1971.

104. Wands, J. R., Mann, E., Alpert, E., and Isselbacher, K. J. The pathogenesis of arthritis associated with acute hepatitis-B surface antigen-positive hepatitis. Complement activation and characterization of circulating immune complexes. *J. Clin. Invest.* 55:930, 1975.

105. Wands, J. R., Perrotto, J. L., and Isselbacher, K. J. Circulating immune complexes and complement sequence activation in infectious mononucleosis. *Am. J. Med.* 60:269, 1976.

106. Ward, P. A., and Kibukamusoke, J. W. Evidence for soluble immune complexes in the pathogenesis of the glomerulonephritis of quartan malaria. *Lancet* 1:283, 1969.

107. White, R. H. R. Quartan malarial nephrotic syndrome. *Nephron* 11:147, 1973.

108. Wickbom, B., and Winberg, J. Coincidence of congenital toxoplasmosis and acute nephritis with nephrotic syndrome. *Acta Paediatr. Scand.* 61:470, 1972.

109. Wiggelinkhuizen, J., Kaschula, R. O. C., Uys, C. J., Kuijten, R. H., and Dale, J. Congenital syphilis and glomerulonephritis with evidence for immune pathogenesis. *Arch. Dis. Child.* 48:375, 1973.

110. Williams, R. C., and Kunkel, H. C. Rheumatoid factor, complement, and conglutinin aberrations in patients with subacute bacterial endocarditis. *J. Clin. Invest.* 41:666, 1962.

111. Wilson, C. B., and Smith, R. C. Goodpasture's syndrome associated with influenza A2 virus infection. *Ann. Intern. Med.* 76:91, 1972.

112. Wing, A. J., Hutt, M. S. R., and Kibukamusoke, J. W. Progression and remission in the nephrotic syndrome associated with quartan malaria in Uganda. *Q. J. Med.* 163, 273, 1972.

113. Woodroffe, A. J., Row, P. G., Meadows, R., and Lawrence, J. R. Nephritis in infectious mononucleosis. *Q. J. Med.* 43, 451, 1974.

114. Yuceoglu, A. M., Berkovich, S., and Minkowitz, S. Acute glomerulonephritis associated with ECHO virus type 9 infection. *J. Pediatr.* 69:603, 1966.

115. Yuceoglu, A. M., Tresser, G., Wasserman, E., and Lange, K. The glomerulopathy of congenital syphilis. A curable immune-deposit disease. *J.A.M.A.* 229, 1085, 1974.

116. Zelazko, M., and Feldman, G. Behavior of the complement system in the nephropathy of congenital syphilis. *J. Pediatr.* 88:359, 1976.

117. Ziegler, E. E. Infectious mononucleosis. Report of a fatal case with autopsy. *Arch. Pathol.* 37:196, 1944.

67. Macroglobulinemia, Cryoglobulinemia, and Dysglobulinemia

Edmund C. Burke

Macroglobulinemia

Macroglobulinemia has been associated with renal disease in myeloma, lymphoma, other malignancies, immunodeficiency states, and Waldenström's macroglobulinemia, although this coexistence has been infrequent. Macroglobulinemia has occurred in the pediatric age group, but there have been no reports of renal lesions associated with the disorder in children. Nonetheless, the nephropathologic changes described in adults with macroglobulinemia should be considered. In the nephrotic syndrome, alpha-2-macroglobulinemia occurs but is not the cause of the nephropathy [1].

Macroglobulins have a sedimentation constant of 19S to 20S, as compared with the normal 7S globulins (Fig. 67-1). The macroglobulins may be monoclonal (M-type), as in Waldenström's disease, or polyclonal, as in autoimmune and collagen diseases.

The macroglobulins migrate as beta globulins or gamma globulins on free electrophoresis (Fig. 67-2). The M-component globulins may belong to any class, that is, IgG, IgA, IgE, or IgM, and an M-component may be associated with kappa or lambda chains. Whereas the plasma cell is involved in the formation of 7S gamma globulin, the lymphocytoid cell produces macroglobulin. The macroglobulins sometimes behave like cryoglobulins, that is, they precipitate with cold.

In Waldenström's macroglobulinemia, renal changes are uncommon; the passive deposition of circulating IgM has been suggested as the cause of the renal lesion [35]. Renal lesions also have been associated with abnormal immunoglobulins in lymphoproliferative disease, the abnormality being dysproteinemia [9, 14, 36]. Lin and associates [24] described a 56-year-old man with Waldenström's macroglobulinemia, mesangiocapillary glomerulonephritis, angiitis, and myositis in whom the primary disease was dysproteinemia. A renal biopsy specimen from this patient showed increased mesangium and thickening and splitting of the basement membranes in the lobulated glomerular tufts. Endothelial and epithelial cells were hypertrophied, and focal tubular atrophy and interstitial fibrosis were seen. Electron microscopy

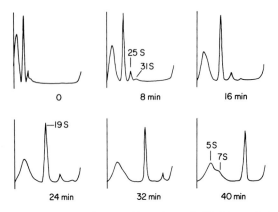

Figure 67-1. Ultracentrifugation of Waldenström's macroglobulinemia serum at 44,770 RPM (serum diluted 1 : 8). Macroglobulin (19S) peak is tallest spike at each time interval.

showed electron-dense granular material in the mesangium and glomerular basement membrane. Aggregates of basement membrane–like material extending between the endothelium and the basement membrane accounted for the splitting of the basement membrane that was seen on light microscopy. Capillary lumens were occasionally occluded by strands of fibrin, hypertrophic endothelial cells, and cellular debris.

Immunofluorescence studies showed anti-β1A, anti-C3, and anti-IgM in the basement membranes and occasionally in the mesangium. A moderate reaction with anti-IgA and a weak reaction with anti–gamma globulin, antifibrin, and antifibrinogen were visible.

Lin and associates' [24] report is the only one concerning mesangiocapillary glomerulonephritis associated with Waldenström's macroglobulinemia,

although similar renal alterations have been described in a patient with adenocarcinoma and monocytic leukemia, as well as in another patient with reticulum cell sarcoma. Lin and associates admitted that the pathogenesis of the renal lesion was inconclusive, but they implicated an immune mechanism as having a role in the renal damage.

Morel-Maroger et al. [35] studied 16 patients who had Waldenström's macroglobulinemia and renal disease and noted 3 with amyloidosis. However, the other 13 patients had nonamyloid deposits in the glomeruli; the deposits were always on the endothelial aspect of the basement membrane. These deposits were sometimes so voluminous that they occluded the capillary lumens either partially or completely and were considered thrombi. In the interstitium, cellular infiltration was usually confined to the superficial cortex, but at times it was perihilar, spreading around the renal hilus. In all patients, renal tubules were separated by the infiltrates, tubular basement membranes were thickened, and tubular epithelial cells showed nonspecific degenerative lesions.

Immunofluorescence studies showed intraglomerular thrombi and endomembranous deposits staining strongly with anti-IgM serum. In some thrombi the fixation was most striking at the periphery, whereas smaller endomembranous deposits showed homogeneous staining. One patient had a thready fixation of anti-IgM serum in the glomerular lumens, arterioles, and peritubular capillaries, which was interpreted as indicating circulating IgM.

Morel-Maroger et al. [35] stated that the immunofluorescent patterns of the IgM deposition in the kidneys of their patients were strikingly different from those described by Dixon (antigen-antibody complexes), suggesting that the circulating pathologic proteins may precipitate in glomerular capillary lumens because of increased viscosity. With regard to the viscosity theory, the renal lesions of Waldeström's macroglobulinemia differ from those of myeloma [41] in that, in the former, intraglomerular thrombi are found without tubular lesions, whereas in myeloma, tubular casts with macrophagic reaction occur without glomerular thrombi. Morel-Maroger et al. [35] concluded that the finding of IgM exclusively in glomerular thrombi is the characteristic renal lesion of Waldenström's macroglobulinemia.

Despite the statement that M-component disorders in infants and children are only of theoretical interest to the pediatrician, because most of the patients with multiple myeloma and macroglobulinemia are adults, there have been several reports of macroglobulinemia occurring in chil-

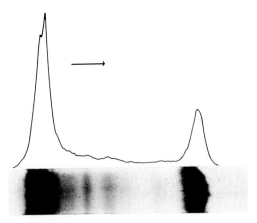

Figure 67-2. Paper electrophoresis of serum in Waldenström's macroglobulinemia (120 v, 18 hr; pH 8.6). Macroglobulin fraction is peak on left.

dren. Čejka et al. [8] noted macroglobulinemia in a 12-year-old boy with leukemia. The boy had an IgM-type kappa chain and Bence Jones proteinuria, which occurred as free kappa chains. In the serum and urine, increased amounts of beta-2-microglobulins were found. Renal biopsy was not done, and renal studies were not done at autopsy. Kyle [21] contends that Čejka and associates' patient had monoclonal gammopathy of the IgM type rather than the adult type of macroglobulinemia. However, they believed that the same relationship existed between lymphoid cell type and the monoclonal macroglobulin production as exists in Waldenström's macroglobulinemia. Their patient differed from 2 other patients with leukemia whose cases were reported by Lindqvist et al. [25] and Stoop et al. [43] in that neither of the latter 2 patients had IgM gammopathy.

Weinberg et al. [48] reported on an 8-month-old infant with monoclonal macroglobulinemia and cytomegalic inclusion disease. The infant had a kappa-chain monoclonal macroglobulinemia that was noted first when the child was 4 months old. The congenital cytomegalovirus infection may have induced the immunologic abnormalities in this infant. Such an explanation was also offered by Hancock et al. [17], who found an IgM macroglobulinemia in an infant with congenital rubella syndrome.

In support of the passive deposition capillary obstruction theory of Morel-Maroger and colleagues [35], Merrill [34] stated that in Waldenström's macroglobulinemia there is no evidence for participation of an immune mechanism in the glomerular lesion. However, other investigators believe that the generalized angiitis in Waldenström's macroglobulinemia is due to the accumulation of unidentified circulating immune complexes or to the passive deposition of IgM.

Cryoglobulinemia

Cryoglobulins, which are proteins that precipitate with cold, were first observed in patients with multiple myeloma. Subsequently, cryoproteins were observed in leukemia, lymphosarcoma, infectious mononucleosis, and syphilis and in collagen disorders such as systemic lupus erythematosus, polyarteritis nodosa, rheumatoid arthritis, and purpura-arthralgia–rheumatoid factor syndrome [23]. Patients with cryoglobulinemia and renal involvement, in addition to hypertension, proteinuria, and hematuria, may have purpura, arthralgia, or rheumatoid factor syndrome. They also may have anemia, hypergammaglobulinemia, antinuclear antibodies, rheumatoid factor, and a depression of serum complement levels. The renal histologic findings are characterized by proliferation and swelling of intracapillary cells and mild-to-moderate infiltration of neutrophils in the glomeruli. The axial regions show a slight-to-moderate increase in basement membrane–like material [4]. A rapidly progressive and fatal diffuse proliferative glomerulonephritis, with hypertension, hematuria, and proteinuria, has been found in some patients.

Some investigators have suggested that cryoglobulins represent antigen-antibody complexes deposited in the glomeruli, thus producing vasculitis in small vessels and glomerulonephritis. Compatible with this concept is the demonstration, by immunohistologic studies, of the deposition of IgM and IgG in target tissues [1, 10, 13].

Although as early as 1933 cold-precipitable proteins were reported to be associated with clinical disease [49] (the term *cryoglobulin* was introduced by Lerner and Watson [22] in 1947), cryoglobulins have been observed as incidental findings in many diseases, including those that involve the kidney [16, 33, 39, 44, 45, 47].

In 1968, Grupe [15] provided one of the first reports of cryoglobulins in children with acute glomerulonephritis. Although Grupe was uncertain as to the significance of the cryoglobulinemia, the presence of a cold-precipitable complex of IgG in the serum in association with the same immunoglobulins in the glomerulus suggested that cryoglobulins could be of immunopathologic importance. To confirm that immune complexes participate in renal injury, however, it must be shown that an antigen exists in the cryoglobulin.

In 1970, McIntosh et al. [31] studied the incidence and nature of cryoglobulins and assessed their clinical and prognostic significance in renal disease. Cryoglobulins were not detected in 19 patients without renal disease, nor in 10 patients with childhood nephrotic syndrome; 22 patients with proliferative glomerulonephritis had clinical, laboratory, and morphologic findings related to the presence of cryoglobulin. In 7 other patients with mild-to-severe renal structural and functional abnormalities, only 1 had cryoglobulins. These 7 patients, none of whom was more than 16 years of age, were followed from 1 to 10 years; several had been treated with corticosteroids and antimetabolites. Finally, of 3 patients with membranous nephropathy, 2 had cryoprecipitates; all 3 had the nephrotic syndrome, and 2 of the 3 were 15 years old. McIntosh et al. noted that there was no correlation between the isolation of cryoprecipitates and either the decreased levels of serum total hemolytic complement and C3 or the cause of the disease. None of the cryoglobulins of 5 of their patients with streptococcal infection and high titers of antistreptolysin O and type 12M protein showed evidence of antibody activity to these antigens. McIntosh et al. suggested that cryoproteins are common in several types of immune complex nephritis and are associated with the activity of the disease, that the exact immunopathologic significance of cryoglobulins was unclear, but that they may be complexes of specific antibody and antigen or altered gamma globulins with the biologic properties of immune complexes. They concluded that the significance of cryoglobulins in glomerulonephritis had not been clarified by their investigation, but that the prognostic significance indicated that the findings of these cryoprecipitates may be more than a coincidence.

McIntosh et al. [32], in 1971, delineated further the role of biologic and chemical properties of cryoproteins in acute poststreptococcal glomerulonephritis to determine whether cryoprecipitates were (1) antigen and antibody-specific complexes, (2) immune complexes that were formed secondary to the primary immunologic process, or (3) immunoglobulins that were altered by either the disease process or an antimocrobial agent. They isolated cryoglobulins from 3 patients with acute poststreptococcal glomerulonephritis. Each of three guinea pigs received (at different sites) intradermal injections of cryoglobulin solution and of supernatant IgG from the 3 individual patients. In addition, each guinea pig received intradermal injections of a buffer plus pooled human IgG instead of supernatant IgG. The effects of the IV administration of cryoglobulins were studied in a group of male New Zealand white rabbits: four subgroups of six rabbits received intravenous solutions containing cryoglobulin, supernatant IgG, pooled human IgG, and the buffer respectively. Other guinea pigs either received cryoglobulins administered IV or were studied to evaluate the complement-fixing properties of cryoglobulins. McIntosh et al. [32] determined that the cold-insoluble precipitates had biologic characteristics attributed to immune complexes or aggregated gamma globulin, based on their findings that skin-reactive and complement-fixing properties were associated with cryoproteins, that human IgG localized on glomerular basement membranes, and that anaphylactic shock occurred after IV administration of the cryoproteins. Therefore, cryoprecipitates may represent complexes of specific antigen and antibody, the antigen being a foreign protein, such as streptococcal products, or an autologous protein, such as altered serum or tissue component. Cryoglobulins may be of primary immunopathologic importance in glomerulonephri-

tis, or their production may be secondary to some other immunologic phenomenon, their presence producing further renal injury.

Barnett et al. [5], in commenting on cryoglobulinemia and disease, stated that immunoglobulin constituents so far identified as cryoglobulins sometimes have been either IgG or IgM alone, but more frequently they consist of mixtures of immunoglobulins and complement components. Although IgG may be demonstrated solely as a cryoprecipitate, part of the IgG population may consist of antigens, and other IgG molecules may represent antibodies. The precipitation of immunoglobulins at reduced temperatures suggests that the IgG components may be autoantigens, and that IgM, IgG, or IgA components may be antibodies plus certain cofactors, including complement, which may precipitate at reduced temperatures.

Barnett et al. [5] stated that, since cryoglobulins are associated with unusual infectious diseases, in diseases of unknown cause a relationship may be found in the future among uncommon infectious agents, the heteroantigens of persistent infectious processes, DNA, RNA, or viruses, and the antibodies to these heteroantigens plus cofactors. They added that, whereas some IgG-IgM cryoglobulin complexes containing DNA have been described, the quantity of cryoglobulins is small, and definitive studies on the role of DNA within them are most difficult to conduct.

In 1971, McIntosh and Grossman [30] described the case of a 13-year-old boy with acute glomerulonephritis whose serum contained fibrinogen or fibrinogen products (or both) in the cryoprecipitates, a situation previously unreported. He experienced rapidly progressive renal failure, persistently low serum complement, and persistent cryoproteins despite cyclophosphamide therapy. Immunofluorescence study of a renal biopsy specimen showed nodular deposits of IgG and C3 on glomerular basement membranes and large amounts of fibrinogen in the mesangium. Electron microscopy showed large subendothelial deposits of a granular material separating the lamina densa and the reactive intracapillary cells. Some glomeruli showed extensive collagenization. Numerous large subepithelial humps were demonstrated. Light microscopy showed large hypercellular glomeruli, extensive glomerular ischemia, and conspicuous eosinophilic thickening of capillary loops. Central lobular distortion, mesangial hyperplasia, and widening of the stalk were also seen. In this patient, cryoprecipitates of IgG, C3, and fibrinogen may have played a role in the development of severe glomerular disease.

Porush and associates [38] reported glomerulonephritis associated with the nephrotic syndrome in which the serum contained a paraprotein and mixed cryoglobulin with a positive rheumatoid factor. They suggested that the mixed cryoglobulins represented antigen-antibody complexes.

In 1971, Lewis and Couser [23] noted that denatured DNA was found to be a component of some mixed cryoglobulins to which it is tightly bound both in solution and in precipitate. These complexes have been observed in lupus erythematosus, and the authors suggested that mixed cryoglobulins represent soluble antigen-antibody complexes.

Cryoglobulins have been found in association with several renal diseases, including lupus nephritis, poststreptococcal nephritis, and rapidly progressive glomerulonephritis, as well as the nephritis in NZB mice. Although much recent interest has focused on the role of cryoglobulins in glomerulonephritis in man, it has yet to be demonstrated that cryoglobulins representing immune complexes have a role in the pathogenesis of glomerulonephritis.

Burman et al. [7] described the case of a 5½-year-old boy with hemophilia and factor VIII deficiency who was treated with cryoprecipitate. After 10 ml of cryoprecipitate was given, the patient began to cough, and after an additional 5 ml, he became pale and sweaty and was in shock. He experienced an anaphylactoid reaction, with pulmonary edema and intravascular hemolysis, which was followed by hemoglobinuria that persisted for 16 hours. Subsequent investigation showed that the reactions were probably due to a high titer of anti-IgA in the plasma of one of the donors. These authors therefore warned against injecting cryoprecipitates into hemophiliac patients; specifically, the use of blood from donors with high anti-IgA titers should be avoided.

Druet et al. [11] studied cryoglobulinemia in a large series of 76 patients with renal diseases. They also studied cryoglobulins in 597 patients who had primary renal disease or an illness that could be complicated by renal disease. (The report does not specify the number of children included.) A group of 200 patients with arteriosclerosis obliterans of the lower extremities were used as controls, because glomerular disease is not usually found in this disorder. Druet et al. found that cryoglobulin was relatively rare in membranous glomerulopathies and in glomerulonephritis with mesangial deposits, minimal glomerular changes, and focal hyalinosis, but was found frequently in lupus erythematosus with morphologic renal involvement. They noted 5 patients with cryoprecipitates among 10 patients with acute streptococcal proliferative glomerulonephritis. In contrast, only 1 patient with cryoglobulin was found among 12 patients with acute proliferative glomerulonephritis without evidence of streptococcal infection.

There was no statistically significant difference among the serum levels of IgG, IgA, or IgM whether a cryoglobulin was present or absent. A search was made for anti–gamma globulin activity, that is, rheumatoid factor activity, in the sera of 417 patients. High concentrations were found in 1 patient with primary membranoproliferative glomerulonephritis and in 1 with acute proliferative glomerulonephritis (both of whom had mixed cryoglobulinemia), in 2 patients with lupus erythematosus (1 of whom had a cryoglobulin), and in 1 patient with cirrhosis of the liver with cryoglobulin and glomerular disease. No anti–gamma globulin activity was found in 6 patients with isolated cryoglobulins. Although there was no significant relationship between cryoglobulin levels and complement, a negative correlation was suggested. All these patients, however, probably were adults.

McIntosh et al. [29] produced serum sickness nephritis in 25 rabbits, half of whom were nephrectomized on the ninth day after the injection. Cryoprecipitates were noted in significant quantities in 15 of the 25 rabbits, and all 15 had glomerular changes or positive immunohistologic findings. The major increase in the cryoprecipitate after nephrectomy suggests that cryoproteins were immune complexes. McIntosh and coworkers suggested that the isolation of the cryoprecipitates may aid in the decision regarding the time and the method of renal transplantation.

Törnroth and Skrifvars [46] studied the ultrastructural changes in a 61-year-old man who had acute nonstreptococcal glomerulonephritis associated with mixed cryoglobulinemia. Renal biopsy showed focal proliferation of endothelial and mesangial cells, focal increase in the mesangial matrix, and various electron-dense deposits, including discrete subepithelial deposits. Such deposits had not been noted previously in this syndrome. This suggests that immune complexes are implicated in the pathogenesis of glomerulonephritis and that the cryoglobulins may be contributing to the immune complexes.

Pien et al. [37] noted cryoglobulins in an infant with congenital cytomegalovirus infection. Although the patient continued to excrete cytomegalovirus in the urine, there was no evidence of nephritis.

Druet et al. [12] stated that to determine the role of cryoglobulinemia in the pathogenesis of

glomerulonephritis, one would have to characterize the antigen and the antibody in the cryoglobulin and in the glomerular tuft. In streptococcal
glomerulonephritis, a streptococcal antigen is present in the glomerular deposits, but it could not be
detected in the cryoglobulin, according to McIntosh et al. [32]. In addition, anti-IgG activity has
not been reported. Most of the serum cryoglobulins seen in glomerulonephritis are of the mixed
type. As in lupus erythematosus, leprosy, infectious mononucleosis, cytomegalovirus infection,
and normal subjects, one of the constituents of
cryoglobulin may have anti-IgG activity, which
could be identified only in the isolated cryoglobulin at 4°C. Conversely, since IgM is not found
in the glomerular tuft of acute endocapillary proliferative glomerulonephritis, in such cases cryoglobulin may be unrelated to the glomerular disease.

Thus, although more than 6 years have elapsed
since a concerted effort was made to identify
the specific contribution of cryoproteins in renal
disease, and most studies to date suggest that cryoglobulinemia is an antiimmune manifestation, the
problem still has not been solved, although the
work of Adam et al. [1] strongly suggests that
cryoglobulin plays a causal role. Surprisingly,
there are few reports in the pediatric literature on
cryoglobulinemia and childhood renal disease.

Dysglobulinemia

Dysglobulinemia includes all disorders of the
globulins, ranging from the complete absence of
globulins, or agammaglobulinemia, to elevated
levels of globulins, or hyperglobulinemia.

The immunoglobulins are IgA, IgG, IgM, IgD,
and IgE; the other globulins are alpha and beta
globulins. Two of the complement factors are also
globulins, namely C3 (β1C-β1A globulin) and
C4 protein (β1E globulin). Various renal diseases
are associated with reduced serum levels of complement, such as lupus nephritis, poststreptococcal
glomerulonephritis, and membranoproliferative
glomerulonephritis [3, 18, 42]. Some renal diseases may be associated with elevated levels of
alpha-2-globulin and macroglobulin, as in some
types of nephrotic syndrome. Immunologic aspects
of various nephropathies are discussed in detail in
Chap. 3.

Globulin disorders are listed in Table 67-1. Renal disease is rare in congenital agammaglobulinemia, except as the consequence of superimposed
or intercurrent infection.

In hyperglobulinemia, renal disease is also uncommon unless the primary cause is a systemic
disease, such as anaphylactoid purpura or lupus

Table 67-1. Globulin Disorders

Agammaglobulinemia
  Congenital
    Burton's
    Nezelof-DiGeorge
    Swiss type
  Acquired
    Hodgkin's disease, lymphomas, and leukemias
    Homograft recipients (on immunosuppressive
      treatment)

Hyperimmunoglobulinemia
  Elevated levels of one or two immunoglobulins
    Immunodeficiency diseases
      Immunodeficiency with hyper-IgM
      Wiskott-Aldrich (IgA)
    Infections
      Congenital
      Infectious mononucleosis
      Trypanosomiasis
    Miscellaneous
      Anaphylactoid purpura (IgA)
      Extrinsic allergy (IgE)
  High levels of all immunoglobulins
    Infections
      Collagen diseases (lupus erythematosus, rheumatic
        fever, rheumatoid arthritis, regional enteritis, ul-
        cerative colitis)
    Liver disease
    Miscellaneous (Down's syndrome, hypergammaglob-
      ulinemic purpura, pulmonary hypersensitivity dis-
      eases)

erythematosus. The role of the immunologic system is difficult to define, although lupus nephritis
is a result of immune complex deposition.

Recently, reports have appeared concerning a
nephropathy associated with immunologic deposits
in the mesangium of the glomeruli [19, 26, 28].
None of the patients had evidence of a systemic
disease and all had normal levels of gamma globulin. These so-called IgA nephropathies might be
considered dysglobulinemias. These patients are
not all children, but the adults as well as the children have hematuria and usually a benign clinical
course (see Chap. 46).

Berger and Hinglais [6] were the first to report glomerular mesangial localization of IgA,
with less intense localization of IgG and C3. Their
patients had normal renal function, gross or microscopic hematuria, no systemic disease, and usually a focal glomerulonephritis. Often, the microhematuria was exacerbated by upper respiratory
infections. McEnery et al. [28] described IgA,
IgG, and C3 localization without IgM in 9 similar patients. Lowance et al. [26] reported the
cases of 15 patients in whom IgA was the predominant immunoglobulin in the glomerular
mesangium, but IgM, IgG, and C3 also were

present. Berger and Hinglais [6] noted the occurrence of this nephropathy in 18 percent of 300 biopsy specimens.

McCoy and associates [27] reviewed 470 biopsy specimens and noted that 20 had IgA as the predominant localizing immunoglobulin. Eleven of their patients were less than 16 years of age. In the study, there were 54 bilateral nephrectomies, but none of the kidneys that had been removed exhibited IgA. In half of the patients, IgA was the most intensely localized globulin, but IgG was found with IgG and IgM. Localization of C3, frequently of substantial intensity, was seen in 17 of 20 specimens, and 14 of 15 specimens were positive for properdin. The immunoglobulins were localized predominantly in the mesangium; C3 was distributed in axial regions of the glomerulus and along the basement membrane of Bowman's capsule.

Light microscopy showed a generalized proliferative glomerulonephritis in 2 patients, but most showed focal proliferative glomerulonephritis. Several patients had repeat biopsy specimens taken; only one showed progressive global sclerosis of the glomeruli.

Electron microscopy showed that the most striking alterations were found in the mesangial regions, where there was an increase in mesangial matrix deposits and an increase in mesangial cellularity. Electron-dense deposits were prominent in the mesangial matrix, in the axial or hilar regions of the glomerulus, and in the intramembranous position along Bowman's capsule.

Roy et al. [40] were not sure of the immunologic pathogenesis of IgA in the mesangium. They stated that immunoglobulins and complement components in the mesangium in recurrent macroscopic hematuria may be associated with an antigen of an immune complex, but that the immune reactants may be a nonspecific consequence of injury due to other mechanisms.

Hyman et al. [19] regard the immunologic role of IgA as unclear. IgA seldom is the only localized immunoglobulin in diseased glomeruli; therefore, if IgG and IgM do have a pathogenetic role in glomerulopathies, it is difficult to implicate IgA itself as a single or major cause of glomerular lesions.

Lowance and associates [26] believed that IgA was pathogenetically involved in the nephritis of their patients because of the uniformity of IgA distribution in involved kidneys and its presence with or without other immunoglobulins or serum proteins. They also admitted that IgA could be a secondary passive phenomenon but that it was the only immunoglobulin in 3 patients and that the distribution of IgA was constant and not random in all 15 of their patients.

McCoy et al. [27] insisted that this nephropathy should be designated as IgA nephropathy because IgA is the only constant immunoglobulin, inasmuch as C3 is not confined to the mesangium.

Kaplan and Kaplan [20] reported nephritis associated with gammopathies: a 49-year-old coal miner presented with the nephrotic syndrome and was noted later to have a monoclonal gammopathy of the IgG type. His renal lesion was a proliferative glomerulonephritis that progressed to a chronic glomerulonephritis and renal failure, which necessitated chronic dialysis.

We are unaware of any additional reports of gammopathies producing childhood renal disease.

References

1. Adam, C., Morel-Maroger, L., and Richet, R. Cryoglobulins in glomerulonephritis not related to systemic disease. *Kidney Int.* 3:334, 1973.
2. Ado, M. A., Polyantseva, L. R., Mukhin, N. A., Tareeva, I. E., and Dvoretskova, L. K. α_2-macroglobulin in patients with the nephrotic syndrome. *Ter. Arkh.* 45:94, 1973.
3. Alexander, J. W., and Good, R. A. *Immunology for Surgeons.* Philadelphia: Saunders, 1970.
4. Anttila, R. Renal involvement in juvenile rheumatoid arthritis: A clinical and histopathologic study. *Acta Paediatr. Scand.* [Suppl.] 227:1, 1972.
5. Barnett, E. V., Bluestone, R., Cracchiolo, A., III, Goldberg, L. S., Kantor, G. L., and McIntosh, R. M. Cryoglobulinemia and disease. *Ann. Intern. Med.* 73: 95, 1970.
6. Berger, J., and Hinglais, N. Les dépôts intercapillaires d'IgA-IgG. *J. Urol. Nephrol. (Paris)* 74:694, 1968.
7. Burman, D., Hodson, A. K., Wood, C. B. S., and Brueton, N. F. W. Acute anaphylaxis, pulmonary oedema, and intravascular haemolysis due to cryoprecipitate. *Arch. Dis. Child.* 48:483, 1973.
8. Čejka, J., Bollinger, R. O., Schuit, H. R. E., Lusher, J. M., Chang, C.-H., and Zuelzer, W. W. Macroglobulinemia in a child with acute leukemia. *Blood* 43:191, 1974.
9. Costea, N., Yakulis, V. J., Libnoch, J. A., Pilz, C. G., and Heller, P. Two myeloma globulins (IgG & IgA) in one subject and one cell line. *Am. J. Med.* 42:630, 1967.
10. Dall'Aglio, P., Olivetti, G., and Migone, L. Correlazioni fra reperti immunoistochimici ed ultrastrutturali in nefrologia. *Minerva Nefrol.* 20:211, 1973.
11. Druet, P., Letonturier, P., Contet, A., and Mandet, C. Comparaison entre la composition des dépôts glomérulaires et celle des cryoprotéines sériques. *Minerva Nefrol.* 20:193, 1973.
12. Druet, P., Letonturier, P., Contet, A., and Mandet, C. Cryoglobulinemia in human renal diseases: A study of seventy-six cases. *Clin. Exp. Immunol.* 15:483, 1973.
13. Feizi, T., and Gitlin, N. Immune-complex disease of the kidney associated with chronic hepatitis and cryoglobulinaemia. *Lancet* 2:873, 1969.
14. Ghosh, L., and Muehrcke, R. C. The nephrotic syn-

drome: A prodrome to lymphoma. *Ann. Intern. Med.* 72:379, 1970.

15. Grupe, W. E. IgG-B$_1$C cryoglobulins in acute glomerulonephritis. *Pediatrics* 42:474, 1968.

16. Hanauer, L. B., and Christian, C. L. Studies of cryoproteins in systemic lupus erythematosus. *J. Clin. Invest.* 46:400, 1967.

17. Hancock, M. P., Huntley, C. C., and Sever, J. L. Congenital rubella syndrome with immunoglobulin disorder. *J. Pediatr.* 72:636, 1968.

18. Humphrey, J. H., and White, R. G. *Immunology for Students of Medicine* (3rd ed.). Oxford: Blackwell, 1970.

19. Hyman, L. R., Wagnild, J. P., Beirne, G. J., and Burkholder, P. M. Immunoglobulin-A distribution in glomerular disease: Analysis of immunofluorescence localization and pathogenetic significance. *Kidney Int.* 3:397, 1973.

20. Kaplan, N. G., and Kaplan, K. C. Monoclonal gammopathy, glomerulonephritis, and the nephrotic syndrome. *Arch. Intern. Med.* 125:696, 1970.

21. Kyle, R. A. Personal communication.

22. Lerner, A. B., and Watson, C. J. Studies of cryoglobulins. I. Unusual purpura associated with the presence of a high concentration of cryoglobulin (cold precipitable serum globulin). *Am. J. Med. Sci.* 214:410, 1947.

23. Lewis, E. J., and Couser, W. G. The immunologic basis of human renal disease. *Pediatr. Clin. North Am.* 18:467, 1971.

24. Lin, J. H., Orofino, D., Sherlock, J., Letteri, J., and Duffy, J. L. Waldenström's macroglobulinemia, mesangio-capillary glomerulonephritis, angiitis, and myositis. *Nephron* 10:262, 1973.

25. Lindqvist, K. J., Ragab, A. H., and Osterland, C. K. Paraproteinemia in a child with leukemia. *Blood* 35:213, 1970.

26. Lowance, D. C., Mullins, J. D., and McPhaul, J. J., Jr. Immunoglobulin A (IgA) associated glomerulonephritis. *Kidney Int.* 3:167, 1973.

27. McCoy, R. C., Abramowsky, C. R., and Tisher, C. C. IgA nephropathy. *Am. J. Pathol.* 76:123, 1974.

28. McEnery, P. T., McAdams, A. J., and West, C. D. Glomerular morphology, natural history, and treatment of children with IgA-IgG mesangial nephropathy. *Perspect. Nephrol. Hypertension* 1:305, 1973.

29. McIntosh, R. M., Gross, M., Laplante, M., Kaufman, D. B., and Kulvinskas, C. Cryoproteins in immune complex disease: Role of nephrectomy and implications in recurrent glomerulonephritis in human transplants. *Exp. Med. Surg.* 29:108, 1971.

30. McIntosh, R. M., and Grossman, B. IgG, β_1C, fibrinogen, cryoprotein in acute glomerulonephritis. *N. Engl. J. Med.* 285:1521, 1971.

31. McIntosh, R. M., Kaufman, D. B., Kulvinskas, C., and Grossman, B. J. Cryoglobulins. I. Studies on the nature, incidence, and clinical significance of serum cryoproteins in glomerulonephritis. *J. Lab. Clin. Med.* 75:566, 1970.

32. McIntosh, R. M., Kulvinskas, C., and Kaufman, D. B. Cryoglobulins. II. The biological and chemical properties of cryoproteins in acute post-streptococcal glomerulonephritis. *Int. Arch. Allergy Appl. Immunol.* 41:700, 1971.

33. Meltzer, M., Franklin, E. C., Elias, K., McCluskey, R. T., and Cooper, N. Cryoglobulinemia—a clinical and laboratory study. II. Cryoglobulins with rheumatoid factor activity. *Am. J. Med.* 40:837, 1966.

34. Merrill, J. P. Glomerulonephritis (second of three parts). *N. Engl. J. Med.* 290:313, 1974.

35. Morel-Maroger, L., Basch, A., Danon, F., Verroust, P., and Richet, G. Pathology of the kidney in Waldenström's macroglobulinemia. *N. Engl. J. Med.* 283:123, 1970.

36. Muggia, F. M., and Ultmann, J. E. Glomerulonephritis or nephrotic syndrome in malignant lymphoma, reticulum-cell type. *Lancet* 1:805, 1971.

37. Pien, F. D., Smith, T. F., Taswell, H. F., and Hable, K. A. Cold-reactive antibodies in a case of congenital cytomegalovirus infection. *Am. J. Clin. Pathol.* 61:352, 1974.

38. Porush, J. G., Grishman, E., Alter, A. A., Mandelbaum, H., and Churg, J. Paraproteinemia and cryoglobulinemia associated with atypical glomerulonephritis and the nephrotic syndrome. *Am. J. Med.* 47:957, 1969.

39. Richet, G., Adam, C., and Morel-Maroger, L. Cryoglobulines au cours de glomérulonéphrites prolifératives diffuses. *Minerva Nefrol.* 20:243, 1973.

40. Roy, L. P., Fish, A. J., Vernier, R. L., and Michael, A. F. Recurrent macroscopic hematuria, focal nephritis, and mesangial deposition of immunoglobulin and complement. *J. Pediatr.* 82:767, 1973.

41. Schubert, G. E. Die Plasmocytomniere. I. Häufigkeit pathologisch-anatomischer Veranderungen. II. Vergleich von Struktur und Funktion unter besonderer Berücksichtigung des akuten Nierenversagens. *Klin. Wochenschr.* 52:763, 771, 1974.

42. Stiehm, E. R., and Fulginiti, V. A. *Immunologic Disorders in Infants and Children.* Philadelphia: Saunders, 1973. Pp. 46–47.

43. Stoop, J. W., Zegers, B. J. M., van der Heiden, C., and Ballieux, R. E. Monoclonal gammopathy in a child with leukemia. *Blood* 32:774, 1968.

44. Strauss, J., Koss, M., Griswold, W., Chernack, W., Pardo, V., and McIntosh, R. M. Cryoprecipitable immune complexes, nephropathy, and sickle-cell disease (letter to the editor). *Ann. Intern. Med.* 81:114, 1974.

45. Tarantino, A., Barbiano Di Belgiojoso, G., Durante, A., Imbasciati, E., and Bazzi, C. Caratterizzazione immuno-istologica delle nefropatie glomerulari, valutata mediante la metodica diretta ed indiretta. *Minerva Nefrol.* 20:199, 1973.

46. Törnroth, T., and Skrifvars, B. Ultrastructural changes in acute nonstreptococcal glomerulonephritis associated with mixed cryoglobulinemia. *Exp. Mol. Pathol.* 19:160, 1973.

47. Wager, O., Mustakallio, K. K., and Räsänen, J. A. Mixed IgA-IgG cryoglobulinemia: Immunological studies and case reports of three patients. *Am. J. Med.* 44:179, 1968.

48. Weinberg, A. G., McCracken, G. H., Jr., LoSpalluto, J., and Luby, J. P. Monoclonal macroglobulinemia and cytomegalic inclusion disease. *Pediatrics* 51:518, 1973.

49. Wintrobe, M. M., and Buell, M. V. Hyperproteinemia associated with multiple myeloma: With report of a case in which an extraordinary hyperproteinemia was associated with thrombosis of the retinal veins and symptoms suggesting Raynaud's disease. *Bull. Johns Hopkins Hosp.* 52:156, 1933.

68. The Kidney in Lysosomal Storage Diseases

G. A. Grabowski
and R. J. Desnick

The lysosomal storage diseases constitute a family of more than 30 disorders related by their molecular pathology. Each of these recessively inherited diseases is characterized by hypertrophied lysosomes engorged with a particular substrate(s) resulting from the defective activity of a specific lysosomal enzyme (Table 68-1). Normally, these hydrolytic enzymes completely degrade complex macromolecules, such as glycosphingolipids, glycoproteins, glycogen, and mucopolysaccharides, to their simple components (amino acids, monosaccharides, fatty acids, etc.) [17]. In each of these inborn errors of metabolism, the accumulation of a particular substrate is dependent on its occurrence in specific tissues and its normal rate of metabolic turnover.

Pathophysiologically, the continued deposition of substrate in the lysosomes of a particular cell or tissue leads to lysosomal hypertrophy and hyperplasia. The accumulation of these engorged lysosomes eventually cause impairment of normal cellular and physiologic processes. For example, the early and progressive neurologic involvement in Tay-Sachs disease, G_{M2} gangliosidosis, type 1, results from the accumulation of G_{M2} ganglioside in neural tissues, where it is rapidly synthesized and normally catabolized. Analogously, the cardiovascular-renal manifestations in Fabry's disease result from the deposition of trihexosyl ceramide in the visceral endothelium. The neurologic involvement in these patients is secondary to cerebrovascular disease, since the Fabry glycosphingolipid substrate does not normally occur in neural tissues. Patients with certain disorders, e.g., Sandhoff's disease and G_{M2} gangliosidosis, type 2, exhibit systemic manifestations, reflecting the generalized deposition of the pathologic substrate(s) in both neural and visceral tissues.

Renal accumulation of substrate in almost all the lysosomal storage diseases can be demonstrated by histochemical, ultrastructural, or biochemical techniques. In some of these disorders, the lysosomal abnormalities result in clinically manifest renal disease; the others rarely are associated with

renal failure, explainable perhaps by the absence of glomerular sclerosis in the latter group. It is the objective of this chapter to present the major biochemical and morphologic abnormalities in each of these disorders, with primary emphasis on those with clinically significant renal involvement. More comprehensive reviews are available on the structure and function of the lysosomal apparatus [27] and the molecular pathology of the lysosomopathies [27, 38].

Disorders of Glycosphingolipid Metabolism

FABRY'S DISEASE

Fabry's disease (defective α-galactosidase A activity) is an inborn error of glycosphingolipid metabolism (Fig. 68-1) resulting from the defective activity of the lysosomal enzyme, α-galactosidase A (see [22] for a comprehensive review). The enzymatic defect, transmitted by an X-linked gene, leads to the progressive deposition of trihexosyl ceramide in the lysosomes of endothelial, perithelial, and smooth-muscle cells of the cardiovascular-renal system and, to a lesser extent, in reticuloendothelial, myocardial, and connective-tissue cells. Epithelial cells of the cornea, kidney, and other tissues contain accumulations, as do the ganglion and perineural cells of the autonomic nervous system.

The clinical manifestations of Fabry's disease are the sequelae of the anatomic and physiologic alterations produced by the progressive deposition of glycosphingolipids in the tissues. Onset of the disease in hemizygous males usually occurs during childhood or adolescence, with periodic crises of severe pain in the extremities, the appearance of vascular cutaneous lesions, angiokeratoma, hypohidrosis, and the characteristic corneal dystrophy. With increasing age, the major morbid symptoms of the disease result from the progressive infiltration of glycosphingolipid in the cardiovascular-renal system. Death usually occurs in the third or fourth decade of life from renal, cardiac, or cerebral complications of the vascular disease. Hetero-

The experimental work described in this review was supported in part by grants from The National Foundation–March of Dimes (I-273 and C-174), the American Heart Association (74-915), the National Institutes of Health (AM 15174), and the Clinical Research Centers Program of the Division of Research Resources, National Institutes of Health (RR-400).

Table 68-1. *Inherited Disorders of the Lysosome*

Disease	Defective Enzyme(s)	Major Accumulated Substrates or Lysosomal Defects	Major Phenotypic Manifestations	Major Renal Manifestations
		Defects of Specific Lysosomal Hydrolases		
I. Lipidoses				
A. *Glycosidase deficiencies*				
1. Ceramidetrihexosidosis (Fabry)	α-Galactosidase A [8]	Galactosyl-galactosyl-glucosylceramide; digalactosylceramide	Juvenile onset; angiokeratoma; corneal opacity; acroparathesias; renal and cardiovascular insufficiency; death usually in 4th decade; X-linked inheritance	Endothelial and epithelial glycosphingolipid deposits in glomerulus and renal blood vessels resulting in end-stage kidney disease
2. Glucocerebrosidoses				
a. Type 1 (adult Gaucher)	β-Glucosidase [11]	Glucosylceramide; glucosylsphingosine; sialyl lactosylceramide	Juvenile or adult onset; hepatosplenomegaly; thrombocytopenia; bone erosion and pain; avascular necrosis of hip; Gaucher cells in bone marrow	Large, pale Gaucher cells scattered in glomerulus and interstitium of cortex and medulla
b. Type 2 (infantile Gaucher)	β-Glucosidase [9]	Same as type 1	Infantile onset; severe psychomotor retardation; hepatosplenomegaly; Gaucher cells in bone marrow; death by 2 yr	Same as type 1
c. Type 3 (juvenile Gaucher)	β-Glucosidase [29]	Same as type 1	Juvenile onset; hepatosplenomegaly; moderate neurologic involvement; Gaucher cells in bone marrow	Same as type 1
3. Galactocerebrosidosis (Krabbe)	β-Galactosidase [83]	Galactosylceramide Galactosyl-sphingosine	Infantile onset; severe psychomotor retardation; progressive spasticity; seizures rare; failure to thrive; death by 2 yr	Normal
4. G$_{M2}$ gangliosidoses				
a. Type 1 (Tay-Sachs)	β-N-acetyl-hexosaminidase A [64]	G$_{M2}$ ganglioside; asialo-G$_{M2}$ ganglioside	Infantile onset before 1 yr; severe psychomotor retardation; seizures; blindness; startle response to sound; cherry-red macula; Jewish predilection; no visceromegaly; death by 5 yr	Minimal glomerular deposition
b. Type 2 (Sandhoff)	β-N-acetyl-hexosaminidase A and B [73]	G$_{M2}$ ganglioside; asialo-G$_{M2}$ ganglioside; globoside	Same as type 1; no Jewish predilection; in addition, hepatosplenomegaly; cardiomyopathy	PAS(+) granules in glomerulus, capsular and tubular epithelium. Eosinophilic bodies in collecting tubules
c. Type 3 (juvenile)	β-N-acetyl-hexosaminidase A (partial deficiency?) [58]	G$_{M2}$ ganglioside; asialo-G$_{M2}$ ganglioside	Late infantile onset (2–6 yr); progressive psychomotor retardation; seizures; blindness; startle response to sound; death by 15 yr	Not reported
5. G$_{M1}$ gangliosidoses				
a. Type 1 (Landing disease)	β-Galactosidase [63]	G$_{M1}$ ganglioside; asialo-G$_{M1}$ ganglioside; keratan sulfate–like mucopolysaccharide; asialo-glycoproteins.	Onset in infancy; severe psychomotor retardation; blindness; cherry-red macula; startle response to sound; dysostosis multiplex; vacuolated lymphocytes; hepatosplenomegaly; death by 2 yr	Keratan sulfate–like deposits in glomerular and tubular epithelium. Vacuolization of tubules. Late renal dysfunction

Disease	Enzyme deficiency	Stored material	Clinical manifestations	Pathology
b. Type 2	β-Galactosidase [91]	Same as type 1	Onset at 6–20 months; same as type 1, but milder or attenuated manifestations	Not reported
B. Sulfatase deficiencies				
1. Metachromatic leukodystrophies				
a. Late infantile	Arylsulfatase A [3]	Galactosylsulfatide; lactosylsulfatide	Onset between 12 and 18 months; progressive neurologic deterioration; weakness; incoordination; spasticity; death by 15 yr	Glomerulus normal. Metachromatic granules in proximal convoluted tubule, loop of Henle. Metachromatic casts
b. Juvenile	Arylsulfatase A [80]	Same as late infantile	Juvenile onset; progressive neurologic deterioration; spasticity; loss of deep tendon reflexes	Not reported
c. Adult	Arylsulfatase A [1]	Same as late infantile	Onset in adolescence or adult life; neurologic deterioration; associated with psychosis; corticobulbar involvement	Not reported
2. Multiple sulfatase deficiency	Arylsulfatases A and B Sterol sulfatase [2]	Sulfatides; sulfated glycosaminoglycans; steroid sulfate	Infantile onset; progressive psychomotor deterioration; seizures; hepatomegaly; dysostosis multiplex	Not reported
C. Esterase and deacylase deficiencies				
1. Ceramidosis (Farber)	Ceramidase [81]	Ceramide	Infantile onset; psychomotor retardation; arthropathy; swollen joints with subcutaneous nodules; death by 2 yr	Not reported
2. Sphingomyelinoses (Niemann-Pick)				
a. Type A	Sphingomyelinase [10]	Sphingomyelin; lyso-bis-phosphatidic acid; cholesterol	Infantile onset; severe psychomotor retardation; cherry-red macula (50%); hepatosplenomegaly; vacuolated lymphocytes; marrow foam cells; Jewish predilection; death by 4 yr	Rare vacuolated glomerular cell. Swollen epithelial cells of glomerulus
b. Type B	Sphingomyelinase [74]	Same as type A	Infantile onset; no CNS involvement; hepatosplenomegaly; some patients may live into adulthood	Not reported
c. Type C	Unknown	Sphingomyelin, cholesterol	Onset 1–6 yr; psychomotor retardation; hepatosplenomegaly; foam cells; death between 5 and 15 yr	Not reported
d. Type D	Unknown	Same as type C	Nova Scotian variant of type C with infantile onset; early jaundice	Not reported
3. Acid esterase deficiency (Wolman)	Acid esterase [66]	Cholesterol esters; triglycerides; cholesterol	Infantile onset; hepatosplenomegaly; adrenal calcification; death by 6 months	Not reported

Table 68-1. (Continued)

Disease	Defective Enzyme(s)	Major Accumulated Substrates or Lysosomal Defects	Major Phenotypic Manifestations	Major Renal Manifestations
		Defects of Specific Lysosomal Hydrolases		
II. Mucopolysaccharidoses				
1. MPS I-H (Hurler)	α-L-Iduronidase [5]	Dermatan sulfate; heparan sulfate	Infantile onset; characteristic craniofacial dysmorphism; mental retardation; dysostosis multiplex; growth retardation; corneal opacities; hepatosplenomegaly; death by 20 yr	Metachromatic granules in glomerular epithelium
2. MPS I-S (Scheie)	α-L-Iduronidase [4]	Same as I-H	Same as MPS I-H, except normal intelligence; moderate short stature; normal life span	Not reported
3. MPS II (Hunter)				
a. Type A	Sulfoiduronate sulfatase [4]	Dermatan sulfate; heparan sulfate	Similar to, but milder than, B; normal-to-mild retardation; survival up to 60 yr; X-linked inheritance	Not reported
b. Type B	Sulfoiduronate sulfatase [4]	Same as type IIA	Infantile onset; mental retardation; hepatosplenomegaly; dysostosis multiplex; no corneal opacities; death by 20 yr; X-lined inheritance	Not reported
4. MPS III (Sanfilippo)				
a. Type A.	Heparan-N-sulfate sulfatase [44]	Heparan sulfate	Onset noted by 4 yr; severe neurologic involvement; dysostosis multiplex; hepatosplenomegaly; clear corneas; death by 20 yr	Not reported
b. Type B	α-N-acetylglucosaminidase [60]	Same as type IIIA		
5. MPS IV (Morquio)	Chondroitin-6-sulfate sulfatase [50]	Keratan sulfate	Severe growth retardation by 2 yr; severe skeletal abnormalities; corneal opacities; normal intelligence	Not reported
6. MPS VI (Maroteaux-Lamy)				
a. Type A	Chondroitin-4-sulfate sulfatase [61]	Dermatan sulfate	Mild form of type B	Not reported
b. Type B	Chondroitin-4-sulfate sulfatase [61]	Same as type VI A	Infantile onset, type I-H-like phenotype; mild dysostosis multiplex; growth retardation; normal intelligence	Not reported
7. MPH VII (Sly)	β-Glucuronidase [35]	Chondroitin-4-sulfate Chondroitin-6-sulfate	Onset noted by age 2 yr; moderate psychomotor retardation; dysostosis multiplex; short stature; hepatosplenomegaly	Not reported
III. Glycoproteinoses				
1. Mannosidosis	α-Mannosidases A and B [62]	Mannose-rich oligosaccharides and glycopeptides	Infantile-to-juvenile onset; psychomotor retardation; deafness; dysostosis multiplex; recurrent infections; vacuolated lymphocytes	Not reported

Disorder	Enzyme defect [ref]	Substance accumulated	Clinical features	Morphology
2. Fucosidosis	α-L-Fucosidase [88]	Fucose-rich glycolipids; glycoproteins and glycosaminoglycans	Infantile onset; progressive psychomotor retardation; spasticity; mild dysostosis multiplex; hepatomegaly; angiokeratoma	Not reported
3. Aspartylglycosaminuria	4-L-Aspartylglycosylamine aminohydrolase [41]	Aspartylglycosylamine; aspartylglycosylamine-containing oligosaccharides	Infantile onset; mental retardation; mild dysostosis multiplex; recurrent infections; vacuolated lymphocytes	Not reported
IV. Glycogenosis Type II (Pompe)	α-Glucosidase [37]	Glycogen	Infantile onset; cardiomegaly; muscular weakness; failure to thrive	Lysosomal and cytoplasmic monoparticulate glycogen in epithelium of glomerulus and tubules. Some foot processes destroyed. Renal function normal
V. Other				
1. Lysosomal acid phosphatase deficiency	Acid phosphatase [55]	Not characterized	Failure to thrive; seizures; hepatomegaly	Not reported
2. Total acid phosphatase deficiency	Acid phosphatase [56]	Not characterized	Onset in newborn; lethargy; opisthotonus; death in first days of life	Not reported
3. Cystinosis	Unknown	Cystine	Infantile onset; renal failure; rickets; growth retardation by 1 yr; corneal cystine deposits; death before puberty	See Chap. 81

Defects of Lysosomal Apparatus

Disorder	Enzyme defect	Substance accumulated	Clinical features	Morphology
I. Mucolipidoses				
A. Type II (I-cell; Leroy disease)	Unknown	Inclusion bodies and most lysosomal hydrolases decreased in cultured skin fibroblasts with concomitantly increased lysosomal hydrolases in culture media; elevated plasma levels of most lysosomal hydrolases	Infantile onset; dysostosis multiplex; short stature (<80 cm); mild-to-severe psychomotor retardation; gingival hypertrophy; death usually in childhood	Vacuoles in glomerulus and proximal convoluted tubule epithelium. Basement membrane normal. Foot processes normal. Vacuolated interstitial fibroblasts
B. Type III (pseudo-Hurler polydystrophy)	Unknown	Similar to mucolipidosis II	Juvenile onset; mild mental retardation; dysostosis multiplex; restriction of joint mobility; ± corneal opacities	Not reported
II. Chediak-Higashi	Unknown	Increased rate of phagocytosis by granulocytes, melanocytes and Schwann cells; decreased rate of intralysosomal degradation	Susceptibility to infection; peripheral neuropathy; seizures and retardation; albinism common; death before adulthood	Not reported

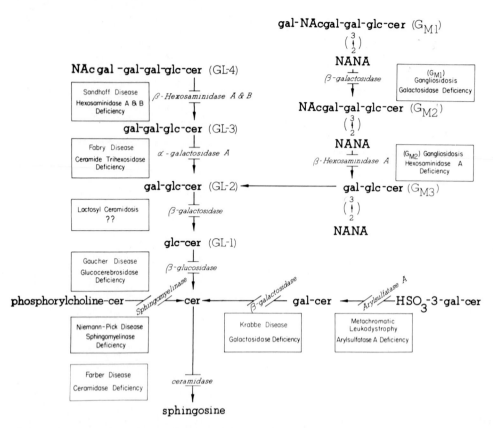

Figure 68-1. Catabolism of glycosphingolipids and the inborn glycosphingolipidoses. (Cer = ceramide; gal = galactose; glc = glucose; NAcgal = N-acetylgalactosamine; NANA = N-acetylneuraminic acid.)

zygous females, who may exhibit the disease in an attenuated form, are most likely to show only corneal opacities.

Early glycosphingolipid deposits antedate clinical signs and symptoms; the lesions of the renal vasculature are less prominent than those of the nephron, and renal architecture is maintained. The early abnormalities in renal function have their basis in these lesions; the later and more severe renal changes are the result of glomerular sclerosis, progressive vascular lesions, and hypertension. During childhood and adolescence, proteinuria occurs, and casts, red cells, and desquamated kidney and urinary tract cells may appear in the urinary sediment. Birefringent, lipid globules with characteristic "Maltese crosses" within and outside cells can be observed in the urine and sediment by polarization microscopy. Mild proteinuria may be explained by alteration of the glomerular epithelial cells and their foot processes [51] or by increased desquamation of lipid-laden tubular epithelial cells.

With advancing age, progressive renal impairment is evidenced by significant proteinuria, decreased glomerular filtration rate, and alterations of renal tubular function [65]. Loss of renal concentrating ability, with polyuria [14, 36] and polydypsia [36, 89, 90], may occur well in advance of a significant decrease in glomerular filtration or evidence of renal failure [65]. The occasional development of a diabetes insipidus–like syndrome, which is not related to faulty electrolyte transfer in the distal tubules, may be the result of tubular insensitivity to antidiuretic hormone [36] or to combined dysfunction of the renal tubular cells and lesions of the glycosphingolipid-laden supraoptic nucleus, an antidiuretic center of the hypothalamus [65].

The progressive deposition of glycosphingolipid in the kidney results in gradual deterioration of renal function and development of azotemia in the second to fourth decade of life. Death most often results from uremia unless chronic hemodialysis or renal transplantation is undertaken.

On pathologic examination, the accumulation of glycosphingolipids in the kidney is seen as a progressive process, the earliest documentation of which was found in the examination of a 3-year-old heterozygote [84]. The early lesions are due to the accumulation of glycosphingolipid in endothelial and epithelial cells of the glomerulus and of Bowman's space and in the epithelium of the loops of Henle and of the distal tubules (Fig. 68-2). In later stages and to a lesser degree, the proximal tubules [51, 90], interstitial histiocytes, and fibrocytes [70] may show an accumulation of lipid (Fig. 68-3). Lipid-laden distal tubular epithelial cells desquamate and may be detected in the urinary sediment [20].

Concurrently, renal blood vessels are also involved progressively and often extensively. Other histologic changes in the kidney are the sequelae of nonspecific, severe end-stage renal disease, with evidence of severe arteriolosclerosis, glomerular atrophy and fibrosis, pseudotubular proliferation of residual glomerular epithelium, tubular atrophy, and diffuse interstitial fibrosis. Ultrastructural studies of the lipid inclusions in the kidney have been reported, and reviews of the renal involvement are available [30, 36, 47, 51, 53, 65].

All suspect hemizygotes should be confirmed biochemically by the demonstration of markedly deficient α-galactosidase A activities in plasma or serum [18], leukocytes [7, 18, 33, 43], tears [42], biopsy specimens, or cultured skin fibroblasts [6, 18, 39, 72, 92]. Alternatively, glycosphingolipid analyses can be accomplished to demonstrate the increased levels of trihexosyl ceramide in urinary sediment [21, 25, 33, 47, 69], plasma [22], or cultured skin fibroblasts [15]. Suspect heterozygotes should be biochemically identified by the intermediate levels of α-galactosidase activity in the preceding sources.

Prenatal diagnosis of Fabry's disease has been accomplished by amniocentesis at approximately 14 weeks of gestation, by biochemical analysis of the amniotic fluid components [12, 23, 24]. The minimal requirements for the prenatal diagnosis of an affected hemizygous male fetus are the demonstration of deficient α-galactosidase A activity and an XY karyotype in cultured amniotic cells.

Since renal insufficiency is the most frequent late complication in patients with this disease, chronic hemodialysis and renal transplantation have become lifesaving procedures. In addition to treatment of the renal failure, kidney transplantation has been undertaken to determine if the allo-

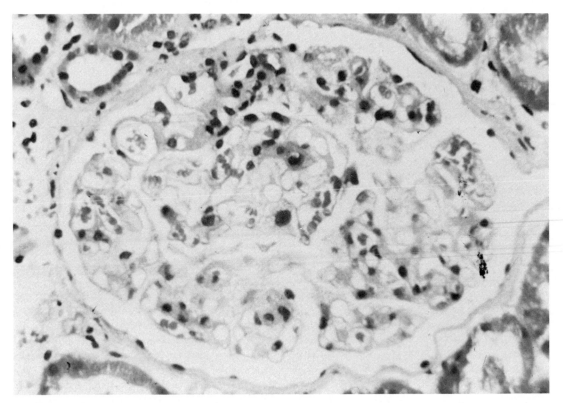

Figure 68-2. Photomicrograph of a glomerulus from a hemizygote with Fabry's disease. The epithelial cells of the parietal and visceral layers of Bowman's capsule show multiple vacuoles from which the accumulated glycosphingolipid substrate was extracted. (×500.) (Courtesy Dr. J. G. White, University of Minnesota.)

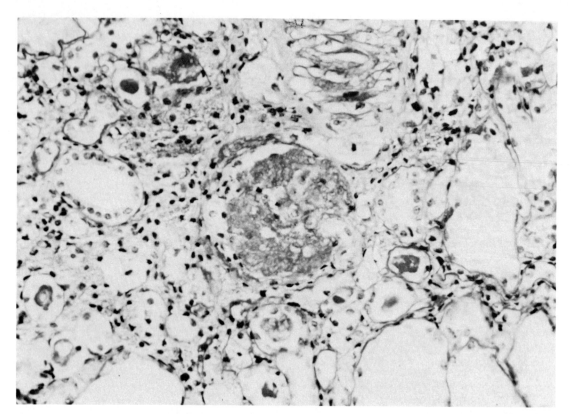

Figure 68-3. Photomicrograph of a section of renal tissue from a hemizygote with Fabry's disease showing end-stage renal disease. (×250.)

graft could provide normal α-galactosidase A for substrate metabolism [19]. Hypothetically, the normal kidney might metabolize the accumulated substrate by uptake and catabolism within the allograft, or by the release of the active enzyme into the circulation for uptake and metabolism in other tissues, such as the vascular endothelium. Although biochemical and clinical improvement has been reported in several recipients [19, 67], no biochemical effect could be demonstrated in others [78, 86]. Thus, the use of renal allografts to alter the rate of progressive accumulation of substrate remains controversial, and further studies are required to determine the long-term biochemical effects of this strategy. In view of these results, renal transplantation should be undertaken only in patients with clinically significant renal failure. At present, the most practical and effective therapy is preventive. Therefore, screening of all suspect heterozygotes, genetic counseling, and prenatal diagnostic studies should be made available to all families at risk.

G_{M1} GANGLIOSIDOSIS, TYPE 1
G_{M1} gangliosidosis, type 1 (defective β-galactosidase activity), presents a unique phenotype among the lysosomal storage disorders. Many of the clinical manifestations are reminiscent of both the cerebral lipidoses and the mucopolysaccharidoses. The presentation of neonatal seizures or poor feeding, a "Hurler-like" facial dysmorphia, and cherry-red maculae signal the clinical diagnosis. These infants suffer from severe psychomotor retardation and usually die by 2 years of age [59, 87]. Hepatosplenomegaly, dysostosis multiplex, and bone marrow macrophages are present at birth, indicating the systemic accumulation of G_{M1} ganglioside and a keratan sulfate–like mucopolysaccharide [57, 64, 77]. Diagnostic confirmation requires the demonstration of deficient β-galactosidase activity in peripheral blood leukocytes; prenatal diagnosis has been accomplished.

The renal pathologic findings in G_{M1} gangliosidosis are attributable to the lysosomal accumulation in the glomerular epithelial cells of the amorphous keratan sulfate–like mucopolysaccharide and asialo-glycoproteins [45, 52, 57, 75]. On histologic examination, cytoplasmic ballooning of epithelial cells is variably present in the proximal convoluted tubule and loop of Henle [45, 52], and the severity is age-related [75], as is renal mass [45]. The glomerular lesions of G_{M1} gangliosidosis are remarkably reminiscent of those in Fabry's disease (Fig. 68-4).

Ultrastructural studies [52, 75, 76] reveal substrate-engorged lysosomes that are extensive in the glomerular epithelium and proximal convoluted tubule, with less involvement of arteriolar smooth muscle [52]. In addition, small amounts of lamellar, lipidlike material have been found in the epithelial cells of the glomerulus and proximal convoluted tubule [52, 57, 59].

G_{M1} ganglioside is increased twentyfold to fiftyfold in the liver and spleen [82]. Presumably, the primary accumulated substrates in the kidney are the keratan sulfate–like material and asialoglycoproteins; these substrates are consistent with the histochemical and morphologic observations of large amounts of amorphous, PAS-positive material in renal lysosomes.

Although the renal histologic lesions are extensive, impairment of renal function is not typically described in G_{M1} gangliosidosis. Only one case report [52] has documented preterminal decreases in creatinine clearance, with glycosuria and aminoaciduria, presumably due to proximal tubular dysfunction. More severe renal abnormalities may possibly be found if these children survive longer, as suggested by the renomegaly in the older children who have died from this disease [45].

G_{M2} GANGLIOSIDOSIS, TYPE 2 (SANDHOFF'S DISEASE)

Sandhoff's disease (defective β-hexosaminidase A and B activities) presents at 3 to 9 months of age with failure to thrive. While many clinical features are shared by Sandhoff's and Tay-Sachs diseases, the organomegaly secondary to the storage of globoside clearly distinguishes Sandhoff's disease. Death usually occurs by 5 years of age due to intercurrent pulmonary infections [26].

On pathologic examination, small granules that stain positive with Luxol fast blue, hematoxylin and eosin, Sudan IV, and PAS are seen in the glomerulus, tubules, and vascular endothelial cells. The epithelial cells of the glomerulus and tubules have patchy granular involvement, except for sparing of the lower collecting tubules [28]. Near the papilla, large round eosinophilic bodies are described as being larger than the nuclei and staining

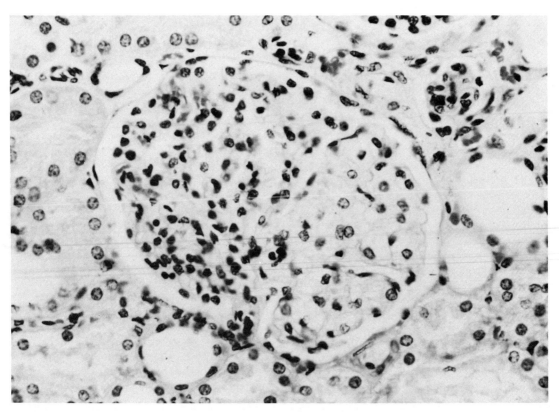

Figure 68-4. Photomicrograph of a glomerulus from a homozygote with G_{M1} gangliosidosis, type 1, showing the cytoplasmic vacuolation of the epithelial cells. Note the similarity to the glomerular pathologic findings in Fabry's disease, Fig. 68-2. ($\times$500.) (Courtesy Dr. J. H. Sung, University of Minnesota.)

faintly with Sudan IV. Ultrastructurally, these inclusions are lysosomes containing membranous lamellar osmophilic concretions similar to the cytoplasmic inclusion bodies observed in neurons from Tay-Sachs disease [28].

The deficient activities of β-hexosaminidase A and B (see Fig. 68-1) in the kidney correlate well with the reported accumulation of globoside and the abnormal excretion of N-acetylneuraminic acid and galactosamine-rich oligosaccharides [73]. There is no functional impairment.

METACHROMATIC LEUKODYSTROPHY

Metachromatic leukodystrophy (defective arylsulfatase A activity) is an insidious disease of the nervous system that presents with difficulties with gait or coordination in the first to fourth year of life [2]. While early development is normal, involvement of the nervous system leads to progression to a vegetative state by 7 to 10 years of age; death occurs some years later [34].

The major clinical pathologic changes are confined to the nervous system; however, on pathologic examination, lesions have been found in the liver, gallbladder, adrenal glands, pituitary, and kidney. Renal lesions characteristically are confined to the tubular system; the proximal convoluted tubules, loops of Henle, and collecting tubules have a patchy distention of the cytoplasm by metachromatic granules [2]. Resibois's [71] elegant ultrastructural study documented lamellar and prismatic inclusions of a lipid nature in the distal tubules. The collecting ducts, however contain fewer, but much larger, cytoplasmic inclusions of membranous, lamellar material. These lamellated structures represent accumulated renal sulfatide [71], which results from a deficiency of lysosomal arylsulfatase A (see Fig. 68-1). Although the monohexosyl sulfatide that is found primarily in the brain is present in the kidney, much larger quantities of dihexosyl sulfatide accumulate in the kidney; the latter sulfatide occurs only in certain other visceral tissues [48]. These data suggest that the source of the accumulated renal sulfatides is endogenous [54, 68, 79]. Despite the striking morphologic changes, there are no functional abnormalities.

GAUCHER'S DISEASE

The major clinical features of the three forms of Gaucher's disease (defective β-glucosidase activity) are given in Table 68-1. The pathologic descriptions have focused on the infantile (type 2) and the adult (type 1) forms of the disease. Occasionally, the kidney is involved with either typical Gaucher cells in the glomerulus or cells scattered

either singularly or as groups throughout the interstitium [13]. In addition, tubular epithelial cell involvement and Gaucher cells in the tubular lumens have been described [13]. There are no reports of clinically significant renal dysfunction in children [16, 29].

Disorders of Glycogen Metabolism

Pompe's disease or glycogenosis type II (defective α-glucosidase activity) has the unique distinction of being the only lysosomal glycogen storage disease. Pompe's disease presents early in infancy with signs and symptoms of congestive heart failure and marked failure to thrive. Death usually occurs by 1 year of age.

The systemic deficiency of acidic α-glucosidase activity leads to generalized glycogen accumulation, predominantly in the skeletal muscle, myocardium, liver, and kidney [40]. On histologic examination, glomerular and tubular epithelial cells appear ballooned due to glycogen accumulation [31, 40]. Ultrastructural examination reveals interstitial cells containing vacuoles of monoparticulate glycogen in the cytoplasm, within lysosomes and occasionally in mitochrondria. In addition, tubular and glomerular epithelial cells contain glycogen-engorged lysosomes [40], and the foot processes are vacuolated, with occasional complete loss of their architecture. Clinically manifest renal dysfunction has not been noted.

Disorders of the Lysosomal Apparatus

Since its original description in 1965 [46], I-cell disease (Leroy's disease) has presented a challenge and vexation to investigators of disorders of the lysosomal apparatus. Unlike most of the lysosomal storage diseases, which result from a single defective enzyme activity, I-cell disease is characterized by multiple deficiencies of lysosomal hydrolase activities in certain tissues (particularly of mesenchymal origin) and marked elevations of these activities in the plasma and urine of affected patients [85]. Clinically, patients with I-cell disease have progressive psychomotor retardation, severe growth failure, gingival hypertrophy, dysostosis multiplex, and a Hurler-like facial dysmorphia. Renal function is not impaired. Death usually occurs before the fourth year of life.

Striking foamy transformation of the visceral cells of Bowman's capsule is evident in the renal glomerulus [49], while only a few vacuoles are noted in the proximal convoluted tubule. Ultrastructurally, extensive lesions of the glomerular epithelium are seen; however, it is noteworthy that the foot processes are spared or slightly vacuolated (Fig. 68-5). The interstitial cells, presumably fibroblasts, may have extensive vacuolation [49].

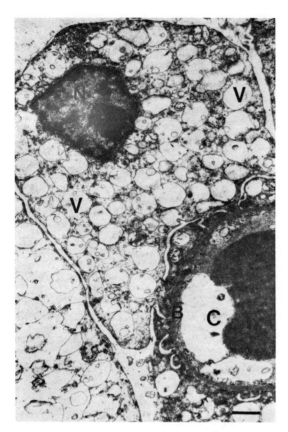

Figure 68-5. Electron micrograph showing the glomerular changes in I-cell disease. The visceral cells of Bowman's capsule are markedly distended by membrane-bound cytoplasmic vacuoles (V). The foot processes adjacent to the basal membrane (B) of a capillary (C) are not similarly ballooned. (×20,000.) (From J. J. Martin et al., Acta Neuropathol. *33:285, 1975.)*

Martin et al. [49] found that the vacuolated cells did not stain with PAS, Fiel-Nielsen, alcian blue, toluidine blue O, Sudan black B, Sudan III, or oil red O, after use of any fixative [49]. In addition, they found that no lysosomal hydrolase activity could be demonstrated in the visceral cells of Bowman's capsule, whereas the loops of Henle and collecting ducts were histochemically stained for acid phosphatase, β-glucuronidase, and nonspecific esterase [49].

Diagnosis and Management of Lysosomal Storage Diseases

Further biochemical and morphologic characterization of these "experiments of nature" [32] may provide insights into the functional roles of these stored renal compounds in health and disease. However, the renal manifestations of the lysosomal storage diseases are only a reflection of their systemic involvement. The debilitation of these patients from lesions in the nervous system and cardiovascular-renal system necessitates the exploitation of multiple sociomedical resources. Although inroads have been made into specific enzyme replacement therapy [20, 27], supportive care of affected persons and precise enzymatic diagnosis remain the foundation of patient management. Presumptive diagnosis can be made by quantitative urinary determination of glycosphingolipids, glycoproteins, and mucopolysaccharides; the specific confirmatory enzyme diagnosis is available for each of these disorders. Education of families of affected children, heterozygote detection, and prenatal diagnosis are prerequisites for the management of these devastating disorders.

References

1. Austin, J., Armstrong, D., Fouch, S., Nutchell, C., Stumpf, D., Shearer, L., and Briner, O. Metachromatic leucodystrophy (MLD) VIII. MLD in adults; diagnosis and pathogenesis. *Arch. Neurol.* 18:225, 1968.
2. Austin, J., Armstrong, D., and Shearer, L. Metachromatic form of diffuse cerebral sclerosis V. The nature and significance of low sulfatase activity: A controlled study of brain, liver and kidney in four patients with metachromatic leucodystrophy. *Arch. Neurol.* 13:593, 1965.
3. Austin, J., Balasubramanian, A., Pattabiraman, T., Sarswathi, S., Basu, D., and Bachhawat, B. A controlled study of enzyme activities in three human disorders of glycolipid metabolism. *J. Neurochem.* 10: 805, 1963.
4. Bach, G., Eisenberg, F., Jr., Cantz, M., and Neufeld, E. F. The defect in the Hunter syndrome: Deficiency of sulfoiduronate sulfatase. *Proc. Natl. Acad. Sci. U.S.A.* 70:2134, 1973.
5. Bach, G., Friedman, R., Weissman, B., and Neufeld, E. F. The defect in the Hurler and Scheie syndromes: Deficiency of α-L-iduronidase. *Proc. Natl. Acad. Sci. U.S.A.* 69:2048, 1972.
6. Beutler, E., and Kuhl, W. Purification and properties of human α-galactosidases. *J. Biol. Chem.* 247: 7195, 1972.
7. Beutler, E., Kuhl, W., Matsumoto, F., and Pangalis, G. Acid hydrolases in leukocytes and platelets of normal subjects and in patients with Gaucher's and Fabry's disease. *J. Exp. Med.* 143:975, 1976.
8. Brady, R. O., Gal, A. E., Bradley, R. M., Martensson, E., Warshaw, A. L., and Laster, L. Enzymatic defect in Fabry's disease; ceramidetrihexosidase deficiency. *N. Engl. J. Med.* 276:1163, 1967.
9. Brady, R. O., Kanfer, J. N., Bradley, R. M., and Shapiro, D. Demonstration of a deficiency of glucocerebrosidase-cleaving enzyme in Gaucher's disease. *J. Clin. Invest.* 45:1112, 1966.
10. Brady, R. O., Kanfer, J. N., Mock, M. B., and Fredrickson, D. S. The metabolism of sphingomyelin. II. Evidence of an enzymatic deficiency in Niemann-Pick disease. *Proc. Natl. Acad. Sci. U.S.A.* 55:366, 1966.
11. Brady, R. O., Kanfer, J. N., and Shapiro, D. Metabolism of glucocerebrosides. II. Evidence of an

enzymatic deficiency in Gaucher's disease. *Biochem. Biophys. Res. Commun.* 18:221, 1965.

12. Brady, R. O., Uhlendorf, B. W., Jacobson, C. B. Fabry's disease: Antenatal diagnosis. *Science* 172:172, 1971.

13. Chang-Lo, M., Yam, L. T., and Rubenstone, A. I. Gaucher's disease. *Am. J. Med. Sci.* 254:303, 1967.

14. Colley, J. R., Miller, D. L., Hutt, M. S. R., Wallace, H. J., and de Wardner, H. E. The renal lesion in angiokeratoma corporis diffusum. *Br. Med. J.* 1:1266, 1958.

15. Dawson, G., Matalon, R., and Dorfman, A. Glycosphingolipids in cultured human fibroblasts. II. Characterization and metabolism in fibroblasts from patients with inborn errors of glycosphingolipid and mucopolysaccharide metabolism. *J. Biol. Chem.* 247:5951, 1972.

16. DeBrito, T., DosReis, V. G., Penna, D. O., and Camargo, M. E. Glomerular involvement in Gaucher's disease. A light, immunofluorescent, and ultrastructural study based on kidney biopsy specimens. *Arch. Pathol.* 95:1, 1973.

17. DeDuve, C. From cytases to lysosomes. *Fed. Proc.* 23:1045, 1964.

18. Desnick, R. J., Allen, K. Y., Desnick, S. J., Raman, M. K., Bernlohr, R. W., and Krivit, W. Enzymatic diagnosis of hemizygotes and heterozygotes with Fabry's disease. *J. Lab. Clin. Med.* 81:157, 1973.

19. Desnick, R. J., Allen, K. Y., Simmons, R. L., Woods, J. E., Anderson, C. F., Najarian, J. S., and Krivit, W. Correction of enzymatic deficiencies by renal transplantation: Fabry's disease. *Surgery* 72:203, 1972.

20. Desnick, R. J., Bernlohr, R. W., and Krivit, W. (eds.). *Enzyme Therapy in Genetic Diseases.* Baltimore: Williams & Wilkins, 1972.

21. Desnick, R. J., Dawson, G., Desnick, S. J., Sweeley, C. C., and Krivit, W. Diagnosis of glycosphingolipidoses by urinary sediment analysis. *N. Engl. J. Med.* 284:739, 1971.

22. Desnick, R. J., Klionsky, B., and Sweeley, C. C. Fabry's Disease: α-Galactosidase A Deficiency. In J. B. Stanbury, J. B. Wyngaarden, and N. S. Fredrickson (eds.), *The Metabolic Basis of Inherited Disease* (4th ed.). New York: McGraw-Hill, 1977.

23. Desnick, R. J., Raman, M. K., Bendel, R. P., Kersey, J., Lee, L. C., and Krivit, W. Prenatal diagnosis of glycosphingolipidoses: Sandhoff's and Fabry's disease. *J. Pediatr.* 83:149, 1973.

24. Desnick, R. J., and Sweeley, C. C. Prenatal Detection of Fabry's Disease. In A. Dorfman (ed.), *Antenatal Diagnosis.* Chicago: University of Chicago Press, 1971.

25. Desnick, R. J., Sweeley, C. C., and Krivit, W. A method for the quantitative determination of the neutral glycosphingolipids in urine sediment. *J. Lipid Res.* 11:31, 1970.

26. Desnick, R. J., Synder, P. D., Desnick, S. J., Krivit, W., and Sharp, H. L. Sandhoff's disease: Ultrastructural and biochemical studies. *Adv. Exp. Med. Biol.* 19:351, 1972.

27. Desnick, R. J., Thorpe, S. R., and Fiddler, M. B. Toward enzyme therapy for lysosomal storage diseases. *Physiol. Rev.* 56:57, 1976.

28. Dolman, C. L., Chang, E., and Duke, R. J. Pathologic findings in Sandhoff disease. *Arch. Pathol.* 96:272, 1973.

29. Fredrickson, D. S., and Sloan, H. R. Glucosylceramide Lipidoses: Gaucher's Disease. In J. B. Stanbury,

J. B. Wyngaarden, and D. S. Fredrickson (eds.), *The Metabolic Basis of Inherited Disease* (3rd ed.). New York: McGraw-Hill, 1972.

30. Funck-Brentano, J. L., Dorman, J., Mery, J. P., De Montera, H., and Moreira, M. Les lesions renales de l'angiokeratose de Fabry: A propos d'une observation. *J. Urol. Nephrol.* 70:826, 1964.

31. Garancis, J. Type II glycogenosis: Biochemical and electron microscopic study. *Am. J. Med.* 44:289, 1968.

32. Garrod, A. E. Inborn errors of metabolism (Croonian lectures). *Lancet* 2:2,73,142,214, 1908.

33. Goto, I., Tabira, T., Nawa, A., Kurokawa, T., and Kuroiwa, Y. Biochemical and genetic studies in two families with Fabry disease. *Arch. Neurol.* 31:45, 1974.

34. Hagberg, B., Svennerholm, L., and Wranne, B. The excretion of urinary sulfatides in health and neurological disease. *Acta Paediatr. Scand.* 54:409, 1965.

35. Hall, C., Cantz, M., and Neufeld, E. F. A β-glucuronidase deficiency mucopolysaccharidosis: Studies in cultured fibroblasts. *Arch. Biochem. Biophys.* 155:32, 1973.

36. Henry, E. W., and Rally, C. R. The renal lesion in angiokeratoma corporis diffusum (Fabry's disease). *Can. Med. Assoc. J.* 89:206, 1963.

37. Hers, H. G. α-Glucosidase deficiency in generalized glycogen-storage disease (Pompe's disease). *Biochem. J.* 86:11, 1963.

38. Hers, H. G., and Van Hoof, F. (eds.). *Lysosomes and Storage Diseases.* New York: Academic, 1973.

39. Ho, M. W., Beutler, S., Tennant, L., and O'Brien, J. S. Fabry's disease: Evidence for a physically altered α-galactosidase. *Am. J. Hum. Genet.* 24:256, 1972.

40. Hug, G., and Schubert, K. Glycogenosis type II. *Arch. Pathol.* 84:141, 1967.

41. Jenner, F. A., and Pollitt, R. J. Large quantities of 2-acetamido-1 (β-l-aspartamido)-1,2 dideoxyglucose in the urine of mentally retarded siblings. *Biochem. J.* 103:48p, 1967.

42. Johnson, D. L., Del Monte, M. A., Cotlier, E., and Desnick, R. J. Fabry disease: Diagnosis of hemizygotes and heterozygotes by α-galactosidase A activity in tears. *Clin. Chim. Acta* 63:81, 1975.

43. Kint, J. A. Fabry's disease, alpha-galactosidase deficiency. *Science* 167:1268, 1970.

44. Kresse, H., and Neufeld, E. F. The Sanfilippo A corrective factor. Purification and mode of action. *J. Biol. Chem.* 247:2164, 1972.

45. Landing, B., Silverman, F., Craig, J., Jacoby, M. D., Lahey, M. E., and Chadwick, D. L. Familial neurovisceral lipidosis. *Am. J. Dis. Child.* 108:503, 1964.

46. Leroy, J., and Demars, R. I. Mutant enzymatic and cytological phenotypes in cultured fibroblasts. *Science* 157:804, 1967.

47. Malmquist, E., Ivemach, B. I., Lindsten, J., Maunsbach, A. B., and Martensson, E. Pathologic lysosomes and increased urinary glycosylceramide excretion in Fabry's disease. *Lab. Invest.* 25:1, 1971.

48. Martensson, E. Sulfatides of human kidney isolation, identification and fatty acid composition. *Biochim. Biophys. Acta* 116:521, 1966.

49. Martin, J. J., Leroy, J. G., Farrioux, J. P., Fontaine, G., Desnick, R. J., and Cabello, A. I-cell disease (mucolipidosis II): A report on its pathology. *Acta Neuropathol.* 33:285, 1975.

50. Matalon, R., Arbogast, B., Justice, P., Brandt, I. K.,

and Dorfman, A. Morquio's syndrome: Deficiency of a chondroitin sulfate N-acetyl-hexosamine sulfate sulfatase. *Biochem. Biophys. Res. Commun.* 61:759, 1975.

51. McNary, W., and Lowenstein, L. M. A morphological study of the renal lesion in angiokeratoma corporis diffusum universale (Fabry's disease). *J. Urol.* 93:641, 1965.

52. Mihatsch, M., Ohnacker, H., Riede, U. N., Remagen, W., Bassewitz, D. B., Schuppler, J., and Meier-Ruge, W. G_{M1} gangliosidosis part II: Morphological aspects and review of the literature. *Helv. Paediatr. Acta* 28:521, 1973.

53. Morel-Maroger, L., Ganter, P., Ardailow, R., Cathelineau, G., and Richet, G. Des rapports avec l'angiokeratose de Fabry et la cytodystrophie renale familiale. *Bull. Soc. Med. Hop. Paris* 117:49, 1966.

54. Moser, H., Moser, A., and McKhann, G. The dynamics of a lipidosis: Turnover of sulfatide, steroid sulfate, and polysaccharide sulfate in metachromatic leukodystrophy. *Arch. Neurol.* 17:494, 1967.

55. Nadler, H. L. Genetic heterogeneity in acid phosphatase deficiency. *Pediatr. Res.* 5:421, 1971.

56. Nadler, H. L., and Egan, T. J. Deficiency of lysosomal acid phosphatase: A new familial metabolic disorder. *N. Engl. J. Med.* 282:302, 1970.

57. O'Brien, J. Generalized gangliosidosis. *J. Pediatr.* 75:167, 1969.

58. O'Brien, J. S. Five gangliosidoses. *Lancet* 2:805, 1969.

59. O'Brien, J. S. The Gangliosidoses. In J. B. Stanbury, J. B. Wyngaarden, and D. S. Fredrickson (eds.), *The Metabolic Basis of Inherited Disease* (4th ed.). New York: McGraw-Hill, 1978.

60. O'Brien, J. S. Sanfilippo syndrome: Profound deficiency of alpha-acetylglycosaminidase activity in organs and skin fibroblasts from type B patients. *Proc. Natl. Acad. Sci. U.S.A.* 69:1720, 1972.

61. O'Brien, J. S., Cantz, M., and Spranger, J. Maroteaux-Lamy disease (mucopolysaccharidosis VI), subtype A: Deficiency of an N-acetyl-galactosamine-4-sulfatase. *Biochem. Biophys. Res. Commun.* 60:1170, 1974.

62. Öckerman, P. A. A generalized storage disorder resembling Hurler's syndrome. *Lancet* 2:239, 1967.

63. Okada, S., and O'Brien, J. S. Generalized gangliosidosis: β-Galactosidase deficiency. *Science* 160:1002, 1968.

64. Okada, S., and O'Brien, J. S. Tay-Sachs disease: Generalized absence of a β-D-N-acetylhexosaminidase component. *Science* 165:698, 1969.

65. Pabico, R. C., Atanacio, B. C., McKenna, B. A., Pamurcoglu, T., and Yodaiken, R. Renal pathologic lesions and functional alterations in a man with Fabry's disease. *Am. J. Med.* 55:415, 1973.

66. Patrick, A. D., and Lake, B. D. Deficiency of an acid lipase in Wolman's disease. *Nature* 222:1067, 1969.

67. Philippart, M., Franklin, S. S., and Gordon, A. Reversal of an inborn sphingolipidosis (Fabry's disease) by kidney transplantation. *Ann. Intern. Med.* 77:195, 1972.

68. Philippart, M., Sarlieve, L., Meurant, C., and Mechler, L. Human urinary sulfatides in patients with sulfatidosis (metachromatic leukodystrophy). *J. Lipid Res.* 12:434, 1971.

69. Pilz, H., and Denden, A. Glycolipidausscheidung in Urin bei einer Sippe mit Fabryscher Krankheit (Angiokeratoma Corporis diffusum). *Dtsch. Me Wochenschr.* 97:120, 1973.

70. Rae, A. F., Lee, J. C., and Hopper, J. Clinical and electron microscopic studies of a case of glycolipid lipidosis. *J. Clin. Pathol.* 20:21, 1967.

71. Resibois, A. Electron microscopic studies of metachromatic leucodystrophy. IV. Liver and kidney alterations. *Eur. Pathol.* 6:278, 1971.

72. Romeo, G., and Migeon, B. R. Genetic inactivation of the α-galactosidase locus in carriers of Fabry's disease. *Science* 170:180, 1970.

73. Sandhoff, K., Andreae, U., and Jatzkewitz, H. Deficient hexosaminidase activity in an exceptional case of Tay-Sachs disease with additional storage of kidney globoside in visceral organs. *Pathol. Eur.* 3:278, 1968.

74. Schneider, P. B., and Kennedy, E. P. Sphingomyelinase in normal human spleen and in spleens from subjects with Niemann-Pick disease. *J. Lipid Res.* 8:202, 1967.

75. Scott, R., Lagunoff, D., and Trump, B. Familial neurovisceral lipidosis. *J. Pediatr.* 71:357, 1967.

76. Seringe, P., Plainfosse, B., Lautmann, F., Lorilloux, J., and Watchi, J. M. Precoce, et place ausein des lipidoses, de la gangliosidose type Normal-Landing, a G_{M1}. *Soc. Med. Hop. Paris* 119:179, 1960.

77. Severi, F., Marguini, V., Tettamanti, G., Bianchi, E., and Lanzi, G. Infantile G_{M1} gangliosidosis. Histochemical, ultrastructural and biochemical studies. *Helv. Paediatr. Acta* 2:192, 1971.

78. Spense, M. W., Mackinnon, K. E., Burgess, J. K., d'Entoremont, D. M., Belitsky, P., Lannon, S. G., and McDonald, A. S. Failure to correct the metabolic defect by renal allotransplantation in Fabry's disease. *Ann. Intern. Med.* 84:13, 1976.

79. Stinshoff, K. Kinetic properties of the arylsulfatase A from human kidneys. *Biochim. Biophys. Acta* 276:475, 1972.

80. Stumpf, D., and Austin, J. Metachromatic leukodystrophy (MLD). IX. Qualitative and quantitative differences in urinary arylsulfatases A in different forms of MLD. *Arch. Neurol.* 24:117, 1971.

81. Sugita, M., Dulaney, J. T., and Moser, H. W. Ceramidase deficiency in Farber's disease (lipogranulomatosis). *Science* 178:110, 1972.

82. Suzuki, K. Cerebral G_{M1} gangliosidosis: Chemical pathology of visceral organs. *Science* 159:1471, 1968.

83. Suzuki, K., and Suzuki, Y. Globoid cell leucodystrophy (Krabbe's disease): Deficiency of galactocerebroside β-galactosidase. *Proc. Natl. Acad. Sci. U.S.A.* 66:320, 1970.

84. Tondeur, M. Fabry's disease in children: An electron microscopic study. *Virchows Arch.* (Zellpathol.) 2:239, 1969.

85. Tondeur, M., Vamos-Hurwitz, E., Mockel-Pohl, S., Dereume, J. P., Crimer, N., and Loeb, H. Clinical, biochemical, and ultrastructural studies in a case of chondrodystrophy presenting the I-cell phenotype in tissue culture. *J. Pediatr.* 79:366, 1971.

86. Van den Bergh, F. A. J. T. M., Rietra, P. J. G. M., Kolk-Vegter, A. J., Bosch, E., and Tager, J. M. Therapeutic implications of renal transplantation in a patient with Fabry's disease. *Acta Med. Scand.* 200:249, 1976.

87. Van Hoof, F. G_{M1} Gangliosidosis. In H. G. Hers and F. Van Hoof (eds.), *Lysosomes and Storage Diseases*. New York: Academic, 1973.

88. Van Hoof, F., and Hers, H. G. Mucopolysacchari-

sis by absence of α-L-fucosidase. *Lancet* 2:1198, 968.

on Gemmingen, G., Kierland, R. R., and Opitz, J. M. Angiokeratoma corporis diffusum (Fabry's disease). *Arch. Dermatol.* 91:206, 1965.

. Wallace, H. J. Angiokeratoma corporis diffusum. *Br. J. Dermatol.* 70:354, 1958.

91. Wolfe, L. S., Callahan, J., Fawcett, J. S., Andermann, F., and Scriver, C. R. G_{M1} gangliosidosis without chondrodystrophy or visceromegaly. *Neurology* 20:23, 1970.

92. Wood, S., and Nadler, H. L. Fabry's disease: Absence of an α-galactosidase isozyme. *Am. J. Hum. Genet.* 24:250, 1972.

Section Four. Treatment of Glomerular Diseases

 Treatment of Glomerular Diseases: Immunosuppressive and Antiinflammatory Therapy   *Clark D. West*

Specific therapy of the glomerulonephritides has been an obvious goal of nephrologists for many years, and numerous approaches to therapy have been tried. In recent years, therapeutic efforts have been greatly influenced by the concept that most cases of acquired glomerulonephritis are produced by the phlogogenic effects of circulating immune complexes deposited in the glomeruli or, in a minority of instances, from the reaction of circulating antibody with fixed glomerular antigen. It was therefore logical that attempts at therapy should employ cytotoxic agents and corticosteroids as a means of inhibiting antibody formation. More sophisticated and precise manipulations that might lead to specific inhibition of antibody formation have not been employed, because in most forms of nephritis the composition of the complexes is not known with respect to the nature and origin of the antigen.

A second possible approach to therapy is by inhibition of complex deposition. From studies in animals, it appears that circulating complexes are removed from the circulation in large part by the reticuloendothelial system. If deposition of complexes in the glomerulus could be inhibited or prevented, leaving circulating complexes to be removed entirely by the reticuloendothelial system, the nephritis presumably would heal. Although some light has been shed in recent years on the factors that promote the deposition of complexes subendothelially in capillaries and venules, application of the observations to man has not, in general, been rewarding.

A third approach to therapy is the use of antiinflammatory agents. Immunosuppressive therapy often has an antiinflammatory effect in addition to inhibiting antibody formation. Purine analogues and, more especially, corticosteroids, inhibit the inflammatory response; thus, when improvement is noted with regimens that include these agents, it is often difficult to determine the relative contributions of the two effects. A nonsteroidal antiinflammatory agent, indomethacin, has also been used, especially by European workers, as primary therapy in chronic glomerulonephritis, with variable results.

A fourth approach to therapy has been the attempt to blunt the glomerular deposition of fibrin, one of the by-products of immune complex deposition and glomerular inflammation that may contribute to glomerular malfunction. Immunofluorescence techniques often reveal abundant deposits of fibrin in the glomeruli in nephritis, and further circumstantial evidence for fibrin deposition is provided by the observation that fibrin degradation products may be found in the serum and urine. Fibrin deposition is probably especially important in the production of glomerular crescents. In animals injected with nephrotoxic serum, anticoagulants have been shown to reduce the severity of the nephritis, but their use in human subjects has given variable results, and their place in treatment is not established.

This chapter deals with immunosuppressive therapy, antiinflammatory agents, and attempts to prevent immune complex deposition. Anticoagulant therapy is the subject of Chap. 70.

The Immune System

Agents used for immunosuppression in glomerulonephritis act on the immune system at different sites and in different ways. Although much remains to be learned about their effects and how they are produced, full appreciation of what is known requires an understanding of the nature of the immune system.

NATURE OF THE IMMUNE SYSTEM

The immune system consists of an afferent, a central, and an efferent limb [32], each of which is highly complex and as yet incompletely understood. This complexity allows for the very diverse functional capacity and flexibility that is essential to protect the organism from invaders from the environment. It also makes for multiple sites at which immunosuppressive drugs can and do act.

The afferent limb of the system is concerned with the transport of antigen to the potentially reactive cell. In the central limb, antibody is formed by the immunocompetent cell, and the immune response is expressed via the efferent limb.

The important component of the afferent limb is the macrophage. This cell participates in variable ways and degrees, depending on the nature of the antigen and its presentation. In general, the macrophage could be said to ingest and catabolize potential antigen and, at the same time, to allow a small amount of the antigen or of antigenic fragments to become bound to its plasma membrane; the latter is thought to be responsible for the induction of immunity [32].

In the central limb, lymphocytes "recognize" the macrophage-bound antigenic determinants and become sensitized to them. The primordial source of the lymphocyte is the bone marrow stem cell. From the bone marrow, some lymphocytes travel to the thymus and some to the structures that are the equivalent in man to the bursa of Fabricius in the chicken. In these structures they are thought to undergo a programming that influences their future function. Lymphocytes from the thymus, the T cells, take up residence in paracortical or marginal areas of the lymph nodes and spleen. They also constitute the majority of the lymphocytes of the peripheral blood and the thoracic duct lymph. Lymphocytes from the bursal system, the B cells, are concentrated in the corticomedullary and medullary cord areas of the lymph nodes and in the germinal centers; they are not abundant in the circulation. Both T cells and B cells are found in the bone marrow. When sensitized by antigen, T cells respond by blast transformation and after sensitization are responsible for cell-mediated immunity. They often have a long life span and are the carriers of immunologic memory; being motile, they are available to react locally with antigen at many sites. For their sensitization by antigen, B cells require the presence of thymus-derived "helper" cells, which may serve as handlers of antigen.

The steps involved in the sensitization of B cells are not clear. Presumably, the antigen or a fragment of it is transferred to a receptor site on the cell and triggers the cell to produce antibody; at the same time, it stimulates the cell to proliferate into other antibody-forming cells that amplify the antibody response. These antibody forming cells differentiate into plasma cells. B lymphocytes are relatively nonmotile and have a short life span. The period over which antibody is formed in this system is therefore relatively short. The system, however, is capable of responding rapidly to a second contact with the same antigen, even if the contact is minimal, with the production of large quantities of highly specific antibody. This is the so-called anamnestic reaction. It may be the result of the fact that a population of long-lived T cells with an immunologic memory for that antigen is already present and allows a minimal antigenic stimulus to be amplified markedly.

The efferent limb of the immune response consists of the modalities derived from the central limb, namely, sensitized cells and humoral antibodies, which directly protect the integrity of the host by recognizing antigen. In addition to protecting the host, this limb is also responsible for the tissue injury and hypersensitivity that occurs in disease. Reaction of humoral antibody with antigen results in the formation of immune complexes, which in turn activate the complement system to form anaphylatoxins and agents chemotactic for polymorphonuclear leukocytes.

The role of complement in producing glomerular inflammation has been studied extensively. Whereas activation of the complement system in the relatively stagnant interstitial fluid or in the glomerular mesangium may produce an inflammatory reaction, the phlogogenic products of a reaction occurring in the glomerular capillary wall may be swept rapidly into the circulation and be ineffective [19]. The reaction could, however, confer on the walls the property of immune adherence, due to the deposition of C3b. Immune adherence would result in stickiness and cause accumulation of passing polymorphonuclear leukocytes. It is important to note that, in the absence of an intact complement system in the experimental animal, transient proteinuria but not overt glomerulonephritis follows the administration of nephrotoxic serum [19, 21a]. On the other hand, glomerulonephritis will develop in mice injected with complexes formed with avian antibody even though avian antibody is a poor activator of the complement system [59].

Immunosuppressive Therapy

The means of suppressing the formation of cell-mediated or humoral antibody take diverse forms, some which are not applicable to glomerulonephritis. The function of the afferent limb may be blocked or blunted by administration of more than one antigen simultaneously or within an interval of a few days. Similarly, passive administration of preformed antibody blocks the immunogenic qualities of homologous antigen presented simultaneously. Advantage is taken of this effect, for example, in preventing Rh sensitization of mothers at the time of delivery by administering antibody to the Rh factor. Since, in glomerulonephritis, the nature of the antigen often is not known, and antibody induction has already occurred when the patient is first seen, neither of these maneuvers holds promise in the therapy of this disease.

Blockage of the central limb can be induced by tolerance. However, induction of tolerance in glomerulonephritis is not possible for two reasons: (1) it can be produced only in the preinduction phase of antibody formation; and (2) it can be induced only by the administration of antigen, and the nature of the antigen is not known in most forms of glomerulonephritis. The central limb can also be prevented from functioning optimally in the production of cellular immunity by depleting it of T cells by thoracic-duct drainage. This procedure has not been attempted in glomerulonephritis. Antilymphocyte serum also blocks the system centrally, mainly by its effect on cell-mediated immunity; it has had only limited use in the treatment of glomerulonephritis.

Because antibody formation is already under way when the patient with glomerulonephritis is first seen, and because the nature of the antigen is not known, the approach to therapy of glomerulonephritis has usually been the nonspecific use of cytotoxic drugs that inhibit antibody formation by various means and with variable degrees of success. Recently, to reduce the concentration of circulating antibody in the Goodpasture syndrome and of circulating immune complexes in the nephritis of systemic lupus, multiple plasmaphoreses have been employed. Success in the treatment of patients with the Goodpasture syndrome was reported [56a] when this procedure was combined with immunosuppressive agents to inhibit antibody formation; in patients with lupus, plasmaphoresis alone may be effective [51a].

ACTIONS OF CYTOTOXIC AGENTS USED FOR IMMUNOSUPPRESSION

As a result of the complexity of the immune system, the action of cytotoxic agents is often at more than one site. Most of the agents currently in use are by-products of the effort to develop cancer chemotherapeutic agents. Because they interfere with more than one biochemical pathway, all of them have complex actions. In general, they are cell poisons that prevent the rapid proliferation of cells, an event that is central to the induction of immunity.

If the immune complex theory of the causation of glomerulonephritis is correct, the ideal immunosuppressive agent would be one that, in a dose that produces no toxicity or acceptable toxicity, would interfere with the ongoing production of humoral antibody induced by an unknown antigen some time in the past. To be safe, it should not interfere with the induction of antibody to new antigens encountered by the host or with the anamnestic response to antigens already encountered, so that the patient would not be at risk of infection. It should thus act on the central limb to inhibit antibody formation already in progress and not affect the stage of rapid cellular proliferation characteristic of the induction of antibody formation or of the anamnestic reaction. The agent would have added value if it modified the activity of the efferent limb in a way that reduced the inflammatory reaction in the glomerulus. Since it has not been proved that cell-mediated antibody plays a role in the production or progression of glomerulonephritis, an effect on this system might not be beneficial and, in fact, might be harmful in that immunosuppression would be too profound and endanger the host.

Only two of the several classes of immunosuppressive agents have been used to any extent in the therapy of glomerulonephritis. These are the *alkylating agents,* in the form of cyclophosphamide, nitrogen mustard, and chlorambucil, and the *antipurines,* of which 6-mercaptopurine, azathioprine, and 6-thioguanine are prototypes. The complex actions of these agents are incompletely understood. In general, it can be said that the first group of agents alkylate and cross-link DNA and protein, thus interfering with the proliferation and differentiation of cells, which occurs, for example, with activation of the central limb of the immune system. They are also lympholytic and cause lymphocyte counts to decrease. The antipurines block the synthesis and interconversion of purine nucleotides, thus preventing nucleic acid synthesis. Studies of the drugs in both groups have shown, however, that their actions go beyond those expected from these basic effects, illustrating again that they block several biochemical pathways.

A highly detailed literature has developed concerning the effects of these drugs on the immune system, and the subject has been frequently reviewed [1, 12, 57]. Background information pertinent to the use of immunosuppressive drugs in disease is provided by the wealth of information that has accumulated concerning their effects in animals. It should be noted, however, that application of animal experiments to man is clouded by many factors. Not only are there species differences in response, but also the experiments in animals often have employed near-lethal doses of immunosuppressants for a short time, whereas clinically they are used in much lower dose over long periods. The results in animals—and presumably also in human subjects—often differ, depending on the nature of the antigen employed. It is easier to suppress the antibody response to soluble protein antigens, which are relatively weak stimulators of the immune system, than it is to depress the response to potent antigens, such as viruses and heterologous erythrocytes, which are potent immunogens. Since, in the patient with glomerulonephritis, the nature of the antigen is not known, these considerations make it difficult to use the information obtained from animal experiments in choosing an immunosuppressive drug and the regimen to employ in a patient. Thus, careful clinical observations are of great importance.

Immunosuppressive drugs can be classified according to the timing of their immunosuppressive effects in relation to the time of giving the antigen [57]. Some are effective if given just before antigenic stimulation; others are most effective when given a day or two afterward; and still others are effective when given either before or after the antigenic stimulation. Corticosteroids are the only commonly used immunosuppressants that are most effective when given before the antigenic stimulus. Most of the cytotoxic agents are most effective if given within a short time after antigenic stimulation, when cell proliferation in the central limb in response to the antigenic stimulation is most rapid. The purine analogues, including 6-mercaptopurine, azathioprine, and 6-thioguanine, and the pyrimidine analogues, the *Vinca* alkaloids, methotrexate, and the alkylating agents (except for cyclophosphamide) are in this group. To be truly effective in inhibiting antibody formation, these drugs must be given immediately after antigen administration. In some situations, if the period of drug administration is relatively short, antibody will be formed as soon as administration is stopped. Only two agents, procarbazine and cyclophosphamide, are effective if given either before or after antigen administration. In human subjects cyclophosphamide is not as reproducibly immunosuppressive if given a day or two before the antigenic stimulation as

it is if administration is started a day or two later [57].

In animals, it has been noted that, given at certain times in relation to antigen administration, immunosuppressive drugs will *enhance* antibody formation. Thus, in the rat, administration of nitrogen mustard before or busulfan before or after immunization enhances antibody production [77]. The rabbit responds to a small antigenic stimulation with production of large amounts of antibody if 6-mercaptopurine is given for several days and then stopped several days before antigen is administered [79]. Enhancement of the primary antibody response has also been observed occasionally in patients receiving methotrexate and azathioprine [88].

In man as well as in animals, a drug (e.g., 6-mercaptopurine) may inhibit 7S but not 19S antibody formation [77]. Thus, in patients with autoimmune disorders, treatment with methotrexate or azathioprine started at the time of administration of a foreign protein (keyhole limpet hemocyanin) resulted in little production of antibody to the foreign protein of the IgG class; however, a number of patients responded over a prolonged period with the production of antibody of the IgM class [88].

Studies in patients with autoimmune disorders have indicated no correlation between the therapeutic effectiveness of an immunosuppressive regimen and the ability of the regimen to inhibit the antibody response to a foreign protein [88]. The immunosuppressive therapy may ameliorate the disease in patients who have a vigorous antibody response to immunization with a foreign protein. The effectiveness may be due in part to the fact that the agents significantly alter the activity of the efferent limb by an antiinflammatory effect. The purine analogues 6-mercaptopurine and azathioprine may be especially effective in this way. These observations would indicate that effective therapy will not necessarily endanger the patient with respect to inability to ward off intercurrent infection.

In choosing a cytotoxic drug for use in glomerulonephritis, the risks as well as the efficacy of the agent in question must be considered. All the agents have potentially serious side effects, and, particularly if the dose is large, patients receiving them should be observed carefully. Under certain conditions the drugs may be ineffective and the risk of serious side effects potentiated. More detailed information concerning specific drugs frequently used for immunosuppression in glomerulonephritis with respect to their effect on the immune system, their metabolism and their toxicity is given in the following sections.

CORTICOSTEROIDS

Mechanism of Action

Of all agents, corticosteroids are used most frequently in the therapy of autoimmune disorders in general and of glomerulonephritis in particular. They act at all three limbs of the immune system [99]. In large doses they inhibit macrophage activity, thus reducing uptake of antigen and inhibiting at the efferent limb. In addition, they act centrally through their lympholytic action, although there is evidence that lymphocytes already programmed to make antibody or to mediate cellular immunity, as well as thymus-derived "helper" cells, are resistant to lysis by corticosteroids. Thus, corticosteroids are more effective when given in the induction phase of antibody formation than after sensitization has occurred. In man, antibody synthesis is not greatly affected by corticosteroid administration, although studies to test this have not employed large doses [79]. An important function of corticosteroids is the blunting of the effect of efferent-limb activity by inhibiting inflammatory reactions. This is apparently accomplished in two ways [99]. First, sensitized T cells in contact with antigen liberate the migration inhibitory factor, which normally serves to reduce the motility of passing nonsensitized cells so that they accumulate at the site; corticosteroids antagonize this effect. Second—and perhaps of more importance in glomerulonephritis—is their action in stabilizing the lysosomal granules of cells, thus preventing the tissue destruction that otherwise would occur when granules are liberated from lymphocytes and polymorphonuclear leukocytes attracted to the site of an immune reaction. It is obvious that these effects also potentiate the risk of overwhelming infection.

Commonly Used Corticosteroids

The corticosteroids most frequently employed for immunosuppression are prednisone, prednisolone, and methylprednisolone. Cortisol and cortisone, when given in amounts producing the same antiinflammatory effect as prednisone and prednisolone, cause considerable sodium retention and foster potassium excretion. The synthetic fluoro derivatives of the corticosteroids are almost devoid of sodium-retaining effects and, on a weight basis, are potent antiinflammatory agents. However, the spectrum of toxic effects they produce, other than sodium retention, is the same as that for prednisone, prednisolone, and methylprednisolone, and no advantage has been seen in their use.

Corticosteroid Regimens

Certain aspects of therapy with corticosteroids are unique and must be borne in mind by the clinician in balancing toxicity and effectiveness. The regimen of administration is as important as the size of the dose. A single dose of a corticosteroid, even a large one, is virtually without harmful effects if given for only a few days. The greatest toxicity occurs when corticosteroids are given daily over a long period, and the extent of the toxicity is dose-dependent. Furthermore, if the daily dosage is divided into three or four doses, toxicity, as well as effectiveness, is greater than if the medication is given once daily.

The administration of corticosteroids depresses the secretion of corticotropin (ACTH) by the adenohypophysis; ACTH stores in the adenohypophysis are reduced, and hyalinization of the basophils may occur. The adrenal cortex also undergoes atrophy. As a result, symptoms of adrenal insufficiency may develop in the form of fever, myalgia, arthralgia, headache, and malaise when corticosteroid therapy is abruptly terminated. Therefore, if daily corticosteroid therapy has been given for more than a few weeks, the daily dosage may need to be reduced gradually before discontinuing the drug [27]. When corticosteroids have been given over very long periods, concentrations of both ACTH and cortisol in plasma remain below normal for 1 to 2 months [34]. Then, the ACTH level becomes elevated, but the level of cortisol remains low for several more months before it returns into the normal range. At about 9 months, ACTH levels fall to normal, suggesting complete return of adrenocortical responsiveness. Since production of corticosteroids by the pituitary-adrenal axis is an important element of homeostasis, particularly in times of stress, patients who are receiving corticosteroids or who have recently terminated a long course of therapy should receive exogenous corticosteroids when they undergo surgery or are subjected to trauma, to avoid the hazard of relative adrenal insufficiency.

Since 1963 [44], it has been known that administration of a single large dose of corticosteroids every other day will minimize adrenal and adenohypophyseal suppression, generate little toxicity, and yet in a number of situations produce antiinflammatory and other therapeutic effects. Corticosteroids are now widely used on this alternate-day schedule. To avoid upsetting the diurnal cycle of adrenocortical activity, the dose should be given in the morning. Children on such a regimen often gradually gain weight and have some degree of growth suppression, especially if the dose is high. Teenagers often exhibit few signs of toxicity. Since the regimen has little effect on adrenocortical activity, administration of corticosteroids to patients subject to surgery or trauma may not be necessary, although usually it is done. Under usual circumstances, alternate-day therapy can be terminated abruptly without development of withdrawal symptoms. However, in changing a patient who has received corticosteroids daily for a long period to an alternate-day regimen, the administration of a small dose of prednisone in the late afternoon on days that a morning dose is not given will make for a symptomless transition. The afternoon dose may be decreased gradually and discontinued over a 7-day to 10-day period.

High doses of methylprednisolone (15 to 30 mg per kilogram) given IV as a "pulse" have been extensively used in the treatment of renal transplant rejection [91]. After such a "pulse" dose, prednisolone achieves a very high level in serum, but the half-life is relatively short (2.3 ± 0.7 hr). Within 12 hr, prednisolone has virtually disappeared from the circulating fluids and none is detectable at 24 hr. With a similar dose of prednisone given orally, the peak concentration in serum is much lower but the level is sustained longer, and at 24 hr a significant concentration is still present. The depression of white blood cell and lymphocyte counts is similar with the two drugs. Successful use of pulse therapy with methylprednisolone has been reported in a few patients with severe (rapidly progressive) glomerulonephritis [20].

Toxic Effects

The toxic effects of corticosteroids are well known (Table 69-1); signs of Cushing's syndrome are most common. Significant or bothersome fluid retention or hypokalemia is uncommon with the derivatives in use today. Diabetes induced by corticosteroids may disappear if the drug can be withdrawn. Growth suppression is of particular concern in the treatment of children, although catch-up growth may occur with cessation of therapy, especially if corticosteroids have not previously been given over very long periods. The growth-suppresssing effect is less if an alternate-day regimen is used. Leukocytosis occurs fairly consistently; the high white cell counts negate the value of such counts as indicators of infection. Leukocytosis is an advantage in the management of patients concurrently receiving agents that suppress the bone marrow, in that counts appear to mirror more precisely the status of the bone marrow than when the cytotoxic agents are given without concurrent use of corticosteroids. Ecchymoses, muscular weakness, and atrophy are seen only in children receiving high doses over long periods; psychological changes, although occasionally observed, are relatively uncommon and seldom contraindicate the use of corticosteroids in children. Posterior

Table 69-1. Toxic Effects of Long-Term Corticosteroid Therapy

Cushingoid appearance
  Moon facies
  Obesity
  Acne
  Striae
	Psychological
	  Euphoria
	  Irritability
	  Insomnia

Fluid retention
  Edema
  Hypokalemia
	Circulatory
	  Hypertension
	  Cerebral edema

Endocrine abnormalities
  Diabetogenic in the
    latent diabetic
  Exacerbation of
    existing diabetes
  Suppression of
    adrenal function
  Growth suppression
	Osseous
	  Osteoporosis
	  Pathologic and com-
	    pression fracture

Hematologic changes
  Leukocytosis
  Ecchymosis
	Gastrointestinal
	  Peptic ulcer
	  Acute pancreatitis

Muscular system
  Weakness
  Atrophy
	Immunologic
	  Fungal infection
	  Activation of tuberculosis

Ophthalmologic Cataract	

subcapsular cataracts may develop in children who have received corticosteroids over long periods. In the absence of severe renal disease, corticosteroids produce only mild hypertension; however, severe hypertension with encephalopathy may be produced by these agents in the patient with significant glomerulonephritis, particularly, certain patients with membranoproliferative glomerulonephritis. The blood pressure of such patients should be closely monitored for several weeks after initiation of corticosteroid therapy, particularly if therapy is given daily in divided dosage. The hypertension usually can be controlled with prompt use of appropriate antihypertensives. Osseous changes and pathologic fractures are rare unless the corticosteroids are given daily over long periods. Peptic ulceration and pancreatitis are also uncommon in children.

Increased susceptibility to infection and rapid dissemination and masking of infections were feared when these agents first became available; however, widespread use has largely dissipated these concerns. Increased susceptibility and lowered resistance to infection usually become a hazard only in patients who are receiving cytotoxic drugs concurrently with corticosteroids. With the advent of infection in a patient receiving corticosteroids, the dose should be maintained or increased while the infection is being treated. Chickenpox may be fatal in the patient with severely depressed adrenal function, but no fatalities have been reported in children receiving corticosteroids on the alternate-day regimen.

PURINE ANALOGUES

The purine analogues produce maximal suppression of antibody response if given in the first 3 days after administration of antigen; they are probably most effective in aborting the early central phase of antibody production [12]. As previously noted, their use in the preinduction phase may, in animals, stimulate antibody formation [79, 88]. This stimulatory effect is probably confined to humoral antibody production, since use of azathioprine before renal transplantation in man does not enhance rejection of the graft. The purine analogues appear to have little effect on established antibody production. They do, however, have a marked effect on the manifestations of the immune state, that is, on the efferent limb. Thus, in the rabbit, without influencing the level of antibody to a foreign protein, 6-mercaptopurine will abolish the Arthus reaction when the foreign protein is given intradermally [11]. However, the animals in which this effect was demonstrated received doses of 6 to 10 mg per kilogram, which are considerably higher than those used therapeutically.

Azathioprine, the imidazole derivative of 6-mercaptopurine, is probably one of the best tolerated of the immunosuppressive agents, and, with its wide use in patients with organ transplants, considerable information has accumulated concerning its characteristics. It is probable that metabolites of the drug rather than azathioprine itself produce the immunosuppression as well as the toxic effects. The formation of 6-mercaptopurine during metabolism may account for some of the drug effects, but it is probable that other metabolites play a larger role. The drug is rapidly absorbed, but formation of active products does not occur until about 30 min after ingestion; the active metabolites are degraded in about 4 hr [43]. Very little azathioprine or 6-mercaptopurine is excreted in the urine, and the metabolites that are excreted are largely inactive. This circumstance should make the agent well tolerated in renal failure, since inactivation would occur normally. In practice, however, it is often found that leukopenia develops with the advent of renal failure when the usual dosage is maintained, necessitating a reduction in dosage if bone marrow depression is to be avoided. This effect may be due to an increased sensitivity of the bone marrow to the active metabolites, since with many of the cytotoxic agents, azotemia predisposes to leukopenia.

Since the biochemical pathways of activation and degradation of azathioprine are complex, there is considerable variation in tolerance to the drug [43]. Persons with a genetic constitution predisposing them to gout are said to have extreme sensitivity to the bone marrow–depressing effects of azathioprine. A similar increase in toxicity, together with a reduction in effectiveness, is seen in patients given allopurinol concurrently with azathioprine. In patients with hepatitis or cirrhosis, the metabolism of the drug is inhibited, with the result that it is not efficacious and in addition may be poorly tolerated. Azathioprine is not only of little value in patients with hepatic disease but also is hepatotoxic itself in some patients; cholestatic jaundice has occurred in a few patients, apparently as a direct toxic effect, contraindicating its use.

Bone marrow depression with azathioprine varies in its severity. Rarely, thrombocytopenia occurs. In some patients, anemia without leukopenia may develop at dosages that are usually well tolerated. In others, both anemia and leukopenia occur. The anemia and usually the leukopenia are easily reversed by discontinuing the drug for a time, but on other occasions, especially when the dose has been high, leukopenia may occur suddenly and herald dangerous, relatively long-standing bone marrow depression.

Infection is always a danger in patients being treated with cytotoxic drugs; its incidence and severity are increased in those concurrently receiving corticosteroids. With severe immunosuppression, ordinary pyogenic infections may occur, such as furuncles, abscesses, and wound infection. More frequently seen, however, are disseminated infections with opportunistic organisms that rarely cause disease in normal subjects. These may occur in patients only moderately suppressed immunologically and include active infection with the cytomegalovirus or with the protozoan *pneumocystis carinii*. Among the fungi, *Aspergillus, Nocardia,* and *Candida* may become invaders, and defense against the tuberculosis bacillus is also reduced. With the advent of such infection, the dose of immunosuppressive agents should be reduced or the drugs discontinued and specific treatment given if available. The lack of defense against these organisms is probably due primarily to the effect of the immunosuppressive regimen on cellular immunity.

Experience with 6-mercaptopurine as an immunosuppressive agent is not as extensive as with azathioprine. Its metabolism is similar, but it appears to produce a more profound bone marrow depression, and peripheral white cell counts may continue to fall for several days after the drug is discontinued. Thus, frequent blood counts are necessary, and the drug should be discontinued immediately when the count begins to fall. 6-Mercaptopurine also may produce gastrointestinal symptoms, especially when the drug has caused bone marrow depression.

ALKYLATING AGENTS

Mechlorethamine

Mechlorethamine, or nitrogen mustard, was for a time largely replaced by other alkylating agents that were more convenient to administer. Its use, however, has been increasing because of evidence of its efficacy and because the toxicity of the other agents has become more fully appreciated. It is the parent compound of a large series of cytotoxic agents, of which chlorambucil and cyclophosphamide are those most frequently used for immunosuppression.

Mechlorethamine is highly reactive with tissue and must be administered IV. Extravasation into tissue produces local necrosis and slough. After injection, it rapidly undergoes transformation and deactivation; almost none of the active material is excreted in the urine. It has an almost immediate lympholytic effect, a reduction in lymphocyte counts being noted within a few hours after administration; the nadir of the count is reached in 6 to 7 days. Granulocytopenia develops more slowly and lasts for 10 to 20 days. In patients with normally functioning bone marrow, the therapeutic dose neither produces significant thrombocytopenia nor predisposes to intercurrent infection. Nausea and vomiting may occur, the incidence of which is dose-dependent; thus, the total dose of 0.4 mg per kilogram is often divided into three or four daily doses. The agent does not produce alopecia or cystitis.

Cyclophosphamide

As noted previously, cyclophosphamide is most effective as an immunosuppressive agent if given immediately after antigenic stimulation; however, it also has some effect if given in the preinduction phase. It does not alter the function of macrophages as they participate in the efferent limb, but it does affect the central limb, possibly by interfering with the differentiation and replication of antigen-activated lymphocytes [12]. It is possibly by this latter means that it has some effect on established immunity and hence is of value in the therapy of autoimmune disorders in man.

Cyclophosphamide contains the same bis-(2-chloroethyl) grouping as nitrogen mustard but is relatively inert in vitro because of the stabilizing effect of the cyclic phosphamide that substitutes for the methyl group in nitrogen mustard. The compound was synthesized as an antitumor agent on the presumption that it would enter tumor cells. Since tumor cells supposedly contain phosphamidases, it was thought that in the cell the stabilizing phosphamide bond would be split, making it an active intracellular alkylating agent. The compound proved effective against many tumors, but subsequent studies indicated that its mechanism of action was more complex. Experimental tumors that in the host respond to cyclophosphamide therapy do not respond to the addition of cyclophosphamide to the medium when grown in vitro. Subsequent studies have shown that metabolites are largely responsible for the antitumor effects, and that these are produced in the microsomal mixed-function oxidase system of the liver on which the oxidative metabolism of many drugs depends. In man the drug is metabolized slowly, and the metabolites persist for a long period at relatively low levels, whereas in animals the rate of metabolism is rapid and high levels of metabolites are achieved. The active metabolites are thought to be aldophosphamide and carboxyphosphamide [47]. Both are alkylating agents and are effective in vitro against cultured neoplastic cells. Over a 2-day period after cyclophosphamide administration, two-thirds of the dose is excreted in the urine, most of it in the form of active metabolites [4]. In renal insufficiency, the active metabolites may be retained, resulting in toxicity at a lower dose [4]. Administration of inducers of the hepatic mixed-function microsomal enzyme system prior to the administration of cyclophosphamide causes the serum levels of metabolites to achieve a high level rapidly, but their rapid excretion makes the product of concentration × time approximately the same as in subjects without induced enzymes, so that the antitumor effect of the drug is not enhanced, nor is there significant enhancement of toxicity under the usual conditions [4, 50, 83]. Conversely, drugs that inhibit the mixed-function microsomal enzyme system reduce the levels of metabolites of concurrently administered cyclophosphamides. No studies of the effect of enzyme inducers or inhibitors on the immunosuppressive qualities of cyclophosphamide have been carried out.

Numerous toxic effects occur with cyclophosphamide therapy. The most serious of these are sterility and reduced resistance to certain viral infections. Sperm counts may fall within 3 weeks of starting treatment [30] and continue to fall for many months after the drug is discontinued. Permanent azoospermia is usually considered a hazard with treatment periods in excess of 60 to 80 days

[29], although patients treated for 7 to 9 months may have only reduced sperm counts and mild abnormalities on testicular biopsy [71]. Further observations must be made to determine the effect on spermatogenesis of multiple, widely spaced courses of the drug and the total dose-time relationships. The effect on the immature testis also needs further study, although there is evidence that subsequent spermatogenesis may be inhibited by treatment of prepubertal boys.

Reduced resistance to viral infection is a serious hazard of cyclophosphamide therapy, and several deaths have been attributed to it. Deaths from measles [64] and varicella infection [28, 78] have been reported in patients treated with cyclophosphamide. Severe varicella with recovery has also occurred [36]. The mortality and morbidity are not correlated with a high dose of cyclophosphamide, with the presence of leukopenia, or with the concurrent use of large amounts of prednisone.

Bone marrow depression occurs with large doses of cyclophosphamide. Clinically, it is expressed most commonly by a fall in leukocyte count with little change in hemoglobin or in the platelet count. The leukocyte count returns to normal relatively rapidly when administration is stopped or when the dose is reduced. Thus, the patient with a severely depressed leukocyte count is at risk of developing intercurrent infection for only a short time. Very often after prolonged use there is a marked lymphocytopenia.

Hemorrhagic cystitis and bladder fibrosis can also occur with cyclophosphamide administration. Hemorrhagic cystitis can occur acutely and is manifested by symptoms of bladder irritation and hematuria that gives a positive three-glass test. Acute hemorrhagic cystitis occurs in 10 percent of patients receiving the drug orally and in a somewhat higher percentage of those receiving it parenterally. It is apparently the result of the action of metabolites of cyclophosphamide on the bladder mucosa and can to some extent be prevented by maintaining a high fluid intake and by having the patient void frequently. In children, this is most easily accomplished by giving the dose in the morning or at noon and encouraging a high fluid intake. If hematuria or symptoms of bladder irritation develop, therapy should be immediately discontinued; it can be reinstituted again with greater attention to prophylactic measures when the symptoms subside. Continuing administration despite the hematuria can result in severe, possibly life-threatening bleeding. Bladder fibrosis can occur in the absence of hematuria or other symptoms and is more common in patients receiving the drug

IV. Its production is apparently dependent both on the dose and duration of therapy. A cumulative dose in excess of 6 gm per square meter predisposes to this complication [51]. It may develop without symptoms, but if bleeding should occur once fibrosis has developed, it may be severe and difficult to control, due to the marked telangiectasia of the bladder mucosa that accompanies the fibrosis.

Loss of hair that is continuously growing, e.g., that on the scalp, is a frequent accompaniment of cyclophosphamide administration. It is apparently due to a toxic effect of the cyclophosphamide itself on the rapidly dividing cells at the base of the hair follicle rather than to an effect of its metabolic products [9]. Alopecia appears to be dose-dependent; it does not usually occur when 2.5 mg per kilogram is given daily for 90 days [60]. Even with very large doses, some patients are not affected. In patients receiving the drug IV in large doses, a scalp tourniquet applied at the time of IV administration and left in place for 10 or 15 minutes thereafter will largely prevent hair loss. In some patients, regrowth of hair occurs despite continuing administration of the drug.

Nausea and vomiting may occur 8 to 12 hours after drug administration. It is especially frequent in older children who take a large total dose. The symptoms are best controlled with cyclizine.

Chlorambucil

Chlorambucil is another alkylating agent reported to be useful in the therapy of renal disease. Like cyclophosphamide it may be given orally. The bone marrow depression it produces responds quickly to withdrawal of the drug and in many respects it is the safest of the alkylating agents. Although in patients with neoplasms, bone marrow depression may occur after cumulative doses of 6.5 mg per kilogram, in patients with nephrosis, cumulative doses as high as 31 mg per kilogram have been given during a course of therapy without untoward effects [37]. The drug produces azoospermia, as does cyclophosphamide [76], but the incidence of alopecia, cystitis and gastrointestinal symptoms is very low [37, 37a]. Although potentiation of morbidity and mortality in patients with measles and chickenpox has not been described, chlorambucil apparently predisposes to herpes zoster [85] and herpes simplex.

Nonsteroidal Antiinflammatory Drugs

Indomethacin is the nonsteroidal antiinflammatory drug most often used in the treatment of glomerulonephritis, mainly by European nephrologists.

Like other antiinflammatory agents, one of its primary effects is depression of the synthesis of the prostaglandins. There is also evidence that it impedes the release of lysosomal granules by neutrophils during phagocytosis [92] and reduces the mobility of the polymorphonuclear leukocytes [72]. One of its striking effects when used for the treatment of nephritis is the reduction in proteinuria. Ultrastructural studies of the glomeruli of normal rats receiving indomethacin over periods of several weeks indicate that the drug increases the cellular activity of the epithelial cells [80]. Since epithelial cells are considered to be responsible for the synthesis of basement membrane material, their stimulation by indomethacin in nephritis could conceivably be responsible for the reduction in proteinuria.

In general, there is considerable dissociation between the clinical effects of indomethacin and changes in glomerular morphology. Thus, although the patient is improved clinically, renal biopsies may indicate no change or even progression of the glomerular lesion [86]; and when therapy is stopped, signs and symptoms of active disease often promptly return. The possible effectiveness of this drug must be balanced against the frequent side effects associated with its prolonged use, mainly gastrointestinal hemorrhage and perforation.

Antagonists of Vasoactive Amines in Prevention of Immune Complex Deposition

Interest in agents that have antiserotonin-antihistamine activity in the therapy of glomerulonephritis derives from studies of experimental nephritis in animals. Observations of Benacerraf et al. [6], and later of Cochrane [17, 18], indicated that when histamine was given to a mouse or a guinea pig, colloidal carbon, injected simultaneously, was deposited beneath the endothelium of small vessels in the lung, heart, stomach, and, in the mouse, beneath the glomerular endothelium. If histamine was not given, the carbon was quickly removed from the circulation by the reticuloendothelial system. Subendothelial localization also occurred if antigen-antibody complexes were given with the carbon in sufficient amounts to produce anaphylaxis. Serotonin, even in high dosage, caused no subendothelial deposition, and when deposition was produced by anaphylaxis with antigen-antibody complexes, antihistamines were effective in preventing deposition but antiserotonins were not.

The role of histamine in the genesis of serum sickness nephritis in the rabbit produced by the injection of foreign protein was subsequently investigated by Kniker and Cochrane [56]. Although anaphylactic shock does not occur in this disease, histamine is apparently liberated from platelets at the time of immune elimination of the antigen. The release is apparently leukocyte-dependent [46]. In the presence of the protein, rabbit basophils sensitized with homocytotropic antibody to the injected protein generate a soluble factor that causes platelet release of vasoactive amines that foster subendothelial deposition of concurrently formed complexes. It has also been found that this form of experimental nephritis can be ameliorated by depleting the animal of platelets or by the use of antihistamines. Kniker and Cochrane [55, 56] reported that acute and chronic serum sickness nephritis could be largely prevented by use of antihistamines; given after chronic serum sickness nephritis had developed, antihistamines caused amelioration of the disease [55]. The antihistamine most effective was chlorpheniramine maleate or the combination of chlorpheniramine with methysergide maleate, an antiserotonin. Cyproheptadine, which is both an antiserotonin and an antihistamine, was less effective. Least effective was methysergide alone.

These observations in themselves would appear to have limited applicability to nephritis in man. In contrast to the rabbit, man has no histamine in his platelets and only small amounts of serotonin. Thus, if a platelet-releasing mechanism were functional in man, release of histamine would not occur, and, judging from the observations in animals, the release of serotonin would not be effective in producing immune complex deposition. It should be noted, however, that studies by Bolton et al. [10] of autologous immune complex (Heymann) nephritis in the rat have shown that the administration of cyproheptadine delays the onset and reduces the severity of the proteinuria. The rat, like man, has no histamine and only small amounts of serotonin in platelets, and the question arises as to whether or not histamine release in immune complex nephritis in species in which it is not found in platelets might be from another source. Although these observations open possibilities for therapy, evidence is as yet lacking that antihistamines are effective in any form of human glomerulonephritis.

Problems Encountered in the Development of Specific Therapy of the Glomerulonephritides

Although a number of publications have reported the use of regimens of therapy designed specifically for glomerulonephritis, the information that has accumulated does not allow unequivocal definition of optimal therapy for any form of the disease. With few exceptions, the efficacy of a treatment regimen as claimed by one group of observers has not been verified by others. As pointed out by Skinner and Schwartz [82], the literature is confusing and difficult to analyze, and, in some reports, insufficient information is given to allow the reader to draw independent conclusions.

In part, the difficulty in developing successful regimens of therapy and proving that they are efficacious is the combined result of the nature of glomerulonephritis and the characteristics of the therapeutic agents employed. Some of the factors that complicate the problem are enumerated in the following sections.

Heterogeneity of Glomerulonephritis

Glomerulonephritis is a blanket term that encompasses a number of disease entities (Chap. 43). It seems unlikely that any form of therapy will emerge that will be applicable to all forms of the disease. Hence, use of a therapeutic regimen for all patients with glomerulonephritis without regard to type often results in data that are difficult to interpret. With modern techniques and expanded criteria for identifying disease, treatment trials in recent reports have often been confined to one entity, and, by such efforts, progress will eventually be made.

Variable Natural History of Glomerulonephritis

Many forms of glomerulonephritis undergo spontaneous remission, making evaluation of therapeutic regimens used anecdotally difficult. Thus, in membranous glomerulopathy and membranoproliferative glomerulonephritis, particularly in children, spontaneous improvement in the clinical course is not unusual. Hence, unless the therapy is consistently and unquestionably efficacious, demonstration of the efficacy of a regimen using clinical and laboratory observations as criteria demands a controlled trial.

Time at Which Therapy is Initiated

In several diseases, a demonstrable improvement might occur if therapy were initiated early in the course of the disease, but with time, damage may occur that is irreparable and unresponsive to any treatment. A prime example is rapidly progressive glomerulonephritis. Another may be the nephritis of anaphylactoid purpura. Some disease may have a "silent" onset, so that the stage at which therapy is initiated is not known with certainty. Heterogeneity of patients with respect to time of onset thus

may constitute a variable of unknown magnitude in judging the effectiveness of therapy, especially when data emanating from a referral hospital are compared with those from a primary care center.

Basis for Judgment of Efficacy of Therapy

In diseases in which the patients uniformly exhibit renal insufficiency at the initiation of treatment, improvement in function as determined by clearance and other functional studies may be taken as evidence of success. Similarly, in diseases characterized by a nephrotic syndrome, reduction or clearing of proteinuria would demonstrate efficacy. However, in conditions in which proteinuria is not excessive and renal impairment is not uniform, as in many cases of membranoproliferative glomerulonephritis, in the early stages of membranous glomerulopathy, or in long-standing cases of the nephritis of anaphylactoid purpura, the only measure of success may be changes observed on renal biopsy. Thus, an important basis for judgment in many trials would be comparison of pretreatment and posttreatment biopsy findings. Data on this aspect of the disease are often meager or absent.

It is to be hoped that the methods for measurement of immune complexes in serum that are now being developed will provide a measure of the efficacy of an immunosuppressive regimen that is quickly available and more direct than criteria currently employed.

Simultaneous Use of Multiple Therapeutic Agents

It is rare for treatment trials to employ one agent; some regimens consist of as many as four agents. Assuming some efficacy is shown for the regimen, many questions arise. Are the effects the result of synergism among agents, or could agents producing dangerous side effects or complications be eliminated? Comparison with other trials employing different combinations or the same agents in a different regimen or dosage is often not possible, especially when all the other variables are considered.

The Regimen of Therapy and Dose

It is within the realm of possibility that a given agent in a low dose may be of no value in therapy, but given intensively over a short period at the onset of the disease, a therapeutic advantage might be achieved. Thus, a trial may indicate that an agent is of no benefit when, had a different regimen been used, effectiveness could have been demonstrated. The regimen is particularly important in the case of corticosteroids. The therapeutic effect of giving a dose once daily may be entirely different than that observed when the same dosage is divided into three or four doses daily. Similarly, duration of therapy is of prime importance; courses of short duration may give no information about the value of a drug. Improvement may not be discernible during a short course of therapy, since some time may be required for areas of the glomerulus that are not irreversibly damaged to improve their functional capacity. It is well known that even in situations in which the immune complexes that generate nephritis are rapidly and completely eliminated from the circulation, as is possible in the nephritis of chronic bacteremia, the glomerular deposits may persist for months, and proteinuria may continue over long periods [95]. Since therapeutic trials seldom last more than 1 year and usually are of shorter duration, drugs that may be potentially of benefit may be classed as ineffective.

Although many of these circumstances in themselves do not constitute insurmountable obstacles to the design of treatment regimens or the interpretation of their results, when considered together, many difficulties arise. The solution may lie in the use of controlled trials. However, many disadvantages attend such controlled trials. Not only are suitable protocols often difficult to formulate from the information available, but also the small number of patients with a single disease at a given institution requires that expensive and often cumbersome collaboration be instituted among several centers to provide sufficient patients and that the study extend for long periods. The ethics of denying therapy or using a regimen thought to be less efficacious to one group must always be considered. Changes in the protocol that experience might suggest would be advantageous cannot easily be made. Despite those difficulties, it is the opinion of many investigators that properly designed controlled trials provide the only acceptable means of determining the balance between clinical efficacy and toxicity of therapeutic agents. Others, including the author, believe that, in view of the present state of knowledge about many of the nephritides and their therapy, it would appear more advantageous in these instances to continue with anecdotal observations, modifying the regimen if there are signs of efficacy, until firmer impressions are gained that one or more regimens with the greatest benefit and the least toxicity have been identified. At this stage, if some of the variables that have been mentioned prevent clear interpretation of results, a controlled trial would be indicated.

Status of Specific Therapy of Glomerulonephritis

PRIMARY GLOMERULAR DISEASE

Rapidly Progressive Glomerulonephritis
Rapidly progressive glomerulonephritis is a descriptive term often applied to a syndrome characterized by rapid deterioration of glomerular function and with crescent formation in a large proportion of the glomeruli. Although many diseases have been known to evolve in this manner, in a large proportion of the cases, a disease entity cannot be identified [3]. The therapy of patients with this syndrome has been markedly influenced by the observation that in experimental animals the nephritis produced by nephrotoxic serum, characterized also by rampant crescent formation, can be prevented by anticoagulation of the animals with heparin [42], warfarin [94], or the defibrinating agent ancrod [68]. Because crescents are produced by a leakage of fibrinogen into Bowman's space with formation of fibrin, anticoagulant therapy would appear logical. A platelet inhibitor (dipyridamole), a cytotoxic agent and/or corticosteroids are frequently added to the anticoagulant therapy.

Although the usefulness of anticoagulants has been stressed by a number of observers, no controlled study has been undertaken to evaluate their effect critically; their use is by no means universal, in part because of their hazard (Chap. 70) [87]. In rabbits, anticoagulants are effective in preventing or ameliorating the experimental disease only when given in very high, potentially dangerous dosage. Thus, in a study of Vassalli and McClusky [94] employing warfarin, the effective dose was such that 75 percent of the rabbits died of intrathoracic or intraperitoneal hemorrhage before the conclusion of the experiment. In the study of Halpern et al. [42], the dose of heparin was 20 to 40 mg per kilogram, four to eight times the dose usually employed clinically. Thomson et al. [90] recently showed that heparin in doses up to 8 mg per kilogram had no effect on the development of the nephritis, and that doses of 16 mg per kilogram, producing virtually unclottable blood, ameliorated but did not prevent renal damage.

Recently, success with therapy consisting of large IV doses of methylprednisolone has been reported [20].

Membranoproliferative (Mesangiocapillary)
Glomerulonephritis
Because an immunologic origin of membranoproliferative glomerulonephritis seems likely, as evidenced by the frequent presence of a low serum complement level and of glomerular deposits of

complement and immunoglobulin, a number of therapeutic trials employing immunosuppressive agents and corticosteroids have been reported. When evaluated by changes in the clinical course, the results of these trials indicate that neither immunosuppressive agents, corticosteroids, nor combinations of the two, are efficacious [41].

A criticism of these trials is that judgment of efficacy was largely based on the clinical course [16]. Improvement in glomerular morphology, rarely occurring spontaneously [58], would be a better criterion [16]. Analysis according to survival rate is impractical because of the long duration of the disease before irreversible renal failure develops. A second criticism is that the therapy may not have been continued over sufficiently long periods. It seems likely, in view of the severity of the renal lesion and from experience with shunt nephritis [95], that improvement in glomerular morphology would occur slowly.

Kincaid-Smith [53, 54] has described a regimen consisting of cyclophosphamide, an anticoagulant, and a platelet inhibitor (dipyridamole). Given over periods of 4 to 53 months to patients with varying degrees of renal failure, it produced striking improvement in the glomerular morphologic picture, at least in certain patients; survival also appeared to be prolonged, although no acceptable comparison group was available. The data do not permit dissection of the regimen to determine which component(s) was necessary for the apparent therapeutic effect.

McAdams et al. [58] have observed in 8 patients who did not have end-stage disease that prednisone given on alternate days for periods of 3.5 to 10 years produced improvement in the glomerular morphologic findings, with amelioration of many of the clinical signs of the disease. Intramembranous deposits persisted despite overall improvement in morphology, whereas subendothelial deposits diminished or disappeared.

Long-term therapy with indomethacin alone [66, 86] or combined with small doses of cyclophosphamide [93] has also been used in this disease. Indomethacin alone was reported to slow deterioration of renal function and, in combination with cyclophosphamide, to improve it. With both regimens, proteinuria diminished. Indomethacin alone caused no improvement in the glomerular morphologic picture.

Membranous Glomerulonephropathy

Spontaneous symptomatic remission of membranous nephropathy is not unusual, especially in children [40]. The renal lesion also may spontaneously improve or, occasionally, completely resolve,

although in adults, progression is more commonly observed [33].

The variability of the course of the disease makes assessment of the effectiveness of therapy from anecdotal observations difficult. In adults, remissions have been observed during or after corticosteroid therapy [26, 31, 33], but a number of patients have not responded. In a number the disease has worsened during therapy, and one patient who went into remission during daily corticosteroid therapy had a relapse while still receiving the drug [33]. Despite occasional unfavorable responses, a retrospective study of the outcome of 103 cases [26a] strongly suggested that adequate steroid therapy is beneficial, especially when the changes in the basement membrane are not severe.

The results of anecdotal use [33] and of a controlled trial [23] of cyclophosphamide have been reported. In the trial, no advantage of this therapy was evident.

Since the disease is probably the result of deposition of immune complexes in the glomerulus, there is a theoretical basis for the use of antihistamines [55, 56]. Bolton et al. [10] have shown that in experimental autologous glomerulonephritis in rats, a disease in which glomerular morphology is similar to that seen in human membranous glomerulopathy, continuous administration of cyproheptadine following injection of autologous renal tissue slowed the appearance of and reduced the severity of the proteinuria. However, there have been no reports of successful use of antagonists of vasoactive amines in the human disease.

IgA-IgG Mesangial Nephropathy

The only reported attempt at therapy of IgA-IgG mesangial nephropathy, which is characterized by mesangial proliferation apparently secondary to mesangial deposits of IgA, IgG, and C3 [8], has been the use of alternate-day prednisone over long periods [62]. With five courses of such treatment given to 4 patients, the urinary abnormalities disappeared to a large extent. However, microhematuria recurred in 12 to 29 months in 2 patients. Further experience with this therapy in our hands has given similar results. However, 1 patient who had been free of urinary abnormalities for 2 years after cessation of therapy had on repeat renal biopsy immunofluorescence findings and mesangial proliferation unchanged from the pretreatment biopsy.

GLOMERULAR DISEASE ACCOMPANYING SYSTEMIC DISEASE

Nephritis of Systemic Lupus Erythematosus

The principles of humoral immunosuppression described earlier in this chapter should be especially applicable to glomerular disease accompanying systemic lupus erythematosus, since deposition of circulating immune complexes in the glomerulus appears to play a central role in its pathogenesis [74]. Corticosteroids have been long employed in treating this condition, particularly after the observations of Pollak et al. [73] indicating that survival was increased in patients receiving a relatively high dose for 6 months (40 to 60 mg of prednisone daily in the adult) in comparison with that in patients receiving a lower dose. Corticosteroids are still considered to have the highest therapeutic index in ameliorating this form of nephritis, but therapeutic failures in some patients and excessive toxicity from high doses given over long periods have stimulated trials of supplementation of corticosteroid therapy with cytotoxic agents such as 6-mercaptopurine, azathioprine, cyclophosphamide, and mechlorethamine [22, 24, 25, 84, 89] and of multiple plasmaphoreses to eliminate circulating complexes [51a]. Cytotoxic agents may be combined with corticosteroids either in the beginning of the illness or later as a means of "covering" gradual reduction in the corticosteroid dosage [69]. At the present time, an optimal therapeutic regimen has not been established.

Nephritis of Anaphylactoid Purpura
The variable clinical course and relatively few predictors of outcome in the acute phase of the nephritis of anaphylactoid purpura render judgment of the efficacy of therapy very difficult [52, 63]. Patients with acute nephritic or nephrotic syndromes or both at onset are the only ones who need to be treated; and to demonstrate benefits statistically, many would have to be treated needlessly, since few of these patients suffer permanent renal impairment. The time after onset that therapy is initiated might also be a factor in its success. Since the disease in severe form is not common, significant results would be demonstrable with a given regimen only by pooling cases from a large number of centers. Both corticosteroids and cytotoxic drugs have been used for therapy, but their effectiveness has not been convincingly demonstrated, either alone or in combination [52, 56a, 63].

Wegener's Granulomatosis
Numerous case reports of therapy in Wegener's granulomatosis indicate quite uniformly that corticosteroids are of little value, except perhaps in the mild case before the development of severe pulmonary and renal lesions. On the other hand, many cytotoxic agents appear to be effective, including azathioprine, methotrexate, and the alkylating agents mechlorethamine, chlorambucil, and cyclophosphamide [2]. Of these, azathioprine, cyclophosphamide, and methotrexate have been used most frequently. Methotrexate is said to be most rapidly effective and hence useful in acutely ill or moribund patients [15], but the results with azathioprine and cyclophosphamide have been highly satisfactory [49, 70]. It appears unnecessary to combine the cytotoxic agent with corticosteroid therapy [49].

The Goodpasture Syndrome
Although the Goodpasture syndrome is not invariably fatal [7, 75], very few patients in whom significant renal insufficiency develops recover [21, 67]. Corticosteroid therapy has, in some patients, seemed to suppress the pulmonary hemorrhage [7], but has had little or no effect on the progression of the renal lesion. Success with cytotoxic agents on the renal lesion has been variable; those reported effective when initiated after the development of renal insufficiency are azathioprine [45, 65] and mechlorethamine [21]; however, failures with such agents have also been reported [21, 45]. Recently, efforts to reduce circulatory antibody to basement membrane by combining multiple plasmaphoreses with immunosuppression have been reported [56b] to improve the prognosis.

Nephrotic Syndrome of Childhood
Minimal Change
In the absence of a known pathogenesis of minimal change nephrotic syndrome, it cannot be assumed that therapy is effective because it is immunosuppressive. Yet certain agents that are immunosuppressive do alter its course. Corticosteroid therapy not only produces a remission in about 90 percent of patients, but also, used when the disease is in remission, often prevents relapses. Alkylating agents are also effective in producing prolonged remissions, even if the course of therapy is administered while the disease is in remission. The three modalities that appear to influence the course of this disease, namely, corticosteroids, alkylating agents [5, 13, 36, 37, 37a, 48, 60, 61], and infection with the measles virus, produce lysis or functional alterations of lymphocytes; this observation has led Shalhoub [81] to the attractive hypothesis that the basic abnormality is a disorder of T lymphocytes. Until more information is available on this point, nephrologists must, unfortunately, use trial-and-error experience to formulate optimal therapy in this disease. There are currently no guidelines other than relapses of the disease that can serve as an index of the effectiveness of therapy.

Nephrotic Syndrome with Mesangial Proliferation

Some patients with slight to moderate mesangial proliferation will respond to corticosteroid therapy, as do patients with nil disease [35, 98]. In these patients the mesangial proliferation may disappear with time [35]. Those with more severe degrees of mesangial proliferation are less frequently corticosteroid-responsive [96, 98] and probably gain little benefit from the use of alkylating agents [96]. In those initially unresponsive, an intermittent or alternate-day prednisone regimen is often instituted and, with time, because of or despite such a regimen, they may eventually lose their proteinuria and the prognosis may be good [98].

Focal Glomerulosclerosis

A rare child with focal glomerulosclerosis may respond to conventional corticosteroid therapy [97]. In one series [39], complete responsiveness to corticosteroid was observed in 23 percent, and in another, none responded [14]. Some authors [14, 38, 39] have observed partial (diminution of proteinuria) or complete response in a few patients receiving cytotoxic therapy, but others [97] have seen no response to these agents. Those most responsive to cytotoxic drug therapy are largely from the group who are partially responsive to corticosteroid therapy [39].

References

1. Aisenberg, A. C. An introduction to immunosuppressants. *Adv. Pharmacol. Chemother.* 8:31, 1970.
2. Aldo, M. A., Benson, M. D., Comerford, F. R., and Cohen, A. S. Treatment of Wegener's granulomatosis with immunosuppressive agents. *Arch. Intern. Med.* 126:298, 1970.
3. Bacani, R. A., Valasquez, F., Kanter, A., Pirani, C. L., and Pollak, V. E. Rapidly progressive (nonstreptococcal) glomerulonephritis. *Ann. Intern. Med.* 69:463, 1968.
4. Bagley, C. M., Jr., Bostick, F. W., and DeVita, V. T., Jr. Clinical pharmacology of cyclophosphamide. *Cancer Res.* 33:226, 1973.
5. Barratt, T. M., Bercowsky, A., Osofsky, S. G., Soothill, J. F., and Kay, R. Cyclophosphamide treatment in steroid-sensitive nephrotic syndrome of childhood. *Lancet* 1:55, 1975.
6. Benacerraf, B., McClusky, R. T., and Patras, D. Localization of colloidal substances in vascular endothelium. A mechanism of tissue damage. I. Factors causing the pathologic deposition of colloidal carbon. *Am. J. Pathol.* 35:75, 1959.
7. Benoit, F. L., Rulon, D. B., Theil, G. B., Doolan, P. D., and Watter, R. H. Goodpasture's syndrome. A clinicopathologic entity. *Am. J. Med.* 37:424, 1964.
8. Berger, J. IgA glomerular deposits in renal disease. *Transplant. Proc.* 1:939, 1969.
9. Bergsagel, D. E. Toxicity with Cyclophosphamide. In M. E. Vancil (ed.), *Workshop on Immunosup-*

pressive Properties of Cyclophosphamide. Evansville, Ind.: Mead Johnson, 1971.
10. Bolton, W. K., Spargo, B. A., and Lewis, E. J. Chronic autologous immune complex glomerulopathy: Effect of cyproheptadine. *J. Lab. Clin. Med.* 83:695, 1974.
11. Borel, Y., and Schwartz, R. Inhibition of immediate and delayed hypersensitivity in the rabbit by 6-mercaptopurine. *J. Immunol.* 92:754, 1964.
12. Bradley, J., and Elson, C. J. Suppression of the immune response. *J. Med. Genet.* 8:321, 1971.
12a. Brown, C. B., Wilson, D., Turner, D., Cameron, J. S., Ogg, C. S., Chantler, C., and Gill, B. Combined immunosuppression and anticoagulation in rapidly progressive glomerulonephritis. *Lancet* 2:1166, 1974.
13. Cameron, J. S., Chantler, C., Ogg, C. S., and White, R. H. R. Long-term stability of remission in nephrotic syndrome after treatment with cyclophosphamide. *Br. Med. J.* 4:7, 1974.
14. Cameron, J. S., Ogg, C. S., Turner, D. R., and Weller, R. O. Focal Glomerulosclerosis. In P. Kincaid-Smith, T. H. Mathew, and E. L. Becker (eds.), *Glomerulonephritis: Morphology, Natural History and Treatment.* New York: Wiley, 1973. Pp. 249–261.
15. Capizzi, R. L., and Bertano, J. R. Methotrexate therapy of Wegener's granulomatosis. *Ann. Intern. Med.* 74:74, 1971.
16. Chirawong, P., Nanra, R. S., and Kincaid-Smith, P. Fibrin degradation products and the role of coagulation in "persistent" glomerulonephritis. *Ann. Intern. Med.* 74:853, 1971.
17. Cochrane, C. G. Studies on the localization of antigen-antibody complexes and other macromolecules in vessels. I. Structural studies. *J. Exp. Med.* 118:489, 1963.
18. Cochrane, C. G. Studies on the localization of antigen-antibody complexes and other macromolecules in vessels. II. Pathogenic and pharmacodynamic studies. *J. Exp. Med.* 118:503, 1963.
19. Cochrane, C. G. Mediation of immunologic glomerular injury. *Transplant. Proc.* 1:949, 1969.
20. Cole, B. R., Brocklebank, J. T., Kienstra, R. A., Kissane, J. M., and Robson, A. M. "Pulse" methylprednisolone therapy in the treatment of severe glomerulonephritis. *J. Pediatr.* 88:307, 1976.
21. Couser, W. G. Goodpasture's syndrome: A response to nitrogen mustard. *Am. J. Med. Sci.* 268:175, 1974.
21a. Couser, W. G., Stilmant, M. M., and Jermanovich, N. B. Complement independent nephrotoxic nephritis in the guinea pig. *Kidney Int.* 11:170, 1977.
22. Dillard, M. G., Dujovne, I., Pollak, V. E., and Pirani, C. L. The effect of treatment with prednisone and nitrogen mustard on the renal lesions and life span of patients with lupus glomerulonephritis. *Nephron* 10:273, 1973.
23. Donadio, J. V., Holley, K. E., Anderson, C. F., and Taylor, W. F. Controlled trial of cyclophosphamide in idiopathic membranous nephropathy. *Kidney Int.* 6:431, 1974.
24. Donadio, J. V., Holley, K. E., Wagoner, R. D., Ferguson, R. H., and McDuffie, F. C. Treatment of lupus nephritis with prednisone and combined prednisone and azathioprine. *Ann. Intern. Med.* 77:829, 1972.
25. Drinkard, J. P., Stanley, T. M., Dornfeld, L., Austin,

R. C., Barnett, E. V., Pearson, C. M., Vernier, R. L., Adams, D. A., Latta, H., and Gonick, H. C. Azathioprine and prednisone in the treatment of adults with lupus nephritis. *Medicine (Baltimore).* 49:411, 1970.

26. Ehrenreich, T., and Churg, J. Pathology of membranous nephropathy. *Pathol. Annual* 3:145, 1968.

26a. Ehrenreich, T., Porush, J. G., Churg, J., Garfinkel, L., Glabman, S., Goldstein, M. G., Grishman, E., and Yunis, S. L. Treatment of idiopathic membranous nephropathy. *N. Engl. J. Med.* 295:741, 1976.

27. Ensign, D. C., Sigler, J. W., and Wilson, G. M., Jr. Steroids in rheumatoid arthritis: A challenge to the internist. *Arch. Intern. Med.* 104:949, 1959.

28. Etteldorf, J. N., Roy, S. III, Summitt, R. L., Sweeney, M. J., Wall, H. P., and Berton, W. M. Cyclophosphamide in the treatment of idiopathic lipoid nephrosis. *J. Pediatr.* 70:758, 1967.

29. Etteldorf, J. N., West, C. D., Pitcock, J. A., and Williams, D. L. Gonadal function, testicular histology, and meiosis following cyclophosphamide therapy in patients with nephrotic syndrome. *J. Pediatr.* 88:206, 1976.

30. Fairley, K. F., Barrier, J. U., and Johnson, W. Sterility and testicular atrophy related to cyclophosphamide therapy. *Lancet* 1:568, 1972.

31. Forland, M., and Spargo, B. H. Clinicopathological correlations in idiopathic nephrotic syndrome with membranous nephropathy. *Nephron* 6:498, 1969.

32. Frenkel, E. P., and Stone, M. J. The rationale and approach to immunosuppressive therapy. *Adv. Intern. Med.* 17:21, 1971.

33. Gluck, M. C., Gallo, G., Lowenstein, J., and Baldwin, D. Membranous glomerulonephritis: Evolution of clinical and pathological features. *Ann. Intern. Med.* 78:1, 1973.

34. Graber, A. L., Ney, R. L., Nicholson, W. E., Island, D. P., and Liddle, G. W. Natural history of pituitary-adrenal recovery following long-term suppression with corticosteroids. *J. Clin. Endocrinol. Metab.* 25:11, 1965.

35. Grishman, E., and Churg, J. Pathology of Nephrotic Syndrome with Minimal or Minor Glomerular Changes. In P. Kincaid-Smith, T. H. Mathew, and E. L. Becker (eds.), *Glomerulonephritis: Morphology, Natural History and Treatment.* New York: Wiley, 1973. Pp. 165–181.

36. Grunberg, J. Cyclophosphamide therapy for nephrosis. *J. Pediatr.* 73:641, 1968.

37. Grupe, W. E. Chlorambucil in steroid dependent nephrotic syndrome. *J. Pediatr.* 82:598, 1973.

37a. Grupe, W. E., Makker, S. P., and Ingelfinger, J. R. Chlorambucil treatment of frequently relapsing nephrotic syndrome. *N. Engl. J. Med.* 295:746, 1976.

38. Habib, R. Focal glomerular sclerosis (editorial). *Kidney Int.* 4:355, 1973.

39. Habib, R., and Gubler, M.-C. Focal Sclerosing Glomerulonephritis. In P. Kincaid-Smith, T. H. Mathew, and E. L. Becker (eds.), *Glomerulonephritis: Morphology, Natural History and Treatment.* New York: Wiley, 1973. Pp. 263–278.

40. Habib, R., Kleinknecht, C., and Gubler, M.-C. Extramembranous glomerulonephritis in children: Report of 50 cases. *J. Pediatr.* 82:754, 1973.

41. Habib, R., Kleinknecht, C., Gubler, M.-C., and Levy, M. Idiopathic membranoproliferative glomerulonephritis in children. Report of 105 cases. *Clin. Nephrol.* 1:194, 1973.

42. Halpern, B., Milliez, P., Lagrue, G., Fray, A., and Morard, J. C. Protective action of heparin in experimental immune nephritis. *Nature* 205:257, 1965.

43. Hamburger, J., Crosnier, J., Dormont, J., and Bach, J. F. *Renal Transplantation, Theory and Practice.* Baltimore: Williams & Wilkins, 1972. Pp. 77–99.

44. Harter, J. G., Reddy, W. J., and Thorn, G. W. Studies on an intermittent corticosteroid dosage regimen. *N. Engl. J. Med.* 269:591, 1963.

45. Hayslett, J. P., Berte, J. B., and Kashgarian, M. Successful treatment of renal failure in Goodpasture's syndrome. *Arch. Intern. Med.* 127:953, 1971.

46. Henson, P. M., and Cochrane, C. G. Immune complex disease in rabbits. The role of complement and of a leukocyte dependent release of vasoactive amines from platelets. *J. Exp. Med.* 133:554, 1971.

47. Hill, D. L., Laster, W. R., Jr., and Struck, R. F. Enzymatic metabolism of cyclophosphamide and nicotine and production of a toxic cyclophosphamide metabolite. *Cancer Res.* 32:658, 1972.

48. International Study of Kidney Disease in Children. Prospective, controlled trial of cyclophosphamide therapy in children with the nephrotic syndrome. *Lancet* 2:423, 1974.

49. Israel, H. L., and Patchefsky, A. S. Wegener's granulomatosis of lung: Diagnosis and treatment. Experience with 12 cases. *Ann. Intern. Med.* 74:881, 1971.

50. Jao, J. Y., Jusko, W. J., and Cohen, J. L. Phenobarbitol effects on cyclophosphamide pharmacokinetics in man. *Cancer Res.* 32:2761, 1972.

51. Johnson, W. W., and Meadows, D. C. Urinary-bladder fibrosis and telangiectasia associated with long-term cyclophosphamide therapy. *N. Engl. J. Med.* 284:290, 1971.

51a. Jones, J. V., Bucknall, R. C., Cammin, R. H., Asplin, C. M., Fraser, I. D., Bothamley, J., Davis, P., and Hamblin, T. J. Plasmaphoresis in the management of acute systemic lupus erythematosus? *Lancet* 1:709, 1976.

52. Kalowski, S., and Kincaid-Smith, P. Glomerulonephritis in Henoch-Schönlein Syndrome. In P. Kincaid-Smith, T. H. Mathew, and E. L. Becker (eds.), *Glomerulonephritis: Morphology, Natural History and Treatment.* New York: Wiley, 1973. Pp. 1123–1132.

53. Kincaid-Smith, P. The treatment of chronic mesangio-capillary (membranoproliferative) glomerulonephritis with impaired renal function. *Med. J. Aust.* 2:587, 1972.

54. Kincaid-Smith, P. The Natural History and Treatment of Mesangio-Capillary Glomerulonephritis. In P. Kincaid-Smith, T. H. Mathew, and E. L. Becker (eds.), *Glomerulonephritis: Morphology, Natural History and Treatment.* New York: Wiley, 1973. Pp. 591–609.

55. Kniker, W. T. Modulation of the Inflammatory Response in Vivo: Prevention or Amelioration of Immune Complex Disease. In I. H. Lepow and P. A. Ward (eds.), *Inflammation: Mechanisms and Control.* New York: Academic, 1972. Pp. 335–363.

56. Kniker, W. T., and Cochrane, C. G. The localization of circulating immune complexes in experimental serum sickness. The role of vasoactive amines and hydrodynamic forces. *J. Exp. Med.* 127:119, 1968.

56a. Levy, M., Broyer, M., Arsan, A., Levy-Bentolila, D., and Habib, R. Anaphylactoid purpura nephritis in childhood: Natural history and immunopathology. *Adv. Nephrol.* 6:183, 1977.

56b. Lockwood, C. M., Pearson, T. A., Rees, A. V., Evans, D. J., Peters, D. K., and Wilson, C. B. Immunosuppression and plasma-exchange in the treatment of Goodpasture's syndrome. *Lancet* 1:711, 1976.

57. Makinodan, T., Santos, G. W., and Quinn, R. P. Immunosuppressive drugs. *Pharmacol. Rev.* 22:189, 1970.

58. McAdams, A. J., McEnery, P. T., and West, C. D. Mesangio-capillary glomerulonephritis: Changes in glomerular morphology with long-term alternate day prednisone therapy. *J. Pediatr.* 86:23, 1975.

59. McClusky, R. T., Benacerraf, B., Potter, J. L., and Miller, F. The pathologic effects of intravenously administered soluble antigen-antibody complexes. I. Passive serum sickness in mice. *J. Exp. Med.* 111: 181, 1960.

60. McCrory, W. W., Shibuya, M., Lu, W. H., and Lewy, J. E. Therapeutic and toxic effects observed with different dosage programs of cyclophosphamide in treatment of steroid-responsive but frequently relapsing nephrotic syndrome. *J. Pediatr.* 82:614, 1973.

61. McDonald, J., Murphy, A. V., and Arneil, G. C. Long-term assessment of cyclophosphamide therapy for nephrosis in children. *Lancet.* 2:980, 1974.

62. McEnery, P. T., McAdams, A. J., and West, C. D. Glomerular Morphology, Natural History and Treatment of Children with IgA-IgG Mesangial Nephropathy. In P. Kincaid-Smith, T. H. Mathew, and E. L. Becker (eds.), *Glomerulonephritis: Morphology, Natural History and Treatment.* New York: Wiley, 1973. Pp. 305–320.

63. Meadow, S. R., Glasgow, E. F., White, R. H. R., Moncrieff, M. W., Cameron, J. S., and Ogg, C. S. Schönlein-Henoch nephritis. *Q. J. Med.* 41:241, 1972.

64. Meadow, S. R., Weller, R. O., and Archibald, R. W. R. Fatal systemic measles in a child receiving cyclophosphamide for nephrotic syndrome. *Lancet* 2:876, 1969.

65. Michael, A. F., Vernier, R. L., Drummond, K. N., Levitt, J. I., Herdman, R. C., Fish, A. J., and Good, R. A. Immunosuppressive therapy of chronic renal disease. *N. Engl. J. Med.* 276:817, 1967.

66. Michielsen, P., Van Damne, B., Dotremont, G., Verberckmoes, R., Oei, L. S., and Vermylen, J. Indomethacin Treatment of Membranoproliferative and Lobular Glomerulonephritis. In P. Kincaid-Smith, T. H. Mathew, and E. L. Becker (eds.), *Glomerulonephritis: Morphology, Natural History and Treatment.* New York: Wiley, 1973. Pp. 611–631.

67. Munro, J. F., Geddes, A. M., and Lamb, W. L. Goodpasture's syndrome: Survival after acute renal failure. *Br. Med. J.* 4:95, 1967.

68. Naish, P., Pesces, G. B., Evans, D. J., and Peters, D. K. The effect of defibrination on nephrotoxic serum nephritis in rabbits. *Clin. Sci.* 42:643, 1972.

69. Nanra, R. S., and Kincaid-Smith, P. Lupus Nephritis: Clinical Course in Relation to Treatment. In P. Kincaid-Smith, T. H. Mathew, and E. L. Becker (eds.), *Glomerulonephritis: Morphology, Natural History and Treatment.* New York: Wiley, 1973. Pp. 1193–1210.

70. Novack, S. N., and Pearson, C. M. Cyclophosphamide therapy in Wegener's granulomatosis. *N. Engl. J. Med.* 284:938, 1971.

71. Penso, J., Lippe, B., Ehrlich, R., and Smith, F. G., Jr. Testicular function in prepubertal and pubertal male patients treated with cyclophosphamide for nephrotic syndrome. *J. Pediatr.* 84:831, 1974.

72. Phelps, P., and McCarty, D. J. Suppressive effects of indomethacin on crystal induced inflammation at canine joints and on neutrophilic motility in vitro. *J. Pharmacol. Exp. Ther.* 158:546, 1967.

73. Pollak, V. E., Pirani, C. L., and Kark, R. M. Effect of large doses of prednisone on the renal lesions and life span of patients with lupus glomerulonephritis. *J. Lab. Clin. Med.* 57:495, 1961.

74. Pollak, V. E., Pirani, C. L., and Schwartz, F. D. The natural history of the renal manifestations of systemic lupus erythematosus. *J. Lab. Clin. Med.* 63: 537, 1964.

75. Proskey, A. J., Weatherbee, L., Easterling, R. E., Greene, J. A., Jr., and Weller, J. M. Goodpasture's syndrome. A report of five cases and review of the literature. *Am. J. Med.* 48:162, 1970.

76. Richter, P., Calamera, J. C., Morgenfeld, M. C., Kierszenbaum, A. L., Lavieri, J. C., and Mancini, R. E. Effect of chlorambucil in spermatogenesis in the human with malignant lymphoma. *Cancer* 25: 1026, 1970.

77. Santos, G. W. Immunosuppressive drugs I. *Fed. Proc.* 26:907, 1967.

78. Scheinman, J. I., and Stamler, F. W. Cyclophosphamide and fatal varicella. *J. Pediatr.* 74:117, 1969.

79. Schwartz, R. S. Immunosuppressive Drug Therapy. In F. T. Rapaport and J. Dausset (eds.), *Human Transplantation.* New York: Grune & Stratton, 1968. Pp. 440–471.

80. Sessa, A., Allaria, P. M., Conte, F., Cioffi, A., and D'Amico, G. Ultrastructural changes of the glomeruli of the rat induced by indomethacin. *Nephron* 10:238, 1973.

81. Shalhoub, R. J. Pathogenesis of lipoid nephrosis: A disorder of T-cell function. *Lancet* 2:556, 1974.

82. Skinner, M. D., and Schwartz, R. S. Immunosuppressive therapy (second of two parts). *N. Engl. J. Med.* 287:281, 1972.

83. Sladek, N. E. Therapeutic efficacy of cyclophosphamide as a function of its metabolism. *Cancer Res.* 32:535, 1972.

84. Steinberg, A. D., Kaltreider, H. B., Staples, P. J., Goetzl, E. J., Talal, N., and Decker, J. L. Cyclophosphamide in lupus nephritis: A controlled trial. *Ann. Intern. Med.* 75:165, 1971.

85. Steinberg, A. D., Plotz, P. H., Wolff, S. M., Wong, V. G., Agus, S. G., and Decker, J. L. Cytotoxic drugs in treatment of non-malignant diseases. *Ann. Intern. Med.* 76:619, 1972.

86. Suc, J. M., Conte, J., and Conte, M. Treatment of Glomerulonephritis with Indomethacin and Heparin. In P. Kincaid-Smith, T. H. Mathew, and E. L. Becker (eds.), *Glomerulonephritis: Morphology, Natural History and Treatment.* New York: Wiley, 1973. Pp. 927–947.

87. Suc, J. M., Durand, D., Conte, J., Mignon-Conte, M., Orfila, C., and Ton That, H. The use of heparin in the treatment of idiopathic rapidly progressive glomerulonephritis. *Clin. Nephrol.* 5:9, 1976.

88. Swanson, M. A., and Schwartz, R. S. Immunosuppressive therapy. The relation between clinical response and immunologic competence. *N. Engl. J. Med.* 277:163, 1967.

89. Sztejnbok, M., Stewart, A., Diamond, M., and Kaplan, D. Azathioprine in the treatment of systemic lupus erythematosus. A controlled study. *Arthritis Rheum.* 14:639, 1971.

90. Thomson, N. M., Simpson, I. J., and Peters, D. K. A quantitative evaluation of anticoagulants in experimental nephrotoxic nephritis. *Clin. Exp. Immunol.* 19:301, 1975.

91. Turcotte, J. G., Feduska, N. J., Carpenter, E. W., McDonald, F. D., and Bacon, G. E. Rejection crisis in human renal transplant recipients: Control with high dose methylprednisolone therapy. *Arch. Surg.* 105:230, 1972.

92. Van Arman, C. G., Carlson, R. P., Brown, W. R., and Itkin, A. Indomethacin inhibits the local Shwartzman reaction. *Proc. Soc. Exp. Biol. Med.* 134:163, 1970.

93. Vanreterghem, Y., Roels, L., Verberckmoes, R., and Michielsen, P. Treatment of chronic glomerulonephritis with a combination of indomethacin and cyclophosphamide. *Clin. Nephrol.* 4:218, 1975.

94. Vassalli, P., and McClusky, R. T. The pathogenic role of the coagulation process in rabbit Masugi nephritis. *Am. J. Pathol.* 45:653, 1964.

95. Wegmann, W., and Leumann, E. P. Glomerulonephritis associated with (infected) ventriculo-atrial shunt. *Virchows Arch. (Pathol. Anat.)* 359:185, 1973.

96. White, R. H. R. Mesangial Proliferative Glomerulonephritis in Childhood. In P. Kincaid-Smith, T. H. Mathew, and E. L. Becker (eds.), *Glomerulonephritis: Morphology, Natural History and Treatment.* New York: Wiley, 1973. P. 383.

97. White, R. H. R., Glasgow, E. F., and Mills, R. J. Focal Glomerulosclerosis in Childhood. In P. Kincaid-Smith, T. H. Mathew, and E. L. Becker (eds.), *Glomerulonephritis: Morphology, Natural History and Treatment.* New York: Wiley, 1973. P. 231.

98. White, R. H. R., Glasgow, E. F., and Mills, R. J. Clinicopathological study of nephrotic syndrome in childhood. *Lancet* 1:1353, 1970.

99. Zurier, R. B., and Weissman, G. Anti-immunologic and anti-inflammatory effects of steroid therapy. *Med. Clin. North Am.* 57:1295, 1973.

70. Treatment of Glomerular Diseases: Anticoagulant and Fibrinolytic Therapy

Jerry Michael Bergstein

In certain experimental models of intravascular coagulation and immune-related glomerulonephritis, the coagulation process plays a significant role in the pathogenesis of the glomerular lesions. Treatment with anticoagulants and fibrinolytic agents results in significant improvement in glomerular abnormalities. The major benefit, however, occurs when therapy is initiated at the time of, or shortly after, injection of the inciting agent. Unfortunately, it is rare for patients to come forward during this important time interval.

Currently, the value of anticoagulant or fibrinolytic therapy in human renal disease is unknown. Although controlled studies are lacking, several recent reports suggest that these forms of therapy may be of value in certain types of human renal disease.

Intravascular Coagulation

The renal lesion in the hemolytic-uremic syndrome most resembles that seen in experimental models of intravascular coagulation. Although a localized rather than a disseminated form of intravascular coagulation appears to be operant in the hemolytic-uremic syndrome, the renal pathologic changes are characterized primarily by arteriolar and glomerular deposition of fibrin. Therefore, it seems reasonable that inhibition of the coagulation process would have a beneficial effect on the progression of the renal disease.

In the absence of carefully controlled studies, it is difficult, if not impossible, to interpret the results of any type of therapy for the hemolytic-uremic syndrome. This is due to the marked variability in the natural history of the disease. For example, a study from California revealed that 19 of 21 patients, followed 2 to 10 years, recovered completely, with normal blood pressure and renal function [47]. On the other hand, a 1- to 8-year follow-up of 76 patients from Argentina revealed that 20 percent had hypertension and 30 percent had chronic renal insufficiency [15]. The apparent great variability in the natural history of the hemolytic-uremic syndrome must be considered in assessing the results of studies utilizing anticoagulant and fibrinolytic therapy.

ANTICOAGULANT THERAPY

Heparin therapy has been utilized in over 100 patients with the hemolytic-uremic syndrome [5, 6, 10–12, 14, 17, 18, 22, 24, 26, 31–34, 36–38, 40, 41, 46, 47, 49, 52]. Because of differences in diagnostic criteria and severity of the disease, variations in the dose, time of initiation, duration, and means of administration of heparin, the concomitant use of other drugs, and the absence of controlled studies with long-term follow-up, the value of heparin therapy for the patient with hemolytic-uremic syndrome remains an open issue. Several authors [11, 14, 24, 33, 42, 49] have concluded on the basis of their own experience, including one controlled trial, that heparin does not significantly alter the course of the disease. On the other hand, after an extensive review of all reported series, Powell and Ekert [38] concluded that patients treated with heparin generally did better than those who were not so treated.

Recently, 3 patients were described in whom drugs that inhibit platelet function (aspirin and dipyridamole) were added to heparin therapy [2]. Following addition of these agents, a prompt rise in platelet count was noted. The ultimate value of this type of therapy remains to be determined.

FIBRINOLYTIC THERAPY
The clinical manifestations of the hemolytic-uremic syndrome appear to result from a single event that injures the kidneys by an etiologic agent as yet unidentified. Studies suggest that by the time the patient is seen initially, the renal lesion is already established, and intravascular coagulation is no longer taking place [19, 25]. If true, the ultimate prognosis would be a function of the degree of fibrin deposition and the ability of the kidney to remove fibrin. Patients whose kidneys can remove deposited fibrin, including those in whom fibrin deposition may have been diminished by early treatment with heparin, would ultimately recover. On the other hand, cortical necrosis may develop in patients whose kidneys are stressed beyond their capacity to remove fibrin. In these patients, fibrinolytic therapy might be of value in removing previously formed thrombi.

Urokinase would be the appropriate enzyme to use. However, since it has not been available, the fibrinolytic activator *streptokinase* has been used in the treatment of the hemolytic-uremic syndrome. Streptokinase, obtained from filtrates of cultures of group C β-hemolytic streptococci, indirectly activates a circulating inactive precursor (plasminogen) to form the active fibrinolytic agent plasmin [39]. Plasmin is a nonspecific proteolytic enzyme acting on a number of protein substrates, including fibrin, fibrinogen, coagulation factors V, VIII, XII, and prothrombin. Besides activating the *circulating* fibrinolytic system, streptokinase penetrates into thrombi, converting plasminogen to plasmin within the clot [1]. Plasminogen appears to be in higher concentration in

the clot than in the blood, and the plasmin formed in the clot is not subject to the circulating antiplasmins alpha-1-antitrypsin and alpha-2-macroglobulin. Thus, lysis occurs both from within and without the clot.

Although streptokinase is clearly of value in removing various types of arterial and venous thrombi, little is known as to its effect on removing clots from the microvasculature, such as that found in the kidney. In uncontrolled studies, several centers have used streptokinase in the treatment of patients with hemolytic-uremic syndrome. In the largest series, from the Netherlands, 25 patients, 12 of whom were initially anuric, received streptokinase [35], and 22 survived. Of the 3 deaths, 2 were from the anuric group. In only 1 of these 3 deaths was cortical necrosis detected. Further follow-up data are not available.

We have treated 6 patients with streptokinase, 3 of whose cases have been reported [4]. All patients were anuric; 4 recovered completely, with normal blood pressure and renal function. In 1 patient who was not treated until 9 days after the onset of renal disease, chronic renal insufficiency developed. This poor response may be explained by the fact that, as shown in patients with peripheral vascular occlusions treated with streptokinase, clots are most susceptible to fibrinolytic therapy during the first few days following development, and the chance of recovery diminishes as the clot becomes organized. Our sixth patient died of pulmonary infection following streptokinase therapy. No evidence of renal cortical necrosis was detected at autopsy.

Experiences with small numbers of patients in other countries, including Australia [38], England [42], France [16], and Germany [20, 45] generally have been similar, and suggest that fibrinolytic therapy may be of value in the hemolytic-uremic syndrome.

Glomerulonephritis
Little information is available with regard to anticoagulant treatment of children with glomerulonephritis. Recent uncontrolled studies have been primarily in adults and also involve the use of other therapeutic agents.

In 1968, Kincaid-Smith et al. [30] reported the results of anticoagulant therapy in 6 patients with acute renal failure secondary to various types of renal disease. Therapy consisted of heparin infusion, in addition to corticosteroids and immunosuppressive agents. Of 6 patients, 5 had a rapid increase in urine output following treatment with heparin; 3 patients suffered a decline in renal function when heparin was stopped. The same group has suggested that anticoagulant therapy (heparin followed by coumadin plus the platelet inhibitor dipyridamole) and, in some instances, immunosuppressive agents may be of value in patients with the following diseases: acute renal failure secondary to glomerulonephritis or tubular necrosis, malignant hypertension, hemolytic-uremic syndrome, thrombotic thrombocytopenic purpura, acute and chronic glomerulonephritis, and renal homograft rejection [29]. Wardle and Uldall [50] have also demonstrated that heparin may improve renal function in patients with hypertension, glomerulonephritis, and renal homograft rejection.

Other reports on the use of heparin in small numbers of patients with chronic proliferative glomerulonephritis [8], various forms of glomerulonephritis associated with intravascular coagulation [39a, 51], and rapidly progressive glomerulonephritis [3, 7, 9, 13a, 30, 43, 44] have suggested that such therapy may have some value. Kincaid-Smith [27, 28] has reported improvement in renal function and histologic findings and increased survival in patients with mesangiocapillary glomerulonephritis treated with cyclophosphamide, dipyridamole, and anticoagulants. On the other hand, Freedman et al. [13] reported that heparin therapy failed to benefit 6 patients with chronic glomerulonephritis and 1 patient with diabetic nephropathy.

In the single study in children, Herdman et al. [21] used heparin or Warfarin in the treatment of 13 patients having a variety of chronic renal diseases. Five patients appeared to improve (two with idiopathic rapidly progressive glomerulonephritis, one with anaphylactoid purpura nephritis, one with mesangiocapillary glomerulonephritis, and one with Wegener's granulomatosis, who also received immunosuppressive agents).

These preliminary studies, many of which suggest benefit from anticoagulant therapy in various forms of glomerulonephritis, should set the stage for well-defined controlled therapeutic trials.

References

1. Alkjaersig, N., Fletcher, A. P., and Sherry, S. The mechanism of clot dissolution by plasmin. *J. Clin. Invest.* 38:1086, 1959.
2. Arenson, E. B., Jr., and August, C. S. Preliminary report: Treatment of the hemolytic-uremic syndrome with aspirin and dipyridamole. *J. Pediatr.* 86:957, 1975.
3. Arieff, A. I., and Pinggera, W. F. Rapidly progressive glomerulonephritis treated with anticoagulants. *Arch. Intern. Med.* 129:77, 1972.
4. Bergstein, J. M., Edson, J. R., and Michael, A. F., Jr. Fibrinolytic treatment of the haemolytic-uraemic syndrome. *Lancet* 1:448, 1972.
5. Berman, W., Jr. The hemolytic-uremic syndrome: Initial clinical presentation mimicking ulcerative colitis. *J. Pediatr.* 81:275, 1972.
6. Brain, M. C., Baker, L. R. I., McBride, J. A., Rubenberg, M. L., and Dacie, J. V. Treatment of patients with microangiopathic haemolytic anemia with heparin. *Br. J. Haematol.* 15:603, 1968.
7. Brown, C. B., Wilson, D., Turner, D., Cameron, J. S., Ogg, C. S., Chantler, C., and Gill, D. Combined immunosuppression and anticoagulation in rapidly progressive glomerulonephritis. *Lancet* 2:1166, 1974.
8. Cade, J. R., de Quesada, A. M., Shires, D. L., Levin, D. M., Hackett, R. L., Spooner, G. R., Schlein, E. M., Pickering, M. J., and Holcomb, A. The effect of long term high dose heparin treatment on the course of chronic proliferative glomerulonephritis. *Nephron* 8:67, 1971.
9. Cameron, J. S., Gill, D., Turner, D. R., Chantler, C., Ogg, C. S., Vosnides, G., and Williams, D. G. Combined immunosuppression and anticoagulation in rapidly progressive glomerulonephritis. *Lancet* 2:923, 1975.
10. Chan, J. C. M., Eleff, M. G., and Campbell, R. A. The hemolytic-uremic syndrome in nonrelated adopted siblings. *J. Pediatr.* 75:1050, 1969.
11. Clarkson, A. R., Lawrence, J. R., Meadows, R., and Seymour, A. E. The haemolytic uraemic syndrome in adults. *Q. J. Med.* 39:227, 1970.
12. Egli, F., Stalder, G., Gloor, F., Duckert, F., Killer, F., and Hottinger, A. Heparin therapie des haemolytisch-uramischen syndroms. *Helv. Paediatr. Acta* 24:13, 1969.
13. Freedman, P., Meister, H. P., De La Paz, A., and Ronaghy, H. The clinical, functional, and histologic response to heparin in chronic renal disease. *Invest. Urol.* 7:398, 1970.
13a. Fye, K. H., Hancock, D., Moutsopoulos, H., Humes, H. D., and Arieff, A. I. Low-dosage heparin in rapidly progressive glomerulonephritis. *Arch. Intern. Med.* 136:995, 1976.
14. Gervais, M., Richardson, J. B., Chiu, J., and Drummond, K. N. Pathology of the hemolytic-uremic syndrome. *J. Pediatr.* 47:352, 1971.
15. Gianantonio, C. A., Vitacco, M., Mendilaharzu, F., and Gallo, G. The hemolytic-uremic syndrome. Renal status of 76 patients at long-term follow-up. *J. Pediatr.* 72:757, 1968.
16. Guillin, M. C., Boyer, C., Beaufils, F., and Lejeune, C. Utilisation de streptokinase dans deux cas de syndrome hemolytique et urémique. *Arch. Fr. Pediatr.* 30:401, 1973.
17. Habib, R., Courtecuisse, V., Leclerc, F., Mathieu, H., and Royer, P. Etude anatomo-pathologique de 35 observations du syndrome hemolytique et urémique de l'enfant. *Arch. Fr. Pediatr.* 26:391, 1969.
18. Habib, R., Leclerc, R., Mathieu, H., and Royer, P. Comparison clinique et anatomo-pathologique entre les formes mortelles et curables du syndrome hemolytique et urémique. *Arch. Fr. Pediatr.* 26:417, 1969.
19. Harker, L. A., and Slichter, S. J. Platelet and fibrinogen consumption in man. *N. Engl. J. Med.* 287:999, 1972.
20. Heimsoth, V. H., Blumcke, S., Bohlmann, H. G., Haupt, H., and Kuster, F. Erfolgreiche thrombolytische Therapie bei bilateralen Nierenrindennekrosen. *Dtsch. Med. Wochenschr.* 98:1895, 1973.
21. Herdman, R. C., Edson, J. R., Pickering, R. J., Fish, A. J., Marker, S., and Good, R. A. Anticoagulants

in renal disease in children. *Am. J. Dis. Child.* 119: 27, 1970.

22. Hitzig, W. H. Therapie mit Antikoagulantien in der Pediatrie. *Helv. Paediatr. Acta* 19:213, 1964.

23. Jones, F. E., Black, P. J., Cameron, J. S., Chantler, C., Gill, D., Maisey, M. N., Ogg, C. S., and Saxton, H. Local infusion of urokinase and heparin into renal arteries in impending renal cortical necrosis. *Br. Med. J.* 4:547, 1975.

24. Kaplan, B. S., Katz, J., Krawitz, S., and Lurie, A. An analysis of the results of therapy in 67 cases of the hemolytic-uremic syndrome. *J. Pediatr.* 78:420, 1971.

25. Katz, J., Krawitz, S., Sacks, P. V., Levin, S. E., Thomson, P., Levin, J., and Metz, J. Platelet, erythrocyte, and fibrinogen kinetics in the hemolytic-uremic syndrome of infancy. *J. Pediatr.* 83:739, 1973.

26. Kibel, M. A., and Barnard, P. J. Treatment of acute haemolytic-uraemic syndrome with heparin. *Lancet* 2:259, 1964.

27. Kincaid-Smith, P. The treatment of chronic mesangiocapillary (membranoproliferative) glomerulonephritis with impaired renal function. *Med. J. Aust.* 2:587, 1972.

28. Kincaid-Smith, P. The Natural History and Treatment of Mesangiocapillary Glomerulonephritis. In P. Kincaid-Smith, T. H. Mathew, and E. L. Becker (eds.), *Glomerulonephritis.* New York: Wiley, 1973. P. 591.

29. Kincaid-Smith, P., Laver, M. C., and Fairley, K. F. Dipyridamole and anticoagulants in renal disease due to glomerular and vascular lesions. *Med. J. Aust.* 1: 145, 1970.

30. Kincaid-Smith, P., Saker, B. M., and Fairley, K. F. Anticoagulants in irreversible acute renal failure. *Lancet* 2:1360, 1968.

31. Kunzer, W., and Aalam, F. Treatment of the acute haemolytic-uraemic syndrome with heparin. *Lancet* 1:1106, 1964.

32. Lieberman, E. Hemolytic-uremic syndrome. *J. Pediatr.* 80:1, 1972.

33. McCredie, D. A., and Dixon, S. R. The Hemolytic-Uremic Syndrome. In P. Kincaid-Smith, T. H. Mathew, and E. L. Becker (eds.), *Glomerulonephritis.* New York: Wiley, 1973. P. 1069.

34. Moncrieff, M. W., and Glasgow, E. F. Haemolytic-uraemic syndrome treated with heparin. *Br. Med. J.* 3:188, 1970.

35. Monnens, L., Kleynen, F., Van Munster, P., Schretlen, E., and Bonnerman, A. Coagulation studies and streptokinase therapy in the haemolytic-uraemic syndrome. *Helv. Paediatr. Acta* 27:45, 1972.

36. Monnens, L., and Schretlen, E. Haemolytic-uraemic syndrome. *Lancet* 2:735, 1968.

37. Piel, C. F., Goodman, J. R., and Beck, J. Ultramicroscopic glomerular lesions in hemolytic uremia. *Clin. Res.* 18:225, 1970.

38. Powell, H. R., and Ekert, H. Streptokinase and anti-

thrombotic therapy in the hemolytic-uremic syndrome. *J. Pediatr.* 84:345, 1974.

39. Rickli, E. E. The biochemistry of the fibrinolytic enzyme system in man. *Angiologica* 5:66, 1968.

39a. Robson, A. M., Cole, B. R., Kienstra, R. A., Kissane, J. M., Alkjaersig, N., and Fletcher, A. P. Severe glomerulonephritis complicated by coagulopathy: Treatment with anticoagulant and immunosuppressive drugs. *J. Pediatr.* 90:881, 1977.

40. Seiler, G., and Tietze, H. U. Haemolytisch-uramisches Snydrom. *Z. Kinderheilkd.* 106:249, 1969.

41. Sharpstone, P., Evans, R. G., O'Shea, M., Alexander, L., and Lee, H. A. Haemolytic-uraemic syndrome: Survival after prolonged oliguria. *Arch. Dis. Child.* 43:711, 1968.

42. Stuart, J., Winterborn, M. H., White, R. H. R., and Flinn, R. M. Thrombolytic therapy in haemolytic-uraemic syndrome. *Br. Med. J.* 2:217, 1974.

43. Suc, J. M., Conte, J., and Conte, M. Treatment of Glomerulonephritis with Indomethacin and Heparin. In P. Kincaid-Smith, T. H. Mathew, and E. L. Becker (eds.), *Glomerulonephritis.* New York: Wiley, 1973. P. 927.

44. Suc, J. M., Durand, D., Conte, J., Mignon-Conte, M., Orfila, C., That, H. T., and Duchet, J. P. The use of heparin in the treatment of idiopathic rapidly progressive glomerulonephritis. *Clin. Nephrol.* 5:9, 1976.

45. Sutor, A. H., Schindera, F., Jacobi, H., and Kunzer, W. Haemolytic-uraemic syndrome; thrombocyturia after treatment with streptokinase and aspirin. *Lancet* 2:762, 1972.

46. Troelstra, J. A., and Visser, H. K. A. Haemodialysis in the haemolytic-uraemic syndrome. *Lancet* 1:770, 1965.

47. Tune, B. M., Leavitt, T. J., and Gribble, T. J. The hemolytic-uremic syndrome in California: A review of 28 nonheparinized cases with long-term follow-up. *J. Pediatr.* 82:304, 1973.

48. Uttley, W. S. Serum levels of fibrin/fibrinogen degradation products in the haemolytic-uraemic syndrome. *Arch. Dis. Child.* 45:587, 1970.

49. Vitacco, M. J., Avalos, S., and Gianantonio, C. A. Heparin therapy in the hemolytic uremic syndrome. *J. Pediatr.* 83:271, 1973.

50. Wardle, E. M., and Uldall, P. R. Effect of heparin on renal function in patients with oliguria. *Br. Med. J.* 3:135, 1972.

51. Whitaker, A. M., Bunce, I. H., Nicoll, P., and Emmerson, B. T. Disseminated Intravascular Coagulation and Intravascular Hemolysis in Glomerular Disease: The Response to Heparin Therapy. In P. Kincaid-Smith, T. H. Mathew, and E. L. Becker (eds.), *Glomerulonephritis.* New York: Wiley, 1973. P. 845.

52. Willoughby, M. L. N., Murphy, A. V., McMorris, S., and Jewell, F. G. Coagulation studies in haemolytic uraemic syndrome. *Arch. Dis. Child.* 47:766, 1972.

Section Five. Other Nephropathies

71. The Interstitial Nephritides (Interstitial Renal Inflammation)

Lawrence R. Freedman

The term *interstitial nephritis* indicates a *type of renal reaction to injury* characterized by a non-suppurative inflammatory response in the potential space between nephrons and the renal vasculature [117]. An acute inflammatory response consists of edema and cellular exudate, predominantly lymphocytes and eosinophils, with generally few though variable numbers of polymorphonuclear leukocytes. The acute response may be generalized or localized to foci of inflammation distributed through the kidney. The kidney may be normal in size or swollen with a tense capsule. This histologic pattern is referred to as acute interstitial nephritis.

Chronic interstitial nephritis is characterized by atrophy and disappearance of renal tubules from zones of inflammation and the deposition of collagen (scarring). The inflammatory exudate is generally composed of lymphocytes and macrophages, but varying numbers of eosinophils also may be seen. The distribution of lesions may be diffuse, focal and widely distributed, or focal and localized. The kidney may be normal in size, with a smooth capsule, or considerably decreased in size, with scars evident on gross examination. One kidney may be much more severely involved than the other; in fact, one kidney may be normal in the presence of severe involvement of the other.

In their pure forms interstitial nephritides are not accompanied by changes in the renal pelvis, glomeruli, or renal blood vessels. However, glomerular fibrosis or sclerosis and vascular thickening may occur in regions of scarring and are distinguished from primary diseases, which they might mimic, by their absence in undamaged portions of the renal parenchyma. The problem is more complicated, however, since important interstitial damage in the presence of minor glomerular lesions is being described in disorders traditionally considered to be primary glomerular diseases [25]. Of course renal pelvic changes may also be seen if the patient simultaneously has a bacterial urinary infection.

Renal papillary injury is a common finding in chronic interstitial nephritis. The most dramatic form of this damage is frank anemic necrosis with sloughing of one or many renal papillae. These papillae may be excreted in the urine or they may cause ureteral obstruction. In addition, there is a spectrum of many more subtle degrees of renal papillary damage [15, 16]. Papillary sclerosis may result rarely in ossification of the renal papillae [31].

The frequency of renal papillary damage is difficult to estimate, since it depends on the criteria used to define it. It is likely that until recently renal papillary disease was not searched for systematically at autopsy. The frequency of this finding will also vary with the type and definition of the underlying disease state. For example, in some reported series papillary necrosis is taken as an essential criterion for the diagnosis of analgesic nephropathy, whereas in others it is found in only about 20 percent of patients with clinical evidence of chronic interstitial nephritis and a history of excessive analgesic ingestion [33].

Pronounced inflammatory changes in the interstitium of the kidney may accompany any primary renal disease. The ability, therefore, to determine whether a given renal disease began in the glomeruli or blood vessels or in the interstitium depends on the stage of disease at the time the kidney is examined. Far-advanced renal disease is often not susceptible to this type of morphologic analysis. Renal biopsies are not suitable for excluding interstitial nephritis in the genesis of a particular renal disease except when a specific diagnosis of primary glomerular or vascular disease can be made.

There are two major problems in considering the definitions of interstitial nephritis just presented: (1) When does an interstitial infiltrate, seen in almost all diseased kidneys, become interstitial nephritis? (2) At what point in the evolution of an interstitial reaction does the definition shift from acute to chronic? Since these infiltrates may be focal and may not be visible upon gross examination of the kidney at autopsy, how many kidney sections must be examined to exclude the diagnosis of interstitial nephritis?

It is evident that all subsequent considerations of incidence, clinical manifestations, and other characteristics will depend on these definitions; at present, they lack precision. In general, acute interstitial nephritis refers to the recent onset of changes in renal function or to urinary abnormalities associated with easily detectable inflammation in the kidney; and chronic interstitial nephritis indicates a prominent histologic change of indeterminate duration often associated with long-standing renal functional abnormalities and evidence of renal scarring. There is a need to reconsider this system of classification.

HISTORIC ASPECTS OF NEPHRITIDES TERMINOLOGY

The meaning of the terms *acute* and *chronic interstitial nephritis* has changed considerably during the past 60 years. Prior to the classification of renal diseases by Volhard and Fahr in 1914, *chronic interstitial nephritis* was synonymous with chronic Bright's disease. Subsequently the term was virtually discarded until the study of Weiss and Parker in 1939, when it became synonymous with chronic pyelonephritis [111].[1]

Today the term *chronic interstitial nephritis* is reemerging, hopefully to be recognized for what it should be: a way of *describing a pattern of reaction* in the kidneys with many possible causes [32]. The term *interstitial nephritis* is no more or less useful than terms such as *fever* or *congestive heart failure*. Interstitial nephritis is always secondary to some underlying injury; thus we should speak of acute or chronic interstitial nephritis due to a specific etiologic agent or process; if none can be identified, "cause undetermined" or "etiology unknown" should be appended.[2]

The fundamental confusion arising from the use of these terms today stems from the fact that until recently it was the rule to label all renal disease characterized principally by an interstitial inflammatory response as pyelonephritis, even in the absence of evidence for a pathogenetic role of bacterial infection in the production of the renal disease. This custom has had two major consequences: first, it generated an exaggerated fear of the risk of renal damage due to bacterial infections of the urinary tract; and second, it discouraged the search for possible causes of the renal lesions other than bacterial infection.

It is difficult to overestimate the impact of the inappropriate use of the term *pyelonephritis* on medical thinking and practice. In one major university hospital in the United States it was found that the majority of children treated in the emergency room for acute urinary infections were found on the basis of urine culture to have had sterile urine specimens before treatment was started. Large numbers of children are referred for complete urologic investigation of pyelonephritis, often including general anesthesia, without documented evidence of bacterial urinary infection. How many surgical procedures have been carried out to correct ill-defined "abnormalities" (meatal stenosis, urethral stenosis, bladder neck obstruction, megalocystis) in the absence of data demonstrating the efficacy of these procedures on the long-term course of the illness—all because of an unwarranted fear of the consequences of urinary tract infection? How many refluxing ureters have been reimplanted in order to prevent the consequences of urinary infections when, in reality, the reflux was a result of infection and would disappear with proper treatment of the infection? Thus the names we apply have an important impact on medical practice and require close scrutiny.

Ideally we should discard the terms *acute* and *chronic interstitial nephritis* and replace them by the specific entity responsible for the renal damage, as suggested by Heptinstall and Kincaid-Smith [47, 47a, 56]. In reality, however, the process by which we determine the etiology of a renal disease is usually first to characterize the broad type of renal injury and then to search for possible etiologic agents. It would seem reasonable, therefore, in considering the clinical problem to separate glomerular diseases from what in broadest terms can be called the *tubulointerstitial renal disorders*. The tubulointerstitial renal disorders could then be characterized in functional (e.g., nephrogenic diabetes insipidus) and morphologic (e.g., interstitial renal inflammation) terms. This system of classification would avoid the term *interstitial nephritis* and the implication of a specific renal disease, would stimulate the search for all possible etiologic factors, would allow for the presence of multiple pathogenic factors and the

---

[1] Renal disease due to the immediate or late effects of bacterial infection of the kidney.

[2] Some authors prefer the classification wherein all chronic interstitial nephritis is called chronic pyelonephritis, with further subdivision into bacterial and abacterial forms [91]. Since the term *pyelonephritis* is well accepted as one indicating a specific pathogenesis, however, and since the pathogenesis of chronic interstitial nephritis is so often in doubt, my preference is to use *chronic interstitial nephritis* as the generic term, reserving *chronic pyelonephritis* for those examples of interstitial nephritis in which there is positive evidence for a pathogenic role of bacterial infection [32].

presence of simultaneous glomerular disease of similar or different etiology. For the remainder of this chapter the term *interstitial renal inflammation* (IRI) will replace *interstitial nephritis* to describe the nonspecific inflammatory (acute or chronic) reaction seen in a wide variety of tubulointerstitial renal disorders.

Etiologies and Pathogenesis

It is customary to classify IRI as acute or chronic according to the type of histologic response. However, it is likely that the type of inflammatory exudate and the degree of tubular atrophy and scarring are more a reflection of the chronicity of the process than an indication of different disease mechanisms. Although there is, of course, some relation between etiology and chronicity, it seems more useful to discuss these entities from the standpoint of pathogenesis.

Interstitial inflammation and tubular atrophy and fibrosis are commonly seen in a variety of renal diseases. It is evident that the pathogenesis of the renal lesions will vary according to the nature of the underlying disease process; however, it is possible to distinguish five major categories of disease that are associated with IRI: (1) those associated with immunologic mechanisms; (2) congenital lesions; (3) those associated with papillary necrosis or papillary injury; (4) a miscellaneous group; and (5) bacterial infection of the kidney (Table 71-1).

Immunologic Reaction in the Kidney (Table 71-1, Group 1). This is one of the means by which tubular injury and IRI are produced. Drug reactions and the rejected kidney allograft produce acute IRI. The immunologic mechanism that may account for the production of these interstitial

Table 71-1. Classification of Interstitial Renal Inflammation

Group & Etiology	Reference No.	Group & Etiology	Reference No.
Group 1. Immunologic reactions		Aplastic anemia	113
Transplantation rejection	85	Hemorrhagic fever	106
Drug hypersensitivity		Balkan nephropathy	47, 56, 89, 114
Methicillin	10, 98	Analgesic mixture abuse—	8, 15, 16, 56
Rifampin	29, 73	phenacetin, phenylbutazone,	76
Penicillin	18, 38	other	81
Ampicillin	38, 73	Transplantation rejection	36, 52a, 110a
Other antibiotics	4a, 68	Aging	11, 54
Anticonvulsant drugs	44, 47, 68	Alcoholism	23, 65
Glafenine	22	Unilateral xanthogranulomatous	47, 59a
Diuretics	27, 45, 67	change with pyelonephritis	
Phenindione	47, 68	B. Papillary injury	
Allopurinol	37a, 70	Uric acid deposition	
Lupus erythematosus	70	Gout	7, 42, 102, 105
Glomerulonephritis	70	Lesch-Nyhan syndrome	68
Sjögren's syndrome	110	Nephrocalcinosis	66
Sarcoidosis	47	Potassium depletion	75
Granulomatous disease,	21a	Hyperphosphatemia	51
unknown etiology		Sulphonamides	44, 47, 93
		Heavy metal poisoning	24, 32, 44, 109
		Amyloidosis	47
Group 2. Congenital lesions		Group 4. Miscellaneous causes	
Cystinosis	20	Choline deficiency	6
Oxalosis	20	Irradiation	5, 84, 99, 112
Wilson's disease	20	Disseminated intravascular	13
Alport's syndrome	83	coagulation	
? Ask-Upmark kidney	97	Systemic infection	
Medullary cystic disease and/or	17a, 37	Scarlet fever	68
nephronophthisis		Typhoid fever	68
Other congenital lesions	9, 17, 86, 87, 101	Toxoplasmosis	43
		Leptospirosis	115
Group 3. Association with papillary		Brucellosis	78
damage		Bacterial sepsis	68, 115
A. Papillary necrosis		Viral infection	103
Urinary obstruction	34, 45	? Syphilis	
Vesicoureteral reflux	48–50, 94	Heat stroke	55
Diabetes mellitus	88	Acute tubular necrosis	47
Vascular disease of the kidney	60	Group 5. Bacterial infection	32, 33
Sickle cell disorders	1, 33, 53, 77	of the kidney	

lesions, as well as for the lesions found in lupus erythematosus and various forms of glomerulonephritis, have recently been discussed in detail by McCluskey and Klassen [70]. In one instance of acute IRI due to methicillin, anti-tubular basement membrane antibodies were found in the serum. These antibodies were thought to have developed in response to dimethoxyphenylpenicilloyl–tubular basement membrane "hapten-protein conjugate" [10]. Elevated IgE levels have been noted in patients with IRI attributable to a variety of medications [82].

Congenital Causes. Congenital lesions producing IRI are listed as Group 2 in Table 71-1.

Renal Papillary Damage (Table 71-1, Group 3). This damage is a feature of many of the disorders underlying chronic interstitial inflammation of the kidney. This long list of conditions can be further divided into those that are associated with frank papillary necrosis and those associated with papillary injury as an important feature of the renal insult. It is well known that frank anemic papillary necrosis is associated with disease states that compromise the blood supply to the renal papilla; these include urinary obstruction, diabetes mellitus, vascular diseases of the kidney, sickle cell disorders and aplastic anemia, hemorrhagic fever, and shock and dehydration. There is evidence that a similar process is operative in the pathogenesis of the renal lesions arising from abuse of analgesic mixtures [81]. Balkan nephropathy remains a disease of unknown origin; however, the frequent finding in these patients of papillary necrosis and renal pelvic cancer suggests that some toxin is involved with effects similar to analgesic abuse, in which papillary necrosis is common and renal pelvic cancer has also been observed. The suggestion that alcoholism is also associated with frank papillary necrosis is of interest; however, alcoholics frequently ingest large quantities of analgesic mixtures. It is likely that many other toxins that reach high concentrations in the renal papilla will be found responsible for the production of renal papillary necrosis and tubulointerstitial renal disorders [22a]. The diseases in Group 3B are often associated with direct damage to renal papillary tubules.

The hypothesis is put forward that all of these disorders, because of their ability to injure the renal papilla, establish a process whereby sudden necrosis or gradual injury to the renal papilla produces inflammatory interstitial and tubular change in the renal cortex. Support for this view comes from observations in man by Burry [15, 16] showing clearly the development of papillary disease in analgesic nephropathy in the absence of renal cortical abnormalities. In addition, animal studies have demonstrated a primary diminution of papillary blood flow in animals fed analgesics [81].

Renal papillary injury (necrosis) resulting from anoxemia or direct papillary injury has also been shown in animals to produce the changes of chronic interstitial nephritis in the cortex [30, 34, 41]. Thus it is clear that renal papillary injury leads to changes that produce IRI in man and animals. It is not necessary, however, to postulate that all forms of IRI are a result of renal papillary damage.

Diffuse Renal Tubular Damage (Table 71-1, Group 4). This damage results from a variety of miscellaneous mechanisms. Irradiation to the kidney (see Chap. 77) produces fatal renal disease associated with IRI as late as 7 years following in utero irradiation. Acute IRI is sometimes seen in various systemic infections. The pathogenesis of these lesions is not well understood. Toxoplasmosis is of interest in that it has been associated also with glomerulonephritis and the nephrotic syndrome [39], suggesting that the mechanism of IRI might prove to be immunologic rather than a result of direct injury. The fact that diffuse intravascular coagulation in animals has been shown to result in lesions of IRI raises the interesting possibility that systemic infections might injure the kidney by this mechanism [13].

Bacterial Infection of the Kidney (Table 71-1, Group 5). Bacterial infection *as a primary causative agent of chronic IRI has yet to be demonstrated convincingly.* More than 1,000 adult patients with urinary infections have been followed for long periods of time, approximately 300 for about 5 years and 100 for longer periods. Despite the fact that about 30 percent of these patients have had persistent infection or frequent reinfections throughout the period of follow-up, it has not yet been possible to document the development or the progression of renal disease attributable to the effects of infection alone.[3] The arguments to support this statement have been presented in detail elsewhere [32, 33].

The results of prospective studies of urinary infections in children have been similar to those in adults. Neither Kunin nor Smellie and Normand were able to document the development or progression of renal disease in children with recurrent urinary infections followed as long as 10 years except in a few children with severe vesico-

---

[3] By *infection alone* is meant infection in the absence of underlying disease known to be capable by itself of causing the lesions of IRI.

ureteral reflux [61, 62, 104]. It has been shown, however, that renal damage resulting from severe vesicoureteral reflux may progress even in the absence of urinary infection [2, 48, 49, 50, 71, 95]. Lesser degrees of reflux are also frequently associated with renal scars in children, but these scars are present when infection is first diagnosed and have not been seen to develop under observation.

The nature and the pathogenesis of the renal scars found in association with reflux and urinary infection are under considerable study. It has not been proved that these scars are a result of infection. For example, the scarred kidneys found by Andersen et al. [4] and by Stickler et al. [107] in children with hypertension and vesicoureteral reflux were not associated with bacteriologic evidence of urinary infection (although Andersen et al. found high *E. coli* antibody titers) and are indistinguishable from the cases of Royer et al., who judged similar renal lesions to be those of the Ask-Upmark kidney [97].

Thus the renal scars found in the upper and lower poles may result from severe reflux alone or they may be congenital in origin. If these scars are congenital, it is interesting to speculate that their association with reflux may also be determined by congenital factors [3, 14, 90, 92]. Particularly interesting in this regard is the association of renal scarring in vesicoureteral reflux with the phenomenon of intrarenal reflux [2, 94]. Recent observations suggest that susceptibility to intrarenal reflux may be attributable to developmental characteristics of the upper and lower pole renal papillae [90, 90a].

It is important to emphasize, however, that renal changes due to bacterial infection of the kidney are nonspecific [32]. Furthermore, it is well known that renal papillary damage is one of the most effective means of increasing the susceptibility of the kidney to infection and that the consequences of the combination of infection plus urinary obstruction are catastrophic for the kidney [32]. Thus it would seem logical to search for the consequences of urinary infection in patients with underlying conditions known to be capable of producing renal papillary damage and chronic IRI. Stated another way, *it might be useful to presume the presence of underlying renal papillary damage in all patients with renal scarring attributable to urinary infection.*

For many years it has been hypothesized that the means by which bacterial infection of the kidney produces chronic IRI is by an immunologic reaction. Following an initial infection, the deposition of bacterial or bacterial-kidney protein antigen in the kidney provokes an antibody response that over many years, even in the absence of continued infection, produces chronic inflammation and progressive kidney damage.

Although it has been shown that bacterial antigen does persist in the kidney of animals after the disappearance of viable bacteria [19, 93] and that local antibody production against bacterial antigen does take place in the kidney [63], evidence for the progression of sterile or even infected lesions has not been shown until recently. A report by Glassock et al. [40] has demonstrated an increase in the size, number, and intensity of fibrosis and tubular lesions 77 to 94 weeks after the production of enterococcal pyelonephritis in the rat, a model in which viable bacteria persist in the kidneys for years. Penicillin treatment with resulting sterilization of the infection 23 to 35 weeks after infection had no effect, compared with untreated controls, on the progression of the lesions. Thus Glassock et al. concluded that "some of the histopathologic lesions of chronicity developing 6 months or longer after infection are independent of continued bacterial infection."

Although these studies demonstrate a progressive chronic interstitial renal inflammation after injury in rats, it has not been shown that this progression has anything to do with the bacterial nature of the initial injury. For example, Fox has demonstrated the progressive nature of chronic IRI in mice following unilateral anoxemia [28]. In addition, Mayor et al. have recently shown that correction of urinary obstruction in infants with renal insufficiency less than 1 year of age is associated with progressive improvement of renal function, whereas if urinary obstruction is corrected after 2 years of age, there is a slow but progressive decline in renal function despite technical success of the operative procedure [69]. Thus it would appear that the duration of renal obstruction prior to correction or amelioration is an important factor in the natural history of the lesion. It is not known whether this critical period is different for different varieties of renal injury.

It must be emphasized that insofar as it is possible to measure progression with available clinical techniques, recurrent or persistent urinary tract infection in man has not yet been shown to be a progressive process in the absence of underlying disorders capable themselves of producing renal disease [32, 33, 41a]. It may be that current clinical techniques are not sufficiently sensitive to measure this "progression" or that patients have not been followed for a sufficient period of time.

Alternatively, it is possible that progression occurs in only a very small proportion of the large number of patients with urinary infections and that means for identifying these few patients are not at hand.

Whatever the outcome of these continuing investigations, it is evident today that, in the absence of underlying renal disease, the risk, if any, of progressive renal disease resulting from bacterial infection of the kidney is sufficiently small to obviate the need for therapeutic procedures that have their own complications and that have not been shown unequivocally to be beneficial to the patient.

Epidemiology

PREVALENCE

There is no way to estimate the frequency of IRI in the general spectrum of renal disease; its frequency in specific renal diseases with which it is associated is discussed in the appropriate chapters. The frequency of any specific disease will, of course, depend on a variety of factors involved in its development. For example, analgesic nephropathy was first described in Switzerland and then in Scandinavia [117]. In Australia the first known case was recognized in 1957, and by 1969 analgesic nephropathy was recorded as the cause of renal failure in 10 percent of renal transplantations. In Australia it is now considered the most common cause of renal scarring in adults and the most common cause of renal calcification [56, 58]. In a survey conducted in Scotland, 5 percent of the population over 16 years of age took analgesics daily, women more frequently than men. There was also a difference according to social class in the preparation taken [79]. Similar findings were noted in a Boston survey [63].

A particularly interesting report was recently presented by Murray and Goldberg [80]. They surveyed 320 patients at the Hospital of the University of Pennsylvania newly diagnosed as having renal disease (serum creatinine > 1.3 mg per deciliter) during a 4-year period. After excluding all patients with biopsy-proved glomerulonephritis, red blood cell casts in the urine sediment, a protein excretion >4.0 gm per day, or the presence of systemic disease commonly associated with glomerulopathy (e.g., diabetes mellitus, necrotizing vasculitis, etc.), 101 patients who fulfilled their criteria for tubulointerstitial renal disease remained. All 37 patients in whom renal biopsies were obtained had evidence of chronic IRI. The etiologic factors assigned primary and secondary roles in the pathogenesis of renal disease in these patients are shown in Table 71-2.

Table 71-2. *Etiologic Factors in Chronic Interstitial Nephritis in 101 Patients*

Factor	Primary Cause[a]	Secondary Factor[b]
Anatomic abnormalities	31	0
Analgesic abuse	20	0
Hyperuricemia	15	0
Nephrosclerosis	10	10
Stones	9	3
Sickle cell disease	1	1
Renal tuberculosis	1	0
Bacterial urinary tract infection	0	27
Multiple	3	0
Idiopathic	11	0
Total	101	41

[a] Primary cause: single or initial etiologic factor.
[b] Secondary factor: Occurred subsequent to primary cause.
Source: Data from T. Murray and M. D. Goldberg [80].

There are no comparable studies of renal disease in children. There is evidence, however, that IRI as a result of antibiotic treatment may be much more common than is presently suspected [98].

FAMILIAL OCCURRENCE

The familial occurrence of IRI depends, of course, upon the nature of the underlying process. Congenital lesions (see Table 71-1, group 2) must always be considered. Familial occurrences in cases of abuse of analgesics are difficult to interpret [80]. In 2 of 20 cases in the series of Murray and Goldberg [80], family histories were positive. In one family the abuse of analgesics was detected in four generations and was judged to be responsible for renal disease in three of the four members of the third generation. The index case was a 48-year-old woman with a history of analgesic abuse since her teenage years. The second patient's history included extensive abuse of analgesics, and mild renal impairment was found in his only two children. Analgesic abuse has also been reported in families with migraine headache. It must be emphasized that it is often extremely difficult to obtain a history of analgesic abuse in adults, and suspicion of it must be pursued with vigor. Patients are often reluctant to admit to taking large quantities of medications and many do not consider analgesics to be medicines.

Although well-developed analgesic nephropathy is rare in children, it has been noted that the analgesic habit may begin in childhood [35], reflecting familial behavior. Also, although papillary necrosis in children is usually attributable to the consequences of infection and dehydration, it is not unreasonable to assume that nephrotoxins such as analgesic mixtures would increase this tendency [108].

Clinical Manifestations

Patients with *acute* IRI may present with a systemic infection or systemic allergic reaction to a drug, perhaps with oliguria.

Patients with *chronic* IRI usually come to the attention of the physician because of symptoms of chronic renal insufficiency. However, the presenting symptoms may also be those of (1) a primary underlying disorder (e.g., gout, diabetes mellitus, renal colic); (2) renal papillary necrosis (severe fulminating pyelonephritis, often with sepsis); (3) renal colic or gross hematuria due to passage of a renal papilla; or (4) simple urinary tract infection. The patient also may be seen because of symptoms of salt wasting or nephrogenic diabetes insipidus associated with tubular dysfunction as a consequence of predominant damage to renal tubules. Finally, some patients are seen first with urinary abnormalities detected on routine examination.

The course and complications of the disease depend upon the nature of the causative lesion. Acute IRI resulting from an allergic drug reaction may subside with return of renal function to normal following treatment with corticosteroids; however, the process may progress to renal failure and death. Mathieu describes a patient with iridocyclitis and acute IRI who responded well to corticosteroids [68]. Patients with analgesic nephropathy may have an excellent prognosis if they can stop the habit of taking analgesics. Some patients with severe renal insufficiency have recovered sufficiently after stopping analgesics that they no longer required maintenance hemodialysis [58].

Clinical Pathology

In acute IRI patients may be seen with the sudden onset of oliguria and acute renal insufficiency. Urinary abnormalities include small amounts of protein, many leukocytes, and occasionally gross hematuria. Red blood cell casts are not seen. It has recently been noted that eosinophils were present in the urine of a patient with acute IRI due to methicillin hypersensitivity [18]. This finding might prove an extremely useful clinical diagnostic tool.

Chronic IRI may be the responsible process in any renal disease resulting in renal scarring, overall diminution of renal function, or hypertension. It should be suspected particularly in those clinical states characterized by tubular functional abnormalities out of proportion to changes in glomerular function. Urinary findings are nonspecific. Large amounts of protein in the urine (>3.0 gm/ 24 hr) in the absence of malignant hypertension or congestive heart failure or the finding of red blood cell casts indicates the presence of renal disease in addition to or other than IRI.

Management

Aside from measures directed toward specific disease problems, the treatment of IRI does not differ from the general management of patients with other renal disorders. However, two factors deserve special attention: urinary infection and the use of analgesics.

It is of greatest importance to maintain a sterile urine in patients with IRI. The combination of chronic IRI frequently associated with actual or potential primary renal papillary disease and infection may precipitate acute papillary necrosis leading to life-threatening sepsis or chronic renal insufficiency. On the other hand, there is no evidence to support the practice of treating sterile pyuria with antibiotics. An exception may be selected patients with well-documented primary renal papillary disease, due, for example, to analgesic nephropathy, who continue to have pyuria and bacteriuria following initial treatment of a bacterial infection [26]. A search must be made for urinary tract tuberculosis in patients with sterile pyuria. Furthermore, during the recovery phase of renal papillary necrosis, sterile pyuria is a regular finding; it persists for weeks or months after treatment of the original infection and ultimately disappears spontaneously [59].

In view of the potential risks of serious renal damage due to superimposed urinary infection in these patients, the indications for diagnostic studies that carry the risk of introducing infection must be critically assessed. For example, it is frequently debated whether to perform a voiding cystourethrogram in all children to detect urinary reflux as an etiologic factor in the production of renal scarring. Although many physicians would recommend this procedure, in my own view it should not be done routinely. It has been clearly pointed out by Rolleston, Smellie, and Hodson and their coworkers that the risk of progressive renal damage as a result of reflux is seen only in those children with the most severe grades of reflux [48–50, 95, 104] resulting in obvious ureteral dilatation and perhaps hydronephrosis. Most children with this degree of reflux have changes visible on the usual intravenous pyelogram. Furthermore, I suspect that the application of pressure to the bladder during an intravenous pyelogram would be likely to demonstrate ureteral dilatations in advanced cases if such dilatations are not already visible in the usual series of films. Special procedures are available to demonstrate reflux during an intravenous pyelogram [21, 72].

Discontinuing the use of all analgesics is an essential objective in the management of patients with analgesic nephropathy; in some instances renal function has improved sufficiently to permit discontinuing hemodialysis. "All proprietary analgesics should at present be regarded as potentially dangerous" [57]. In some countries elimination of phenacetin from analgesic preparations has had a dramatic effect in decreasing the incidence of analgesic nephropathy [52]. Kincaid-Smith has pointed out that aspirin may be responsible for serious deterioration of renal function in patients with analgesic nephropathy [57]. It is not known if patients with any underlying renal disease are more susceptible to renal damage from analgesic mixtures. That this may be the case in some patients with renal disease is suggested by the ease with which papillary necrosis is produced by analgesics in the Gunn rat, an animal model in which there is underlying renal papillary damage due to chronic hyperbilirubinemia [6a].

Summary

Tubulointerstitial renal disorders exhibiting the morphologic changes of IRI constitute a major component of the spectrum of kidney diseases. Except for special cases, neither the morphologic nor the functional pattern of renal damage is capable of establishing the etiology or pathogenesis of the disorder. In addition, several injurious processes may be operating simultaneously. Identification of etiologic factors is of the utmost importance, since their removal may be associated with significant improvement in renal function. It is likely that many pathogenetic mechanisms and injurious agents capable of producing IRI remain to be discovered.

References

1. Akinkugbe, O. O. Renal papillary necrosis in sickle-cell haemoglobinopathy. *Br. Med. J.* 3:283, 1967.
2. Amar, A. D. Colicotubular backflow with vesicoureteral reflux: Relation to pyelonephritis. *J.A.M.A.* 213:293, 1970.
3. Ambrose, S. S. Reflux pyelonephritis in adults secondary to congenital lesions of the ureteral orifice. *J. Urol.* 102:302, 1969.
4. Andersen, H. J., Jacobsson, B., Larsson, H., and Winberg, J. Hypertension, asymmetric renal parenchymal defect, sterile urine, and high *E. coli* antibody titre. *Br. Med. J.* 3:41, 1973.
4a. Appel, G. B., and Nev, H. C. Nephrotoxicity of antimicrobial agents. *N. Engl. J. Med.* 296:663, 772, 784, 1977.
5. Arneil, G. C., Harris, F., Emmanuel, I. G., Young, D. G., Flatman, G. E., and Zachary, R. B. Nephritis in two children after irradiation and chemotherapy for nephroblastoma. *Lancet* 1:960, 1974.
6. Ashworth, C. T., and Grollman, A. Renal lesions in experimental hypertension: Morphological changes in the kidney of rats rendered chronically hypertensive following a period of choline deficiency. *Arch. Pathol.* 67:375, 1959.
6a. Axelsen, R. A. Analgesic-induced renal papillary necrosis in the Gunn rat: The comparative nephrotoxicity of aspirin and phenacetin. *J. Pathol.* 120: 145, 1976.
7. Barlow, K. A., and Beilin, L. J. Renal disease in primary gout. *Q. J. Med.* 37:79, 1968.
8. Bengtsson, U. A comparative study of chronic nonobstructive pyelonephritis and renal papillary necrosis. *Acta Med. Scand.* [Suppl. 338] 172:4, 1962.
9. Bois, E., and Royer, P. Association de nephropathie tubulo-interstitielle chronique et de dégénérescence tapeto-rétinienne. *Arch. Fr. Pediatr.* 27:471, 1970.
10. Border, W. A., Lehman, D. H., Egan, J. D., Sass, H. J., Glade, J. E., and Wilson, C. B. Antitubular basement-membrane antibodies in methicillin-associated interstitial nephritis. *N. Engl. J. Med.* 291: 381, 1974.
11. Bras, G. Age-associated kidney lesions in the rat. *J. Infect. Dis.* 120:131, 1969.
12. Brass, H., Lapp, H., and Heintz, R. Akute interstitielle nephritis—mögliche Ursache eines akuten Nierenversagens. *Dtsch. Med. Wochenschr.* 99: 2335, 1974.
13. Brentjens, J. R. H., Vreeken, J., Feltkamp-Vroom, T., and Helder, A. W. Pyelonephritis-like lesions as a late effect of diffuse intravascular coagulation. *Acta Med. Scand.* 183:203, 1968.
14. Burger, R. H., and Smith, C. Hereditary and familial vesicoureteral reflux. *J. Urol.* 106:845, 1971.
15. Burry, A. F. The evolution of analgesic nephropathy. *Nephron* 5:185, 1967.
16. Burry, A. F. The Pathology and Pathogenesis of Renal Papillary Necrosis. In P. Kincaid-Smith and K. F. Fairley (eds.), *Renal Infection and Renal Scarring.* Melbourne: Mercedes Publication Services, 1970. Pp. 335–344.
17. Claireaux, A. E., and Pearson, M. G. Chronic nephritis in a newborn infant. *Arch. Dis. Child.* 30: 366, 1955.
17a. Coles, G. A., Robinson, K., and Branch, R. A. Familial interstitial nephritis. *Clin. Nephrol.* 6:513, 1976.
18. Colvin, R. B., Burton, J. R., Hyslop, M. E., Jr., Spitz, L., and Lichtenstein, N. S. Penicillin-associated interstitial nephritis. *Ann. Intern. Med.* 81: 404, 1974.
19. Cotran, R. S. The renal lesion in chronic pyelonephritis: Immunofluorescent and ultrastructural studies. *J. Infect. Dis.* 120:109, 1969.
20. Darmady, E. M. The Renal Changes in Some Metabolic Diseases. In F. K. Mostofi and D. E. Smith (eds.), *The Kidney.* Baltimore: Williams & Wilkins, 1966. Pp. 253–268.
21. Davis, P. H. Demonstration of Vesico-ureteric Reflux Following an Intravenous Pyelogram. In P. Kincaid-Smith and K. F. Fairley (eds.), *Renal In-*

fection and Renal Scarring. Melbourne: Mercedes Publication Services, 1970. Pp. 261–264.

21a. Dobrin, R. S., Vernier, R. L., and Fish, A. J. Acute eosinophilic interstitial nephritis and renal failure with bone marrow-lymph node granulomas and anterior uveitis. *Am. J. Med.* 59:325, 1975.

22. Duplay, H., Mattei, M., Barillon, D., Bavza, R., Gaillot, M., Kermarec, J., and Duplay, H. Néphrite tubulo-interstitielle aiguë par intoxication à la glafénine. *Therapie* 29:593, 1974.

22a. Editorial. Curry kidney. *Br. Med. J.* 2:69, 1976.

23. Edmondson, H. A., Reynolds, T. B., and Jacobson, A. Renal papillary necrosis with special reference to chronic alcoholism (a report of 20 cases). *Arch. Intern. Med.* 118:255, 1966.

24. Emerson, B. T. Metals and the Kidney. In D. A. K. Black (ed.), *Renal Disease* (2nd ed.). Oxford: Blackwell, 1964. P. 561.

25. Epstein, F. H., and McCluskey, R. T. Systemic lupus erythematosus with renal failure and unusual urinary findings. *N. Engl. J. Med.* 294:100, 1976.

26. Fairley, K. F., and Butler, H. M. Sterile Pyuria as a Manifestation of Occult Bacterial Pyelonephritis with Special Reference to Intermittent Bacteriuria. In P. Kincaid-Smith and K. F. Fairley (eds.), *Renal Infection and Renal Scarring.* Melbourne: Mercedes Publication Services, 1970. Pp. 51–68.

27. Fialk, M. A., Romankiewicz, J., Perrone, F., and Sherman, R. L. Allergic interstitial nephritis with diuretics. *Ann. Intern. Med.* 81:403, 1974.

28. Fox, M. Progressive renal fibrosis following acute tubular necrosis: An experimental study. *J. Urol.* 97:196, 1967.

29. Frankel, H. J., and Grasso, M. A. Rifampicin-induced nephropathy. *Kidney Int.* 8:411, 1975.

30. Freedman, L. R. Experimental pyelonephritis: XII. Changes mimicking "chronic pyelonephritis" as a consequence of renal vascular occlusion in the rat. *Yale J. Biol. Med.* 39:113, 1966.

31. Freedman, L. R. Chronic pyelonephritis at autopsy. *Ann. Intern. Med.* 66:697, 1967.

32. Freedman, L. R. Urinary Tract Infection, Pyelonephritis, and Other Forms of Chronic Interstitial Nephritis. In M. B. Strauss and L. G. Welt (eds.), *Diseases of the Kidney* (2nd ed.). Boston: Little, Brown, 1971. Pp. 667–733.

33. Freedman, L. R. The natural history of urinary infection in adults. *Kidney Int.* 8S:96, 1975.

34. Freedman, L. R., Werner, A. S., Beck, D., and Paplanus, S. H. Experimental pyelonephritis: IX. The bacteriologic course and morphologic consequences of staphylococcal pyelonephritis in the rat, with consideration of the specificity of the changes involved. *Yale J. Biol. Med.* 34:40, 1961.

35. Frithz, G. Phenacetin nephropathy in a mother and daughter. *Acta Med. Scand.* 181:529, 1967.

36. Fuller, T., Tarrant, D., and Juncos, L. Papillary necrosis—a complication of renal transplantation. *Kidney Int.* 8:497, 1975.

37. Gardner, K. D. Evolution of clinical signs in adult-onset cystic disease of the renal medulla. *Ann. Intern. Med.* 74:47, 1971.

37a. Gelbart, D. R., Weinstein, A. B., and Fajardo, L. F. Allopurinol-induced interstitial nephritis. *Ann. Intern. Med.* 86:196, 1977.

38. Gilbert, D. M., Gourley, R., d'Agostino, A., Goodnight, S. H., Jr., and Worthen, H. Interstitial ne-

phritis due to methicillin, penicillin and ampicillin. *Ann. Allergy* 28:378, 1970.

39. Ginsberg, R. E., Wasserman, J., Huldt, G., and Bergstrand, A. Case of glomerulonephritis associated with acute toxoplasmosis. *Br. Med. J.* 3:369, 1974.

40. Glassock, R. J., Kalmanson, G. M., and Guze, L. B. Pyelonephritis: XVIII. Effect of treatment on the pathology of enterococcal pyelonephritis in the rat. *Am. J. Pathol.* 76:49, 1974.

41. Godley, J. A., and Freedman, L. R. Experimental pyelonephritis: XI. A comparison of temporary occlusion of renal artery and vein on susceptibility of the rat kidney to infection. *Yale J. Biol. Med.* 36:268, 1964.

41a. Gower, P. E. A prospective study of patients with radiological pyelonephritis, papillary necrosis and obstructive atrophy. *Q. J. Med.* 45:315, 1976.

42. Greenbaum, D., Ross, J. H., and Steinberg, V. L. Renal biopsy in gout. *Br. Med. J.* 1:1502, 1961.

43. Guignard, J. P., and Torrado, A. Interstitial nephritis and toxoplasmosis in a 10-year-old child. *J. Pediatr.* 85:381, 1974.

44. Hamburger, J., Richet, G., Crosnier, J., Funck-Brentano, J. L., Antoine, B., Ducrot, H., Mery, J. P., and deMontera, H. *Nephrology.* Philadelphia: Saunders, 1968. P. 780.

45. Harrington, J. T. Acute oliguric renal failure with IgA glomerular deposits. *N. Engl. J. Med.* 290:1365, 1974.

46. Hemholz, H. F., and Field, R. S. Acute changes in rabbit's kidney, particularly pelvis, produced by ligating ureter. *J. Urol.* 15:409, 1926.

47. Heptinstall, R. H. *Pathology of the Kidney* (2nd ed.). Boston: Little, Brown, 1974.

47a. Heptinstall, R. H. Interstitial nephritis. *Am. J. Pathol.* 83:214, 1976.

48. Hodson, C. J. The effects of disturbance of flow on the kidney. *J. Infect. Dis.* 120:54, 1969.

49. Hodson, C. J. The Mechanism of Scar Formation in Chronic Pyelonephritis. In P. Kincaid-Smith and K. F. Fairley (eds.), *Renal Infection and Renal Scarring.* Melbourne: Mercedes Publication Services, 1970. Pp. 327–329.

50. Hodson, C. J. Vesico-ureteric reflux and renal scarring—with and without infection. *Kidney Int.* 5:308, 1974.

51. Holliday, M. A., Winters, R. W., Welt, L. G., MacDowell, M., and Oliver, J. The renal lesions of electrolyte imbalance: II. The combined effect on renal architecture of phosphate loading and potassium depletion. *J. Exp. Med.* 110:161, 1959.

52. Kasanen, A. The effect of the restriction of the sale of phenacetin on the incidence of papillary necrosis established at autopsy. *Ann. Clin. Res.* 5:369, 1973.

52a. Kaude, J. V., Stone, M., Fuller, T. J., Cade, J. R., Tarrant, D. G., and Juncos, L. I. Papillary necrosis in kidney transplant patients. *Radiology* 120:69, 1976.

53. Kay, C. J., Rosenberg, M. A., Fleisher, P., and Small, J. Renal papillary necrosis in hemoglobin SC disease. *Radiology* 90:897, 1968.

54. Keresztury, S., and Megyeri, L. Histology of renal pyramids with special regard to changes due to aging. *Acta Morphol. Acad. Sci. Hung.* 11:205, 1962.

55. Kew, M. C., Abrahams, C., and Seftal, H. C.

Chronic interstitial nephritis as a consequence of heat stroke. *Q. J. Med.* 39:189, 1970.

56. Kincaid-Smith, P. Interstitial nephritis—is it an entity? *Kidney* 6:1, 1973.

57. Kincaid-Smith, P. The Prevention of Renal Failure. In *Proceedings of the 5th International Congress of Nephrology, Mexico City, 1972–3.* Basel: Karger, 1974. Pp. 100–118.

58. Kincaid-Smith, P., and Fairley, K. F. (eds.). *Renal Infection and Renal Scarring.* Melbourne: Mercedes Publication Services, 1970.

59. Kincaid-Smith, P., Nanra, R. S., and Fairley, K. F. Analgesic Nephropathy: A Recoverable Form of Chronic Renal Failure. In P. Kincaid-Smith and K. F. Fairley (eds.), *Renal Infection and Renal Scarring.* Melbourne: Mercedes Publication Services, 1970. Pp. 385–400.

59a. Klugo, R. C., Anderson, J. A., Powell, I., and Cerny, J. C. Xanthogranulomatous pyelonephritis in children. *J. Urol.* 117:350, 1977.

60. Koletsky, S. Hypertensive vascular disease produced by salt. *Lab. Invest.* 7:377, 1958.

61. Kunin, C. M. The natural history of recurrent bacteriuria in school-girls. *N. Engl. J. Med.* 282:1443, 1970.

62. Kunin, C. M. A ten-year study of bacteriuria in school-girls: Final report of bacteriologic, urologic, and epidemiologic findings. *J. Infect. Dis.* 122:382, 1970.

63. Lawson, D. H. Analgesic consumption and impaired renal function. *J. Chronic Dis.* 26:39, 1973.

64. Lehmann, J. D., Smith, J. W., Miller, T. E., Barnett, J. A., and Sanford, J. P. Local immune response in experimental pyelonephritis. *J. Clin. Invest.* 47:2541, 1969.

65. Longacre, A. M., and Popky, G. L. Papillary necrosis in patients with cirrhosis: A study of 102 patients. *J. Urol.* 99:391, 1968.

66. Lowe, G. K., Henderson, J. L., Park, W. W., and McGreal, D. A. The idiopathic hypercalcemia syndromes of infancy. *Lancet* 2:101, 1954.

67. Lyons, H., Pinn, V. W., Cortell, S., Lohen, J. J., and Harrington, J. T. Allergic interstitial nephritis: Reversible renal failure in nephrotic syndrome. *N. Engl. J. Med.* 288:124, 1973.

68. Mathieu, H. Néphrites Interstitielles Non Microbiennes. In P. Royer, R. Habib, H. Mathieu, and M. Broyer (eds.), *Néphrologie Pédiatrique.* Paris: Flammarion, 1973. Pp. 130–135.

69. Mayor, G., Genton, N., Torrado, A., and Guignard, J. P. Renal function in obstructive nephropathy: Long-term effect of reconstructive surgery. *Pediatrics.* 50:740, 1975.

70. McCluskey, R. T., and Klassen, J. Immunologically mediated glomerular, tubular and interstitial renal disease. *N. Engl. J. Med.* 288:564, 1973.

71. McRae, C. V., Shannon, F. T., and Utley, W. L. F. Effect on renal growth of reimplantation of refluxing ureters. *Lancet* 1:1310, 1974.

72. Mellins, H. Z. (Moderator). A Panel on the Role of Radiology in the Diagnosis of Abnormalities of the Urinary Conduit System. In J. F. Glenn (ed.), *Proceedings of a Workshop on Ureteral Reflux in Children.* Washington, D.C.: National Academy of Sciences–National Research Council, 1967. P. 89.

73. Méry, J. P., and Morel-Maroger, L. Acute Interstitial Nephritis. A Hypersensitivity Reaction to

Drugs. In *Proceedings of the 6th International Congress of Nephrology.* Basel: Karger, 1976. P. 524.

74. Michie, A. J. Chronic pyelonephritis mimicking ureteral obstructions. *Pediatr. Clin. North Am.* 6:1117, 1959.

75. Milne, M. D., and Muehrcke, R. C. Potassium deficiency and kidney. *Br. Med. Bull.* 13:15, 1957.

76. Morales, A., and Steyn, J. Papillary necrosis following phenylbutazone ingestion. *Arch. Surg.* 103:420, 1971.

77. Mostofi, F. K., Verder, Brugge, C. F., and Diggs, L. W. Lesions in kidneys removed for unilateral hematuria in sickle-cell disease. *Arch. Pathol.* 63:336, 1957.

78. Muehrcke, R. C. *Acute Renal Failure: Diagnosis and Management.* St. Louis: Mosby, 1969.

79. Murray, R. M. The use and abuse of analgesics. *Scott. Med. J.* 17:393, 1972.

80. Murray, T., and Goldberg, M. D. Etiologies of chronic interstitial nephritis. *Ann. Intern. Med.* 82:453, 1975.

81. Nanra, R. S., Chirawong, P., and Kincaid-Smith, P. Medullary ischaemia in experimental analgesic nephropathy—the pathogenesis of renal papillary necrosis. *Aust. N.Z. J. Med.* 3:580, 1973.

82. Ooi, B. S., First, M. R., Pesce, A. J., and Pollak, V. E. IgE levels in interstitial nephritis. *Lancet* 1:1254, 1974.

83. Perkoff, G. T. Hereditary Chronic Nephritis. In E. L. Quinn and E. H. Kass (eds.), *Biology of Pyelonephritis* (Henry Ford Hospital International Symposium). Boston: Little, Brown, 1960. P. 259.

84. Phemister, R. D., Thomassen, R. W., Norrdin, R. W., and Jaenke, R. S. Renal failure in perinatally irradiated beagles. *Radiat. Res.* 55:399, 1973.

85. Porter, K. A. Renal Transplantation. In R. H. Heptinstall, *Pathology of the Kidney* (2nd ed.). Boston: Little, Brown, 1974. Pp. 977–1041.

86. Porter, K. A., and Giles, H. A pathological study of 5 cases of pyelonephritis in the newborn. *Arch. Dis. Child.* 31:303, 1956.

87. Potter, W. Z., Trygstad, C. W., Helmer, O. M., Nance, W. E., and Jodson, W. E. Familial hypokalemia associated with renal interstitial fibrosis. *Am. J. Med.* 57:971, 1974.

88. Raaschou, F. Discussion. In E. H. Kass (ed.), *Progress in Pyelonephritis.* Philadelphia: Davis, 1965. P. 373.

89. Radonic, M., Radošević, Z., and Županić, V. Endemic Nephropathy in Yugoslavia. In F. K. Mostofi and D. E. Smith (eds.), *The Kidney.* Baltimore: Williams & Wilkins, 1966. Pp. 503–522.

90. Ransley, P. G., and Risdon, R. A. Renal papillae and intrarenal reflux in the pig. *Lancet* 2:1114, 1974.

90a. Ransley, P. G., and Risdon, R. A. Renal papillary morphology in infants and young children. *Urol. Res.* 3:111, 1975.

91. Relman, A. S. Pyelonephritis. In D. A. K. Black (ed.), *Renal Disease* (3rd ed.). Oxford: Blackwell, 1972. Pp. 399–415.

92. Retik, A. B. Urinary reflux in children: An approach to management. *Hosp. Pract.* 9:125, 1974.

93. Rocha, H., Guze, L. B., and Beeson, P. B. Experimental pyelonephritis: V. Susceptibility of rats to hematogenous pyelonephritis following chemical injury of the kidneys. *Yale J. Biol. Med.* 32:120, 1959.

94. Rolleston, G. L., Maling, T. M. J., and Hodson, C. J. Intrarenal reflux and the scarred kidney. *Arch. Dis. Child.* 49:531, 1974.

95. Rolleston, G. L., Shannon, F. T., and Utley, W. L. F. Relationship of infantile vesicoureteral reflux to renal damage. *Br. Med. J.* 1:460, 1970.

96. Rom, W. N. Tumors of renal pelvis and analgesics. *N. Engl. J. Med.* 292:47, 1975.

97. Royer, P., Habib, R., Broyer, M., and Novaille, Y. Segmental hypoplasia of the kidney in children. *Adv. Nephrol.* 1:145, 1971.

98. Sanjad, S. A., Haddad, G. G., and Nassar, V. H. Nephropathy—an underestimated complication of methicillin therapy. *J. Pediatr.* 84:873, 1974.

99. Schärer, K., Mühlethaler, J. P., Stettler, M., and Bosch, H. Chronic radiation nephritis after exposure in utero. *Helv. Paediatr. Acta* 23:489, 1968.

100. Schwartz, M. M., and Cotran, R. S. Common enterobacterial antigen in human chronic pyelonephritis and interstitial nephritis. *N. Engl. J. Med.* 289:830, 1973.

101. Senior, B. Familial renal-retinal dystrophy. *Am. J. Dis. Child.* 125:442, 1973.

102. Siller, W. G. Avian nephritis and visceral gout. *Lab. Invest.* 8:1319, 1959.

103. Siller, W. G., and Cumming, R. B. Histopathology of an interstitial nephritis in the fowl produced experimentally with infectious bronchitis virus. *J. Pathol.* 114:163, 1974.

104. Smellie, J. M., and Normand, I. C. S. Experience of Follow-up of Children with Urinary Tract Infection. In F. O'Grady and W. Brumfitt (eds.), *Urinary Tract Infection* (Proceedings of the 1st National Symposium on Urinary Tract Infection, London, April 1968). London: Oxford University Press, 1968. P. 123.

105. Smith, J. F., and Lee, Y. C. Experimental uric acid nephritis in the rabbit. *J. Exp. Med.* 105:615, 1957.

106. Steer, A. Pathogenesis of Renal Changes in Epidemic Hemorrhagic Fever. In F. K. Mostofi and D. E. Smith (eds.), *The Kidney.* Baltimore: Williams & Wilkins, 1966. Pp. 476–487.

107. Stickler, G. B., Kelalis, P. P., Burke, E. C., and Segar, W. E. Primary interstitial nephritis with reflux. *Am. J. Dis. Child.* 122:144, 1973.

108. Storling, G. A. Renal papillary necrosis in childhood. *J. Clin. Pathol.* 11:296, 1958.

109. Stowe, H. D., Wilson, M., and Goyer, R. A. Clinical and morphological effects of oral cadmium toxicity in rabbits. *Arch. Pathol.* 94:389, 1972.

110. Tu, W. H., Shearn, M. A., Lee, J. C., and Hopper, J., Jr. Interstitial nephritis in Sjögren's syndrome. *Ann. Intern. Med.* 69:1163, 1968.

110a. Tuma, S., Chaimowitz, C., Erlik, D., Gellei, B., Rosenberger, A., and Better, O. S. Fatal papillary necrosis in a kidney graft. *J.A.M.A.* 235:754, 1976.

111. Weiss, S., and Parker, F., Jr. Pyelonephritis: Its relation to vascular lesions and to arterial hypertension. *Medicine* 18:221, 1939.

112. Wilson, C., Ledingham, J. M., and Cohen, M. Hypertension following x-irradiation of the kidneys. *Lancet* 1:9, 1958.

113. Wind, E. S., and Platt, N. Renal papillary necrosis in aplastic anemia. *N.Y. State J. Med.* 70:2117, 1970.

114. Wolstenholme, G. E. W., and Knight, J. (eds.). *The Balkan Nephropathy* (Ciba Foundation Study Group No. 30). Boston: Little, Brown, 1967.

115. Zech, P., Bouletreau, R., Moskovtchenko, J. F., Bervard, M., Favre-Bulle, S., Blanc-Brunat, N., and Traeger, J. Infection in acute renal failure. *Adv. Nephrol.* 1:231, 1971.

116. Zollinger, H. U. Chronic Abuse of Phenacetin and Kidney Lesions. In F. K. Mostofi and D. E. Smith (eds.), *The Kidney.* Baltimore: Williams & Wilkins, 1966. Pp. 523–528.

117. Zollinger, H. U. Interstitial Nephritis. In F. K. Mostofi and D. E. Smith (eds.), *The Kidney.* Baltimore: Williams & Wilkins, 1966. Pp. 269–281.

72. Medullary Sponge Kidney

*John P. Hayslett**

Medullary sponge kidney (MSK) is a cystic disorder characterized by the formation of cysts or the dilatation of collecting ducts or both in the medullary pyramids, especially in the inner papillary portions. Histologic changes do not extend beyond the corticomedullary junction, and the columns of Bertin are normal unless altered by infection or obstruction. Since the initial radiologic and histologic description of this entity 30 years ago [3, 12], several published series [1, 2, 5, 6] have provided clinicopathologic correlations distin-guishing MSK disease from other renal cystic disorders. Although there are a few documented cases of MSK in children [9, 11, 12, 14, 18], the disease is usually diagnosed in adults. Other terminologies applied to MSK, to avoid confusion with progressive types of renal cystic disease involving medullary portions of the kidney, include *precalyceal canalicular ectasia* and *cystic dilatation of renal collecting tubules.* Neither term, however, has gained popularity in the English-language literature.

* Established Investigator of the American Heart Association.

Incidence

The incidence of MSK is unknown because the diagnosis is dependent upon intravenous pyelography, a procedure that is unlikely to be performed in asymptomatic cases. It is of interest that in the years 1950–1965 76 cases of MSK were discovered at the Karolinska Hospital in Stockholm [6] and 12 cases were recognized in a consecutive series of 2,600 excretion urograms performed in the Exeter Hospitals, England [16]. In the United States 29 cases were diagnosed in a 1-year-period at the University of California Medical Center in San Francisco [19]. In most series the sex distribution has been approximately equal, and diagnosis is most commonly made in patients between the ages of 20 and 50 years, when clinical symptoms first appear.

Pathogenesis

The pathogenesis of MSK is unclear, although it seems likely that it is developmental in origin. The collecting tubule system is known to be embryologically derived from a branch of the mesonephric duct, which inflexes and arborizes into the cortex producing metanephric anlage. In MSK, early generations of the ductal arborizations become dilated or undergo a cystic transformation. This view is supported by the constancy of radiographic changes that have been documented in the few cases followed serially over many years; however, it cannot be proved because of the absence of similar information on the existence of the same alterations in the newborn. Most reported cases occur sporadically, although MSK has been described in two siblings [3] and in six members of one family [23]. It should be noted that the characteristic radiologic appearance and histologic changes associated with MSK have also been reported in other disorders, including kinships with polycystic disease and other hereditable disorders. For example, Reilly and Neuhauser [24] reported a series of 11 children, including 5 siblings, with collecting duct dilatation in association with polycystic disease of the liver and kidney. Morris and associates [17] described a group of 20 patients with a diverse spectrum of congenital disorders in whom typical radiographic findings of MSK were found. It is evident, therefore, that the diagnosis of MSK by clinical and radiologic criteria may be difficult.

Pathologic Findings

There is a paucity of information on the histopathologic changes in MSK. The most relevant data are derived from the elegant series of Ekstrom and coworkers [5, 6], who reported morphologic examinations of 15 specimens from partial or total nephrectomies. The changes in uncomplicated cases are characteristic and are confined, as denoted by radiographic studies, to the inner renal pyramids. On gross examination the papillary region contains varying numbers of cavities filled with an opaque liquid and usually numerous smooth-surfaced calculi. Dilatation of collecting ducts and cysts connected to tubules or appearing as isolated lesions are found microscopically. Cysts are lined with one or more layers of cells of the transitional type. Sometimes cysts communicate with one another to form a ductal system that runs radially. The lumens of cavities contain a gelatinous substance and cell detritus as well as concrements. Ekstrom et al. [6] demonstrated that stones were most often formed of pure apatite. Interstitial tissue surrounding involved collecting tubules and cysts is infiltrated with round cells. Typical histologic changes of pyelonephritis are found in cases with that complication.

Urographic Appearance

The diagnosis of MSK depends mainly upon radiologic examination, usually performed either for reasons unrelated to urologic symptoms or because of the not infrequent complications of infection or nephrolithiasis. On plain films radiopaque calculi varying in size from barely visible to 5 to 7 mm and occurring as solitary stones or in clusters of several hundred are usually found in one or both kidneys [7, 15, 19]. On the intravenous pyelogram the outlines of the kidneys are smooth; moderate enlargement is found in about one-third of the cases. The pathologic changes seen radiographically are confined to the pyramids, mainly in the papillary portion, and are characterized by discrete ectatic dilated collecting tubules and rounded or irregularly shaped cavities. One or both organs may be involved, and cyst formation may be localized to a single pyramid or may include all pyramids. The cortex and columns of Bertin appear normal.

Typically the cavities are the first structures to visualize on an intravenous pyelogram; they retain contrast material after the renal pelvis has emptied. Since fewer cavities are seen by retrograde pyelography than by intravenous pyelography, it seems likely that sphincters at the aperture of tubules continue to function in a normal manner to prevent reflux. Within papillae, cavities vary in size and shape, as shown in Figs. 72-1 and 72-2. In some involved kidneys the cavities are striated and resemble dilated collecting tubules passing from the tip to the base of the papillae. In others, cavities are rounded and cystlike,

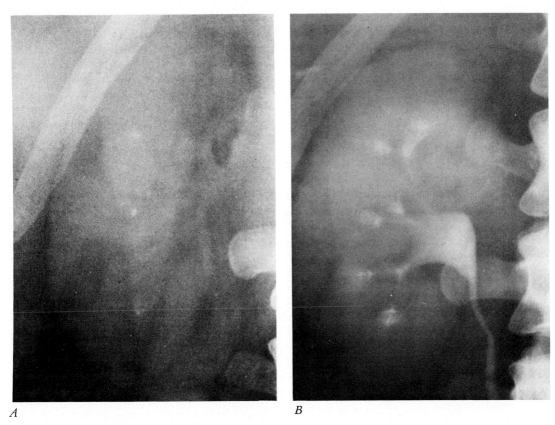

A   *B*

Figure 72-1. A. Medullary sponge kidney with scattered groups of small round calculi. B. Same kidney during pyelography. Dye-filled striated cavities are seen in all papillae. Disappearance of calculi during pyelographic phase suggests that calculi lie in either cysts or calyces.

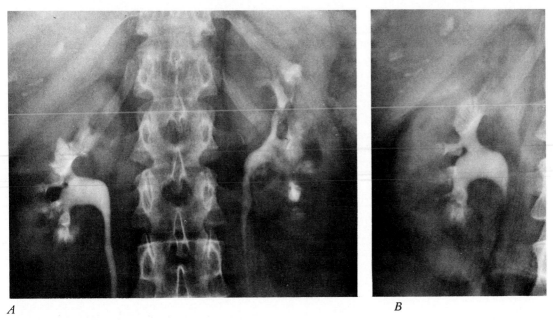

A   *B*

Figure 72-2. A. Bilateral medullary sponge kidneys with characteristic striated cavities involving papillae. An irregular cyst is shown in the area of the left upper pole calyx. B. Right kidney from same patient demonstrating striated cavities in papillae in more detail.

varying in size. Use of contrast material helps to demonstrate that calculi are within cavities rather than in the interstitium, an important distinction in the differential diagnosis of MSK. Palubinskas [20] has demonstrated the spectrum of changes that may be found by intravenous pyelography in normal kidneys and in MSK, from the pyramidal blush or sunburst appearance of the normal pyramid to the classic findings of ectasia and cystic change in MSK. In mild or moderate ectasia it may not be possible to visualize pathologic alterations.

Several reports of long-term urographic follow-up indicate that the pattern of pyramidal opacification in individual cases tends to remain constant [8, 11]. In instances in which changes in size or shape do occur, they appear to be sequelae to infection or obstruction from stones. Moreover, there is neither evidence that cyst formation follows microcalculus formation nor evidence that papillary blush progresses to more florid cyst patterns. In contrast to the constancy of collecting duct abnormalities, an increase in the number or size of calculi occurs in approximately 40 to 60 percent of patients [7, 8].

Differential Diagnosis

The diagnosis of MSK is made by demonstration of radiographic features that are regarded as characteristic of the disease and by the exclusion of other types of renal cystic disease and acquired renal disease that may be associated with cavitation within the medullary portion of the kidney. A general outline for the classification of renal cysts is provided in Chap. 40. With the exception of a few cases in which overlapping features may prohibit a precise diagnosis, separation of MSK from polycystic kidney disease, renal dysplasia, and the various hereditary disorders often associated with microcysts in the renal cortex is made by the distinctive clinical and radiologic characteristics of each of the other entities. Infantile polycystic disease of the autosomal recessive type, however, is characterized by medullary ductal ectasia, and differentiation of infantile polycystic disease and MSK may be impossible on clinical and radiographic grounds. The other renal medullary cystic disorder, medullary cystic disease or familial juvenile nephronophthisis, is confusing only because of terminology, since this complex is associated with a progressive decline in renal function and medullary cysts do not fill with dye on pyelography.

The major problems in differential diagnosis, therefore, concern those disorders in which cavitation in or about the renal papillae may occur in ways similar to the findings in MSK. The more important entities include:

1. Calyceal diverticula or cysts are usually solitary and are situated between pyramids. They often arise from a narrow channel at the fornix or neck of a calyx. In contrast to MSK, calyceal diverticula are as demonstrable on retrograde pyelography as they are on intravenous pyelography.

2. Pyelonephritic cysts may occur as the result of cavitation of microabscesses. Characteristic distortion of calyces due to interstitial scarring is usually an important associated feature.

3. Renal papillary necrosis may be difficult to distinguish from MSK. Coexisting radiologic features such as the calyceal ring sign and clinical features may provide important clues.

4. Renal tuberculosis with cavitation and calcification of necrotic tuberculous tissue may resemble the medullary changes in MSK, but the changes in renal tuberculosis are usually not confined to the medulla. Moreover, cavities in this condition are usually best seen on delayed films and by retrograde pyelography. Nevertheless, the possibility of renal tuberculosis should be considered in patients with radiologic changes of MSK, and appropriate tests, including urine culture, chest films, and skin testing, may be required.

5. Nephrocalcinosis involves primarily medullary calcification and can result from diverse causes. Stones may be seen in the calyceal system or renal pelvis as well as in the interstitium of the kidney, but they generally are not present as intracavitary calculi. In individual patients with bilateral disease, however, the distinction between MSK and nephrocalcinosis may be quite difficult. Stella and associates [25] have reported hyperparathyroidism in two patients with recurrent nephrolithiasis and X-ray findings characteristic of MSK. It was not clear whether the medullary cavities resulted from nephrocalcinosis or whether two separate and relatively uncommon diseases occurred concomitantly.

Excellent reviews of the important radiologic features of these different types of renal diseases are available [6, 10, 15].

Clinical Course

The clinical features of MSK have been described in the large series of Ekstrom et al. [5, 6] and of Abeshouse and Abeshouse [1]. The high incidence of symptomatic patients in each of these series probably reflects the criteria used in identifying the disorder. It is generally understood that the changes in the collecting duct, whether dilatation or cyst formation, do not cause symptoms by themselves, and that symptoms occur as the consequence of pyelonephritis or nephrolithiasis. Renal colic was the presenting symptom in more than one-half of cases, gross hematuria in 10 to 18 percent, and urinary tract infection in approximately one-third [6]. While long asymptomatic intervals are the rule for a large number of patients, many experience frequent recurrences of infection or renal colic. The most complete long-term follow-up is provided by Ekstrom's series, in which 34 patients were studied for an interval of at least 2 years and 25 for 5 or more years. Prognosis was determined mainly by the frequency of complications due to extensive pyramidal calculi, the occurrence of infection, and the presence of free renal pelvic calculi. In 29 cases pyramidal calculi increased in number and size, and hydronephrosis developed in 8 of the 34 cases. Of the 25 patients followed clinically, 12 underwent palliative nephrectomy; 8 of these were considered cured by surgery. The remaining 13 cases were free from infection or had attacks of acute pyelonephritis with infection-free intervals and unimpaired renal function.

Renal function has been found to be normal in most patients with bilateral disease as well as in those with unilateral disease. As would be expected in patients with pathologic damage of the medullary collecting duct, an impairment in urinary concentrating ability [4, 8, 13, 17] and impaired net acid excretion following ammonium chloride administration [17] have been reported. The likelihood of these functional abnormalities occurring in individual patients probably is related to the extent of medullary damage.

References

1. Abeshouse, B. S., and Abeshouse, G. H. Sponge kidney: A review of the literature and a report of five cases. *J. Urol.* 84:252, 1960.
2. Cacchi, R. *Il rene a spugna: O malattia cistica delle piramidi renali.* Capelli: Maggio, 1960.
3. Cacchi, R., and Ricci, V. Sopra una rara e forse ancora non descritta affezione cistica delle pyramidi renali "rene a spugna." *Atti. Soc. Ital. Urol.* 5:59, 1948.
4. Deck, N. D. F. Medullary sponge kidney with renal tubular acidosis: A report of 3 cases. *J. Urol.* 94:330, 1965.
5. Ekstrom, T., Engfeldt, B., Lagergren, C., and Lindvall, N. Medullary sponge kidney. Stockholm: Almqvist and Wiksell, 1959.
6. Ekstrom, T., Engfeldt, B., Lagergren, C., and Lindvall, N. Medullary Sponge Kidney. In *Proceedings of the 3rd International Congress of Nephrology, Washington, D.C., 1966.* Basel: Karger, 1966. Vol. 2, pp. 54–64.
7. Evans, J. A. Medullary sponge kidney. *Am. J. Roentgenol. Radium Ther. Nucl. Med.* 86:119, 1961.
8. Granberg, P. O., Lagergren, C., and Theve, N. O. Renal function studies in medullary sponge kidney. *Scand. J. Urol. Nephrol.* 5:177, 1971.
9. Habib, R., Mouzet-Mazzo, M. T., Courteciusse, V., and Roger, P. L'ectasie tubulaire precalicielle chez l'enfant. *Ann. Pediatr. (Paris)* 12:288, 1965.
10. Lagergren, C., and Lindvall, N. Renal papillary necrosis. *Acta Radiol.* 49:249, 1958.
11. Lalli, A. F. Medullary sponge kidney disease. *Radiology* 92:92, 1969.
12. Lenarduzzi, G. Reporto pielografico poco commune dilataziane delle vie urinarie intrarenali. *Radiol. Med. (Torino)* 26:346, 1939.
13. Levin, N. W., Rosenberg, B., Zwi, S., and Reid, F. P. Medullary cystic disease of the kidney, with some observations on ammonium excretion. *Am. J. Med.* 30:807, 1961.
14. Lindgren, I. Dilated renal collecting ducts in a newborn infant as a precursor to medullary sponge kidney: Report of a case. *Acta Pathol. Microbiol. Scand.* 58:295, 1963.
15. Lindvall, N. Roentgenologic diagnosis of medullary sponge kidney. *Acta Radiol.* 51:193, 1959.
16. Mayall, G. F. The incidence of medullary sponge kidney. *Clin. Radiol.* 21:171, 1970.
17. Morris, R. C., Yamauchi, N., Palubinskas, A. J., and Howenstine, J. Medullary sponge kidney. *Am. J. Med.* 38:883, 1965.
18. Murisasco, A., DeBelsance, N., and Barnovin, F. L'ectasie canaliculaire precalisielle. *Presse Med.* 79:2367, 1971.
19. Palubinskas, A. J. Medullary sponge kidney. *Radiology* 76:911, 1961.
20. Palubinskas, A. J. Renal pyramidal structure opacification in excretory urography and its relation to medullary sponge kidney. *Radiology* 81:963, 1963.
21. Potter, E. L. *Normal and Abnormal Development of the Kidney.* Chicago: Year Book, 1972.
22. Potter, E. L., and Osathanondh, V. Medullary sponge kidney: Two cases in young infants. *J. Pediatr.* 62:901, 1963.
23. Pyrah, L. N. Medullary sponge kidney. *J. Urol.* 95:274, 1966.
24. Reilly, B. J., and Neuhauser, E. B. D. Renal tubular ectasia in cystic disease of the kidneys and liver. *Am. J. Roentgenol. Radium Ther. Nucl. Med.* 84:566, 1960.
25. Stella, F. J., Massry, S. G., and Kleeman, C. R. Medullary sponge kidney associated with parathyroid adenoma. *Nephron* 10:332, 1973.

73. Urate Nephropathy

William L. Nyhan

An increase in the concentration of uric acid in body fluids leads to a variety of impressive clinical manifestations. In pediatric patients with hyperuricemia the most common of these involve the kidneys and urinary tract. Urate nephropathy may be considered in its narrowest sense to be the result of microtophaceous deposits of crystals of urate in the interstices of the pyramids of the kidneys, which may, as they increase, lead to obstruction and atrophy of the nephrons and a considerable inflammatory reaction. Ultimately this process yields a scarred end-stage kidney with advanced renal failure. Urate nephropathy more broadly may include any effect on the kidneys or urinary tract of the presence of large amounts of urate in the urine. Urinary tract stones and sludge are common, and these lead to obstruction and infection. Pediatric patients with hyperuricemia tend to have unusually large amounts of urate in the urine. They are especially susceptible to episodes of complete urinary obstruction under conditions of intercurrent infection when fluid intake is reduced. These processes too, unless treated promptly and vigorously, may lead to hematuria, crystalluria, renal colic, and, ultimately, renal failure.

Gout, the classic expression of hyperuricemia, was recognized by Hippocrates as early as 460–357 B.C. [24]. Hippocrates recognized also that gout was essentially a disease of the adult male, affecting the female only after menopause. These concepts have stayed with us over the years, and only recently have infants and children been considered candidates for hyperuricemia.

The effectiveness of colchicine as a specific anti-inflammatory agent in acute gouty arthritis was recognized by the early Greek physicians. Its use was described by Alexander of Tralles in the fifth century [16, 18, 23]. Uric acid was first isolated in 1776 by the Swedish chemist Scheele [63]; his starting material was a renal stone. In 1797 a British chemist, Wollaston, isolated uric acid from a tophus that is said to have been removed from his own ear [76]. It was half a century later that Alfred B. Garrod, a British physician, demonstrated that gout was associated with hyperuricemia [16]. He did this by suspending a thread overnight in acidified plasma and weighing the crystals of uric acid that accumulated on the fiber. This was the first demonstration of a chemical abnormality in the blood of a patient with a metabolic disease. Archibald Garrod, the son of Alfred, first classified gout among the inborn errors of metabolism [17].

Chemistry of Uric Acid and the Biochemistry of Its Formation

CHEMISTRY

Uric acid is a purine that is oxidized at each of its free carbon atoms. Its structure is 2,6,8-trioxypurine [14] (Fig. 73-1). Uric acid is weakly acidic. It ionizes particularly at the hydrogen atom on nitrogen of position 9. The pK_a is 5.75. The hydrogen of position 3 may also ionize ($pK_a = 10.3$). The other hydrogen atoms at positions 1 and 7 do not ionize. In body fluids of pH 7.4 uric acid is found almost entirely in the form of its monovalent sodium salt (see Fig. 73-1). The urate in the tophi of patients with gout is virtually all monosodium urate monohydrate.

The clinical manifestations that characterize gout are a consequence of a limited solubility of uric acid in body fluids. Sodium urate has a solubility in water of 120 mg per deciliter. Free uric acid has a solubility of only 65 mg per deciliter. It has been calculated [68] from the sodium content of serum at about 0.13 M and the solubility product of monosodium urate in water of 4.9×10^{-5} that the concentration of urate at which serum should be saturated is 6.4 mg per deciliter. It is true, of course, that considerably higher concentrations are found clinically, since it is possible to produce supersaturated solutions. Concentrations as high as 400 mg per deciliter have been obtained briefly by dissolving uric acid in serum. Stable supersaturated solutions of 50 mg per deciliter or even higher are regularly encountered in patients with rapidly growing neoplasms, such as acute leukemia or lymphoma, and particularly under conditions of rapid cell destruction during chemotherapy. Incubation of uric acid with plasma at 37°C yields supersaturated solutions of 100 mg per deciliter or more that are stable for a while but fall in 24 hours at this temperature to about 13 mg per deciliter with precipitation of sodium urate [68]. By 96 hours, concentrations of 8.5 mg per deciliter are found. Actual determinations of the solubility of sodium urate in human plasma

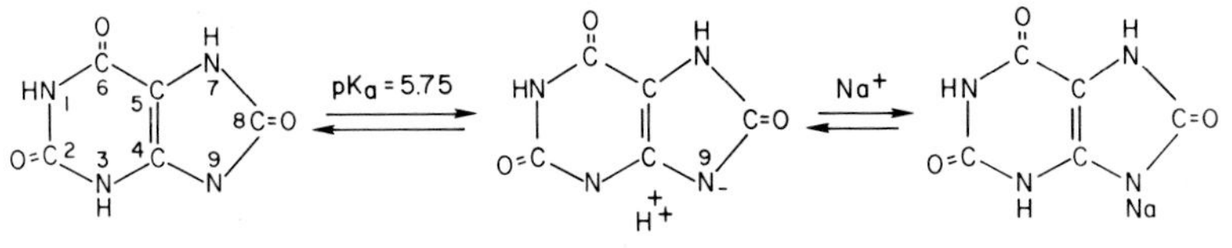

Figure 73-1. The structure and ionization of uric acid and the formation of monosodium urate. The numbers indicate the conventional nomenclature. (Reprinted, by permission, from the New England Journal of Medicine *268:712, 1963 [68].)*

indicate a saturation concentration of 7 mg per deciliter [64]. These data are all consistent with clinical observations in patients with chronic hyperuricemia. With treatment, tophi dissolve, but only when concentrations in the serum are below 7 mg per deciliter. Patients with gout tend to maintain serum concentrations of uric acid over 6 mg per deciliter, and those with the most severe forms, the ones that are overproducing purine, generally maintain serum concentrations between 8.5 and 12 mg per deciliter.

Solubility in urine is a very different matter. The pH of urine is substantially lower than the pH of serum, and therefore more of the molecules in urine are in the form of free uric acid (see Fig. 73-1). Concentrations of uric acid in urine two to three times the solubility in water or plasma are readily achieved, and this has been attributed to the presence of solubilizing substances. Urinary tract calculi occur in patients with gout at a rate one thousand times that of the general population. The deposits found in the kidney tubules and urinary tract are those of free uric acid, not sodium urate [57].

BIOCHEMISTRY

Uric acid is the end product of purine metabolism in man. As such it may be considered metabolically inert, a poorly soluble metabolic waste product that the system must excrete. It may be derived from preformed purines, which may be of dietary origin, or it may come from the turnover and breakdown of cells and their nucleic acids. It may also be synthesized de novo from small molecules such as glutamine, glycine, formate, and bicarbonate. A series of studies using labeled precursors [77] has shown that glycine is incorporated whole to form carbons 4 and 5 and the 7 nitrogen of the purine ring. Formate is the precursor of carbon atoms 2 and 8, and carbon dioxide is the precursor of carbon 6. Nitrogen atoms 3 and 9 come from the amide nitrogen of glutamine, and N_1 comes from the amino group of aspartic acid.

A key reaction in the biosynthesis of the purine ring is the glutamine amidotransferase reaction (Fig. 73-2) in which the amide nitrogen of glutamine is transferred to phosphoribosyl pyrophosphate (PRPP, PP-ribose-P) to form phosphoribosylamine. This is the first committed step in the synthesis of purines. It is an irreversible reaction and an important control point. This reaction is the site of feedback inhibitory control by adenine and guanine ribonucleotides (AMP and GMP). If concentrations of PRPP increase, the rate of purine synthesis increases. It is also possible for the concentration of glutamine to be rate limiting for purine synthesis [60]. The inhibitory effects of AMP and GMP together are more than additive. Thus there is a cooperative form of end-product control of purine biosynthesis. As intracellular purine nucleotide concentrations fall through the removal of nucleotides serving as precursors of RNA and DNA synthesis or through degradation, the activity of the amidotransferase is released and de novo synthesis yields more inosine monophosphate (IMP). Then, as concentrations of AMP and GMP increase, the amidotransferase is modulated down.

Once formed, phosphoribosylamine reacts with glycine to form glycinamide ribotide, which reacts in turn with a one-carbon tetrahydrofolate derivative to form formylglycinamide ribotide (FGAR). This compound reacts to receive another amide of glutamine. The amidine that results then undergoes a carbon dioxide fixation reaction that is followed by a reaction with aspartic acid, yielding aminoimidazole carboxamide ribotide (AICR). Following the addition of another formyl moiety, the ring closes to produce IMP.

Inosine monophosphate is a central compound in the interrelation of purine nucleotides (Fig. 73-3). The branch that leads to the formation of GMP proceeds with IMP dehydrogenase to xanthosine monophosphate. In the subsequent xanthosine monophosphate aminase reaction the amide nitrogen of glutamine is added to the ring to form GMP. This reaction is catalyzed by ATP (adenosine triphosphate). Similarly, the conversion

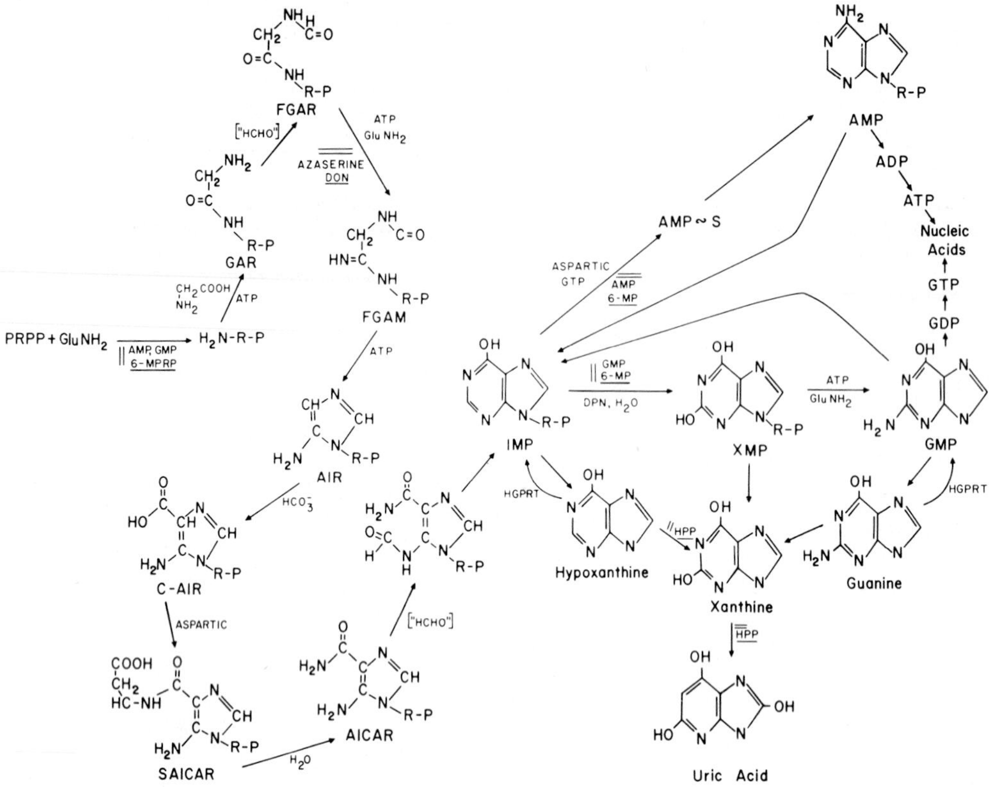

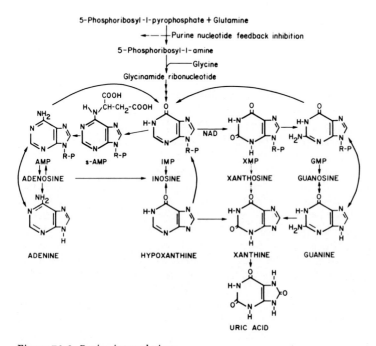

Figure 73-2. Pathways of the de novo biosynthesis of purines.

Figure 73-3. Purine interrelations.

of IMP to adenylosuccinate, which is then converted to AMP, is catalyzed by GTP (guanosine triphosphate).

The reutilization of purines, whether of dietary origin or resulting from catabolism of nucleic acids, involves their conversion to their respective nucleotides in reactions catalyzed by phosphoribosyl transferases, of which there are two. Hypoxanthine guanine phosphoribosyl transferase (HGPRT) catalyzes the reaction of hypoxanthine or guanine with PRPP to form the nucleotides IMP and GMP. This enzyme catalyzes the formation of nucleotides from a number of other purine bases, including xanthine, 6-mercaptopurine, 6-thioguanine, 8-azaguanine, and allopurinol. The other enzyme is known as adenine phosphoribosyl transferase. It catalyzes the formation of AMP from adenine. Aminoimidazole carboxamide (AIC), 8-azaadenine, and 2,6-diaminopurine also serve as substrates for this enzyme. The activity of adenine phosphoribosyl transferase is elevated in the newborn to levels 150 to 200 percent of those seen in adults [7]. Current information indicates that there is a considerable reutilization of purine bases with recycling back into nucleotide pools through the action of the phosphoribosyl transferases. As discussed below, deficiency of HGPRT leads to enormous consequences for the metabolic economy of the body. In contrast, deficiency of adenine phosporibosyl transferase (at least partial deficiency) appears to be of little consequence [33].

A second pathway for the reutilization of purine bases involves first a nucleoside phosphorylase reaction. In this reaction the purine base reacts with ribose 1-phosphate to form the nucleoside plus phosphate. The nucleoside may then react with ATP in the presence of adenosine kinase, inosine kinase, or guanosine kinase to form the nucleotide. It appears that these pathways for the reutilization of purines are much less active than the phosphoribosyl transferases.

In nucleic acid catabolism the initial products of the nucleases ribonuclease and deoxyribonuclease are oligonucleotides. These are further cleaved by phosphodiesterases to yield mononucleotides. These compounds are split by a variety of specific and nonspecific phosphatases to the nucleosides. Nucleoside phosphorylase is active at this stage in the presence of inorganic phosphate in converting the nucleoside to the free purine base and ribose 1-phosphate. Adenosine and AMP are also converted by specific enzymes adenosine deaminase and adenylic deaminase to inosine and IMP. The free bases that result are adenine, guanine, hypoxanthine, and xanthine. Adenine is not further broken down, and a small amount is excreted. The rest is reutilized by conversion to AMP or adenosine. The other purine bases are catabolized to uric acid. Guanine is deaminated in a reaction catalyzed by guanase to yield xanthine. Hypoxanthine and xanthine are oxidized by a single enzyme, xanthine oxidase, to xanthine and uric acid, respectively.

Xanthine oxidase is found in man only in the liver and the intestinal mucosa. It appears, therefore, that most uric acid is made in the liver. This distribution of the enzyme accounts for the very low concentration of uric acid in the central nervous system. It cannot be made there, and its passage from blood to brain is very inefficient. A casual reading of the metabolic map would suggest that if this enzyme were inhibited, the purine ordinarily excreted as uric acid would be excreted as hypoxanthine. This would be therapeutically advantageous, as hypoxanthine is much more soluble than uric acid. Unfortunately this is not the case. When xanthine oxidase is inhibited virtually completely by large doses of allopurinol in individuals with normal purine metabolism, essentially all of the oxypurine excreted is xanthine [72]. This is consistent with the fact that patients with an inherited deficiency of xanthine oxidase have xanthinuria [9, 10], not hypoxanthinuria. From the point of view of therapy this is a problem, because xanthine is even less soluble than uric acid. From the point of view of metabolism, it indicates that under normal conditions the purine found in the urine as uric acid is formed from xanthine that does not come from hypoxanthine. Presumably it comes from guanine.

Pathophysiologic Effects of Hyperuricemia

The concentration of urate in the serum aproximates 5 mg per deciliter in the normal adult male [68]. In general the level in the premenopausal female is about 1 mg per deciliter lower.

Infants and children tend to have lower concentrations of urate in the serum than adults. In the first few days of life considerable variability is encountered [48]. The mean concentration in cord blood is about 4.5 mg per deciliter and the level rises in the next 12 to 24 hr to a mean of 5.7, with a range of 3.9 to 8.8 mg per deciliter. Thereafter there is a progressive decrease to a steady state after 3 days. Perinatal complications regularly raise concentrations of urate in the serum of the infant. Therefore, testing of infants for inborn errors of purine metabolism should be done after 3 days of life, when the mean becomes 1.9 with a range of 1.3 to 3.4 mg per deciliter. In childhood, concentrations over 6 mg per deciliter are distinctly abnormal.

The excretion of uric acid in the urine is the easiest way in which to evaluate the overall metabolism of purines. Among adult patients with gout there are two general populations: those who excrete normal or reduced amounts of urate in the urine and those with clear metabolic abnormalities in whom the urinary excretion is excessive. It has been estimated that 20 to 25 percent of adults with gout are hyperexcretors [68]. The classification is usually based on an excretion of over 600 mg per 24 hr while the patient is receiving a purine-free diet, in contrast to normal subjects, who excrete less than 500 mg of urate per 24 hr. Children generally excrete smaller quantities of uric acid than adults; on the other hand, there is a greater excretion per unit of mass, reflecting a greater turnover of cells and nucleic acids with growth [51]. The excretion of uric acid relative to body weight decreases progressively throughout childhood. Similarly, when the excretion of uric acid per milligram of creatinine is plotted against age, a significant negative regression is observed.

Infants and children with hyperuricemia may also be found to have increased or decreased excretion of uric acid in the urine. However, those that have renal stone disease or urate nephropathy are almost all hyperexcretors. Generally the patients are those with an increased rate of purine synthesis de novo or those with some cellular proliferative disorder such as leukemia. Therefore an assessment of rates of excretion of urate is even more valuable in hyperuricemic pediatric populations than it is in adults.

Some pediatric patients produce so much uric acid that they would be clearly recognized even by adult standards, for they excrete more than 600 mg of uric acid per 24 hr. Normal children seldom excrete more than 10 mg per kilogram of body weight [51], while patients may range from 40 to 60 mg per kilogram [54]. A more useful approach is to express the excretion of uric acid in milligrams per milligram of urinary creatinine [32, 51, 54]. This approach also compensates for inadequacy of collection. It can be done using random samples of urine and a regular diet [32]. For the most precise results, however, it is preferable to employ a 24-hr collection in a patient who has not been receiving purines for at least 3 days. Normal individuals over 1 year of age excrete less than 1 mg of uric acid per milligram of creatinine. Patients with increased rates of purine biosynthesis de novo usually excrete 3 to 4 mg per milligram of creatinine.

The metabolism of purines has been studied by determining the rate at which uric acid is synthesized from glycine following administration of ^{14}C-labeled glycine [40, 56]. In patients with increased rates of de novo synthesis there is a rapid peak of specific activity in the urine in the first 24 hr. At the peak, it is easy to distinguish patients from controls. In studies of this sort in adults, it has not been possible to distinguish gouty from control populations. Therefore, it has become conventional to express the data as the cumulative percent of administered glycine converted to uric acid. Adults with overproduction gout convert about twice as much glycine to uric acid as do controls. In children with the Lesch-Nyhan syndrome a mean of over 2 percent of the glycine administered has been recovered in uric acid [40]. When compared with control children, the difference was of the order of twentyfold [52], and this represents the highest rate of overproduction of purine reported in any condition.

The crystallization of uric acid is critical to the pathogenesis of the clinical consequences of hyperuricemia. Uric acid crystallizes in rhombic plates in pure solution. However, crystals that form in urine may take a variety of shapes and colors that confound easy identification. Monosodium urate crystallizes in the monohydrate form in monoclinic or triclinic forms that are needle- or bar-shaped. In cases of very rapid precipitation or impurity, sodium urate precipitates in the form of an amorphous fine powder without crystalline structure. This is the form in which urate is usually seen in a tophus.

Garrod's original idea was that the deposition of crystals as a consequence of hyperuricemia was the cause of the pathophysiology of gout. Over the years this idea was widely accepted for all the manifestations of the disorder except for the acute attack of gouty arthritis. It is now clear that the original conceptualization was correct, even for acute gouty arthritis.

The deposition of sodium urate in tophi is obviously a function of the limited solubility of urate in body fluids. The choice of sites reflects the relatively avascular nature of the cartilaginous areas in which these deposits occur. In such an area, a predominance of anaerobic metabolism permits accumulation of lactic acid formed from glucose, and this accounts for the low pH actually found in tophi [27]. A decrease in pH favors increased crystallization of urate.

In urate nephropathy, crystals of sodium urate are found in renal interstitial tissue and uric acid crystals are deposited in tubular lumina [66]. The urate crystals in the renal pyramids are long and needle-like, and they may be seen with polarized

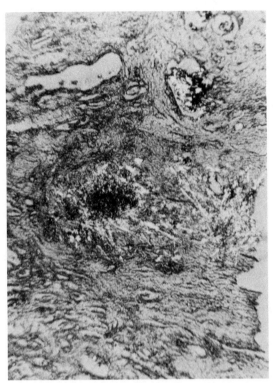

Figure 73-4. Urate crystals in the renal parenchyma of a patient with gout and nephropathy. The tissue was unstained and photographed under polarized light. (Reprinted with permission from J. E. Seegmiller and P. D. Frazier, Ann. Rheum. Dis. *[66].)*

light (Fig. 73-4). Inflammatory reaction, necrosis, and scarring are seen in the areas of crystal deposition. The ultimate result of this process is a scarred, shrunken kidney. The crystals of uric acid within the tubules represent a different type of renal lesion. These deposits occur at times of increased uric acid excretion, as occurs in myeloproliferative disorders or during periods of decreased fluid intake in a patient with metabolic hyperuricemia and uricosuria. The result is the same whether the accumulations are sludge or actual stones. They occur anywhere from the tubule to the urethra and tend to produce obstruction. This may present as acute renal shutdown, or, if asymmetric, as unilateral dilatation of the calyceal system. Infection often supervenes, resulting in chronic obstructive uropathy and pyelonephritis. These changes doubtless lead to further deposits of urate in the parenchyma.

The mechanism of the acute inflammation of a joint that makes up the acute attack of gouty arthritis is a function of the crystalline structure of urate. Urate crystals have been found in the synovial fluid of patients undergoing an attack of acute gouty arthritis, and these crystals are actively phagocytized by leukocytes in the fluid [43]. However, if amorphous sodium urate is injected under the skin or even into a joint, there is no inflammatory reaction. It has now been convincingly demonstrated [11, 44, 67] that when sodium urate is carefully crystallized so that the crystals take the long needle-like form of crystalline urate rather than the amorphous powder, it produces a distinct inflammatory response in man and experimental animals, whether injected subcutaneously or intraarticularly. The degree of inflammatory response is proportional to the amount injected. It seems likely that a similar inflammatory response to urate crystals underlies the nephropathy of sodium urate.

Clinical Manifestations of Hyperuricemia

Hyperuricemia may remain asymptomatic for many years. In the average adult male destined to have "garden-variety" gout, the serum uric acid may become elevated in late adolescence, but the patient may be 40 years of age before his first attack of gouty arthritis occurs. Similarly, we see children hyperuricemic from birth who are making enormous amounts of urate. They seldom have arthritis before 15 to 20 years of age. It is also true that even after clinical manifestations have surfaced, untreated hyperuricemia may have long asymptomatic periods.

In infants and children with hyperuricemia the most common clinical consequences are renal. In patients in whom the process starts at birth, a history of deposits of orange crystals in the diaper is frequently obtained. Renal stone disease may develop within the first days of life or at any time thereafter. Such a patient may have an asymptomatic stone completely obstructing one ureter for months and present to the physician only when a stone or sludge plugs the other ureter, producing complete renal shutdown.

Urinary tract infections are common in all patients with stones. Pure urate stones are radiolucent and are often seen only when there is contrast medium in the urinary tract (Fig. 73-5). However, a urate stone may incorporate calcium salts and be radiopaque.

As nephropathy develops, patients develop proteinuria. Some develop hypertension. Limitations in concentration and dilution of the urine are common, although some patients may continue to dilute well. Some patients have severe enough concentrating defects to exhibit frank polyuria and polydipsia. The amount of water ingested is important with regard to the development of complications; urolithiasis occurs in about 20 percent

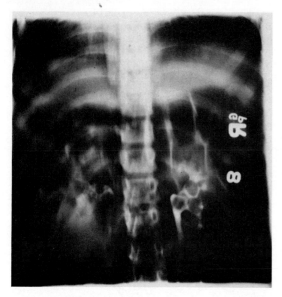

Figure 73-5. Intravenous pyelogram of a patient with the Lesch-Nyhan syndrome. Radiolucent stones are clearly illustrated in the right kidney pelvis. Stones are present bilaterally. (Reprinted, by permission, from Actualités Nephrologiques de l'Hôpital Necker *[54].)*

of patients with gout in the United States but in 75 percent of patients in Israel [2].

The classic description of the acute attack of gouty arthritis was that of Sydenham [74]. The first attack is in the great toe in about 50 percent of adults and is known as podagra. In children the joint chosen is much more variable, and any joint in the body may be involved. Arthritis does not make up much of the clinical picture in pediatric patients, and chronic gouty arthritis is rare.

Tophi may be seen in pediatric patients, but they are rare. Nearly all of those I have seen in children have been in the ears. The others have been in unusual locations such as subcutaneous sites on an upper arm or on the abdominal wall. The skin over such a subcutaneous deposit of urate may appear bluish. On biopsy it may turn out to contain hard scale or soft, amorphous urate.

Tests of renal function in patients with gout usually reveal normal or low-normal values for the glomerular filtration rate. The clearance of para-aminohippurate (PAH) regularly reveals a significant reduction. The transport maximum (Tm_{PAH}) is reduced from a mean of 77 to 62 mg/min/1.73 m^2 [22, 70].

Disorders in Which Hyperuricemia Occurs

THE LESCH-NYHAN SYNDROME

The Lesch-Nyhan syndrome is a genetically determined disorder of purine metabolism [40]. It was the first disorder of purine metabolism that was definitively localized to a defect in a single enzyme. The responsible gene is on the X chromosome, and the phenotype is expressed as an autosomal recessive characteristic. The molecular site of the defect is the enzyme HGPRT (E.C.2.4.2.8) [69]. The most prominent metabolic consequence of this defect is an enormous overproduction of purine [40, 56], which leads to the accumulation of large amounts of uric acid in body fluids. Patients with the Lesch-Nyhan syndrome have a remarkable disorder of central nervous system function, and they regularly display extraordinary self-mutilative, aggressive behavior [40, 45, 50, 52]. The large quantities of uric acid encountered in children with this syndrome may lead to any of the clinical manifestations of gout, including nephropathy [26, 52].

Clinical Manifestations

The cardinal clinical characteristics of the Lesch-Nyhan syndrome are mental retardation, spastic cerebral palsy, choreoathetosis, and self-mutilative behavior [53]. These patients also have hyperuricemia, gouty arthritis, tophi, urolithiasis, and nephropathy.

The Lesch-Nyhan syndrome occurs exclusively in males. Involved infants appear normal at birth and usually develop normally for the first 6 to 8 months. Crystalluria, hematuria, or urolithiasis may develop during these early months of life, but in most patients the neurologic examination is negative.

The onset of cerebral manifestations is with athetosis. Involuntary movements of both choreic and athetoid type are prominent. Choreoathetoid cerebral palsy may be the most consistent feature of the syndrome, but aggressive, self-mutilating behavior is the most striking aspect [40, 53] and may begin as early as the eruption of the teeth. Sensation is intact, and these children scream in pain when they bite themselves.

Manifestations of Hyperuricemia. A number of the clinical manifestations of these patients are related directly to the accumulation of uric acid in the body fluids. Patients with the Lesch-Nyhan syndrome have hyperuricemia from the neonatal period. They are subject to all of the clinical abnormalities of gout, but acute attacks of arthritis develop only after a number of years. Three of our older patients have had acute arthritis. An involved cousin of one patient was said to have died at 21 years and to have had repeated episodes of arthritis in his last year.

Hematuria and crystalluria are common in Lesch-Nyhan syndrome. Very early there may be masses of orange crystalline material in the diapers. A number of patients have had urinary tract stones [26, 56]. Infantile colic and recurrent abdominal pains in older children may relate to the presence of large amounts of insoluble material in the urine. Urinary tract infections have been common only in those with stones. Marie, Royer, and Rappaport [41, 42] have emphasized the occurrence of a renal concentrating defect associated with Pitressin-resistant polyuria. While I have some doubt that their 18-year-old patient had the Lesch-Nyhan syndrome, he certainly had a related disorder, and we have seen polyuria, polydipsia, and failure to concentrate in typical examples of the syndrome. These patients may have real trouble satisfying their thirst in a large, busy institution. This tubular concentrating defect is clearly related to uric acid. Early in its course it may respond to alkalinization or allopurinol. Later, permanent renal changes are found as glomeruli are affected as well. Urate nephropathy may lead to renal failure, and this has probably been the most common cause of early death. Autopsies have revealed urate crystallinization in the kidneys, with changes typical of urate nephropathy [8, 62].

Tophi also develop, and we have seen this in three patients. One patient had a tophus on his ear that was as large as a golf ball. Another had tophi that broke down and drained solid white urate.

Metabolic Abnormalities

In most patients with Lesch-Nyhan syndrome the first evidence of metabolic abnormality is the elevated concentration of uric acid in the blood, usually approximating 10 mg per deciliter, although in some patients normal concentrations are found occasionally and in a very few normal concentrations are found regularly.

The excretion of uric acid in the urine is always elevated. Children often excrete over 600 mg per day, which would permit classification as a hyperexcretor even in an adult. Patients generally excrete from 40 to 60 mg/kg/24 hr, or 3 to 4 mg of uric acid per milligram of creatinine.

One would expect that an overproduction of purine of the magnitude seen in this syndrome would lead to an accumulation of compounds other than uric acid. These patients excrete xanthine in about the quantities found in normal urine. However, the amounts of hypoxanthine are markedly increased [4, 72]. In most individuals the molar ratio of hypoxanthine to xanthine is less than 1. In these patients the ratio is considerably greater than 1, and it may be as high as 8. When the patient is treated with allopurinol, which inhibits xanthine oxidase, urate excretion decreases and

the other oxypurines remain as the major products of the overproduction. The hypoxanthine-xanthine ratio decreases with small doses of allopurinol, but as the degree of the block is increased, more and more purine ends up in hypoxanthine. In controls treated with allopurinol most of the oxypurine excreted is xanthine.

The Molecular Defect—Deficiency of Hypoxanthine Guanine Phosphoribosyl Transferase

The primary site for the expression of the abnormal gene in the Lesch-Nyhan syndrome is the enzyme HGPRT (Fig. 73-6). This enzyme converts the purine bases, hypoxanthine and guanine, to their respective nucleotides, IMP and GMP. Deficiency in the activity of HGPRT in the Lesch-Nyhan syndrome was first reported by Seegmiller, Rosenbloom, and Kelley [69]. This important observation has been confirmed by a number of investigators [3, 6, 73]. The enzyme is normally present in all tissues of the body, and in involved patients activity is deficient in all tissues. It is most conveniently measured in the erythrocyte; values obtained in patients cannot be distinguished from zero.

Genetics. The Lesch-Nyhan syndrome is found exclusively in males and is transmitted as an X-linked recessive trait [57]. Establishment of the deficiency of HGPRT activity permitted the molecular exploration of the genetics of the condition. In an X-linked recessive the fathers should have normal activity of the enzyme; this is the case. The Lyon hypothesis specifies that the mothers, as heterozygotes, should exhibit mosaicism with two populations of cells, one completely normal and one completely deficient. This has now

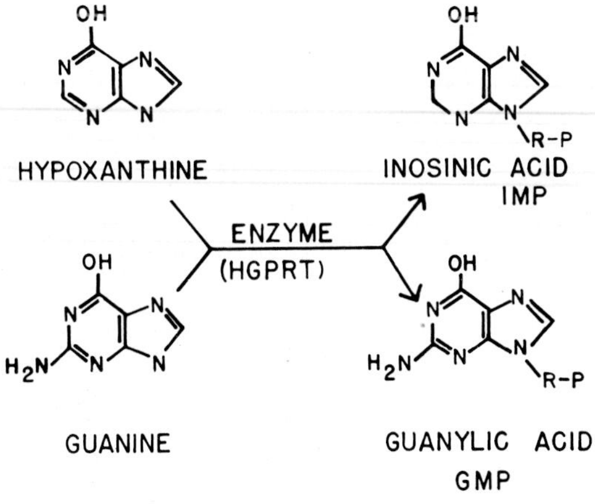

Figure 73-6. The reaction catalyzed by hypoxanthine guanine phosphoribosyl transferase (HGPRT). This is the defect in the Lesch-Nyhan syndrome.

been demonstrated by experiments in which fibroblasts in cell culture were cloned [47, 61].

Assessment of HGPRT activity in the erythrocytes and leukocytes of obligate heterozygotes for this condition has always revealed a normal activity of HGPRT. This problem of hemizygous expression has complicated the process of heterozygote detection. Molecular diagnosis is essential for precise genetic counseling. It is clear that heterozygosity cannot be detected using the blood.

The presence of both cell types in cultures derived from skin permits the use of fibroblasts in culture for diagnosis, in which heterozygosity can be demonstrated by cloning [47, 61]. The time and attention involved, however, precludes the use of cloning as a routine method for the diagnosis of the carrier of the gene. Pharmacologic methods of cell selection [12, 46] provide the cell culture method of choice for heterozygote detection. The best and the most practical method for heterozygote detection is the hair root assay [15].

PARTIAL DEFECTS OF HYPOXANTHINE GUANINE PHOSPHORIBOSYL TRANSFERASE
A number of patients and families have now been described in whom there is an abnormality in the activity of HGPRT, but quantitative assay indicates that the activity of the enzyme is greater than zero. The phenotype in these instances is different from that of the Lesch-Nyhan syndrome.

Patients with partial deficiency of HGPRT are generally found among male patients with clinical gout. These individuals have large amounts of uric acid in both blood and urine. Among pediatric patient populations these patients present with renal stone disease [37]. They usually do not develop urate nephropathy in childhood, although they may present initially with acute renal failure due to obstruction, particularly at times of dehydration and intercurrent illness. Acute attacks of gouty arthritis and tophaceous deposits of urate may occur, and hyperuricemia has been present from birth. In this, as in other forms of hyperuricemia, many years of increased concentrations of urate seem to be required before the onset of the arthritic manifestations that are ultimately the hallmark of gout.

A number of these patients have had some abnormality of the nervous system [34]. This has been occasionally in the form of mild mental retardation and more often in the form of spinocerebellar degeneration. It is not at all clear that these associations are anything but chance. Behavioral abnormalities and self-mutilation have been conspicuous by their absence.

Hyperuricemia, overproduction of purine de novo, and gout have been described in patients in whom PRPP synthetase activity is increased [5, 71]. The gene for this enzyme appears to be autosomal. These observations are consistent with the importance of PRPP concentrations in regulating the rate of synthesis of purines de novo. Patients with the Lesch-Nyhan syndrome have markedly increased concentrations of PRPP in their erythrocytes [20]. It is also consistent that a patient recently described from Japan with a deficiency of PRPP synthetase had hypouricemia [75].

OVERPRODUCTION OF PURINE IN CHILDHOOD WITH NORMAL HYPOXANTHINE GUANINE PHOSPHORIBOSYL TRANSFERASE
Review of the literature from 1823 to the time of the description of the Lesch-Nyhan syndrome revealed only 15 patients less than 10 years of age with hyperuricemic disorders [40]. Some of these may, of course, have had HGPRT deficiency, some may have had glycogen storage disease (although there was no recorded evidence of this), and some probably had normal HGPRT, because 5 of them were girls.

Hyperuricemic children are now being diagnosed in increasing numbers, and it is clear that some of them have normal HGPRT activity. We reported a boy with hyperuricemia, increased urinary urate, and an increased rate of incorporation of ^{14}C-labeled glycine into urate, although the activity of HGPRT in both erythrocytes and fibroblasts was normal [55]. This boy had a number of other abnormalities which may or may not be related. He was mildly mentally retarded, had small, dysplastic teeth, and failed to cry with tears. His behavior was abnormal in that he did not speak and had some other autistic features.

A girl has been reported from the Netherlands in whom there was increased production of uric acid, choreoathetosis, and self-mutilation [25]. The enzyme activity of HGPRT has not been assayed in this patient. However, the kinetics of incorporation of ^{14}C-labeled glycine into uric acid were so different from those of patients with HGPRT deficiency that we would expect the activity of her HGPRT to be normal.

We and others are studying a number of patients as yet unreported in whom hyperuricemia and increased urinary urate accompany normal activity of HGPRT. In our view, the variety of hyperuricemic disorders has only begun to be defined.

OBESITY
Extremely high concentrations of urate are often found in the serum of children who are very obese. Renal manifestations have not been re-

ported, but these children tend to have large quantities of uric acid in the urine. The levels are proportional to total body mass, however, and their urinary excretion rate per mg of creatinine is normal [1, 34, 51].

HYPERURICEMIA AS A CONSEQUENCE OF DIMINISHED URATE EXCRETION

Any disorder in which there is diminished excretion of uric acid can lead to hyperuricemia. Patients with complete renal failure maintained on hemodialysis may develop extensive tophaceous deposits, since uric acid dialyzes poorly. Patients with renal insufficiency as a consequence of glomerulonephritis or pyelonephritis may develop hyperuricemia, although these states usually are not associated with the clinical consequences of hyperuricemia. Patients with nephrogenic diabetes insipidus may also develop hyperuricemia [19].

Among the most common causes of hyperuricemia is the inhibition of tubular secretion of uric acid by other organic molecules. Some are endogenous metabolic products; many are drugs such as salicylates, pyrazinamide, or ethanol. In the case of ethanol the problem appears to be the production of increased quantities of lactic acid as a consequence of increased amounts of reduced NAD. Beta-hydroxybutyric acid, which accumulates in ketosis, also effectively reduces urate clearance. Thus hyperuricemia may be seen in starvation ketosis, in diabetes, in methylmalonic acidemia, and in propionic acidemia.

One of the classic situations in which hyperuricemia occurs is glycogen storage disease due to glucose-6-phosphatase deficiency. Patients with this disorder cannot convert phosphorylated carbohydrates to glucose and have severe hypoglycemia. Glycogenolysis leads directly to high concentrations of lactic acid. These patients also are very ketotic and have high concentrations of β-hydroxybutyrate. As a consequence renal clearance of uric acid is low [29]. Glycogen storage disease type I is complicated in that the turnover of the urate pool [36] and the rate of incorporation of ^{14}C-labeled-1-glycine into urate [28, 30] is excessive, indicating that the rate of de novo biosynthesis of purine is increased.

Patients with this disorder may develop clinical gout and urate nephropathy. Gouty arthritis may develop by the end of the first 10 years of life [13, 28, 31, 36, 65].

SECONDARY HYPERURICEMIA IN LEUKEMIA AND OTHER CELLULAR PROLIFERATIVE DISORDERS

Hyperuricemia is seen in a variety of situations in which cells are turning over faster than normally. The most common cause in pediatric patients is acute leukemia. These patients have large amounts of uric acid in the blood and in the urine. At times of effective cytotoxic therapy, large amounts of cellular material may break down at once, and the amounts of urate may exceed those that can be processed. The uric acid that must be excreted in the urine crystallizes in the tubules and ureters. Acute renal failure may result.

This type of hyperuricemia may occur in a wide variety of proliferative disorders, including polycythemia vera, multiple myeloma, and psoriasis. The experimental drug 2-ethyl-amino-1,3,4-thiadiazole regularly leads to overproduction of purine de novo [38, 39, 58]. Hyperuricemia may also be seen in infectious mononucleosis and in hemolytic anemia.

Investigation of the Patient with Hyperuricemia, Urate Nephropathy, and Urolithiasis

The investigation of an infant or child found to have a high concentration of urate in the blood can follow a logical progression. It is important to identify early patients with chronic renal disease; often that diagnosis is obvious. Nevertheless, some children with chronic renal disease present initially with an acute episode in which one finds a high concentration of urate in the serum along with a high blood urea nitrogen and creatinine, making it difficult to determine which abnormality is the primary one. Examination of the urine for crystals of uric acid and the presence of infection may be helpful. In cases in which the diagnosis is not apparent, it is important to treat the patient and follow the levels of uric acid, creatinine, and urea nitrogen. If crystallization of urate was the primary event in a child presenting for the first time, it will usually be possible with hydration and alkalinization to return renal function to normal while the serum concentration of urate remains elevated. In patients with chronic renal disease, the reverse usually holds.

In the patient with documented hyperuricemia and an established steady state, the next step is to study the excretion of uric acid in the urine. A quantitative assessment of the amounts of urate and creatinine in the urine will distinguish patients who are hyperexcretors from those with normal or reduced excretion. For those patients who are hyperexcretors, the next distinction is to rule out the presence of a neoplasm or some other proliferative state. This seldom proves difficult, for the patients who present with hyperuricemia in childhood are those with enormous numbers of abnormal cells. Once this form of secondary hyperuricemia has been ruled out, the rest of the hyperexcretors may be assumed to have an inborn error of purine metabolism. Among these patients the most common in children are those with a partial or complete deficiency of HGPRT; therefore, blood should be collected in heparin or ACD solution for analysis of the activity of HGPRT and APRT in erythrocytes. Patients found to have a deficiency of HGPRT will have elevated activity of APRT. Their HGPRT should then be studied carefully in order to determine the nature of the variant. Any female found to have an abnormal HGPRT should probably have an analysis of the karyotype to determine whether she has cells that carry only one X chromosome.

Patients with overproduction hyperuricemia and normal HGPRT activity may have elevated levels of APRT. This may be another clue to the presence of a metabolic abnormality. Erythrocytes should be analyzed for the level of PRPP and the activity of PRPP synthetase. Those that do not have an elevated activity of PRPP synthetase must represent new disorders of purine metabolism as yet undefined at the molecular level. It may be of interest in such a patient to establish that there is in fact an overproduction of purine de novo. This can be done in vivo by studying the rate of conversion of ^{14}C-labeled glycine or ^{13}C-labeled glycine to urinary uric acid. It can be done using fibroblasts in cell culture using ^{14}C-labeled formate, which accumulates in formylglycinamide ribotide in the presence of an azaserine block. It may also be useful in such a patient to fractionate the purines excreted in the urine.

Patients not in renal failure found to have normal or low excretion of uric acid in the urine are best examined first for some type of drug treatment that interferes with urate excretion. If this can be rigorously excluded, such a patient is a candidate for the detection of an inborn error of metabolism that leads to an accumulation of something that interferes with urate excretion. The manifestations of glycogen storage disease should lead readily to its diagnosis. On the other hand, documentation of the deficiency of glucose-6-phosphatase requires a liver biopsy. Other metabolic disorders to be considered include maple syrup urine disease, methylmalonic acidemia, propionic acidemia, and fructose intolerance. These patients should be investigated using a routine screen of the urine for metabolic disease. Urine should be examined for the presence of unusual organic acids.

Treatment

Currently no treatment ameliorates the central nervous system manifestations of the Lesch-Nyhan syndrome. On the other hand, the other manifestations of this disease, those that are related directly to uric acid itself, and the manifestations which pediatric patients have in common with adults with gout, are effectively managed using allopurinol. Oral administration in a dose of 200 to 400 mg per day causes a reduction of plasma and urinary levels of uric acid and a concomitant increase in the oxypurines, hypoxanthine and xanthine [4, 72]. In control individuals and in most adults with gout, the total excretion of oxypurines, that is, the sum of uric acid, xanthine, and hypoxanthine, is less after treatment with allopurinol than under control conditions. In patients with a deficiency of HGPRT, this decrease in oxypurine excretion is not seen [35, 41].

Following treatment with allopurinol and effective reduction of uric acid levels, we have seen rapid resorption of tophi as well as improvement in renal function. Thirst decreases, and crystalluria, hematuria, stone formation, and urinary tract infection may be prevented. We have not seen stones resorb, but they have decreased in size and have been passed, although large radiopaque stones may contain too much calcium to be affected by therapy. It would thus appear that arthritis and nephropathy are preventable by early and continued treatment.

Xanthine stones have been observed in patients with the Lesch-Nyhan syndrome [21, 49] during therapy with allopurinol. However, this complication is rare, even with massive doses of the drug [72]. If the patient with HGPRT deficiency behaved metabolically like other individuals, xanthinuria and xanthine stones would be a common complication of allopurinol therapy. However, these patients are unable to reutilize hypoxanthine, and most of their purine leak appears in the urine as hypoxanthine [72]. As the block is increased with increasing dosage of allopurinol, these patients become increasingly hypoxanthinuric. While xanthinuria is even more likely to lead to stones than uric aciduria, hypoxanthinuria is much less likely to do so because hypoxanthine is much more soluble than these other two purines. These factors, along with the fact that the purine load that was excreted primarily as uric acid prior to treatment is now directed to two or three purines, make the likelihood of stone formation much less.

Probenecid and other uricosuric agents have been used in the management of hyperuricemic patients. This is an excellent agent in those patients with normal or reduced quantities of urate in the urine. I believe that uricosuric agents are contraindicated in patients with overproduction hyperuricemia. These individuals are already processing an enormous amount of renal urate. A uricosuric agent could lead to renal shutdown and death.

Alkali therapy with sodium citrate or sodium bicarbonate is effective in many patients who drink sufficient water to prevent crystalluria and stones and to maintain a normal level of urea nitrogen in the blood. However, this form of management is much more difficult than allopurinol therapy, particularly at times of intercurrent illness.

References

1. Acheson, R. M., and Florey, C. D. Body-weight, ABO blood-groups, and altitude of domicile as determinants of serum-uric-acid in military recruits in four countries. *Lancet* 2:391, 1969.
2. Atsmon, A., deVries, A., and Frank, M. *Uric Acid Lithiasis.* Amsterdam: Elsevier, 1963.
3. Bakay, B., Telfer, M. A., and Nyhan, W. L. Assay of hypoxanthine-guanine and adenine phosphoribosyl transferases, a simple screening test for the Lesch-Nyhan syndrome and related disorders of purine metabolism. *Biochem. Med.* 3:230, 1969.
4. Balis, M. E., Krakoff, I. H., Berman, P. H., and Dancis, J. Urinary metabolites in congenital hyperuricosuria. *Science* 156:1122, 1967.
5. Becker, M. A., Meyer, L. J., and Seegmiller, J. E. Gout with purine overproduction due to increased phosphoribosylpyrophosphate synthetase activity. *Am. J. Med.* 55:232, 1973.
6. Berman, P. H., Balis, M. E., and Dancis, J. Diagnostic test for hyperuricemia with central nervous system dysfunction. *J. Lab. Clin. Med.* 71:247, 1968.
7. Borden, M., Nyhan, W. L., and Bakay, B. Increased activity of adenine phosphoribosyltransferase in erythrocytes of normal newborn infants. *Pediatr. Res.* 8:31, 1974.
8. Crussi, F. G., Robertson, D. M., and Hiscox, J. L. The pathological condition of the Lesch-Nyhan syndrome. *Am. J. Dis. Child.* 118:501, 1969.
9. Dent, C. E., and Philpot, G. R. Xanthinuria, an inborn error (or deviation) of metabolism. *Lancet* 1: 182, 1954.
10. Dickinson, D. J., and Smellie, J. M. Xanthinuria. *Br. Med. J.* 2:1217, 1959.
11. Faires, J. S., and McCarty, D. J., Jr. Acute synovitis in normal joints of man and dog produced by injections of microcrystalline sodium urate, calcium oxalate and corticosteroid esters. *Arthritis Rheum.* 5:295, 1962.
12. Felix, J. S., and DeMars, R. Detection of females heterozygous for the Lesch-Nyhan mutation by 8-azaguanine-resistant growth of cultured fibroblasts. *J. Lab. Clin. Med.* 77:596, 1971.
13. Fine, R. N., Strauss, J., and Donnell, G. N. Hyperuricemia in glycogen storage disease Type I. *Am. J. Dis. Child.* 112:572, 1966.
14. Fischer, E. *Untersuchungen in der Puringruppe.* Berlin: Springer, 1907.
15. Francke, U., Bakay, B., and Nyhan, W. L. Detection of heterozygous carriers of the Lesch-Nyhan syndrome by electrophoresis of hair root lysates. *J. Pediatr.* 82:472, 1973.
16. Garrod, A. B. *A Treatise on Gout and Rheumatic Gout (Rheumatic Arthritis)* (3rd ed.). London: Longmans, Green, 1876.
17. Garrod, A. E. *The Inborn Factors in Disease: An Essay.* Oxford, England: Clarendon, 1931.
18. Ghaliounguy, P. Rheumatic disorders in ancient Egyptian papyri. *Egypt. Rheumatol.* 1:4, 1964.
19. Gorden, P., Robertson, G. L., and Seegmiller, J. E. Hyperuricemia: A concomitant of congenital vasopressin-resistant diabetes insipidus in the adult. *N. Engl. J. Med.* 284:1057, 1971.
20. Greene, M. L., Boyle, J. A., and Seegmiller, J. E. Substrate stabilization: Genetically controlled reciprocal relationship of two human enzymes. *Science* 167:887, 1970.
21. Greene, M. L., Fujimoto, W. Y., and Seegmiller, J. E. Urinary xanthine stones, a rare complication of allopurinol therapy. *N. Engl. J. Med.* 280:426, 1969.
22. Gutman, A. B., and Yü, T.-F. Renal function in gout with a commentary on the renal regulation of urate excretion, and the role of the kidney in the pathogenesis of gout. *Am. J. Med.* 23:600, 1957.
23. Hartung, E. F. Historical considerations. *Metabolism* 6:196, 1957.
24. Hippocrates. *The Genuine Works of Hippocrates,* Vols. I and II. Translated from the Greek with a preliminary discourse and annotations by Francis Adams. New York: Wood, 1886.
25. Hooft, C., Van Nevel, C., and De Schaepdryver, A. F. Hyperuricosuria encephalopathy without hyperuricaemia. *Arch. Dis. Child.* 43:734, 1968.
26. Howard, R. S., and Walzak, M. P. A new cause for uric acid stones in childhood. *J. Urol.* 98:639, 1968.
27. Howell, D. S. Preliminary observations on local pH in gouty tophi and synovial fluid. *Arthritis Rheum.* 8:736, 1965.
28. Howell, R. R. The interrelationship of glycogen storage disease and gout. *Arthritis Rheum.* 8:780, 1965.
29. Howell, R. R., Ashton, D. M., and Wyngaarden, J. B. Glucose-6-phosphatase deficiency glycogen storage disease: Studies on the interrelationships of carbohydrate, lipid, and purine abnormalities. *Pediatrics* 29: 553, 1962.
30. Jakovcic, S., and Sorensen, L. B. Studies of uric acid metabolism in glycogen storage disease associated with gouty arthritis. *Arthritis Rheum.* 10:129, 1967.
31. Jeune, M., Charrat, A., and Bertrand, J. Polycorie hepatique, hyperuricemie et goutte. *Arch. Fr. Pediatr.* 14:897, 1957.
32. Kaufman, J. M., Green, M. L., and Seegmiller, J. E. Urine uric acid to creatinine ratio: A screening test for inherited disorders of purine metabolism. *J. Pediatr.* 73:583, 1968.
33. Kelley, W. N., Fox, I. H., and Wyngaarden, J. B. Further evaluation of adenine phosphoribosyltransferase deficiency in man: Occurrence in a patient with gout. *Clin. Res.* 18:53, 1970.
34. Kelley, W. N., Greene, M. L., Rosenbloom, F. M., Henderson, J. F., and Seegmiller, J. E. Hypoxanthine-guanine phosphoribosyltransferase deficiency in gout. *Ann. Intern. Med.* 70:155, 1969.
35. Kelley, W. N., Rosenbloom, F. M., Miller, J., and Seegmiller, J. E. An enzymatic basis for variation in response to allopurinol. *N. Engl. J. Med.* 278:286, 1968.
36. Kelley, W. N., Rosenbloom, F. M., Seegmiller, J. E., and Howell, R. R. Excessive production of uric acid in Type I glycogen storage disease. *J. Pediatr.* 72:488, 1968.
37. Kogut, M. D., Donnell, G. N., Nyhan, W. L., and Sweetman, L. Disorder of purine metabolism due to

partial deficiency of hypoxanthine-guanine phosphoribosyltransferase. *Am. J. Med.* 48:148, 1970.

38. Krakoff, I. H., and Balis, M. E. Studies on the uricogenic effect of 2-substituted thiadiazoles in man. *J. Clin. Invest.* 38:907, 1959.

39. Krakoff, I. H., and Magill, G. B. Effects of 2-ethylamino-1,3,4-thiadiazole HCl on uric acid production in man. *Proc. Soc. Exp. Biol. Med.* 91:470, 1956.

40. Lesch, M., and Nyhan, W. L. A familial disorder of uric acid metabolism and central nervous system function. *Am. J. Med.* 36:561, 1964.

41. Marie, J., Royer, P., and Rappaport, R. Hyperuricemie congenitale avec troubles neurologiques, renaux et sanguins (abstract). *Arch. Fr. Pediatr.* 23:970, 1966.

42. Marie, J., Royer, P., and Rappaport, R. Hyperuricemie congenitale avec troubles neurologiques, renaux et sanguins. *Arch. Fr. Pediatr.* 24:501, 1967.

43. McCarty, D. J. Phagocytosis of urate crystals in gouty synovial fluid. *Arthritis Rheum.* 4:425, 1961.

44. McCarty, D. J. The inflammatory reaction to microcrystalline sodium urate. *Arthritis Rheum.* 8:726, 1965.

45. Michener, W. M. Hyperuricemia and mental retardation with athetosis and self-mutilation. *Am. J. Dis. Child.* 113:195, 1967.

46. Migeon, B. R. X-linked hypoxanthine-guanine phosphoribosyl transferase deficiency: Detection of heterozygotes by selective medium. *Biochem. Genet.* 4:377, 1971.

47. Migeon, B. R., Der Kaloustian, V. M., Nyhan, W. L., and Young, W. J. X-linked hypoxanthine guanine phosphoribosyl transferase deficiency: Heterozygote has two clonal populations. *Science* 160:425, 1968.

48. Monkus, E. St. J., Nyhan, W. L., Foget, B. J., and Yankow, S. Concentrations of uric acid in the serum of neonatal infants and their mothers. *Am. J. Obstet. Gynecol.* 108:91, 1970.

49. Nyhan, W. L. Unpublished data, 1977.

50. Nyhan, W. L. A disorder of uric acid metabolism and cerebral function in childhood. *Arthritis Rheum.* 8:659, 1965.

51. Nyhan, W. L. Purine Metabolism as Reflected in Uric Acid Excretion. In D. B. Cheek (ed.), *Human Growth, Body Composition, Cell Growth, Energy, and Intelligence.* Philadelphia: Lea & Febiger, 1968. Pp. 396–416.

52. Nyhan, W. L. Introduction—Clinical and Genetic Features. In J. H. Bland (ed.), Seminars on the Lesch-Nyhan Syndrome. *Fed. Proc.* 27:1027, 1968.

53. Nyhan, W. L. Clinical features of the Lesch-Nyhan syndrome. *Arch. Intern. Med.* 130:186, 1972.

54. Nyhan, W. L. Le Syndrome de Lesch-Nyhan. In *Actualités Nephrologiques de l'Hôpital Necker.* Paris: Flammarion, 1973. Pp. 59–70.

55. Nyhan, W. L., James, J. A., Teberg, A. J., Sweetman, L., and Nelson, L. G. A new disorder of purine metabolism with behavioral manifestations. *J. Pediatr.* 74:20, 1969.

56. Nyhan, W. L., Oliver, W. J., and Lesch, M. A familial disorder of uric acid metabolism and central nervous system function: II. *J. Pediatr.* 67:257, 1965.

57. Nyhan, W. L., Pesek, J., Sweetman, L., Carpenter, D. G., and Carter, C. H. Genetics of an X-linked disorder of uric acid metabolism and cerebral function. *Pediatr. Res.* 1:5, 1967.

58. Nyhan, W. L., Sweetman, L., and Lesch, M. Effects of the uricogenic agent, 2-ethylamino-1,3,4-thiadiazole

in hypoxanthine-guanine phosphoribosyl transferase deficiency. *Metabolism* 17:846, 1968.

59. Prien, E. L. Crystallographic analysis of urinary calculi: A 25-year survey study. *J. Urol.* 89:917, 1963.

60. Raivio, K. O., and Seegmiller, J. E. Role of glutamine in purine synthesis and interconversion. *Clin. Res.* 19:161, 1971.

61. Salzmann, J., De Mars, R., and Benke, P. Single-allele expression at an X-linked hyperuricemia locus in heterozygous human cells. *Proc. Natl. Acad. Sci. U.S.A.* 60:545, 1968.

62. Sass, J. K., Itabashi, H. H., and Dexter, R. A. Juvenile gout with brain involvement. *Arch. Neurol.* 13:639, 1965.

63. Scheele, K. W. *Examen Chemicum Calculi Urinarii, Opuscula II.* 1776, p. 73. Cited from P. A. Levene and L. W. Bass, *Nucleic Acids.* New York: Chemical Catalog Co., 1931.

64. Seegmiller, J. E. The acute attack of gouty arthritis. *Arthritis Rheum.* 8:714, 1965.

65. Seegmiller, J. E. Diseases of Purine and Pyrimidine Metabolism. In P. K. Bondy (ed.), *Duncan's Diseases of Metabolism.* Philadelphia: Saunders, 1969. P. 516.

66. Seegmiller, J. E., and Frazier, P. D. Biochemical considerations of the renal damage of gout. *Ann. Rheum. Dis.* 25:668, 1966.

67. Seegmiller, J. E., Howell, R. R., and Malawista, S. E. Inflammatory reaction to sodium urate: Its possible relationship to genesis of acute gouty arthritis. *J.A.M.A.* 180:468, 1962.

68. Seegmiller, J. E., Laster, L., and Howell, R. R. Biochemistry of uric acid and its relation to gout. *N. Engl. J. Med.* 268:712, 764, and 821, 1963.

69. Seegmiller, J. E., Rosenbloom, F. M., and Kelley, W. N. Enzyme defect associated with a sex-linked human neurological disorder and excessive purine synthesis. *Science* 155:1682, 1967.

70. Smith, H. W. *The Kidney.* Oxford, England: Oxford University Press, 1951.

71. Sperling, O., Boer, P., Persky-Broch, S., Kanarek, E., and deVries, A. Altered kinetic property of erythrocyte phosphoribosylpyrophosphate synthetase in excessive purine production. *Eur. J. Clin. Biol. Res.* 17:703, 1972.

72. Sweetman, L., and Nyhan, W. L. Excretion of hypoxanthine and xanthine in a genetic disease of purine metabolism. *Nature* 215:859, 1967.

73. Sweetman, L., and Nyhan, W. L. Further studies of the enzyme composition of mutant cells in X-linked uric aciduria. *Arch. Intern. Med.* 130:214, 1972.

74. Sydenham, T. *The Works of Thomas Sydenham,* Vol. II. Translated by R. G. Latham. London: Sydenham Society, 1850. P. 214.

75. Wada, Y., and Arakawa, T. Hypouricemia, Mentally Retarded Infant with a Defect of 5-Phosphoribosyl-1-pyrophosphate Synthetase of Erythrocytes. In *Pediatria XIV, Genetics-Metabolism* (14th International Congress of Pediatrics Oct. 3–9, 1974, Buenos Aires, Argentina). Pp. 210–216.

76. Wollaston, W. H. On gouty and urinary concretions. *Phil. Trans. (London)* 87:386, 1797.

77. Wyngaarden, J. B., and Kelley, W. N. Gout. In J. B. Stanbury, J. B. Wyngaarden, and D. S. Fredrickson (eds.), *The Metabolic Basis of Inherited Disease* (4th ed.). New York: McGraw-Hill, 1978. Pp. 916–1010.

74. Hypercalcemia, Hypercalciuria, and Renal Disease

Gunnar B. Stickler and Wolfgang W. Hagge

Many different conditions seen in pediatric practice are associated with hypercalcemia. These conditions are so uncommon that prevalence figures are not available. They include the following: vitamin D intoxication, idiopathic hypercalcemia, immobilization hypercalcemia, primary hyperparathyroidism, hypercalcemia in hypothyroidism, hypercalcemia in hyperthyroidism, hypercalcemia associated with fat necrosis, and miscellaneous causes (sarcoidosis, hypercalcemia associated with parenteral nutrition, benign familial hypercalcemia, blue diaper syndrome).

Although all of the hypercalcemic states are associated with either functional or morphologic renal changes, the nature of these relationships has not been answered conclusively. The renal changes may be due to an alteration of vitamin D metabolism. In most conditions associated with hypercalcemia, there is the possibility that the primary disease process renders the kidney more reactive to vitamin D or its metabolites or that more vitamin D metabolites than normal are formed. A brief review of vitamin D metabolism may allow a better understanding of the concept of vitamin D sensitivity.

The precursor of vitamin D_3 in the skin is activated by ultraviolet light. Vitamin D_3 from either this source or the diet is hydroxylated primarily in the liver by the enzyme vitamin D_3 25-hydroxylase to 25-$(OH)D_3$. This product is further metabolized in the kidney to more polar metabolites, primarily 1,25-$(OH)_2D_3$. The 1,25-$(OH)_2D_3$ is metabolically the most active form of vitamin D in intestinal calcium transport and in the mobilization of calcium from the bone [63]. Regardless of the amount of vitamin D produced in the skin or contained in the diet, the amount of vitamin D_3 converted to 25-$(OH)D_3$ in the liver depends on the disappearance rate of 25-$(OH)D_3$ rather than on the concentration of its precursor, vitamin D_3 [102]. Thus, the pathogenesis of the so-called vitamin D hypersensitivity in some hypercalcemic conditions may be an abnormal feedback control system in the liver, resulting in a greater than normal synthesis of vitamin D_3 to 25-$(OH)D_3$. Another possibility may be some alteration of vitamin D metabolism in the kidney. In hyperparathyroidism, excessive secretion of parathyroid hormone, which controls the renal synthesis of 1,25-$(OH)_2D_3$ [102], may yield excessive amounts of 1,25-$(OH)_2D_3$ and therefore result in vitamin D intoxication.

In discussing hypercalcemia, normal values for serum calcium for various age groups must be defined. The mean total serum calcium is 10.2 mg per deciliter in children less than 2 years of age, decreases to near 9.8 mg per deciliter by the age of 6 to 8 years, and reaches the adult level of 9.6 mg per deciliter at the age of 16 to 20 years [6]. The range of normal values at each age is similar, namely 1.4 mg per deciliter.

Vitamin D Intoxication

Vitamin D intoxication was first described in two infants by Hess and Lewis in 1928 [65].

PATHOGENESIS AND ETIOLOGY

Vitamin D intoxication causes initial hypercalciuria, which is followed by hypercalcemia, decreased renal blood flow and glomerular filtration rate, and loss of renal concentrating ability. Brunette and coworkers [22] have shown in dogs that hypercalcemia and particularly vitamin D intoxication causes a redistribution of intrarenal blood flow, possibly contributing to hyposthenuria. They also confirmed that hypercalcemia decreases the osmotic corticomedullary gradient, an observation previously made by Eigler and associates [40] and Manitius and coworkers [87]. Stickler, Beabout, and Riggs [116] have reported decreased stool excretion and increased urinary excretion of calcium and phosphorus. David and Anast [33] were unable to detect calcitonin in two patients with hypervitaminosis D.

Vitamin D intoxication has become rare in the United States because there is virtually no indication for the medical use of pharmacologic doses of vitamin D other than in the treatment of hypoparathyroidism, familial hypophosphatemic rickets, and renal osteodystrophy. Most physicians do not use large doses of vitamin D in these conditions. Ergocalciferol, cholecalciferol, 25-$(OH)D_3$, and dihydrotachysterol in toxic doses have similar effects; $1\alpha,25$-$(OH)_2D_3$ probably should be added to this list.

Many authors have suggested that the sensitivity of persons to vitamin D varies widely. In a large study in 1937, Steck and associates [114] gave

773 persons different doses of vitamin D and found that, at each level of intake, only a certain number manifested toxic symptoms. None of the patients in the series of Stickler et al. [116] developed hypercalcemia with daily doses of less than 1,500 IU per kilogram, whereas Steck et al. found no toxic signs when the intake was less than 3,000 IU/kg/day. Anning and associates [5] considered 1,100 IU/kg/day to be the lower limits of a toxic dose. In the Stickler study [116], all patients with intakes more than 7,000 IU per kilogram developed hypercalcemia, but in the Steck series [114], toxic signs in patients receiving 7,000 to 15,000 IU/kg/day occurred in only 15.7 percent. Furthermore, Stickler et al. noted that younger children tolerated much higher doses of vitamin D per unit of weight before hypercalcemia developed than did older children. Steck's patients developed symptoms 87 days after doses of from 3,000 to 5,000 IU/kg/day were given and 60 days after doses of from 3,000 to 7,000 IU/kg/day were given.

The largest series of children with vitamin D intoxication (21 patients) was reported in 1948 by Debré [34]. In that series, large doses of vitamin D were used for the treatment of tuberculosis. The most recent series was reported from Lebanon [91] (infants 7 to 19 months old).

A high calcium diet enhances the risk of vitamin D intoxication, as does exposure to the sun or to ultraviolet light; excessive exposure to ultraviolet light may produce all the signs and symptoms of vitamin D intoxication [88]. Seelig [111] noted a racial difference, with fair-skinned persons having a lower threshold to vitamin D intoxication than dark-skinned persons.

CLINICAL MANIFESTATIONS

The first symptom of vitamin D intoxication is usually anorexia [34]; it often appears suddenly, and parents generally can point out the specific time. Nausea is noted at about the same time, and vomiting, which may be severe, occurs a few days later. Increased thirst and polyuria are noted, and there is constipation. Many other symptoms develop, such as pain in the extremities, headache (which may be severe), abdominal pain, and muscle cramps. These symptoms disappear quickly if vitamin D is discontinued at this stage. If vitamin D is continued, the children become anemic and lose weight, primarily because of the loss of subcutaneous fat. The skin and mucous membranes become dry, and the child experiences irritability, depression, indifference to surroundings, and eventually stupor. Usually hypertension occurs. Deposits of calcium may be seen in the con-

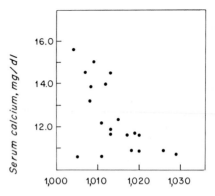

Figure 74-1. Relationship between hypercalcemia and urine specific gravity in vitamin D intoxication (random A.M. urine specimen).

junctiva and in the tympanic membrane. Patients who are more severely affected suffer hypotonia, loss of reflexes, and ataxia. Seizures have been observed, and hearing acuity may be decreased.

The calcium level may be as high as 20.5 mg per deciliter; the serum phosphate level is normal or elevated; the alkaline phosphatase concentration is normal or low. Various degrees of azotemia occur, aggravated in part by dehydration. Renal plasma flow and glomerular filtration rate are decreased. Urinary specific gravity is inversely related to the serum calcium level (Fig. 74-1). The urine may contain protein, erythrocytes, and casts.

The skeletal roentgenograms show evidence of large deposits of mineral in the metaphyses of long bones and occasional demineralization of the epiphysis. Roentgenographic demonstration of nephrocalcinosis or nephrolithiasis is rare.

Renal biopsy or tissue examined at autopsy usually shows periglomerular fibrosis or complete sclerosis of glomeruli. There are tubular atrophy and calcium deposits in the interstitium. The lymphocytic infiltrate is striking (Fig. 74-2).

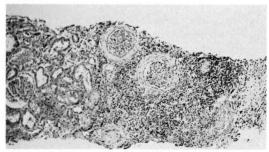

Figure 74-2. Renal biopsy in vitamin D intoxication. Note periglomerular fibrosis and interstitial lymphocytic infiltrate. (H&E, ×70, before 29% reduction.)

Idiopathic hypercalcemic-aortic stenosis syndrome and hyperparathyroidism, as well as the other conditions discussed in this chapter, should be considered in the differential diagnosis.

TREATMENT

The treatment of vitamin D intoxication consists in prompt withdrawal of vitamin D therapy and institution of a low calcium diet. The oral or parenteral intake of fluids must be ample, and furosemide may be given if the patient is well hydrated. This therapy can lower the serum calcium level rapidly. Most frequently, steroids have been used to lower the level of calcium, and this has been accomplished in 5 to 7 days; however, sometimes the effect is delayed for 2 to 3 weeks. Buckle and coworkers [23] reported what probably is the most promising treatment. They infused calcitonin into three adults who had vitamin D intoxication. The serum calcium level decreased within 2 to 3 days in two patients and 7 days in the other. No well-controlled studies of these various forms of treatment are available.

PROGNOSIS

The prognosis in vitamin D intoxication varies. Among Debré's 21 patients, 2 died [34], whereas 5 of 111 patients reported by Chaplin and coworkers died [29]. In a series recently reported by Najjar and Yasigi [91], 1 of 15 children died.

In milder hypercalcemia, vomiting abates in 8 to 15 days after discontinuing vitamin D, the thirst decreases in 10 days, and the blood urea level decreases within 2 to 4 months. The serum calcium level returns to normal in 1 to 3 months if the patient is not treated. However, the serum calcium level has remained elevated for more than 2 years and hypertension has remained unchanged for 10 years [116]. The renal injury appears to be permanent. One of Debré's patients [34] remained hemiplegic and had serious mental deficiencies. Amann [3] described a patient who was mentally retarded and continued to have seizures and suggested that vitamin D intoxication can cause the hypercalcemia-mental retardation-aortic stenosis syndrome; however, in reviewing the findings in the report, we could not detect the characteristic facial features of that syndrome or any cardiac abnormalities.

Idiopathic Infantile Hypercalcemia

Idiopathic infantile hypercalcemia is characterized by hypercalcemia in infancy, with laboratory findings not dissimilar from those observed in vitamin D intoxication. In severe forms the child has a characteristic facial appearance, supravalvular aortic stenosis or other vascular malformations, and mental retardation.

HISTORIC ASPECTS

The severe form of idiopathic infantile hypercalcemia was reported in 1951 by Butler and Schlesinger [25] and in 1952 by Fanconi and Girardet [44] and Schlesinger, Butler, and Black [110]. In 1961 Williams and coworkers [122] first called attention to patients who had mental and growth retardation, supravalvular aortic stenosis, and a characteristic facial appearance. This combination is now called the Williams triad. Black, who had collaborated with Butler and Schlesinger on the earlier report of the infant with idiopathic hypercalcemia [110], noted with Bonham-Carter in 1963 [19] the similarity of the appearance of an 11-year-old survivor of hypercalcemia to that of the children reported by Williams et al. [122]. In 1965 Black and coauthors [20] reported the autopsy findings of supravalvular stenosis of the child originally described in 1951 [25]. The biochemical evidence of the association of the Williams triad—that is, mental retardation, supravalvular aortic stenosis, and a characteristic facial appearance—with the hypercalcemia in infancy was supplied by Garcia and coworkers [55] in 1964. It now seems questionable whether all of the patients with the Williams triad had hypercalcemia. In one patient (one of two siblings), Black [18] found no hypercalcemia in early life but noted that the patient later had the Williams triad.

In their review in 1966, Fraser and associates [52] supported the concept that the Williams triad is the late normocalcemic stage of severe idiopathic hypercalcemia. Subsequently investigators have pointed out the great variation in the severity of the hypercalcemia-aortic stenosis syndrome, ranging from children with supravalvular aortic stenosis alone to children who also have pulmonary stenosis and variations in the degree of mental retardation.

PATHOGENESIS AND ETIOLOGY

In their description of mild hypercalcemia, Lightwood and Stapleton [81–83] suggested that a hypersensitivity to vitamin D exists. After Beuren had observed the frequent occurrence of this syndrome in Germany [15, 16, 16a], he suggested that patients with supravalvular aortic stenosis may respond abnormally to vitamin D. This high incidence may have been related to the widespread practice in Germany of preventing rickets by the "Vitamin-D-Stoss"—giving 400,000 to 600,000 units one to three times at intervals of 6 to 12 weeks, beginning at 1 month of age. Taussig [117] suggested that a variation in the metabolism of vitamin D in affected children may be responsible for the development of the supravalvular aortic stenosis syndrome.

On the basis of her exhaustive review, Seelig [111] stated that there is strong evidence that hypercalcemia of infancy is caused by hyperreactivity to vitamin D, as indicated by (1) the increased incidence of disease in England during a period of overdosage with vitamin D; (2) its occurrence in infants given massive doses of vitamin D; (3) the demonstration of increased antirachitic activity of the blood of affected infants; and (4) the metabolic evidence of increased response to vitamin D by such infants.

The possibility that there may be a familial hypersensitivity to vitamin D was pointed out by Hooft and coworkers [68], who described an 8-month-old infant who had mild hypercalcemia after receiving only 15 mg of vitamin D on two separate occasions. The infant's father had sarcoidosis with hypercalcemia; yet, familial cases of idiopathic hypercalcemia have been rare. Illig and Prader [71] observed familial idiopathic hypercalcemia in a set of fraternal twins; Forfar [50] noted it in two sets of siblings in 11 families; and Kenny et al. [78] described a patient with asymptomatic hypercalcemia who had a severely affected sibling. Among 137 patients seen by Beuren with supravalvular aortic stenosis, he found 54 patients in 11 different families [16a]. Méhes and coauthors reported a patient with possible autosomal-dominant inheritance [89a].

In a review of patients with idiopathic hypercalcemia reported up to 1969, Seelig [111] found only one black child. This observation supported her thesis that fair-skinned children may be more sensitive to vitamin D than black children. Furthermore, the observation that black children develop rickets more easily than white children under similar environmental conditions may point again to some difference in vitamin D metabolism.

Seelig's concept [111] that the benign and severe forms of hypercalcemia are expressions of the same pathophysiologic process on two extremes of a spectrum has been questioned by other authors. Fraser and coworkers [52] believe clinical evidence favors the concept that severe hypercalcemia has its inception in utero because the facial appearance has been noted at birth and because hypercalcemic children tended in retrospect to have a low birth weight.

Most of the clinical and laboratory findings in mild and severe infantile hypercalcemia are similar to those found in vitamin D intoxication. The facial appearance, cardiac findings, and mental retardation, however, as well as the low birth weight, would be difficult to explain on the basis of either vitamin D intoxication or increased vitamin D sensitivity alone.

After reviewing all the evidence, we propose the following summary. First, the benign form of hypercalcemia seen in Britain during the 1950s was probably caused by the relatively high vitamin D intake and had clinical expression only in relatively vitamin-D-sensitive persons. Second, increased vitamin D sensitivity may be due to an increased end-organ response, to delayed turnover or degradation of active metabolites of vitamin D, or to disturbance in cholesterol metabolism. Third, the Williams triad (mental retardation, peculiar facies, and supravalvular aortic stenosis) is a congenital abnormality either inherited or acquired in utero, with most persons being particularly sensitive to vitamin D. The observation by Forbes and coworkers [49] that patients with the Williams triad who are normocalcemic have a prolonged hypercalcemic phase after the intravenous administration of calcium (in contrast to normal controls but similar to patients with hypothyroidism) suggested to these investigators the possibility that patients with the Williams triad have a deficiency of calcitonin. This may be the reason for the vitamin D sensitivity similar to that seen in hypothyroidism. This hypothesis is supported by the fact that hypercalcemia has not been observed in patients with the Williams triad in the newborn period and that the Williams triad may not be associated with hypercalcemia. Our interpretation of the case report by Amann [3] and of the reports of many other patients who have early, severe vitamin D intoxication without later development of the Williams triad suggests that vitamin D sensitivity is a result rather than a cause of the Williams triad.

On the basis of the British Paediatric Association survey [95], Fraser and coworkers [52] estimated that the prevalence of hypercalcemia is 1 per 20,000 births, at least during the time that the child is receiving milk with high vitamin D fortification. Based on their experience in Toronto, the same authors believed that the prevalence of hypercalcemia-aortic stenosis syndrome is 1 per 150,000 births.

CLINICAL MANIFESTATIONS

The patient with idiopathic infantile hypercalcemia initially has anorexia, vomiting, loss of weight, and constipation. Polydipsia, polyuria, episodes of dehydration, and fever are seen. Failure to thrive usually appears between the ages of

3 and 6 months. Frequently the patient has difficulty in swallowing. The patient has a prominent forehead (but the head circumference is usually below normal limits), a marked epicanthal fold, frequent esotropia, a flat nasal bridge, and a short, upturned nose. The upper lip is prominent, and the mouth is wide. Pediatricians have described the facies as elfin-like. Hayles and Nolan [64] originally published the representative photograph of a child with this syndrome (Fig. 74-3). The patient had a significant heart murmur during the hypercalcemic phase and underwent operation for supravalvular aortic stenosis at the age of 8 years. Dental abnormalities included malocclusion, hypodontia, and microdontia. Abnormalities of the voice have been noted frequently, and the voice has been described as coarse or deep, with a metallic quality.

The patients have growth failure during the period of hypercalcemia and remain shorter than normal throughout life. They are usually mentally retarded, with intelligence quotients between 40 and 70. Papilledema has been noted in a few instances. The blood pressure is usually elevated during the hypercalcemic phase. In reviewing the cardiac findings, Rashkind and coworkers [101] stated that significant systolic heart murmurs were usually heard in the left upper parasternal region during the hypercalcemic phase. Neurologic findings include muscular hypotonia and increase in deep tendon reflexes. Seizures have been observed.

The roentgenographic findings include cranial synostosis and a generalized increased bone density in long bones and the skull, primarily in the base and orbit. Deposits of calcium can be seen in the kidneys, blood vessels, brains, muscles, and bronchi.

At autopsy of patients who died during the hypercalcemic phase, various cardiovascular abnormalities have been found, such as calcified atrioventricular valves, coronary subintimal proliferations, myocardial calcification, and left ventricular hypertrophy. Garcia and coworkers [55] noted angiographic evidence of supravalvular aortic stenosis and pulmonic stenosis during the hypercalcemic phase in a 9-month-old infant.

The calcium level may vary from 12 to 23 mg per deciliter, and there may be normal or high values for serum phosphate and normal or lowered values for alkaline phosphatase. The cholesterol level may be elevated, and Forfar [50] reported a positive linear relationship between cholesterol levels and the degree of hypercalcemia in 19 patients.

Balance studies have shown decreased fecal excretion of calcium and increased calcium retention [60, 69, 78]. Hypercalciuria and hyperphosphaturia are present as in vitamin D intoxication. A reduction of renal plasma flow has been shown by Fellers and Schwartz [46] and Hövels and Stephan [69]. The glomerular filtration rate is lowered, and there is azotemia. The concentrating ability of the kidneys is decreased, protein is found in the urine, and leukocytes and granular

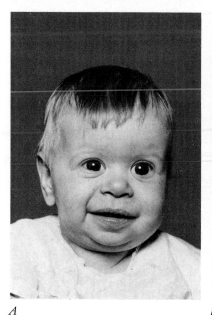 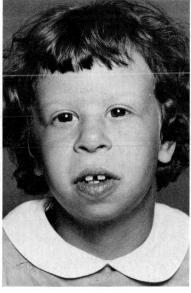

A   *B*

Figure 74-3. Patient with severe idiopathic hypercalcemia. A. Four months old. B. Eight years old.

casts are present. The ability to produce an acid urine is impaired. One-fifth of the patients cannot produce urine with a pH below 5.0. In one report [77] a patient had prolonged acidosis and no titratable acidity in two 24-hr urine specimens.

The histologic findings in the kidney in idiopathic infantile hypercalcemia are indistinguishable from those seen in other renal diseases during the hypercalcemic state. The findings include nephrocalcinosis, tubular atrophy, interstitial lymphocytic infiltration, and focal sclerosis. There may be periglomerular fibrosis.

PROGNOSIS

The prognosis of untreated patients with the severe form of idiopathic infantile hypercalcemia is grave. Of the 44 patients reviewed by Hövels and Stephan in 1962 [69], one-fourth died between the ages of 11 months and $3\frac{1}{2}$ years. The usual cause of death was renal failure.

The hypercalcemia may last as long as 4 years, and the serum cholesterol level may remain elevated even longer. Growth usually remains retarded, and mental retardation is almost invariably present.

The usual cardiovascular abnormalities include supravalvular stenosis of the aorta or the pulmonary arteries (or both), although peripheral artery stenoses and peripheral pulmonary artery stenoses also have been reported [101].

The differential diagnosis includes all the many forms of hypercalcemic renal disease, but the facial appearance, mental retardation, and cardiac manifestations should permit reliable differentiation.

TREATMENT

Controlled treatment trials in idiopathic infantile hypercalcemia have not been done. Vitamin D must be eliminated from the diet, and Fraser and coworkers [52] suggested a severe reduction in calcium intake, to between 25 and 35 mg per day. Exposure to the sun should be avoided. Steroid administration has become standard treatment. The use of furosemide may be indicated in the acute phase, but this agent should be given only if the patient is well hydrated. While there are no data available regarding the levels of calcitonin in these patients, we suspect that the levels are low, and the administration of calcitonin probably should be considered in future treatment trials.

Immobilization Hypercalcemia

Hypercalcemia due to immobilization may be more common than has been documented because the levels of serum calcium often are not determined in such patients.

The first patient with immobilization hypercalcemia was described by Albright et al. in 1941 [2]. Since that time at least 10 additional patients have been reported [13, 35, 70, 80, 115]. In retrospect this syndrome was probably described first by Mawson [89] in the 25 children she reported in 1932; she failed to relate the hypercalcemia to immobilization but did relate it to exposure to the sun.

PATHOGENESIS AND ETIOLOGY

Most typically, immobilization hypercalcemia occurs in an active adolescent who, after trauma, is suddenly immobilized in a cast. The pathogenesis has been considered by Hyman and associates [70]. Immobilization hypercalciuria has been observed in human volunteers [59]. The hypercalciuria, which is followed by hypercalcemia, has been explained on the basis of an increased resorption from the bone rather than of increased dietary calcium intake or decreased renal calcium excretion; in fact, urinary calcium excretion is increased.

The resultant hypercalcemia affects renal function in a manner similar to that observed in vitamin D intoxication. Investigations of vitamin D metabolism in this syndrome have not been made, but we believe that one or more of the metabolic products of vitamin D is increased in order to account for all the manifestations. This hypothesis is supported by a review of the high incidence of hypercalcemia and urolithiasis reported by Mawson [89] in immobilized children with bone or joint tuberculosis who were exposed to prolonged solar irradiation and who regularly took cod-liver oil. During the phase of hypercalcemia, low levels of parathyroid hormone are found. Immobilization hypercalcemia has been observed not only in growing boys but also in adults, including two 58-year-old patients with Paget's disease [65].

CLINICAL MANIFESTATIONS

Most of the immobilization hypercalcemia patients reported had suffered fractures or burns during the spring of the year, and their hypercalcemic symptoms appeared 1 to 3 months later. Mawson [89] found calcium levels that ranged between 11.7 and 25 mg per deciliter in 34 children who had been immobilized for various periods. The patient complains of abdominal discomfort, nausea, and vomiting and may suffer headaches. Polydipsia and polyuria are usually seen, and constipation is present. Loss of weight occurs, and Mawson [89] commented on the impressive loss of subcutaneous fat. Loss of hearing has been noted in one patient [89]. Muscle wasting, severe muscular weakness, hyporeflexia, and lethargy are also present. Hypertension, including hypertensive encephalopathy, has been noted.

The pertinent laboratory findings, in addition to the hypercalcemia, are not different from those seen in hyperparathyroidism and were difficult to evaluate in the past. Determinations of parathyroid hormone allow for an easy diagnosis, however, the levels being normal or low in immobilization hypercalcemia. Roentgenograms of the skeleton show evidence of demineralization.

The effects on renal function are also similar to those described for vitamin D intoxication. With diminished urinary concentrating ability, the specific gravity is inversely proportional to the degree of hypercalcemia, as seen in vitamin D intoxication (see Fig. 74-1). The glomerular filtration rate is reduced, and there is hypercalciuria. Nephrocalcinosis has been reported, and we have observed one such patient with nephrolithiasis. Many of the patients reported by Mawson [89] had kidney stones.

TREATMENT
Mobilization at the earliest possible time is the treatment of choice for immobilization hypercalcemia. The hypercalcemia responds quickly to weight bearing. If mobilization is impossible, a hypercalcemic crisis should be treated with furosemide, but dehydration must be avoided. For long-term treatment, the oral administration of phosphate is effective, at least during the first 12 weeks. Prednisone in a dose of 25 to 40 mg per square meter of body surface area for 1 to 2 weeks can be used. So far there are no reports on the use of calcitonin in this condition.

Primary Hyperparathyroidism
Primary hyperparathyroidism is a rare endocrine disorder in childhood; it is a generalized disorder of calcium and phosphate metabolism that results from an abnormally high secretion of parathyroid hormone. Since the first pediatric patient was described in 1930 [96], more than 50 patients have been reported [17, 26, 30, 57, 93]. Diffuse hyperplasia of all parathyroid glands is the cause of primary hyperparathyroidism in infancy. In the older child, primary hyperparathyroidism results from the neoplastic transformation of one parathyroid gland. All neoplasms are benign adenomas; carcinomas of the parathyroid gland have not been noted to occur in children.

Familial hyperparathyroidism in combination with other endocrine abnormalities (Zollinger-Ellison syndrome, Wermer's syndrome) has received wide attention. Less frequently, hyperparathyroidism without other endocrine involvement has been found in families [54, 58, 86, 112]. Parathyroid hyperplasia in infancy occurring in more than one family member has been reported [32, 57, 66]; such hyperplasia is probably inherited as an autosomal-recessive trait. About 75 percent of patients were between the ages of 6 and 15 years when the diagnosis was made; the remainder had the onset of the disease in early infancy, usually before the fourth month. Primary hyperparathyroidism with onset at an older age occurs more often in the male, whereas the sex distribution is equal when the onset is in infancy.

CLINICAL MANIFESTATIONS
The clinical signs and symptoms of primary hyperparathyroidism in the older child are similar to those seen in the adult. The symptoms are primarily related to hypercalcemia, to changes in the bone and metastatic calcifications [121], and to renal disease. The dominating presenting signs are weakness, anorexia, and irritability, which are seen in about half of the patients [17, 26]. Less common manifestations are polydipsia, polyuria, and vomiting (25 percent).

In 50 to 75 percent of patients the typical bone changes of primary hyperparathyroidism may be present on roentgenographic examination: demineralization of the bone, thinning of the cortex, subperiosteal cortical erosions on the phalanges, disappearance of the lamina dura surrounding the roots of the teeth, and osteitis fibrosa. The long bones, vertebrae, pelvis, skull, jaw, thorax, and carpal and tarsal bones are also involved. The bone involvement is found often on roentgenographic examination, whereas clinical symptoms of bone involvement are relatively rare. Bone pain, fractures, and deformities are found in less than 10 percent of children and usually are late manifestations.

Impairment of renal function is transitory in most pediatric patients with primary hyperparathyroidism and may be related to hypercalcemia; most patients have a serum calcium concentration of more than 15 mg per deciliter. As shown in dog experiments by Brunette et al. [22], hypercalcemia per se may impair kidney function, with reduced glomerular filtration rate, lowered extraction of para-aminohippurate, and a redistribution of renal blood flow. The last may be responsible for a decrease of the corticomedullary gradient and the hyposthenuria. There have been only a few reports of kidney function tests in children.

Reduction in concentrating ability with polyuria, polydipsia, and transient azotemia is seen in about one-fourth of the patients. In most adults with hyperparathyroidism, inulin and para-aminohippurate clearances are decreased before operation. In advanced disease with more severe renal impairment, the filtration fraction is elevated [39]. There is hypercalciuria, with calcium excretion usually exceeding 400 mg per 24 hr. The tubular resorption of calcium, expressed as a percentage of filtered load, is high [85]. Serum phosphate concentrations are low and are accompanied by increased phosphaturia, high phosphate clearance, and elevation of the alkaline phosphatase [119].

Patients with hyperparathyroidism may show a slight acidosis and excrete an alkaline urine [8, 99]. Some adult patients cannot acidify the urine normally after an ammonium chloride load [51] —a defect that seems to be directly related to parathyroid hormone. Parathyroid hormone increases the excretion of bicarbonate and decreases the urinary excretion of hydrogen and ammonium ions. Large amounts of parathyroid hormone may produce a pattern similar to that seen in renal tubular acidosis [8, 99].

Hyperaminoaciduria has been noted in an infant with hyperplasia of the parathyroid glands [66]. The excretion of the free amino acids—hydroxyproline, proline, and glycine—were especially increased; in contrast, the "bound" amino acids in the urine were normal. A few hours after subtotal parathyroidectomy, the aminoaciduria of this patient disappeared completely.

Hypertension has been noted in only a few instances. In advanced renal disease, the hypertension may be due to renal damage [62]. However, Vazquez [119] observed a patient with hypertension who had no significant impairment of kidney function. The hypertension was of short duration and may have been related to hypercalcemia alone.

Nephrolithiasis may be the presenting sign in primary hyperparathyroidism and has been noted in about one-third of pediatric patients. In contrast, nephrocalcinosis is rare, being reported on postmortem examination in only two cases [97, 98] and in only one case on roentgenographic examination [104]. In nephrocalcinosis, the calcium deposits may be so small that there is no evidence on roentgenographic examination, as demonstrated in Vazquez's patient, in whom deposits were seen only on microscopic examination of the kidney [119]. The deposits in patients with hyperparathyroidism and nephrocalcinosis occur pre-

dominantly in the medulla [12]. After the injection of parathyroid hormone, these deposits have been demonstrated by microdissection studies of animals to localize early in the ascending loop of Henle, the distal convoluted tubule, and the collecting system. Obstructions by calcified casts caused dilatation of the tubule proximal to the obstruction [27]. Proximal convoluted tubules are usually not involved. In long-standing hyperparathyroidism, interstitial reaction is present [4].

Nephrocalcinosis was studied after the injection of parathyroid hormone in animal experiments by the use of electron microscopy [14, 28] and electron microprobe analysis [14]. Calcium deposits were found in three regions of the kidney of the mouse and dog. In the cytoplasm, needle-like deposits that contained phosphorus, calcium, magnesium, and oxygen were seen. Intraluminar deposits appeared to be arc-shaped and contained sulfur in addition to the other elements, whereas the deposits in the basement membrane were round and contained calcium and phosphate only. Similar lesions were found in a patient with primary hyperparathyroidism [14]. The calcium deposits in the kidney after vitamin D intoxication are similar, but the needle-like deposits in the cytoplasm are localized in vacuoles and contain only calcium and phospate [56, 109].

Primary hyperparathyroidism in infancy is a rare autosomal-recessive disease caused by diffuse hyperplasia of the parathyroid glands. In the 11 cases reported [31, 45, 57, 66, 90, 97, 98, 100, 104], the disease usually had its onset during the newborn period or the first few months of life. The clinical features resemble those of idiopathic infantile hypercalcemia: failure to thrive, feeding difficulties, anorexia, constipation, dehydration, irritability, and hypotonia. Despite hypotonia, the tendon reflexes are increased greatly. Polyuria, polydipsia, hepatomegaly, splenomegaly, and seizures have been noted.

Hypercalcemia ranging from 15 to 30 mg per deciliter was prominent in all of the 11 cases of primary hyperparathyroidism that have been reported. Hypophosphatemia and increased urinary phosphate and calcium excretion have been found in most patients. Severe bone demineralization was a constant roentgenographic finding. Fractures of several bones were found in 3 of the 11 patients [31, 45, 66]. Evidence of nephrocalcinosis was seen in 5 patients either on roentgenographic examination [104] or at autopsy. The prognosis of this rare condition is poor; only 4 infants have survived infantile primary hyperparathyroidism after subtotal or total parathyroidectomy.

Hypercalcemic crisis was rarely observed in

children [47, 62, 103]. This complication of primary hyperparathyroidism seems to have an abrupt onset and is caused by a rapid elevation of the calcium concentration. In the three children reported, the calcium concentrations were 17, 20, and 22 mg per deciliter, respectively. Immobilization may be a factor in precipitating a hypercalcemic crisis. Polyuria, dehydration, azotemia, vomiting, nausea, and coma are the clinical manifestations, and sometimes a toxic psychosis may be present.

The differential diagnosis of primary hyperparathyroidism includes the other causes of hypercalcemic renal disease mentioned in this chapter. Hyperparathyroidism in the older child should be considered when hypercalcemia, nephrolithiasis, and bone disease are present. Hypercalcemia associated with a low serum phosphate concentration is also suggestive of hypercalcemic renal disease. In adults, several diagnostic therapeutic tests are used. After administration of hydrocortisone for 10 days, the calcium level is not lowered in hyperparathyroidism as it is in other hypercalcemic states. Thiazides, however, may produce severe hypercalcemia in patients with borderline calcium concentrations. False-positive and false-negative results of these tests are not uncommon. The most reliable test is the radioimmunoassay of parathyroid hormone.

TREATMENT
The treatment of choice in primary hyperparathyroidism is surgery. In infantile hyperplasia, the treatment may be a surgical emergency [57]. Total and subtotal parathyroidectomies have been performed. The initial medical treatment of a hypercalcemic crisis is infusion of saline and glucose solutions to correct the dehydration. If renal function is adequate, infusion of large amounts of saline in combination with the administration of furosemide will facilitate urinary calcium excretion and lower the serum calcium concentration. The intravenous administration of phosphate also lowers serum calcium, but it has the risk of producing metastatic calcium deposits. Corticosteroids do not lower serum calcium concentration in primary hyperparathyroidism.

The prognosis in the older child is good. Most of the reported patients had no significant impairment of kidney function after removal of the parathyroid adenoma.

Hypercalcemia and Disorders of Thyroid Function
During the past 20 years, hypercalcemia or nephrocalcinosis (or both) in infants, children, and adults with hypothyroidism has been reported [9, 43, 75, 76, 84, 92, 106, 121]. These patients either were athyrotic or had deficient thyroid function. Royer et al. [107] investigated 37 children who had insufficient thyroid function and found that most had roentgenographic evidence of a mild or moderate localized density of the bones; 3 children had sclerosis of the bones. The bone changes were most prominent in the vertebrae and the base of the skull. Of 37 children with hypothyroidism, 7 had elevation of the serum calcium above 11 mg per deciliter. The serum phosphate concentration was either normal or slightly decreased. Two patients had roentgenographic evidence of nephrocalcinosis. Three others had nephrocalcinosis found at autopsy. In addition to nephrocalcinosis, 1 patient had nephrolithiasis. All degrees of nephrocalcinosis were seen [76, 106]. In most patients, the hypercalcemia and nephrocalcinosis were found incidentally. The impairment of renal function was dependent on the degree and duration of hypercalcemia or nephrocalcinosis. In mild disease, only a defect in concentrating ability has been found, but in long-lasting hypercalcemia, decreased creatinine clearance and azotemia have been reported [107].

In thyroxine deficiency, the calcium balance is strongly positive because of increased intestinal calcium absorption [21, 73, 74, 79]. The oral administration of calcium to hypothyroid patients induces a significant increase in serum calcium level. A similar effect was demonstrated in hypothyroid rats [84]. In addition, the calcium infusion test performed in hypothyroid children [107] showed an abnormal increase in the serum calcium concentration with a slow return to normal.

Bone remodeling is significantly decreased in hypothyroidism. A marked decrease of osteolytic osteolysis, surface formation, and resorption has been found [102]. The increased absorption of calcium and the decreased bone remodeling could be the cause of hypercalcemia, but, as stated by Rasmussen and Bordier [102], the calcium concentration is usually normal in hypothyroidism as well as in hyperthyroidism. Therefore additional factors may be responsible for the hypercalcemia that is occasionally observed in hypothyroid patients, such as vitamin D hypersensitivity [43, 61, 67, 75, 84, 106, 121], calcium intake [84], or a defect in vitamin D metabolism or catabolism [102]. At present no experimental data are available.

The treatment of the hypothyroidism corrects the hypercalcemia and the bone changes, and the nephrocalcinosis may be decreased. Vitamin D administration should be avoided. In patients with severe hypercalcemia, which is rarely seen, calcitonin may be tried. The early diagnosis and treatment of hypothyroidism prevent the development of hypercalcemia and nephrocalcinosis.

In hyperthyroidism, quantitative study of bone shows an increased bone resorption surface and an increase in osteolytic osteolysis [102]. In addition, a negative calcium balance is found because of decreased intestinal calcium absorption [21]. Usually the serum calcium concentration in hyperthyroidism is normal, but in some adult patients, hypercalcemia with mild nephrocalcinosis and transitory renal insufficiency has been noted [1, 10, 41, 53].

There are several possible explanations for the hypercalcemia in hyperthyroidism. These include the accelerated bone turnover because of immobilization, the potentiation of vitamin D or parathyroid hormone action, the imbalance between bone resorption and bone formation, and the effect of thyroxine on vitamin D metabolism [102].

Hypercalcemia Associated with Neonatal Fat Necrosis

A curious association of subcutaneous fat necrosis of the newborn followed by symptomatic hypercalcemia has been noted in a group of about 20 patients [7, 24, 113, 120]. We have also seen such a patient. Our patient at the age of 7 weeks had sclerema involving the cheeks, back, buttocks, and thighs (Fig. 74-4). A biopsy specimen of the involved regions revealed sclerosis of the subcutaneous fat. The estimated vitamin D intake of our patient before admission was 275 to 325 IU per day. Our patient failed to thrive, began to vomit, and was dehydrated when hospitalized. There was hypercalcemia with a calcium level of 19.1 mg per deciliter, and the blood urea level was 45 mg per deciliter. The specific gravity of the urine was initially 1.004, but this increased as serum calcium levels decreased. There were proteinuria, minimal erythrocyturia, and occasional granular casts. A vitamin D assay on serum showed less than 1.0 USP unit per milliliter. The urinary excretion of calcium and phosphate was initially high, and the stool calcium and phosphate contents were low. The patient continued to improve after the administration of a milk-free electrolyte solution and the avoidance of vitamin D. There was no rebound when milk was reintroduced after a few days. At 6 months, reexamination showed complete resolution of the skin lesions, and the patient was normocalcemic. The most likely explanation for the hypercalcemic stage in patients with fat necrosis is an excessive production of a metabolite of vitamin D_3.

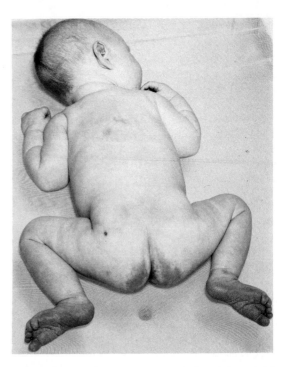

Figure 74-4. Sclerema in 7-week-old patient with hypercalcemia. Note involvement over upper thoracic spine and sacral region. Skin biopsy was taken from left lateral edge of area involved.

Hypercalcemia from Other Causes

Hypercalcemia has been noted to be associated with sarcoidosis. Hypercalcemia is a frequent complication of malignant disease in the adult, and it may result from osteolytic metastasis, for example, from carcinoma of the breast, prostate, kidney, or thyroid; from ectopic production of parathyroid hormone; or from production of parathyroid hormone-like substances. Hypercalcemia in malignancy has not been observed often in children.

Hypercalcemia due to overdosage of calcium has been described in children who have parenteral alimentation [118]. A familial benign hypercalcemia was described in 1972 by Foley and associates [48]: 12 members of this family had mild hypercalcemia without any symptoms and a low urinary calcium excretion. The levels of parathyroid were normal, and exploration of the parathyroid glands of the proband showed normal parathyroid histologic structure.

Drummond and coworkers [38] reported two brothers who had severe hypercalcemia, all the symptoms of hypercalciuria, and significant renal involvement identical to that seen in vitamin D intoxication or idiopathic hypercalcemia. They found a specific defect in the absorption of tryptophan, with high urine excretion of indican and indole derivatives, and they called the condition the blue diaper syndrome.

Idiopathic Hypercalciuria in Children

This rare disorder (about 17 cases have been reported [11, 36, 37, 42, 72, 94, 105]) was first described by Royer and associates in 1962 [108]. Besides the hypercalciuria without hypercalcemia, the affected children showed severe growth retardation, polyuria, decreased urinary concentrating ability, and a mild or moderate proteinuria. Of 10 children investigated by the French group [105], 8 had hypercalciuria with calcium levels higher than 10 mg/kg/day; one-half of the children had proteinuria of the tubular type. The maximal concentrating ability in the urine was between 170 and 178 mOsm per liter. No additional tubular defects were found, and the glomerular filtration rate as measured by creatinine clearance was within normal limits. Renal biopsy revealed interstitial nephritis [105] and nephrocalcinosis [42] in some patients. Roentgenographic evidence of nephrocalcinosis in combination with nephrolithiasis has been found occasionally [11, 42]. Osteoporosis or rickets also has been seen. In 4 of the 17 cases a familial occurrence was noted [11, 36, 105], but the mode of inheritance was not established.

For the treatment of idiopathic hypercalciuria in children, hydrochlorothiazide [42] and a diet low in calcium (300 mg/day) and low in sodium (10 mEq/day) have been recommended [105].

References

1. Adams, P. H., Jowsey, J., Kelly, P. J., Riggs, B. L., Kinney, V. R., and Jones, J. D. Effects of hyperthyroidism on bone and mineral metabolism in man. *Q. J. Med.* 36:1, 1967.
2. Albright, F., Burnett, C. H., Cope, O., and Parson, W. Acute atrophy of bone (osteoporosis) simulating hyperparathyroidism. *J. Clin. Endocrinol. Metab.* 1:711, 1941.
3. Amann, L. Vitamin D-Überdosierung und chronische idiopathische Hypercalcämie. *Monatsschr. Kinderheilkd.* 107:5, 1959.
4. Anderson, W. A. D. Hyperparathyroidism and renal disease. *Arch. Pathol.* 27:753, 1939.
5. Anning, S. T., Dawson, J., Dobly, D. E., and Ingram, J. T. The toxic effects of calciferol. *Q. J. Med.* (n.s.) 17:203, 1948.
6. Arnaud, S. B., Goldsmith, R. S., and Stickler, G. B. Serum parathyroid hormone and blood minerals: Interrelationships in normal children. *Pediatr. Res.* 7: 485, 1973.
7. Barltrop, D. Hypercalcaemia associated with neonatal subcutaneous fat necrosis. *Arch. Dis. Child.* 38:516, 1963.
8. Barzel, U. S. Parathyroid hormone, blood phosphorus, and acid-base metabolism. *Lancet* 1:1329, 1971.
9. Bateson, E. M., and Chander, S. Nephrocalcinosis in cretinism. *Br. J. Radiol.* 38:581, 1965.
10. Baxter, J. D., and Bondy, P. K. Hypercalcemia of thyrotoxicosis. *Ann. Intern. Med.* 65:429, 1966.
11. Beilin, L. J., and Clayton, B. E. Idiopathic hypercalciuria in a child. *Arch. Dis. Child.* 39:409, 1964.
12. Bell, E. T. *Renal Diseases* (2nd ed.). Philadelphia: Lea & Febiger, 1950. P. 408.
13. Berliner, B. C., Shenker, I. R., and Weinstock, M. S. Hypercalcemia associated with hypertension due to prolonged immobilization: An unusual complication of extensive burns. *Pediatrics* 49:92, 1972.
14. Berry, J. P. Néphrocalcinose expérimentale par injection de parathormone: Etude au microanalyseur à sonde électronique. *Nephron* 7:97, 1970.
15. Beuren, A. J. Cited by H. B. Taussig, Possible injury to the cardiovascular system from vitamin D. *Ann. Intern. Med.* 65:1195, 1966.
16. Beuren, A. J., Apitz, J., Stoermer, J., Kaiser, H., Schlange, H., Berg, W., and Jörgensen, G. Vitamin D-hypercalcämische Herz- und Gefasserkrankung. *Monatsschr. Kinderheilkd.* 114:457, 1966.
16a. Beuren, A. J. Supravalvular aortic stenosis: A complex syndrome with and without mental retardation. *Birth Defects* 8:45, 1972.
17. Bjernulf, A., Hall, K., Sjögren, I., and Werner, I. Primary hyperparathyroidism in children: Brief review of the literature and a case report. *Acta Paediatr. Scand.* 59:249, 1970.
18. Black, J. A. Familial "hypercalcaemia" facies with other unusual features and normal serum calcium in two brothers. *Proc. R. Soc. Med.* 66:1072, 1973.
19. Black, J. A., and Bonham-Carter, R. E. Association between aortic stenosis and facies of severe infantile hypercalcaemia. *Lancet* 2:745, 1963.
20. Black, J. A., Butler, N. R., and Schlesinger, B. E. Aortic stenosis and hypercalcaemia (letter to the editor). *Lancet* 2:546, 1965.
21. Bordier, P., Miravet, L., Matrajt, H., Hioco, D., and Ryckewaert, A. Bone changes in adult patients with abnormal thyroid function: With special reference to ^{45}Ca kinetics and quantitative histology. *Proc. R. Soc. Med.* 60:1132, 1967.
22. Brunette, M. G., Vary, J., and Carrière, S. Hyposthenuria in hypercalcemia: A possible role of intrarenal blood-flow (IRBF) redistribution. *Pfluegers Arch.* 350:9, 1974.
23. Buckle, R. M., Gamlen, T. R., and Pullen, I. M. Vitamin D intoxication treated with porcine calcitonin. *Br. Med. J.* 3:205, 1972.
24. Buffa, V., Tancredi, F., and Vetrella, M. Sulla sindrome ipercalcemia-adiponecrosi sottocutanea nel neonato. *Pediatria (Napoli)* 81:603, 1973.
25. Butler, N. R., and Schlesinger, B. Generalized retardation, with renal impairment, hypercalcaemia and osteosclerosis of skull. *Proc. R. Soc. Med.* 44: 296, 1951.
26. Canlorbe, P., Lagrue, G., and Bader, J.-C. Adénomes parathyroïdiens de l'enfant opérés. *Sem. Hop. Paris* 45:2373, 1969.
27. Carone, F. A., Epstein, F. H., Beck, D., and Levitin, H. The effects upon the kidney of transient hypercalcemia induced by parathyroid extract. *Am. J. Pathol.* 36:77, 1960.
28. Caulfield, J. B., and Schrag, P. E. Electron microscopic study of renal calcification. *Am. J. Pathol.* 44:365, 1964.
29. Chaplin, H., Jr., Clark, L. D., and Ropes, M. W.

Vitamin D intoxication. *Am. J. Med. Sci.* 221:369, 1951.

30. Chavez-Carballo, E., and Hayles, A. B. Parathyroid adenoma in children: Report of three cases, with unusual articular manifestations in one case. *Am. J. Dis. Child.* 112:553, 1966.

31. Corbeel, L., Casaer, P., Malvaux, P., Lormans, J., and Bourgeois, N. Hyperparathyroidie congenitale. *Arch. Fr. Pediatr.* 25:879, 1968.

32. Cutler, R. E., Reiss, E., and Ackerman, L. V. Familial hyperparathyroidism: A kindred involving eleven cases, with a discussion of primary chief-cell hyperplasia. *N. Engl. J. Med.* 270:859, 1964.

33. David, L., and Anast, C. Studies of immunoreactive parathyroid hormone (IPTH) and calcitonin (ICT) in infants and children (abstract). *Pediatr. Res.* 8:128, 1974.

34. Debré, R. Toxic effects of overdosage of vitamin D_2 in children. *Am. J. Dis. Child.* 75:787, 1948.

35. Deitrick, J. E., Whedon, G. D., and Shorr, E. Effects of immobilization upon various metabolic and physiologic functions of normal men. *Am. J. Med.* 4:3, 1948.

36. De Luca, R., and Guzzetta, F. L'ipercalciuria idiopatica infantile: Osservazione in quattro fratelli. *Pediatria (Napoli)* 73:613, 1965.

37. Dent, C. E., and Friedman, M. Hypercalciuric rickets associated with renal tubular damage. *Arch. Dis. Child.* 39:240, 1964.

38. Drummond, K. N., Michael, A. F., Ulstrom, R. A., and Good, R. A. The blue diaper syndrome—familial hypercalcemia with nephrocalcinosis and indicanuria: A new familial disease, with definition of the metabolic abnormality. *Am. J. Med.* 37:928, 1964.

39. Edvall, C. A. Renal function with hyperparathyroidism: A clinical study of 30 cases with special reference to selective renal clearance and renal vein catheterization. *Acta Chir. Scand.* [*Suppl.*] 229:1, 1958.

40. Eigler, J. O. C., Salassa, R. M., Bahn, R. C., and Owen, C. A., Jr. Renal distribution of sodium in potassium-depleted and vitamin D-intoxicated rats. *Am. J. Physiol.* 202:1115, 1962.

41. Epstein, F. H., Freedman, L. R., and Levitin, H. Hypercalcemia, nephrocalcinosis and reversible renal insufficiency associated with hyperthyroidism. *N. Engl. J. Med.* 258:782, 1958.

42. Fanconi, A. Idiopathische Hypercalciurie im Kindesalter. *Helv. Paediatr. Acta* 18:306, 1963.

43. Fanconi, G., and Chastonay, E. Die D-Hypervitaminose im Säuglingsalter. *Helv. Paediatr. Acta* 5 [Suppl.]:5, 1950.

44. Fanconi, G., and Girardet, P. Chronische Hypercalcämie, kombiniert mit Osteosklerose, Hyperazotämie, Minderwuchs und kongenitalen Missbildungen: Zürcher Fall. *Helv. Paediatr. Acta* 7:314, 1952.

45. Farriaux, J. P., Maillard, E., Tahon, A., du Bois, R., Dupont, A., and Fontaine, G. Étude d'une nouvelle observation d'hyperparathyroïdie primitive par hyperplasie chez une enfant de un mois. *Sem. Hop. Paris* 44:2752, 1968.

46. Fellers, F. X., and Schwartz, R. Etiology of the severe form of idiopathic hypercalcemia of infancy: A defect in vitamin D metabolism. *N. Engl. J. Med.* 259:1050, 1958.

47. Fentz, V. Hypertensive encephalopathy in a child. *Acta Neurol. Scand.* 38:307, 1962.

48. Foley, T. P., Jr., Harrison, H. C., Arnaud, C. D., and Harrison, H. E. Familial benign hypercalcemia. *J. Pediatr.* 81:1060, 1972.

49. Forbes, G. B., Bryson, M. F., Manning, J., Amirhakimi, G. H., and Reina, J. C. Impaired calcium homeostasis in the infantile hypercalcemic syndrome. *Acta Paediatr. Scand.* 61:305, 1972.

50. Forfar, J. O. Cited by F. M. Kenny et al. [78].

51. Fourman, P., McConkey, B., and Smith, J. W. G. Defects of water reabsorption and of hydrogen-ion excretion by the renal tubules in hyperparathyroidism. *Lancet* 1:619, 1960.

52. Fraser, D., Kidd, B. S. L., Kooh, S. W., and Paunier, L. A new look at infantile hypercalcemia. *Pediatr. Clin. North Am.* 13:503, 1966.

53. Frizel, D., Malleson, A., and Marks, V. Plasma levels of ionized calcium and magnesium in thyroid disease. *Lancet* 1:1360, 1967.

54. Frohner, R. N., and Wolgamot, J. C. Primary hyperparathyroidism: Five cases in one family. *Ann. Intern. Med.* 40:765, 1954.

55. Garcia, R. E., Friedman, W. F., Kaback, M. M., and Rowe, R. D. Idiopathic hypercalcemia and supravalvular aortic stenosis. *N. Engl. J. Med.* 271:117, 1964.

56. Giacomelli, F., Spiro, D., and Wiener, J. A study of metastatic renal calcification at the cellular level. *J. Cell Biol.* 22:189, 1964.

57. Goldbloom, R. B., Gillis, D. A., and Prasad, M. Hereditary parathyroid hyperplasia: A surgical emergency of early infancy. *Pediatrics* 49:514, 1972.

58. Goldman, L., and Smyth, F. S. Hyperparathyroidism in siblings. *Ann. Surg.* 104:971, 1936.

59. Goldsmith, R. S., Killian, P., Ingbar, S. H., and Bass, D. E. Effect of phosphate supplementation during immobilization of normal men. *Metabolism* 18:349, 1969.

60. Hagge, W. Über den Einfluss des Prednisolons auf die Ca- und HPO_4-Bilanz bei der idiopathischen Hypercalcaemie. *Arch. Kinderheilkd.* 160:216, 1959.

61. Handovsky, H., and Goormaghtigh, N. D_2-Vitamin, Schilddrüse und Arteriosklerose. *Arch. Int. Pharmacodyn. Ther.* 56:376, 1937.

62. Harmon, M. Parathyroid adenoma in a child: Report of a case presenting as central nervous system disease and complicated by magnesium deficiency. *Am. J. Dis. Child.* 91:313, 1956.

63. Haussler, M. R. Vitamin D: Mode of action and biomedical applications. *Nutr. Rev.* 32:257, 1974.

64. Hayles, A. B., and Nolan, R. B. Idiopathic hypercalcemia. *Proc. Staff Meet. Mayo Clin.* 33:367, 1958.

65. Hess, A. F., and Lewis, J. M. Clinical experience with irradiated ergosterol. *J.A.M.A.* 91:783, 1928.

66. Hillman, D. A., Scriver, C. R., Pedvis, S., and Shragovitch, I. Neonatal familial primary hyperparathyroidism. *N. Engl. J. Med.* 270:483, 1964.

67. Hooft, C., and Vermassen, A. Hypersensibilité à la vitamine D. *Acta Paediatr. Belg.* 16:71, 1962.

68. Hooft, C., Vermassen, A., Eeckels, R., and Vanheule, R. Familial incidence of hypercalcaemia: Extreme hypersensitivity to vitamin D in an infant whose father suffered from sarcoidosis. *Helv. Paediatr. Acta* 16:199, 1961.

69. Hövels, O., and Stephan, U., III. Das Krankheitsbild der "idiopathischen" Hypercalcämie, eine

chronische Vitamin D-Intoxikation. *Ergeb. Inn. Med. Kinderheilkd.* 18:116, 1962.

70. Hyman, L. R., Boner, G., Thomas, J. C., and Segar, W. E. Immobilization hypercalcemia. *Am. J. Dis. Child.* 124:723, 1972.

71. Illig, R., and Prader, A. Kasuistische Beiträge zur idiopathischen Hypercalcämie und Vitamin-D-Intoxikation. *Helv. Paediatr. Acta* 14:618, 1959.

72. Jeune, M., Gilly, R., Hermier, M., Frederich, A., Collombel, C., and Raveau, J. L'hypercalciurie idiopathique de l'enfant: A propos d'une observation. *Pediatrie* 22:17, 1967.

73. Jeune, M., and Muller, J.-M. L'ostéopetrose myxoedémateuse: Hyperdensification généralisée du squelette au cours du myxoedème congénital. *Pediatrie* 14:43, 1959.

74. Job, J.-C., Milhaud, G., Antener, I., and Rossier, A. Les anomalies du métabolisme calcique chez les enfants hypothyroïdiens. *Sem. Hop. Paris* 43:2412, 1967.

75. Job, J.-C., Ribierre, M., and Badoual, J. Hypercalcémie, hypercalciurie et diminution du pouvoir concentrateur du rein: Au cours du traitement de l'hypothyroidie congénitale. *Arch. Fr. Pediatr.* 20:1033, 1963.

76. Johnson, F., and White, H. Cretinism and marble bones. *Case Rep. Child. Mem. Hosp. (Chicago)* 10:2030, 1952.

77. Kelly, P. J., Salassa, R. M., Peterson, L. F. A., and Stickler, G. B. The demonstration of osteoid by microradiography in two patients with osteosclerosis. *Surg. Clin. North Am.* 41:1087, 1961.

78. Kenny, F. M., Aceto, T., Jr., Purisch, M., Harrison, H. E., Harrison, H. C., and Blizzard, R. M. Metabolic studies in a patient with idiopathic hypercalcemia of infancy. *J. Pediatr.* 62:531, 1963.

79. Lang, K. Untersuchungen zum Calciumstoffwechsel bei der Hypothyreose im Kindesalter. *Monatsschr. Kinderheilkd.* 108:395, 1960.

80. Lawrence, G. D., Loeffler, R. G., Martin, L. G., and Connor, T. B. Immobilization hypercalcemia: Some new aspects of diagnosis and treatment. *J. Bone Joint Surg. [Am.]* 55:87, 1973.

81. Lightwood, R. Idiopathic hypercalcaemia in infants with failure to thrive. *Arch. Dis. Child.* 27:302, 1952.

82. Lightwood, R. Idiopathic hypercalcaemia with failure to thrive: Nephrocalcinosis. *Proc. R. Soc. Med.* 45:401, 1952.

83. Lightwood, R., and Stapleton, T. Idiopathic hypercalcaemia in infants. *Lancet* 2:255, 1953.

84. Lowe, C. E., Bird, E. D., and Thomas, W. C., Jr. Hypercalcemia in myxedema. *J. Clin. Endocrinol.* 22:261, 1962.

85. Lund, H. T. Primary hyperparathyroidism in childhood. *Acta Paediatr. Scand.* 62:317, 1973.

86. Mandl, F. Klinisches und Experimentelles zur Frage der lokalisierten und generalisierten Ostitis fibrosa: Unter besonderer Berücksichtigung der Therapie der letzteren. *Arch. Klin. Chir.* 143:1, 1926.

87. Manitius, A., Levitin, H., Beck, D., and Epstein, F. H. On the mechanism of impairment of renal concentrating ability in hypercalcemia. *J. Clin. Invest.* 39:693, 1960.

88. Marfan, A.-B., and Dorlencourt, H. Accidents d'hypercalcémie, consécutifs a des applications prolongées de rayóns ultra-violets: Entérolithes et concrétions calcaires sous-cutanées. *Nourrisson* 19:273, 1931.

89. Mawson, E. E. A consideration of some possible factors concerned in the development of urolithiasis in children. *Liverpool Med. Chir. J.* 40:99, 1932.

89a. Méhes, K., Szelid, Z., and Tóth, P. Possible dominant inheritance of the idiopathic hypercalcemic syndrome. *Hum. Hered.* 25:30, 1975.

90. Mühlethaler, J. P., Schärer, K., and Antener, I. Akuter Hyperparathyreoidismus bei primärer Nebenschilddrüsen-hyperplasie. *Helv. Paediatr. Acta* 22:529, 1967.

91. Najjar, S. S., and Yazigi, A. Abuse of vitamin D: A report on 15 cases of vitamin D poisoning. *J. Med. Liban.* 25:113, 1972.

92. Naylor, J. M. A case of hypothyroidism with nephrocalcinosis. *Arch. Dis. Child.* 30:165, 1955.

93. Nolan, R. B., Hayles, A. B., and Woolner, L. B. Adenoma of the parathyroid gland in children: Report of case and brief review of the literature. *Am. J. Dis. Child.* 99:622, 1960.

94. Nordio, S., Gatti, R., and Tambussi, M. Il nanismo ipercalciurico. *Minerva Pediatr.* 18:1221, 1966.

95. Oppé, T. E. Infantile hypercalcaemia, nutritional rickets, and infantile scurvy in Great Britain: A British Paediatric Association report. *Br. Med. J.* 1:1659, 1964.

96. Pemberton, J. de J., and Geddie, K. B. Hyperparathyroidism. *Ann. Surg.* 92:202, 1930.

97. Philips, R. N. Primary diffuse parathyroid hyperplasia in an infant of four months. *Pediatrics* 2:428, 1948.

98. Pratt, E. L., Geren, B. B., and Neuhauser, E. B. D. Hypercalcemia and idiopathic hyperplasia of the parathyroid glands in an infant. *J. Pediatr.* 30:388, 1947.

99. Pyrah, L. N., Hodgkinson, A., and Anderson, C. K. Primary hyperparathyroidism. *Br. J. Surg.* 53:245, 1966.

100. Randall, C., and Lauchlan, S. C. Parathyroid hyperplasia in an infant. *Am. J. Dis. Child.* 105:364, 1963.

101. Rashkind, W. J., Golinko, R., and Arcasoy, M. Cardiac findings in idiopathic hypercalcemia of infancy. *J. Pediatr.* 58:464, 1961.

102. Rasmussen, H., and Bordier, P. *The Physiological and Cellular Basis of Metabolic Bone Disease.* Baltimore: Williams & Wilkins, 1974.

103. Reinfrank, R. F., and Edwards, T. L. Parathyroid crisis in a child. *J.A.M.A.* 178:468, 1961.

104. Roget, J., Beaudoing, A., Bernard, Y., and Jobert: Un cas d'hyperparathyroïdie primitive chez un enfant de 30 mois. *Pediatrie* 14:21, 1959.

105. Royer, P., Habib, R., Mathieu, H., and Broyer, M. *Néphrologie Pédiatrique.* Paris: Flammarion médecine-sciences, 1973.

106. Royer, P., Lestradet, H., and Habib, R. Les hypercalcémies et les néphrocalcinoses au cours du myxoedème congénital. *Arch. Fr. Pediatr.* 15:896, 1958.

107. Royer, P., Mathieu, H., and Balsan, S. Troubles du métabolisme calcique dans l'insuffisance thyroïdienne de l'enfant. *Ann. Endocrinol. (Paris)* 29:610, 1968.

108. Royer, P., Mathieu, H., Gerbeaux, S., Fréderich, A., Rodriguez-Soriano, J., Dartois, A. M., and Cuisinier,

P. Nanisme, atteinte rénale et hypercalciurie chez l'enfant: 1. L'hypercalciurie idiopathique avec nanisme et atteinte rénale chez l'enfant. *Sem. Hop. Paris* 38:147, 1962.

109. Scarpelli, D. G. Experimental nephrocalcinosis: A biochemical and morphologic study. *Lab. Invest.* 14: 123, 1965.

110. Schlesinger, B., Butler, N., and Black, J. Chronische Hypercalcämie, kombiniert mit Osteosklerose, Hyperazotämie, Minderwuchs und kongenitalen Missbildungen: Londoner Fall. *Helv. Paediatr. Acta* 7:335, 1952.

111. Seelig, M. S. Vitamin D and cardiovascular, renal, and brain damage in infancy and childhood. *Ann. N.Y. Acad. Sci.* 147:539, 1969.

112. Shallow, T. A., and Fry, K. E. Parathyroid adenoma: Occurrence in father and daughter. *Surgery* 24:1020, 1948.

113. Sharlin, D. N., and Koblenzer, P. Necrosis of subcutaneous fat with hypercalcemia: A puzzling and multifaceted disease. *Clin. Pediatr. (Phila.)* 9: 290, 1970.

114. Steck, I. E., Deutsch, H., Reed, C. I., and Struck, H. C. Further studies on intoxication with vitamin D. *Ann. Intern. Med.* 10:951, 1937.

115. Steigman, A. J. Treatment of acute phase of poliomyelitis. *Am. J. Dis. Child.* 87:343, 1954.

116. Stickler, G. B., Beabout, J. W., and Riggs, B. L. Vitamin D-resistant rickets: Clinical experience with 41 typical familial hypophosphatemic patients and 2 atypical nonfamilial cases. *Mayo Clin. Proc.* 45:197, 1970.

117. Taussig, H. B. On the evolution of our knowledge of congenital malformations of the heart (T. Duckett Jones memorial lecture). *Circulation* 31:768, 1965.

118. Ulstrom, R. A., and Brown, D. M. Hypercalcemia as a complication of parenteral alimentation (letter to the editor). *J. Pediatr.* 81:419, 1972.

119. Vazquez, A. M. Nephrocalcinosis and hypertension in juvenile primary hyperparathyroidism. *Am. J. Dis. Child.* 125:104, 1973.

120. Wilkerson, J. A. Idiopathic infantile hypercalcemia, with subcutaneous fat necrosis. *Am. J. Clin. Pathol.* 41:390, 1964.

121. Wilkins, L. *The Diagnosis and Treatment of Endocrine Disorders in Childhood and Adolescence* (3rd ed.). Springfield, Ill.: Thomas, 1965.

122. Williams, J. C. P., Barrett-Boyes, B. G., and Lowe, J. B. Supravalvular aortic stenosis. *Circulation* 24: 1311, 1961.

75. Effects of Potassium Deficiency

Oskar H. Oetliker and George B. Haycock

Lesions of the renal tubules in patients dying from prolonged diarrhea were described more than 50 years ago, but it was in 1950 that Perkins and associates [36] postulated a relationship between these histologic changes and total body potassium depletion. During the ensuing decade a comprehensive clinical description of this syndrome emerged, although the intrinsic mechanisms responsible for the morphologic and functional disturbances observed under these circumstances still remain to be unraveled.

Causes of Potassium Deficiency

Potassium deficiency may occur in a variety of clinical conditions. *Renal losses* of potassium occur in the syndromes of Liddle and of Bartter. Primary disturbances of renal tubular function, such as Fanconi's syndrome and renal tubular acidosis, may also be accompanied by potassium loss; in the latter case the hypokalemia may be episodic and profound. Most diuretic agents, including thiazides, furosemide, and ethacrynic acid, increase the urinary excretion of potassium and may lead to

hypokalemia unless adequate supplementation is given. Exceptions are spironolactone, amiloride, and triamterene, which cause potassium retention. The severity of hypokalemia induced by a diuretic is proportional to its natriuretic effect, being a consequence of increased delivery of sodium to the distal nephron, which results in an enhancement of the driving force for potassium secretion. Hypokalemia may occur secondary to structural renal damage in a wide variety of conditions including cystinosis, juvenile nephronophthisis (medullary cystic disease), renal dysplasia, oligomeganephronia, and chronic pyelonephritis; in these diseases hypokalemia is usually, but not always, associated with salt wasting.

The best known example of hypokalemia due to *endocrine* dysfunction is primary hyperaldosteronism (Conn's syndrome), an exceedingly rare disorder in childhood. Hyperaldosteronism secondary to renal, hepatic, and cardiac disease is relatively common and may lead to significant hypokalemia, which is frequently exaggerated by concomitant diuretic therapy. Untreated diabetic

Supported in part by Grant 3.3340.74 of the Swiss National Foundation for Scientific Research and the Kidney Foundation of New York.

ketoacidosis leads to progressive depletion of intracellular potassium, although the plasma level remains relatively normal and increased renal excretion prevents hyperkalemia. During the repair phase of therapy with insulin and fluid, however, potassium rapidly enters the cells, and this may lead to dangerous hypokalemia unless the replacement fluid contains the ion in adequate concentration. The so-called glucocorticoid drugs, with one or two synthetic compounds representing the exception, possess some mineralocorticoid activity and over a period of prolonged use may cause significant potassium depletion. This leads some clinicians to prescribe potassium supplements to patients on long-term steroid therapy. The thyroid gland also influences potassium metabolism, and hypokalemia has been reported as a complication of hyperthyroidism [16].

Familial hypokalemic periodic paralysis is a *genetic* disorder transmitted by an autosomal dominant mode of inheritance with incomplete penetrance. In contrast to most hypokalemic states, this disorder is not associated with total body potassium deficiency; the low plasma potassium concentration is now known to be due to accumulation of the ion within muscle cells [20]. The prognosis is guarded, since up to 10 percent of affected individuals die in respiratory arrest during a hypokalemic crisis.

Hypokalemia is a frequent result of *chronic diarrhea* and has been reported in familial chloride-losing enteropathy [29], ulcerative colitis [12], the diarrhea associated with villous papillomas of the colon [44], and abuse of laxatives [42]. The hypokalemia is due in part to potassium depletion, since the potassium content of diarrheal fluid may be as high as 40 mEq per liter [49], and in part to hyperaldosteronism occurring in response to volume depletion. Excessive intake of licorice (or its active principle, carbenoxolone) is known to induce hyperaldosteronism and hypokalemia [37]. Certain antibiotics (e.g., carbenicillin and gentamicin) are strongly anionic and have been reported as causes of hypokalemia by their action as ion exchangers [30]. Fulminant meningococcal septicemia has been found to be consistently associated with hypokalemia [31]; the mechanism is unknown.

Clinical Effects

The clinical manifestations of hypokalemia reflect abnormalities of neuromuscular, cardiac, and renal functions.

The neuromuscular abnormalities are illustrated by muscle weakness and hypotonia accompanied by depression or absence of tendon reflexes, progressing in severe instances to paralysis and even respiratory arrest. Paradoxically, the same clinical syndrome may be associated with elevation of the plasma potassium concentration (*hyperkalemic* periodic paralysis). Both disorders are characterized by reduced intracellular potassium levels, however, which suggests that the reduction in muscular excitability is a consequence of intracellular sodium-potassium balance and not simply of hypokalemia.

Cardiac effects are manifested mainly in the electrocardiogram. In ascending order of severity, the changes are: flattening of the T wave, depression of the S-T segment, appearance of a U wave, and inversion of the T wave. The Q-T interval is unchanged, but fusion of T and U waves may give the false impression of Q-T prolongation [41]. The electrocardiographic features of hypokalemia are best seen in the precordial leads. Disturbance of atrioventricular conduction may also be observed. Cardiac sensitivity to digitalis is markedly increased by hypokalemia, and signs of intoxication, especially arrhythmias, may appear in patients receiving only moderate doses of the drug [33]. Since patients with heart disease are frequently on diuretic therapy and may in addition have secondary hyperaldosteronism, it is important to monitor plasma potassium concentration in such subjects and to give adequate supplements when indicated.

The clinical manifestations of the renal effects of hypokalemia are polyuria, polydipsia, symptoms of alkalosis (pallor, malaise, vomiting, and sometimes tetany), and proteinuria.

Pathophysiology

Potassium deficiency impairs the capacity to form maximally concentrated urine. The mechanism involved remains obscure; several possible causes appear to have been excluded. Under the conditions of osmotic diuresis, man has been shown to be unable to reabsorb appropriate amounts of osmotically free water (T^cH_2O) [40]; dogs, however, were found to have normal T^cH_2O under similar circumstances [7]. More evidence against a defect at the level of the collecting duct has been reported in at least two other species: Osmotic equilibrium was shown to exist among fluids in the collecting duct, loop of Henle, and vasa recta of potassium-depleted hamsters [19]; and papillary sodium concentration was shown to be low in proportion to urinary osmolality in hydropenic potassium-depleted rats [15]. Diluting capacity likewise is preserved [6], which argues against impaired chloride transport in the thick ascending limb of Henle. Antidiuretic hormone deficiency is probably eliminated as a possible cause by the observation that administration of the hormone produces no increase in urinary concentration [23] and by the finding that medullary cyclic AMP levels are elevated in hypokalemia [8]. The normal ability to form free water also makes unlikely inadequate delivery of solute to the distal nephron. The studies of Kannegiesser and Lee [25] indicate that oxidative metabolism of the outer medulla of potassium-depleted rabbits is impaired when the slice is immersed in a hypertonic solution, but this does not occur in an isotonic solution. This observation may in part explain the contradictory findings with regard to T^{c}H$_2$O; chloride transport might be normal under some experimental diuretic conditions and abnormal under others. In the light of present knowledge, the most likely explanation for the concentration defect of potassium deficiency is that, despite normal chloride transport in the thick ascending limb, the efficiency of the countercurrent multiplier is impaired by some as-yet unidentified defect, probably in the loop of Henle.

It has been known for many years that hypokalemic states are generally accompanied by acid urine in the presence of metabolic alkalosis. Based on the assumption that hydrogen and potassium ions compete for secretion in exchange for reabsorbed sodium, Berliner et al. [9] proposed that potassium deficiency might enhance hydrogen ion secretion in the distal tubule; in turn, this would facilitate distal bicarbonate resorption. Doubt was cast on this interpretation by the observation of Rector et al. [39] that the inhibitory effect of potassium loading on bicarbonate resorption could not be overcome by increasing the supply of hydrogen ions, a finding inconsistent with the idea of simple competition between the two ionic species. It was thought that the volume contraction associated with states of potassium depletion accounts entirely for the increase in bicarbonate resorption and maintenance of metabolic or "contraction" alkalosis. Volume expansion with saline will partially correct the acidosis [4], but careful quantitative studies have shown that complete correction is not possible unless potassium is given also [26]. The demonstration by Kurtzman [27] that potassium depletion induced by a potassium-deficient diet and desoxycorticosterone acetate produces alkalosis even if extracellular volume is controlled confirms the existence of an effect of hypokalemia on renal acid-base regulation apart from that mediated by volume contraction. A clinical study in two hypokalemic children [34], in which extracellular fluid and plasma volumes were controlled, showed that hypokalemia markedly elevates the tubular bicarbonate threshold. Micro-

puncture studies [26] have now clearly demonstrated that proximal tubular bicarbonate resorption is enhanced in hypokalemia, despite the existence of alkalosis.

Two additional effects may contribute to the acid-base disorder of hypokalemia: increased renal tubular production of ammonium, and disturbances in the renin-angiotensin-aldosterone system. Tubular synthesis of ammonium is consistently increased in potassium depletion and depressed in potassium loading; it was first thought that this was mediated by increased tubular glutaminase activity [5], but more recent work does not support this contention [46]. An alternative explanation for which recent experimental evidence exists [11] is that enzymes of the purine nucleotide cycle are stimulated by hypokalemia with the consequent production of ammonia from amino groups of amino acids.

The mode of action of potassium deficiency on hydrogen ion secretion has been formulated by Rector [38], who showed that hypokalemia increases peritubular transmembrane potential, leading to accelerated removal of bicarbonate from the cell, intracellular acidosis, and augmented secretion of hydrogen ion. Recent work [48] indicates that this may be a consequence of increased carbonic anhydrase activity in the proximal tubular epithelial cells. It is postulated that the normal inhibition of carbonic anhydrase by cyclic AMP and ATP is dependent on potassium. Hydrogen ion secretion is probably thus enhanced in both proximal and distal segments.

An interesting, presumably homeostatic effect of potassium deficiency of nonrenal origin is the induction of potassium resorption in the distal tubule, a phenomenon that until recently was thought not to occur. The fraction of filtered potassium appearing in the early distal tubule of rats fed a low potassium diet is about 10 percent, with only 3 percent reaching the final urine [17]. This finding indicates that hypokalemia induces net potassium resorption along the distal tubule or the collecting duct or both. Diezi et al. [14] have shown that during sodium and potassium depletion even the terminal collecting ducts contribute to net potassium resorption. The decrease of intracellular pH and the low peritubular potassium concentration might be responsible for the net resorption, since both retard the active uptake of potassium across the peritubular cell border [18].

Hyperkalemia reduces aldosterone secretion and enhances renin secretion. These effects are part of the hormonal double-cycle feedback system involved in sodium-potassium and extracellular fluid volume homeostasis [28]. It is known that the effect of potassium on aldosterone may be dampened by its effect on renin, yet other studies show that a given level of potassium (slight potassium depletion) may suppress aldosterone secretion but have no effect on renin production [13]. These are subtle quantitative and qualitative interrelationships not fully understood at present.

Proteinuria of less than 1 gm per 24 hr is observed almost constantly in severe potassium deficiency. Electrophoretic studies have disclosed that the predominant fractions are α- and β-globulins [2, 35], and immunologic studies [1, 3] have suggested that they originate from tissues rather than plasma.

Structural changes are commonly seen in potassium depletion; the histopathology of the lesion has been reviewed in detail by Heptinstall [21]. The most consistent change of chronic hypokalemia is vacuolation of the renal tubules affecting principally the proximal convolution but also the distal segment [24, 36]. Electron microscopic studies suggest that the "vacuoles" represent dilatation of the intercellular spaces [10], although true intracytoplasmic vacuoles also have been observed [45]. Interstitial fibrosis has been described in man [32], but a true association between potassium depletion and fibrosis is not established. An association between hypokalemia and chronic pyelonephritis has been postulated, but it remains unconfirmed [22]. Proliferation of droplet-like particles with a positive periodic acid–Schiff reaction located in the cells lining the collecting ducts has been demonstrated in acute experimental potassium depletion in the rat; recent studies [47] appear to confirm the suspicion that these particles are lysosomes. A similarity between these particles and the intracellular vacuoles seen in chronic potassium deficiency in man, although postulated, remains purely speculative. In view of the consistent finding of a concentrating defect in potassium depletion, it is noteworthy that little, if any, histologic alterations are observed in the medullary collecting ducts. With the possible exception of fibrosis, all changes are fully reversible upon correction of hypokalemia [43].

Therapeutic Considerations

In mild cases of potassium deficiency oral administration of foods rich in potassium (such as fresh fruit juices, bananas, or fresh spinach) and correction of hypovolemia will correct hypokalemia and slowly replenish potassium stores. However, in all patients presenting with even minimal clinical symptomatology of potassium deficiency, more aggressive replacement therapy is mandatory.

The fact that the absolute loss of this cation cannot be accurately estimated and that extracellular fluid potassium concentration is low and must be maintained within a relatively narrow range (3 to 6 mEq per liter of plasma) creates major problems in the treatment of a patient with potassium deficiency. Replacement therapy needs to be performed cautiously, particularly if there is associated sodium deficiency, hypocalcemia, or cardiac failure. The rate of administration should correspond initially to 2 to 3 mEq/kg/day. If given intravenously, the potassium concentration should not exceed 40 mEq per liter. During parenteral therapy, plasma potassium levels should be measured at 12- to 24-hr intervals so that the rate of potassium input can be adjusted to meet the patient's needs. In addition, monitoring of the electrocardiogram is a desirable precaution, since it permits the rapid detection of dangerous hyperkalemia.

Although treatment may safely and fully correct hypokalemia within a matter of days, final recovery of the patient depends upon correcting the cause of the disturbance. If this cannot be done, supportive therapy should attempt to minimize the chance of recurrence of symptomatic hypokalemia. For example, if diuretic therapy needs to be continued in a cardiac patient, potassium-sparing diuretics should be used and adequate supplements of potassium given. If hyperaldosteronism persists, aldosterone antagonists should be prescribed (although their practical effectiveness is often disappointing) and fluid balance should be carefully watched. In sodium- or bicarbonate-losing disorders, maintaining normal fluid balance will prevent secondary hyperaldosteronism. Prophylactic administration of potassium is necessary during treatment of diabetic ketoacidosis.

References

1. Antoine, B.   Gel acrylique synthétique pour immunoprécipitation. *Rev. Fr. Etud. Clin. Biol.* 6:612, 1962.
2. Antoine, B., Patte, D., and Barcelo, R.   Consequences Rénales du Manque de Potassium. In *Actualités Néphrologiques de l'Hôpital Necker*. Paris: Flammarion, 1962. Vol. 1, p. 67.
3. Antoine, B., and Rolland, R.   Recherches sur les Antigénicites Rénales. In *Actualités Néphrologique de l'Hôpital Necker*. Paris: Flammarion, 1963. P. 159.
4. Atkins, E. L., and Schwartz, W. B.   Factors governing correction of the alkalosis associated with potassium deficiency: The critical role of chloride in the recovery process. *J. Clin. Invest.* 41:218, 1962.
5. Balagura-Baruch, S.   Renal Metabolism and Transfer of Ammonia. In C. Rouiller and A. F. Muller (eds.), *The Kidney: Morphology, Biochemistry, Physiology.* New York: Academic, 1971. Vol. III.
6. Bank, N., and Aynedjian, H. S.   A micropuncture study of the renal concentrating defect of potassium depletion. *Am. J. Physiol.* 206:1347, 1964.
7. Bennet, C. M.   Urine concentration and dilution in

hypokalemic and hypercalcemic dogs. *J. Clin. Invest.* 49:1447, 1970.

8. Berl, T., Anderson, R., Aisenbrey, G., McDonald, K., and Schrier, R. On the mechanism of abnormal urinary concentration in hypokalemia: Evidence against cAMP and a prostaglandin mediated mechanism (abstract). *Clin. Res.* 24:393A, 1976.

9. Berliner, R. W., Kennedy, T. J., Jr., and Orloff, J. Relationship between acidification of the urine and potassium metabolism. *Am. J. Med.* 11:274, 1951.

10. Biava, C. G., Dyrda, I., Genest, J., and Bensosure, S. A. Kaliopenic nephropathy: A correlated light and electron microscopic study. *Lab. Invest.* 12:443, 1963.

11. Bogusley, R. T., Lowenstein, L. M., Steele, K. A., and Lowenstein, J. M. The purine nucleotide cycle: A new pathway for renal ammonia production in K$^+$ deficiency (abstract). *Clin. Res.* 24:394A, 1976.

12. Broch, O. J. Low potassium alkalosis with acid urine in ulcerative colitis. *Scand. J. Clin. Lab. Invest.* 2:113, 1950.

13. Broyer, M., and Rizzoni, G. Plasma renin activity and aldosterone excretion in normal children on mild potassium restriction. *Biomedicine* 18:538, 1973.

14. Diezi, J., Michoud, P., Aceves, J., and Giebesch, G. Micropuncture study of electrolyte transport across papillary collecting duct of the rat. *Am. J. Physiol.* 224:623, 1973.

15. Eigler, J. O. C., Salassa, R. M., Bahn, R. C., and Owen, C. A., Jr. Renal distribution of sodium in potassium-depleted and vitamin D intoxicated rats. *Am. J. Physiol.* 202:1115, 1962.

16. Gamstorp, I. Intermittierende Muskellahmungen und Kaliumstoffwechsel. *Nervenarzt* 43:1, 1972.

17. Giebisch, G. Renal Potassium Excretion. In C. Rouiller and A. F. Muller (eds.), *The Kidney: Morphology, Biochemistry, Physiology*. New York: Academic, 1971. Vol. III.

18. Giebisch, G. Some Recent Developments in Renal Electrolyte Transport. In L. G. Wesson and G. J. Fanelli, Jr. (eds.), *Recent Advances in Renal Physiology and Pharmacology*. Baltimore: University Park Press, 1974.

19. Gottschalk, C. W., Mylle, M., Jones, N. F., Winters, R. W., and Welt, L. G. Osmolality of renal tubular fluids in potassium depleted rodents. *Clin. Sci.* 29: 249, 1965.

20. Grob, D., Johns, R. J., and Liljestrand, A. Potassium movement in patients with familial periodic paralysis. *Am. J. Med.* 23:356, 1957.

21. Heptinstall, R. H. *Pathology of the Kidney* (2nd ed.). Boston: Little, Brown, 1974. Vol. II, p. 1052.

22. Hollander, W., Jr., and Blythe, W. B. Nephropathy of Potassium Depletion. In M. B. Strauss and L. G. Welt (eds.), *Diseases of the Kidney* (2nd ed.). Boston: Little, Brown, 1971. P. 933.

23. Hollander, W., Jr., Winters, R. W., Williams, T. F., Bradley, J., Oliver, J., and Welt, L. G. Defect in the renal tubular reabsorption of water associated with potassium depletion in rats. *Am. J. Physiol.* 189:557, 1957.

24. Jaffe, R. J., and Stemberg, H. Ueber die vakuolare Nierendegeneration bei chronischer. *Ruhr. Virchows Arch.* 227:313, 1919–1920.

25. Kannegiesser, H., and Lee, J. B. Role of outer medullary metabolism in the concentrating defect of K depletion. *Am. J. Physiol.* 220:1701, 1971.

26. Kunau, R. T., Jr., Frick, A., Rector, F. C., Jr., and Seldin, D. W. Micropuncture study of the proximal tubular factors responsible for the maintenance of alkalosis during potassium deficiency in the rat. *Clin. Sci.* 34:223, 1968.

27. Kurtzman, N. A. Regulation of renal bicarbonate reabsorption by extracellular volume. *J. Clin. Invest.* 49:586, 1970.

28. Laragh, J. H., and Sealey, J. E. The Renin-Angiotensin-Aldosterone Hormonal System and Regulation of Sodium, Potassium and Blood Pressure Homeostasis. In J. Orloff, R. W. Berliner, and S. R. Geiger (eds.), *Handbook of Physiology*. Section 8, *Renal Physiology*. Washington, D.C.: American Physiological Society, 1973. P. 831.

29. Launiala, K., Pasternack, A., and Perhencterpa, J. Familial chloride diarrhea. *Acta Paediat. Scand.* 56: 320, 1967.

30. Lipner, H. I., Ruzany, F., Dasgupta, M., Lief, P. D., and Bank, N. The behaviour of carbenicillin as a non-reabsorbable anion. *J. Lab. Clin. Med.* 86:183, 1975.

31. Mauger, D. C. Hypokalemia as a consistent feature of fulminant meningococcal septicemia. *Aust. Paediatr. J.* 2:84, 1971.

32. Muehrcke, R. C., and Rosen, S. Hypokalemic nephropathy in rat and man: A light and electron microscopic study. *Lab. Invest.* 13:1359, 1964.

33. Nadas, A. S., and Fyler, D. D. *Pediatric Cardiology* (3rd ed.). Philadelphia: Saunders, 1972. P. 272.

34. Oetliker, O., Schultz, S., Schutt, B., Donath, A., and Rossi, E. Hypokalemia—a factor influencing renal bicarbonate reabsorption. *Pediatr. Res.* 5:618, 1971.

35. Patte, D. Recherches sur les conséquences rénales des déficits en potassium. Paris: Thèse Med., 1963. A.G.E.M.P., éd.

36. Perkins, J. G., Peterson, A. B., and Rilery, J. A. Renal and cardiac lesions in potassium deficiency secondary to chronic diarrhea. *Am. J. Med.* 8:115, 1950.

37. Rankin, J., and Scott, M. E. Hypokalaemic paralysis due to carbenoxolone. *Ulster Med. J.* 42:84, 1973.

38. Rector, F. C., Jr. Renal Secretion of Hydrogen Ion. In C. Rouiller and A. F. Muller (eds.), *The Kidney: Morphology, Biochemistry, Physiology*. New York: Academic, 1971. Vol. III.

39. Rector, F. C., Jr., Buttram, H., and Seldin, D. W. An analysis of the mechanism of the inhibitory influence of K$^+$ on H$^+$ secretion. *J. Clin. Invest.* 41:611, 1962.

40. Rubini, M. E. Water excretion in potassium-deficient man. *J. Clin. Invest.* 40:2215, 1961.

41. Schaub, F. A. Dokumenta Geigy. Grundriss der klinischen Elektrokardiographie. In J. R. Geigy (ed.), *Wissenschaftliche Tabellen*, Basel, Switzerland. [Suppl. 1], 1965. P. 71.

42. Schwartz, W. B., and Relman, A. S. Metabolic and renal studies in chronic potassium depletion resulting from overuse of laxatives. *J. Clin. Invest.* 32:258, 1953.

43. Schwartz, W. B., and Relman, A. S. Effects of electrolyte disorders on renal structure and function. *N. Engl. J. Med.* 276:338, 1967.

44. Schrock, L. G., and Polk, H. C. Rectal villous adenoma producing hypokalemia. *Am. Surg.* 40:54, 1974.

45. Spargo, B. H. Renal Changes with Potassium Depletion. In G. L. Becker (ed.), *Structural Basis of Renal Disease*. New York: Harper & Row, 1968. P. 565.
46. Tannen, R. L. The effect of K^+ loading on NH_3 production by cortex and outer medulla (abstract). *Clin. Res.* 24:413A, 1976.
47. Toback, F. G., Aithal, H. N., Spargo, B. H., Dube, S., and Getz, G. S. Induction of renal lysosome forma-

tion during potassium depletion nephropathy (abstract). *Clin. Res.* 24:413A, 1976.
48. Webster, S. K., and Beck, N. Role of carbonic anhydrase in the kidney on the genesis of metabolic alkalosis in K^+ depletion (abstract). *Clin. Res.* 24: 415A, 1976.
49. Winters, R. W. Maintenance Fluid Therapy. In R. W. Winters (ed.), *The Body Fluids in Pediatrics*. Boston: Little, Brown, 1973. P. 130.

76. Hepatorenal Syndrome

John P. Hayslett*

The hepatorenal syndrome is characterized by the occurrence of severe and progressive renal failure in patients with cirrhosis of the liver in the absence of other recognizable causes of renal disease or of physiological factors that might result in reduced renal function. Although renal failure was described as a complication of severe liver disease more than a century ago [16], the etiology and pathogenesis of this condition remain unknown. While other terms have been employed to avoid confusion with diseases that cause simultaneous injury to both the liver and the kidney [36], we have retained the term *hepatorenal syndrome* because of common usage.

Diagnosis requires the exclusion of other causes of hepatic and renal damage, including sepsis [32] and certain toxins such as carbon tetrachloride [29] and methoxyflurane anesthesia [13]. Renal and hepatic failure has also been encountered in certain hereditary disorders such as Wilson's disease [4], congenital hepatic fibrosis, and infantile polycystic disease [28]. In most of these disorders the factor responsible for renal failure is easily recognized. It is of interest that severe hepatic failure in subacute hepatitis and Reye's syndrome has not been associated with clinical evidence of renal involvement [21].

Renal Function in Liver Disease

VIRAL HEPATITIS

Since viral hepatitis is a common disorder in children, it is important to note that renal involvement, if present, is not associated with significant functional impairment. Conrad and associates [11] evaluated renal biopsy specimens from 20 young servicemen with viral hepatitis and re-

ported that transient urinary abnormalities were found in association with focal glomerular hypercellularity and interstitial edema. Eknoyan and associates [12] extended these observations in seven patients with hepatitis (both positive and negative for Australian antigen) and found a focal increase in material with a positive periodic acid–Schiff reaction in the mesangium; immunoglobulin in discrete, focal nodular deposits; and basement membrane thickening with deposition of a homogeneous, finely granular electron-dense material. In both reports the renal histopathologic changes associated with acute hepatitis were mild. Significant impairment of renal function was absent, and there was no evidence of progression to chronic renal failure. Recently, however, the nephrotic syndrome was reported in a patient with persistent Australian (Au) antigenemia after posttransfusion hepatitis [8]. The membranous nephropathy found on biopsy was associated with glomerular deposits of IgG, C3, and Au antigen in a pattern characteristic of immune complex disease.

COMPENSATED CIRRHOSIS

Studies of renal function in patients with compensated cirrhosis, defined as cirrhosis with the absence of edema formation and ascites, have not been extensive. In several reports [7, 19, 25] glomerular filtration rate and "effective" renal plasma flow (C_{PAH}) were found to be normal or only slightly reduced. Nevertheless, in comparison to normal subjects, a modest and variable reduction in diluting ability, concentrating capacity, and sodium excretion was observed. Papper and Rosenbaum [34] found in patients with cirrhosis a

* Established Investigator of the American Heart Association.

moderate but definite reduction in the diuretic response to water loading and a lowered rate of sodium excretion.

DECOMPENSATED CIRRHOSIS

Marked changes in overall renal function and in specific tubular functions are found in this group of cirrhotic patients with ascites or peripheral edema or both. Glomerular filtration rate and renal plasma flow vary from supernormal to low levels [1, 25, 31]. Although renal function tends to be reduced more in the sickest patients, there is only a weak correlation between the extent of renal insufficiency and the severity of the clinical state as judged by clinical appearance, degree of ascites, and serum level of bilirubin or albumin [25]. Most patients with decompensated cirrhosis have an impairment in the natriuretic response to increased sodium intake and an absence or reversal of the usual diurnal pattern in sodium excretion [22]. The tendency toward enhanced sodium resorption occurs independent of the level of the glomerular filtration rate, and consequently patients with normal filtration rates may have extensive ascites and edema.

In addition to the abnormality in the renal handling of sodium, there is often a defect in diluting ability [35] and in urinary concentration [45] in decompensated cirrhosis. The abnormal handling of sodium is of clinical importance because of the tendency of these patients to develop dilutional hyponatremia when dietary intake of sodium is restricted and they are allowed to drink ad lib. Indirect evidence suggests that these changes in tubular function result from increased proximal resorption of sodium [38]. Since both diluting and concentrating mechanisms depend on the resorption of sodium in the ascending limb of Henle, enhanced proximal resorption of this ion would be expected to impair both mechanisms through a reduction in distal delivery.

While most studies have not included sequential observations in patients with cirrhosis, Leslie [27] and Klingler [25] and their associates reported a tendency toward improvement in renal hemodynamics and in renal function as liver function improves.

Renal Failure in Decompensated Cirrhosis

Within the group of patients with decompensated cirrhosis, some patients develop severe, irreversible renal failure. The decline in renal function usually occurs rapidly over the course of a few days and may follow an episode of mild gastrointestinal bleeding or performance of a paracentesis. While the occurrence of renal failure is more

common in patients with deteriorating hepatic function, it may also occur in relatively stable patients and during periods of apparent improvement.

The clinical features of renal failure in cirrhosis are characterized by progressive deterioration in glomerular filtration rate and renal plasma flow in association with moderate or severe hepatic dysfunction and ascites [33, 41]. Hepatic coma is present in more than half the patients. There is a progressive fall in the rate of urinary flow to oliguric levels. The urine is generally acid, may contain small amounts of protein, and has a sodium concentration usually less than 10 mEq per liter, reflecting the marked tendency toward sodium retention. Urinary concentration is variable. Although early in the course of renal failure urinary osmolality is often 2 to 3.5 times that of plasma, concentrating capacity tends to fall as renal function deteriorates. Because of the severe protein deficiency exhibited by most patients with cirrhosis, the blood urea level does not rise in proportion to the fall in the glomerular filtration rate and is therefore a poor index of renal functional status. The serum creatinine also does not reach levels usually found in terminal uremia. The relative importance of renal insufficiency as a major contributor in the death of these patients therefore is often difficult to evaluate. The development of renal failure of cirrhosis has grave prognostic significance, since a fatal outcome is usual. Only a few patients have been reported to recover either spontaneously [18] or after therapeutic maneuvers such as portacaval shunting [40].

Hepatorenal Failure in Children

Hepatorenal syndrome appears to be uncommon in children. In an informal survey of centers interested in this clinical entity, Vaamonde was unable to discover a single case of hepatorenal syndrome occurring in a child [44].

It is likely that the apparent rarity of the syndrome in children reflects the prevalence of cirrhosis in younger age groups. A patient managed recently at the Yale–New Haven Hospital demonstrates that children may develop this complication of severe liver failure and illustrates many of the typical clinical features of the syndrome.

A 14-year-old girl was hospitalized with a 2-month history of abdominal pain; malaise; loose, yellow stools; and emotional lability. Her past medical history had been unremarkable. On admission, she was jaundiced and exhibited drowsiness and incoherence. On physical examination there were generalized edema and ascites; Kayser-Fleischer rings were found on slit lamp examination. Laboratory studies were typical for hepatic failure. Urinalysis showed trace protein and 2 to 4 erythrocytes per high power field; blood urea nitrogen was 43 mg per deciliter; and serum creatinine was 2.4 mg per deciliter. The concentration of sodium in urine was 19 mEq per liter with an osmolality of 406 mOsm per kilogram of water.

The patient subsequently became severely oliguric and obtunded. Efforts to induce a diuretic response with spironolactone (Aldactone) and furosemide were unsuccessful, and she died 1 week later. Postmortem examination showed cirrhosis of the liver with extensive areas of necrosis, increased amounts of fibrous tissue and regenerating lobules, as well as loss of architecture. The concentrations of copper in the liver and the brain were strikingly elevated. Histologic examination of the kidney showed many intraluminal bile casts and mild focal areas of perivascular infiltration with lymphocytes and plasma cells. Histology of the glomeruli was normal.

This child was diagnosed as having Wilson's disease with severe cirrhosis of the liver. In the absence of a recognizable cause of renal failure and because of the demonstration of adequate renal tubular function, it seemed likely that the cause of renal failure was the hepatorenal syndrome. The overall clinical features exhibited in the course of this child's disease were similar to those observed in adult patients with Laennec's cirrhosis.

Pathogenesis

Although the cause of renal failure in the hepatorenal syndrome has not been established, it appears that a disturbance in renal circulation plays an important role. Baldus and associates [2] demonstrated that the fall in total renal blood flow correlated with a significant increase in renal vascular resistance. This observation has been extended in studies by Kew et al. [23] and Epstein et al. [15] using ^{133}Xe washout curves, which showed decreased cortical perfusion. Moreover, by angiographic techniques Epstein et al. [15] demonstrated beading and tortuosity of interlobular and proximal arcuate arteries and a reduced caliber of vessels in the outer cortex. It seems likely that these changes were caused by severe vasoconstriction, since postmortem studies demonstrated a resolution of the morphologic changes. An attractive explanation for the reduction in renal cortical blood flow suggests that blood is shunted toward the medulla [9]. This interpretation, based on ^{133}Xe washout curves, should be viewed with caution, however, because of the potential errors involved in estimating flow rate with this technique.

Efforts to enhance renal blood flow through the short-term administration of vasodilatory agents have not altered the clinical course of patients with hepatorenal syndrome. Infusion of phentolamine directly into the renal artery of four patients did not significantly increase renal blood flow [15], while intravenous administration of dopamine caused a transient improvement in effective renal plasma flow without increasing the glomerular filtration rate [3]. Conn and associates [10] reported a transient increase in renal plasma flow during the infusion of phenylalanine-lysine vasopressin.

It is of interest that the alterations in renal hemodynamics in patients with decompensated cirrhosis are similar to those found in dogs with thoracic caval occlusion [24]. Partial occlusion of the thoracic vena cava causes avid salt retention, significant reduction in blood flow to the superficial renal cortex, and no change or increased flow to the juxtamedullary region. Interruption of the renal nerves and intrarenal infusion of phentolamine blunt but do not prevent the reduction in superficial cortical flow induced by thoracic caval occlusion.

While these data suggest that renal failure is due to a circulatory mechanism resulting from renal vascular constriction, the underlying cause for the increase in vascular resistance remains unknown. There are three major hypotheses. First, as suggested by Schorr et al. [39], renal failure may result from a metabolic disturbance caused by substances either produced by or inadequately detoxified by the diseased liver. There is at present no evidence that this mechanism is operative in human disease. Second, it has been proposed that the renal hemodynamic changes may occur as a consequence of increased abdominal and renal venous pressure from the presence of ascites [42]. Mullane and Gliedman [30] found, however, that increased renal venous pressure may occur in the absence of ascites due to intrahepatic compression of the inferior vena cava. Moreover, renal venous pressure in cirrhotic patients does not increase to levels that have been demonstrated to cause reduction in renal blood flow [5], and relief of intraabdominal pressure through paracentesis does not cause more than transient improvement in renal hemodynamics [18]. The third hypothesis suggests that renal ischemia is due to a reduction in *effective* blood volume [43]. This theory remains unproved, since there are no techniques for estimating this. In most studies in patients with decompensated cirrhosis [29], total plasma or blood volume has been found to be normal or increased, and, in general, cardiac output has been increased. Moreover, efforts to expand plasma volume with infusions of dextran, ascitic fluid, or blood products have not achieved sustained improvement of renal function [37].

While the relative importance of changes in renal hemodynamics remains controversial and an area of active investigation, it is well established that histopathologic changes in the kidney are not severe enough to explain the functional abnormalities. There is no correlation between functional changes and the presence of swollen tubular cells and bile casts. Several investigators [6] have described diffuse glomerular sclerosis, an increase in mesangial tissue, and a mild glomerular hypercellularity in patients with cirrhosis. The clinical significance of these structural changes is unclear, however, since they do not correlate with functional alterations. It is of special interest that kidneys from patients dying with hepatorenal syndrome have been successfully employed as donor organs in cadaveric transplantation [26].

Treatment

Since the diagnosis of hepatorenal syndrome is made, in part, by exclusion, it is important to search carefully for other causes of reversible renal failure [14]. It is common practice to treat cirrhotic patients with renal failure with dialysis until the possibility of acute reversible tubular injury can be reasonably excluded. General supportive measures usually employed in treating patients with uremia are indicated. Specific therapeutic measures, including plasma volume expansion, paracentesis, administration of vasodilating agents, and portacaval anastomosis, have not been shown to be effective in improving renal function except transiently [9]. We are unaware of any extensive trial with hemodialysis in this group of patients, although it is possible that renal function might recover in patients who have slow but eventual improvement of liver function. It seems unlikely that effective and rational specific therapeutic modalities will be developed until a better understanding of the pathogenesis and etiology of the hepatorenal syndrome is established.

References

1. Baldus, W. P., Feichter, R. N., Summerskill, W. H., Hunt, J. C., and Wakins, K. E. The kidney in cirrhosis: II. Disorders of renal function. *Ann. Intern. Med.* 60:366, 1964.
2. Baldus, W. P., Summerskill, W. H., Hunt, J. C., and Maher, F. T. Renal circulation in cirrhosis: Observations based on catheterization of the renal vein. *J. Clin. Invest.* 43:1090, 1964.
3. Barnardo, D. E., Baldus, W. P., and Maher, F. T. Effects of dopamine on renal function in patients with cirrhosis. *Gastroenterology* 58:524, 1970.
4. Bearn, A. G., Yu, T. F., and Gutman, A. B. Renal

function in Wilson's disease. *J. Clin. Invest.* 36:1107, 1957.
5. Blake, W. D., Wegria, R. P., and Keating, R. P. Effect of increased renal venous pressure on renal function. *Am. J. Physiol.* 157:1, 1949.
6. Bloodworth, J. M. B., Jr., and Sommers, S. C. "Cirrhotic glomerulosclerosis," a renal lesion associated with hepatic cirrhosis. *Lab. Invest.* 8:962, 1959.
7. Brandt, J. L., and Caccese, A. The effects of modified human globin on renal function in cirrhosis of the liver. *J. Lab. Clin. Med.* 39:57, 1952.
8. Combes, B., Shorey, J., Barrera, A., Stastny, P., Eigenbrodt, E. H., Hull, A. R., and Carter, H. W. Glomerulonephritis with deposition of Australia antigen-antibody complexes in glomerular basement membrane. *Lancet* 2:234, 1971.
9. Conn, H. O. A rational approach to the hepatorenal syndrome. *Gastroenterology* 65:321, 1973.
10. Conn, J. H., Tristani, F. E., and Katri, I. M. Renal vasodilator therapy in the hepatorenal syndrome. *Med. Ann. D.C.* 39:1, 1970.
11. Conrad, M. E., Schwartz, F. D., and Young, A. A. Infectuous hepatitis—a generalized disease: A study of renal, gastrointestinal, and hematologic abnormalities. *Am. J. Med.* 37:789, 1964.
12. Eknoyan, G., Gyorkey, F., Dichoso, C., Martinez-Maldonado, M., Suki, W. N., and Gyorkey, P. Renal morphological and immunological changes associated with acute viral hepatitis. *Kidney Int.* 1:413, 1972.
13. Elkington, S. G., Goffinet, J. A., and Conn, H. O. Renal and hepatic injury associated with methoxyflurane anesthesia. *Ann. Intern. Med.* 69:1229, 1968.
14. Epstein, F. H. Reversible uremic states. *J.A.M.A.* 161:494, 1956.
15. Epstein, M., Berk, D. P., Hollenberg, N. K., Adams, D. F., Chalmers, T. C., Abrams, H. L., and Merrill, J. P. Renal failure in the patient with cirrhosis: The role of active vasoconstriction. *Am. J. Med.* 49:175, 1970.
16. Flint, A. Clinical report on hydroperitoneum, based on an analysis of forty-six cases. *Am. J. Med. Sci.* 45:306, 1863.
17. Gabuzda, G. J., Traeger, H. S., and Davidson, C. S. Hepatic cirrhosis: Effects of sodium chloride administration and restriction and of abdominal paracentesis on electrolyte and water balance. *J. Clin. Invest.* 33:780, 1954.
18. Galambos, J. T., and Wilkinson, H. A., III. Reversible hyponatremia and azotemia in a patient with cirrhosis and ascites. *Am. J. Dig. Dis.* 7:642, 1962.
19. Goodyer, A. V. N., Relman, A. S., Lawrason, F. D., and Epstein, F. H. Salt retention in cirrhosis of the liver. *J. Clin. Invest.* 29:973, 1950.
20. Guild, W. R., Young, J. V., and Merrill, J. P. Anuria due to carbon tetrachloride intoxication. *Ann. Intern. Med.* 48:1221, 1958.
21. Huttenlocher, P. R., Schwartz, A. D., and Klatskin, G. Reye's syndrome: Ammonia intoxication as a possible factor in the encephalopathy. *Pediatrics* 43:443, 1969.
22. Jones, R. A., McDonald, G. O., and Last, J. H. Reversal of diurnal variation in renal function in cases of cirrhosis with ascites. *J. Clin. Invest.* 31:326, 1952.
23. Kew, M. C., Brunt, P. W., and Varma, R. R. Renal and intrarenal blood flow in cirrhosis of the liver. *Lancet* 2:504, 1971.
24. Kilcoyne, M. M., and Cannon, P. J. Influence of

thoracic caval occlusion on intrarenal blood flow distribution and sodium excretion. *Am. J. Physiol.* 220: 1220, 1971.

25. Klingler, E. L., Jr., Vaamonde, C. A., Vaamonde, L. S., Lancestremere, R. G., Morasi, H. L., Frisch, E., and Papper, S. Renal function changes in cirrhosis of the liver. *Arch. Intern. Med.* 125:1010, 1970.

26. Koppel, M. H., Coburn, J. W., and Mims, M. M. Transplantation of cadaveric kidneys from patients with hepatorenal syndrome: Evidence for the functional nature of renal failure in advanced liver disease. *N. Engl. J. Med.* 280:1367, 1969.

27. Leslie, S. H., Johnston, B., and Ralli, E. P. Renal function as a factor in fluid retention in patients with cirrhosis of the liver. *J. Clin. Invest.* 30:1200, 1951.

28. Lieberman, E., Salinas-Madrigal, L., Gwinn, J. L., Brennan, L. P., Fine, R. N., and Landing, B. H. Infantile polycystic disease of the kidneys and liver. *Medicine* 50:277, 1971.

29. Lieberman, F. L., and Reynolds, T. B. Plasma volume in cirrhosis of the liver: Its relation to portal hypertension, ascites and renal failure. *J. Clin. Invest.* 46:1297, 1967.

30. Mullane, J. R., and Gliedman, M. L. Elevation of the pressure in the abdominal inferior vena cava as a cause of hepatorenal syndrome in cirrhosis. *Surgery* 59:1135, 1966.

31. Mullane, J. R., and Gliedman, M. L. Development of renal impairment in Laennec's cirrhosis. *Ann. Surg.* 174:892, 1971.

32. Papper, S. The role of the kidney in Laennec's cirrhosis of the liver. *Medicine* 37:299, 1958.

33. Papper, S., Belsky, J. L., and Bleifer, K. H. Renal failure in Laennec's cirrhosis of the liver: I. Description of clinical and laboratory features. *Ann. Intern. Med.* 51:759, 1959.

34. Papper, S., and Rosenbaum, J. P. Abnormalities in the excretion of water and sodium in "compensated" cirrhosis of the liver. *J. Lab. Clin. Med.* 40:523, 1952.

35. Papper, S., and Saxon, L. The diuretic response to administered water in patients with liver disease: II. Laennec's cirrhosis of the liver. *Arch. Intern. Med.* 103:750, 1959.

36. Papper, S., and Vaamonde, C. A. The Kidney in Liver Disease. In M. B. Strauss and L. G. Welt (eds.), *Diseases of the Kidney* (2nd ed.). Boston: Little, Brown, 1971. P. 1139.

37. Reynolds, T. B., Lieberman, F. L., and Redeker, A. G. Functional renal failure with cirrhosis: The effect of plasma expansion therapy. *Medicine* 46:191, 1967.

38. Schedl, H. P., and Bartter, F. C. An explanation for an experimental correction of the abnormal water diuresis in cirrhosis. *J. Clin. Invest.* 39:248, 1960.

39. Schorr, E., Zweifach, B. W., and Furchgott, R. F. Hepatorenal factors in circulatory hemostasis; influence of humoral factors of hepatorenal origin on vascular reactions to hemorrhage. *Ann. N.Y. Acad. Sci.* 49:571, 1948.

40. Schroeder, E. T., Numann, P. J., and Chamberlain, B. E. Functional renal failure in cirrhosis: Recovery after portacaval shunt. *Ann. Intern. Med.* 72:923, 1970.

41. Shear, L., Kleinerman, J., and Gabeizda, G. J. Renal failure in patients with cirrhosis of the liver: I. Clinical and pathological characteristics. *Am. J. Med.* 39: 184, 1965.

42. Thorington, J. M., and Schmidt, C. F. A study of urinary output and blood pressure changes resulting in experimental ascites. *Am. J. Med. Sci.* 165:880, 1923.

43. Tristani, F. F., and Cohn, J. N. Systemic and renal hemodynamics in oliguric hepatic failure: Effect of volume expansion. *J. Clin. Invest.* 46:1894, 1967.

44. Vaamonde, C. A. Personal communication, 1976.

45. Vaamonde, C. A., Vaamonde, L. S., Morosi, H. J., Klingler, E. L., and Papper, S. Renal concentrating ability in cirrhosis: I. Changes associated with the clinical status and course of the disease. *J. Lab. Clin. Med.* 70:179, 1967.

77. Radiation Nephritis

A. Madrazo

Radiation nephritis can be defined as the sum of changes induced in the kidney by ionizing radiation. The name is actually a misnomer, because the main changes are degenerative rather than inflammatory. However, it is retained here because it is firmly embedded in the literature and because its clinical manifestations resemble those of other types of nephritis. Radiation nephritis is rather uncommon today because of proper shielding and advanced radiotherapy techniques. The main cause is therapy of malignant tumors close to or within the kidneys. In children this means Wilms' tumor, neuroblastoma, and malignant lymphomas [1, 6, 10, 14, 23, 24, 27, 28, 30].

Radiation nephritis was recognized shortly after the introduction of x-ray therapy for tumors [29], though there was considerable debate about the sensitivity of the kidneys to radiation and about the relative importance of the primary disease in the production of symptoms. The first clear descriptions of human radiation nephritis were given by Domagk and by Doub et al. in 1927 [3, 4]. These authors found proteinuria, hypertension, and uremia in patients who had previously normal kidneys. Domagk described tubular necrosis, glomerular hyalinization, and thickening of arterial walls. Following these first articles a number of reports appeared dealing with early and late radiation injury [5, 8, 22]. In children, kidney damage after radiotherapy for Wilms' tumor was recognized by Mertz et al. [19], who observed glomerular hyalinization, tubular atrophy, and vascular sclerosis and occlusion in the *opposite* kidney. Zuelzer et al. [30] described early glomerular lesions in children who died 3 to 7 months after radiation. The history of radiation nephritis has been reviewed by Mostofi [20] and by Madrazo et al. [16].

Clinical Manifestations

It has been calculated that radiation nephritis is likely to occur when the dose to the kidneys exceeds 2300 rads given over a period of 5 weeks [10]. This figure is approximate, of course, and it is very likely that radiation nephritis in children can occur with appreciably lower doses, especially if chemotherapy is also used [23]. Cases have been reported to occur 20 years after receiving 1400 rads at age $3\frac{1}{2}$ months [24].

The clinical manifestations of radiation injury of the kidneys become apparent after a latent period of several months to several years. The main features are proteinuria, hypertension, and renal insufficiency, although edema, anemia, and microscopic hematuria also may be present. A threefold increase in urinary tract infection as compared to normal children has been reported [23]. The best analysis of clinical symptoms has been given by Luxton [12] and by Luxton and Baker [13]. Luxton, in a long-term study of 58 patients, described five clinical types of radiation nephritis. These differ in the length of the latent period and in the severity of clinical manifestations, and they include (1) acute radiation nephritis, (2) chronic radiation nephritis, (3) asymptomatic proteinuria, (4) benign hypertension, and (5) late malignant hypertension.

ACUTE RADIATION NEPHRITIS. This type of nephritis develops after a latent period ranging from 6 to 13 months in adults but usually shorter in children. The commonest early symptoms are edema, dyspnea on exertion, and hypertensive headaches. Urinalysis shows proteinuria that is usually of moderate degree but sometimes is severe enough to cause the nephrotic syndrome. Edema is more often due to cardiac insufficiency than to renal involvement, and it may be associated with serous effusions. Severe edema is usually a poor prognostic sign. Hypertension is almost always present and is usually moderate, but malignant hypertension occurs in 30 to 40 percent of the patients and carries a grave prognosis: Most patients die within several months after onset of malignant hypertension. Those with moderate hy-

pertension may improve, though one-half of them will experience progression to chronic radiation nephritis. Renal insufficiency is also a constant finding; in about two-thirds of the patients blood urea levels may be over 80 mg per deciliter, and 30 percent have urea clearance values below 25 percent of normal. Anemia is normochromic and normocytic and is generally severe and resistant to therapy. It may be accompanied by thrombocytopenia.

CHRONIC RADIATION NEPHRITIS. This nephritis may follow acute radiation nephritis, as mentioned above, or it may develop insidiously. The symptoms are similar to those of acute radiation nephritis but are milder. They consist of persistent proteinuria, anemia, and impairment of renal function. Moderate hypertension occurs in about half the patients. The disease runs a prolonged course, with one-half of the patients dying in renal insufficiency within 10 years.

ASYMPTOMATIC PROTEINURIA AND BENIGN ESSENTIAL HYPERTENSION. These are really mild forms of chronic radiation nephritis. Patients have normal renal function but impaired renal reserve. Benign hypertension develops 2 to 5 years after radiation and resembles benign essential hypertension. It may lead to the usual complications, or it may end in malignant hypertension.

LATE MALIGNANT HYPERTENSION. This may develop in patients with chronic radiation nephritis. If it occurs after injury to only one kidney, a cure can be achieved by removing the affected organ [2]. Careful studies are necessary to exclude significant disease in the opposite kidney.

Pathology

The early descriptions of pathologic changes in radiation nephritis by Domagk [3] and by Zuelzer et al. [30] depicted glomerular endothelial damage together with basement membrane thickening, obstruction of capillary loops, and focal necrosis. Many glomeruli were obsolete. There were also extensive tubular necrosis, interstitial fibrosis, and fibrinoid necrosis and thrombosis of small arteries and arterioles.

Most of the early published work on the subject of radiation nephritis pathology was based on light microscopy and gross examination. More recent reports by Rosen et al. [25], Guttman and Kohn [7], Madrazo et al. [15, 17, 18], and Keane and associates [9] include electron microscopic studies in humans and animals.

The extent of the lesion depends, among other factors, upon the dose given and the elapsed time. There is generally a good correlation between the degree of damage and the type of clinical presen-

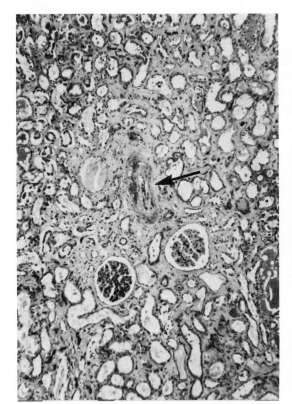

Figure 77-1. Acute radiation nephritis after treatment (4,400 rads) for retroperitoneal lymphoma. Light microphotograph shows tubular atrophy and early interstitial fibrosis. Glomeruli show mesangial thickening and capillary collapse. Note small artery with early fibrinoid necrosis (arrow). (H&E, ×140.)

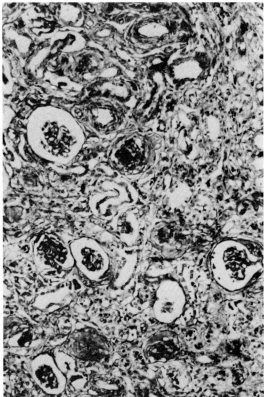

Figure 77-2. Chronic radiation nephritis 12 months after treatment of massive hepatoma. Light microphotograph shows extensive destruction and collapse of renal tubules and marked interstitial fibrosis. Some glomeruli show advanced changes with marked sclerosis. (Trichrome stain, ×140.)

tation. The most severe changes accompany acute radiation nephritis and malignant hypertension, and the mildest are observed in cases with asymptomatic proteinuria or benign hypertension. Nevertheless, the lesions are essentially similar. All renal structures are involved, but the tubules and glomeruli are affected early, while the vascular changes appear later. The tubular lesions are severe and involve mostly the proximal segments. They consist of cellular degeneration, necrosis, and desquamation, followed by partial regeneration, basement membrane thickening, and eventually by tubular atrophy (Fig. 77-1). Later, complete destruction of the tubules may occur with ensuing chronic interstitial fibrosis (Fig. 77-2). As a rule, only a few inflammatory cells are seen in the interstitium. The glomerular lesions consist of fusion of the foot processes, tortuosity of the basement membranes, detachment of endothelial cells, and collapse of glomerular loops (Fig. 77-3). Mesangial thickening and, to a lesser degree, basement membrane thickening occurs later and

progresses to complete glomerular sclerosis (Fig. 77-4). Glomerular necrosis is often seen if malignant hypertension develops. In the later stages of the pathologic process, the arteries show medial and intimal thickening that may be accompanied by fibrinoid necrosis and thrombosis (Fig. 77-5).

There are two descriptions of electron microscopic changes in human radiation nephritis in the literature [9, 25]. These studies found endothelial and epithelial cell degeneration in the glomeruli. The glomerular basement membranes were thickened and split, with subendothelial deposits of basement membrane-like and electron-lucent material. Degenerative changes of tubular cells and tubular basement membrane thickening were noted. There was moderate interstitial increase in connective tissue.

Pathogenesis

The nature of radiation injury at the cellular level will not be discussed here. The mode of development of radiation nephritis is not clear, and, as

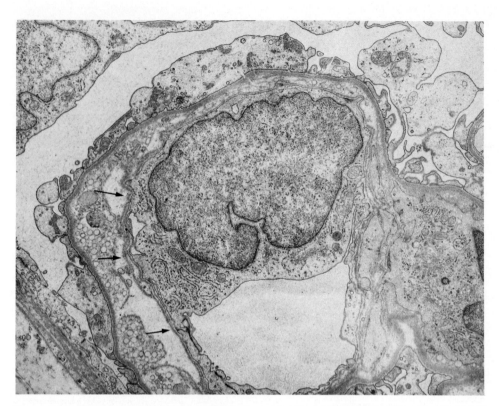

Figure 77-3. Experimental radiation nephritis 4 months after a single dose of 2,000 rads. Swollen endothelial cell with bizarre nucleus is partially detached from basement membrane. Note widening of subendothelial space. New basement membrane (arrows) *is being formed, presumably by endothelial cell. (×7,200.) (Reprinted, by permission, from the* American Journal of Pathology *6:1, 1970.)*

pointed out by Mostofi and Berdjis [21], the terminology is inappropriate since it implies an inflammatory process, while the lesion is essentially degenerative and involves all the elements of the kidney, leading to progressive sclerosis. Because human kidneys are seldom examined early in the asymptomatic phase of disease, it is difficult to follow the development of the process. Some authors state the fundamental lesion is localized to the fine interstitial vasculature and that tubules and glomeruli are only destroyed as the result of vascular damage [11, 26]. Others believe that the tubules are markedly sensitive to radiation and that tubular degeneration and necrosis result in interstitial fibrosis and lead eventually to renal sclerosis [20].

The mechanism by which the vascular and glomerular lesions occur is not completely understood. Some investigators have suggested that radiation may affect the ground substance of the basement membrane, with resultant endothelial cell detachment. Others have speculated that endothelial cells, which control in part the replacement of the ground substance, may be injured.

This would result in an anatomic and functional disruption of the normal endothelial cell barrier and allow platelets to come in contact with the basement membrane proper, thus leading to the activation of the coagulation system. Thrombosis following endothelial cell damage could explain to some extent the functional and circulatory abnormalities seen in radiation nephritis. However, such early thrombosis has not been actually observed. Alternatively, endothelial cell detachment and epithelial cell damage might in themselves lead to progressive capillary damage.

To clarify the pathogenesis of radiation nephritis, one has to resort to experimental studies. Such studies by Madrazo et al. [15, 17, 18] were carried out in rats, with doses ranging from 1500 to 10,000 rads. Serial light and electron microscopic examinations demonstrated that the vascular endothelium in the glomeruli and the epithelial tubular cells were equally sensitive to radiation. After large doses (5000 to 9600 rads), epithelial tubular cells showed degeneration, necrosis, and desquamation, with eventual collapse and atrophy of the tubules (see Fig. 77-1). The glomerular

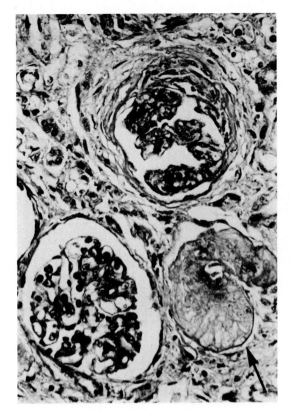

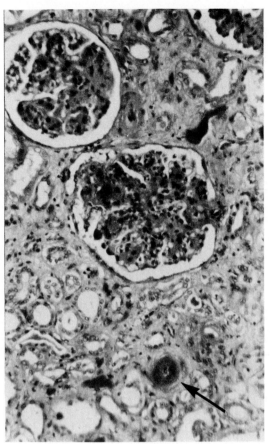

Figure 77-4. Human radiation nephritis, same case as in Figure 77-2. Glomeruli show mild to marked changes with complete sclerosis as final stage (arrow). There are tubular atrophy and interstitial fibrosis. Note lack of inflammatory reaction. (Trichrome stain, ×350.)

Figure 77-5. Acute human radiation nephritis, same case as in Figure 77-1. Light microphotograph shows glomerular mesangial thickening and capillary collapse. There is tubular atrophy. Note arteriolar fibrinoid necrosis (arrow). (H&E, ×350.)

endothelial cells showed cytoplasmic degeneration and detachment from the basement membrane, which underwent progressive tortuosity leading to collapse of the capillary walls and sclerosis (see Fig. 77-3). These changes could result in complete destruction of the glomeruli. The third important and relatively late change was the injury to the walls of small- and medium-sized arteries, with degeneration of basement membrane material in the endothelial and muscular layers followed by degeneration of smooth muscle cells, fibrinoid necrosis and thrombosis. The interstitial capillaries showed minimal changes, usually limited to moderate endothelial swelling.

The end result of these experimental nephritic processes was the destruction of the renal parenchyma, with marked shrinkage of kidneys and diffuse fibrosis of all renal structures. These changes were similar to those seen in acute radiation nephritis in man. The lesions observed with low and high doses were not different. If kidneys radiated with doses ranging from 1500 to 2500

rads were examined serially by electron microscopy over a number of months, the same glomerular and tubular changes were seen, although the lesions were of lesser degree and slower in development. They were not detectable by light microscopy until the late stages, when their morphogenesis was impossible to unravel. Given enough time, extensive destruction of renal parenchyma could occur, resembling the outcome of chronic radiation nephritis in man.

It can be seen that lesions of radiation nephritis form a continuous spectrum in which the immediate early tubular and glomerular lesions lead to a latent clinical period, during which rapid or gradual progression of anatomic changes takes place. This eventually results in the anatomic and physiologic abnormalities known as acute or chronic radiation nephritis. The changes are the same in all instances, the only difference being in the extent and degree of involvement of the individual components. In the clinical setting, interpretation of some of the lesions may be complicated by the development of hypertension, vascular damage and repair, and secondary bacterial infection.

Therapy

In acute radiation nephritis, stress must be laid upon carrying the patient through the severe phase of illness in the hope of spontaneous improvement. Hypertension, edema, and cardiac complications are treated specifically. Hemodialysis or peritoneal dialysis may be needed.

In chronic radiation nephritis attempts are made at maintaining the patient's general health and treating the complications of uremia. When renal failure becomes chronic, dialysis and transplantation should be considered.

As discussed under Pathogenesis, there is suggestive evidence of abnormal coagulation processes in the damaged kidneys. Heparin has been used with some success in treating radiation damage of the liver, and possibly it should be tried in radiation nephritis.

References

1. Cogan, S. R., and Ritter, I. I. Radiation nephritis: Clinicopathologic correlation of three surviving cases. *Am. J. Med.* 24:530, 1958.
2. Dean, A. L., and Abels, J. C. Study by newer renal function tests of an unusual case of hypertension following irradiation of one kidney and the relief of the patient by nephrectomy. *J. Urol.* 52:497, 1944.
3. Domagk, G. Die Roentgenstrahlenwirkung auf das Gewebe, im besonderen betrachet an den Nieren: Morphologische und funktionelle Veranderungen. *Bietr. Pathol. Anat.* 77:525, 1927.
4. Doub, H. P., Hartman, F. W., and Bollinger, A. The relative sensitivity of kidney to irradiation. *Radiology* 8:142, 1927.
5. Elward, J. F., and Belair, J. F. Relative degrees of radiosensitivity of tissue. *Radiology* 33:450, 1939.
6. Grossman, B. J. Radiation nephritis. *J. Pediatr.* 47:424, 1955.
7. Guttman, P. H., and Kohn, H. I. Age at exposure and acceleration of intercapillary glomerulosclerosis in mice. *Lab. Invest.* 12:250, 1963.
8. Hagner, F. R., and Coleman, S. R. Nephrectomy for malignant disease of the kidney: Suppression of urine and death following massive doses of x-ray. *J. Urol.* 32:27, 1934.
9. Keane, W. F., Crosson, J. T., Staley, N. A., Anderson, W. R., and Shapiro, F. L. Radiation-induced renal disease: A clinicopathologic study. *Am. J. Med.* 60:127, 1976.
10. Kunkler, P. B., Farr, R. F., and Luxton, R. W. Limit of renal tolerance to x-rays: Investigation into renal damage occurring following treatment of tumors of testes by abdominal baths. *Br. Med. J.* 2:910, 1956.
11. Ljunquist, A., Urge, G., Lagergren, C., and Notter,

G. The intrarenal vascular alterations in radiation nephritis and their relationship to the development of hypertension. *Acta Pathol. Microbiol. Scand.* [A] 79:629, 1971.
12. Luxton, R. W. Effects of Irradiation on the Kidney. In M. B. Strauss and L. G. Welt (eds.), *Diseases of the Kidney* (2nd ed.). Boston: Little, Brown, 1971. Pp. 1040–1070.
13. Luxton, R. W., and Baker, S. B. deC. Radiation Nephritis. In E. L. Becker (ed.), *Structural Basis of Renal Disease.* New York: Harper & Row, 1969. Pp. 620–656.
14. Mackay, E. V., and Biggs, S. S. G. Late sequelae of radiotherapy for Wilms's tumor in infancy. *Aust. Radiol.* 10:356, 1966.
15. Madrazo, A., and Churg, J. Radiation nephritis: Chronic changes following moderate doses of radiation. *Lab. Invest.* 34:283, 1976.
16. Madrazo, A., Schwarz, G., and Churg, J. Radiation nephritis: A review. *J. Urol.* 114:822, 1975.
17. Madrazo, A., Suzuki, Y., and Churg, J. Radiation nephritis: Acute changes following high dose of radiation. *Am. J. Pathol.* 54:507, 1969.
18. Madrazo, A., Suzuki, Y., and Churg, J. Radiation nephritis: II. Chronic changes after high doses of radiation. *Am. J. Pathol.* 61:37, 1970.
19. Mertz, H. O., Howell, R. D., and Hendricks, J. W. The limitations of irradiation of solid renal tumors in children. *J. Urol.* 46:1103, 1941.
20. Mostofi, F. K. Radiation Effects on the Kidney. In F. K. Mostofi and D. E. Smith (eds.), *The Kidney* (International Academy of Pathology Monograph). Baltimore: Williams & Wilkins, 1966. Pp. 338–386.
21. Mostofi, F. K., and Berdjis, C. C. Radiopathology of Kidney. In C. C. Berdjis (ed.), *Pathology of Irradiation.* Baltimore: Williams & Wilkins, 1971. Pp. 597–635.
22. Munger, A. D. Irradiation of malignant renal neoplasms, with special reference to the effects of irradiation on the acquired single kidney. *J. Urol.* 37:68, 1937.
23. Nitus, A., Tefft, M., and Fellers, X. F. Long term follow-up of renal functions of 108 children who underwent nephrectomy for malignant disease. *Pediatrics* 44:912, 1969.
24. O'Malley, B., D'Augio, J. G., and Vauter, F. G. Late effects of roentgen therapy given in infancy. *Am. J. Roentgenol. Radium Ther. Nucl. Med.* 89:1067, 1963.
25. Rosen, S., Swerdlow, M. A., Muehrcke, R. C., and Pirani, C. L. Radiation nephritis: Light and electron microscopic observations. *Am. J. Clin. Pathol.* 41:487, 1964.
26. Scanlon, G. T. Vascular alterations in the irradiated rabbit kidney. *Radiology* 94:401, 1970.
27. Schreiner, B. F., and Greendyke, R. M. Radiation nephritis: Report of a fatal case. *Am. J. Med.* 26:146, 1959.
28. Vaeth, J. M., Levitt, S. H., Jones, M. D., and Holtfreter, C. Effects of radiation therapy in survivors of Wilms' tumor. *Radiology* 79:562, 1962.
29. Warthin, A. S. Changes produced in kidneys by roentgen irradiation. *Am. J. Med. Sci.* 113:736, 1907.
30. Zuelzer, W. W., Palmer, H. D., and Newton, W. A., Jr. Unusual glomerulonephritis in young children, probably radiation nephritis: Report of three cases. *Am. J. Pathol.* 26:1019, 1950.

78. Effects of Drugs and Toxins on the Kidney

Edward J. Cafruny

The kidney is exceedingly vulnerable to the deleterious effects of chemicals. Its transport systems (both active and passive), which permit the excretion of solutes in relatively small volumes of fluid, create gradients favoring the resorption of filtered chemicals into and through renal cells. In addition, many chemicals foreign to the body (xenobiotics) are actively transported across the tubular epithelium. This chapter deals with some of the major nephrotoxic drugs and toxins. Some of these exert extrarenal actions that ultimately affect renal function and structure; others act directly on nephrons and thus produce lesions in all or most tubules [14].

As used here, *drug* refers to a medicinal and *toxin* to a nonmedicinal xenobiotic. It should be noted, however, that no sharp distinction between these two categories is possible. Drugs are incomplete toxins, effective as medicines because they selectively alter normal biochemical events. When the alterations become intolerable, as for example when the administered dose is excessive, a drug becomes a complete toxin. The first part of this chapter deals with conceptual and theoretical aspects. The second part contains information on potentially nephrotoxic chemicals that are most likely to be encountered in pediatric practice. Lead poisoning is discussed in Chap. 79. Heavy metals and drugs that induce systemic lupus erythematosus or the nephrotic syndrome are discussed in Chaps. 58 and 52, respectively. Drug- or toxin-induced acute renal failure is discussed in Chap. 91.

Renal Accumulation of Drugs and Toxins

There are no specific criteria on which to base a set of rules about the nephrotoxic potential of a given chemical. The propensity for causing damage must be related to molecular structure, although the actual occurrence of damage is based simply on clinical experience. It is prudent, therefore, to consider suspect all chemicals foreign to the body in the same way that all drugs are viewed as capable of producing side effects. Renal accumulation is the decisive factor in nephrotoxicity. Cellular injury occurs when sufficient molecules of a drug or toxin are in contact with the cells for a sufficient period of time; this *threshold concentration* and the time of exposure vary over a wide range from one agent to another.

The renal accumulation of toxic agents is dependent on a host of physiologic factors, both renal and extrarenal, some of which vary with age. Although there is general agreement on what these factors are, their significance is subject to interpretation.

EXTERNAL FACTORS

Plasma Protein Binding. The renal accumulation of foreign compounds is influenced considerably by physicochemical factors that govern extrarenal distribution and disposition. Foremost among these is plasma protein binding, largely to serum albumin. This not only reduces glomerular filtration of the substance but also increases its time of retention in plasma. Rate of passage of the substance through the kidney, and consequently the concentration to which the renal epithelium is exposed, are diminished. On the other hand, renal excretion may be rapid if the substance, like phenol red, is secreted by the tubules (see below). The fractional plasma protein binding of many drugs and toxins has been found to be lower in infants than in adults, even when the lower level of albumin in the serum of the infant is taken into account [4, 11].

Hepatic Biotransformation. Metabolizing systems of the hepatic endoplasmic reticulum catalyze a variety of reactions that convert drugs into derivative products. The reactions are mostly oxidative, but other types of transformations (e.g., conjugative, reductive) occur also. The resultant products invariably are more polar and less soluble in lipid than the original molecules, and these properties restrict penetration into cells and hasten renal excretion. The liver of newborn mammals is deficient in the enzymes and cytochrome elements necessary to carry out these important reactions [5, 8], although recent data indicate that the differences between the adult and newborn are not as striking as the earlier reports indicated [13], particularly when the relatively greater weight of the neonatal liver is considered. When differences are encountered, other variables such as hepatic uptake and clearance [13] must be considered.

Volume of Extracellular Fluid. The size of the extracellular fluid compartment can markedly affect the rate of passage of drugs through the kidney. Since most drugs have molecular weights of 500 or less, molecules that are not protein bound in plasma readily diffuse into the interstitial fluid. Entry into cells is governed by lipid solubility, electrochemical gradients, and cellular water concentration and protein binding.

The extracellular water volume (ECW) of a young infant of 4.5 kg is approximately 150 times the magnitude of the glomerular filtration rate ($\frac{ECW}{C_{IN}} = \frac{1,500}{10}$), while that of a 70-kg adult is about 100 times the glomerular filtration rate ($\frac{13,000}{130}$).* Using the equation

$$t\frac{1}{2} = \frac{0.7\ V_D}{C}$$

where $t\frac{1}{2}$ = apparent half-life in the body for a substance
V_D = volume of distribution of the substance
C = its renal clearance,

Rane and Wilson [15] have calculated that the $t\frac{1}{2}$ for any drug that is excreted only by glomerular filtration, such as inulin, would be about 67 minutes in adults and 100 minutes in young infants. The authors suggest that immaturity of renal excretory mechanisms in the infant is responsible for the larger $t\frac{1}{2}$. It appears, however, that the chief reason is the expanded ECW in infants. Although this factor undoubtedly slows the rate of renal excretion of xenobiotics, it is not entirely responsible for the large delays noted in some cases. For example, Gladtke and Heimann [6] found that the elimination half-life for thiosulfate, a substance handled much like inulin, was almost three times longer in newborns than in older children. Clearly a prolongation of elimination half-life of such magnitude cannot be explained by a difference in ECW alone, and differences in glomerular clearance most likely play a role.

RENAL FACTORS
Immaturity of Renal Function. In the young infant, and particularly the low birth weight infant,

* Numerical values used to calculate ECW/C_{IN} are taken from Rane and Wilson [15] and are rounded off to permit ease of calculation.

rates of glomerular filtration and renal blood flow are lower than in older infants and children (Chap. 2). Immaturity of renal function thus plays an important role in the renal accumulation of drugs and toxins, as discussed in the next section. In addition, different rates of tubular resorption and secretion in the immature kidney will influence the rate of entry of drugs or toxins into renal cells (see Tubular Transport).

Glomerular Filtration Rate and Renal Blood Flow. The rate of entry of a drug or toxin into the kidney and ultimately into renal cells is controlled by the rates of renal blood flow and glomerular filtration and the capacity of the kidney to extract the drug from the peritubular capillaries. In the mature kidney, about 20 percent of the renal plasma flow is filtered; this percentage of the drug present free in renal plasma is extracted continuously. The remainder of the drug or toxin, or a fraction of it, may or may not be extracted by the proximal tubules as blood flows through the peritubular capillaries. With the notable exception of creatinine and perhaps a few other neutral substances, secreted drugs and endogenous compounds are bases or weak organic acids. It should be noted that plasma protein binding generally does not prevent tubular extraction, although it may retard it, because the extracting system (active secretory transport system) shuttles free drug across the tubular cell rapidly enough to permit the equilibrium between protein-bound and free drug to be reestablished. Strong binding, however, does limit the rate of tubular secretion under certain conditions [18].

Tubular Transport. A drug or toxin may enter renal cells or their membranes from the peritubular blood, the glomerular filtrate, or both. Passive transport of drug molecules into renal cells from the tubular lumen is probably the major mechanism by which the elimination of drugs is slowed and renal accumulation is achieved. Factors that govern the passive resorption of foreign substances include the lipid solubility of such substances and the concurrent fractional excretion of water, which affects the concentration of foreign substances in the tubular fluid.

Most drugs are weak electrolytes. At physiologic pH they are present in ionized and un-ionized forms. Cell membranes are relatively impermeable to the lipid-insoluble ionized form, but they retard the passage of lipid-soluble un-ionized molecules far less. The rate of diffusion of many drugs thus is dependent on the pH of the fluid (urine or blood) in which they are dissolved, since the concentration of the un-ionized form varies with the pH.

For weak acids,

$$pH - pK = \log \frac{\text{(ionized drug)}}{\text{(un-ionized drug)}}$$

For weak bases,

$$pH - pK = \log \frac{\text{(un-ionized drug)}}{\text{(ionized drug)}}$$

where pK = negative logarithm of the acidic dissociation constant

where pH = negative logarithm of the H^+ concentration

Non-ionic diffusion across renal membranes varies strikingly with the pH only for acidic drugs that have pK values between 3 and 7.5 and for basic drugs with pK values between 7.5 and 10.5 [12]. The urinary excretion of drugs such as acetylsalicylic acid (pK = 3.5) and phenobarbital (pK = 7.2) may be accelerated considerably by procedures that increase urinary pH. Maintenance of a high rate of urine flow will further facilitate the excretion of these drugs.

Active transport of drugs across the proximal tubule takes place by both secretion and resorption. With the exception of ascorbic acid [10] and possibly urate [3], there is no evidence for active transport of organic molecules across the distal tubule. At least two secretory systems have been recognized in the proximal tubule, one for organic acids and one for organic bases. In addition, there is abundant evidence that certain substances undergo bidirectional carrier-mediated transport in this segment of the nephron [1, 2, 9, 19]. Active transport in the resorptive direction has been demonstrated for a variety of substances, for example, glucose and amino acids.

A large number of drugs, including penicillins, diuretics, morphine, cephalosporins, and phenylbutazone, are actively transported across the proximal tubule. The secretory transport systems of newborn and young animals are functionally immature [16] and can be stimulated by repeated exposure to transportable molecules such as penicillin [7]. There is no evidence, however, that tubular immaturity amplifies the response to nephrotoxic chemicals. It may well be that cellular trapping is prevented in part because weaker secretory transport limits the delivery of offending molecules.

On theoretical grounds and in the absence of firm data there does not appear to be any greater susceptibility of the newborn or young infant to the nephrotoxic action of xenobiotics. The fact that the half-life of potential toxins in the body is prolonged does not warrant the conclusion a priori that the risk of renal injury is multiplied as are the pharmacologic responses and attendant side effects. In fact, there appears to be justification for the notion that renal immaturity constitutes a defense against renal injury (Table 78-1).

Nephrotoxicity of Chemicals
SYSTEMS FOR CLASSIFYING NEPHROTOXINS
Ideally a system of classification should be heuristic, helpful in establishing an accurate diagnosis,

Table 78-1. Renal Consequences of Immature Functions or Conditions in the Newborn and Young Infant Exposed to a Drug

Function or Condition	Results
Lower filtration rate per glomerulus	Less drug in the nephron at any given time
Limited proximal tubular active transport of acids or bases	Reduced trapping in proximal tubular cells and lower concentration of drug in urine (most drugs are acids or bases)
Less efficient countercurrent multiplier system	Lower concentration of drug in renal medulla
Reduced plasma protein binding	More rapid delivery of drug to kidney
Delayed hepatic metabolism	Slower renal excretion and enhanced cycling of drug between tubular lumen and blood
Larger fractional volume of extracellular fluid	Larger volume of distribution and slower rate of renal excretion

Table 78-2. Classification of Nephrotoxins

Class	Effect of Toxin	Examples
1	Direct effect on renal cells leading to morphologic or persisting functional changes	Mercurials, carbon tetrachloride, bacitracin
2	Immune reaction resulting in nephrotic or nephritic syndrome	Various pollens, animal venoms, trimethadione
3	Sensitivity reaction of the angiitis or vasculitis type involving the renal vasculature	Sulfonamides
4	Chronic nephropathy developing over months or years; evidence remains largely epidemiologic or circumstantial	Lead, cadmium
5	Aggravation of preexisting renal disease or involvement in the production of secondary renal disease such as pyelonephritis	Drugs that increase uric acid excretion or produce potassium deficiency

Source: Modified from Schreiner and Maher [17].

Table 78-3. Selected Potential Nephrotoxins in Children

Toxin Classification and Effect	Reference
Analgesics (nonnarcotic)	
Acetaminophen	See text for references
Salicylates (see Chap. 71)	
Phenacetin	
Antimicrobial drugs	
Sulfonamides—obstructive uropathy, necrotizing angiitis, tubular necrosis, interstitial nephritis	Kutscher et al., *J. Allergy* 25:135, 1954
Antibiotics	
Aminoglycosides—acute tubular necrosis	Bobrow et al., *J.A.M.A.* 222: 1546, 1972; Opitz et al., *Med. Welt Berl.* 22:434, 1971
Cephalosporins—acute tubular necrosis, interstitial nephritis	Weinstein and Kaplan, *Ann. Intern. Med.* 72:729, 1970
Polypeptides	
Bacitracin—degeneration of tubular epithelium	Miller et al., *J. Clin. Invest.* 29:389, 1950
Polymyxin B—acute tubular necrosis	Yow and Moyer, *Arch. Intern. Med.* 92:248, 1953; Nord and Hoeprich, *N. Engl. J. Med.* 270:1030, 1964
Polymyxin E (colistin)—acute tubular necrosis	
Others	
Deteriorated tetracyclines—Fanconi syndrome	Frimpter et al., *J.A.M.A.* 184:111, 1963
Amphotericin B—glomerular damage, tubular atrophy	Douglas and Healy, *Am. J. Med.* 46:154, 1969
Glycols	
Diethylene glycol—acute cortical necrosis	Cornish. In Casarett and Doull (eds.), *Toxicology.* New York: Macmillan, 1975, Chap. 19
Ethylene glycol—obstructive uropathy (oxalate crystals), tubular destruction	
Propylene glycol—hemoglobin casts, acute tubular necrosis	
Organic solvents	
Carbon tetrachloride—acute cortical necrosis (especially outer band)	Oettingen, Public Health Service Publication No. 414. Washington, D.C.: U.S. Govt. Printing Office, 1955
Turpentine—glomerular and tubular degeneration	In Thienes and Haley (eds.), *Clinical Toxicology* (5th ed.). Philadelphia: Lea & Febiger, 1972
Trichloroethylene—acute tubular necrosis	Defalque, *Clin. Pharmacol. Ther.* 2:665, 1961
Metals (See also Chap. 79)	
Bismuth—tubular necrosis (especially proximal tubules)	Karelitz and Freedman, *Pediatrics* 8:772, 1951
Lead—Fanconi syndrome, tubular necrosis	Hirsch, *Toxicol. Appl. Pharmacol.* 25:84, 1973
Mercury—tubular necrosis (especially proximal tubules), renal ischemia	Miller and Clarkson (eds.), *Mercury, Mercurials, and Mercaptans.* Springfield, Ill.: Thomas, 1973; Valek, *Acta Med. Scand.* 177:63, 1965
Miscellaneous	
Ethylenediaminotetraacetic acid (EDTA)—acute tubular necrosis	Reubes and Bradley, *J.A.M.A.* 174:263, 1960
Oxalates—obstructive uropathy	Salyer and Keren, *Kidney Int.* 4:61, 1973
Drugs associated with lupus erythematosus	See Chap. 58
Drugs associated with the nephrotic syndrome	See Chap. 52

and useful in directing therapy. No classification of nephrotoxins achieves these ends, and the reasons for this are clear. Chemicals can generate lesions by interfering with blood supply, by acting directly on renal cells, by blocking tubular lumens, or by changing the internal milieu of the kidney. Because of the interrelationships among these factors, a drug or toxin that initially involves one factor subsequently may involve others, resulting in a combined effect. Oliver et al. [14] point out that the renal lesions associated with traumatic or toxic injury may involve any or all parts of nephrons indiscriminately. Localization of the primary site of damage on the basis of specific functional characteristics of a particular tubular segment may occur, but even in such instances the lesions are usually more widely scattered. For example, although certain mercurial compounds are secreted by the proximal tubule and produce their worst effects there, lesions are detectable in other segments as well. The probable reason for this is that urine processed by the proximal tubule passes through and delivers mercury to all succeeding segments. This nonspecificity renders any classification based on pathologic features relatively valueless. A classification based on clinical features has only limited value for the same reasons. Diagnosis thus depends largely on a complete review of the history.

SCHREINER-MAHER CLASSIFICATION OF NEPHROTOXINS

Schreiner and Maher [17] have classified the major nephrotoxins encountered in clinical practice. A slightly modified version is presented in Table 78-2. Class 1 nephrotoxins act directly on renal epithelium to produce acute nephropathies. Classes 2 and 3 cause injury by evoking immunologic responses. Class 4 includes agents that produce chronic nephropathies on repeated exposure. Class 5 substances are not ordinarily nephrotoxic, but, under appropriate circumstances, aggravate existing disorders or adversely affect the renal concentration of endogenous substances so that lesions develop. Although class 5 does not constitute a well-defined category, it is a necessary one, if only to emphasize two points: that some chemicals that are usually innocuous can be injurious in disease, and that drugs that increase or deplete endogenous electrolytes can produce renal lesions.

The main virtue of the Schreiner-Maher classification is that it attempts to relate cause and effect. The main difficulty with the classification is its lack of precision, since many chemicals belong to two or more classes.

NEPHROTOXIC DRUGS AND TOXINS

Some of the more important nephrotoxins that are most likely to be encountered in a pediatric practice are arranged in Table 78-3 according to the chemical or therapeutic class to which they belong. The incidence of nephrotoxicity is low for all the drugs listed, but it is increased in the child who is dehydrated or poorly nourished. The toxic response, like the pharmacologic response, is dose-dependent. Renal injury is not apt to occur with any of these drugs unless the therapeutic dose is exceeded or is inappropriate because of the clinical state of the child. (Hypersensitivity reactions are obvious exceptions to these general rules.) Although nonnarcotic analgesic nephropathy does not appear to be a problem in the pediatric age group, it is mentioned in Table 78-3 because the drugs involved are among those most commonly used in children (see Chap. 71).

References

1. Beechwood, E. C., Berndt, W. O., and Mudge, G. H. Stop-flow analysis of tubular transport of uric acid in rabbits. *Am. J. Physiol.* 207:1265, 1964.
2. Cho, K. C., and Cafruny, E. J. Renal tubular reabsorption of *p*-aminohippuric acid (PAH) in the dog. *J. Pharmacol. Exp. Ther.* 173:1, 1970.
3. Davis, B. B., Field, J. B., Rodnan, G. P., and Kedes, L. H. Localization and pyrazinamide inhibition of distal transtubular movement of uric acid-2-C14 with a modified stop-flow technique. *J. Clin. Invest.* 44:716, 1965.
4. Ehrnebo, M., Agurell, S., Jalling, B., and Boreus, L. O. Age differences in drug binding by plasma proteins: Studies on human foetuses, neonates and adults. *Eur. J. Clin. Pharmacol.* 3:189, 1971.
5. Fouts, J. R. Hepatic Microsomal Drug Metabolism in the Perinatal Period. In *Diagnosis and Treatment of Fetal Disorders.* Berlin: Springer, 1968. P. 291.
6. Gladtke, E., and Heimann, G. The rate of development of elimination functions in kidney and liver of young infants. In P. L. Morselli, S. Garattini, and F. Sereni (eds.), *Basic and Therapeutic Aspects of Perinatal Pharmacology.* New York: Raven Press, 1975. Pp. 393–403.
7. Hirsch, G. H., and Hook, J. B. Maturation of renal organic acid transport: Substrate stimulation by penicillin and *p*-aminohippurate (PAH). *J. Pharmacol. Exp. Ther.* 171:103, 1970.
8. Jondorf, W., Maikel, R., and Brodie, B. Inability of newborn mice and guinea pigs to metabolize drugs. *Biochem. Pharmacol.* 1:352, 1958.
9. Kinter, W. B. Renal tubular transport of diodrast-I131 and PAH in necturus; evidence for simultaneous reabsorption and secretion. *Am. J. Physiol.* 196:1141, 1959.
10. Kleit, S., Levin, D., Perenich, T., and Cade, R. Renal excretion of ascorbic acid by dogs. *Am. J. Physiol.* 209:195, 1965.
11. Krasner, J., Giacoia, G. P., and Yaffe, S. J. Drug-protein binding in the newborn infant. *Ann. N.Y. Acad. Sci.* 226:101, 1973.
12. Milne, M. D. Influence of acid-base balance on efficacy and toxicity of drugs. *Proc. R. Soc. Med.* 58:961, 1965.
13. Mirkin, B. L. Drug disposition and therapy in the developing human. *Pediatr. Ann.* 5:542, 1976.
14. Oliver, J., MacDowell, M., and Tracy, A. The pathogenesis of acute renal failure associated with traumatic and toxic injury: Renal ischemia, nephrotoxic damage and the ischemuric episode. *J. Clin. Invest.* 30:1307, 1951.
15. Rane, A., and Wilson, J. T. Clinical pharmacokinetics in infants and children. *Clin. Pharmacokinetics* 1:2, 1976.
16. Rennick, B., Hamilton, B., and Evans, R. Development of renal tubular transports of TEA and PAH in the puppy and piglet. *Am. J. Physiol.* 201:743, 1961.
17. Schreiner, G. E., and Maher, J. F. Toxic nephropathy. *Am. J. Med.* 38:409, 1965.
18. Weiner, I. M. Mechanisms of drug absorption and excretion. *Annu. Rev. Pharmacol.* 7:39, 1967.
19. Zins, G. R., and Winer, I. M. Bidirectional urate transport limited to the proximal tubule in dogs. *Am. J. Physiol.* 215:411, 1968.

The purpose of this chapter is to categorize metals according to their effects upon the kidney, to explain their mechanism of action, and to elaborate upon the more common metal nephropathies encountered by pediatricians. Comprehensive reviews of heavy metal nephropathies have been presented elsewhere [53, 105, 136, 137].

The growing concern for the environment, combined with the increasing exposure to biologically active drugs, chemicals, and pollutants, has led to a heightened awareness of the effects of these agents on the body. Since the kidneys receive 20 percent of the cardiac output and have an extremely high ratio of blood flow to tissue mass; a high rate of oxygen consumption; a large endothelial surface area; a countercurrent multiplication system; and a high capacity to bind, transport, and metabolize various substances; the kidneys' vulnerability to toxins is apparent [105, 160]. The cortex, which receives over 90 percent of the renal blood flow, is particularly susceptible.

Nephrotoxicity can assume four discrete clinical patterns: acute renal failure (tubular necrosis), the Fanconi syndrome, chronic nephropathy, and the nephrotic syndrome [53]. In general, the greater the exposure to a metallic toxin, the more likely it is that acute renal failure will result. Lesser degrees of exposure may cause injury limited to the proximal tubule, leading occasionally to the Fanconi syndrome, or injury confined to the glomerulus, sometimes resulting in the nephrotic syndrome. The nephrotic syndrome may also result from a hypersensitivity reaction, presumably through immune mechanisms. Chronic nephropathy may occur after prolonged exposure to toxins such as lead. Finally, acute renal failure may result secondary to hemolysis or to dehydration; the latter may be induced by vomiting or excessive urinary losses caused, for instance, by mercurial diuretics.

Cases of metal nephropathy have been described in children for most of the metals listed in Table 79-1; however, the type of exposure was usually different from that encountered in adults. With the exception of lead, children are rarely in continuous contact with metals, as occurs in adults subjected to occupational hazards. Many of the early cases reported in children resulted from administration of drugs subsequently found to be nephrotoxic, such as mercuric chloride and sodium bis-

muth thioglycollate. The use of most of these harmful drugs and toxins has been abandoned. Screening the child and his surroundings for lead was a large step in prevention of metal poisoning, as was the institution of child-proof containers for medications. Consequently, fewer cases of metal nephropathy have been reported in the last 15 years.

In view of the multitude of more common causes of renal injury and the frequent difficulty of documenting a history of heavy metal exposure, the diagnosis of heavy metal nephropathy requires a strong suspicion. It is essential to inquire about recent medications taken by the patient or family members, changes in the general health and behavior of the child, pica, housing conditions (an old house with peeling paint, a house 1 mile from a smelting plant), hobbies and activities that might result in undue exposure to metals (basement chemistry laboratory), history of allergy, and, in the adolescent, a motivation for "drug kicks" or suicide.

General Aspects of Metal Nephropathy

Renal damage caused by metals may be considered in terms of three pathogenetic mechanisms [146]. The first is the interaction of the metal with cell membranes, such interaction affecting the surface-active properties of cell-membrane lipids and thus altering membrane permeability and carrier transport mechanisms. The second mechanism is the binding of metal to certain ligands within the cell, such as protein-sulfhydryl groups. By binding to enzymes having functional groups, by displacing essential metals from metalloenzymes, or by binding to coenzymes or substrates, toxic metals may inhibit enzyme activity. The result is a disruption in metabolic and synthetic activity of the cell. Moreover, by binding to nonenzymic proteins or by complexing with nucleic acids, metals may affect the functions of these vital molecules. Third, by acting as haptens bound to proteins, some metal-protein antigens cause a hypersensitivity reaction that occasionally may be manifested as a nephrotic syndrome.

Toxic injury usually involves the tubular segment most concerned with a particular metal's handling [119], and the characteristic structural lesion is apparent in each affected nephron. The

Table 79-1. Manifestations of Metal Nephropathies

Metal	Acute Nephropathy		Chronic Nephropathy	Nephrotic Syndrome
	Tubular Necrosis	Fanconi Syndrome		
Lead	+	+	+	0
Cadmium	+	+	+	0
Mercury	+	0	+	+
Gold	+	0	0	+
Uranium	+	+	+	0
Copper	+	+	+	0
Bismuth	+	+	+	0
Thallium	+	0	0	+
Arsenic	+	0	0	0
Iron	±	0	0	+
Chelating agents	+	0	0	+

Source: Modified from B. T. Emmerson, Metals and the Kidney. In D. A. K. Black (ed.), *Renal Disease* (2nd ed). Philadelphia: Davis, 1967. Pp. 561–593.

histopathologic severity of the lesion, however, bears little correlation with the duration or severity of renal functional impairment [58, 118].

In a review of the causes of acute renal failure in infants and children reported in the literature from 1941–1957, Robinson and Wong [128] found that nephrotoxic agents accounted for 21 of 37 cases; 7 of 21 intoxications involved heavy metals, including 6 cases of bismuth and one of mercuric bichloride poisoning. In a review of 130 cases of acute renal failure admitted at l'Hôpital des Énfants Malades, a major pediatric hospital in Paris, Broyer [20] attributed only 14 (11 percent) to nephrotoxins, and of these, only 1 each to arsenic and mercury (for a total of 1.4 percent). Lieberman [101] noted that nephrotoxins were rare causes of acute renal failure at Children's Hospital of Los Angeles.

Acute renal failure attributed to metal intoxication in children has been described for bismuth [9, 17, 26, 79, 93, 97, 108, 117, 120, 142, 150, 165] and mercury [92, 127, 141]; additional cases have resulted from the use of chelating agents in the treatment of metal intoxication [45, 124], but this form appears to be more common in adults [61, 111, 159, 164].

Less extensive renal damage, attributed to acute exposure to smaller quantities, to more chronic exposure, or to exposure to substances with lower toxicity, may explain the clinical picture of Fanconi syndrome. Histologic damage is demonstrable in proximal tubules and is more likely associated with disrupted cell metabolism along that portion

of the nephron. The Fanconi syndrome has been found in children with lead poisoning [30, 32, 44] and copper intoxication due to Wilson's disease [12, 51, 113].

The nephrotic syndrome associated with exposure to certain metals appears to be the result of marked alterations in glomerular capillary permeability to protein due to deposition of metal-protein immune complexes, rather than to the cumulative effect of the metal per se [53]. Nephrotic syndrome has been reported in children exposed to mercurous compounds such as calomel powders [56, 168] and to the chelating agent penicillamine [57, 95]. Gold salts used in the treatment of rheumatoid arthritis have been reported to cause the nephrotic syndrome in adults [78, 99, 123, 140, 152, 155] but not in children, although proteinuria and hematuria occur rather frequently in children receiving gold therapy [5, 46, 131].

Types of Metal Nephropathy
LEAD
Acute Lead Nephropathy
Epidemiology. Lead is one of the oldest metals to have served mankind [18], yet there is "none with a greater literature cataloguing its ill effects on those who come into contact with it" [161]. Although it is a preventable affliction, lead poisoning exists in epidemic proportions in many cities of the United States, especially among children between 1 and 3 years of age [23, 34]. Of the nearly 400,000 children screened by 67 Childhood Lead Poisoning Prevention programs during fiscal year 1976, 33,000 were found to have blood lead levels above 40 μg per deciliter, and 4,000 required chelation therapy [55]. The usual source of lead is paint on plaster walls, windowsills, and woodwork of dilapidated pre-World War II dwellings. As of 1970, nearly 6 million buildings were considered to have potentially dangerous quantities of lead present on surfaces accessible to young children [30]; almost 23,000 dwelling units inspected during fiscal 1976 were found to have this hazard [55].

Clinical Manifestations. Undue lead absorption, indicated by a blood lead concentration of 40 or more μg per deciliter of whole blood, represents the preclinical or asymptomatic phase of lead poisoning, which may be associated with deleterious effects in the absence of overt clinical toxicity [102]. A substantial number of children with undue lead absorption develop clinical manifestations of poisoning [102], of whom 25 percent or more sustain permanent damage to the nervous system and 5 to 10 percent die despite chelation therapy

[23, 34, 112]. Symptoms of lead intoxication relate to the gastrointestinal and central nervous systems: vomiting, abdominal pain, anorexia, constipation, irritability, drowsiness, incoordination, and seizures. A history of pica frequently can be elicited [30, 34]. Signs include pallor, muscle weakness, weight loss, coma, convulsions, papilledema, hyperreflexia, and ataxia [31, 34].

Laboratory Findings. Laboratory findings in lead poisoning include anemia, frequently with basophilic, stippled erythrocytes; presence of delta-aminolevulinic acid, lead, and coproporphyrin III in the urine; high blood levels of lead and delta-aminolevulinic acid and reduced levels of delta-aminolevulinic acid dehydratase; roentgenographic evidence of radiopaque material in the gut and condensation of lines of provisional calcification in the long bones; elevations in cerebrospinal fluid pressure and protein concentration [23, 31, 132].

The renal response in lead poisoning characteristically reflects proximal tubular dysfunction. Isolated glycosuria may be found in 10 to 20 percent of children with lead intoxication and may be associated with aminoaciduria [34, 66, 167]. The full Fanconi syndrome is observed only in patients with severe manifestations [27]. The triad of aminoaciduria, glycosuria, and hypophosphatemia was observed in 9 of 23 children with acute lead intoxication, and in 9 of 19 children with lead encephalopathy. The finding of fructosuria and citraturia in some patients with lead poisoning has not been recorded in any other disease giving rise to the Fanconi syndrome [27], and it may reflect injury to the proximal tubule, where these substances are reabsorbed. Rickets has been described with the Fanconi syndrome and lead poisoning, and it is found in the absence of the typical lead lines in the long bones [24, 32]; such rachitic changes may often accompany the hypophosphatemic state. The Fanconi syndrome usually disappears within 2 months following treatment [27]. Severe intoxication may result in azotemia [35, 44, 107, 167].

Pathologic Findings. Morphologic evidence for acute lead nephropathy is apparent principally in the proximal convoluted tubules, the epithelial cells of which show nonspecific degenerative changes, mitochondrial swelling, increased intertubular connective tissue, thickened tubular basement membranes, and some round cell infiltration; regenerative signs in epithelial cells are found later [53, 146]. Glomeruli may show fusion of foot processes and increased epithelial cytoplasmic density adjacent to a normal-appearing basement membrane [35, 104].

The characteristic response to the ingestion of large quantities of lead is the formation of eosinophilic, dense-staining intranuclear inclusion bodies in the epithelial cells of the proximal convoluted tubule [4, 16, 33, 40, 72, 146]. The dose-response relationship is not established in humans [146], although blood levels in the range of 40 to 80 μg per deciliter are associated with inclusion bodies in renal tubular epithelium. A single dose of lead (0.05 mg per gram body weight) caused the formation of intranuclear inclusions in rat proximal-tubule epithelium within 1 to 6 days [33]. These bodies are composed of a lead-protein complex in which the metal is bound by sulfhydryl groups [98] in a nondiffusible form [25, 75]. They are formed during periods of increased lead accumulation and enable the kidney to excrete large amounts of lead, while minimizing toxic injury to the mitochondria [72, 76, 161]. It has not been determined in humans whether these bodies are formed prior to the appearance of proximal tubular dysfunction, as has been shown for rats [72, 76]. The inclusions may be demonstrated within the tubular epithelial cells that are shed into the urine [98]. Chelation therapy with calcium disodium ethylenediaminetetraacetic acid (CaNa$_2$ EDTA) mobilizes the lead within the inclusions, causing it to be excreted in the urine [77]. No nuclear inclusions could be demonstrated in kidneys of lead-poisoned rats after 3 days of CaNa$_2$ EDTA therapy. The morphologic and functional changes in the proximal tubule are at least partially reversible following chelation therapy [77, 146, 161].

Experiments in animals have provided suggestive evidence that lead poisoning interferes with cellular metabolism [71, 73, 74]. There is a decreased rate of respiration and partially uncoupled oxidative phosphorylation in mitochondria isolated from lead-intoxicated rats, which is largely reversed when CaNa$_2$ EDTA is added to the medium [74]. Incubation of suspensions of rat mitochondria in a medium containing lead (final concentration, $1 \times 10^{-3}M$) results in diminished oxidative decarboxylation of pyruvate and alpha-ketoglutarate and inhibition of fatty acid oxidation [7]. Electron microscopy reveals that these mitochondria are swollen and have an increased number of ruptured outer membranes [74], indicating that the structural and functional alterations might be related. Examination of enzyme activities in the kidneys of lead-poisoned animals reveals marked increases in isoenzymes of lactate dehydrogenase, LDH$_4$ and LDH$_5$, and of glucose 6-phosphate dehydrogenase, along with a decrease in glutamate dehydrogenase [138]. These changes are similar to those found in hypoxia. Another finding, the markedly reduced Na^+-K^+-activated ATPase in kidney [139], supports the conclusion that lead poisoning limits energy production by the cell and inhibits the active transport processes.

It is of interest to note one study in which experimental lead nephropathy could not be produced in adult animals unless the kidney was undergoing hypertrophy as a result of unilateral nephrectomy [147]. This phenomenon may account for the vulnerability of the growing kidney to lead and may explain the high incidence of chronic renal disease in persons exposed to lead during childhood (see Chronic Lead Nephropathy and references 115, 116). Rats given lead in their drinking water for a period of 6 weeks following weaning failed to grow, had a blunting of the age-related rise in GFR, and developed hypertension in adulthood [6].

Therapy. Treatment of lead poisoning requires avoidance of further exposure and the administration of a substantial molar excess of chelating agent over lead [18]. Should inadequate doses be given, the result might be a redistribution of the metal in the body and an increase in toxic effects [28]. For this reason, combined therapy with $CaNa_2$ EDTA, 12.5 mg/kg/4 hr IM, and 2, 3-di-mercapto-1-propanol (BAL), 4 mg/kg/4 hr IM for 5 days, is indicated whenever the blood lead levels are in excess of 80 μg per deciliter [28, 31]. Oral penicillamine at 40 mg/kg/day given for 2 months following the initial therapy has been recommended to prevent "rebound" [31, 157].

It should be noted that chelating agents, although relatively safe, are not without their own renal toxicity. The administration of $CaNa_2$ EDTA to rats at doses of 250 mg/kg/day for 16 days caused severe hydropic degeneration of the most proximal portion of the proximal convoluted tubules [61]. Subsequently, it was found that simultaneous administration of cortisone enhanced the severity and extent of proximal tubular degeneration [124]. Accordingly, if endogenous corticosteroids were elevated in a patient with concurrent infection, the potential for $CaNa_2$ EDTA-induced renal injury might be increased [124]. The finding that the stable compound, chromium $CaNa_2$ EDTA, was not injurious to dog kidney suggested that any toxicity attributable to $CaNa_2$ EDTA is due to its chelative properties rather than to some effect of the $CaNa_2$ EDTA moiety per se [2]. As might be expected, acute renal failure has followed $CaNa_2$ EDTA therapy in adults [21, 61, 111, 159, 164] as well as children [45, 125], many of whom had concurrent infection.

D-Penicillamine has been most widely employed in the treatment of Wilson's disease, although it now is also recommended for lead poisoning, as discussed. It has caused nephrotic syndrome in children [57, 95] and adults [1, 87, 89, 135], presumably due to a hypersensitivity reaction rather than to direct glomerular damage. Moreover, cases of focal glomerulitis [81], a systemic lupus erythematosuslike syndrome [51], and Goodpasture syndrome [65, 143] have occurred following penicillamine therapy.

Chronic Lead Nephropathy
A possible link between exposure to lead in early childhood and development of chronic renal disease in adulthood was first suggested by Nye [115, 116] on the basis of a retrospective study performed in Queensland, Australia. The typical home built in that area at the end of the last century had an open veranda surrounded by painted railing. Because of the tropical climate, the paint, which contained lead, was transformed to a powder that was easily ingested by the children confined on the verandas during hot days. Twenty to thirty years later, Nye observed that the incidence of chronic renal failure was three times higher in Queensland than in other areas of the country and attributed this finding to previous exposure to lead.

Support for the hypothesis was provided by Henderson [82, 83] in a follow-up study of 401 persons hospitalized for plumbism in Brisbane between 1915 and 1935. Thirty years later, 27 percent of these patients were dead from renal or vascular disease, and 5 percent of the survivors had hypertension, albuminuria, or both [82]. The incidence of gouty arthritis was as high as 50 percent among this population and was attributed to defective uric acid secretion by the diseased kidney [52]. Patients dying of this "cryptogenic nephritis" had more lead in their bodies than those dying of renal diseases of recognized etiology [84]. The response of the renin-aldosterone system to salt deprivation was found to be blunted [133]. The significance of this finding in the development of hypertension has not been established. With the subsequent introduction of lead-free paint, the incidences of plumbism and chronic "nephritis" gradually declined to those of other Australian states [82, 84].

Similar follow-up studies conducted in the United States failed to show an increased incidence of renal injury in patients with a history of lead intoxication [28, 149]. This result has been attributed both to a less prolonged exposure and a more temperate climate [149]; other factors that would mitigate or delay the clinical manifestations of lead-poisoning disease [54], such as higher levels of dietary calcium, lesser degrees of iron deficiency, and lower exposures to sunlight and vitamin D, have also been implicated.

The kidney of chronic lead nephropathy is granular with marked cortical atrophy and interstitial fibrosis. The number of glomeruli is reduced, and the remaining tubules are hypertrophied. Severe arteriosclerosis is apparent [53, 54].

MERCURY

Epidemiology

An uncommon type of poisoning among children [173], mercury intoxication has become still rarer as the use of harmful and generally ineffective calomel teething powders, ammoniated mercury ointments, and mercuric chloride tablets has vanished. The new and more potent diuretics have practically eliminated the use of mercurial compounds in the treatment of edema, although mercury continues to be used in many industries, including chemical, electrical, and agricultural. As residues of industrial processing are discarded in rivers and the sea, fish and other living forms become contaminated with organic mercury [156, 169].

Pathophysiology

Mercury can reach the human either as inorganic compounds, mercury vapor (which is oxidized in the body to inorganic mercuric salts [69]), or as organic compounds, of which alkyl mercury and phenyl-methyl and methoxy-methyl mercury are a few examples. The phenyl-methyl and methoxy-methyl compounds are degraded to inorganic mercury, and their toxicity is similar to inorganic salts, whereas the alkyl mercury compounds maintain the covalent carbon-mercury bond [40, 91, 156].

Following injection, inorganic salts and mercurial diuretics are rapidly cleared from plasma, and they accumulate in high concentrations in the renal cortex. Excretion of inorganic and phenyl mercury compounds is by renal tubular secretion into the urine, and also by fecal, sweat, and salivary routes. Distribution of alkyl mercury compounds, primarily ethyl and methyl mercury compounds, is more uniform in the body, perhaps because of their greater solubility in lipids and their stable covalent mercury-carbon bond. Hence, higher concentrations are attained in liver, blood, brain, hair, and epidermis [91]. Elimination of alkyl mercury from the body is slow and mainly through the feces; less than 10 percent appears in the urine [91]. Thus, the urinary excretion of mercury does not correlate well with exposure to alkyl mercury.

Toxicity is the result of mercury's high affinity for sulfhydryl groups, the majority of which are found in proteins [130]. This affinity leads to disintegration of mitochondria, nuclear karyorrhexis, necrosis, and loss of enzyme activity [105]. The specific proteins and enzymes affected by mercury are unknown [69]. In the kidney most of the non-alkyl mercury is bound to a soluble protein of 8,000 to 13,000 MW; organic mercury is bound to larger protein fractions [50]. The rate of release depends on the form in which the mercury is administered.

In animals, mercurials cause necrosis of the middle and terminal portion of the proximal convoluted tubule [15, 38, 41, 43, 109, 119, 148], although larger doses affect the entire segment [43, 59, 148]. Microscopically there is vacuolization of the cytoplasm and destruction of mitochondria, followed by coagulation necrosis [53, 105, 148]. Regeneration begins rapidly, with surviving cells originating from the zone of necrosis and effecting a complete repair by 4 to 5 days [38, 109]. If the dose of mercury is so large as to leave few surviving cells in the necrotic zone, the injury is not repaired [38]. Glomerular structures [10, 141] and superficial single-nephron GFRs are not greatly affected [60], even though whole-kidney GFR is markedly reduced [43]. This discrepancy might be due to tubular obstruction by debris and artifactual "venting" by the micropuncture technique [60, 118] or to tubular back leakage of filtrate [8, 15] (see also Chap. 7).

Clinical Features

Acute inorganic mercury poisoning, which is found in accidental or suicidal ingestions, causes severe gastrointestinal intolerance, central nervous system symptoms, and acute renal failure [146, 156], with anuria developing within 24 hr after exposure and lasting 10 days on the average [63, 153]. The mortality rate in a series of 48 patients was 21 percent, although hemodialysis prevented any deaths from uremia [154]. The survivors recovered full renal function by 5 months [153]. Similar observations were reported by Schreiner and Maher [137]. A child who ingested mercuric chloride and was anuric for 3 days recovered gradually and attained nearly normal function within 2 months [92]. Acute renal failure has also been reported in an infant with cyanotic congenital heart disease who received excessive amounts of a mercurial diuretic [127]. Similar acute effects have been noted experimentally [10] as well as in adults [63].

Nephrotic syndrome has followed prolonged mercury administration, particularly in calomel teething powders [56, 168], mercury-containing ointments [14, 106, 166], mercurial diuretics [114, 122], and industrial exposure [96]. The mechanism is presumed to be a hypersensitivity reaction to a mercury-protein complex formed in the kidney, but specific proof is lacking. Glomerular changes on light microscopy have been minimal [95, 114], although membranous glomerulonephropathy was found in some cases [14].

Chronic mercury intoxication in children is the cause of acrodynia. This disease, also thought to be a hypersensitivity reaction [86, 162, 163, 173], is characterized by irritability, anorexia, insomnia, salivation, sweating, cold and pink extremities, stomatitis, hypertension [173], and occasionally, albuminuria [163]. Since the use of mercury has been declared medically worthless, harmful, or of less value than newer agents, iatrogenic acrodynia should remain confined to the history of medicine. A child who lived in a house in which mercury had been incorporated into paint to prevent the growth of molds, however, developed acrodynia half a year after exposure [86].

Acute or chronic organic alkyl mercury poisoning may follow ingestion of contaminated fish or grain, and it causes central nervous system manifestations such as peripheral neuropathies, seizures, spasticity, mental disturbances, and retardation [88, 91, 110, 156]. Epidemic alkyl-mercury poisoning involving fetuses, infants, and children has been reported from Minamata, Japan [110]. Neurologic manifestations associated with high levels of mercury in the brain, liver, and kidneys indicated that methyl mercury was the toxic agent [91 110]. The renal pathology was unremarkable [110]. The urinary content of renal tubular antigen and beta-2-microglobulin was found to be elevated in these patients, indicating renal tubular dysfunction [88a].

Treatment
Treatment of all inorganic mercury poisoning should include, in addition to precipitating the mercury and removing it, the use of BAL, beginning with 3 mg/kg/4 hr IM [173]. Should anuria ensue, a combination of BAL and hemodialysis is recommended [135]. The use of *N*-acetyl-D, L-penicillamine is effective in mercury poisoning, particularly in chronic poisoning [86, 94]. The nephrotic syndrome may remit when exposure to the metal ceases, or it may respond to BAL therapy [168] or corticosteroids [63].

GOLD
Gold remains an important nephrotoxin in childhood because of its role as an antiinflammatory agent in severe cases of juvenile rheumatoid arthritis. Toxic reactions following gold-salt therapy have occurred in the majority of adults receiving gold therapy, although most are mild cutaneous hypersensitivity reactions, reversible blood dyscrasias, and lesions of the buccal mucosa [62]. The incidence of nephrotoxicity, which is manifested by albuminuria, hematuria, and casts, was reported to be around 10 percent [62, 140]. Mild proteinuria may disappear while gold therapy is continued [85]. In children, renal complications have followed administration of gold in 28 to 50 percent of cases [37, 46, 131]; proteinuria and hematuria have been found in 5 to 50 percent of the patients [5, 46, 131]. An impairment in tubular function, as measured by phenolsulfonphthalein excretion, with no change in GFR or concentrating-diluting capacity, was noted in some of these children [5]. In general, the urinary findings disappear following discontinuation of gold administration. One report, however, describes a case of acute renal failure leading to anuria and death in a 39-year-old woman receiving her third course of gold therapy. The pathology revealed acute tubular necrosis with metallic inclusions in tubular cells, precipitates in the tubular lumens, and glomerular hyalinization [42]. A 17-year-old girl [144] with proteinuria and hematuria recovered when gold was discontinued and BAL was administered for 10 days. The authors suggested that early recognition of renal involvement and prompt therapy might account for the recovery.

Hypersensitivity to gold resulting in nephrotic syndrome has been extensively reported in adults receiving gold therapy [78, 99, 123, 140, 152, 155, 163a, 172]. No differences in blood and urinary gold levels or site of renal gold deposition could be distinguished among patients who did or did not develop nephrotic syndrome [140]. Biopsy studies confirmed the presence of basement-membrane thickening in two-thirds of patients, the remainder of whom showed minimal changes [99, 123, 140, 152]. Renal biopsies performed at various intervals after gold administration show that the metal is found initially in the cytoplasm of proximal tubules and then disappears from this site within months. Glomerular deposits are always observed, irrespective of the interval from the last administration [22]. In three-quarters of cases, the nephrotic syndrome disappears following the use of prednisone, immunosuppressive agents, chelating agents, or simply discontinuation of gold treatment. A gold-salt hapten may cause the renal lesion [99].

After parenteral injection in animals, gold is demonstrable in the reticuloendothelial system, kidney, spleen, liver, lung, and in the adrenal glands [105], with the highest concentration in the kidneys [90]. Gold may get into proximal tubule cells via the tubular capillaries or the glomerular filtrate [145]. Within hours of injection, it accumulates in globular deposits in the apical cytoplasm and then in laminated inclusions throughout the cytoplasm [64]. Using electron-probe analysis, Stuve and Galle [145] and Yarom et al. [172] were able to show that the primary site of gold concentration is the proximal tubule cell mitochondrion, and that this accumulation results in destruction of the mitochondrion and expulsion of the gold into the tubular lumen. The greater the quantity of gold injected, the greater the number of proximal tubular cells containing gold inclusions. These granules appear to be nontoxic, but their accumulation in increasing numbers in the mitochondria ultimately compromises the cell's energy supply [145]. The significance of these findings has not been fully determined in regard to human cases of nephrotoxicity.

PLATINUM
Certain platinum compounds have been found to have antineoplastic effects and have been tried in patients failing to respond to conventional therapy. Changes in BUN and serum creatinine values have suggested a deleterious effect on renal function [103]. Dose-related nephrotoxicity was observed in rats and monkeys, beginning with vacuolization of proximal convoluted tubule mitochondria and followed by loss of brush border and ultimately cell necrosis. No platinum deposition in tubular epithelial cells was detected [100].

COPPER
Ingestion of copper sulfate has been used as a means of committing suicide. It causes severe gastrointestinal symptoms, hepatic necrosis, acute hemolytic anemia, and renal damage. Fatal acute renal failure occurred in two young men shortly after the development of sulfhemoglobinemia, suggesting that anoxia due to the latter caused acute tubular necrosis [134]. Similarly, an infant dying after inhaling bronze gilding powder developed acute renal failure with proximal tubular necrosis [80]. In none of these cases was it determined whether kidney damage was caused by a direct effect of copper or by secondary phenomena, such as shock, anoxia, and hemoglobinuria.

In mice, Vogel has found reversible degenerative changes occurring in the proximal convoluted tubules following intraperitoneal injection of a copper-albumin complex [158]. In rats receiving multiple intraperitoneal injections of cupric chloride, Wolff has demonstrated degeneration and sloughing of proximal convoluted tubule cells and histochemical evidence of copper deposition in the cytoplasm of these cells [170]. More recently, the renal effects of low-dose copper poisoning were demonstrated in sheep [70]. Prior to acute hemolytic crisis, copper levels rose in the kidney, and eosinophilic intracytoplasmic granules became numerous in the proximal convoluted tubule epithelium. No functional impairment was seen. Once hemolysis occurred, there was cell degeneration and vacuolization and loss of enzyme activity in the proximal convoluted tubule associated with decreased GFR. Signs of tubular regeneration were apparent subsequently. It was suggested that the combination of hemoglobinemia and hypercupremia acting on renal tubular cells already loaded with copper caused the damage.

Wilson's disease (hepatolenticular degeneration) is a hereditary disorder of copper metabolism associated with increased copper absorption from the gut, reduced levels of ceruloplasmin (the copper-carrying protein), reduced total serum copper, and increased copper content of the body, namely in brain, liver, and kidneys [11]. Urinary copper excretion is also increased, usually in conjunction with a generalized aminoaciduria [11, 36, 151] or the Fanconi syndrome [11, 113]. The Fanconi syndrome with hypercalciuria in association with rickets remains a unique presentation of Wilson's disease [113]. The kidneys of patients with Wilson's disease show injury to and degeneration of proximal convoluted tubular cells and mitochondria, with histochemical evidence of copper deposition in the damaged cells [126, 171]. With time and progression of the renal lesion, the morphologic and functional abnormalities no longer remain confined to the proximal tubule, and decreases in GFR and renal plasma flow [12], along with mild proteinuria, become apparent. The reversibility of hepatic and central nervous system damage by chelation therapy with D-penicillamine [129] suggests that a similar improvement may occur in renal function.

BISMUTH
Bismuth salts have been used in the treatment of warts, wounds, gingivostomatitis, tonsillitis, and upper respiratory infections. Although the last case of nephrotoxicity reported in children was in 1966 [150], and the efficacy of bismuth in any of the aforementioned ailments has long since fallen into disrepute, it is possible that subsequent intoxications will occur, since the drug is still available [121].

The characteristic response of children receiving toxic doses of bismuth salts is the development of acute renal failure. Following parenteral, oral, or rectal administration, the onset is within 48 hr;

after topical use the interval is longer [150]. Pathologically, the chief finding is proximal tubular cell degeneration with dense, sharply circumscribed spherical, nuclear, and cytoplasmic inclusions [13]. The period of oligoanuria lasts 5 to 10 days, and the survivors recover full renal function [93, 108, 117, 120, 150]. The use of BAL and dialysis, if necessary, is recommended [137]. The mortality rate was nearly 50 percent for the series reported by Urizar and Vernier [150], although the majority of deaths occurred before the wide availability of hemodialysis.

IRON

The widespread use of medicinal iron compounds has led to a substantial increase in the incidence of acute iron poisoning in children [3]. Clinical manifestations follow a predictable chronology. The first phase occurs within 30 to 40 min of ingesting the tablets and is characterized by vomiting, bloody diarrhea, and metabolic acidosis. Cardiovascular collapse may ensue, accounting for almost half the fatalities. The second phase represents a period of improvement following supportive therapy; it may last 10 to 14 hr and leads to eventual recovery for most children. In some children, however, a third phase of rapid deterioration occurs 20 hr after ingestion; it leads to irreversible shock and accounts for the other half of the deaths. The overall mortality rate after ingestion of large amounts of iron is approximately 50 percent. Children who recover may develop severe gastric scarring requiring surgery 1 or 2 months later [3].

The changes noted in kidneys of autopsied patients have been nonspecific: edema, cloudy swelling, and areas of hemorrhage [3]. Such lesions are found in many other organs and suggest that iron is not severely nephrotoxic and that acute renal failure following iron poisoning is more likely due to renal ischemia. There is, however, one report of extensive renal tubular degeneration and necrosis in a child who died during the third phase of iron poisoning [39]. The histology was consistent with anoxia due to circulatory collapse, except for the finding of iron in the renal tubules. In another case of iron poisoning, the authors noted the transient appearance of generalized aminoaciduria [19].

In rabbits, the administration of large doses of parenteral saccharated iron compounds results in the deposition of iron within glomerular capillary endothelial cells and often causes thrombosis [48, 68]. Signs of acute glomerular injury then appear, and massive proteinuria is present within a week of administration; the full nephrotic syndrome

follows repeated doses. Electron microscopy shows loss of foot processes but normal basement membranes [49]. Animals surviving massive administration of iron recovered fully within 3 months and 1 year later showed no renal pathology apart from siderosis [67, 68]. It is possible that the nephrotoxicity seen in the rabbit is due to its relatively hypoactive reticuloendothelial system, which allows serum iron levels to rise to very high levels [68]. The role of the potentially antigenic saccharated iron complex in causing nephrotic syndrome in these animals must also be considered.

Kidney damage from acute iron poisoning can result from cardiovascular collapse, which is more likely to occur if the serum iron level exceeds 500 μg per deciliter within 6 hr of ingestion [47]. For these reasons, circulatory support combined with desferrioxamine (a highly effective iron-binding agent), 90 mg per kilogram of body weight over 6 hr, given IV, is recommended [47]. The excretion of orange-brown urine, indicating the presence of ferrioxamine, necessitates continued desferrioxamine therapy. Dialysis is indicated if acute renal failure ensues.

References

1. Adams, D. A., Goldman, R., Maxwell, M. H., and Latta, H. Nephrotic syndrome associated with penicillamine therapy of Wilson's disease. *Am. J. Med.* 36:330, 1964.
2. Ahrens, F. A., and Aronson, A. L. A comparative study of the toxic effects of calcium and chromium chelates of ethylenediaminetetraacetate in the dog. *Toxicol. Appl. Pharmacol.* 18:10, 1971.
3. Aldrich, R. A. Acute Iron Toxicity, 1957. In R. O. Wallerstein and S. R. Mettier (eds.), *Iron In Clinical Medicine.* Berkeley and Los Angeles: University of California Press, 1958. Pp. 93–104.
4. Angevine, J. M., Kappas, A., DeGowin, R. L., and Spargo, B. H. Renal tubular nuclear inclusions of lead poisoning: A clinical and experimental study. *Arch. Pathol.* 73:486, 1962.
5. Anttila, R. Renal involvement in juvenile rheumatoid arthritis: A clinical and histopathological study. *Acta Paediatr. Scand.* [Suppl.] 227:3, 1972.
6. Aviv, A., John, E., Goldsmith, D. I., and Spitzer, A. The effect of lead intoxication during development upon the kidney (abstract). *Pediatr. Res.* 11:547, 1977.
7. Baier, H., Bassler, K. H., and Lang, K. Über Wirkungen von Blei im Intermediärstoff wechsel. *Arch. Exp. Pathol. Pharmakol.* 229:495, 1956.
8. Bank, N., Mutz, B. F., and Aynedjian, H. S. The role of "leakage" of tubular fluid in anuria due to mercury poisoning. *J. Clin. Invest.* 46:695, 1967.
9. Barnett, R. N. Reactions to a bismuth compound. *J.A.M.A.* 135:28, 1947.
10. Barrett, M. Chronic and acute effects of Mercuhydrin and Thiomerin on renal tubular function in the dog. *J. Pharmacol. Exp. Ther.* 100:502, 1950.
11. Bearn, A. G., and Kunkel, H. G. Abnormalities of copper metabolism in Wilson's disease and their re-

lationship to the aminoaciduria. *J. Clin. Invest.* 33: 400, 1954.

12. Bearn, A. G., Yu, T. F., and Gutman, A. B.   Renal function in Wilson's disease. *J. Clin. Invest.* 36: 1107, 1957.

13. Beaver, D. L., and Burr, R. E.   Electron microscopy of bismuth inclusion. *Am. J. Pathol.* 42:609, 1963.

14. Becker, C. G., Becker, E. L., Maher, J. F., and Schreiner, G. E.   Nephrotic syndrome after contact with mercury. *Arch. Intern. Med.* 110:178, 1962.

15. Biber, T. U. L., Mylle, M., Baines, A. D., Gottschalk, C. W., Oliver, J. R., and MacDowell, M. C.   A study by micropuncture and microdissection of acute renal damage in rats. *Am. J. Med.* 44:664, 1968.

16. Blackman, S. S., Jr.   Intranuclear inclusion bodies in the kidney and liver caused by lead poisoning. *Bull. Johns Hopkins Hosp.* 58:384, 1936.

17. Boyette, D. P.   Bismuth nephrosis with anuria in an infant: Report of a case. *J. Pediatr.* 28:493, 1946.

18. Browing, E.   *Toxicity of Industrial Metals.* London: Butterworth, 1961. Pp. 149–172.

19. Brown, R. J. K., and Gray, J. D.   The mechanism of acute ferrous sulphate poisoning. *Can. Med. Assoc. J.* 73:192, 1955.

20. Broyer, M.   Acute Renal Failure. In P. Royer, R. Habib, H. Mathieu, M. Broyer, and A. Walsh (eds.), *Pediatric Nephrology.* Philadelphia: Saunders, 1974. Pp. 343–357.

21. Brugsch, H. G.   Fatal nephropathy during edathamil therapy in lead poisoning. *Arch. Ind. Health* 20:285, 1959.

22. Brun, C., Olsen, S., Raaschou, F., and Sorensen, A. W. S.   The localization of gold in the human kidney following chrysotherapy: A biopsy study. *Nephron* 1:265, 1964.

23. Byers, R. K.   Lead poisoning: Review of the literature and report on 45 cases. *Pediatrics* 23:585, 1959.

24. Caffey, J.   Lead poisoning associated with active rickets: Report of a case with absence of lead lines in the skeleton. *Am. J. Dis. Child.* 55:798, 1938.

25. Carroll, K. G., Spinelli, F. R., and Goyer, R. A.   Electron probe microanalyser localization of lead in kidney tissue of poisoned rats. *Nature* 227:1056, 1970.

26. Chamberlain, J. L., III, and Franks, R. C.   Nephropathy resulting from bismuth. *South. Med. J.* 56:509, 1963.

27. Chisholm, J. J., Jr.   Aminoaciduria as a manifestation of renal tubular injury in lead intoxication and a comparison with patterns of aminoaciduria seen in other diseases. *J. Pediatr.* 60:1, 1962.

28. Chisholm, J. J., Jr.   The use of chelating agents in the treatment of acute and chronic lead intoxication in childhood. *J. Pediatr.* 73:1, 1968.

29. Chisholm, J. J., Jr.   Acute and Chronic Effects of Lead on the Kidney. Presented at the *Lead Conference,* Mayaguez, Puerto Rico, 1970. Quoted in R. A. Goyer, Lead and the kidney. *Curr. Top. Pathol.* 55:147, 1971.

30. Chisholm, J. J., Jr.   Management of increased lead absorption and lead poisoning in children. *N. Engl. J. Med.* 289:1016, 1973.

31. Chisholm, J. J., Jr.   Lead Poisoning. In H. L. Barnett and A. H. Einhorn (eds.), *Pediatrics* (16th ed.). New York: Appleton-Century-Crofts, 1977. Pp. 797–806.

32. Chisholm, J. J., Jr., Harrison, H. C., Eberlein, W. R., and Harrison, H. E.   Aminoaciduria, hypophosphatemia, and rickets in lead poisoning: Study of a case. *Am. J. Dis. Child.* 89:159, 1955.

33. Choie, D. D., and Richter, G. W.   Lead poisoning: Rapid formation of intranuclear inclusions. *Science* 177:1194, 1972.

34. Cohen, G. J., and Ahrens, W. E.   Chronic lead poisoning: A review of seven years' experience at the Children's Hospital, District of Columbia. *J. Pediatr.* 54:271, 1959.

35. Cohen, S., Sweet, A. Y., Mautner, W., Churg, J., and Grishman, E.   Light and electron microscopy of lead nephropathy (abstract). *Am. J. Dis. Child.* 100:559, 1960.

36. Cooper, A. M., Eckhardt, R. D., Faloon, W. W., and Davidson, C. S.   Investigation of the aminoaciduria in Wilson's disease (hepatolenticular degeneration): Demonstration of a defect in renal function. *J. Clin. Invest.* 29:265, 1950.

37. Coss, J. A., Jr., and Boots, R. H.   Juvenile rheumatoid arthritis: A study of fifty-six cases with a note on skeletal changes. *J. Pediatr.* 29:143, 1946.

38. Cuppage, F. E., Chiga, M., and Tate, A.   Cell cycle studies in the regenerating rat nephron following injury with mercuric chloride. *Lab. Invest.* 26:122, 1972.

39. Curtiss, C. D., and Kosinski, A. A.   Fatal case of iron intoxication in a child. *J.A.M.A.* 156:1326, 1954.

40. Dallenbach, F.   Die Aufnahme von radioaktivem Blei^{210} durch die Tubulusepithelien der Niere. *Verh. Dtsch. Ges. Pathol.* 49:179, 1965.

41. Darmady, E. M., and Stranack, F.   Autoradiography of the isolated nephron. *Proc. Soc. Exp. Biol. Med.* 100:658, 1959.

42. Derot, M., Kahn, J., Mazalton, A., and Peyrafort, J.   Néphrite anurique aiguë mortelle après traitement aurique, chrysocyanose associée. *Bull. Mem. Soc. Med. Hop. (Paris)* 70:234, 1954.

43. DiBona, G. F., McDonald, F. D., Flamenbaum, W., Dammin, G. J., and Oken, D. E.   Maintenance of renal function in salt loaded rats despite severe tubular necrosis induced by $HgCl_2$. *Nephron* 8:205, 1971.

44. Dillard, M. G., Pesce, A. J., Pollak, V. E., and Boreisha, I.   Proteinuria and renal protein clearances in patients with renal tubular disorders. *J. Lab. Clin. Med.* 78:203, 1971.

45. Dudley, H. R., Ritchie, A. C., Schilling, A., and Baker, W. H.   Pathologic changes associated with the use of sodium ethylene diamine tetra-acetate in the treatment of hypercalcemia: Report of two cases with autopsy findings. *N. Engl. J. Med.* 252:331, 1955.

46. Edstrom, G., and Gedda, P. O.   Clinic and prognosis of rheumatoid arthritis in children. *Acta Rheumatol. Scand.* 3:129, 1957.

47. Einhorn, A. H.   Iron Poisoning. In H. L. Barnett and A. H. Einhorn (eds.), *Pediatrics* (16th ed.). New York: Appleton-Century-Crofts, 1977. Pp. 790–793.

48. Ellis, J. T.   Glomerular lesions and the nephrotic syndrome in rabbits given saccharated iron oxide intravenously: With special reference to the part played by intracapillary precipitates in the pathogenesis of the lesions. *J. Exp. Med.* 103:127, 1956.

49. Ellis, J. T.   Glomerular lesions in rabbits with ex-

perimentally induced proteinuria as disclosed by electron microscopy (abstract). *Am. J. Pathol.* 34: 559, 1958.

50. Ellis, R. W., and Fang, S. C. The in vivo binding of mercury to soluble proteins of the rat kidney. *Toxicol. Appl. Pharmacol.* 20:14, 1971.

51. Elsas, L. J., Hayslett, J. P., Spargo, B. H., Durant, J. L., and Rosenberg, L. E. Wilson's disease with reversible renal tubular dysfunction: Correlation with proximal tubular ultrastructure. *Ann. Intern. Med.* 75:427, 1971.

52. Emmerson, B. T. Chronic lead nephropathy: The diagnostic use of calcium EDTA and the association with gout. *Aust. Ann. Med.* 12:310, 1963.

53. Emmerson, B. T. Metals and the Kidney. In D. A. K. Black (ed.), *Renal Disease* (2nd ed.). Philadelphia: Davis, 1967. Pp. 561–593.

54. Emmerson, B. T. Chronic lead nephropathy. *Kidney Int.* 4:1, 1973.

55. Environmental Health Services Division, C.D.C. Surveillance of childhood lead poisoning—United States. *Morbid. Mortal. Weekly Rep.* 25:318, 323, 1976.

56. Farquhar, H. G. Mercurial poisoning in early childhood. *Lancet* 2:1186, 1953.

57. Fellers, F. X., and Shahidi, N. T. The nephrotic syndrome induced by penicillamine therapy (abstract). *Am. J. Dis. Child.* 98:669, 1959.

58. Finckh, E. S., Jeremy, D., and Whyte, H. M. Structural renal damage and its relation to clinical features in acute oliguric renal failure. *Q.J. Med.* 31:429, 1962.

59. Flamenbaum, W., Kotchen, T. A., Nagle, R., and McNeil, J. S. Effect of potassium on the renin-angiotensin system and $HgCl_2$-induced acute renal failure. *Am. J. Physiol.* 224:305, 1973.

60. Flamenbaum, W., McDonald, F. D., DiBona, G. F., and Oken, D. E. Micropuncture study of renal tubular factors in low dose mercury poisoning. *Nephron* 8:221, 1971.

61. Foreman, H., Finnegan, C., and Lushbaugh, C. C. Nephrotoxic hazard from uncontrolled edathamil calcium-disodium therapy. *J.A.M.A.* 160:1042, 1956.

62. Fraser, T. N. Gold treatment in rheumatoid arthritis. *Ann. Rheum. Dis.* 4:71, 1945.

63. Freeman, R. B., Maher, J. F., Schreiner, G. E., and Mostofi, F. K. Renal tubular necrosis due to nephrotoxicity of organic mercurial diuretics. *Ann. Intern. Med.* 57:34, 1962.

64. Ganote, C. E., Beaver, D. L., and Moses, H. L. Renal gold inclusions: A light and electron microscopic study. *Arch. Pathol.* 81:429, 1966.

65. Gibson, T., Burry, H. C., and Ogg, C. Goodpasture syndrome and D-penicillamine (letter). *Ann. Intern. Med.* 84:100, 1976.

66. Goettsch, E., and Mason, H. H. Glycosuria in lead poisoning: Report of a case and study of pathogenesis. *Am. J. Dis. Child.* 59:119, 1940.

67. Goldberg, L. Pharmacology of Parenteral Iron Preparations, 1957. In R. O. Wallerstein and S. E. Mettier (eds.), *Iron in Clinical Medicine.* Berkeley and Los Angeles: University of California Press, 1958. Pp. 74–92.

68. Goldberg, L., Smith, J. P., and Martin, L. E. The effects of intensive and prolonged administration of iron parenterally in animals. *Br. J. Exp. Pathol.* 38: 297, 1957.

69. Goldwater, L. J., and Clarkson, T. W. Mercury. In D. H. K. Lee (ed.), *Metallic Contaminants and Human Health.* New York: Academic, 1972. Pp. 17–56.

70. Gopinath, C., Hall, G. A., and Howell, J. McC. The effect of chronic copper poisoning on the kidneys of sheep. *Res. Vet. Sci.* 16:57, 1974.

71. Goyer, R. A. The renal tubule in lead poisoning: I. Mitochondrial swelling and aminoaciduria. *Lab. Invest.* 19:71, 1968.

72. Goyer, R. A., and Chisholm, J. J. Lead. In D. H. K. Lee (ed.), *Metallic Contaminants and Human Health.* New York: Academic, 1972. Pp. 57–97.

73. Goyer, R. A., and Krall, R. C. Ultrastructural transformation in mitochondria isolated from kidneys of normal and lead intoxicated rats. *J. Cell Biol.* 41:393, 1969.

74. Goyer, R. A., Krall, A., and Kimball, J. P. The renal tubule in lead poisoning: II. In vitro studies of mitochondrial structure and function. *Lab. Invest.* 19:78, 1968.

75. Goyer, R. A., May, P., Cates, M., and Krigman, M. R. Lead and protein content of isolated inclusion bodies from kidneys of lead-poisoned rats. *Lab. Invest.* 22:245, 1970.

76. Goyer, R. A., Moore, J. F., Rhyne, B., and Krigman, M. R. Lead dosage and the role of the intranuclear inclusion body. *Arch. Environ. Health* 20:705, 1970.

77. Goyer, R. A., and Wilson, M. H. Lead-induced inclusion bodies: Results of ethylenediaminetetraacetic acid treatment. *Lab. Invest.* 32:149, 1975.

78. Grégoire, F., Malmendier, C., and Lambert, P. P. Syndrome néphrotique après traitement aux sels d'or. *J. Urol. Med. Chir.* 62:140, 1956.

79. Gryboski, J. D., and Gotoff, S. P. Bismuth nephrotoxicity: Report of a case. *N. Engl. J. Med.* 265: 1289, 1961.

80. Harris, G. B. C., and Haggerty, R. J. Toxic hazards-bronze powder inhalation. *N. Engl. J. Med.* 256:40, 1957.

81. Hayslett, J. P., Bensch, K. G., Kashgarian, M., and Rosenberg, L. E. Focal glomerulitis due to penicillamine. *Lab. Invest.* 19:376, 1968.

82. Henderson, D. A. A follow-up of cases of plumbism in children. *Aust. Ann. Med.* 3:219, 1954.

83. Henderson, D. A. The aetiology of chronic nephritis in Queensland. *Med. J. Aust.* 1:377, 1958.

84. Henderson, D. A., and Inglis, J. A. The lead content of bone in chronic Bright's disease. *Aust. Ann. Med.* 6:145, 1957.

85. Hersperger, W. G. Gold therapy for rheumatoid arthritis: A current evaluation. *Ann. Intern. Med.* 36:571, 1951.

86. Hirschman, S. Z., Feingold, M., and Boylen, G. Mercury in house paint as a cause of acrodynia: Effect of therapy with N-acetyl-D,L-penicillamine. *N. Engl. J. Med.* 269:889, 1963.

87. Hirschman, S. Z., and Isselbacher, K. J. The nephrotic syndrome as a complication of penicillamine therapy for hepatolenticular degeneration (Wilson's disease). *Ann. Intern. Med.* 62:1297, 1965.

88. Hook, O., Lundgren, K. D., and Swensson, A. On alkyl mercury poisoning with a description of two cases. *Acta Med. Scand.* 150:131, 1954.

88a. Iesato, K., Wakashin, M., Wakashin, Y., and Tojo, S.: Renal tubular dysfunction in Minamata disease: Detection of renal tubular antigen and beta-

2-microglobulin in the urine. *Ann. Intern. Med.* 86: 731, 1977.

89. Jaffe, I. A., Treser, G., Suzuki, Y., and Ehrenreich, T.   Nephropathy induced by D-penicillamine. *Ann. Intern. Med.* 69:549, 1968.

90. Jeffrey, M. R., Freundlich, H. F., and Bailey, D. M. Distribution and excretion of radiogold in animals. *Ann. Rheum. Dis.* 17:52, 1958.

91. Joselow, M. M., Louria, D. B., and Browder, A. A. Mercurialism: Environmental and occupational aspects. *Ann. Intern. Med.* 76:119, 1972.

92. Kaplan, S. A., and Fomon, S. J.   Function recovery pattern in acute renal failure following ingestion of mercuric chloride. *Am. J. Dis. Child.* 85:633, 1953.

93. Karelitz, S., and Freedman, A. D.   Hepatitis and nephrosis due to soluble bismuth. *Pediatrics* 8:772, 1951.

94. Kark, R. A. P., Poskanzer, D. C., Bullock, J. D., and Boylen, G.   Mercury poisoning and its treatment with N-acetyl-D,L-penicillamine. *N. Engl. J. Med.* 285:10, 1971.

95. Karp, M., Lurie, M., and Yonis, Z.   Nephrotic syndrome in the course of treatment of Wilson's disease with DL-penicillamine. *Arch. Dis. Child.* 41: 684, 1966.

96. Kazantzis, G., Schiller, K. F. R., Asscher, A. W., and Drew, R. G.   Albuminuria and the nephrotic syndrome following exposure to mercury and its compounds. *Q.J. Med.* 31:403, 1962.

97. Krige, H. N.   Bismuth poisoning: A case report. *S. Afr. Med. J.* 37:1005, 1963.

98. Landing, B. H., and Nakai, H.   Histochemical properties of renal lead-inclusions and their demonstration in urinary sediment. *Am. J. Clin. Pathol.* 31:499, 1959.

99. Lee, J. C., Dushkin, M., Eyring, E. J., Engleman, E. P., and Hopper, J., Jr.   Renal lesions associated with gold therapy: Light and electron microscopic studies. *Arthritis Rheum.* 8:1, 1965.

100. Leonard, B. J., Eccleston, E., Jones, D., Todd, P., and Walpole, A.   Antileukaemic and nephrotoxic properties of platinum compounds. *Nature* 234:43, 1971.

101. Lieberman, E.   Acute Renal Failure. In E. Lieberman (ed.), *Clinical Pediatric Nephrology.* Philadelphia: Lippincott, 1976. Pp. 272–293.

102. Lin-Fu, J. S.   Undue absorption of lead among children—a new look at an old problem. *N. Engl. J. Med.* 286:702, 1972.

103. Lippman, A. J., Helson, C., Helson, L., and Krakoff, I. H.   Clinical trials of cis-diaminedichloroplatinum (NSC-119875). *Cancer Chemother. Rep.* 57:191, 1973.

104. Macadam, R. F.   The early glomerular lesion in human and rabbit lead poisoning. *Br. J. Exp. Pathol.* 50:239, 1969.

105. Maher, J. F.   Toxic Nephropathy. In B. M. Brenner and F. C. Rector, Jr. (eds.), *The Kidney.* Philadelphia: Saunders, 1976. Pp. 1355–1395.

106. Mandema, E., Arends, A., van Zeijst, J., Vermeer, G., vander Hem, G. K., and vander Slikke, L. B. Mercury and the kidney (letter). *Lancet* 1:1266, 1963.

107. Marsden, H. B., and Wilson, V. K.   Lead poisoning in children: Correlation of clinical and pathological findings. *Br. Med. J.* 1:324, 1955.

108. McClendon, S. J.   Toxic effects with anuria from a

single injection of a bismuth preparation: Report of two cases. *Am. J. Dis. Child.* 61:339, 1941.

109. McCreight, C. E., and Witcofski, R. L.   Sequence of Morphological and Functional Changes in Renal Epithelia Following Heavy Metal Poisoning. In W. W. Nowinski and R. J. Goss (eds.), *Compensatory Renal Hypertrophy.* New York: Academic, 1969. Pp. 251–268.

110. Medical Study Group of Minamata Disease. Minamata Disease. Kumamoto University, Minamata, Japan, 1968.

111. Moeschlin, S. Zur Klinik und therapie der Bleivergiftung mit Bericht über eine tödliche toxische nephrose durch Ca-EDTA (Calcium-versenat). *Schweiz. Med. Wochenschr.* 87:1091, 1957.

112. Moncrieff, A. A., Koumides, O. P., Clayton, E., Patrick, A. D., Renwick, A. G. C., and Roberts, G. E.   Lead poisoning in children. *Arch. Dis. Child.* 39:1, 1964.

113. Morgan, H. G., Stewart, W. K., Lowe, K. G., Stowers, J. M., and Johnstone, J. H.   Wilson's disease and the Fanconi syndrome. *Q.J. Med.* 31:361, 1962.

114. Munck, O., and Nissen, N. I.   Development of nephrotic syndrome during treatment with mercurial diuretics. *Acta Med. Scand.* 153:307, 1956.

115. Nye, L. J. J.   An investigation of the extraordinary incidence of chronic nephritis in young people in Queensland. *Med. J. Aust.* 2:145, 1929.

116. Nye, L. J. J.   *Chronic Nephritis and Lead Poisoning.* Sydney, Australia: Angus and Robertsen, 1933.

117. O'Brien, D.   Anuria due to bismuth thioglycollate. *Am. J. Dis. Child.* 97:384, 1959.

118. Oken, D. E.   On the passive back flow theory of acute renal failure. *Am. J. Med.* 58:77, 1975.

119. Oliver, J., MacDowell, M., and Tracy, A.   The pathogenesis of acute renal failure associated with traumatic and toxic injury: Renal ischemia, nephrotoxic damage and the ischemuric episode. *J. Clin. Invest.* 30:1307, 1951.

120. Petersilge, C. L.   Prolonged anuria following a single injection of a bismuth preparation: Possible response to therapy with BAL. *J. Pediatr.* 31:580, 1947.

121. *Physicians' Desk Reference.*   Oradell, N.J.: Medical Economics, 1977.

122. Preedy, J. R. K., and Russell, D. S.   Acute salt depletion associated with the nephrotic syndrome developing during treatment with a mercurial diuretic. *Lancet* 2:1181, 1953.

123. Renier, J. C., Boasson, M., Bernat, M., and Fresinaud, P.   Syndrome néphrotique dû aux sels d'or: A propos de quatre cas. *Sem. Hôp. Paris* 49:881, 1973.

124. Reuber, M. D.   Accentuation of Ca edetate nephrosis by cortisone. *Arch. Pathol.* 76:382, 1963.

125. Reuber, M. D., and Bradley, J. E.   Acute versenate nephrosis: Occurring as the result of treatment for lead intoxication. *J.A.M.A.* 174:263, 1960.

126. Reynolds, E. S., Tannen, R. L., and Tyler, H. R. The renal lesion in Wilson's disease. *Am. J. Med.* 40:518, 1966.

127. Robillard, J. E., Rames, L. K., Jensen, R. L., and Roberts, R. J.   Peritoneal dialysis in mercurial diuretic intoxication. *J. Pediatr.* 88:79, 1976.

128. Robinson, G. C., and Wong, L. C.   Acute tubular necrosis in infancy and childhood. *Am. J. Dis. Child.* 95:417, 1958.

129. Rosen, F. S., and Alper, C. A. Anomalies of Protein Metabolism: Serum and Metal-Binding Proteins. In H. L. Barnett and A. H. Einhorn (eds.), *Pediatrics* (15th ed.). New York: Appleton-Century-Crofts, 1972. Pp. 386–391.

130. Rothstein, A. Mercaptans, the Biological Targets for Mercurials, 1971. In M. W. Miller and T. W. Clarkson (eds.), *Mercury, Mercurials and Mercaptans*. Springfield, Ill.: Thomas, 1973. Pp. 68–108.

131. Sairanen, E., and Laaksonen, A.-L. The toxicity of gold therapy in children suffering from rheumatoid arthritis. *Ann. Paediatr. Fenn.* 8:105, 1962.

132. Salick, B. Heavy metal poisoning: Mercury and lead. J. S. Felton (moderator). *Ann. Intern. Med.* 76:779, 1972.

133. Sandstead, H. H., Michelakis, A. M., and Temple, T. E. Lead intoxication, its effect on the renin aldosterone response to sodium deprivation. *Arch. Environ. Health* 20:356, 1970.

134. Sanghvi, L. M., Sharma, R., Misra, S. N., and Samuel, K. C. Sulfhemoglobinemia and acute renal failure after copper sulfate poisoning: Report of two cases. *Arch. Pathol.* 63:172, 1957.

135. Scheinberg, I. H. D-Penicillamine with particular relation to Wilson's disease. *J. Chronic Dis.* 17:293, 1964.

136. Schreiner, G. E. Toxic Nephropathy. In E. L. Becker (ed.), *Structural Basis of Renal Disease*. New York: Harper and Row, 1968. Pp. 703–756.

137. Schreiner, G. E., and Maher, J. F. Toxic nephropathy. *Am. J. Med.* 38:409, 1965.

138. Secchi, G. C., Alessio, L., and Cirla, A. The effect of experimental lead poisoning on some enzymatic activities of the kidney. *Clin. Chim. Acta* 27:467, 1970.

139. Secchi, G. C., Alessio, L., and Geruasini, N. Ricerche sulla Na$^+$–K$^+$-ATPase renale nella intossicazione saturina sperimentale. *Med. del Lavoro.* 60:674, 1969.

140. Silverberg, D. S., Kidd, E. G., Shnitka, T. K., and Ulan, R. A. Gold nephropathy: A clinical and pathologic study. *Arthritis Rheum.* 13:812, 1970.

141. Stejskal, J. Acute renal insufficiency in intoxication with mercury compounds: III. Pathological findings. *Acta Med. Scand.* 177:75, 1965.

142. Sterne, T. L., Whitaker, C., and Webb, C. H. Fatal cases of bismuth intoxication. *J. La. State Med. Soc.* 107:332, 1955.

143. Sternlieb, I., Bennett, B., and Scheinberg, I. H. D-Penicillamine induced Goodpasture's syndrome in Wilson's disease. *Ann. Intern. Med.* 82:673, 1975.

144. Strauss, J. F., Jr., Barrett, R. M., and Rosenberg, E. F. BAL treatment of toxic reactions to gold: A review of the literature and report of two cases. *Ann. Intern. Med.* 37:323, 1952.

145. Stuve, J., and Galle, P. Role of mitochondria in the handling of gold by the kidney. *J. Cell Biol.* 44:667, 1970.

146. Subcommittee on Toxicology of Metals of the Permanent Commission and International Association of Occupational Health, Tokyo, 1974. In G. F. Nordberg (ed.) *Effects and Dose-Response Relationships of Toxic Metals.* New York: Elsevier, 1976. Pp. 7–111.

147. Tange, J. D., Hayward, N. J., and Brenner, D. A. Renal lesions in experimental plumbism and their clinical implications. *Aust. Ann. Med.* 14:49, 1965.

148. Taylor, N. S. Histochemical studies of nephro-toxicity with sublethal doses of mercury in rats. *Am. J. Pathol.* 46:1, 1965.

149. Tepper, L. B. Renal function subsequent to childhood plumbism. *Arch. Environ. Health* 7:76, 1963.

150. Urizar, R., and Vernier, R. L. Bismuth nephropathy. *J.A.M.A.* 198:187, 1966.

151. Uzman, L., and Denny-Brown, D. Amino-aciduria in hepato-lenticular degeneration (Wilson's disease). *Am. J. Med. Sci.* 215:599, 1948.

152. Vaamonde, C. A., and Hunt, F. R. The nephrotic syndrome as a complication of gold therapy. *Arthritis Rheum.* 13:826, 1970.

153. Valek, A. Acute renal insufficiency in intoxication with mercury compounds: I. Aetiology, clinical picture, renal function. *Acta Med. Scand.* 177:63, 1965.

154. Valek, A. Acute renal insufficiency in intoxication with mercury compounds: II. Treatment and prognosis. *Acta Med. Scand.* 177:69, 1965.

155. Vanden Broek, H., and Han, M. T. Gold nephrosis. *N. Engl. J. Med.* 274:210, 1966.

156. Van Natta, F. C. Heavy metal poisoning: Mercury and lead. J. S. Felton (moderator). *Ann. Intern. Med.* 76:779, 1972.

157. Vitale, L. F., Rosalinas-Bailon, A., Folland, D., Brennan, J. F., and McCormick, B. Oral penicillamine therapy for chronic lead poisoning in children. *J. Pediatr.* 83:1041, 1973.

158. Vogel, F. S. Nephrotoxic properties of copper under experimental conditions in mice, with special reference to the pathogenesis of the renal alterations in Wilson's disease. *Am. J. Pathol.* 36:699, 1960.

159. Vogt, W., and Cottier, H. Nekrotisierende Nephrose nach Behandlung einer subakutchronischen Bleivergiftung mit Versenat in holen Dosen. *Schweiz. Med. Wochenschr.* 87:665, 1957.

160. Vostal, J., and Heller, J. Renal excretory mechanisms of heavy metals: I. Transtubular transport of heavy metal ions in the avian kidney. *Environ. Res.* 2:1, 1968.

161. Waldron, H. A., and Stofen, D. *Sub-clinical Lead Poisoning.* New York: Academic, 1974.

162. Warkany, J., and Hubbard, D. M. Mercury in the urine of children with acrodynia. *Lancet* 1:829, 1948.

163. Warkany, J., and Hubbard, D. M. Adverse mercurial reactions in the form of acrodynia and related conditions. *Am. J. Dis. Child.* 81:335, 1951.

163a. Watanabe, I., Whittier, F. C., Jr., Moore, J., and Cuppage, F. E. Gold nephropathy: Ultrastructural, fluorescence, and microanalytic studies of two patients. *Arch. Pathol. Lab. Med.* 100:632, 1976.

164. Weinig, E., and Schwerd, W. Nil nocere! Gefahren bei der Behandlung der Bleintoxikation mit Calcium versenat ("mosatil Komplexon") *Munch. Med. Wochenschr.* 100:1788, 1958.

165. Weinstein, I. Fatalities associated with analbis suppositories. *J.A.M.A.* 133:962, 1947.

166. Williams, N. E., and Bridge, H. G. T. Nephrotic syndrome after the application of mercury ointment. *Lancet* 2:602, 1958.

167. Wilson, V. K., Thomson, M. L., and Dent, C. E. Amino-aciduria in lead poisoning: A case in childhood. *Lancet* 2:66, 1953.

168. Wilson, V. K., Thomson, M. L., and Holzel, A. Mercury nephrosis in young children with special reference to teething powders containing mercury. *Br. Med. J.* 1:358, 1952.

169. Wobeser, G. Mercury poisoning from fish (letter). *Can. Med. Assoc. J.* 102:1209, 1970.
170. Wolff, S. M. Copper deposition in the rat. *Arch. Pathol.* 69:223, 1960.
171. Wolff, S. M. Renal lesions in Wilson's disease. *Lancet* 1:843, 1964.
172. Yarom, R., Stein, H., Peters, P. D., Slavin, S., and

Hall, T. A. Nephrotoxic effect of parenteral and intraarticular gold. *Arch. Pathol.* 99:37, 1975.
173. Zavon, M. R. Mercury Poisoning. In H. L. Barnett and A. H. Einhorn (eds.), *Pediatrics* (15th ed.). New York: Appleton-Century-Crofts, 1972. Pp. 548–550.

80. Balkan Nephropathy

Hayim Boichis

In the late 1950s an endemic nephropathy of familial distribution causing renal failure was described independently in Bulgaria, Roumania, and Yugoslavia [5, 11, 12]. This disease has been referred to as Balkan nephropathy (BN), endemic Balkan nephropathy, or endemic Danubian nephropathy. Balkan nephropathy occurs in a well-defined area 220 km long and 50 km wide where the three states of Bulgaria, Roumania, and Yugoslavia share common borders and the Danube intersects the southern Carpathian Mountains. The regional climate is humid, and the flora and fauna are abundant. Balkan nephropathy is restricted to a hilly zone 150 to 300 meters in altitude, and it affects mostly people in the villages situated in eroded valleys created by fast-flowing rivers. The incidence of BN varies from 0.5 percent of the inhabitants of some villages to 38 percent in others; it is only sporadically found in hilltop villages and is practically nonexistent in towns.

In most communities, 10 to 75 percent of households are affected. The patients are mainly agricultural workers and their families. In some families most members of one or more generations have the disease.

The disease occurs either in resident natives or among strangers who have stayed in the endemic area for more than 10 years. Those who left the area as children were considered free of the disease. However, BN was recently reported among adults who left the endemic area in childhood, as well as in second-generation subjects born outside the affected area [4, 11].

The disease is rare in the first two decades of life (about 8 percent of known cases). The incidence increases with age, the peak occurring in the fifth and sixth decades (41 percent of known cases). About 15 percent of the cases occur after age 60. Women are more frequently and more severely affected than men. This sex difference is extreme in the younger age group (5 : 1 in the twenties), but it tends to diminish with age. Morbidity and mortality seem to fluctuate seasonally and are enhanced by profuse rainfall.

Balkan nephropathy is probably not a new disease, since numerous cases of uremia were reported by Volhard in Serbia during World War I. Moreover, the average life expectancy of agricultural workers in the area before 1945 was less than 40 years; many may have died before the disease was manifest.

Although screening programs have yielded large numbers of asymptomatic patients, the incidence of overt cases remains at 1 to 3 per 100 inhabitants per year.

Etiology

The etiology and pathogenesis of this disease have not been elucidated. The idea that exogenous toxic agents caused the interstitial nephritis and the tumors that are frequently associated (see under Clinical Features) and that cohabitation was a predominant epidemiologic factor has prompted numerous studies by local and international agencies [4, 11, 12].

Danilovic discovered evidence of chronic lead ingestion among patients in one region, but laborious studies failed to demonstrate lead accumulation in other endemic areas [12]. Repeated spectrographic analyses of water, soil, and foods have shown acceptable levels of most trace elements. Although the local concentration of cadmium in fertilizer and plants is higher than usual, it is below toxic levels. Increased concentrations of several metals, particularly aluminum, tin, nickel, and chromium, have been found in the organs of some patients at autopsy; these results, however, remain uninterpretable. Investigation of infectious agents, including streptococci, leptospirae, and fungi, has been unrewarding, and urinary tract infections are only a minor complication of the disease. Morbidity and mortality from all other causes in the endemic area are comparable to the rest of the country, and so are living and housing conditions, hygiene, alcohol distilling techniques and consumption, foods and their storage, and use of herbal remedies, insecticides, and pesticides [11, 12].

Several old horses, dogs, and cats have recently been found to have a renal disease similar to BN, but most animal species studied so far have not been affected.

Bulic has suggested that the familial distribution may be the result of some factor that occurred in the past, producing a genetic inability to detoxify exogenous environmental agents [12]. The existence of an asymptomatic phase and the late appearance of the disease render complete ascertainment very difficult; moreover, genetic factors alone cannot explain the appearance of BN in more than 50 percent of members of many consecutive sibships. Cytogenetic studies of patients with BN showed a 40 percent incidence of structural chromosomal abnormalities in uremic subjects [2], compared to only 3.4 percent in uremic patients with other diseases. A visible chromosomal aberration affects multiple genes and produces birth defects in several organ systems. The chromosomal abnormalities observed in patients with BN are probably not constitutional but are acquired. Such changes could result, however, from a viral infection, maintained by an autoimmune system, or from continuous low-dose ionizing radiation [2].

The finding of low C3 complement levels and of cryoglobulins in the sera of several patients with BN [8] suggests that an immune process may operate in this disease; this warrants further investigation. The correlation of peak BN morbidity and mortality following heavy rainfall is subject to various interpretations. The resultant high humidity favors the growth of molds, and fungal toxins have been considered as the possible cause of BN [4, 7, 11]. On the other hand, it has been suggested that the erosion of the volcanic rock by heavy rain could increase to toxic levels the content of silicic acid in the drinking water; moreover, radioisotopes released by the decomposition of silicon could contribute to the genesis of both the renal disease and the frequently associated urothelial malignancies [9]. However, the long-term addition of silicic acid to the drinking water of guinea pigs failed to reproduce the renal disease [1], and no signs of increase of radioactive elements in the endemic area have been discovered [11]. Multifactorial investigations of the BN disease continue.

Clinical Features

An asymptomatic stage of varying duration may precede the onset of clinical disease. Community screening by immunoelectrophoresis of urinary proteins has revealed a tubular pattern of proteinuria in many asymptomatic subjects, including children. Their daily protein excretion varied little from normal, and many had no detectable proteinuria on routine testing [6]. Renal biopsies performed on individuals with tubular proteinuria only, with no clinical evidence of renal disease, show abnormalities [5].

The clinical onset of BN usually is insidious; headache, lassitude, weakness, anorexia, pallor, loss of weight, polydypsia, and polyuria are common, as well as abdominal pain and lumbar pain and tenderness. Xanthochromia, an ochre pigmentation of the skin that appears particularly on the face, palms, and soles, may precede renal failure by several years.

Edema, the nephrotic syndrome, and acute oliguric renal failure have not been described in this disease, and elevation of blood pressure until terminal stages is uncommon.

Slowly developing malignancies of the urinary tract are very common in the endemic area and are found in 35 percent of patients with BN [9, 12]. These tumors are occasionally multiple or bilateral and do not metastasize to other organs. They are frequently heralded by profuse hematuria and severe lumbar pain.

Laboratory Findings

At the onset of the symptomatic stage urinary findings are scant, consisting of a few erythrocytes, leukocytes, and casts, and proteinuria in the range of 0.5 to 1 gm per day. The proteinuria is usually of the classic tubular type [12]. Its principal proteins are below 50,000 in molecular weight and consist of relatively little albumin; much α-1-, α-2-, and β-1-globulin; β-2-microglobulin; and fast γ-globulin, such as some components of light chains.

Another type of tubular proteinuria that is detected early in the asymptomatic state is found in many subjects of all ages. It consists of proteins of less than 30,000 molecular weight, mainly β-2- and fast γ-globulins (muramidase [lysozyme], ribonuclease, β-glucuronidase, and amylase), all of which are normally filtered at the glomerulus and metabolized or reabsorbed by the tubules [6]. Patients may fluctuate seasonally from a normal state, through the early type of tubular proteinuria, on to the classic pattern, and vice versa. In the more advanced stages of BN, however, the classic tubular pattern is fixed. As the disease progresses further, a mixed type of proteinuria emerges due to enhanced glomerular permeability combined with tubular dysfunction.

Early in the course of BN, while the glomerular

filtration rate is normal or minimally decreased, tubular functions are impaired; urinary excretion of α-aminonitrogen, glucose, and phosphate is higher than normal; Tm_{PAH}, PAH (para-amino-hippurate) clearance, and urinary concentration are low; and the patient fails to increase ammonium production appropriately in response to an acid load [6]. High uric acid clearances and increased potassium excretion continue well into the state of uremia.

Anemia precedes renal failure. It is usually normochromic, with normal red cell fragility and no basophilic stippling; toxic changes in leukocytes and a moderate thrombocytopenia are common. Some liver functions are disturbed; bromsulphalein excretion is low, and serum levels of alkaline phosphatase, guanase [10], and several free amino acids [3] are usually elevated irrespective of the degree of renal failure. Osteoporosis is seen in one-third of the patients, but renal osteodystrophy is rare, probably because of the swift evolution of the disease. A hippuran (^{131}I-labeled sodium iodohippurate) renogram is similar in pattern to that found in other forms of interstitial nephritis.

Pathology

The earliest histologic lesions of BN are seen on renal biopsies of children in affected families or in asymptomatic subjects with tubular proteinuria [4, 5, 11, 12]. These lesions are seen as focal mesangial thickening of the glomerular basement membrane and minimal changes in the tubules consisting of focal areas of atrophy and interstitial fibrosis, with electron-dense deposits in the mitochondria of proximal tubular cells. Renal biopsies performed in the symptomatic stage show varying degrees of axial glomerular sclerosis and mesangial proliferation, as well as more pronounced tubular atrophy with regenerations, thickening of the tubular basement membrane, and a progressive, acellular interstitial sclerosis. At autopsy, the kidneys are symmetrically very contracted with moderate sparing of the poles. The outer cortex is uniformly atrophied and fibrosed and contains only hyalinized glomeruli and atrophic tubules. The inner zone contains atrophic and dystrophic tubules, some regenerating tubules, few inflammatory cells, and both hyalinized and nearly normal glomeruli. There are no calcium deposits in the areas of atrophy, and the juxtaglomerular apparatus is not hypertrophied. Papillary scars are common. Other findings at autopsy are a hypoplastic, nonregenerating bone marrow and, in 40 percent of cases, periportal proliferation of connective tissue with round cell infiltration.

Treatment, Course, and Prognosis

Treatment is symptomatic, since no form of therapy has been shown to influence the course of the disease. Survival after recognition of clinical signs is short; the usual experience has been that more than 50 percent of patients with BN die within 2 years and 95 percent within 4 years. Recent follow-up of several thousand inhabitants of the endemic region, however, has shown a decrease in the number of severe cases among the younger subjects along with an increase in the number of suspects of all ages (discovered by screening). Many of the milder cases with tubular proteinuria alone, particularly in the younger age group, have shown no evidence of deterioration, suggesting that the disease may occasionally follow a slow course with low lethality.

References

1. Benninger, J. L., Graepel, P., and Hodler, J. Failure to produce renal changes in the guinea-pig by chronic administration of silicic acid: An experiment concerning the etiology of Balkan nephropathy. *Res. Exp. Med.* 162:215, 1974.
2. Bruckner, I., and Motoiu, I. Chromosome changes in Balkan nephropathy. *Lancet* 1:348, 1971.
3. Dotchev, D., Hugerland, H., and Liappis, N. Free amino acids in blood serum of patients with endemic (Balkan) nephropathy. *Klin. Wochenschr.* 50:614, 1972.
4. Endemic nephropathy (editorial). *Lancet* 1:472, 1973.
5. Hall, P. W., III, Dammin, G. J., Griggs, R. C., Fajgelj, A., Zimonjic, B., and Goan, J. Investigation of chronic endemic nephropathy in Yugoslavia. *Am. J. Med.* 39:210, 1965.
6. Hall, P. W., III, Piscator, M., Vasiljevic, M., and Popovic, N. Renal function studies in individuals with the tubular proteinuria of endemic Balkan nephropathy. *Q. J. Med.* 41:385, 1972.
7. Krogh, P., Hald, B., and Pedersen, E. J. Occurrence of ochratoxin A and citrinin in cereals associated with mycotoxic porcine nephropathy. *Acta Pathol. Microbiol. Scand.* [B] 81:689, 1973.
8. Macanovic, M. Endemic nephropathy. *Lancet* 1:720, 1973.
9. Markovic, B. Endemic nephropathy and cancer of the upper urinary tract urothelium in Yugoslavia. *Isr. J. Med. Sci.* 8:540, 1972.
10. Prodarov, K., and Astrug, A. Guanase activity in endemic Balkan nephropathy. *Clin. Chim. Acta* 35: 445, 1971.
11. Puchlev, A. R. Problem of Endemic Nephropathy. W.H.O. Mimeographed Report, Geneva, 1971.
*12. Wolsterholme, G. E. W., and Knight, J. (eds.). *The Balkan Nephropathy* (Ciba Foundation Study Group No. 30). London: Churchill, 1967.

* The reader is particularly referred to this work. For reasons of brevity the various authors and sections of this book have not been referred to individually. The reader will find in it references to many earlier publications on this subject.

81. The Fanconi Syndrome

Johannes Brodehl

Definition

The renal Fanconi syndrome (de Toni-Debré-Fanconi syndrome) is characterized by generalized dysfunction of the proximal tubule leading to excessive urinary loss of amino acids, glucose, phosphate, bicarbonate, and other substances handled by the proximal tubule. The distal tubule can be disturbed in a similar way; glomerular filtration is not affected initially. The metabolic consequences of the renal dysfunctions are acidosis, polyuria, dehydration, hypokalemia, hypophosphatemia, rickets, osteoporosis, and growth retardation. This syndrome may be either congenital or acquired, and it may be either primary or secondary.

Remarks on History

A special type of renal hypophosphatemic rickets was first postulated by de Toni [77], who in 1933 reported on a 5-year-old girl with severe renal rickets accompanied by hypophosphatemia and renal glucosuria. A similar case was observed independently by Debré and coworkers [72] 1 year later in an 11-year-old girl with glucosuria and rickets, who, in addition, showed an excessive urinary loss of organic acids bound to fixed bases and ammonia. In 1936 Fanconi [91] described three additional cases of "nephrotic-glucosuric dwarfism with hypophosphatemic rickets," including a patient who had already been mentioned by him in 1931 [90]. Fanconi described an excessive urinary loss of organic acids in one of his cases and postulated that these organic compounds could possibly be amino acids. In 1943 McCune et al. [217] demonstrated that 82 percent of the organic acids excreted in a patient with this syndrome were indeed free amino acids. Finally, in 1947 Dent [74] demonstrated the renal origin and described the generalized type of hyperaminoaciduria in this syndrome.

Many of the facets of the Fanconi syndrome were described earlier under different headings that later could be recognized as parts of this syndrome. This relationship is true for Milkman's case [220] and especially for the cystine storage disease described first by Abderhalden [2] in

1903 and by Lignac [199] in 1924 and shown to be accompanied by the Fanconi syndrome by Beumer and Wepler [24] in 1937. For many years after Bickel and coworkers [28] published their extensive studies on cystinosis, it was assumed that both entities were identical and that only a few cases of Fanconi syndrome occurred "without cystinosis." With the wide application of chromatographic procedures in clinical medicine, however, it became evident (1) that many diseases and conditions lead to the Fanconi syndrome and (2) that each generalized hyperaminoaciduria is not accompanied by the fully developed Fanconi syndrome but may occur as an isolated abnormality. Fanconi syndromes were found to be caused or accompanied by Wilson's hepatolenticular degeneration [66, 307], glycogenosis [92], galactosemia [150, 160], Lowe's oculocerebrorenal dystrophy [73, 203], hereditary fructose intolerance [193, 195], and tyrosinemia [7, 110]. Furthermore, in some acquired diseases the syndrome could be produced by endogenous products such as proteins of multiple myeloma [83, 292] or nephrotic syndrome [154, 305] or by exogenous toxic substances and drugs such as lead [121, 322], cadmium [57, 121], uranium [57], mercury [191], Lysol [295], outdated tetracycline [84, 102], and methyl 3-chromone [243]. In experimental studies it was shown that the Fanconi syndrome can be produced by many substances, including maleic acid [22, 137], outdated tetracycline [19, 201, 204], and heavy metals [99, 118–120, 311]. A few cases, however, failed to reveal any detectable cause for this syndrome and therefore were classified as idiopathic [18, 167, 185, 187].

The Fanconi syndrome must be separated from other tubular syndromes that also are accompanied by excessive losses of some amino acids, glucose, phosphate, and other substances. For example, cystinuria was recognized as an independent entity by Dent and Rose [76] in 1949, and X-linked hypophosphatemic rickets was recognized as a separate disease by Albright, Butler, and Bloomberg [3] in 1937. Through the development of new methods for quantitative measurements of biologic functions, it has become possible to delineate the Fanconi syndrome and to recognize its characteristic features. For a more detailed description of the intricate ways in which the definition of this syndrome evolved, see de Toni [78], McCune et al. [217], Bickel [27], Woolf [328], Leaf [190], Milne [221], and Royer [265].

Renal Symptoms in the Fanconi Syndrome

Although there is a wide spectrum of diseases that are accompanied by the Fanconi syndrome, the main features common to all entities are due to renal tubular impairment. These cardinal symptoms will be described in the following section; specific findings in individual types of the syndrome, including the morphology, will be discussed separately.

HYPERAMINOACIDURIA

The excretion of free amino acids is increased in the Fanconi syndrome, resulting in a hyperaminoaciduria considered to be due to diminished rates of tubular resorption. In Fig. 81-1 the urinary excretion rates of free amino acids in a child with glycogenosis and Fanconi syndrome are compared with normal rates of excretion standardized for age. All amino acids are involved in the hyperexcretion; however, the pattern of excretion of individual amino acids is similar to that of normal children of the same age. The hyperaminoaciduria is of renal origin and is not due to increased concentrations of plasma amino acids, which are normal or slightly reduced. Therefore the clearance rates of free amino acids (C_{AA}) are increased, and the rates of percentage tubular resorption (percent T_{AA}) are correspondingly decreased. The latter is shown in Fig. 81-2, where the percent T_{AA} of the same child is compared with the normal ranges.

The degree of hyperaminoaciduria varies considerably from one case to another and from one type of Fanconi syndrome to another. In Fig. 81-3 the clearance rates of 7 patients with the Fanconi syndrome due to different etiologies are depicted. Their mean values are used in Chap. 86 to demonstrate the pattern of generalized hyperaminoaciduria. This pattern is typical for the Fanconi syndrome. It is recognized best when clearances, rather than rates of urinary excretion, are estimated. Also, short periods of urine collection are preferable to 24-hr collection periods, since changes in concentrations of individual amino acids in plasma influence the pattern of hyperaminoaciduria considerably over a 24-hr period [298]. Plasma amino acids are increased by extrarenal factors such as underlying enzymatic defects, hepatic failure, or a high intake of protein-rich foods. The pattern of hyperaminoaciduria can be easily distorted by those influences, which must be considered when comparing data in the literature.

The mechanism by which generalized hyper-

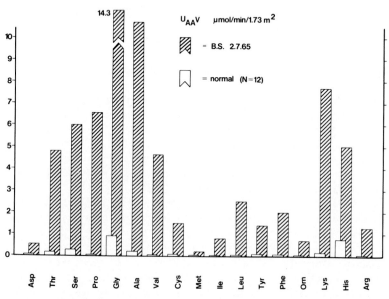

Figure 81-1. Endogenous urinary excretion rates of free amino acids in an 8-year-old boy (B. S.) with glycogenosis and Fanconi syndrome as compared with normal values (blank columns). *(Normal values from Brodehl and Gellissen [39].)*

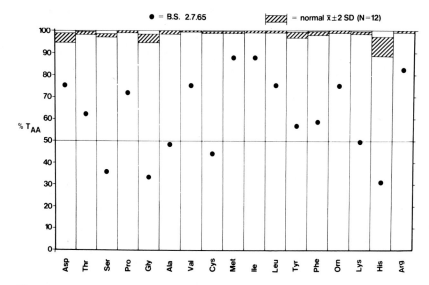

Figure 81-2. Percentage of tubular resorption of free amino acids [percent $T_{AA} = 100 \ (1 - C_{AA}/C_{In})$] in an 8-year-old boy (B. S.) with glycogenosis and Fanconi syndrome as compared with normal values. (Normal values from Brodehl and Gellissen [39].)

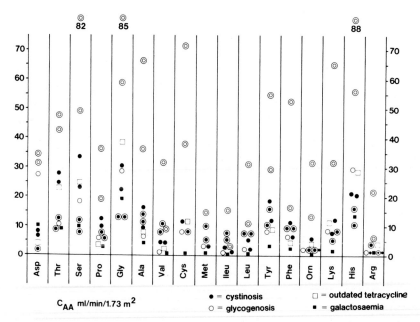

Figure 81-3. Clearance rates of free amino acids in seven children with Fanconi syndrome due to various etiologies. The double-circled symbols indicate the same patient investigated twice.

aminoaciduria is produced is not thoroughly understood. Estimation of tubular net resorption (T_{AA}) in patients with the Fanconi syndrome indicates that it is not a saturation of tubular resorptive capacity which leads to hyperaminoaciduria; rather the degree of impairment in T_{AA} seems to be independent of the tubular load of amino acids. As shown in Fig. 81-4, the endogenous rates of tubular glycine resorption (T_{Gly}) are plotted against the load filtered through the glomeruli ($C_{In} \times P_{Gly}$). Six children with the Fanconi syndrome due to cystinosis and glycogenosis are compared with normal values derived from 34 children (author's unpublished data). The normal values are just below the line of identity regardless of the endogenous filtered load, indicating that

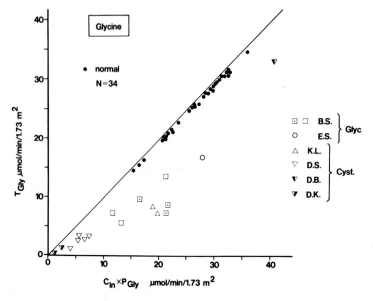

Figure 81-4. The tubular resorption of glycine (T_{Gly}) in normal children (dark dots, N = 34) and six children with Fanconi syndrome (two with glycogenosis, four with cystinosis). The values of T_{Gly} are plotted against the filtered load of glycine ($C_{In} \times P_{Gly}$).

this amino acid is reabsorbed rather completely over a wide range. In the patients with the Fanconi syndrome, the rates of resorption are variable but also are unrelated to the filtered loads. The same mechanism applies for all amino acids: There is no indication of either surpassing the saturation capacity of individual amino acids or of inhibition of specific carrier systems; instead, the data indicate a generalized cellular defect that may be related to either (1) the energy-regenerating or energy-transferring systems of the cells, or (2) the luminal membranes, leading to increased leakage of amino acids from the intracellular pool to the luminal fluid. The presence of a cellular defect was first suggested by Fellers et al. [94], who demonstrated in a case of cystinosis that hyperaminoaciduria increased with greater rates of urine flow.

Experimental data also seem to support the Fellers' hypothesis. Maleic acid produces in rat kidney slices an impaired influx and accelerated efflux of amino acids [261]. In vivo, intoxication with maleic acid is followed by an increased transfer of leucine from the peritubular space into the luminal fluid, while the net resorption of this amino acid is not decreased in the proximal convoluted tubule [21]. It is possible, therefore, that generalized hyperaminoaciduria may be produced by increased leakage of cellular amino acids into the tubular lumen, a mechanism that still has to be confirmed for the different types of Fanconi syndrome.

From the clinical point of view, renal loss of amino acids, even when severe, does not seem to have a great influence on general protein metabolism of the affected organism. The concentration of amino acids in plasma is usually lower than normal, but otherwise no metabolic deficiency can be recognized. It may be speculated that amino acid loss contributes to the severe osteoporosis and growth retardation that are encountered in some patients with the Fanconi syndrome. However, hard data are not available to support this opinion. The nephrolithiasis occasionally reported in patients with the Fanconi syndrome is probably not due to increased cystine excretion. In some cases defects in the intestinal absorption of some amino acids have been reported [5, 12, 63].

GLUCOSURIA
Glucosuria is the second cardinal symptom of the Fanconi syndrome. It is also of renal origin, as first pointed out by de Toni [77]. The amount of glucose excreted is variable and seems to be pathognomonic of some types of this syndrome, as discussed later.

The renal threshold for glucose is reduced or completely abolished. This is shown in Fig. 81-5, in which the rate of tubular resorption of glucose (T_G) is plotted against the tubular load ($C_{In} \times P_G$). In the four children with the Fanconi syndrome there is overt glucosuria even in the very low range of tubular load (author's unpublished

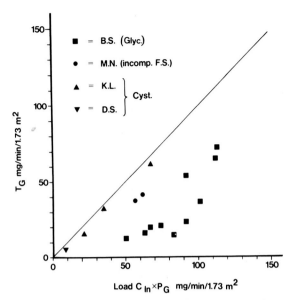

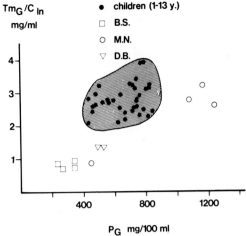

Figure 81-5. The endogenous tubular resorption of glucose (T$_G$) in relation to tubular load (C$_{In}$ × P$_G$) in four children with the Fanconi syndrome. The diagonal line of identity represents complete resorption as found normally.

Figure 81-6. The maximal tubular resorption of glucose corrected for glomerular filtration rate (Tm$_G$/C$_{In}$) in three children with Fanconi syndrome in comparison with normal values (hatched area). Tm$_G$/C$_{In}$ is plotted against the filtered load (C$_{In}$ × P$_G$). (Normal values from Brodehl et al. [38a.].)

data). When the tubules are loaded with more glucose, there is a gradual increase in the rate of resorption. These findings indicate that there is both a very low or even absent renal threshold for glucose and no saturation of the glucose resorptive capacity, at least within the range of endogenous loads.

The tubular maximum for resorption of glucose (Tm$_G$) can be determined only by loading tests. Due to their hypokalemic effects [30, 51, 72, 87, 92], however, such loading tests can be dangerous in some types of the Fanconi syndrome, especially in cystinosis. Only few data are available, therefore, on Tm$_G$ in the Fanconi syndrome. My own experience is shown in Fig. 81-6. In moderately loaded states, with plasma glucose (P$_G$) between 300 and 500 mg per deciliter, the tubular maximum for glucose per milliliter of glomerular filtrate (Tm$_G$/C$_{In}$) is significantly lower than normal; however, with very large filtered loads (P$_G$ = 900 to 1,200 mg per deciliter), it is within the normal range. Similar findings are reported by Bradley [35] and Bauer [13]. In adults with Fanconi syndrome, thresholds and low or normal values for Tm$_G$ are also reported, the latter obviously depending on the amount of glucose used for loading [253]. Occasionally, however, Tm$_G$ was found to drop after prolonging the glucose loading test [253], perhaps because of volume expansion.

The mechanism of glucosuria in the Fanconi

syndrome is comparable neither with the type A of Reubi [254] (true renal glucosuria of Govaerts [117]), nor with type B or pseudorenal glucosuria. The cellular pathophysiology is still unknown; the findings can be interpreted best by an inability of the tubular cell to maintain a gradient across the luminal membrane after having reabsorbed the filtered glucose. In this respect the pathophysiology of glucosuria in the Fanconi syndrome could be similar to that postulated for the hyperaminoaciduria. Another possibility is that tubular gluconeogenesis could be so accelerated that glucose could leak into both the luminal and peritubular sides of the tubular cell. Experimental data are not available to clarify this issue.

Clinical consequences of the glucosuria are usually mild or even absent. It is only in patients with very severe glucosuria, especially in those with glycogenosis, that hypoglycemia and ketonemia are encountered, both of which do respond to dietary treatment.

DECREASED TUBULAR RESORPTION OF PHOSPHATE

The impairment in renal handling of inorganic phosphate is considered to be the main cause of the skeletal changes in the Fanconi syndrome [65, 167, 185, 191, 321]. It is often called phosphate diabetes, although the actual amount of phosphate excreted in the urine is not higher than in normal subjects (Fig. 81-7). Higher values are found only when a patient is just in the state of

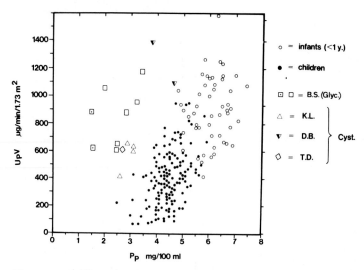

Figure 81-7. The urinary excretion rates of phosphate (U_pV) *in relation to plasma phosphate concentration* (P_p) *in normal infants and children* (open and black dots) *and in four children with Fanconi syndrome (three with cystinosis and one with glycogenosis). Infant D. B. with cystinosis was 6 months old and was in the state of just developing hypophosphatemia. (Normal values author's own unpublished data.)*

developing hypophosphatemia, as shown for a 6-month-old infant (D. B.) with cystinosis in Fig. 81-7. Otherwise, rates of excretion of phosphate in urine reflect only the phosphate intake [296, 321], a circumstance that is also found in X-linked hypophosphatemic rickets [180] and vitamin D deficiency [181].

The most important finding is hypophosphatemia, which is apparent in the data shown in

Figs. 81-7 and 81-8. In normal states the plasma phosphate level is regulated predominantly by the rate of tubular resorption; there is a very close correlation between plasma phosphate concentration (P_p) and fractional phosphate resorption (T_p/C_{In}). This correlation obtains also in the Fanconi syndrome, as shown in Fig. 81-8 (author's unpublished data). It indicates that hypophosphatemia is determined mainly by impaired

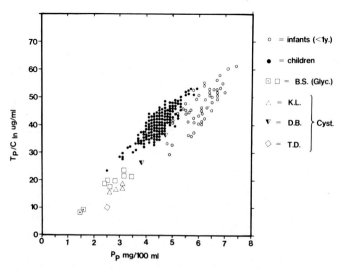

Figure 81-8. The correlation between fractional phosphate resorption (T_p/C_{In}) *and plasma phosphate concentration* (P_p) *in infants and children* (white and black dots) *in comparison with four children with the Fanconi syndrome. (Normal values author's own unpublished data.)*

tubular resorption of phosphate and that severe hypophosphatemia reflects severe reduction of phosphate resorption.

Loading with phosphate to demonstrate a maximal rate of phosphate resorption (Tm_p) fails to increase the actual level of phosphate resorption (T_p or T_p/C_{In}), as shown in Fig. 81-9 (author's unpublished data). It may be added that the same is true in our experience with normal infants and children, demonstrating that phosphate resorption is already maximal in endogenous states and therefore actually determines the plasma phosphate level. Net tubular secretion of phosphate was never observed in our patients with Fanconi syndrome [321].

In long-term studies of the Fanconi syndrome the impairment in phosphate resorption seems to be fairly constant (Fig. 81-10), although it can be modified by extrarenal factors such as changes in extracellular fluid volume; vitamin D intake; acidosis; and hormonal activity, especially parathormone activity. For a long time it had been postulated that secondary hyperparathyroidism might be the primary cause for the decrease of phosphate resorption in this syndrome, and there were reports that seemed to support this hypothe-

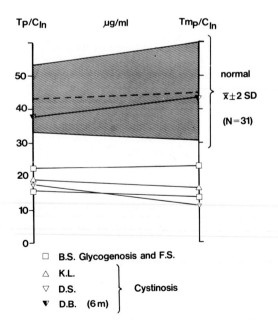

□ **B.S. Glycogenosis and F.S.**

△ **K.L.**

▽ **D.S.** ⎫
⎬ **Cystinosis**
▼ **D.B.** (6 m) ⎭

Figure 81-9. The effect of acute phosphate loading on fractional phosphate resorption (T_p/C_{In}) in 31 normal children and four children with Fanconi syndrome. T_p/C_{In} = endogenous values; Tm_p/C_{In} = maximal values after loading. D. B. (▼) was a 6-month-old child with cystinosis before hypophosphatemia developed. (Author's own unpublished data.)

sis [230]. Recent measurements, however, have revealed that patients with the Fanconi syndrome and unimpaired glomerular filtration rate have values of immunoreactive parathormone in serum within the range of normal [93]. Bone biopsy specimens confirm this finding [37].

The results of calcium loading on renal phosphate resorption in the Fanconi syndrome have been conflicting; some observations showed no or subnormal effects [101, 258, 321], and others demonstrated a definite increase of phosphate resorption [48, 94, 133]. Since the rate of glomerular filtration, the state of acidosis, the intake of phosphate, the extracellular volume, secretion of parathormone and other hormones, and the age of patients all have influences on tubular phosphate handling, it is not surprising to find such divergent reports in the literature. There seems to be no defect in the intestinal absorption of phosphate in the Fanconi syndrome [321].

Hypophosphatemia is the major factor contributing to the alterations in the skeletal system in the Fanconi syndrome [167, 185, 274, 321]. The bones show a wide spectrum of involvement, including defective mineralization and demineralization (rarefications), rickets, and osteoporosis. Only patients with glomerular insufficiency show signs of azotemic osteodystrophy with secondary hyperparathyroidism. These changes produce growth retardation, fractures and pseudofractures, and crippling deformities of the bone; most of them can be prevented by early and continuous treatment. Phosphate depletion due to other causes is accompanied by similar skeletal changes [33, 202].

OTHER TUBULAR SYMPTOMS

Renal Acidification

Acidosis is a frequent finding in the Fanconi syndrome. It is caused mainly by a defect in bicarbonate resorption in the proximal tubule. The renal threshold for bicarbonate is thereby reduced, leading to metabolic acidosis with low plasma bicarbonate characteristic of the findings in proximal renal tubular acidosis [227, 257]. At plasma bicarbonate levels below the renal threshold, the urinary pH can be lowered to 5.4 or less, demonstrating the ability of the distal tubule to establish a normal hydrogen ion gradient [171, 252, 257]. In some advanced cases, however, distal acidification is also disturbed, as shown by an inability to lower urinary pH even in the presence of severe metabolic acidosis [71, 191, 257]. This mixed type of tubular acidosis might be related to long-standing potassium depletion. Tubular ammoniagenesis seems to be unimpaired as long as no global renal insufficiency is present [48, 157, 167,

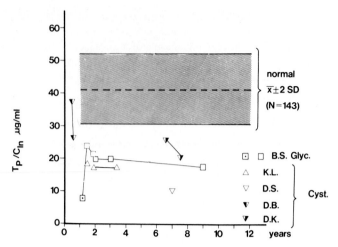

Figure 81-10. Long-term observations of fractional phosphate resorption in five children with Fanconi syndrome in comparison with normal values. (Author's unpublished data.)

171]. In many cases there is even an abundant excretion of ammonia. The metabolic consequence of the tubular dysfunction is a sustained metabolic acidosis that is associated with hyperchloremia and may produce hypercalciuria; it requires large amounts of alkali for compensation.

Urate Resorption
Hypouricemia occurs commonly in the Fanconi syndrome [16, 18, 253, 292, 316, 320, 321], mainly in adults. The incidence in children [157] is not known, due to incomplete reporting [235]. Low plasma urate levels are due to increased clearance rates. Since the exact mechanism of the renal handling of urate is not clarified for humans, it is not known whether decreased proximal resorption or increased distal secretion is involved. The clinical significance of low serum urate and increased excretion of uric acid is unknown [235]. There are no reports on urate lithiasis in the Fanconi syndrome.

Urinary Concentration
Polyuria, polydipsia, and episodes of dehydration are prominent clinical features of Fanconi syndrome. However, data on maximal urinary concentrating ability [18, 34, 71, 92, 191] are rare, since water deprivation can be hazardous to these patients. Polyuria is due both to the osmotic diuresis of glucosuria and hyperaminoaciduria and to a concentrating defect of the distal tubules and collecting ducts that is demonstrable by mannitol-induced diuresis with vasopressin. Fanconi syndromes due to light-chain proteinuria and multiple myeloma seem to be especially prone to develop distal concentrating defects [315]. Dehydration

is accompanied by episodes of fever and vomiting, which, in severe cases, is a frequent finding, especially in young infants and children.

Hypokalemia
Hypokalemia is a serious, constant threat to patients with the Fanconi syndrome [30, 71, 155]. The application of loading tests, especially with glucose, therefore can be dangerous [30, 51, 72, 87, 92]. Hypokalemia is due mainly to increased renal loss of potassium [286, 287]. The clearance rates for potassium can be elevated to more than twice the glomerular filtration rate, demonstrating thereby net tubular secretion [42]. The disturbances are related not only to acidosis, since the correction of acidosis does not necessarily reestablish renal potassium conservation [287]. Proximal tubular resorption of sodium is disturbed [157] and the distal tubules are overloaded with sodium, leading to an increased resorption of sodium and an enhanced secretion of potassium. The potassium loss may be aggravated by impaired hydrogen ion secretion and by increased plasma renin activity and hyperaldosteronism that is often found [114, 286]. The balance of potassium may become negative [71], leading to severe symptoms of potassium depletion such as constipation, muscle weakness, growth retardation, and further disturbances of kidney function.

Sodium Loss
Sodium wasting represents another defect present in the Fanconi syndrome. In some cases the renal salt wasting is so severe that hyponatremia with metabolic alkalosis develops despite the low bicarbonate threshold [157]. Supplementation

with sodium chloride will increase weight, extracellular volume, and glomerular filtration rate, with the reappearance of acidosis. The alkalosis is obviously related to contraction of the extracellular fluid volume, which stimulates aldosterone secretion. Patients with severe renal salt loss complain of orthostatic hypotonicity and exhibit signs of salt craving.

Calcium

Calcium concentration in the blood is normal or slightly reduced, while the rates of excretion of urinary calcium are variable, depending on the degree of acidosis, the state of bone mineralization, and the intakes of sodium [157] and vitamin D [258]. It was originally postulated [30, 296, 300] that there is an impairment in intestinal absorption of calcium in the Fanconi syndrome which might be responsible for the development of rickets. This concept could not be confirmed, however; oral calcium loading is followed by a rise of calcium in the plasma [321], and a high calcium diet renders the calcium balance positive [258]. Furthermore, the finding of normal parathormone activities [93] supports the latter view. The low rate of intestinal calcium absorption could even be explained in the reverse way; it could be an adaptive mechanism of the mucosa to the reduced uptake of calcium in the bone, which probably is caused by lack of available phosphate. An increase in plasma phosphate is followed by increased intestinal calcium absorption [191, 233]. It is still questionable whether the apparent skeletal resistance to vitamin D is due to a defect in the activation of vitamin D to its active metabolites or to the low phosphate. Treatment with 25-hydroxycholecalciferol or 1,25-dihydroxycholecalciferol has no advantage over treatment with ordinary vitamin D [10].

Secretion of Para-aminohippurate

Tubular secretion of para-aminohippurate (PAH) may be impaired in some patients with Fanconi syndrome out of proportion to the depressed glomerular filtration rate, especially in cystinosis [38, 42, 94, 331], in multiple myeloma [292], and in intoxications [41]. In other patients with equally severe tubular symptomatology, as in glycogenosis [13, 40, 188] or Wilson's disease [16], there is no such disproportionate impairment of PAH secretion, indicating differences in handling of PAH in these entities. The C_{PAH} and Tm_{PAH} are affected similarly, producing high values for filtration fraction (C_{In}/C_{PAH}) and very low fractional maximal PAH secretion (Tm_{PAH}/C_{In}), respec-

tively. Since renal extraction of PAH is extremely low in those cases [94], it cannot be used to estimate renal plasma flow.

Proteinuria

Almost all patients with the Fanconi syndrome have abnormal proteinuria, as indicated by the early name for the syndrome—nephrotic-glucosuric dwarfism [91]. Using more sophisticated methods for determining urinary protein, it became evident that there are at least three types of proteinuria that have to be differentiated: the first of prerenal origin, as in multiple myeloma; the second of glomerular origin, as occurs in later stages of cystinosis or chronic intoxications; and the third of tubular origin, which is derived either from the tubular cells or from impaired resorption of filtered proteins. The amount of tubular proteins excreted in the urine is markedly increased in generalized tubulopathies such as the Fanconi syndrome [11, 45, 79, 135, 138, 313]. The tubular proteins are characterized by low molecular weight (10,000 to 50,000) and electrophoretic mobility, mainly in the α-2 and β range. They represent a heterogeneous group of proteins including enzymes, immunoglobulin light chains, and small protein hormones. The clinical significance of tubular proteinuria is still uncertain.

Types of Fanconi Syndrome

Today the Fanconi syndrome is considered to represent a rather uniform response of the renal tubules to various exogenous and endogenous insults that initially do not affect the glomeruli. Although the underlying molecular or enzymatic changes are not well understood, different types of this syndrome can be classified according to their etiology and pathophysiology. The classification has therapeutic implications, since treatment may be different for the various types. Some of them represent hereditary errors of metabolism that can be distinguished by their genetic transmission. These therefore have to be included in the classification as markers of distinct disease entities. Age, however, seems not to be a discriminating factor; there are no basic differences between the Fanconi syndrome of infants or adults. There are, of course, certain diseases that do occur exclusively during infancy and childhood and never in adulthood, and vice versa, but the pathophysiology of the disease and the principles of treatment remain the same.

In Table 81-1 the different types of Fanconi syndrome are listed according to their etiology and pathogenesis. In this classification there are some uncertainties and possibly overlappings, due

Table 81-1. Types of Fanconi Syndrome

Primary
  Hereditary (AD, AR?, XLR?)
  Sporadic
Secondary
  In inborn errors of metabolism
    Cystinosis* (AR)
    Glycogenosis* (AR)
    Lowe's syndrome* (XLR)
    Galactosemia (uridyl transferase deficiency) (AR)
    Fructose intolerance (fructose 1-phosphate aldolase) (AR)
    Tyrosinemia (parahydroxyphenylpyruvic acid oxidase (?) (AR)
    Wilson's diease* (AR)
  In acquired diseases
    Multiple myeloma
    Nephrotic syndrome
    Transplanted kidney
  In intoxications
    Heavy metals (mercury, uranium, lead, cadmium)
    Maleic acid, Lysol
    Outdated tetracycline, methyl 3-chromone

* Enzymatic defect unknown.
Note: Inheritance is shown by AD = autosomal dominant; AR = autosomal recessive; XLR = X-linked recessive.

mainly to the fact that in some types neither the exact mechanism nor an enzymatic defect is known. Two main types are distinguished: the primary Fanconi syndrome and the secondary Fanconi syndrome. In the primary Fanconi syndrome no underlying cause or systemic disease is recognized; however, there is, of course, the possibility that these will be detected in the future. The primary type can occur as a hereditary disease or sporadically. In the secondary type, metabolites derived from inborn errors of metabolism, acquired diseases, or intoxications disturb processes that are responsible for normal tubular transport. In some diseases both kidney and other organs have the defective enzyme, while in others these are located only in extrarenal tissues. Recognition of these types is important, since it may influence the therapeutic approach.

No attempts are made in this classification to include all incomplete types of the Fanconi syndrome, in which at least one of the cardinal features (hyperaminoaciduria, glucosuria, reduced phosphate resorption, proximal tubular acidosis) is not apparent. Such cases probably represent two different groups, one of which may be incomplete expressions of the Fanconi syndrome in which the tubular disturbances are not fully developed. This state could be due to transitional stages of the disease, lesser toxicity of the dam-

aging metabolites, or higher resistance of some unknown intracellular mechanisms to the toxins. These conditions therefore have to be considered as formes frustes of the Fanconi syndrome. They are found in intoxications leading only to gluco-hyperaminoaciduria or in the Luder-Sheldon syndrome, which may later turn out to be a fully developed Fanconi syndrome [291], such a sequential appearance of symptoms being not uncommon [34]. The other group of incomplete Fanconi syndrome types seems to represent defects of more than one specific carrier system of the tubular cell membrane. Their pathophysiology is different from the first group and comparable with that of the primary tubulopathies. This is probably true for glucoglycinuria [173], glucophosphaturia [75], or even glucoaminoaciduria [239]. Both groups have to be observed with special scrutiny, since they could give keys for a better understanding of the basic pathophysiology in the Fanconi syndromes.

PRIMARY FANCONI SYNDROME
The primary type of the Fanconi syndrome is diagnosed by exclusion of all known causes leading to the secondary appearance of the syndrome. It was first considered to occur only in adults, in whom more than 40 cases have been reported [18, 190, 219, 221, 296, 316, 321]. From the histories of those cases, however, it was obvious that in some the symptoms had started early in life [316], which meant that the primary Fanconi syndrome could also occur in children. Indeed, since 1961 reports have appeared in the literature describing children with the primary Fanconi syndrome [55, 157, 167, 234, 291], and it has to be assumed that a few of the original cases described by de Toni [77, 78], Debré et al. [72], Fanconi [91], and McCune et al. [217] might also have been primary. However, this possibility is difficult to assess from the old case reports, as it is difficult today to classify reported cases properly. This problem can be demonstrated by the history of twin girls first described by Luder and Sheldon [206] as having familial glucoaminoaciduria; their father and grandfather were suspected of having the same disease. Six years later the follow-up in these patients was reported by Sheldon [291]. In the interval, both girls had developed hypophosphatemic rickets and had now to be considered as having complete Fanconi syndrome (see also reference 328). Thirteen years later their father had gone into chronic renal failure and both girls were also showing slightly reduced rates of glomerular filtration [49]. This family history demonstrates how important long-term observa-

tions are in order to avoid drawing false conclusions prematurely.

The primary type of Fanconi syndrome is not age specific; it may occur at any age and can continue over a long life. Some cases are familial with an autosomal dominant trait [18, 164, 206, 291], an autosomal recessive trait [167], or even an X-linked recessive trait [234]; but most of them occur sporadically without any evidence of inheritance [34, 36, 55, 157, 191]. The primary type is certainly a heterogeneous group and will remain so as long as the enzymatic defects in the tubular cell are unknown. It has to be kept in mind that many of these apparently primary types may really be secondary types in which the extrarenal cause has not been detected.

The children usually present with the history of failure to thrive, anorexia, polydipsia and polyuria, episodes of vomiting, dehydration and unexplained fever, rickets despite adequate supplementation with vitamin D, and growth retardation. There is moderate to severe metabolic acidosis with low bicarbonate and hyperchloremia, hypokalemia, hypophosphatemia, and urinary findings of hyperaminoaciduria and glucosuria. The glomerular filtration rate is usually normal, but it may decline later in the course. Tubular PAH secretion is not severely affected.

Reports on renal morphology are rare. In one renal biopsy [157], no specific alterations could be detected by light microscopy. Three members of a family with idiopathic Fanconi syndrome revealed changes of interstitial nephritis, but specific lesions could be detected neither by light microscopy nor by electron microscopy [234]. In an autopsy specimen, marked changes in the tubular epithelium and interstitium were found [164]. Zones of tubular atrophy associated with interstitial fibrosis and lymphocytic infiltration alternated with areas of tubular dilatation. In our own observation of a 7-year-old girl with the idiopathic Fanconi syndrome, the renal biopsy showed dilatation of the tubules on light microscopy. The diameters of the tubules measured up to 300 μ, which means that some were as wide as Bowman's capsules (see reference 37). The proximal tubular epithelium was partly swollen and contained a fine granular material, while other parts were completely normal. On electron microscopy grossly enlarged mitochondria were found that contained laterally or marginally dislocated cristae and occasional electron-dense material [37].

The prognosis is variable but may be uncertain in regard to life expectancy. Some patients develop chronic renal insufficiency in a period of 10 to 30 years [36, 49, 164, 191].

Treatment is nonspecific (see under Principles of Treatment), the response depending on the severity of the tubular defects. In some cases it seems to be impossible to compensate adequately for the excessive loss of bicarbonate and phosphate, and consequently acidosis and bone changes persist. Kidney transplantation has been reported in one case [36]. Although this maternal renal allograft was functioning well after 24 months, the patient had developed all the renal symptoms of the Fanconi syndrome; there was no evidence of rejection. This finding suggests that the basic abnormality in this patient with primary Fanconi syndrome was indeed extrarenal and that the kidney was only affected secondarily. Again, the search for metabolites causing the Fanconi syndrome has to continue in each case of the primary type.

CYSTINOSIS

Cystinosis, or cystine storage disease, is a rare metabolic disease inherited as an autosomal recessive trait and characterized by intracellular accumulation of free cystine in many organs, including the kidney. The cystine is thought to accumulate in lysosomes [163, 245], but the primary enzymatic defect is still unknown. It seems likely that the patients are unable to maintain cystine in its reduced form in their cells (for more details see references 182, 279, 283, 285). Cystinosis has to be distinguished from cystinuria, which is a completely different disorder with no deposition of cystine in the tissues and no Fanconi syndrome (see Chap. 86).

There are different types of cystinosis, depending on the degree of involvement of certain organ systems: infantile (nephropathic) cystinosis is the most severe, with progressive tubular and later glomerular impairment leading to renal insufficiency in early life [26, 28, 42, 267, 331]. The adolescent (intermediate) type is characterized by a mild nephropathy presenting clinical signs in the second decade of life and progressing slowly [116, 151]. The adult (benign) type of cystinosis seems to have no renal involvement, with cystine crystals located only in the cornea, bone marrow, and leukocytes [43, 62, 198, 281].

The diagnosis of cystinosis can be made (1) shortly after birth, by determining the cystine content of leukocytes or fibroblasts, in which it is elevated up to eighty to one hundred times normal [278], and (2) later, by detection of pigment degeneration in the retina [327] and of cystine crystals in the bone marrow, lymph nodes, conjunctiva, or rectal mucosa [149]. Crystals can be seen in the cornea by slit lamp examination. Occasionally an early morphologic diagnosis can be achieved only by electron microscopy ([324]; author's observation). A prenatal diagnosis is also possible by finding increased concentration of cystine in amniotic fluid cells [280].

The clinical signs of Fanconi syndrome do not appear in cystinosis before the age of 3 to 6 months, when affected infants start with episodes of unexplained fever, vomiting, anorexia, and polydipsia; they show signs of dehydration, failure to thrive, and rickets. They usually are blond due to a defect in melanin synthesis. The tubular defects develop at the same age [26, 42, 127, 267, 331], at which time the glomerular filtration rate is still normal. Generalized hyperaminoaciduria is massive; however, cystine excretion is not more prominent than in other types of Fanconi syndrome. Glucosuria is only mild to moderate, phosphate resorption is severely impaired, and the bicarbonate threshold is significantly lowered. The excretion of nonaminated organic acids is markedly increased [275]. The renal PAH secretion is severely reduced very early [38, 42, 94, 331], the renal extraction of PAH being minimal [94]. At this stage the tubular dysfunctions present a mortal danger for the patient, since the high glomerular filtration rates can provoke rapid decompensation of electrolyte and fluid homeostasis (electrolyte crisis). The plasma amino acids are generally within the normal range, although cystine and proline may be slightly increased in the later stages of the disease. The glomerular filtration rate falls progressively, and chronic renal insufficiency develops within the first decade of life. At this time the tubular symptoms become less prominent, and the hyperaminoaciduria, with its typical pattern, may disappear completely. Children in the end stage of nephropathic cystinosis show very severe growth retardation [299] and may develop signs of hypothyroidism [50].

The kidneys are found to be without any characteristic changes in the very early phases of cystinosis. In more advanced stages, renal biopsy specimens examined by light and electron microscopy reveal severe though mainly nonspecific alterations of both tubules and glomeruli as seen by light and electron microscopy [168, 294]. The proximal and distal tubules are altered to about the same degree. They show irregularities with marked differences in caliber as well as variations in size and shape. Many cells are swollen with pleomorphic, often clustered nuclei; others are small and flattened. The appearance of the glomeruli varies considerably. Epithelial cells are prominent, with occasional formation of peripheral multinucleated clusters. The interstitium shows a variable degree of focal increase in fibrous tissue that is not associated with significant inflammatory reactions. Groups of birefringent crystals are seen in the interstitial tissue between the tubules but are sometimes recognizable only by electron microscopy [324]. In addition, unusual dark cells are visible that probably contain a reaction product of osmium tetroxide and cystine. In the tubular cells, however, cystine crystals can scarcely be detected [293, 324]. In far-advanced stages of cystinosis the kidneys are small and contracted and the majority of glomeruli are sclerosed, with interstitial fibrosis dominating. By microdissection the so-called swan neck lesion can be demonstrated, which is an atrophy and shortening of the proximal tubuli just beneath the glomeruli [58, 70]. This lesion is not specific for cystinosis, as it may be found in other types of Fanconi syndrome and in chronic interstitial nephritis. By correlating the functional and morphologic disturbances, it is evident that the pathophysiology precedes considerably the pathomorphology.

Treatment of cystinosis can only be symptomatic (see under Principles of Treatment). Trials with low methionine and low cystine diets [14, 54, 275, 289] have been disappointing [31, 67, 267]. Neither penicillamine [59, 131] nor anabolic hormones [318] has long-term effectiveness. Cystine can be mobilized in vitro by dithiothreitol [115] and ascorbic acid [183], and therapeutic trials with these agents are underway.

For patients with end stage disease, hemodialysis and kidney transplantation are recommended. Hemodialysis does not succeed in removing excess cystine from the organism [207]. Renal transplantation is successful [36, 130, 205, 208], although cystine accumulates again in the transplanted kidney. The cystine reaccumulation occurs in a different fashion than before, however, and so far there are no reports of the Fanconi syndrome reappearing in the transplanted kidney. This is an indication that the principal pathophysiology of the kidney damage is not cystine overloading per se; rather, it may be related to an enzymatic defect within the tubular cells. The ultimate outcome of transplanted patients is still uncertain; there may be late sequelae of the disease (eye, brain) that so far have not been observed.

GLYCOGENOSIS WITH FANCONI SYNDROME

The great majority of patients with glycogen storage disease do not develop the Fanconi syndrome [142, 158, 232]. The enzymatic defect in those patients who do develop Fanconi syndrome has not been identified. However, it is clear that these cases do not belong to any one of the nine or ten known types of glycogenosis, and especially not to type I (hepatic glucose 6-phosphatase deficiency [143]), as claimed by some. It seems to be a special type of glycogenosis in which both liver and kidneys are involved in the enzymatic or membrane transport defect. It is inherited as an autosomal recessive trait. Since glucose resorption is most severely affected in these cases, it has been proposed that the condition be called renal glucose-losing syndrome in order to distinguish it from other types of Fanconi syndrome [40].

At least 10 patients with glycogenosis and the Fanconi syndrome have been reported in the literature, most of them from Europe [13, 40, 92, 95, 108, 188, 237, 264]. Their disease is characterized by the combination of hepatic accumulation of glycogen (more than 8 gm/100 gm wet tissue) and a severe renal Fanconi syndrome. First symptoms have been recognized as early as $1\frac{1}{2}$ months of age [108], at which time the Fanconi syndrome but not the hepatomegaly is present. The symptoms of the Fanconi syndrome are usually pronounced and include all the characteristic laboratory findings. Hyperaminoaciduria is massive (see Fig. 81-3 and patient B. S. in Figs. 81-1 and 81-4), and phosphate resorption is severely impaired (see B. S. in Figs. 81-7 to 81-10), resulting in rickets, osteoporosis, and growth retardation. The acidosis is moderate to severe and the excretion of organic nonaminated acids is greatly increased; however, the tubular secretion of PAH is not affected.

The most disturbed function in glycogenosis with Fanconi syndrome is glucose resorption (see B. S. in Figs. 81-5 and 81-6). The rates of glucose excretion in several of these patients are listed in Table 81-2. They are certainly higher than in other types of Fanconi syndrome or renal glucosurias. These high rates occur while the patients are normoglycemic or even hypoglycemic. The ratio of endogenous glucose clearance to inulin clearance (C_G/C_{In}) in our case stayed constantly at 0.7 and did not change under glucose loads between 50 and 350 mg/min/1.73 m^2. These values indicate that only 30 percent of filtered glucose is reabsorbed, which could possibly occur by nonactive processes. Fellers et al. [95], comparing the glucose loss in these patients with the effects of phlorhizin, called this syndrome pseudophlorhizin diabetes. We prefer the term *renal glucose-losing* syndrome [40]. Glucose tolerance tests show curves similar to those seen in diabetes; glucagon produces only a slight increase in blood glucose but a steep increase in renal glucose excretion. Galactose tolerance is also impaired. Blood lactate is often found to be normal or only slightly increased; often there is ketonemia and ketonuria.

The morphologic findings are disappointing in view of the severe pathophysiologic changes; there is some glycogen accumulation in the proximal tubules and ascending limb of Henle's loop, but it is not as severe as in type I glycogenosis. Electron microscopy reveals giant mitochondria in the proximal tubular cells; the triple-layered mitochondrial cristae are displaced and found just beside the membrane [37]. In addition, there are many glycogen granules visible in nuclei and cytoplasm. The glomeruli are not essentially altered.

The treatment of glycogenosis with Fanconi syndrome is symptomatic (see under Principles of Treatment), there being no specific therapy available. Hypoglycemia has to be treated with frequent protein-enriched feedings. The prognosis

Table 81-2. Maximal Urinary Glucose Excretion in Glycogenosis with Fanconi Syndrome (Renal Glucose-losing Syndrome)

Author	Patient's Age (yr)	Maximum U_G (gm/100 ml)	$U_G V$ gm/24 hr	$U_G V$ gm/24 hr/ 1.73 m^2
Fanconi and Bickel [92]	4	6.0	64	240
Rotthauwe et al. [264]	4	5.8	55	206
Odièvre [237]				
Patient R. L.	2	?	50	210
Patient B. B.	6	?	21	74 (average)
Lampert and Mayer [188]	4	8.0	73	230
Bauer [13]	5	?	53	178
Brodehl et al. [40]	1	5.4	43	200
Garty et al. [108]	3	?	35–50	173

Note: U_G = urinary glucose concentration; $U_G V$ = rate of excretion of glucose.

of this type of Fanconi syndrome is fairly good as long as acute decompensation during infections or surgical procedures (even as minor as a liver biopsy) can be prevented by intravenous administration of alkali and fluid. There seems to be no impairment of glomerular filtration, and the tubular defects tend to improve with age. Our patient has been under observation for 10 years and is doing well; and the original patient described by Fanconi and Bickel [92] is reported to be enjoying an active life [26a].

OCULOCEREBRORENAL DYSTROPHY (LOWE)

The oculocerebrorenal syndrome, first reported by Lowe and coworkers [203] in 1952, is characterized by congenital changes in the eyes (cataract, glaucoma, buphthalmos), cerebral dysfunction leading to severe mental retardation, muscular hypotonicity and hyporeflexia, and functional abnormalities of the kidney. The last findings are initially those of the Fanconi syndrome; later there is impairment of glomerular filtration rate with acidosis, rickets, and growth retardation. The underlying metabolic defect is unknown. It is transmitted as an X-linked recessive trait appearing almost exclusively in males. A few females have been reported [269, 304]; however, their disease can be explained by Lion's hypothesis. In the mothers of affected boys a higher incidence of

cataracts [321] and corneal opacities [256] has been reported, although this finding has not been confirmed [147]. More than 100 cases of oculocerebrorenal dystrophy have been reported in the literature.

The Fanconi syndrome is usually not very severe. Hyperaminoaciduria is a constant finding. It usually appears after the first few months of life [132] and tends to decrease after the sixth year [1, 132, 210]. The pattern of hyperaminoaciduria is generalized, although the dibasic aminoacids ornithine, lysine, and arginine seem to be relatively more involved than the others, as reported first by Jagenburg [169]. This finding was confirmed in six cases studied by short-term amino acid clearance techniques in our laboratory [210], as shown in Fig. 81-11. The resorption of arginine seems to be most affected. Whether or not this is of any significance with regard to the underlying metabolic defect remains doubtful. It has been postulated [284] that this syndrome may be related to defective ornithine metabolism, since ornithine loading produced an increase in hyperaminoaciduria in one propositus and his mother. In another family, however, ornithine had the same effect on the propositus and his father [215], and Chutorian and Rowland [56] have shown that ornithine and other amino acids could do the same in a patient with Wilson's disease. It was concluded, therefore, that ornithine has only a nonspecific ef-

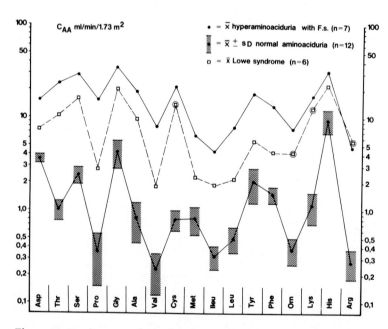

Figure 81-11. Average values of amino acid clearance rates in six children with Lowe syndrome [210] compared with normal rates [39] and with children with generalized hyperaminoaciduria due to various other causes (see Fig. 81-3). Dibasic amino acids and cystine are relatively more involved in the Lowe syndrome.

fect. The intestinal absorption of dibasic amino acids also seems to be impaired [5, 12, 63], since those amino acids are found in increased amounts in the stool. The plasma amino acids are within the normal range.

Glucosuria is usually only slight and intermittently detectable in oculocerebrorenal dystrophy. The defect in phosphate resorption is variable, but it can be very pronounced [306]. The tubular acidosis is due mainly to proximal bicarbonate wasting related to extracellular volume, as shown by Oetliker and Rossi [240] in two patients with Lowe's syndrome. Excretion of organic acid, mainly citric acid, is also increased [166]. Proteinuria is often present from early infancy, and it can become so pronounced that the nephrotic syndrome develops. In this stage glomerular filtration rate usually is reduced; further deterioration can lead to chronic renal insufficiency.

The morphology of the kidney in the early stage of oculocerebrorenal dystrophy is normal on light microscopy [308, 325]. Electron microscopy, however, reveals very early distinct changes in the glomeruli; these consist of slight swelling of the endothelial cells, with vacuolization, thickening, and splitting in the capillary basement membranes and fusion of the epithelial foot processes [308]. In the proximal tubules shortening of the brush borders is seen; there is also enlargement of the mitochondria and distortion or complete disappearance of mitochondrial cristae [242, 269]. In later stages, advanced glomerular changes with membrane thickening, increased glomerular cellularity, and glomerular fibrosis are observed; there is also scattered thickening of renal tubular basement membranes, multifocal tubular atrophy with dilatation, and interstitial fibrosis [126, 256, 308, 325]. Microdissection has revealed no swan neck abnormalities, but segmental dilatation in the distal convoluted tubule has been seen [308].

The treatment of oculocerebrorenal dystrophy is symptomatic (see under Prinicples of Treatment), since no specific therapy is available. It is directed mainly toward correcting acidosis and treating rickets. In the natural course of the disease three stages are recognized: (1) in the early infantile stage the major problems are related to the eyes and central nervous system; (2) in the next stage, from late infancy to middle childhood, the metabolic abnormalities due to the Fanconi syndrome are prominent; (3) these metabolic abnormalities are disappearing in the last stage, in which patients may die from renal insufficiency or intercurrent infection. No attempts at maintenance dialysis or renal transplantation have been reported, probably because mental retardation is usually so severe.

GALACTOSEMIA

Galactosemia is an inherited disease of galactose metabolism transmitted as an autosomal recessive trait; it is due to deficient activity of galactose 1-phosphate uridyltransferase. This enzyme catalyzes the reaction of galactose 1-phosphate with uridine-diphosphate glucose (UDP-glucose) to give UDP-galactose and glucose 1-phosphate (for more details see references 81, 159, 288). With deficient activity of this enzyme, galactose 1-phosphate cannot be converted to glucose, and consequently, when galactose is ingested in the form of milk lactose, it accumulates and produces toxic alterations in many tissues, mainly in liver, brain, kidney, and lens. The clinical features in untreated patients are hepatomegaly with jaundice, mental retardation, renal tubular syndromes, and bilateral cataracts. These signs are not seen in variants of galactosemia.

Early detection of transferase deficiency is possible in newborns [25, 124], in whom the incidence ranges from 1 in 18,000 to 1 in 110,000 [213].

Galactosemia can also be produced by galactokinase deficiency (galactokinase catalyzes the first step of galactose to galactose 1-phosphate). In order to differentiate the two types, one is termed *transferase deficiency galactosemia* and the other *galactokinase deficiency galactosemia* [288]. The latter defect is not associated with liver, kidney, or brain damage but only with bilateral cataracts [113, 223], suggesting that accumulation of galactose 1-phosphate plays a role in the pathogenesis of the disturbances in transferase deficiency galactosemia.

The clinical expression of galactosemia is variable [161]. It may appear after a week of milk intake in newborn babies as an acute intoxication leading to anorexia, vomiting, diarrhea, severe jaundice with hepatomegaly and hypoprothrombinemia, and cerebral symptoms suggesting septicemia [139, 161, 165, 175, 303]. On the other hand, the course may be more protracted, with failure to thrive, development of cataracts, hepatomegaly, and mental retardation; in a few cases the disorder is discovered only by chance.

The renal symptoms start early in the disease. They are characterized by hyperaminoaciduria, impaired phosphate and possibly bicarbonate resorption, tubular proteinuria, and slight to moderate reduction of the glomerular filtration rate. There is a generalized pattern of hyperaminoacid-

Table 81-3. Renal Function in a 6-month-old Boy[a] with Transferase Deficiency Galactosemia in Whom Treatment Was Started July 10, 1966

Measure of Function	Normal		July 4, 1966	July 28, 1966	September 21, 1966
C_{In} (ml/min/1.73 m²)	99	± 18[b]	44	66	80
C_{PAH} (ml/min/1.73 m²)	437	± 87[b]	156	352	347
FF (C_{In}/C_{PAH}) (%)	22.9	± 1.9[b]	28.2	18.8	23.0
C_P (ml/min/1.73 m²)	14.9	± 3.9[c]	12.1	13.1	19.1
T_P (mg/min/1.73 m²)	3.49	± 1.31[c]	1.28	3.01	3.96
T_P/C_{In} (μg/ml)	47.2	± 6.6[c]	28.0	45.6	49.5
T_{mG} (mg/min/1.73 m²)	213	± 71[d]	114	221	233
T_{mG}/C_{In} (mg/ml)	2.9	± 0.7[d]	2.0	2.3	2.6

[a] Patient R.N., born July 1, 1966.
[b] Normal values in author's laboratory for infants 3 to 12 months ($\overline{X} \pm$ S.D.).
[c] Normal values of author's laboratory for infants 2 weeks to 12 months ($\overline{X} \pm$ S.D.).
[d] Normal values for infants 2 to 24 weeks (Brodehl et al. [38a].)
Note: C_{In} = insulin clearance; C_{PAH} = para-aminohippurate clearance; FF = filtration fraction; C_P = phosphate clearance; T_P = tubular resorption of phosphate; T_{mG} = maximum tubular glucose resorption.

uria [29, 68, 69, 150]. The degree of hyperaminoaciduria is usually not as severe as it is in cystinosis or glycogen storage disease (see Fig. 81-3), although the reduction in tubular resorption may be considerable. My findings in a 6-month-old infant with transferase deficiency galactosemia before and after treatment are given in Table 81-3 (renal functions) and Fig. 81-12 (amino acid resorption). Levels of amino acids

in plasma are not elevated, unless there is severe hepatic failure [309]. As can be seen, the glomerular filtration rate and C_{PAH} are significantly reduced, the latter relatively more and leading to an increase in filtration fraction. The tubular resorption of phosphate, especially T_p/C_{In}, is significantly reduced, reflected by the plasma phosphate of 4.0 mg per deciliter, which is low for the age. The tubular resorption of glucose, however,

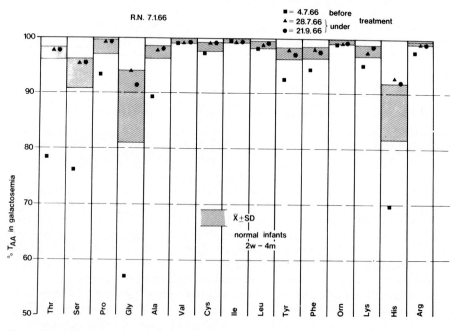

Figure 81-12. Percentage of tubular amino acid resorption in an infant with transferase deficiency galactosemia before and after dietary treatment (see also Tables 81-4, 81-5). (Normal values from Brodehl and Gellissen [39].)

seems not to be impaired, which corresponds with the fact that mellituria in galactosemic infants is due exclusively to galactosuria [69]. Therefore, nonspecific reducing tests (Benedict's test, Clinitest tablets) are positive in the urine, while specific glucose tests (Clinistix, Combistix) remain negative. After starting treatment with a galactosefree diet, all renal symptoms improve rapidly (Table 81-3 and Fig. 81-12). It takes about 1 to 2 weeks for the hyperaminoaciduria to develop after exposing the child to galactose [68, 175] and a similar period to normalize amino acid excretion after discontinuing galactose intake [160, 175]. This time course is longer than in hereditary fructose intolerance.

Proteinuria is a constant finding in untreated patients with transferase-deficiency galactosemia [175]. It is of the tubular type and improves shortly after starting a galactose-free diet [45]. Metabolic acidosis is probably due to diminished bicarbonate resorption [175], although studies to document this have not been reported. In acutely ill patients, acidosis may also be due to intestinal loss of alkali.

Thus the overt tubular symptoms of transferase deficiency galactosemia are hyperaminoaciduria and proteinuria; the defects in phosphate and possibly in bicarbonate resorption and of tubular PAH secretion can be recognized only by special investigations. Glucose resorption seems to be either not affected or only minimally so; therefore the Fanconi syndrome in galactosemia is incomplete and not fully developed. Yet galactosemia is included in this list because the pathophysiology of its development and reversal are typical of the secondary types of the Fanconi syndrome.

In experimental studies in rats high galactose intake was shown to produce hyperaminoaciduria; however, the pattern was different from that in human galactosemia [262]. The oxidation of glucose in kidney slices is not inhibited by galactose. In human beings the infusion of 10% galactose solution was followed by an increase in the excretion of phosphate and amino acids, which was not seen with xylose [100]. Whether or not the mechanisms responsible for this effect are comparable to those in transferase deficiency remains questionable (see reference 159).

The treatment of galactosemia consists in elimination of galactose from the diet, which is relatively simple, since galactose is not an essential nutrient. It is accomplished primarily by avoiding milk and milk products [80], following which all symptoms of galactose intoxication disappear and normal physical growth and development are achieved. Mental development, however, may depend on the degree of intrauterine damage due to fetal exposure to galactose.

HEREDITARY FRUCTOSE INTOLERANCE

Hereditary fructose intolerance is a familial disorder of fructose metabolism that is transmitted as an autosomal recessive trait due to deficient activity of fructose 1-phosphate aldolase [103, 246]. This enzyme catalyzes the splitting of fructose 1-phosphate to D-glyceraldehyde and phosphodihydroxyacetone. With deficiency of this enzyme, fructose 1-phosphate cannot be metabolized and consequently accumulates in those tissues that normally extract fructose briskly and convert it to glucose; in liver, kidney, and small bowel, excess fructose 1-phosphate exerts its toxic effects by blocking other enzyme systems. Ingestion of fructose, therefore, is followed by severe, life-threatening attacks of vomiting, hypoglycemia, and coma in patients with fructose intolerance, especially in infants. Chronic fructose ingestion leads to failure to thrive, vomiting, hepatomegaly with jaundice progressing to liver cirrhosis, and renal dysfunction; the condition may end in cachexia and death. Patients beyond infancy seem to increase their tolerance for fructose. They usually develop a strong aversion to fruits and sweets, thereby avoiding intoxication. Hereditary fructose intolerance has to be differentiated from essential fructosuria (fructose kinase deficiency), galactosefructose intolerance, and hereditary fructose 1,6-diphosphatase deficiency. With the exception of one report [9], none of these produces renal dysfunction.

Disturbance of renal function in hereditary fructose intolerance consists mainly of hyperaminoaciduria, proximal tubular acidosis, and proteinuria. Hyperaminoaciduria was first mentioned in the original report by Froesch et al. [105] in 1957 and was especially emphasized by Levin et al. [195] in 1963. It is of renal origin and of a generalized pattern [170, 193, 196]. However, in severe hepatic involvement, plasma amino acids may be elevated also, especially tyrosine and methionine, and the urinary pattern may be misinterpreted as acute tyrosinosis [122, 200]. The onset of hyperaminoaciduria after exposure to fructose is rapid, almost instantaneous [196, 226, 228, 229]; normalization of amino acid excretion after a fructose-free diet occurs within 2 weeks [195, 196].

Glucosuria is usually absent or mild [195, 196]. Measurements of maximal tubular glucose resorption are not known to the author. Fructose is excreted only when the patient is exposed to it. Phosphate resorption may be disturbed in this syndrome, as suggested by hypophosphatemia with chronic sucrose ingestion [196]. Acute fructose loading is followed by a sharp decline in plasma phosphate level. This is produced by a rapid phosphate uptake by those tissues that accumulate fructose 1-phosphate and are unable to metabolize it further. Phosphate excretion is not increased after acute fructose loading [229, 247] but remains unchanged or is even decreased. Rickets has not been reported in this syndrome. Proteinuria can also be related to the acute intoxicating effect of fructose [196].

The most striking effect of fructose loading is the prompt alteration in renal acidification [226, 228, 229]. Acute fructose loading produces a 20 to 30 percent reduction in tubular bicarbonate resorption at normal plasma bicarbonate levels and a reduction of maximal bicarbonate resorption (Tm_{HCO_3}); in moderately severe acidosis, however, bicarbonate disappears from the urine and normal pH minima can be achieved. These findings are typical of proximal tubular acidosis and are in agreement with the clinical observations of severe metabolic acidosis in acutely ill infants [105, 193, 196, 200]. In adults, chronic tubular acidosis may lead to nephrocalcinosis and urolithiasis [144, 212], although these are expected to be found in the distal type of tubular acidosis.

The acute proximal tubular effects of fructose in hereditary fructose intolerance can be explained by the enzymatic composition of the proximal tubule cells. It can be shown that only the proximal tubules, along with liver and small intestine, contain the whole set of fructokinase, fructose 1-phosphate aldolase, and triokinase enzymes and are therefore capable of rapidly converting fructose to glucose. The renal medulla lacks this enzymatic system [179, 231]. Therefore, if fructose is given to patients with aldolase deficiency, only the proximal tubular cells are enriched with fructose 1-phosphate, while the distal tubular cells are not involved. These biochemical events correspond to the clinical findings and provide a fascinating model for the pathogenetic mechanisms by which tubular disturbances can be produced.

Treatment of hereditary fructose intolerance is simple as soon as the diagnosis is established and the acute phase of intoxication is overcome [104]. It consists in omission of all fructose- and sucrose-containing foods and sweets; most patients beyond infancy have developed a strong aversion to sucrose and avoid foods containing it. Affected newborns and young infants should never be exposed to foods or infusions containing fructose or sucrose [104].

HEREDITARY TYROSINEMIA
Hereditary tyrosinemia is a familial disorder of tyrosine metabolism; it is transmitted as an autosomal recessive trait and apparently is due to a deficiency in *p*-hydroxyphenylpyruvic acid oxidase, which normally catalyzes the second step in tyrosine oxidation, the oxidation of *p*-hydroxyphenylpyruvic acid to homogentisic acid. It is still undecided, however, whether hereditary tyrosinemia represents a nosologic entity or, instead, a syndrome in which the alleged enzyme defect is not primary but secondary to other unknown metabolic defects (see references 186, 285). There are reports of cases with unusual features that do not fit into the typical clinical picture [9, 109, 146, 148, 312]. Hereditary tyrosinemia, however, can be differentiated clearly from the transient neonatal hypertyrosinemia and from the benign "tyrosinosis" originally described by Medes [218] in 1932. There are various names used synonymously to describe the clinical condition of hereditary tyrosinemia, including tyrosyluria with hypermethioninemia, hypermethioninemia, tryosinosis, tyrosinose congenitale, and hepatorenal dysfunction.

Hereditary tyrosinemia is expressed clinically in two types, acute and chronic. Symptoms in the acute type start very early in infancy with severe metabolic disturbances, including jaundice, hepatomegaly, vomiting, melena, ascites, edema, and sepsis-like fever. Death occurs rapidly in hepatic failure in most untreated patients [129, 189, 244, 248].

The chronic type of hereditary tyrosinemia is characterized by the appearance of symptoms in childhood, with failure to thrive, rickets resistant to vitamin D, growth retardation, nodular liver cirrhosis, hypoglycemic attacks associated with hypertrophied islets of Langerhans, and, in some cases, mild to moderate mental retardation [7, 110, 129, 192, 248, 271]. Death occurs mostly in acute exacerbations of electrolyte and water disturbance, liver cirrhosis, or hepatoma, but not in chronic renal insufficiency. Biochemically the disease is characterized by high plasma levels of tyrosine, sometimes accompanied by high plasma methionine and by urinary excretion of large amounts of tyrosyl compounds (mainly *p*-hydroxyphenyllactic acid, pHP-pyruvic acid, and pHP-acetic acid).

The renal symptoms in hereditary tyrosinemia are usually severe, especially in the later stage, and

Table 81-4. *Clearance Values in a 5-week-old Infant (R. S.) with Tyrosinemia*

Clearance Value	Patient R. S.	Normal
C_{In} (ml/min/1.73 m^2)	78	63 ± 17[a]
C_{PAH} (ml/min/1.73 m^2)	168	257 ± 67[a]
FF (C_{In}/C_{PAH}) (%)	46.7	24.4 ± 3.1[a]
C_p (ml/min/1.73 m^2)	25.2	14.9 ± 3.9[b]
TRP (%)	67.7	78 ± 8
T_p (mg/min/1.73 m^2)	1.67	3.49 ± 1.31[b]
T_p/C_{In} (μg/ml)	21.6	47.2 ± 6.6[b]
Glucosuria	2.5 mg/dl	

[a] Normal values in author's laboratory for infants 0 to 3 months ($\overline{X}$ ± S.D.).
[b] Normal values in author's laboratory for infants 2 weeks to 12 months ($\overline{X}$ ± S.D.).
Note: C_{In} = inulin clearance; C_{PAH} = para-aminohippurate clearance; FF = filtration fraction; C_p = phosphate clearance. TRP = percent tubular resorption of phosphate; T_p = tubular resorption of phosphate.

Table 81-5. *Clearance Values for Free Amino Acids in a 5-week-old Infant with Tyrosinemia (R. S.)*[*]

Amino Acid	P_{AA} (mg/100 ml)	C_{AA} (ml/min/ 1.73 m^2)	T_{AA} (%)
Asp	0.21	19.4	75.2
Thr	3.73	9.1	88.3
Ser	1.36	15.6	80.0
Pro	2.64	2.3	97.0
Gly	1.94	23.3	70.1
Ala	2.30	3.9	95.0
Val	1.14	0.5	99.3
(Cys)$_2$	1.20	4.7	94.0
Met	6.00	0.4	99.5
Tyr	19.48	1.9	97.5
Phe	1.25	1.5	98.1
Orn	1.33	1.1	98.6
Lys	4.68	4.5	94.2
His	0.96	18.9	75.8
Arg	1.79	0.5	99.3

[*] Very low excretion rates for isoleucine and leucine. See also Table 81-4.
Note: P_{AA} = plasma concentrations amino acids; C_{AA} = amino acid clearance; T_{AA} = percent tubular resorption of amino acid.

present the fully developed Fanconi syndrome. Glomerular filtration rates are reported to be normal ([272]; see Table 81-4).

Hyperaminoaciduria in the acute stage reflects both the tubular defect and the increased plasma amino acids that occur in acute liver damage ([7, 109, 189]; author's unpublished observation). As a consequence, the typical pattern of generalized hyperaminoaciduria may be obscured. In a 5-week-old infant observed by us, methionine and tyrosine were reabsorbed as completely as normal, despite the fact that they were elevated ten to twenty times normal, indicating that there is no real "overflow" hyperaminoaciduria (see Table 81-5). In later stages the hyperaminoaciduria is generalized but is still overlapped by high tyrosine excretion [110, 271, 272], since plasma tyrosine remains elevated, sometimes accompanied by high methionine. In high doses, vitamin D is reported to improve the lowered resorption rate of free amino acids to a certain extent [110]. Dietary treatment with low phenylalanine and tyrosine may be followed by complete normalization (vide infra). In some cases increased excretion of δ-aminolevulinic acid was described [111, 172], which otherwise is found in lead poisoning and intermittent porphyria. The pathophysiologic relevance is unknown.

Glucosuria is mild and can sometimes be detected only intermittently [110, 192, 236, 272]. Plasma glucose levels often are low. The tubular resorption of phosphate is severely impaired, even in the acute stage (Table 81-4). Plasma phosphate levels are low, and vitamin-D-resistant

rickets is one of the most prominent clinical signs beyond early infancy [6, 110, 236, 272]. Acidification defects have not been intensively investigated, but their presence can be deduced from the severe metabolic acidosis encountered in this syndrome.

Proteinuria is of tubular origin and is mostly mild [110, 192, 272]. The urinary concentrating capacity can be severely impaired due to vasopressin (Pitressin) resistance of the distal tubules [110, 192, 272], and this resistance may be aggravated by renal potassium loss.

The kidneys are enlarged on radiography and at autopsy, mostly due to interstitial edema and marked dilatation of the tubules [110, 244, 251]. Glomeruli are occasionally found to be hyalinized, and the tubules show degenerative alterations, atrophy, and dystrophic calcification. Renal biopsy specimens show dilated proximal tubules with swelling and vacuolization of the epithelium [6].

Treatment with the low phenylalanine and tyrosine diet first reported by Halvorsen and Gjessing [128] produces dramatic improvement in hereditary tyrosinemia: plasma tyrosine drops to normal levels, tyrosyluria stops, and all tubular symptoms can revert to normal [6, 88, 134, 145, 236, 273]. The final prognosis, however, depends on the degree of liver dysfunction when treatment is started. There are cases, especially the acute forms, in which treatment no longer has any beneficial effect. The response to treatment indicates that some unknown metabolites related to tyrosine are responsible for the severe changes in the liver and tubular cells that occur when these patients receive tyrosine in excess of their needs.

WILSON'S DISEASE

Wilson's disease (hepatolenticular degeneration) is a familial disease of copper metabolism that is inherited as an autosomal recessive trait. The primary enzymatic defect is unknown. The disease is characterized by degenerative changes in the brain, particularly in the basal ganglia; cirrhosis of the liver; alterations of kidney function; and Kayser-Fleischer rings; the last are greenish-brown deposits at the limbus of the cornea and are pathognomonic of the disease [15, 317]. Biochemically there is an accumulation of copper in many tissues that seems to be responsible for the cellular disturbances; in most instances there is a reduction of ceruloplasmin, by which copper is transported in the blood. Low concentrations of copper and ceruloplasmin in the blood and increased rates of copper excretion are therefore the most characteristic findings in this disease. The clinical signs rarely start before the age of 6 years. In childhood the presenting symptom is usually hepatic disease [32, 89, 238], with the cerebral symptoms appearing later.

Although the renal symptoms can occur at any stage of Wilson's disease [16, 32, 66, 194, 255, 320], they are rarely described in children. The glomerular filtration rate decreases as the disease progresses. Chronic renal insufficiency is not seen, however, because the extrarenal complications are fatal before this occurs. Para-aminohippurate clearance and maximal tubular PAH secretion are even more impaired than the glomerular filtration rate, which indicates the preponderance of tubular disturbance [16, 194]. Amino acid excretion is greatly increased in some cases [17, 32, 66, 194, 222, 282, 298, 307]. The hyperaminoaciduria is of the generalized type and of renal origin, since plasma amino acids are not elevated unless there is a severe hepatic failure. The degree of hyperaminoaciduria parallels the duration of the overt disease [16]. Glucose resorption seems to be less impaired. At normal blood glucose levels, glucosuria is not always seen [66, 222], although Tm_G has been found to be reduced [16]. Phosphate resorption is also impaired, leading to hypophosphatemia and osteomalacia in some patients [16, 66, 96, 222]. Urate excretion is increased [16, 194, 282, 320], and the ability to

acidify the urine is reduced [16, 107, 194, 255]. Proteinuria is usually only slight.

Morphologic studies in the early stage of Wilson's disease reveal either no significant alterations by light microscopy [112] or only a slightly flattened, faintly staining tubular epithelium without recognizable brush borders [255]. On electron microscopy the brush borders are sparse or absent, the cellular network is destroyed, and electron-dense bodies are seen in the subapical areas of the tubular cytoplasm [85, 255]; these probably represent metalloproteins. The mitochondria show increased density, and their cristae are usually not well preserved. In postmortem specimens the tubular epithelium is damaged, and staining with rubeanic acid reveals intracytoplasmic copper granules [326]. The copper content of kidney tissue is greatly increased [32, 326].

Treatment of the deranged copper metabolism can be achieved successfully with D-penicillamine or other chelating substances [317]. D-Penicillamine therapy produces a striking increase in copper excretion that is associated with marked clinical improvement, particularly when treatment is started early in the disease [17, 85, 89, 162, 194, 222, 282]. If they are not too far advanced, all renal dysfunctions can be reversed to normal. There are, however, occasionally serious side effects of D-penicillamine therapy of Wilson's disease [85]. The prognosis depends on the response to treatment and the time of onset. Treatment is recommended in asymptomatic sibs in whom the diagnosis is established by biochemical means.

FANCONI SYNDROME IN ABNORMAL PROTEINURIAS

Most acquired diseases leading to the Fanconi syndrome are related to abnormal proteinuria. The proteinuria is caused either by extrarenal production of abnormal proteins of low molecular weight or by increased basement membrane permeability to proteins in glomerular disease. Synthesis of abnormal proteins associated with the Fanconi syndrome has been observed in multiple myeloma [64, 87, 140, 191, 209, 270, 292, 316], hypergammaglobulinemia [171], immunoglobulin light-chain disease [136], Sjögren's syndrome [227, 290, 314], and amyloidosis [97]. These diseases are extremely rare during infancy and childhood. They are often not accompanied by the complete Fanconi syndrome but merely by renal tubular acidosis [290] and other renal abnormalities, including acute [44] and chronic renal failure [211]. The appearance of Bence Jones protein in the urine is a constant finding, although this is not necessarily accompanied by renal dysfunction [184].

Multiple Myeloma. This malignancy was first recognized to be associated with the Fanconi syndrome by Sirota and Hamerman [292] in 1954; since then a number of cases have been described [209, 270], although none in children. The appearance of the Fanconi syndrome can precede the diagnosis of myeloma by many years, the longest period of premyeloma reported being 16½ years [209]. Thus it is possible that some of the cases of "idiopathic" Fanconi syndrome reported in adults could subsequently be found to be due to multiple myeloma.

The renal symptoms are often severe and typical of the Fanconi syndrome. Tubular PAH secretion is grossly impaired; although glomerular filtration is affected to a lesser extent, chronic renal failure is rather common in the later stages [211]. On histologic examination there are degenerative changes in the tubular cells, particularly of the proximal convolution [64, 83, 87, 191, 209, 270]. Crystalline inclusion bodies can be visualized by electron microscopy. These are similar to those seen in plasma cells. In experimental studies, the in vivo uptake of PAH by rabbit renal cortex slices is markedly inhibited by the presence of Bence Jones protein in the incubating fluid [249]. Similar results were obtained in rat cortex slices, in which the effect of Bence Jones protein and urinary proteins derived from nephrotic patients was compared. Bence Jones protein inhibited the uptake of hippurate and tetraethylammonium considerably and reduced ammoniagenesis and gluconeogenesis; these effects were not observed with proteins from nephrotic patients [250]. Kappatype Bence Jones protein injected in vivo induced proximal tubular lesions in rats [61]. Electron microscopy revealed inclusion bodies, which were shown by immunofluorescence to be κ-chain proteins. These findings support the hypothesis that the Fanconi syndrome in multiple myeloma is produced by filtered and reabsorbed abnormal proteins that impair tubular cell function by mechanisms still unknown.

Nephrotic Syndrome. The occurrence of the Fanconi syndrome in patients with the nephrotic syndrome is reported much less frequently than in myeloma and related diseases. There are only 11 well-documented cases in the literature [82 154, 155, 266, 297, 301, 302, 305]. In one additional adult case the Fanconi syndrome appeared after treatment with 6-mercaptopurine, which was considered to be the primary cause [46]. In almost all patients the nephrotic syndrome started in early childhood and was resistant to steroid therapy, although it was not familial. Renal biopsy in one case revealed only minimal glomerular lesions but dilatation and atrophy of the proximal tubules, thickening of the basement membranes, and interstitial fibrosis [266]. The tubular symptoms appear 1 to 4 years after the onset of the nephrotic syndrome. They are characterized by the Fanconi syndrome and lead to polyuria, renal acidosis, severe renal potassium loss, rickets, and growth retardation. In addition, a prominent feature is severe hypocalcemia with tetany. In the late stage the biopsy shows marked tubular and interstitial lesions and advanced glomerular hyalinization. Although exceptions exist [156], the course generally is unaffected by therapy, and death occurs usually 2 to 8 years after onset.

In these cases it is an open question whether the glomerular disease is the primary event and pathogenetic for the Fanconi syndrome, or whether the patients suffer from an unknown systemic disease that produces both glomerular proteinuria and later the Fanconi syndrome.

The features of the Fanconi syndrome in the nephrotic syndrome reveal a pronounced involvement of the distal tubules, with polyuria (despite edema), severe potassium loss, and distal tubular acidosis; these are symptoms seen in patients with dysproteinemic types of the Fanconi syndrome. This similarity could indicate that in these nephrotic patients some of the excessively filtered proteins might be responsible for the Fanconi syndrome. It is interesting to note that in one case histologic examination revealed birefringent crystals, mainly in the distal convolutions [155].

Following the early description of the combination of nephrotic syndrome with the Fanconi syndrome, the excretion of amino acids in other patients with the nephrotic syndrome was studied extensively [152, 153, 277, 329]. It was found that amino acid secretion is normal in most nephrotic patients. Only a few show variably increased excretion of some neutral amino acids, and these variations are related mainly to high protein intake and treatment with corticotropin (ACTH) or steroids [153, 277].

Transplantation. A Fanconi syndrome can also appear in a transplanted kidney. This event may be caused either by (1) the existence of an unknown systemic metabolic disturbance leading to an idiopathic Fanconi syndrome in the original kidneys [36], or (2) by ischemia, graft rejection, hyperparathyroidism, or immunosuppressive therapy [214, 310], which could also produce other less complex tubular dysfunctions such as tubular acidosis [23, 125, 197, 214, 224], severe phosphate leak [141, 225], and polyuria [23, 125].

FANCONI SYNDROME DUE TO EXOGENOUS INTOXICATIONS

Various toxic substances have been described that produce disturbances in tubular function without primarily affecting the glomerular filtration rate. The degree of tubular dysfunction shows great variation and is dependent on the kind and severity of exposure to the toxic substance. While severe intoxication usually produces acute renal failure due to tubular necrosis, less severe insults are followed by many types of proximal and distal tubulopathies; these could exist as singular or multiple defects and do not necessarily lead to a complete Fanconi syndrome. The defects are mostly reversible after exposure to the toxin is stopped. It is therefore of great importance to take very careful histories to exclude the possibility of exogenous intoxication in all patients with tubular dysfunction.

The main groups of substances leading to tubular intoxication are heavy metals, organic compounds, and drugs. In human beings heavy metals such as lead [52, 53, 57, 121, 322], cadmium [57, 121, 174], uranium [57, 263], and mercury [57, 191, 268] have been incriminated as causing acute and chronic tubular disturbances. Acute lead poisoning in children may lead to the complete Fanconi syndrome [52, 53, 322] accompanied by the well-known systemic signs of intoxication. The renal symptoms are reversible. A mild Fanconi syndrome has been reported in a 1½-year-old infant [268] following long-term application of a mercury-containing solution used for difficult teething. Chronic thallium intoxication can produce hyperaminoaciduria, due mainly to glycine excretion [98]. Although many organic compounds are nephrotoxic, reports on tubulopathies in humans are rare; aminoaciduria and glycosuria have been reported during the polyuric phase after 10 days of anuria in a patient with Lysol intoxication; however, these are nonspecific dysfunctions seen in many patients after acute tubular necrosis [86].

Tetracycline. Some drugs are also reported to produce the Fanconi syndrome under certain conditions. Outdated or degraded tetracycline was found in 1963 to be the cause of a reversible Fanconi syndrome in both children and adults, even when taken in recommended dosages [84, 102, 123]. Since then a few more cases have been described [41, 60, 106, 216, 319, 332]. The clinical picture is characterized by the development of polyuria, dizziness, muscular weakness, acidosis,

and sometimes severe neurologic symptoms. The laboratory investigations reveal the complete Fanconi syndrome, with reduction of PAH secretion, hyperaminoaciduria of a generalized type, renal glucosuria, hypophosphatemia, hypokalemia, renal tubular acidosis, proteinuria, and hypouricemia. In most cases the glomerular filtration rate is moderately reduced, and in two cases the excretion of Bence Jones proteins was noted [102, 216]. The recovery from most of these abnormalities is rapid. In a patient of mine, glucosuria and hypophosphatemia returned to normal after 2 weeks and hyperaminoaciduria ceased after 3 weeks [41]. Another patient, however, needed potassium supplementation for 1 year [106], and a third did not show normalization of renal acidification capacity until 2 years after the incident. Renal biopsies have been reported in two patients; in one patient a striking vacuolization of the distal tubular epithelium was seen 1 week after the appearance of symptoms [106]; a week later there was hypercellularity of the glomerular tufts with prominent capillary loops and basement membrane thickening. Fine hyaline droplets were present in the proximal convoluted cells, and there were signs of regeneration in the distal tubules [106]. In another case [216] biopsy revealed both glomerular and tubular changes. The tubular cells displayed desquamation, cast formation, and obstruction of the lumen as well as marked hyaline and granular changes and irregular cytoplasmic vacuolization.

The intoxicating substance is anhydro-4-epitetracycline formed from tetracycline under the influence of heat, moisture, and low pH. Only this substance was able to produce similar symptoms in dogs and rats [19, 201, 204], while pure tetracycline and anhydrous tetracycline had only minimal effects. Morphologic changes were first seen after 3 days, with progressive loss of stainable mitochondria and brush borders [201]. In spite of continued application of degraded tetracycline, renal function, cellular enzyme histochemistry, and renal morphology returned to normal after 14 days.

Diacrome. Taken in high amounts, methyl 3-chromone (Diacrome) has been reported to produce the Fanconi syndrome in a 3-year-old boy [243]. This substance has some structural similarity to tetracycline, and the clinical course is similar to outdated tetracycline nephropathy. 6-Mercaptopurine has also been reported to produce the Fanconi syndrome in patients with the nephrotic syndrome [46].

Maleic Acid. The experimental model most widely used in the study of the Fanconi syndrome is that produced by maleic acid, the cis isomer of fumaric acid. The first report, by Berliner and co-workers [22] in 1950, showed that the intravenous injection of maleate into acidotic dogs interfered with the renal tubular acidogenesis and produced an increased excretion of sodium, phosphate, and bicarbonate. Harrison and Harrison [137] injected neutralized maleic acid intraperitoneally in rats kept on a low phosphorus diet and observed a marked phosphaturia, aminoaciduria, and glucosuria, while the excretion of citrate and calcium was reduced. Vitamin D administration 3 days prior to the maleic acid injection did not prevent this effect. Resistance to the maleate effect developed within 3 to 5 days, even if the dose of maleate was increased. When the treatment was discontinued for a 5- to 7-day interval, the maleate effect could be elicited again. Since maleic acid is known to be a sulfhydryl inhibitor similar to cystine, copper, and lead, it was suggested that all these substances linked with the Fanconi syndrome might produce tubular intoxication by blocking the sulfhydryl groups of essential enzyme systems [4, 331]. This hypothesis, however, could not be confirmed by further experimental studies, in which the total amount of soluble and insoluble sulfhydryl groups were found not to be significantly reduced in rats treated with maleic acid; there was, however, a reduction of renal cortical succinic dehydrogenase and a profound distortion of renal tubular ultrastructure [330].

In vitro studies by Rosenberg and Segal [261] revealed that maleic acid impaired the uptake of amino acids by renal cortical slices, both by retarding influx and by accelerating efflux from the cells. The inhibitory effect could be elicited in kidney slices but not in intestinal or muscle tissue. The hyperaminoaciduria produced by maleate involved mainly taurine, serine, threonine, glutamic acid, glycine, alanine, valine, lysine, and histidine, while the other amino acids did not participate [261].

Bergeron [20] has shown that the accumulation of radioactive amino acids in the kidney is reduced in vivo after injection of maleate. Microinjection studies in maleate-treated rat kidneys have demonstrated that the luminal uptake of labeled leucine was not reduced, but that the transcellular transport from the peritubular side to the tubular lumen was enhanced, indicating decreased ability of the tubular cell to retain absorbed amino acids [21].

Biochemical studies have shown that the ATP content is reduced in maleate-treated tubular cells [177, 276], which was found to be due to inhibition of tubular Na-K-ATPase activity [177]. Electron microscopic studies demonstrated increased density, shrinking, and blurring of mitochondrial cristae in the proximal convolutions as well as abnormal formation of apical vesicles within the cytoplasm at the luminal cell border [259, 276]. The transport defect of urate, phosphate, calcium, magnesium, and potassium produced by maleate could be related to that of sodium [178]. It was postulated, therefore, that the inhibition of sodium transport may be the primary mechanism in this syndrome, initiating the impairment in transport phenomena that are sodium dependent. The same authors have shown recently that maleic acid as well as cystine inhibit active sodium transport in the isolated frog skin [176].

Other Intoxicants. Uranium [99], mercury [99], lead [118, 119, 120, 311], and other substances have been used in experimental studies attempting to elucidate the pathophysiology of the Fanconi syndrome. There is considerable experimental evidence that the Fanconi syndrome may be related to disturbances in the energy-producing or transporting mechanisms of cells, evoking morphologic changes in the mitochondria and affecting sodium transport and the ability of the cell to maintain its intracellular homeostasis.

Principles of Treatment

Treatment of the Fanconi syndrome can be either specific or symptomatic. Specific treatment is possible in those cases in which the underlying metabolic defect is recognized and the accumulation of toxic metabolites can be avoided, mostly by dietary means, as in transferase deficiency galactosemia, hereditary fructose intolerance, hereditary tyrosinemia, Wilson's disease, and nephropathies due to intoxications, for example. The specific therapies have been discussed under the specific types. These treatments, if followed, usually lead to complete normalization of the tubular symptoms. Each patient with the Fanconi syndrome therefore has to be worked up completely in order not to miss the exact diagnosis and the possibility of specific therapy.

In the other types of Fanconi syndrome (see Table 81-1) only symptomatic therapy is possible; however, it is equally important since it often can ensure almost complete compensation of the deranged homeostasis. Symptomatic therapy not only will prolong survival of the affected children, but also it often can achieve a normal life with full activities and well-being. Further, it will prevent overt rickets and skeletal deformities; disabilities and severe growth retardation can thus be avoided, although normal growth rates rarely can be achieved.

Symptomatic therapy is directed toward preventing or treating disturbances such as acidosis, hypokalemia, hypophosphatemia, polyuria, and vitamin D resistance. Hyperaminoaciduria, glucosuria, and hypouricemia, on the other hand, are usually not associated with overt clinical signs and require no special treatment.

Acidosis is due to proximal tubular bicarbonate loss and lowered bicarbonate threshold; it requires large amounts of alkali. Depending on the degree of tubular impairment, 2 to 10 mmol/kg/day or more of alkali has to be given in the form of sodium bicarbonate or citrate (as Shohl's solution: 140 gm citric acid and 98 gm sodium citrate dissolved in water to a total volume of 1 liter; 1 ml contains 1 mmol sodium). Alkali should be offered in divided doses every 4 to 5 hr during the daytime; the amount needed should be adjusted to the serum bicarbonate level. Since most patients have severe potassium loss, they should receive potassium in addition, which is given as bicarbonate, citrate, lactate, or phosphate, depending on the levels of these anions in plasma. In Eisenberg's solution, sodium and potassium are mixed in equal parts (2 gm citric acid, 3 gm sodium citrate, and 3.3 gm potassium citrate in 30 ml of a palatable, nonalcoholic syrup base; 1 ml contains 1 mmol each of sodium and potassium). The amount of potassium needed is adjusted to the level in serum; it ranges from 2 to 4 mmol/kg/day.

In some cases the amount of alkali needed in order to compensate for the severe bicarbonate loss is more than the patient can tolerate. In such patients the administration of hydrochlorothiazide in a dosage of 2 to 3 mg/kg/day has been tried successfully [48, 252]. This saluretic agent improves acidosis by increasing the bicarbonate threshold, which occurs when the extracellular fluid volume is reduced.

Hypophosphatemia is due to decreased tubular phosphate resorption; it can be compensated partly by oral supplementation of 1 to 3 gm neutral phosphate per day (145 gm $Na_2HPO_4 \cdot 7H_2O$ and 18.2 gm $NaH_2PO_4 \cdot H_2O$ dissolved in 1 liter of water with syrup base). This solution has to be taken regularly every 4 to 5 hr throughout the daytime. It sometimes evokes intestinal discomfort and diarrhea, which will stop after discontinuation of treatment for a short period. In some cases phosphate supplementation may aggravate or produce hypocalcemia and thereby stimulate hyperparathyroidism. Administration of additional oral calcium and vitamin D can prevent hypocalcemia and may therefore be needed.

Treatment with vitamin D is indicated, although the nature of vitamin D resistance in this syndrome is not well understood. The starting dose of vitamin D should be 5,000 units per day, which should be increased gradually (up to 2,000 to 4,000 units/kg/day) until hypocalcemia and rickets are successfully improved. Careful monitoring of vitamin D treatment is necessary to avoid toxic side effects. The best indicator is urinary calcium excretion, which should not exceed 6 mg/kg/day. Hydroxylated metabolites of vitamin D are not more specifically effective than ordinary vitamin D [10].

Polyuria is a frequent finding in the Fanconi syndrome, and sufficient amounts of fluid have to be offered in order to avoid dehydration. It is our practice to have prepared a fixed amount of fluids for the whole day (1 to 2 liters) in which the required salts are dissolved. This fluid is taken regularly in divided doses, while additional fluids are not withheld if desired. Regular intake of fluid with salt supplementation and careful monitoring of this symptomatic therapy are rewarded by a good therapeutic response, and usually the patient can pursue an active life as long as the course of the disease does not progress to renal insufficiency.

References

1. Abbassi, V., Lowe, C. U., and Calcagno, P. L. Oculocerebrorenal syndrome: A review. *Am. J. Dis. Child.* 115:145, 1968.
2. Abderhalden, E. Familiäre Cystindiathese. *Z. Phys. Chem.* 38:557, 1903.
3. Albright, F., Butler, A. M., and Bloomberg, E. Rickets resistant to vitamin D therapy. *Am. J. Dis. Child.* 54:529, 1937.
4. Angielski, S., and Rogulski, J. Significance of lactose in the diet in aminoaciduria caused by maleic acid. *Nature (Lond.)* 184 [Suppl. 5]:276, 1959.
5. Antener, I., Nordio, S., Kaeser, M., and Gatti, R. Etude clinique de l'absorption intestinale des acides aminés: Determination des acides aminés dans les selles. *Ann. Nestle.* 62:18, 1972.
6. Aronsson, S., Engleson, G., Jagenburg, R., and Palmgren, B. Long-term dietary treatment of tyrosinosis. *J. Pediatr.* 72:620, 1968.
7. Baber, M. D. A case of congenital cirrhosis of the liver with renal tubular defects akin to those in the Fanconi syndrome. *Arch. Dis. Child.* 31:335, 1956.
8. Bach, C., Thiriez, H., Jolly, J., Jarlier, H., and Joannides, Z. Une observation de syndrome de Lowe (Etude clinique et biologique). *Sem. Hop. Paris* 42:43, 1966.
9. Bakker, H. D., De Bree, P. K., Ketting, D., Van Sprang, F. J., and Wadman, S. K. Fructose-1,6 diphosphatase deficiency: Another enzyme defect which can present itself with the clinical features of tyrosinosis. *Clin. Chim. Acta* 55:41, 1974.
10. Balsan, S., Garabedian, M., Sorgniard, R., Holick, M. F., and DeLuca, H. F. 1,25-Dihydroxy vitamin D_3 and 1,α-hydroxy vitamin D_3 in children: Biologic and therapeutic effects in nutritional rickets and different types of vitamin D resistance. *Pediatr. Res.* 9:586, 1975.

11. Barratt, T. M., and Crawford, R. Lysozyme excretion as a measure of renal tubular dysfunction in children. *Clin. Sci.* 39:457, 1970.

12. Bartsocas, C. S., Levy, H. L., Crawford, J. D., and Thier, S. O. A defect in intestinal amino acid transport in Lowe's syndrome. *Am. J. Dis. Child.* 117:93, 1969.

13. Bauer, B. Debré-De-Toni-Fanconi-Syndrom mit Glykogenose der Leber. *Klin. Wochenschr.* 46:317, 1968.

14. Bauer, B., and Antener, I. Eine wirksame diätetische und medikamentöse Cystinose-Behandlung. *Helv. Paediatr. Acta* 21:19, 1966.

15. Bearn, A. G. Wilson's Disease. In J. B. Stanbury, J. B. Wyngaarden, and D. S. Fredrikson (eds.), *The Metabolic Basis of Inherited Disease* (3rd ed.). New York: McGraw-Hill, 1972. P. 1033.

16. Bearn, A. G., Yü, T. T., and Gutman, A. B. Renal function in Wilson's disease. *J. Clin. Invest.* 36:1107, 1957.

17. Bell, G. E., Slivka, D. C., and Huston, J. R. The renal clearance of amino acids in a patient with Wilson's disease during penicillamine treatment. *J. Lab. Clin. Med.* 71:113, 1968.

18. Ben-Ishay, D., Dreyfuss, F., and Ullmann, T. D. Fanconi syndrome with hypouricemia in an adult. *Am. J. Med.* 31:793, 1961.

19. Benitz, K. F., and Diermeir, H. F. Renal toxicity of tetracycline degradation products. *Proc. Soc. Exp. Biol. Med.* 115:930, 1964.

20. Bergeron, M. Renal amino acid accumulation in maleate treated rats. *Rev. Can. Biol.* 30:267, 1971.

21. Bergeron, M., and Vadeboncoer, M. Microinjections of L-leucine into tubules and peritubular capillaries of the rat: II. The maleic acid model. *Nephron* 8:367, 1971.

22. Berliner, R. W., Kennedy, T. J., and Hilton, J. G. The effect of maleic acid on renal function. *Proc. Soc. Exp. Biol. Med.* 75:791, 1950.

23. Better, O. S., Chaimovitz, C., Naveh, Y., Stein, A., Nahir, A. M., Barzilai, A., and Erlik, D. Syndrome of incomplete renal tubular acidosis after cadaveric kidney transplantation. *Ann. Intern. Med.* 71:39, 1969.

24. Beumer, H., and Wepler, W. Über die Cystinkrankheit der ersten Lebenszeit. *Klin. Wochenschr.* 16:8, 1937.

25. Beutler, E., and Baluda, M. C. Improved method for measuring galactose-1-phosphate uridyl transferase activity of erythrocytes. *Clin. Chim. Acta* 13:369, 1966.

26. Bickel, H. Entwicklung der biochemischen Läsion bei Lignac-Fanconi'scher Krankheit. *Helv. Paediatr. Acta* 10:259, 1955.

26a. Bickel, H. Personal communication, 1976.

27. Bickel, H. Proximal Tubular Defects. In D. A. K. Black (ed.), *Renal Disease.* Oxford: Blackwell, 1962. P. 347.

28. Bickel, H., Baar, H. S., Astley, R., Douglas, A. A., Finch, E., Harris, H., Harvey, C. C., Hickmans, E. M., Philpott, M. G., Smallwood, W. C., Smellie, J. M., and Teall, C. G. Cystine storage disease with amino-aciduria and dwarfism (Lignac-Fanconi disease). *Acta Paediatr.* [Suppl. 90] 42:1, 1952.

29. Bickel, H., and Hickmans, E. M. Paperchromatographic investigations on the urine of patients R. T. and R. R. *Arch. Dis. Child.* 27:348, 1952.

30. Bickel, H., and Hickmans, E. M. Part 7: Some biochemical aspects of Lignac-Fanconi disease. *Acta Paediatr.* [Suppl. 90] 42:137, 1952.

31. Bickel, H., Lutz, P., and Schmidt, H. The Treatment of Cystinosis with Diet and Drugs. In J. D. Schulman (ed.), *Cystinosis.* Washington, D.C.: National Institutes of Health, Department of Health, Education, and Welfare, 1973. P. 199.

32. Bickel, H., Neale, F. C., and Hall, G. A clinical and biochemical study of hepatolenticular degeneration (Wilson's disease). *Q. J. Med.* 26:527, 1957.

33. Bloom, W. L., and Flinchum, D. Osteomalacia and pseudofractures caused by the ingestion of aluminium hydroxide. *J.A.M.A.* 174:181, 1960.

34. Bloomer, H. A., Canary, J. J., Kyle, L. H., and Auld, R. M. The Fanconi syndrome with renal hyperchloremic acidosis. *Am. J. Med.* 33:141, 1962.

35. Bradley, S. E. Disorders of renal tubular function. *Am. J. Med.* 20:457, 1956.

36. Briggs, W. A., Kominami, N., Wilson, R. E., and Merrill, J. P. Kidney transplantation in Fanconi syndrome. *N. Engl. J. Med.* 286:25, 1972.

37. Brodehl, J. Tubular Fanconi Syndrome with Bone Involvement. In H. Bickel and J. Stern (eds.), *Inborn Errors of Calcium and Bone Metabolism.* Lancaster, England: MTP Press, 1976. P. 191.

38. Brodehl, J., and Bickel, H. Aminoaciduria and hyperaminoaciduria in childhood. *Clin. Nephrol.* 1:149, 1973.

38a. Brodehl, J., Franken, A., and Gellissen, K. Maximal tubular reabsorption of glucose in infants and children. *Acta Paediatr. Scand.* 61:413, 1972.

39. Brodehl, J., and Gellissen, K. Endogenous renal transport of free amino acids in infancy and childhood. *Pediatrics* 42:395, 1968.

40. Brodehl, J., Gellissen, K., and Hagge, W. The Fanconi Syndrome in Hepato-renal Glycogen Storage Disease. In G. Peters and F. Roch-Ramel (eds.), *Progress in Nephrology.* Berlin: Springer, 1969. P. 241.

41. Brodehl, J., Gellissen, K., Hagge, W., and Schumacher, H. Reversibles renales Fanconi-Syndrom durch toxisches Abbauprodukt des Tetrazyklins. *Helv. Paediatr. Acta* 23:373, 1968.

42. Brodehl, J., Hagge, W., and Gellissen, K. Die Veränderungen der Nierenfunktion bei der Cystinose. Teil I: Die Inulin-, PAH- und Elektrolyt-Clearance in verschiedenen Stadien der Erkrankung. *Ann. Paediatr. (Basel)* 205:131, 1965.

43. Brubaker, R. F., Wong, V. G., Schulman, J. D., Seegmiller, J. E., and Kuwabara, T. Benign cystinosis: The clinical, biochemical and morphological findings in a family with two affected siblings. *Am. J. Med.* 49:546, 1970.

44. Bryan, C., and Healy, J. Acute renal failure in multiple myeloma. *Am. J. Med.* 44:128, 1968.

45. Butler, E. A., and Flynn, F. V. The proteinuria of renal tubular disorder. *Lancet* 2:978, 1958.

46. Butler, H. E., Morgan, J. M., and Smythe, C. M. Mercaptopurine and acquired tubular dysfunction in adult nephrosis. *Arch. Intern. Med.* 116:853, 1965.

47. Calcagno, P. L., and Hollerman, C. E. Hereditary Renal Disease and Certain Renal Tubular Disorders. In M. I. Rubin and I. M. Barratt (eds.), *Pediatric Nephrology.* Baltimore: Williams & Wilkins, 1975. P. 668.

48. Callis, L., Castello, F., Fortuny, G., Vallo, A., and Ballabriga, A. Effect of hydrochlorothiazide on

rickets and on renal tubular acidosis in two patients with cystinosis. *Helv. Paediatr. Acta* 25:602, 1970.

49. Cameron, J. S. Renal tubular disorders in childhood. *Turk. J. Pediatr.* 15:1, 1973.

50. Chan, A. M., Lynch, M. J. G., Bailey, J. D., Ezrin, C., and Fraser, D. Hypothyroidism in cystinosis: A clinical, endocrinologic and histologic study involving sixteen patients with cystinosis. *Am. J. Med.* 48: 678, 1970.

51. Cherry, J. D., and Surawicz, B. Unusual effects of potassium deficiency on the heart of a child with cystinosis. *Pediatrics* 30:414, 1962.

52. Chisolm, J. J. Aminoaciduria as a manifestation of renal tubular injury in lead intoxication and a comparison with patterns of aminoaciduria seen in other diseases. *J. Pediatr.* 60:1, 1962.

53. Chisolm, J. J., Jr., Harrison, H. C., Eberlein, W. R., and Harrison, H. E. Aminoaciduria, hypophosphatemia, and rickets in lead poisoning: Study of a case. *Am. J. Dis. Child.* 89:159, 1955.

54. Christensen, M. F., Nielsen, J. A., and Henriksen, O. Treatment of cystinosis with a diet poor in cystine and methionine. *Acta Paediatr. Scand.* 59: 613, 1970.

55. Christiaens, L., Biserte, G., Farriaux, J., Fontaine, G., Walbaum, R., and Dubois, O. La forme idiopathique du syndrome de de Toni-Débre-Fanconi. *Sem. Hop. Paris Ann. Pediatr.* 41:49, 1965.

56. Chutorian, A., and Rowland, L. P. Lowe's syndrome. *Neurology* 16:115, 1966.

57. Clarkson, T. W., and Kench, J. E. Urinary excretion of amino acids by men absorbing heavy metals. *Biochem. J.* 62:361, 1956.

58. Clay, R. D., Darmady, E. M., and Hawkins, M. The nature of the renal lesion in the Fanconi syndrome. *J. Pathol. Bacteriol.* 65:551, 1953.

59. Clayton, B. E., and Patrick, A. D. Use of dimercaprol or penicillamine in the treatment of cystinosis. *Lancet* 2:909, 1961.

60. Cleveland, W. W., Adams, W. C., Mann, J. B., and Nyhan, W. L. Acquired Fanconi syndrome following degraded tetracycline. *J. Pediatr.* 66:333, 1965.

61. Clyne, D. H., Brendstrup, L., and First, M. R. Renal effects of intraperitoneal kappa chain injection: Induction of crystals in renal tubular cells. *Lab. Invest.* 31:131, 1974.

62. Cogan, D. G., Kuwabara, T., Kinoshita, J., Sheehan, L., and Merola, L. Cystinosis in an adult. *J.A.M.A.* 164:394, 1957.

63. Colombo, J.-P. Hinweis auf eine tubuläre und intestinale Malabsorption der Aminosäuren beim Lowe-Syndrom. *Schweiz. Med. Wochenschr.* 101: 968, 1971.

64. Constanza, D. J., and Smoller, M. Multiple myeloma with the Fanconi syndrome. *Am. J. Med.* 34: 125, 1963.

65. Cooke, W. T., Barlay, J. B., Govan, A. D. T., and Nagley, L. Osteoporosis associated with low serum phosphorus and renal glucosuria. *Arch. Intern. Med.* 80:147, 1947.

66. Cooper, A. M., Eckhardt, R. O., Faloon, W. W., and Davidson, C. S. Investigation of the aminoaciduria in Wilson's disease (hepatolenticular degeneration), demonstration of a defect in renal function. *J. Clin. Invest.* 29:265, 1950.

67. Crawhall, J. C., Lietman, P. S., Schneider, J. A., and Seegmiller, J. E. Cystinosis: Plasma cystine and cysteine concentrations and the effect of D-penicil-

lamine and dietary treatment. *Am. J. Med.* 44:330, 1968.

68. Cusworth, D. C., Dent, C. E., and Flynn, F. V. The aminoaciduria in galactosemia. *Arch. Dis. Child.* 30:150, 1955.

69. Darling, S., and Mortensen, O. Aminoaciduria in galactosaemia. *Acta Paediatr.* 43:337, 1954.

70. Darmady, E. M., and Stranack, F. Microdissection of the nephron in disease. *Br. Med. Bull.* 13:21, 1957.

71. Davies, H. E. F., Evans, B., Rees, H. M. N., and Fourman, P. The defective absorption of phosphorus and calcium and the effect of vitamin D in the Fanconi syndrome. *Guys Hosp. Rep.* 107:486, 1958.

72. Debré, R., Marie, J., Cléret, F., and Messimy, R. Rachitisme tardif coexistant avec une néphrite chronique et une glycosurie. *Arch. Med. Enf.* 37: 597, 1934.

73. Debré, R., Royer, P., Lestradet, H., and Straub, W. L'Insuffisance tubulaire congenitale avec arriération mentale, cataracte et glaucome (syndrome de Lowe). *Arch. Fr. Pediatr.* 12:337, 1955.

74. Dent, C. E. The amino-aciduria in Fanconi syndrome: A study making extensive use of techniques based on paper partition chromatography. *Biochem. J.* 41:240, 1947.

75. Dent, C. E. Rickets and osteomalacia from renal tubule defects. *J. Bone Joint Surg. [Br.]* 34:266, 1952.

76. Dent, C. E., and Rose, G. A. Amino Acid Metabolism in Cystinuria. In Abstracts of the 1st International Congress of Biochemistry, Cambridge, England, 1949.

77. De Toni, G. Remarks on the relations between renal rickets (renal dwarfism) and renal diabetes. *Acta Paediatr. (Uppsala)* 16:479, 1933.

78. De Toni, G. Renal rickets with phospho-gluco-amino renal diabetes (de Toni-Debré-Fanconi syndrome). *Ann. Paediatr. (Basel)* 187:42, 1956.

79. Dillard, M. G., Pesce, A. J., Pollak, V. E., and Boreisha, I. Proteinuria and renal protein clearances in patients with renal tubular disorders. *J. Lab. Clin. Med.* 78:203, 1971.

80. Donnell, G. N., and Bergren, W. The Galactosemias. In D. N. Raine (ed.), *Treatment of Inherited Metabolic Disease.* Lancaster, England: Medical and Technical Publishing Co., 1975. P. 91.

81. Donnell, G. N., Bergen, W. R., and Ng, W. G. Galactosemia. *Biochem. Med.* 1:29, 1967.

82. Doolan, P. D., Morris, M. D., and Harper, H. A. Amino aciduria in an elderly man with the nephrotic syndrome and a young man with a variant of the Fanconi syndrome. *Ann. Intern. Med.* 56:448, 1956.

83. Dragsted, P. J., and Wallis, L. A. The association of the Fanconi syndrome with malignant disease. *Dan. Med. Bull.* 3:177, 1956.

84. Ehrlich, L. I., and Stein, W. S. Abnormal urinary findings following administration of Achromycin V. *Pediatrics* 31:339, 1963.

85. Elsas, L. J., Hayslett, J. P., Spargo, B. H., Durant, J. L., and Rosenberg, L. E. Wilson's disease with reversible renal tubular dysfunction: Correlation with proximal tubular ultrastructure. *Ann. Intern. Med.* 75:427, 1971.

86. Emslie-Smith, D., Johnstone, J. H., Thomson, M. B., and Lowe, K. G. Aminoaciduria in acute tubular necrosis. *Clin. Sci.* 15:171, 1956.

87. Engle, R. L., and Wallis, L. A. Multiple myeloma and the adult Fanconi syndrome: I. Report of a case with crystal-like deposits in the tumor cells and in the epithelial cells of the kidney. *Am. J. Med.* 22:5, 1957.

88. Fairney, A., Francis, D., Ersser, R. S., Seakins, J. W. T., and Cottom, D. Diagnosis and treatment of tyrosinosis. *Arch. Dis. Child.* 43:540, 1968.

89. Falkmer, S., Samuelson, G., and Sjölin, S. Penicillamine-induced normalization of clinical signs, and histochemistry in a case of Wilson's disease. *Pediatrics* 45:260, 1970.

90. Fanconi, G. Die nicht diabetischen Glykosurien und Hyperglykämien des älteren Kindes. *Jahrbuch Kinderheilkd.* 133:257, 1931.

91. Fanconi, G. Der frühinfantile nephrotisch-glykosurische Zwergwuchs mit hypophosphatämischer Rachitis. *Jahrbuch Kinderheilkd.* 147:299, 1936.

92. Fanconi, G., and Bickel, H. Die chronische Aminoacidurie (Aminosäurendiabetes oder nephrotisch-glukosurischer Zwergwuchs) bei der Glykogenose und der Cystinkrankheit. *Helv. Paediatr. Acta* 4:359, 1949.

93. Fanconi, A., Fischer, J. A., and Prader, A. Serum parathyroid hormone concentration in hypophosphatemic vitamin D resistant rickets. *Helv. Paediatr. Acta* 29:187, 1974.

94. Fellers, F. X., Ko, K. W., and Nicolaidou, M. A defect of tubular secretory function in the de Toni-Fanconi syndrome. *Am. J. Dis. Child.* 100:588, 1960.

95. Fellers, F. X., Piedrahita, V., and Galan, E. M. Pseudo-Phlorhizin diabetes (abstract). *Pediatr. Res.* 1:304, 1967.

96. Finby, N., and Bearn, A. G. Roentgenographic abnormalities of the skeletal system in Wilson's disease (hepatolenticular degeneration). *Am. J. Roentgenol. Radium Ther. Nucl. Med.* 79:603, 1958.

97. Finkel, P. N., Kronenberg, K., Pesce, A. J., Pollak, V. E., and Pirani, C. C. Adult Fanconi syndrome, amyloidosis and marked X-light chain proteinuria. *Nephron* 10:1, 1973.

98. Fischl, J. Aminoaciduria in thallium poisoning. *Am. J. Med. Sci.* 251:40, 1960.

99. Foulkes, E. C. Effects of heavy metals on renal aspartate transport and the nature of solute movement in kidney cortex slices. *Biochim. Biophys. Acta* 241:815, 1971.

100. Fox, M., Thier, S., Rosenberg, L., and Segal, S. Impaired renal tubular function induced by sugar infusion in man. *J. Clin. Endocrinol. Metab.* 24: 1318, 1964.

101. Fraser, D., Leeming, J. M., and Cerwenka, E. A. Über die Handhabung von Phosphat durch die Nieren bei hypophosphatämischer vitamin D-resistenter Rachitis der einfachen Art und bei Cystinspeicherkrankheit: Reaktion auf verlängerte Calciuminfusion. *Helv. Paediatr. Acta* 14:497, 1959.

102. Frimpter, G. W., Timpanelli, A. E., Eisenmenger, W. J., Stein, W. S., and Ehrlich, L. I. Reversible Fanconi syndrome caused by degraded tetracycline. *J.A.M.A.* 184:111, 1963.

103. Froesch, E. R. Essential Fructosuria and Hereditary Fructose Intolerance. In J. B. Stanbury, J. B. Wyngaarden, and D. S. Fredrickson (eds.), *The Metabolic Basis of Inherited Disease* (4th ed.) New York: McGraw-Hill, 1978. P. 121.

104. Froesch, E. R. Hereditary Fructose Intolerance and Fructose 1,6-Diphosphatase Deficiency. In D. N. Raine (ed.), *The Treatment of Inherited Metabolic Disease.* Lancaster, England: Medical and Technical Publishing, 1975. P. 151.

105. Froesch, E. R., Prader, A., Labhart, A., Stuber, H. W., and Wolf, H. P. Die hereditäre Fruktoseintoleranz, eine bisher nicht bekannte kongenitale Stoffwechselstörung. *Schweiz. Med. Wochenschr.* 87:1168, 1957.

106. Fulop, M., and Drapkin, A. Potassium-depletion syndrome secondary to nephropathy apparently caused by out-dated tetracycline. *N. Engl. J. Med.* 272:986, 1965.

107. Fulop, M., Sternlieb, I., and Scheinberg, I. H. Defective urinary acidification in Wilson's disease. *Ann. Intern. Med.* 68:770, 1968.

108. Garty, R., Cooper, M., and Tabachnik, E. The Fanconi syndrome associated with hepatic glycogenosis and abnormal metabolism of galactose. *J. Pediatr.* 85:821, 1974.

109. Gaull, G. E., Rassin, D. K., Solomon, G. E., Harris, R. C., and Sturman, J. A. Biochemical observations on so-called hereditary tyrosinemia. *Pediatr. Res.* 4:337, 1970.

110. Gentz, J., Jagenburg, R., and Zetterström, R. Tyrosinemia: An inborn error of tyrosine metabolism with cirrhosis of the liver and multiple renal tubular defects (de Toni-Debré-Fanconi-syndrome). *J. Pediatr.* 66:670, 1965.

111. Gentz, J., Johansson, S., Lindblad, B., Lindstedt, S., and Zetterström, R. Excretion of δ-aminolevulinic acid in hereditary tyrosinemia. *Clin. Chim. Acta* 23: 257, 1969.

112. Gilsanz, V., Barrera, A., and Anaya, A. The renal biopsy in Wilson's disease. *Arch. Intern. Med.* 105: 758, 1960.

113. Gitzelmann, R. Hereditary galactokinase deficiency: A newly recognized cause of juvenile cataracts. *Pediatr. Res.* 1:14, 1967.

114. Godard, C., Valloton, M. B., Broyer, M., and Royer, P. A study of the inhibition of the renin-angiotensin system in potassium wasting syndromes, including Bartter's syndrome. *Helv. Paediatr. Acta* 27:495, 1972.

115. Goldman, H., Scriver, C. R., and Aaron, K. Use of dithiothreitol to correct cystine storage in cultured cystinotic fibroblasts. *Lancet* 2:811, 1970.

116. Goldman, H., Scriver, C. R., Aaron, K., Delvin, E., and Canlas, Z. Adolescent cystinosis: Comparisons with infantile and adult forms. *Pediatrics* 47:900, 1971.

117. Govaerts, P. Physiopathology of glucose excretion by the human kidney. *Br. Med. J.* 172:175, 1952.

118. Goyer, R. A. The renal tubule in lead poisoning: I. mitochondrial swelling and aminoaciduria. *Lab. Invest.* 19:71, 1968.

119. Goyer, R. A., Krall, A., and Kimball, J. P. The renal tubule in lead poisoning: II. in vitro studies of mitochondrial structure and function. *Lab. Invest.* 19:78, 1968.

120. Goyer, R. A., and Leonard, D. Aminoaciduria in experimental lead poisoning. *Proc. Soc. Exp. Biol. Med.* 135:767, 1970.

121. Goyer, R. A., Tsuchiya, K., Leonard, D. L., and Kahyo, H. Aminoaciduria in Japanese workers in the lead and cadmium industries. *Am. J. Clin. Pathol.* 57:635, 1972.

122. Grant, D. B., Alexander, F. W., and Seakins,

J. W. T. Abnormal tyrosine metabolism in hereditary fructose intolerance. *Acta Paediatr. Scand.* 59: 432, 1970.

123. Gross, J. M. Fanconi syndrome (adult type) developing secondary to ingestion of out-dated tetracycline. *Ann. Intern. Med.* 56:523, 1963.

124. Guthrie, R. Screening for Inborn Errors of Metabolism in the Newborn Infant—a Multiple Test Program. In D. Bergsma (ed.), *Human Genetics* (Birth Defects Original Article Series, Vol. 4, No. 6). New York: The National Foundation, 1968. P. 92.

125. Györy, A. Z., Stewart, J. H., George, C. R. P., Tiller, D. J., and Edwards, K. D. G. Renal tubular acidosis, acidosis due to hyperkalaemia, hypercalcaemia, disordered citrate metabolism and other tubular dysfunctions following human renal transplantation. *J. Med.* 38:231, 1969.

126. Habib, R., Bargeton, E., Brissaud, H. E., Raynaud, J., and Le Ball, J.-C. Constatations anatomiques chez un enfant atteint d'un syndrome de Lowe. *Arch. Fr. Pediatr.* 19:945, 1962.

127. Hagge, W., and Brodehl, J. Die Veränderungen der Nierenfunktion bei der Cystinose. Teil II: Die Aminosäuren-Clearance. *Ann. Pediatr. (Basel)* 205: 442, 1965.

128. Halvorsen, S., and Gjessing, L. R. Studies on tyrosinosis: 1. Effect of low-tyrosine and low-phenylalanin diet. *Br. Med. J.* 2:1171, 1964.

129. Halvorsen, S., Pande, H., Løken, A. C., and Gjessing, L. R. Tyrosinosis: A study of 6 cases. *Arch. Dis. Child.* 41:238, 1966.

130. Hambidge, K. M., Goodman, S. I., Walravens, P. A., Mauer, S. M., Brettschneider, L., Penn, I., and Starzl, T. E. Accumulation of cystine following renal homotransplantation for cystinosis. *Pediatr. Res.* 3:364, 1969.

131. Hambraeus, L., and Broberger, O. Penicillamine treatment of cystinosis. *Acta Paediatr. Scand.* 56:243, 1967.

132. Hambraeus, L., Pallisgaard, G., and Kildeberg, P. The Lowe syndrome: Observations on the amino acid metabolism in a 2-year-old affected boy. *Acta Paediatr. Scand.* 59:631, 1970.

133. Haquani, A. H., and Mohanram, M. Renal tubular insufficiency. *J. Pediatr.* 61:242, 1962.

134. Harries, D. T., Seakins, J. W., Ersser, R. S., and Lloyd, J. K. Recovery after dietary treatment of an infant with features of tyrosinosis. *Arch. Dis. Child.* 44:258, 1969.

135. Harrison, J. F., and Blainey, J. D. Low molecular weight proteinuria in chronic renal disease. *Clin. Sci.* 33:381, 1967.

136. Harrison, J. F., and Blainey, J. D. Adult Fanconi syndrome with monoclonal abnormality of immunoglobulin light chain. *J. Clin. Pathol.* 20:42, 1967.

137. Harrison, H. E., and Harrison, H. C. Experimental production of renal glucosuria phosphaturia and aminoaciduria by injection of maleic acid. *Science* 120:606, 1954.

138. Harrison, J. F., Lunt, G. S., Scott, P., and Blainey, J. D. Urinary lysozyme, ribonuclease, and low-molecular-weight protein in renal disease. *Lancet* 1:371, 1968.

139. Haworth, J. C., and Coodin, F. J. Liver failure in galactosemia successfully treated by exchange blood transfusion. *Can. Med. Assoc. J.* 105:301, 1971.

140. Headley, R. N., King, J. S., Cooper, M. R., and

Felts, J. H. Multiple myeloma presenting as adult Fanconi syndrome. *Clin. Chem.* 18:293, 1972.

141. Herdman, R. C., Michael, A. F., Vernier, R. L., Kelly, W., and Good, R. Renal function and phosphorus excretion after human renal homotransplantation. *Lancet* 1:121, 1966.

142. Hers, H. G. Glycogen Storage Disease. In R. Levine and R. Luft (eds.), *Advances in Metabolic Disorders.* New York: Academic, 1964. P. 1.

143. Hers, H. G., and Van Hoof, F. Glycogen Storage Disease: Type VI Glycogenosis. In F. Dickens, P. J. Randle, and W. J. Whelan (eds.), *Carbohydrate Metabolism and Its Disorders.* New York: Academic, 1968. P. 161.

144. Higgins, R. B., and Varney, J. K. Dissolution of renal calculi in a case of hereditary fructose intolerance and renal tubular acidosis. *J. Urol.* 95:291, 1966.

145. Hill, A., Norden, P. M., and Zaleski, W. A. Dietary treatment of tyrosinosis. *J. Am. Diet. Assoc.* 56:308, 1970.

146. Hill, A., and Zaleski, W. A. Tyrosinosis: Biochemical studies of an unusual case. *Clin. Biochem.* 4:263, 1971.

147. Holmes, L. B., McGowan, B. L., and Efron, M. L. Lowe's syndrome: A search for the carrier state. *Pediatrics* 44:358, 1969.

148. Holston, J. L., Levy, H. L., Tomlin, G. A., Atkins, R. J., Patton, T. H., and Hosty, T. S. Tyrosinosis: A patient without liver or renal disease. *Pediatrics* 48:393, 1971.

149. Holtzapple, P. G., Genel, M., Yakovac, W. C., Hummeler, K., and Segal, S. Diagnosis of cystinosis by rectal biopsy. *N. Engl. J. Med.* 281:143, 1969.

150. Holzel, A., Komrower, G. M., and Wilson, V. K. Aminoaciduria in galactosaemia. *Br. Med. J.* 1:194, 1952.

151. Hooft, C., Carton, D., de Schrijver, F., Delbecke, M. J., Samyn, W., and Kint, J. Juvenile Cystinosis in Two Siblings. In N. A. Carson and D. N. Raine (eds.), *Inherited Disorders of Sulphur Metabolism.* London: Livingstone, 1971. P. 141.

152. Hooft, C., and Herpol, J. Aminoaciduria in the course of lipoid nephrosis in children: The influence of ACTH. *Acta Paediatr. Scand.* 48:135, 1959.

153. Hooft, C., and Herpol, J. Aminoaciduria in the course of the nephrotic syndrome in children: The influence of hormonal therapy. *Ann. Paediatr. (Basel)* 198:3, 1962.

154. Hooft, C., and Vermassen, A. Syndrome de De Toni-Debré-Fanconi chez un enfant atteint de néphrose lipoidique. *Ann Pediatr. (Basel)* 190:1, 1958.

155. Hooft, C., and Vermassen, A. De Toni-Debré-Fanconi syndrome in nephrotic children: A review. *Ann. Pediatr. (Basel)* 194:193, 1960.

156. Hooft, C., Vermassen, A., and Herpol, J. Reversible gluco-amino-phosphaturia in a child with lipoid nephrosis. *Helv. Paediatr. Acta* 14:1, 1959.

157. Houston, I. B., Boichis, H., and Edelmann, C. M., Jr. Fanconi syndrome with renal sodium wasting and metabolic alkalosis. *Am. J. Med.* 44:638, 1968.

158. Howell, R. R. The Glycogen Storage Disease. In J. B. Stanbury, J. B. Wyngaarden, and D. S. Frederickson (eds.), *The Metabolic Basis of Inherited Disease* (3rd ed.). New York: McGraw-Hill, 1972. P. 149.

159. Hsia, D. Y.-Y. (ed.). *Galactosemia*. Springfield, Ill.: Thomas, 1969.

160. Hsia, D. Y.-Y., Hsia, H.-H., Green, S., Kay, M., and Gellis, S. S. Amino aciduria in galactosemia. *Am. J. Dis. Child.* 88:458, 1954.

161. Hsia, D. Y.-Y., and Walker, F. A. Variability in the clinical manifestations of galactosemia. *J. Pediatr.* 59:872, 1961.

162. Hsia, Y. E., Combs, J. T., Hook, L., and Brandt, I. K. Hepatolenticular degeneration: The comparative effectiveness of D-penicillamine, potassium sulfide, and diethyldithiocarbonate as decoppering agents. *J. Pediatr.* 68:921, 1966.

163. Hummeler, K., Zajal, B. A., Genel, M., Holtzapple, P. G., and Segal, S. Human cystinosis: Intracellular deposition of cystine. *Science* 166:859, 1970.

164. Hunt, D. D., Stearns, G., McKinley, J. B., Frowning, E., Hicks, P., and Bontiglio, M. Long-term study of family with Fanconi syndrome without cystinosis (de Toni-Debré-Fanconi syndrome). *Am. J. Med.* 40:492, 1966.

165. Huttenlocher, P. R., Hillman, R. E., and Hsia, Y. E. Pseudotumor cerebri in galactosemia. *J. Pediatr.* 76:902, 1970.

166. Illig, R., Dummeruth, G., and Prader, A. Das oculocerebro-renale Syndrom (Lowe): Klinische, metabolische und elektroencephalographische Befunde bei 3 Fällen. *Helv. Paediatr. Acta* 18:173, 1963.

167. Illig, R., and Prader, A. Primäre Tubulopathien: II. Ein Fall von idiopathischem Gluko-Amino-Phosphat-Diabetes (De Toni-Debré-Fanconi-Syndrome). *Helv. Paediatr. Acta* 16:622, 1961.

168. Jackson, J. D., Smith, F. G., Litman, N. N., Yuile, C. L., and Latta, H. The Fanconi syndrome with cystinosis: Electron microscopy of renal biopsy specimens from five patients. *Am. J. Med.* 33:893, 1962.

169. Jagenburg, O. R. The urinary excretion of free amino acids and other amino compounds by the human. *Scand. J. Clin. Lab. Invest.* [Suppl. 43]11:5, 1959.

170. Jeune, M., Planson, E., Cotte, J., Bonnefoy, S., Nivelon, J. L., and Skosowsky, J. l'intolerance héréditaire du fructose, à propos d'un cas. *Pediatrie* 16:605, 1961.

171. Kamm, D. E., and Fischer, M. S. Proximal renal tubular acidosis and the Fanconi syndrome in a patient with hypergammaglobulinemia. *Nephron* 9:208, 1972.

172. Kang, E. S., and Gerald, P. S. Hereditary tyrosinemia and abnormal pyrrole metabolism. *J. Pediatr.* 77:397, 1970.

173. Käser, H., Cottier, P., and Antener, I. Glucoglycinuria, a new familial syndrome. *J. Pediatr.* 61:386, 1962.

174. Kazantzis, G., Flynn, F. V., Spowage, J. S., and Trott, D. G. Renal tubular malfunction and pulmonary emphysema in cadmium pigment workers. *Q. J. Med.* 32:165, 1963.

175. Komrower, G. M., Schwarz, V., Holzel, A., and Golberg, L. A clinical and biochemical study of galactosemia: A possible explanation of the nature of the biochemical lesion. *Arch. Dis. Child.* 31:154, 1956.

176. Kramer, H. J., and Burgard, U. G. Further studies on epithelial transport defect in experimental and human Fanconi syndrome: Effect of maleic acid and L-cystine on sodium transport and $(Na^+ \text{-} K^+)$-ATP-ase of the isolated frogskin. *Clin. Chim. Acta* 55:57, 1974.

177. Kramer, H. J., and Gonick, H. C. Experimental Fanconi syndrome: I. Effect of maleic acid on renal cortical Na, K-ATPase activity and ATP levels. *J. Lab. Clin. Med.* 76:799, 1970.

178. Kramer, H. J., and Gonick, H. C. Effect of maleic acid on sodium-linked tubular transport in experimental Fanconi syndrome. *Nephron* 10:306, 1973.

179. Kranhold, J. F., Loh, D., and Morris, R. C. Renal fructose-metabolising enzymes: significance in hereditary fructose intolerance. *Science* 165:402, 1969.

180. Krohn, H.-P., Brandis, M., Brodehl, J., and Offner, G. Tubulärer Phosphattransport bei der Vitamin D resistenten Rachitis. *Monatsschr. Kinderheilkd.* 122:583, 1974.

181. Krohn, H.-P., Brodehl, J., Offner, G., Liappis, N., and Weber, H. P. Über die Veränderung der Nierenfunktion bei der Vitamin D Mangel-Rachitis. *Monatsschr. Kinderheilkd.* 121:327, 1973.

182. Kroll, W., and Lichte, K. H. Cystinosis: A review of the different forms and of recent advances. *Humangenetik* 20:75, 1973.

183. Kroll, W. A., and Schneider, J. A. Decrease in free cystine content of cultured cystinotic fibroblasts by ascorbic acid. *Science* 186:1040, 1974.

184. Kyle, R. A., Maldonado, J. E., and Bayrd, E. D. Idiopathic Bence Jones proteinuria—a distinct entity? *Am. J. Med.* 55:222, 1973.

185. Kyle, L. H., Merony, M. H., and Freemann, H. E. Study of the mechanism of bone disease in hypophosphatemic glycosuric osteomalacia. *J. Clin. Endocrinol. Metab.* 14:365, 1954.

186. LaDu, B. N., and Gjessing, L. R. Tyrosinosis and Tyrosinemia. In J. B. Stanbury, J. B. Wyngaarden, and D. S. Fredrickson (eds.), *The Metabolic Basis of Inherited Disease* (4th ed.). New York: Mc-Graw-Hill, 1978. P. 256.

187. Lambert, P.-P., and de Heinzelin de Braucourt, C. Syndrome de Fanconi—un cas chez l'adulte. *Acta Clin. Belg.* 6:13, 1951.

188. Lampert, F., and Mayer, H. Glykogenose der Leber mit Galaktoseverwertungsstörung und schwerem Fanconi-Syndrom. *Z. Kinderheilkd.* 98:133, 1967.

189. Larochelle, J., Mortezai, A., Belanger, M., Tremblay, M., Claveau, I. C., and Aubin, G. Experience with 37 infants of tyrosinemia. *Can. Med. Assoc. J.* 97:105, 1967.

190. Leaf, A. The Syndrome of Osteomalacia, Renal Glucosuria, Aminoaciduria, and Increased Phosphorus Clearance (the Fanconi Syndrome). In J. B. Stanbury, J. B. Wyngaarden, and D. S. Fredrickson (eds.), *The Metabolic Basis of Inherited Disease* (2nd ed.). New York: McGraw-Hill, 1966. P. 1205.

191. Lee, D. B. N., Drinkard, J. P., Rosen, V. J., and Gonick, H. C. The adult Fanconi syndrome. *Medicine* 51:107, 1972.

192. Lelong, M., Alagille, D., Gentil, C., Colin, J., Letan, V., and Gabilan, J. C. Cirrhose congénitale et familiale avec diabète phospho-gluco-aminé, rachitisme vitamino-resistant et tyrosinurie massive. *Rev. Fr. Etud. Clin. Biol.* 8:37, 1963.

193. Lelong, M., Alagille, D., Gentil, C., Colin, J., Tupin, J., and Bouqvier, J. Cirrhose hépatique et tubulopathie par absence congénitale de l'aldolase hépatique: Intolérance héréditaire du fructose. *Bull. Soc. Med. Hop. Paris* 113:58, 1963.

194. Leu, M. L., Strickland, G. T., and Gutman, R. A. Renal function in Wilson's disease: Response to penicillamine therapy. *Am. J. Med. Sci.* 260:381, 1970.

195. Levin, B., Oberholzer, V. G., Snodgrass, G. J. A. I., Stimmler, L., and Wilmers, M. J. Fructosemia: An inborn error of fructose metabolism. *Arch. Dis. Child.* 38:220, 1963.

196. Levin, B., Snodgrass, G. J. A. I., Oberholzer, V. G., Burgess, E. A., and Dobbs, R. H. Fructosemia: Observation of seven cases. *Am. J. Med.* 45:826, 1968.

197. Libau, G., Müller, R., Schad, H., and Edel, H.-H. Proximal tubuläre Azidose bei nierentransplantierten Patienten. *Klin. Wochenschr.* 48:624, 1970.

198. Lietman, P. S., Frazier, P. D., Wong, V. G., Shotton, D., and Seegmiller, J. E. Adult cystinosis—a benign disorder. *Am. J. Med.* 40:511, 1966.

199. Lignac, G. O. E. Über Störung des Cystinstoffwechsels bei Kindern. *Dtsch. Arch. Klin. Med.* 145:139, 1924.

200. Lindemann, R., Gjessing, L. R., Merton, B., Löken, A. C., and Halvorsen, S. Amino acid metabolism in hereditary fructosemia. *Acta Paediatr. Scand.* 59:141, 1970.

201. Lindquist, R. R., and Fellers, F. X. Degraded tetracycline nephropathy: Functions, morphologic and histochemical observations. *Lab. Invest.* 15:864, 1966.

202. Lotz, M., Zisman, E., and Bartter, F. C. Phosphorus depletion syndrome in man. *N. Engl. J. Med.* 278:409, 1968.

203. Lowe, C. U., Terrey, M., and McLachlan, E. A. Organic-aciduria, decreased renal ammonia production, hydrophthalmus, and mental retardation. *Am. J. Dis. Child.* 83:164, 1952.

204. Lowe, M. B., and Tapp, E. Renal damage caused by anhydro 4-EPI-tetracycline. *Arch. Pathol.* 81:362, 1966.

205. Lucas, Z. J., Kempson, R. L., Palmer, J., Korn, D., and Cohn, R. B. Renal allotransplantation in man: II. Transplantation in cystinosis, a metabolic disease. *Am. J. Surg.* 118:158, 1969.

206. Luder, J., and Sheldon, W. A familial tubular absorption defect of glucose and amino acids. *Arch. Dis. Child.* 30:160, 1955.

207. Mahoney, C. P., Manning, G. B., and Hickman, R. O. Hemodialysis in a patient with cystinosis. *Am. J. Dis. Child.* 112:65, 1966.

208. Mahoney, C. P., Striker, G. E., Hickman, R. O., Manning, G. B., and Marchioro, T. L. Renal transplantation for childhood cystinosis. *N. Engl. J. Med.* 283:397, 1970.

209. Maldonado, J. E., Velosa, J. A., Kyle, R. A., Wagoner, R. D., Holley, K. E., and Salassa, R. M. Fanconi syndrome in adults: A manifestation of a latent form of myeloma. *Am. J. Med.* 58:354, 1975.

210. Manz, F., Bremer, H. J., and Brodehl, J. Renal transport of Amino Acids in Children with Lowe's syndrome (abstract). Presented at the European Society for Pediatric Nephrology, Dublin, October 4–6, 1972.

211. Martinez-Maldonado, M., Yium, J., Suki, W. N., and Eknoyan, G. Renal complications in multiple myeloma: Pathophysiology and some aspects of clinical management. *J. Chronic Dis.* 24:221, 1971.

212. Mass, R. E., Smith, W. R., and Walsh, J. R. The association of hereditary fructose intolerance and renal tubular acidosis. *Am. J. Med. Sci.* 251:516, 1966.

213. Massachusetts Department of Public Health. New-

214. Massry, S., Preuss, H. G., Maher, J. F., and Schreiner, G. E. Renal tubular acidosis after cadaver kidney homotransplantation. *Am. J. Med.* 42:248, 1967.

215. Matsuda, I., Sugai, M., and Kajii, T. Ornithine loading test in Lowe's syndrome. *J. Pediatr.* 77:127, 1970.

216. Mavromatis, F. Tetracycline nephropathy. *J.A.M.A.* 193:191, 1965.

217. McCune, D. J., Mason, H. H., and Clarke, H. T. Intractable hypophosphatemic rickets with renal glycosuria and acidosis (the Fanconi syndrome). *Am. J. Dis. Child.* 65:81, 1943.

218. Medes, G. A. A new error of tyrosine metabolism: Tyrosinosis. The intermediary metabolism of tyrosine and phenylalanine. *Biochem. J.* 26:917, 1932.

219. Metcoff, J. The Fanconi Syndrome. In M. I. Rubin and T. M. Barratt (eds.), *Pediatric Nephrology.* Baltimore: Williams & Wilkins, 1975. P. 729.

220. Milkman, L. A. Multiple spontaneous idiopathic symmetrical fractures. *Am. J. Roentgenol. Radium Ther. Nucl. Med.* 32:622, 1934.

221. Milne, M. D. Renal Tubular Dysfunction. In M. B. Strauss and L. G. Welt (eds.), *Diseases of the Kidney* (2nd ed.). Boston: Little, Brown, 1971. P. 1071.

222. Monro, P. Effect of treatment on renal function in severe osteomalacia due to Wilson's disease. *J. Clin. Pathol.* 23:487, 1970.

223. Monteleone, J. A., Beutler, E., Monteleone, P. L., Utz, C. L., and Casey, E. C. Cataracts, galactosuria and hypergalactosemia due to galactokinase deficiency in a child. *Am. J. Med.* 50:403, 1971.

224. Mookerjee, B., Gault, M. H., and Dossetor, J. B. Hyperchloremic acidosis in early diagnosis of renal allograft rejection. *Ann. Intern. Med.* 71:47, 1969.

225. Moorhead, J. F., Wills, M. R., Ahmed, K. Y., Baillod, R. A., Varghese, Z., Tatler, G. L. V., and Fairney, A. Hypophosphatemic osteomalacia after cadaveric renal transplantation. *Lancet* 1:694, 1974.

226. Morris, R. Fructose induced disruption of renal acidification in patients with hereditary fructose intolerance. *J. Clin. Invest.* 44:1076, 1965.

227. Morris, R. C., Jr. Renal tubular acidosis: Mechanisms, classification and implications. *N. Engl. J. Med.* 281:1405, 1969.

228. Morris, R. C., Jr. An experimental renal acidification defect in patients with hereditary fructose intolerance: I. Its resemblance to renal tubular acidosis. *J. Clin. Invest.* 47:1389, 1968.

229. Morris, R. C., Jr. An experimental renal acidification defect in patients with hereditary fructose intolerance: II. Its distinctions from classic renal tubular acidosis; its resemblance to the renal acidification defect associated with the Fanconi syndrome of children with cystinosis. *J. Clin. Invest.* 47:1648, 1968.

230. Morris, R. C., Jr., McSherry, E., Sherwood, L. M., and Sebastian, A. Evidence of a pathogenetic role of hyperparathyroidism in the renal tubular dysfunction of patients with Fanconi syndrome (abstract). *J. Clin. Invest.* 49:68a, 1970.

231. Morris, R. C., Jr., Ueki, I., Loh, D., Eanes, R. Z., and McLin, P. Absence of renal fructose-1-phosphate aldolase activity in hereditary fructose intolerance. *Nature* 214:920, 1967.

232. Moses, S. W., and Gutman, A. Inborn errors of glycogen metabolism. *Adv. Pediatr.* 19:95, 1972.

born screening for metabolic disorders. *N. Engl. J. Med.* 288:1299, 1973.

233. Nagant de Deuxchaisnes, C., and Krane, M. The treatment of adult phosphate diabetes and Fanconi syndrome with sodium phosphate. *Am. J. Med.* 43: 508, 1967.

234. Neimann, N., Pierson, M., Marchal, C., Rauber, G., and Grignon, G. Nephropathie familial glomerulotubulaire avec syndrome de de Toni-Debré-Fanconi. *Arch. Fr. Pediatr.* 25:43, 1968.

235. Newcombe, D. S. *Inherited Biochemical Disorders and Uric Acid Metabolism.* Aylesburg, England: HM & M Publishers, 1975.

236. Nützenadel, W., Lutz, P., and Bickel, H. Tyrosinose: Primäre und sekundäre biochemische Veränderungen. *Z. Kinderheilkd.* 113:193, 1972.

237. Odièvre, M. Glycogénose hepato-rénale avec tubulopathie complex. *Rev. Int. Hepatol.* 26:1, 1966.

238. Odièvre, M., Vedrenne, J., Landrien, P., and Alagille, D. Le formes hepatiques "Pures" de la maladie de Wilson chez l'enfant. *Arch. Fr. Pediatr.* 31: 215, 1974.

239. Oetliker, O., Käser, H., Donath, A., and Rossi, E. Beitrag zur Familiarität der idiopathischen Gluko-Hyperaminoacidurie. *Helv. Paediatr. Acta* 19:556, 1964.

240. Oetliker, O., and Rossi, E. The influence of extracellular fluid volume on the renal bicarbonate threshold: A study of two children with Lowe's syndrome. *Pediatr. Res.* 3:140, 1969.

241. Oetliker, O. H., Simon, J., and Tietze, H. U. Diagnostic value of mannitol-induced diuresis in children. *Acta Paediatr. Scand.* 63:113, 1974.

242. Ores, R. O. Renal changes in oculo-cerebro-renal syndrome of Lowe. *Arch. Pathol.* 89:221, 1970.

243. Otten, J., and Vis, H. L. Acute reversible renal tubular dysfunction following intoxications with methyl-3-chromone. *J. Pediatr.* 73:422, 1968.

244. Partington, M. W., and Haust, M. D. A patient with tyrosinemia and hypermethioninemia. *Can. Med. Assoc. J.* 97:1059, 1967.

245. Patrick, A. D., and Lake, B. D. Cystinosis: Electron microscopic evidence of lysosomal storage of cystine in lymph node. *J. Clin. Pathol.* 21:571, 1968.

246. Perheentupa, I., and Hallman, N. Hereditary Fructose Intolerance. In L. I. Gardner (ed.), *Endocrine and Genetic Diseases in Childhood.* Philadelphia: Saunders, 1969. P. 844.

247. Perheentupa, J., Pitkänen, E., Nikkila, E. A., Somersalo, O., and Hakosalo, J. Hereditary fructose intolerance: A clinical study of four cases. *Ann. Paediatr. Fenn.* 8:221, 1962.

248. Perry, T. L., Hardwick, D. F., Dixon, G. H., Dolman, C. L., and Hansen, S. Hypermethioninemia: A metabolic disorder associated with cirrhosis, islet cell hyperplasia, and renal tubular degeneration. *Pediatrics* 36:236, 1965.

249. Preuss, H. G., Hammack, W. J., and Murdaugh, H. V. The effect of Bence Jones protein on the in vitro function of rabbit renal cortex. *Nephron* 5: 210, 1967.

250. Preuss, H. G., Weib, F. R., Iammarino, R. M., Hammack, W. J., and Murdaugh, H. V. Effects on rat kidney slice function in vitro of proteins from the urines of patients with myelomatosis and nephrosis. *Clin. Sci. Molec. Med.* 46:283, 1974.

251. Privé, L. Pathological findings in patients with tyrosinemia. *Can. Med. Assoc. J.* 97:1054, 1967.

252. Rampini, S., Fanconi, A., Illig, R., and Prader, A. Effect of hydrochlorothiazide on proximal renal tubular acidosis in a patient with idiopathic de Toni-Debré-Fanconi syndrome. *Helv. Paediatr. Acta* 23: 13, 1968.

253. Reem, G. H., Isaacs, M., and Vanamee, P. Renal transport of urate, phosphate and glucose in the Fanconi syndrome. *J. Clin. Endocrinol. Metab.* 27:1141, 1967.

254. Reubi, F. C. *Clearance Tests in Clinical Medicine.* Springfield, Ill.: Thomas, 1963.

255. Reynolds, E. S., Tannen, R. L., and Tyler, H. R. The renal lesions in Wilson's disease. *Am. J. Med.* 40:518, 1966.

256. Richards, W., Donnell, G. N., Wilson, W. A., Stowens, D., and Perry, T. The oculo-cerebro-renal syndrome of Lowe. *Am. J. Dis. Child.* 109: 185, 1965.

257. Rodriguez-Soriano, J., and Edelmann, C. M., Jr. Renal tubular acidosis. *Ann. Rev. Med.* 20:363, 1969.

258. Rodriguez-Soriano, J., Houston, I. B., Boichis, H., and Edelmann, C. M., Jr. Calcium and phosphorus metabolism in the Fanconi syndrome. *J. Clin. Endocrinol. Metab.* 28:1555, 1968.

259. Rosen, V. J., Kramer, H. J., and Gonick, H. C. Experimental Fanconi syndrome: II. Effect of maleic acid on renal tubular ultrastructure. *Lab. Invest.* 28: 446, 1973.

260. Rosenberg, L. E., and Scriver, C. R. Disorders of Amino Acid Metabolism. In P. K. Bondy (ed.), *Duncan's Diseases of Metabolism* (6th ed.). Philadelphia: Saunders, 1969. P. 366.

261. Rosenberg, L. E., and Segal, S. Maleic acid-induced inhibition of amino acid transport in rat kidney. *Biochem. J.* 92:345, 1964.

262. Rosenberg, L. E., Weinberg, A. N., and Segal, S. Effect of high galactose diets on urinary excretion of amino acids in rat. *Biochim. Biophys. Acta* 48: 500, 1961.

263. Rothstein, A., and Berke, H. J. Aminoaciduria in uranium poisoning; the use of amino-acid nitrogen to creatinine ratio in "spot" samples of urine. *J. Pharmacol. Exp. Ther.* 96:179, 1949.

264. Rotthauwe, H. W., Fichsel, H., Heldt, H. W., Kirsten, E., Reim, M., Schmidt, E., Schmidt, F. W., and Wesemann, W. Glykogenose der Leber mit Aminoacidurie und Glukosurie. *Klin. Wochenschr.* 41: 818, 1963.

265. Royer, P. Chronic Tubular Disease. In J. Hamburger, G. Richet, J. Crosnier, J. L. Funck-Brentano, B. Antoine, H. Ducrot, J. P. Mery, H. de Montera, P. Royer, and A. Walsh. *Nephrology.* Philadelphia: Saunders, 1966. Vol. 1, p. 576.

266. Royer, P., Delaitre, R., Mathieu, H., Gerbeaux, S., Habib, R., and Koegel, R. Le syndrome néphrotique avec insuffisance tubulaire globale et tétanie récidivante. *Ann. Pediatr. (Paris)* 10:583, 1963.

267. Royer, P., Habib, R., Mathieu, H., Broyer, M., and Walsh, A. Pediatric Nephrology. In A. J. Schafer (ed.), *Major Problems in Clinical Pediatrics* Philadelphia: Saunders, 1974. Vol. 11, p. 56.

268. Rützler, L. Passageres tubuläres Syndrom durch Vergiftung mit einer organischen Quecksilberverbindung (Glyceromerfen) bei einem 1 1/2 jährigen Mädchen. *Schweiz. Med. Wochenschr.* 103:678, 1973.

269. Sagel, I., Ores, R. O., and Yuceoglu, A. M. Renal function and morphology in a girl with oculo-cerebro-renal syndrome. *J. Pediatr.* 77:124, 1970.

270. Sanchez, L. M., and Domz, C. A.   Renal patterns in myeloma. *Ann. Intern. Med.* 52:44, 1960.

271. Sass-Kortsak, A., Ficci, S., Paunier, L., Kooh, W. S., Fraser, D., and Jackson, S. H.   Clinical and biochemical study of three patients with tyrosyluria. *Can. Med. Assoc. J.* 97:1056, 1967.

272. Sass-Kortsak, A., Ficci, S., Paunier, L., Kooh, S. W., Fraser, D., and Jackson, S. H.   Secondary metabolic derangements in patients with tyrosyluria. *Can. Med. Assoc. J.* 97:1079, 1967.

273. Sass-Kortsak, A., Ficci, S., Paunier, L., Kooh, S. W., Fraser, D., and Jackson, S. H.   Observations on treatment in patients with tyrosyluria. *Can. Med. Assoc. J.* 97:1089, 1967.

274. Saville, P. D., Nassim, R., Stevenson, F. H., Mulligen, L., and Carey, M.   The Fanconi syndrome: Metabolic studies on treatment. *J. Bone Joint Surg.* [Br.] 37:529, 1955.

275. Schärer, K., and Antener, I.   Zur Biochemie und Therapie der Cystinose. *Ann. Pediatr. (Basel)* [Suppl. 1] 203:1, 1964.

276. Schärer, K., Yoshida, F., Voyer, L., Berlow, S., Pietra, G., and Metcoff, J.   Impaired renal gluconeogenesis and energy metabolism in maleic acid-induced nephropathy in rats. *Res. Exp. Med.* 157:136, 1972.

277. Schmidt, G.-W.   Langfristige Untersuchungen der Aminosäurenausscheidung mit dem Harn beim nephrotischen Syndrom im Kindesalter. *Helv. Paediatr. Acta* 18:525, 1963.

278. Schneider, J. A., Bradley, K., and Seegmiller, J. E.   Increased cystine in leukocytes from individuals homozygous and heterozygous for cystinosis. *Science* 157:1321, 1967.

279. Schneider, J. A., and Seegmiller, J. E.   Cystinosis and the Fanconi Syndrome. In J. B. Stanbury, J. B. Wyngaarden, and D. S. Fredrickson (eds.), *The Metabolic Basis of Inherited Disease* (3rd ed.). New York: McGraw-Hill, 1972. P. 1581.

280. Schneider, J. A., Verroust, F. M., Kroll, W. A., Garvin, A. J., Horger, E. O., Wong, V. G., Spear, G. S., Jacobson, C., Pellett, O. L., and Becker, F. L. A.   Prenatal diagnosis of cystinosis. *N. Engl. J. Med.* 290:878, 1974.

281. Schneider, J. A., Wong, V., Bradley, K., and Seegmiller, J. E.   Biochemical comparisons of the adult and childhood forms of cystinosis. *N. Engl. J. Med.* 279:1253, 1968.

282. Schφnheider, F., Gregersen, G., Hansen, H. E., and Skov, P. E.   Renal clearances of different amino acids in Wilson's disease before and after treatment with penicillamine. *Acta Med. Scand.* 190:395, 1971.

283. Schulman, J. D.   Cystinosis. NIH 72–249. Washington, D.C.: Department of Health, Education and Welfare, 1973.

284. Schwartz, R., Hall, P. W., and Gabuzda, G. J.   Metabolism of ornithine and other amino acids in the cerebro-oculo-renal syndrome. *Am. J. Med.* 36:778, 1964.

285. Scriver, C. R., and Rosenberg, L. E.   Amino Acid Metabolism and Its Disorders. In A. J. Shafer (ed.), *Major Problems in Clinical Pediatrics.* Philadelphia: Saunders, 1973. Vol. 11.

286. Sebastian, A., McSherry, E., and Morris, R. C., Jr.   On the mechanism of renal potassium wasting in renal tubular acidosis—associated with the Fanconi syndrome (type 2 RTA). *J. Clin. Invest.* 50:231, 1971.

287. Sebastian, A., McSherry, E., and Morris, R. C., Jr.   Renal potassium wasting in renal tubular acidosis (RTA). *J. Clin. Invest.* 50:667, 1971.

288. Segal, S.   Disorders of Galactose Metabolism. In J. B. Stanbury, J. B. Wyngaarden, and D. S. Fredrickson (eds.), *The Metabolic Basis of Inherited Disease* (3rd ed.). New York: McGraw-Hill, 1972. P. 174.

289. Seip, M., Steen-Johnsen, J., Vellan, J. E., and Glessing, L. R.   Dietary treatment of cystinosis. *Acta Paediatr. Scand.* 57:409, 1968.

290. Shearn, M. A., and Tu, W. H.   Nephrogenic diabetes insipidus and other defects of renal tubular function in Sjögren's syndrome. *Am. J. Med.* 39:312, 1965.

291. Sheldon, W., Luder, J., and Webb, B. A.   A familial tubular absorption defect of glucose and amino acids. *Arch. Dis. Child.* 36:90, 1961.

292. Sirota, J. H., and Hamerman, D.   Renal function studies in an adult subject with Fanconi syndrome. *Am. J. Med.* 16:138, 1954.

293. Spear, G.   The proximal tubule and the podocyte in cystinosis. *Nephron* 10:57, 1973.

294. Spear, G. S., Slusser, R. S., Tousimis, A. J., Taylor, C. G., and Schulman, J. D.   Cystinosis—an ultrastructural and electron-probe study of the kidney with unusual findings. *Arch. Pathol.* 91:206, 1971.

295. Spencer, A. G., and Franglen, G. T.   Gross aminoaciduria following a Lysol burn. *Lancet* 1:190, 1952.

296. Stanbury, S. W., and Lumb, G. A.   Metabolic studies of renal osteodystrophy: I. Calcium, phosphorus and nitrogen metabolism in rickets, osteomalacia, and hyperparathyroidism complicating chronic uremia and in the osteomalacia of the adult Fanconi syndrome. *Medicine* 41:1, 1963.

297. Stanbury, S. W., and Macaulay, D.   Defects of renal tubular function in the nephrotic syndrome. *Q. J. Med.* 26:7, 1957.

298. Stein, W. H., Bearn, A. G., and Moore, S.   The amino acid content of the blood and urine in Wilson's disease. *J. Clin. Invest.* 33:410, 1954.

299. Stickler, G. B., and Bergen, B. J.   A review: Short stature in renal disease. *Pediatr. Res.* 7:978, 1973.

300. Stickler, G. B., and Burke, E. C.   External calcium and phosphorus balance. *Am. J. Dis. Child.* 106:68, 1963.

301. Stickler, G. B., Hayles, A. B., Power, M. H., and Ulrich, J. A.   Nephrotic syndrome complicated by renal tubular dysfunction. *Am. J. Dis. Child.* 98:127, 1959.

302. Stickler, G. B., Hayles, A. B., Power, M. H., and Ulrich, J. A.   Renal tubular dysfunction complicating the nephrotic syndrome. *Pediatrics* 26:75, 1960.

303. Suzuki, H., Gilbert, E. F., Anido, V., Jones, B., and Klingberg, W. G.   Galactosemia. *Arch. Pathol.* 82:602, 1966.

304. Svorc, I., Masopust, I., Komarkowa, A., Macek, M., and Hyanek, J.   Oculo-cerebro-renal syndrome in a female child. *Am. J. Dis. Child.* 114:186, 1967.

305. Tegelaers, W. H. H., and Tiddens, H. W.   Nephrotic-glucosuric-aminoaciduric dwarfism and electrolyte metabolism. *Helv. Paediatr. Acta* 10:269, 1955.

306. Texier, J. L., Jully, G., and Bach, C.   Syndrome de Lowe. *Ann. Pediatr. (Paris)* 18:825, 1971.

307. Uzman, L., and Denny-Brown, D.   Amino-aciduria in hepatolenticular degeneration (Wilson's disease). *Am. J. Med. Sci.* 215:599, 1948.

308. Van Acker, K. J., Roels, H., Beelaerts, W., Pasternack, A., and Valke, R. The histologic lesions of the kidney in the oculo-cerebro-renal syndrome of Lowe. *Nephron.* 4:193, 1967.

309. Van Geffel, R., Devriendt, A., Dustin, I.-P., Vis, H., and Loeb, H. La maladie du galactose, considérations génétiques, étude de l'amino-acidémie et de l'amino-acidurie. *Arch. Fr. Pediatr.* 16:158, 1959.

310. Vertuno, L. L., Preuss, H. G., Argy, W. P., and Schreiner, G. E. Fanconi syndrome following homotransplantation. *Arch. Intern. Med.* 133:302, 1974.

311. Von Studnitz, W., and Haeger-Aronson, B. Urinary excretion of amino acids in lead poisoned rabbits. *Acta Pharmacol.* 19:36, 1962.

312. Wadman, S. K., van Sprang, F. J., Maas, J. W., and Ketting, D. An exceptional case of tyrosinosis. *J. Ment. Defic. Res.* 12:269, 1968.

313. Waldmann, T. A., Strober, W., and Mogielnicki, R. P. The renal handling of low molecular weight proteins: II. Disorders of serum protein. Catabolism in patients with tubular proteinuria, the nephrotic syndrome or uremia. *J. Clin. Invest.* 51:2162, 1972.

314. Walker, B. R., Alexander, F., and Tannenbaum, P. J. Fanconi syndrome with renal tubular acidosis and light chain proteinuria. *Nephron* 8:103, 1971.

315. Walker, W. G., Harvey, A. M., and Yardley, J. H. Renal Involvement in Myeloma, Amyloidosis, Systemic Lupus Erythematosus and Other Disorders of Connective Tissue. In M. B. Strauss and L. G. Welt (eds.), *Diseases of the Kidney* (2nd ed.). Boston: Little, Brown, 1971. P. 825.

316. Wallis, L. A., and Engle, R. L., Jr. The adult Fanconi syndrome: II. Review of eighteen cases. *Am. J. Med.* 22:13, 1957.

317. Walshe, J. M. Wilson's Disease (Hepatolenticular Degeneration). In D. N. Raine (ed.), *The Treatment of Inherited Metabolic Disease.* Lancaster, England: Medical and Technical Publishing Co., 1975. P. 171.

318. Weber, H., and Hagge, W. Über die erfolgreiche Behandlung der Zystinose mit einem Anabolikum. *Arch. Kinderheilkd.* 168:110, 1963.

319. Wegienka, L. C., and Weller, J. M. Renal tubular acidosis caused by degraded tetracycline. *Arch. Intern. Med.* 114:232, 1964.

320. Wilson, D. M., and Goldstein, N. P. Renal urate excretion in patients with Wilson's disease. *Kidney Int.* 4:331, 1973.

321. Wilson, D. R., and Yendt, E. R. Treatment of adult Fanconi syndrome with oral phosphate supplement and alkali. *Am. J. Med.* 35:487, 1963.

322. Wilson, V. K., Thomson, M. L., and Dent, C. E. Aminoaciduria in lead poisoning: A case in childhood. *Lancet* 2:66, 1953.

323. Wilson, W. A., Richards, W., and Donnell, G. N. Oculo-cerebral-renal syndrome of Lowe: A review of eight cases noting the genetic inheritance. *Arch. Ophthalmol.* 70:5, 1963.

324. Witzleben, C. L., Monteleone, J. A., and Rejent, A. J. Electron microscopy in the diagnosis of cystinosis. *Arch. Pathol.* 94:362, 1972.

325. Witzleben, C. L., Schoen, E. J., Tu, W. H., and McDonald, L. W. Progressive morphologic renal changes in the oculo-cerebro-renal syndrome of Lowe. *Am. J. Med.* 44:319, 1968.

326. Wolff, S. Renal lesions in Wilson's disease. *Lancet* 1:834, 1964.

327. Wong, V. G., Lietman, P. S., and Seegmiller, J. E. Alterations of pigment epithelium in cystinosis. *Arch. Ophthalmol.* 77:361, 1967.

328. Woolf, L. I. *Renal Tubular Dysfunction.* Springfield, Ill.: Thomas, 1966.

329. Woolf, L. I., and Giles, H. M. Urinary excretion of amino acids and sugar in the nephrotic syndrome: A chromatographic study. *Acta Paediatr. Scand.* 45:489, 1956.

330. Worthen, H. G. Renal toxicity of maleic acid in the rat: Enzymatic and morphologic observations. *Lab. Invest.* 12:791, 1963.

331. Worthen, H. G., and Good, R. A. The de Toni-Fanconi syndrome with cystinosis. *Am. J. Dis. Child.* 95:653, 1958.

332. Zimmerman, M. J., and Werther, Z. L. Renal glycosuria, acidosis and dehydration following administration of outdated tetracycline. *J. Mt. Sinai Hosp.* 31:38, 1964.

82. Nephrogenic Defects of Urinary Concentration

Paul Stern

Definitions

The inability to concentrate the urine maximally in the presence of high levels of antidiuretic hormone (ADH, or vasopressin) constitutes a nephrogenic defect of urinary concentration. The renal concentrating defect may be partial or complete. In a *partial* defect the patient, in response to dehydration or the administration of vasopressin, can concentrate his urine, that is, render it hypertonic to plasma, but not to normal maximal levels. A *complete* defect is manifested by unremitting hyposthenuria. Many disease processes can be responsible for a nephrogenic concentrating defect, which is then part of the more complex symptomatology of the basic process. When polyuria and hyposthenuria are the predominant manifestations, however, one can refer to the patient as presenting the *syndrome of nephrogenic diabetes insipidus.* This clinical definition is not universally accepted, and this fact must be borne in mind when reviewing the literature on the subject.

Causes

The causes of nephrogenic defects of urinary concentration can be divided into those which affect primarily either (1) the tubular permeability to water or (2) the medullary solute gradient. In the latter case, there can be osmotic equilibration between the fluid of the collecting duct and the interstitium of the medulla; but the solute concentration of the medulla is reduced so that the highest urinary osmolality that can be achieved will be below a normal maximal osmolality [42]. All the conditions discussed here can produce defects varying in severity from partial to complete.

CONDITIONS THAT AFFECT PRIMARILY THE ACTION OF ADH ON TUBULAR PERMEABILITY TO WATER

In conditions that affect ADH action on tubular water permeability, there is an interference with one of the steps in a presumed chain of events depicted in Fig. 82-1. ADH binds to a receptor in the basolateral (peritubular) cell membrane of specific epithelial cells of the distal convoluted tubule and collecting duct. Through a series of steps, with cyclic AMP (adenosine 3':5'-cyclic phosphate) as a "second messenger," this results in an increase in the permeability to water of the luminal cell membrane [21]. The permeability to urea of cells of the medullary collecting duct is also increased by ADH [36]. Many hormones, such as the renal prostaglandins, influence this chain of events, but they have a variety of renal and extrarenal influences on the renal concentrating mechanism [33, 66]. Calcium also plays a regulatory role in the ADH-cyclic AMP system [46].

Any disorder leading to *hypokalemia* and any disorder associated with *hypercalcemia* may cause partial or complete renal concentrating defects. Hypokalemia and hypercalcemia interfere with ADH-induced generation of cyclic AMP [20]. These electrolyte disturbances also affect renal hemodynamics and the medullary solute concentration, and therefore exert multiple effects on the renal concentrating mechanism [6, 25]. These renal concentrating defects may be reversible if structural damage such as nephrocalcinosis is absent [34].

Many *drugs* such as methoxyflurane [13, 47], propoxyphene, lithium salts, and demeclocycline can interfere with the action of ADH on the tubules and produce a concentrating defect [68]. Because they interfere with ADH, lithium salts and demeclocycline have been used in the treatment of some patients with the syndrome of inappropriate secretion of ADH [12, 18, 81]. The use of these toxic agents should be restricted to patients in whom treatment of the cause of the inappropriate secretion of ADH and water restriction is not possible.

A very rare but classic disorder in the category of defects that interfere directly with the ADH-cyclic AMP system is *hereditary nephrogenic diabetes insipidus* [8, 28]. The mode of inheritance of this disease remains controversial. There is a preponderance of males affected, suggesting X-linked transmission with a variable expression in females [11, 14, 83], but other genetic modes

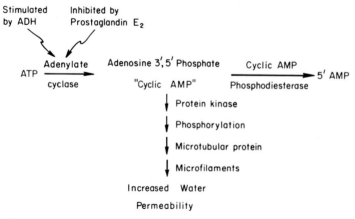

Figure 82-1. Presumed chain of events whereby antidiuretic hormone (ADH) induces an increased water permeability of specific cells of the distal convoluted tubules and collecting ducts. Not depicted is the presence of a receptor for ADH. A defect in water permeability can occur potentially from interference with any of the steps involved. (From Valtin [77]; published with permission.)

have been proposed [10, 60]. Affected females may have either a partial or complete concentrating defect. Generation of cyclic AMP in response to ADH may be impaired in patients with hereditary nephrogenic diabetes insipidus. In contrast with normal individuals, ADH administration has been reported not to increase the excretion of cyclic AMP in the urine in these patients [5, 27, 48], although this has not been a uniform finding [52]. The same discrepancy exists regarding cyclic AMP excretion in the urine of patients with hereditary nephrogenic diabetes insipidus after parathyroid hormone administration [27, 48, 52]. The administration of exogenous cyclic AMP does not improve the concentrating ability of patients with this disorder; it may be that steps beyond ADH-induced generation of cyclic AMP are affected or that the administration of cyclic AMP has other actions, such as hemodynamic and parathyroid hormone-like effects, that obscure its ADH-like action [39, 57, 69]. The availability of animal models [77] may help clarify the pathogenesis of this and other forms of diabetes insipidus.

CONDITIONS THAT AFFECT PRIMARILY THE MEDULLARY SOLUTE CONCENTRATION

Disorders that *primarily* affect the buildup of the corticopapillary gradient of solute concentration do so by interfering with one or more of the elements of the countercurrent mechanism; they do not directly affect the changes in tubular permeability induced by ADH. The disorders in this category, which are reviewed in specific chapters, include chronic renal failure [2, 72]; chronic obstructive nephropathy and postobstructive nephropathy [37, 49, 84]; medullary cystic disease; polycystic kidney disease; interstitial nephropathy associated with pyelonephritis [31] and also with urinary tract infection without evident medullary pathology [41, 61, 84]; nonbacterial interstitial nephropathies due to drugs (acetaminophen, penicillin derivatives) or associated with disorders such as sickle cell anemia [1, 35]; acute renal failure, especially in the diuretic phase; any cause leading to Fanconi syndrome; any cause leading to an osmotic diuresis (glucose, urea, mannitol) [30, 67]; and malnutrition [43]. The relatively diminished concentrating ability of the newborn, when compared to the older infant or adult, should not be considered a defect, but rather a normal stage of development.

One or more of the following elements of the countercurrent mechanism are affected by these disorders: delivery of solutes and water out of the proximal tubules; the functional and anatomic integrity of the loops of Henle; blood flow in the vasa recta; availability of urea; and rate of solute delivery to the distal tubules and collecting ducts [38, 65, 75, 78].

Clinical Manifestations

A partial defect in concentrating ability may not be perceived as a problem either by the patient or the physician. A mild degree of polyuria with rates of urine flow only slightly above the normal range of 50 to 75 ml per 100 kcal metabolized may not be noticed among the more prominent manifestations of the underlying disease. The specific gravity of the urine may rise to the 1.010 to 1.016 range when moderate dehydration is present. Occasionally a specific gravity of 1.025 or above may have been recorded in such a patient after a radiographic study, reflecting the presence of heavy radiographic contrast material in the urine and not renal concentrating capacity.

A patient with a moderate to severe or complete concentrating defect presents more dramatic symptoms. Polyuria, polydipsia, and nocturia are evident. In patients with hereditary nephrogenic diabetes insipidus, polyhydramnios may be present at birth [14]. Hypertonic volume contraction will be a threat to the infant if appropriate water intake is not provided. Hypernatremia and hypertonic volume contraction are associated with potentially severe central nervous system complications and their sequelae [40, 44, 53, 62]. Growth retardation may occur, probably related to caloric deprivation in infants and small children who have to drink water in preference to the ingestion of food with an appropriate caloric content [74, 80]. Fever can occur, particularly in the neonate [64] and small infant. The fever may be due to increased metabolic expenditure because of increased oxygen consumption by cellular sodium pumps when the extracellular environment has a high sodium concentration [54].

In patients with acquired forms of nephrogenic diabetes insipidus, the underlying cause (chronic renal failure for example) will determine the existence of other factors that will impair growth (hormonal factors, metabolic acidosis) [70]. Hyperuricemia not related to treatment with diuretics has been reported in adults with a nephrogenic concentrating defect [32].

Hydronephrosis and dilatation of the collecting system may be found and are thought to be related to a urine flow that is greater than the capacity of the collecting system ("functional obstruction") [45]. Since hydronephrosis itself may be a cause of nephrogenic diabetes insipidus, the problem of determining which was the initiating event may occur in some patients. This may be solved by a careful history and a search for an anatomic obstruction [73, 82].

The polyuria and nocturia and the attendant bed-wetting can be embarrassing to children with complete nephrogenic diabetes insipidus and can cause severe problems in school. Frequently these children cannot sit through an hour of classes without having to excuse themselves in order to urinate and to drink.

Diagnosis

History, physical examination, and pertinent laboratory tests will suggest the underlying cause in most cases. An osmotic diuresis such as that accompanying the glycosuria of diabetes mellitus or of parenteral alimentation of the preterm infant must always be ruled out as a cause of the concentrating defect. In patients who present with hyposthenuria of unclear etiology, three possible alternatives must be considered [78]: (1) primary polydipsia, in which the initiating event is excessive drinking, commonly due to a psychiatric disorder; (2) hypothalamic diabetes insipidus, in which the primary problem is deficient production or release of ADH; or (3) nephrogenic diabetes insipidus.

Several tests based on the classic experiments of E. B. Verney [79] can be employed to distinguish between these alternatives [23, 29]. Increasing plasma osmolality by an infusion of hypertonic saline or by water deprivation is sensed by osmoreceptors in the brain, and ADH is released by the neurohypophysis. As seen in Fig. 82-2A, patients with hypothalamic diabetes insipidus release little or no ADH in response to the osmolar stimulus, whereas patients with primary polydipsia or nephrogenic diabetes insipidus can release ADH comparably to normal individuals. When the concentration of ADH in plasma rises (Fig. 82-2B), patients with partial hypothalamic diabetes insipidus can concentrate their urine to a degree in relation to their ability to release ADH, but patients with nephrogenic diabetes insipidus cannot.

We prefer the water deprivation test over the infusion of hypertonic saline because of the risks associated with the latter in some patients and because the production of an osmotic diuresis of NaCl can obscure the results. In an osmotic diuresis the urine osmolality will tend toward isotonicity. However, water deprivation also has definite risks in a patient who has hypothalamic or nephrogenic diabetes insipidus. The common but objectionable procedure, if a moderate to severe defect is suspected, is an overnight fluid restriction. In a patient with an obligatory loss of water,

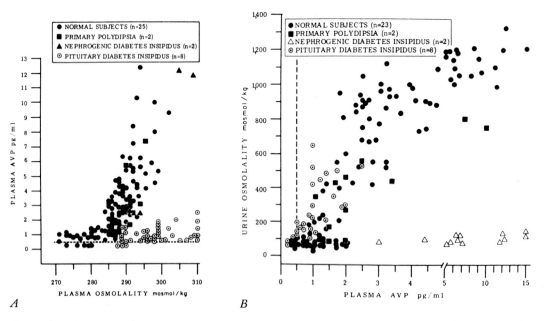

Figure 82-2. Relationship between plasma antidiuretic hormone (ADH; arginine vasopressin, or AVP) concentration and plasma osmolality in the left-hand panel (A) and urine osmolality in the right-hand panel (B) in normal subjects and in subjects with different forms of diabetes insipidus. Note that the patients with hypothalamic (pituitary) diabetes insipidus include some with a complete and others with a partial defect. The broken lines (- - -) indicate the sensitivity limit of the assay employed. (From Robertson et al. [59]; published with permission.)

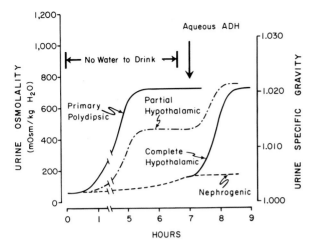

Figure 82-3. Water deprivation test for the differential diagnosis of diabetes insipidus. Not depicted is an example of a patient with a partial nephrogenic defect. (From Valtin [78]; published with permission.)

this practice may lead to dangerous volume contraction. Alternatively, because of the intense thirst, the patient may be prompted to drink surreptitiously, thus rendering the test uninterpretable.

In the test we use, depicted in Fig. 82-3, plasma osmolality is measured and water deprivation is started early in the morning, free access to water having been allowed until then. A patient with primary polydipsia may be overhydrated and have a plasma osmolality below normal (<286 mOsm/kg H_2O). Such a patient may require a more prolonged water deprivation than the one described here. On the other hand, if a patient has clinical evidence of volume contraction at the start of the test or has a plasma osmolality of 295 mOsm per kilogram H_2O or higher in the presence of hyposthenuria, he probably has nephrogenic or hypothalamic diabetes insipidus [56] and should not be subjected to water deprivation; instead, an injection of ADH is given to make the distinction between these two syndromes. If the plasma osmolality is normal or slightly elevated, a period of water deprivation is started. Body weight, vital signs, and urine osmolality are monitored hourly. A urine collector bag can be used in an infant. Measurement of specific gravities, which can be done accurately at the bedside with a refractometer, supplements the measurement of urine osmolalities.

The water deprivation is continued until the patient has lost 3 to 4 percent of body weight, or until urine osmolality has reached a plateau. This usually requires 5 to 7 hr of water deprivation. At that point a second blood sample is drawn for testing plasma osmolality. In patients with pri-

mary polydipsia, plasma osmolality will not have increased detectably; whereas in patients with nephrogenic or hypothalamic diabetes insipidus who cannot concentrate their urine there will be a definite increase over the initial value (usually to above 300 mOsm/kg H_2O) [17]. Approximately 1 unit of aqueous vasopressin per square meter is then injected intramuscularly, and the patient is followed for an additional 1 to 2 hr.

If the urine osmolality reaches a plateau at about 700 to 800 mOsm per kilogram of H_2O before the injection of ADH, it is likely that the ability of both the hypothalamoneurohypophyseal system to release ADH in response to the osmolar stimulus and of the kidneys to respond to ADH is intact. Such a patient has primary polydipsia, and should concentrate his urine no further after the ADH injection. Note that the maximal osmolality achieved is below the normal, which for a school-age child, for example, would be about 1,000 to 1,200 mOsm per kilogram of H_2O [23]. This lower maximal osmolality is so because the solute concentration of the medulla, with which the collecting duct fluid equilibrates in the presence of ADH, is reduced in individuals who have been in a prolonged state of water diuresis [19, 26].

If the urine is still hyposthenuric after a loss of 3 to 4 percent of body weight and the consequent hyperosmolality of plasma, either complete hypothalamic or complete nephrogenic diabetes insipidus is present. The injection of ADH will differentiate between the two.

The major difficulty encountered in interpreting the results of the water deprivation test, aside from technical errors in how the test is conducted, is in the diagnosis of partial defects. Partial nephrogenic defects of concentration are usually associated with a readily identifiable cause, but this may not be so in partial hypothalamic defects. The administration of ADH as described will serve to distinguish partial hypothalamic diabetes insipidus from primary polydipsia. Patients with partial hypothalamic diabetes insipidus can release some ADH in response to the osmolar stimulus, but not enough. These patients may have hypertonic urine after water deprivation but incomplete equilibration of collecting duct fluid with the papillary interstitium. After the dose of ADH, which induces equilibration, a further rise in urine osmolality will occur, usually by more than 50 to 70 mOsm per kilogram of H_2O [50].

When a radioimmunoassay for plasma or urinary ADH is available [51, 59], one can define the diagnosis with more certainty, as can be understood from Fig. 82-2. In a patient with hypothalamic diabetes insipidus the level of ADH in plasma or urine will not increase appropriately in response to elevated plasma osmolality. In patients with primary polydipsia and with nephrogenic diabetes insipidus the level of ADH in plasma will increase, but urine osmolality will increase only in patients with primary polydipsia. This latter increase will not be to the level seen in a normal individual, as mentioned earlier, and the distinction between a patient with primary polydipsia and one with a partial nephrogenic defect may be difficult if based on this test alone. Note in Fig. 82-3 that there may be a slight rise in urine osmolality in a patient with a complete nephrogenic defect. This is due to volume contraction, a drop in the glomerular filtration rate, and a decrease in the availability of solutes and water to the diluting segment of the tubules, coupled with a slower flow rate in the distal nephron that may permit some equilibration with the medullary interstitium [7, 48].

A relatively new development in the conduct of the water deprivation test is the availability of analogues of ADH with minute pressor but high antidiuretic activity [63]. Instead of aqueous ADH, 1-desamino-8-D-arginine vasopressin, DDAVP, can be employed in the test in a dose of 1 or 2 μg given intravenously [3, 24, 71].

Treatment

The most desirable treatment of nephrogenic defects of urinary concentration is of the primary cause. If this is not possible, and if the defect is partial and mild, treatment involves only provision of an adequate water intake in situations in which the patient's thirst cannot be relied on, such as in the infant, the unconscious patient, or the patient on "strict fluid orders."

Treatment of a severe or complete defect is much less satisfactory. It involves (1) early recognition of the defect, particularly in the neonate with hereditary nephrogenic diabetes insipidus; (2) adequate water provision; (3) reduction of the solute load the kidney has to excrete; (4) the use of diuretics such as thiazides, furosemide, or ethacrynic acid; and (5) genetic counseling when appropriate.

The importance of the solute load can be illustrated in the following manner. An average solute load for a 10-kg infant on a standard diet will be approximately 30 mOsm per 100 kcal metabolized, or approximately 300 mOsm. To excrete these 300 mOsm at a urine osmolality of 600 mOsm per kilogram of H_2O, the infant will need to excrete 500 ml of urine in 24 hr, which is in the range of an average urine output for a 10-kg child. If he cannot concentrate his urine over 100 mOsm per kilogram of H_2O, he will need 3 liters of urine to excrete those same 300 mOsm. A reduction in the solute load will lower the volume of urine required; this reduction in solute intake may be difficult to achieve and still provide an adequate protein and caloric intake. In infants, breast milk or a low solute formula should be employed [86].

The use of diuretics such as the thiazides can result in a considerable reduction of the polyuria to as much as 50 percent, albeit with only slight increases in concentration [9, 15]. The mechanism of action of the diuretics probably involves the achievement of extracellular volume contraction, which causes an increase in the fraction of the filtered sodium chloride and water that is reabsorbed in the proximal tubules [16, 22, 58]. Distal tubular flow is decreased as a result. In addition, the thiazides block the resorption of NaCl in the cortical diluting segments. Hydrochlorothiazide in a dosage of 1 to 2 mg/kg/day, can be used. Sodium intake should be reduced simultaneously. Once mild volume contraction is present, the diuretics can be discontinued without abatement of the favorable effect, provided dietary sodium continues to be restricted. It is better, however, not to impose such a strict restriction in salt intake, but rather to combine the long-term use of diuretics with a more moderate restriction of sodium intake (i.e., 1 to 1.5 mEq/kg/day).

The usual precautions involved in the long-term use of diuretics must be observed to avoid complications such as hypokalemia or hyperuricemia. The antihypertensive diazoxide, which increases NaCl and water resorption in the proximal tubules, has also been used [55]; the use of this agent is associated with an increase in plasma volume [4], and hyperglycemia is a frequent complication.

Finally, the course and prognosis of a nephrogenic concentrating defect will be determined more by the underlying disorder that caused it than by the concentrating defect itself, assuming, of course, that the presence of a concentrating defect is suspected and detected early and is managed appropriately to prevent the potentially harmful complications.

References

1. Alleyne, G. A. O., Van Eps, L. W. S., Addae, S. K., Nicholson, G. D., and Schouten, H. The kidney in sickle cell anemia. *Kidney Int.* 7:371, 1975.
2. Anastasakis, S., and Buchborn, E. Störungen der Harnkonzentrierung bei chronischen Nephropathien. *Klin. Wochenschr.* 44:289, 1966.
3. Aronson, A. S., and Svenningsen, N. W. DDAVP test for estimation of renal concentrating capacity in infants and children. *Arch. Dis. Child.* 49:654, 1974.
4. Bartorelli, C., Gargano, N., Leonetti, G., and Zanchetti, A. Hypotensive and renal effects of diazoxide, a sodium-retaining benzothiadiazine compound. *Circulation* 27:895, 1963.
5. Bell, N. H., Clark, C. M., Jr., Avery, S., Sinha, T., Trygstad, C. M., and Allen, D. O. Demonstration of a defect in the formation of adenosine 3′,5′ monophosphate in vasopressin-resistant diabetes insipidus. *Pediatr. Res.* 8:223, 1974.
6. Bennett, C. M. Urine concentration and dilution in hypokalemic and hypercalcemic dogs. *J. Clin. Invest.* 49:1447, 1970.
7. Berliner, R. W., and Davidson, D. G. Production of hypertonic urine in the absence of pituitary antidiuretic hormone. *J. Clin. Invest.* 36:1416, 1957.
8. Bode, H. H., and Crawford, J. D. Nephrogenic diabetes insipidus in North America—the Hopewell hypothesis. *N. Engl. J. Med.* 280:750, 1969.
9. Brown, D. M., Reynolds, J. W., Michael, A. F., and Ulstrom, R. A. The use and mode of action of ethacrynic acid in nephrogenic diabetes insipidus. *Pediatrics* 37:447, 1966.
10. Cannon, J. F. Diabetes insipidus: Clinical and experimental studies with consideration of genetic relationships. *Arch. Intern. Med.* 96:215, 1955.
11. Carter, C., and Simpkiss, M. The "carrier" state in nephrogenic diabetes insipidus. *Lancet* 2:1069, 1956.
12. Cherrill, D. A., Stote, R. M., and Birge, J. R. Demeclocycline treatment in the syndrome of inappropriate antidiuretic hormone secretion. *Ann. Intern. Med.* 83:654, 1975.
13. Crandell, W. B., Pappas, S. G., and MacDonald, A. Nephrotoxicity associated with methoxyflurane anesthesia. *Anesthesiology* 27:591, 1966.
14. Crawford, J. D., and Bode, H. H. Disorders of the Posterior Pituitary in Children. In L. I. Gardner (ed.), *Endocrine and Genetic Diseases of Childhood and Adolescence* (2nd ed.). Philadelphia: Saunders, 1975.
15. Crawford, J. D., and Kennedy, G. C. Chlorothiazid in diabetes insipidus. *Nature* 183:891, 1959.
16. Cutler, R. E., Kleeman, C. R., Maxwell, M. H., and Dowling, J. T. Physiologic studies in nephrogenic diabetes insipidus. *J. Clin. Endocrinol. Metab.* 22:827, 1962.
17. Dashe, A. M., Cramm, R. E., Crist, C. A., Habener, J. F., and Solomon, D. H. A water deprivation test for the differential diagnosis of polyuria. *J.A.M.A.* 185:699, 1963.
18. DeTroyer, A., and Demanet, J. C. Correction of antidiuresis by demeclocycline. *N. Engl. J. Med.* 293:915, 1975.
19. De Wardener, H. E., and Herxheimer, A. The effect of a high water intake on the kidney's ability to concentrate urine in man. *J. Physiol. (Lond.)* 139:42, 1957.
20. Dousa, T. P. Cellular action of antidiuretic hormone in nephrogenic diabetes insipidus. *Mayo Clin. Proc.* 49:188, 1974.
21. Dousa, T. P., and Valtin, H. Cellular actions of vasopressin in the mammalian kidney. *Kidney Int.* 10:46, 1976.
22. Earley, L. E., and Orloff, J. The mechanism of antidiuresis associated with the administration of hydrochlorothiazide to patients with vasopressin-resistant diabetes insipidus. *J. Clin. Invest.* 41:1988, 1962.
23. Edelmann, C. M., Jr., Barnett, H. L., Stark, H., Boichis, H., and Rodriguez-Soriano, J. A standardized test of renal concentrating capacity in children. *Am. J. Dis. Child.* 114:639, 1967.
24. Edwards, C. R. W., Kitau, M. J., Chard, T., and Besser, G. M. Vasopressin analogue DDAVP in diabetes insipidus: Clinical and laboratory studies. *Br. Med. J.* 2:375, 1973.
25. Epstein, F. H. Disorders of renal concentrating ability. *Yale J. Biol. Med.* 39:186, 1966.
26. Epstein, F. H., Kleeman, C. R., and Hendrikx, A. The influence of bodily hydration on the renal concentrating process. *J. Clin. Invest.* 36:629, 1957.
27. Fichman, M. P., and Brooker, G. Deficient renal cyclic adenosine 3′-5′ monophosphate production in nephrogenic diabetes insipidus. *J. Clin. Endocrinol. Metab.* 35:35, 1972.
28. Forssmann, H. The recognition of nephrogenic diabetes insipidus: A very small page from the history of medicine. *Acta Med. Scand.* 197:1, 1975.
29. Frasier, S. D., Kutnik, L. A., Schmidt, R. T., and Smith, F. G., Jr. A water deprivation test for the diagnosis of diabetes insipidus in children. *Am. J. Dis. Child.* 114:157, 1967.
30. Gennari, F. J., and Kassirer, J. P. Osmotic diuresis. *N. Engl. J. Med.* 291:714, 1974.
31. Gilbert, R. M., Weber, H., Turchin, L., Fine, L. G., Bourgoignie, J. J., and Bricker, N. S. A study of the intrarenal recycling of urea in the rat with chronic experimental pyelonephritis. *J. Clin. Invest.* 58:1348, 1976.
32. Gorden, P., Robertson, G. L., and Seegmiller, J. E. Hyperuricemia, a concomitant of congenital vasopressin-resistant diabetes insipidus in the adult. *N. Engl. J. Med.* 284:1057, 1971.
33. Grantham, J. J., and Orloff, J. Effect of prostaglandin E₁ on the permeability response of the isolated collecting tubule to vasopressin, adenosine 3′,5′-monophosphate, and theophylline. *J. Clin. Invest.* 47:1154, 1968.
34. Harrington, J. T., and Cohen, J. J. Clinical dis-

orders of urine concentration and dilution. *Arch. Intern. Med.* 131:810, 1973.

35. Hatch, F. E., Culbertson, J. W., and Diggs, L. W. Nature of the renal concentrating defect in sickle cell disease. *J. Clin. Invest.* 46:336, 1967.

36. Hays, R. M. Antidiuretic hormone. *N. Engl. J. Med.* 295:659, 1976.

37. Jaenike, J. R. The renal functional defect of post-obstructive nephropathy. *J. Clin. Invest.* 51:299, 1972.

38. Jamison, R. L., and Maffly, R. H. The urinary concentrating mechanism. *N. Engl. J. Med.* 295:1059, 1976.

39. Jones, N. F., Barraclough, M. A., Barnes, N., and Cottom, D. G. Nephrogenic diabetes insipidus: Effects of 3,5, cyclic-adenosine monophosphate. *Arch. Dis. Child.* 47:794, 1972.

40. Katzman, R., and Pappius, H. M. Hypernatremia and Hyperosmolarity. In *Brain Electrolytes and Fluid Metabolism.* Baltimore: Williams & Wilkins, 1973.

41. Kaye, D., and Rocha, H. Urinary concentrating ability in early experimental pyelonephritis. *J. Clin. Invest.* 49:1427, 1970.

42. Kettyle, W. M., and Valtin, H. Chemical and dimensional characterization of the renal countercurrent system in mice. *Kidney Int.* 1:135, 1972.

43. Klahr, S., and Alleyne, G. A. O. Effects of chronic protein-calorie malnutrition on the kidney. *Kidney Int.* 3:129, 1973.

44. Macaulay, D., and Watson, M. Hypernatremia in infants as a cause of brain damage. *Arch. Dis. Child.* 42:485, 1967.

45. Manson, A. D., Yalowitz, P. A., Randall, R. V., and Greene, L. F. Dilatation of the urinary tract associated with pituitary and nephrogenic diabetes insipidus. *J. Urol.* 103:327, 1970.

46. Marumo, F., and Edelman, I. S. Effects of Ca^{++} and prostaglandin E_1 on vasopressin activation of renal adenyl cyclase. *J. Clin. Invest.* 50:1613, 1971.

47. Mazze, R. I., Shue, G. L., and Jackson, S. H. Renal dysfunction associated with methoxyflurane anesthesia. *J.A.M.A.* 216:278, 1971.

48. McConnell, R. F., Jr., Lorentz, W. B., Jr., Berger, M., Smith, E. H., Carvajal, H. F., and Travis, L. B. The mechanism of urinary concentration in nephrogenic diabetes insipidus. *Pediatr. Res.* 11:33, 1977.

49. McDougal, W. S., and Wright, F. S. Defect in proximal and distal sodium transport in post-obstructive diuresis. *Kidney Int.* 2:304, 1972.

50. Miller, M., Dalakos, T., Moses, A. M., Fellerman, H., and Streeten, D. H. T. Recognition of partial defects in antidiuretic hormone secretion. *Ann. Intern. Med.* 73:721, 1970.

51. Miller, M., and Moses, A. M. Radioimmunoassay of urinary antidiuretic hormone in man: Response to water load and dehydration in normal subjects. *J. Clin. Endocrinol. Metab.* 34:537, 1972.

52. Monn, E., Osnes, J. B., and Øye, I. Basal and hormone-induced urinary cyclic AMP in children with renal disorders. *Acta Paediatr. Scand.* 65:739, 1976.

53. Morris-Jones, P. H., Houston, I. B., and Evans, R. L. Prognosis of the neurological complications of acute hypernatremia. *Lancet* 2:1385, 1967.

54. Nissan, S., Aviram, A., Czaczkes, J. W., Ullmann, L., and Ullmann, T. D. Increased O_2 consumption of the rat diaphragm by elevated NaCl concentrations. *Am. J. Physiol.* 210:1222, 1966.

55. Pohl, J. E. F., Thurston, H., and Swales, J. D. The antidiuretic action of diazoxide. *Clin. Sci. Mol. Med.* 42:145, 1972.

56. Price, J. D. E., and Lauener, R. W. Serum and urine osmolalities in the differential diagnosis of polyuric states. *J. Clin. Endocrinol. Metab.* 26:143, 1966.

57. Proesmans, W., Eggermont, E., Vanderschueren-Lodeweyckx, M., Tiddens, H., and Eckels, R. The effect of exogenous 3':5'-adenosine monophosphate on urinary output in children with vasopressin-resistant diabetes insipidus. *Pediatr. Res.* 9:509, 1975.

58. Ramos, G., Rivera, A., Peña, J. C., and Díes, F. Mechanism of the antidiuretic effect of saluretic drugs: Studies in patients with diabetes insipidus. *Clin. Pharmacol. Ther.* 8:557, 1967.

59. Robertson, G. L., Mahr, E. A., Athar, S., and Sinha, T. Development and clinical application of a new method for the radioimmunoassay of arginine vasopressin in human plasma. *J. Clin. Invest.* 52:2340, 1973.

60. Robinson, M. G., and Kaplan, S. A. Inheritance of vasopressin-resistant ("nephrogenic") diabetes insipidus. *Am. J. Dis. Child.* 99:164, 1960.

61. Ronald, A. R., Cutler, R. E., and Turck, M. Effect of bacteriuria on renal concentrating mechanisms. *Ann. Intern. Med.* 70:723, 1969.

62. Ruess, A. L., and Rosenthal, I. M. Intelligence in nephrogenic diabetes insipidus. *Am. J. Dis. Child.* 105:358, 1963.

63. Sawyer, W. H., Acosta, M., and Manning, M. Structural changes in the arginine vasopressin molecule that prolong its antidiuretic action. *Endocrinology* 95:140, 1974.

64. Schrager, G. O., Josephson, B. H., Fine, B. F., and Berger, G. Nephrogenic diabetes insipidus presenting as fever of unknown origin in the neonatal period. *Clin. Pediatr. (Phila.)* 15:1070, 1976.

65. Schrier, R. W., and Berl, T. Disorders of Water Metabolism. In R. W. Schrier (ed.), *Renal and Electrolyte Disorders.* Boston: Little, Brown, 1976.

66. Schrier, R. W., and Berl, T. Nonosmolar factors affecting renal water excretion: I. *N. Engl. J. Med.* 292:81, 1975.

67. Seely, J. F., and Dirks, J. H. Micropuncture study of hypertonic mannitol diuresis in the proximal and distal tubule of the dog kidney. *J. Clin. Invest.* 48:2330, 1969.

68. Singer, I., and Forrest, J. N., Jr. Drug-induced states of nephrogenic diabetes insipidus. *Kidney Int.* 10:82, 1976.

69. Stern, P., and Valtin, H. Lack of clearcut antidiuretic effect in vivo, of a new analogue of cyclic AMP, 8(p-chloro-phenyl-thio)-cyclic AMP. *Kidney Int.* 10:600, 1976.

70. Stickler, G. B. Growth failure in renal disease. *Pediatr. Clin. North Am.* 23:885, 1976.

71. Svenningsen, N. W., and Aronson, A. S. Postnatal development of renal concentration capacity as estimated by DDAVP-test in normal and asphyxiated neonates. *Biol. Neonate* 25:230, 1974.

72. Tannen, R. L., Regal, E. M., Dunn, M. J., and Schrier, R. W. Vasopressin-resistant hyposthenuria in advanced chronic renal disease. *N. Engl. J. Med.* 280:1135, 1969.

73. Ten Bensel, R. W., and Peters, E. R. Progressive

hydronephrosis, hydroureter, and dilatation of the bladder in siblings with congenital diabetes insipidus. *J. Pediatr.* 77:439, 1970.

74. Uttley, W. S., Paxton, J., and Thistlethwaite, D. Urinary concentrating ability and growth failure in urinary tract disorders. *Arch. Dis. Child.* 47:436, 1972.

75. Valtin, H. Concentration and dilution of urine: H_2O balance. In *Renal Function: Mechanisms Preserving Fluid and Solute Balance in Health.* Boston: Little, Brown, 1973.

76. Valtin, H. Genetic models in biomedical investigation. *N. Engl. J. Med.* 290:670, 1974.

77. Valtin, H. Genetic Models for Hypothalamic and Nephrogenic Diabetes Insipidus. In T. E. Andreoli, J. J. Grantham, and F. C. Rector, Jr. (eds.), *Disturbances in Body Fluid Osmolality.* Washington: American Physiological Society, 1977.

78. Valtin, H. *Renal Dysfunction: Mechanisms Involved in Fluid and Solute Imbalance.* Boston: Little, Brown, 1978.

79. Verney, E. B. The antidiuretic hormone and the factors which determine its release. *Proc. R. Soc. Lond. [Biol.]* 135:25, 1947.

80. West, C. D., and Smith, W. C. An attempt to elucidate the cause of growth retardation in renal disease. *Am. J. Dis. Child.* 91:460, 1956.

81. White, M. G., and Fetner, C. D. Treatment of the syndrome of inappropriate secretion of antidiuretic hormone with lithium carbonate. *N. Engl. J. Med.* 292:390, 1975.

82. Wiggelinkhuizen, J., Retief, P. J. M., Wolff, B., Fisher, R. M., and Cremin, B. J. Nephrogenic diabetes insipidus and obstructive uropathy. *Am. J. Dis. Child.* 126:398, 1973.

83. Williams, R. H., and Henry, C. Nephrogenic diabetes insipidus: Transmitted by females and appearing during infancy in males. *Ann. Intern. Med.* 27:84, 1947.

84. Wilson, D. R. Micropuncture study of chronic obstructive nephropathy before and after release of obstruction. *Kidney Int.* 2:119, 1972.

85. Winberg, J. Renal function studies in infants and children with acute nonobstructive urinary tract infections. *Acta Paediatr. Scand.* 48:577, 1959.

86. Ziegler, E. E., and Fomon, S. J. Fluid intake, renal solute load, and water balance in infancy. *J. Pediatr.* 78:561, 1971.

83. Renal Tubular Acidosis

J. Rodriguez-Soriano

Definition and Classification

Although it is now accepted that the acidosis of renal disease is always tubular in origin [110], it can be classified conveniently into glomerular acidosis and tubular acidosis on the basis of the underlying pathophysiology. Glomerular acidosis is present in patients with chronic renal insufficiency and is part of the uremic syndrome. Tubular acidosis is a condition in which glomerular function is normal or is comparatively less impaired than tubular function. Used in this general sense, the term *renal tubular acidosis* (RTA) represents a clinical syndrome characterized by a state of tubular insufficiency with regard to the resorption of bicarbonate, the excretion of net hydrogen ion, or both; a large number of etiologies are included.

Renal tubular acidosis was first described by Lightwood et al. [59, 61] and Butler and associates [14] in children and by Baines, Barclay, and Cooke [3] in adults. It was identified as a renal tubular disorder by Albright and coworkers in 1946 [1]. Based on the original studies of Reynolds [96] and Wrong and Davies [131], the characteristic defect in RTA was defined as an inability to establish a normal hydrogen ion gradient between blood and tubular fluid, and the study of urinary pH was for many years the most

valuable test for diagnosis [33]. In the past decade, a number of studies have made it apparent that in many cases the primary defect lies in the tubular resorption of bicarbonate rather than in the establishment of a pH gradient, and thus patients with RTA may exhibit a metabolic hyperchloremic acidosis but be able to excrete a urine of strongly acid pH [70, 102].

On clinical and pathophysiologic grounds, RTA may be classified into two broad categories [100, 102], as follows:

1. *Proximal RTA*, caused by a defect in the tubular resorption of bicarbonate; also called type 2 RTA [70] or rate-limited RTA

2. *Distal RTA*, caused by an inability to establish adequate pH gradients between distal tubular fluid and blood. It corresponds to "classic" RTA, since it was the first form discovered, or type 1 RTA.

Although pH gradients are established throughout the whole length of the nephron and bicarbonate resorption is not confined to the proximal segment, most filtered bicarbonate is reabsorbed in the proximal tubule, whereas maximal urinary acidification is mainly a distal function. Therefore, although the proximal and distal dichotomy may not be entirely precise physiologically, it does have functional validity.

Proximal and distal RTA can be *primary,* that is, isolated and idiopathic, or *secondary,* that is, due to exogenous causes or associated with other renal or generalized disorders. Some organic nephropathies, such as chronic pyelonephritis [51], medullary sponge kidney [22, 77], obstructive uropathy [5], or ureterosigmoidostomy [34], may cause a syndrome of hyperchloremic acidosis but will not be discussed here. Table 83-1 shows the classification and main characteristics of both proximal and distal RTA.

Pathophysiology

Proximal Renal Tubular Acidosis

Under ordinary circumstances virtually all filtered bicarbonate is reabsorbed. If the concentration of bicarbonate in plasma exceeds the level of the renal threshold, bicarbonate resorption is in-

complete and urinary excretion gradually lowers the plasma concentration to a level below the threshold until a new steady state is reached. The level of the renal threshold changes with age: In normal adults bicarbonate appears in the urine in appreciable amounts when the plasma concentration exceeds 25 to 26 mmol per liter [92], whereas in infants bicarbonate is present in the urine when the plasma level exceeds 22 mmol per liter [31]. In patients with proximal RTA there is a depression in the renal bicarbonate threshold, and therefore bicarbonate is present in the urine at lower plasma levels than in normal individuals; accordingly, a steady state is maintained with the plasma bicarbonate in the acidemic range. Figure 83-1 shows data from patients with proximal RTA.

An important feature of these patients is their unimpaired ability to lower urinary pH and to excrete hydrogen ion when bicarbonate concentration in plasma is below their particular renal bi-

Table 83-1. Classification and Characteristics of Renal Tubular Acidosis

Etiology, Diagnosis, and Treatment	Renal Tubular Acidosis	
	Proximal	Distal
Etiology		

Primary	Permanent
	  Familial
	  Isolated (vitamin D deficiency?)
	Transient
	  Infantile
		Permanent
		  Classic adult type
		  Incomplete RTA
		  With bicarbonate wasting
		  With nerve deafness
		Transient (in infancy?)

Secondary	Fanconi syndrome Cystinosis Lowe's syndrome Hereditary fructose intolerance Primary and secondary hyperparathyroidism Vitamin D deficiency Medullary cystic disease Renal transplantation Osteopetrosis Cyanotic congenital heart disease Leigh's syndrome Mineralocorticoid deficiency	Primary hyperthyroidism with nephrocalcinosis Primary hyperparathyroidism with nephrocalcinosis Idiopathic hypercalcemia Vitamin D intoxication Idiopathic hypercalciuria with nephrocalcinosis Amphotericin B nephropathy Toxicity to lithium Hepatic cirrhosis Hyperglobulinemic states Hereditary fructose intolerance with nephrocalcinosis Ehlers-Danlos syndrome Elliptocytosis Medullary sponge kidney Renal transplantation
Diagnosis		
Urine pH	4.5 to 7.8 depending on level of plasma bicarbonate	Always above 6.0 regardless of level of plasma bicarbonate
Bicarbonate threshold	Decreased	Normal
Hydrogen ion excretion	Normal, below bicarbonate threshold	Impaired, below bicarbonate threshold
Therapy	Resistant to alkali therapy; diuretics have effect	Sensitive to alkali therapy; no effect of diuretics

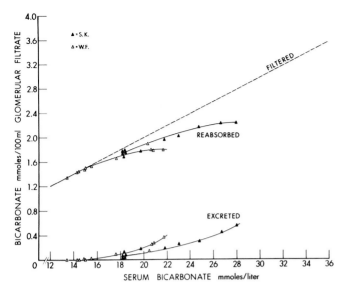

Figure 83-1. Data from patients with proximal renal tubular acidosis. In contrast to normal individuals, bicarbonate is present in the urine at plasma levels as low as 16 to 18 mmol per liter. If hyperchloremic acidosis is corrected by the administration of alkali and the excretion of bicarbonate is studied at normal levels of plasma bicarbonate, these subjects excrete a large percentage of the filtered bicarbonate, frequently as much as 15 to 20 percent. This phenomenon explains the fact that large amounts of alkali are required to correct the acidemia. When therapy is stopped, acidemia quickly reappears, due not only to continuous loss of bicarbonate into the urine but also to inhibition of the distal mechanism of hydrogen ion secretion, since the distal fluid is flooded with a bicarbonate-rich fluid. (From J. Rodriguez-Soriano, H. Boichis, and C. M. Edelmann, Jr. Bicarbonate reabsorption and hydrogen ion excretion in children with renal tubular acidosis, J. Pediatr. 71:802, 1967.)

carbonate threshold. Figure 83-2 demonstrates urine pH as a function of plasma bicarbonate concentration in a group of patients with proximal RTA.

Distal Renal Tubular Acidosis

In this type of RTA the primary defect is an inability to establish adequate gradients of hydrogen ion between blood and tubular fluid despite low levels of plasma bicarbonate. The inability to lower urinary pH appropriately is the most important and characteristic feature, the diminution of the excretion of titratable acid and ammonium being secondary to that phenomenon. Figure 83-3 shows data from a number of patients with distal RTA.

In general, bicarbonate resorption is normal in distal RTA, and the curve of bicarbonate titration is similar to that obtained in normal individuals. However, as a consequence of the elevated urine pH, a certain degree of bicarbonaturia is obligatory. This excretion of bicarbonate, generally less than 3 percent of that filtered, remains almost constant over a wide range of plasma bicarbonate values below the threshold. When the threshold is reached, the usual marked increase in urinary excretion of bicarbonate is noted.

In distal RTA, acidosis results principally from the impaired ability to excrete the usual endogenous load of nonvolatile acid; the loss of bicarbonate is minimal or absent. Patients with distal RTA who can acidify their urine below pH 6.2 do not, in fact, lose significant amounts of bicarbonate when they are acidemic. Hence, correction of the acidosis characteristically is sustained by an amount of alkali slightly greater than the endogenous production of acid, which is on the order of 2 to 3 mEq/kg body weight/day in the infant and young child and 1 mEq/kg/day in the adult.

The possibility that in patients with distal RTA some bicarbonaturia may be the result of a small fixed leak of bicarbonate from the proximal tubule was considered by Seldin and Wilson [116], who examined the effect of water diuresis on urinary pH and bicarbonate excretion in an adult patient. The observation that urinary pH was unchanged and that the rate of excretion of bicarbonate was directly proportional to the rate of urine flow was interpreted as evidence against bicarbonate leakage from the proximal nephron, but it suggested that the factor controlling the amount of bicarbonate excreted was the pH of the tubular fluid and the volume of the final urine. The effect of water diuresis was reexamined by Morris and

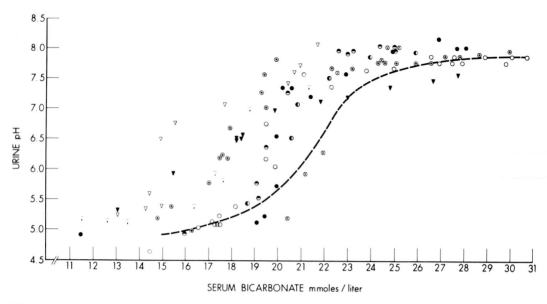

Figure 83-2. Urine pH as a function of plasma bicarbonate concentration in a group of eight patients with proximal renal tubular acidosis (RTA). The broken line represents the response of normal infants and shows a steep decline of urine pH at a level of plasma bicarbonate corresponding to the renal threshold. In adults or older children a smilar curve obtains except that the inflection is at a higher plasma concentration, reflecting the fact that children and adults have a higher threshold for bicarbonate. In every instance the response in patients with proximal RTA is displaced in the left of normal, so that as plasma bicarbonate falls, urine pH eventually reaches the low minimal range, but at a lower bicarbonate concentration than in normal subjects. (From J. Rodriguez-Soriano, and C. M. Edelmann, Jr. Renal tubular acidosis, Annu. Rev. Med. 20: *363, 1969.)*

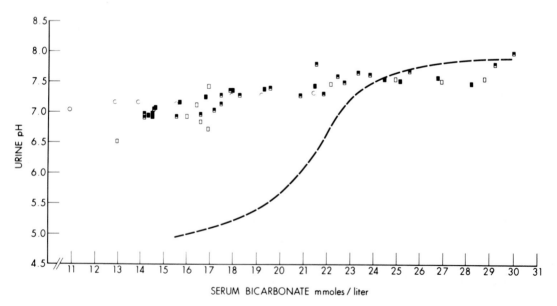

Figure 83-3. Data from four patients with distal renal tubular acidosis (RTA). The decrease of urinary pH is minimal despite a marked reduction in the concentration of plasma bicarbonate; in contrast with normal individuals or patients with proximal RTA, no values below 6.5 were observed. See also legend to Figure 83-2. (From J. Rodriguez-Soriano, and C. M. Edelmann, Jr. Renal tubular acidosis, Annu. Rev. Med. 20:363, *1969.)*

colleagues [74] in six affected patients. In two of these the results were similar to those reported by Seldin and Wilson, but in the remaining four, including two infants and two adults, a significant decrease in urinary pH and bicarbonate concentration occurred as urine flow increased. During acidosis the effect of water diuresis on bicarbonate excretion was more marked than when the patients were studied at normal plasma bicarbonate concentration. As stated by the authors, such studies during water diuresis provide neither evidence for a proximal leak of bicarbonate nor evidence against the existence of a gradient defect in the distal nephron, since the effect on urinary pH and bicarbonate concentration depends on the interaction of several factors, such as hydration of urinary carbon dioxide with generation of hydrogen ion, back-diffusion of this generated hydrogen ion, and dilution of luminal bicarbonate. When the luminal concentration of bicarbonate is high, a reduction of the pH of the urine during water diuresis would not be surprising, even if the presence of bicarbonate was dependent on a fixed elevated urine pH. Conversely, if the initial luminal bicarbonate concentration is only moderately increased, the pH of the urine might remain unchanged during water diuresis even if the presence of bicarbonate in the urine was solely due to a leak of bicarbonate out of the proximal nephron; under these circumstances the small amount of hydrogen ion generated during water diuresis could be dissipated by being both buffered and lost through back-diffusion across the distal nephron.

Combined Proximal and Distal Renal Tubular Acidosis

In some patients the delineation between proximal and distal RTA is difficult to establish, since they share features of both forms. Two patterns of combined RTA have been described. Morris [72, 76, 114] uses the term *hybrid 1,2 RTA* to designate some adult patients with the Sjögren syndrome or renal amyloidosis in whom there is a striking reduction in tubular resorption of bicarbonate at normal plasma levels, but who, in contrast to patients with proximal RTA, are unable to acidify the urine below pH 6.0 despite severe degrees of acidemia.

A second pattern has been observed in some infants with apparently classic distal RTA but with associated bicarbonate wasting [68, 105]. In these patients fractional excretion of bicarbonate may be as large as 5 to 15 percent of the filtered load, and it is constant or increases moderately over a broad range of plasma bicarbonate concentration

(Fig. 83-4). At normal and reduced plasma levels of bicarbonate the urinary loss of base may exceed the net excretion of acid and thus contribute significantly to the development of the acidosis. Although this pattern of distal RTA with bicarbonate wasting could be explained entirely by a distal acidification defect greater than that described in children and adults with this entity [68], there is indirect evidence of an associated impairment of proximal tubular function [105].

Proximal Renal Tubular Acidosis

Primary Proximal Renal Tubular Acidosis

We have described a transient type of primary proximal RTA in a group of nine infants with an isolated defect in bicarbonate resorption that was without identifiable cause or evidence of other renal abnormality or of systemic disease [84, 101, 102]. Eight of the nine patients were boys, and all the cases were diagnosed within the first 18 months of life. The presenting complaint was growth retardation, and except for the constant history of excessive vomiting in early infancy, the infants were free of other symptoms. Physical examination revealed no abnormality other than growth retardation, with length usually far below

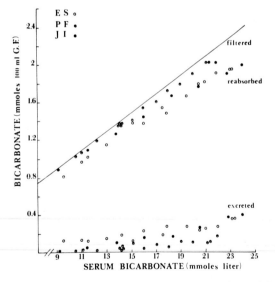

Figure 83-4. A second pattern has been observed in some infants with apparently classic distal renal tubular acidosis but with associated bicarbonate wasting [68, 105]. In these patients fractional excretion of bicarbonate may be as large as 5 to 15 percent of the filtered load, and it is constant or increases moderately over a broad range of plasma bicarbonate concentration. (From J. Rodriguez-Soriano, A. Vallo, and M. Garcia-Fuentes. Distal renal tubular acidosis in infancy: A bicarbonate wasting state, J. Pediatr. 86:524, 1975.)

the third percentile. The only biochemical abnormality was the presence of a metabolic hyperchloremic acidosis, with slightly acid to alkaline urine pH. Other investigations, including a study of other tubular functions, intravenous pyelogram, and renal histology, revealed no abnormalities. The usual complications observed in patients with distal RTA, such as interstitial nephritis, bone lesions, nephrocalcinosis, nephrolithiasis, polyuria, and hypokalemia, were absent. Functional evaluation when the study was performed at a level of plasma bicarbonate below the renal threshold revealed normal glomerular filtration rate, a moderately low bicarbonate threshold (between 18 and 20 mmol per liter), and normal urinary acidification.

The ability of these patients to excrete normal quantities of net acid may explain the absence of secondary complications. Although studies in children have not been performed, it seems likely that at low plasma bicarbonate levels a normal or nearly normal net acid balance is maintained, in contrast to patients with distal RTA or chronic renal insufficiency who are in a continuously positive hydrogen ion balance due to their limitation in net excretion of acid [39, 94, 95]. The presence of an acid urine and, if true, the absence of net retention of acid, might explain why in proximal RTA bone lesions are absent, the calciuria is only slightly elevated or even normal, and nephrocalcinosis is not present radiologically or histologically. It is possible, of course, that persistent acidemia, even in the absence of positive hydrogen ion balance, could cause a gradual dissolution of bone salts. This could be the situation in an adult patient reported by York and Yendt [132], who presented with osteomalacia and an isolated renal loss of bicarbonate. The bone lesions were attributed to chronic acidosis, although the role of vitamin D deficiency or hyperparathyroidism or both could not be excluded.

Recently Brenes et al. [8] have had the opportunity to study a family in which nine members demonstrated chronic hyperchloremic acidosis and growth failure due to proximal RTA. Other renal dysfunction was not found. Despite chronic acidemia, hypercalciuria and bone disease were not present. These findings are similar to those in children with isolated proximal RTA. Metabolic studies performed in two of these patients by Lemann and his associates [54a] showed the patients to be in net acid balance, in striking contrast to studies performed in subjects with distal RTA [39, 94, 95]. Although children have not been studied, these data support our hypothesis that the absence of metabolic complications other than growth re-

tardation in children with proximal RTA relates to their ability to excrete adequate net acid to maintain hydrogen ion balance despite chronic acidemia. These findings also suggest that acidemia per se, in the absence of hydrogen ion retention or disturbance in calcium balance, can lead to growth failure. It is of interest in this regard that the patients of Brenes et al. [8], other than having severe growth retardation, were entirely healthy, leading Brenes to conclude that treatment of acidosis in such adult subjects was not warranted.

Prognosis in the infantile type of primary proximal RTA generally is good. The growth pattern while on alkali therapy has been variable, but usually there is an initial rapid increase in growth that is followed by continued growth at a slower rate. Seven of the nine patients followed by Nash and coworkers [84] maintained normal levels of blood pH and bicarbonate when therapy was discontinued after several years. This self-limited evolution of infantile proximal RTA contrasts with that of primary distal RTA, which appears to be permanent even when the onset is in infancy. Only one case of infantile transient distal RTA has been adequately documented [56].

Donckerwolcke et al. [25, 26] have reported proximal RTA with unusual characteristics in a 20-month-old girl with growth retardation, bilateral band keratopathy, and mild psychomotor retardation. Bicarbonate resorption was severely impaired, and the renal bicarbonate threshold was as low as 10 mmol per liter. Because of the important bicarbonate loss the usual treatment with alkali was ineffective, and adequate correction of acid-base balance was achieved only when a diuretic was added to the therapy. No data were presented about the transient or permanent nature of the disorder.

Secondary Proximal Renal Tubular Acidosis
In the secondary forms of proximal RTA, the tubular defect in bicarbonate resorption is associated with other tubular dysfunctions or it is observed in the context of generalized disease. Proximal RTA is most frequently observed as part of a more generalized proximal tubulopathy. It has been demonstrated in cases of idiopathic Fanconi syndrome [53, 93, 101], cystinosis [15, 101], Lowe's syndrome [50, 66], hereditary fructose intolerance [70, 71], and as part of the tubular dysfunction that follows renal homotransplantation [126, 129] and vascular accidents to the kidney in the newborn period [117]. A similar pathogenesis probably accounts for the acidosis observed in patients with multiple myeloma; gly-

cogen storage disease; galactosemia; tyrosinemia; Wilson's disease; nephrotic syndrome; the Sjögren syndrome; amyloidosis; and intoxication with cadmium, outdated tetracycline, methylchromone, 6-mercaptopurine, and (experimentally induced) maleic and malonic acids [76, 103].

Proximal RTA has also been observed in situations in which there is increased secretion of parathyroid hormone, such as primary hyperparathyroidism [79] or secondary hyperparathyroidism associated with intestinal malabsorption [80] or vitamin-D-deficiency rickets [43]. It may also occur in a number of generalized conditions as diverse as subacute necrotizing encephalomyelopathy (Leigh's syndrome) [41], osteopetrosis [42, 124], tetralogy of Fallot [104], and mineralocorticoid deficiency [88].

NATURE OF THE DISEASE

The pathogenesis of proximal RTA is a matter of speculation. Alteration of either intrinsic or extrinsic renal factors involved in the resorption of bicarbonate may be implicated, depending on the specific etiology.

It is generally accepted that resorption of bicarbonate in the renal tubule (and also the secretion of bicarbonate in the intestine) is interrelated with transport of chloride, sodium, and hydrogen ions via simultaneous double exchange of chloride-bicarbonate and sodium-hydrogen ions. Two independent mechanisms involved in bicarbonate resorption have been proposed: (1) a mechanism dependent on hydrogen ion secretion in which the enzyme carbonic anhydrase, plasma P_{CO_2}, and body potassium stores play important roles, and (2) a mechanism that involves primary anion transport not mediated by hydrogen ion secretion. Bicarbonate resorption is also affected by extrarenal factors modulating the resorptive function of the tubule, such as extracellular fluid volume or circulating levels of parathyroid hormone. Theoretically any of these mechanisms could be defective in patients with proximal RTA.

A deficiency in carbonic anhydrase was excluded in two patients with the primary type of proximal RTA on the basis of a normal response to the administration of the enzyme inhibitor acetazolamide [102], but it was suspected by Donckerwolcke et al. [25, 26], since in their patient bicarbonate resorption was uninfluenced by the administration of acetazolamide. Shapira et al. [117] have described an inactive mutant of the blood cell carbonic anhydrase B in three members of a large kindred with infantile RTA and nerve deafness. Although no bicarbonate titration studies were performed, the data presented are more

in favor of a distal than a proximal type of RTA.

Schoeneman et al. [109] used transintestinal intubation to study bicarbonate transport in the duodenum in an infant with primary proximal RTA. The finding of a marked excess of duodenal secretion of bicarbonate associated with decreased secretion of chloride suggested a defective chloride-bicarbonate pump, both at the renal and intestinal level, due to an impairment in chloride transport, since the patient was able to secrete hydrogen ion in the intestine in a normal fashion. The authors speculate about the role of intestinal loss of bicarbonate in the development of systemic acidosis.

Morris et al. [76] have suggested that the impairment of bicarbonate resorption in many patients with proximal RTA may be due, at least in part, to increased circulating levels of parathyroid hormone, probably mediated by some degree of chronic hypocalcemia. It is known that parathyroid hormone acts directly on the renal tubule to lower bicarbonate resorption by means of activation of the second messenger, cyclic adenosine monophosphate, which has a direct inhibitory effect on the enzyme carbonic anhydrase. This action of parathyroid hormone seems evident in patients with primary or secondary hyperparathyroidism and is probable in many patients with the various types of Fanconi syndrome in whom chronic hypocalcemia is present and plasma concentration of parathyroid hormone is increased [74]. Parathyroid hormone may also modulate the intensity of bicarbonate wasting in patients with hereditary fructose intolerance [73].

DIAGNOSIS

The diagnosis of proximal RTA is established by the demonstration of a low bicarbonate threshold with normal urinary acidification at plasma bicarbonate concentrations below this level. Performance of a bicarbonate titration is useful in the diagnosis of this form of RTA, although it can be clinically suspected when urinary pH levels are plotted against the corresponding values of plasma bicarbonate, as discussed under Pathophysiology (see Figs. 83-2 and 83-3).

This approach to diagnosis has been criticized by Morris [72], who gives special emphasis to the percentage of filtered bicarbonate excreted by the kidney. In his opinion the demonstration of an adequate net acid excretion is unnecessary, and the diagnosis can be established easily by the large requirement of alkali to sustain the plasma bicarbonate concentration at about 22 mmol per liter and by the excretion at this concentration of more than 15 to 20 percent of the filtered bicarbonate load. Undoubtedly, most patients with severe proximal RTA will be identified by this method, but it will miss milder forms of the disorder or the presence of a concomitant distal defect. Patients with distal RTA and a high fixed urinary pH (above 7.0) may excrete more bicarbonate at normal plasma levels than patients with mild proximal RTA and thus may be classified as having proximal RTA if their inability to excrete an adequately acid urine at low plasma levels of bicarbonate is not recognized.

It must be understood that we have proposed the terms *proximal* and *distal* with a pathophysiologic and not a topographic meaning, that is, without implying an exclusive role of either the proximal or the distal tubule in the origin of the disorder. It is evident, as pointed out by Morris [72], that a reduced bicarbonate threshold of 19 mmol per liter, for example, does not implicate the acidifying process of the proximal tubule any more than that of the distal nephron if at normal plasma bicarbonate concentration the resorption of bicarbonate is reduced by less than 10 percent. If such a patient is able to excrete an acid urine, however, it can be assured that the defect, although mild, is in the resorption of bicarbonate and not in the ability to excrete hydrogen ion against a gradient. Using our terminology, such a patient would be classified as having proximal RTA even though there is no documentation of participation of the proximal tubule in the origin of the disorder.

An interesting approach to diagnosis has been proposed by Oetliker et al. [86]. These authors plotted the excretion rates of bicarbonate and of hydrogen ion (as titratable acid plus ammonium) during bicarbonate loading against the corresponding concentrations of bicarbonate in plasma. At the crossing point of the two curves an "equivalent excretion" is present, and the corresponding plasma bicarbonate concentration is very near the value of the renal bicarbonate threshold. The equivalent excretion rate in normal children is on the order of 20 μmol per 100 ml of glomerular filtrate, a figure that corresponds well to the amount of bicarbonate that is excreted at the renal bicarbonate threshold. Patients with proximal RTA present higher equivalent excretion rates, and the corresponding plasma bicarbonate concentration is distinctly higher than the renal bicarbonate threshold. These authors postulate that the plasma bicarbonate concentration at which equivalent excretion of bicarbonate and hydrogen ion occurs represents the metabolic acid-base equilibrium that the kidney is able to maintain.

TREATMENT

In proximal RTA, therapy must compensate for a large urinary loss of bicarbonate, and huge amounts of alkali must be administered at frequent intervals to sustain adequate correction of the acidemia. The starting dosage is between 5 and 10 mEq/kg/day, but often larger doses are needed.

In mild proximal RTA, as observed in the infantile transient type, the administration of potassium is not usually required, since hyperkaliuria and hypokalemia are not regular features of the disorder. In severe proximal RTA, however, as commonly observed in the context of a Fanconi syndrome, administration of potassium may be mandatory. In this group of patients potassium wastage will appear or become greater when acidosis is corrected, and it may persist when correction of the acidosis is sustained [111, 112]. This finding may be explained both by an increased delivery of bicarbonate to the distal nephron and by persistent hyperaldosteronism.

In very severe forms of proximal RTA, alkali therapy alone may be ineffective due to the total loss into the urine of the administered bicarbonate. In this situation diuretic therapy has been used successfully, both in primary [26] and secondary forms [15, 93] of the disorder. Of the diuretics tried, hydrochlorothiazide appears to be the most effective [26, 93]. Initial dosage is about 1.5 to 2 mg/kg/day, but after correction of the acidosis a smaller dose may be sufficient. A low sodium diet is not necessary, but potassium supplements are obligatory to prevent secondary hypokalemia. An additional benefit of hydrochlorothiazide treatment in patients with idiopathic Fanconi syndrome [93] or cystinosis [15] is diminution of urinary calcium excretion and elevation of the tubular resorption of phosphate, with subsequent improvement of osteomalacic lesions.

The increase of tubular resorption of bicarbonate that occurs during administration of hydrochlorothiazide appears to be due to contraction of the extracellular fluid volume [15, 26]. This mechanism of action is suggested also by the observation of Oetliker and Rossi [87] in two patients with Lowe's syndrome that the renal bicarbonate threshold was directly related to the state of the extracellular fluid volume.

An alternative explanation involves the action of the thiazide diuretics in reducing calcium excretion, leading to a rise in plasma calcium level and a consequent diminution in the circulating level of parathyroid hormone. This sequence could answer the question why plasma bicarbonate concentration increases after thiazide therapy, which diminishes calcium excretion, but does not increase after administration of furosemide, which enhances urinary excretion of calcium.

Distal Renal Tubular Acidosis

Primary Distal Renal Tubular Acidosis

The term *primary distal RTA* is applied to those cases of distal RTA in which there are no related antecedent diseases and which are not part of another disease state. Primary distal RTA is almost always permanent, and although it affects both children and adults, it has been called the adult type in distinction to the infantile type, or Lightwood syndrome, which is transient and is observed only within the first year of life. Since the adult type also occurs in infancy and the infantile type constitutes a confusion of several different disorders, the terms *permanent* and *transient distal RTA* are preferred [116].

Permanent Distal Renal Tubular Acidosis (Butler-Albright Syndrome). GENETICS. Most cases of permanent distal RTA are sporadic, but in some instances the disease may be inherited as an autosomal dominant disorder [48, 116]. At least 22 families with several involved members have been reported [12], and in five families the defect was present in three or four consecutive generations [82, 99].

The defect varies considerably in its degree of severity. Some patients do not have systemic acidosis despite the presence of the characteristic acidification defect and other manifestations of the syndrome, such as nephrocalcinosis or nephrolithiasis. This is the so-called incomplete syndrome of distal RTA [131] (see under Incomplete Distal RTA).

CLINICAL FEATURES. Permanent distal RTA occurs in both sexes, with a slight predominance in females. It usually is not diagnosed before 2 years of age and frequently not before adult life. Several cases unquestionably have begun in infancy, however, presenting with vomiting, constipation, anorexia, polyuria, dehydration, and failure to thrive. Growth retardation is most evident beyond early infancy and may represent the only clinical abnormality.

Osteomalacia with bone pain and pathologic fractures is a cardinal sign in adolescents and adults but is rare in children, with no report of this complication occurring in patients below 2 years of age. In children it is more usual to observe a moderately retarded bone age with some degree of generalized bone demineralization.

Nephrocalcinosis is an almost constant finding in permanent distal RTA. Calcium deposits preferentially in the renal medulla, which may become completely petrified. A normal radiologic study, however, does not exclude the presence of nephrocalcinosis, since fine tissue calcification can be demonstrated only by histologic examination. Nephrocalcinosis is more evident in patients in whom therapy is delayed, suggesting that early treatment may reduce the extent of calcium deposition. Urolithiasis is more common in adults than in children.

Polyuria due to a renal concentrating defect is almost always present, but it is not necessarily a feature intrinsic to the disease since in some cases the concentrating defect is absent or reversible. Potassium loss may result in severe hypokalemia and even cause a picture of periodic paralysis. A sudden crisis of dehydration, circulatory collapse, cardiac arrhythmia, vomiting, flaccid paralysis, respiratory difficulty, drowsiness, and coma may endanger the lives of these patients.

Analysis of the blood reveals a low pH and a low concentration of bicarbonate with elevation of chloride in permanent distal RTA. Moderate hyponatremia and a variable degree of hypokalemia may be present, although the serum potassium is not a good index of the degree of potassium deficiency due to the associated acidemia. The concentration of phosphate may be low, with normal or even high levels of calcium. Alkaline phosphatase may be elevated if active osteomalacic lesions are present. Glomerular filtration rate is normal in the young child, but a progressive decrease may take place over the years as a consequence of advancing parenchymal damage. It should be noted that evaluation of glomerular function is best performed after prolonged administration of alkali and sustained correction of the contracted extracellular fluid volume. In some patients the glomerular filtration rate returns to normal only after several years of treatment [84].

Urinary pH is usually 6.0 or 6.5, with low rates of excretion of titratable acid and ammonium. A small degree of proteinuria of the so-called tubular type may be found. Leukocyturia is frequent, even in the absence of urinary tract infection. Other urinary findings are increased rates of excretion of phosphate, calcium, and potassium and reduced excretion of citrate. The urinary excretion of amino acids generally is normal, but there are two reports of amino aciduria that disappeared following correction of the acidosis and hypokalemia [45a].

CLINICAL VARIANTS. "Incomplete" distal RTA was reported by Wrong and Davies [131] in three patients with nephrocalcinosis, but without the presence of systemic acidosis. Although the patients were unable to acidify their urine appropriately, a high rate of excretion of ammonium compensated for their limited excretion of titratable acid. Additional cases subsequently have been reported, detected either because of nephrocalcinosis and lithiasis or as a result of screening families of a propositus with complete RTA [11, 23, 44, 115, 123, 130, 133]. Elkinton and associates [33] have suggested that complete and incomplete RTA are stages of the same disease, the only difference being the ability to excrete ammonium, which in turn may depend on the level of the glomerular filtration rate. Sustaining this hypothesis is the observation in some patients of transition from incomplete to complete RTA, or vice versa, following deterioration or improvement of the glomerular filtration rate, respectively. This interpretation fails to explain the rarity of the incomplete form of distal RTA in children, in whom a normal glomerular filtration rate is the rule.

Distal RTA with bicarbonate wasting in two male infants with apparent primary permanent distal RTA who also demonstrated major wastage of bicarbonate was reported by McSherry et al. [68]. We have reported three infants with identical features [105]. Clinically all these patients are characterized by the early appearance of symptoms: Nephrocalcinosis was detected in one of our patients as early as 1 month of age. Polyuria is also a striking feature, given the young age of the patients.

There is no evidence to classify these cases as a separate entity, and they probably represent cases of primary permanent distal RTA with an unusual degree of bicarbonate loss determined by the special characteristics of bicarbonate resorption during early life. As a matter of fact, bicarbonate wasting appears to be a typical feature of distal RTA during infancy [29, 56, 68, 89, 105], although it is not obligatorily present, as shown by one infant studied by McSherry et al. [68].

There is an indication that bicarbonate wasting may decrease as the infants grow older, since there is a diminution with age in the dose of alkali necessary to correct the acidosis [68, 105]. If this observation is confirmed, a gradual change to the adult type of distal RTA, with minimal bicarbonate loss, is to be expected. A more prolonged follow-up of the reported cases is necessary to investigate this hypothesis.

Distal RTA with nerve deafness was first mentioned by Royer and Broyer [106]. To date at least 14 cases of such an association have been de-

scribed, with four families presenting two or more sibs with the syndrome [20, 24, 49, 83, 128]. The pedigrees of those families strongly suggest that this entity is inherited as an autosomal recessive trait, since the affected individuals are of both sexes, the parents are not affected, and consanguinity was present in three of the families. This genetic pattern identifies this clinical association as a distinct disorder.

Clinically the picture of distal RTA associated with nerve deafness is identical to that previously described, and pathophysiologic studies have shown that the defect is limited to the distal tubule without any associated bicarbonate wasting [24]. In one patient studied by Shapira and associates, however, an important bicarbonate loss appeared to be present, since the requirements of alkali to correct the acidosis were as high as 20 mEq/kg/day [117]. In this patient an inactive mutant form of carbonic anhydrase B was identified in the red cells, and the authors speculate about the possibility that a similar defect might be present in the tubular cells.

There is a great variation in the presentation of deafness, which may occur from birth to late childhood.

PATHOPHYSIOLOGY OF SYMPTOMS. All symptoms of distal RTA are attributable to the primary defect in acidification of the urine and the metabolic abnormalities that follow (Fig. 83-5).

Hyperchloremia is a consequence of the shrinkage of the extracellular space caused by the small, constant loss of sodium bicarbonate without concomitant loss of chloride. Retention of dietary sodium chloride tends to reexpand the extracellular space but in so doing aggravates the hyperchloremia and the acidemia by diluting the plasma bicarbonate and increasing the concentration of chloride relative to that of sodium [116].

Chronic acidosis per se may be responsible for anorexia, lethargy, and dyspnea on exertion and may be an important factor in the failure to achieve normal growth [21]. These patients are in constant positive balance for hydrogen ion, since the endogenously produced acid cannot be excreted and accumulates in the body [94, 95]. Buffering of this excess hydrogen ion by bone salts may result directly in the production of osteomalacia [39]; it has been repeatedly demonstrated that the bone lesions improve after prolonged alkali therapy without any need to increase the administration of vitamin D [36, 97, 107]. Intestinal calcium absorption has been found to be normal [7] or even increased [4], but there is also a study showing a decreased calcium absorption that improved after alkali therapy [40].

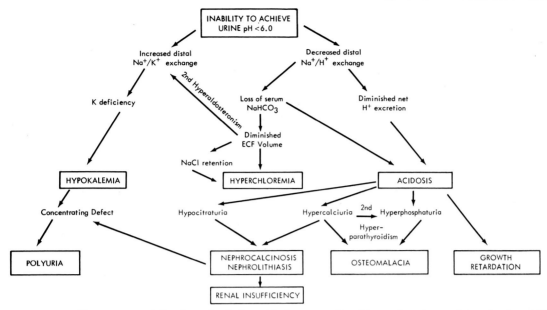

Figure 83-5. All symptoms of distal renal tubular acidosis are attributable to the primary defect in the acidification of the urine and the metabolic abnormalities that follow. (From J. Rodriguez-Soriano, and C. M. Edelmann, Jr. Renal tubular acidosis, Annu. Rev. Med. *20:363, 1969.)*

Studies of chronic acid loading in normal men [55] support the hypothesis that hypercalciuria results from release of skeletal calcium, since the hypercalciuria reverts completely to normal after correction of the acidosis. Secondary hyperparathyroidism has been demonstrated in a few cases [18, 28], contributing, together with hypercalciuria and acidosis, to the development of the bone lesions. The increased level of parathyroid hormone is probably secondary to the hypercalciuria, since chronic acidosis per se is not a primary stimulus to parathyroid hormone secretion [19]. In addition, there is strong evidence that the acidosis may cause tubular wastage of phosphate even in absence of secondary hypeparathyroidism [46, 106].

Nephrocalcinosis and nephrolithiasis have been attributed to the combined effects of hypercalciuria, urine of elevated pH, and decreased urinary excretion of citrate, which is an important factor in the solubilization of urinary calcium. The hypocitraturia, characteristic of distal RTA [9, 23, 78, 85, 107], is probably caused by increased tubular resorption of citrate due to intracellular acidosis, since the factor controlling citrate excretion in acid-base disturbances appears to be the pH of the renal tubular cell rather than the pH of the urine. Correction of hypocitraturia has been observed after prolonged administration of alkali and potassium [78], but in other patients the correction has been incomplete or absent [9, 23, 107].

The defect in urinary concentrating ability may result from both nephrocalcinosis and potassium deficiency. In young children the abnormality can be corrected by combined treatment with sodium and potassium bicarbonate [107], but at later stages the defect becomes permanent, probably due to irreversible tubular damage.

Hyperkaliuria resulting in hypokalemia and intracellular potassium deficiency may be explained as a result of the constant small loss of sodium bicarbonate in the urine, with reduction of the extracellular space, secondary hyperaldosteronism, and increased sodium-potassium exchange in the distal tubule [38]. In many patients urinary excretion of sodium and potassium decrease when acidosis is corrected [38, 112], but in some patients frank renal potassium wastage persists in association with continuing hyperaldosteronism despite sustained correction of the acidosis and provision of a large amount of dietary sodium [112]. This continuing potassium wastage suggests a primary defect in the renal tubular handling of potassium.

PATHOLOGY. The histology of the kidney is normal in the early stages of permanent distal RTA, although nephrocalcinosis may be present as early as 1 month of age. When calcium is deposited in the kidney, it is generally accompanied by a chronic interstitial nephritis of variable degree, with cellular infiltration, tubular atrophy, and glomerular sclerosis.

EVOLUTION AND PROGNOSIS. The prognosis of permanent distal RTA is relatively good, providing that diagnosis is established early enough to prevent severe degrees of nephrocalcinosis, interstitial nephritis, and glomerular damage. The defect is permanent, and any attempt to withdraw therapy is followed by reappearance of metabolic acidosis and related symptoms. With adequate treatment and sustained correction of the acidosis, however, the bone lesions heal, growth rate accelerates, calcium excretion reverts to normal, and further deposition of calcium in the kidneys can be prevented.

Transient Distal Renal Tubular Acidosis (Lightwood Syndrome). Infantile RTA was originally described by Lightwood in 1935 [59, 61] from a retrospective analysis of infants found at autopsy to have nephrocalcinosis, and it was characterized clinically by failure to thrive and muscular weakness. In 1953 Lightwood, Payne, and Black [62] described a second group of infants with a transient variety of RTA. These infants presented with anorexia, vomiting, constipation, and failure to thrive. Most of the infants were male, and rickets and nephrocalcinosis were absent radiologically, features also observed in a similar series of cases subsequently reported by others [10, 16]. The response to alkali therapy was dramatic, and the patients were said to recover by 2 years of age. Although a large number of these infants were diagnosed in various parts of Great Britain in the late 1940s and 1950s, the disease subsequently all but disappeared, suggesting that its frequency at that time was the result of some unrecognized environmental factor. There is evidence that this may have been vitamin D intoxication or toxicity to sulfonamides or mercury, although Lightwood and Butler were unable to implicate any of these factors in many of their infants [60].

The pathophysiology of the acidosis in these infants with transient distal RTA is unclear, since few precise functional studies were performed. Latner and Burnard [52] presented evidence for a defect in bicarbonate resorption in six patients, but despite this the defect became accepted as an inability to acidify the urine. The Lightwood syndrome thus was recognized as a transient, self-limited form of distal RTA in infancy [48, 116].

It is evident now that the patients described by Lightwood and other authors represented a heterogeneous group that probably included both cases of proximal and of distal RTA. It is of interest that many of the patients were male, nephrocalcinosis and rickets were frequently absent, a very high dosage of alkali therapy was required, and the patients had a spontaneous recovery. These features can be recognized as characteristic

of proximal RTA. Some of the infants had nephrocalcinosis, however, a fact never seen in proximal RTA, and they may have been affected with distal RTA, probably secondary to some environmental factor, since they recovered spontaneously. The possibility that some of these patients had primary distal RTA cannot be excluded entirely, since there is at least one such patient in whom recovery has been convincingly demonstrated [56].

Secondary Distal Renal Tubular Acidosis
Distal RTA may be associated with a number of systemic or renal conditions, including starvation [108], malnutrition [119], hyperthyroidism [47], hyperparathyroidism [37], vitamin D intoxication [35], idiopathic hypercalcemia [69], amphotericin B nephropathy [13, 27, 67], toxicity to lithium [91], hepatic cirrhosis [6, 81, 118]; a variety of genetically transmitted disorders such as fructose intolerance with nephrocalcinosis [64], Ehlers-Danlos syndrome [57], and elliptocytosis [2]; and probably also after renal tubular necrosis [54] and homotransplantation [65, 129].

The association of distal RTA and hypergammaglobulinemic states, especially in the adult, is striking. The tubular abnormality has been recognized in cases of idiopathic hypergammaglobulinemia, active chronic hepatitis, hyperglobulinemic purpura, Sjögren's syndrome, cryoglobulinemia, lupus erythematosus, lupoid hepatitis, and fibrosing alveolitis [63, 72, 76, 103].

The finding in a single family of individuals with nephrocalcinosis and distal RTA and individuals with hypercalciuria, but without nephrocalcinosis or distal RTA, suggests that a picture identical to distal RTA may develop as the consequence of long-standing hypercalciuria of genetic origin [12].

NATURE OF THE DEFECT
Distal RTA is characterized functionally by an inability of the cells of the distal nephron to produce a sufficient gradient of hydrogen ion between blood and tubular fluid in the distal nephron, regardless of the degree of the systemic acidosis. The urine pH remains inappropriately high despite the exogenous or endogenous acid load [33, 72, 96, 100, 101, 102, 103, 131] or the intravenous administration of sodium sulfate [75, 107]. Although the absolute rate of excretion of ammonium is low, excretion is adequate when related to the elevated pH of the urine. Excretion of titratable acid also is reduced due to incomplete saturation of urinary buffers.

The exact nature of the acidification defect is

not known. The hypotheses suggested include a defect in the energy mechanism necessary to pump hydrogen ion—or to reabsorb sodium—across the tubular membrane, or an increased rate of passive diffusion of hydrogen ion from the tubular lumen back into the cell. Selective dysfunction of the cells of the distal nephron that secrete hydrogen ion could account for the disorder.

A deficiency in carbonic anhydrase to explain a secretory defect in hydrogen ion is unlikely, since enzyme studies in renal tissue, although not totally satisfactory, have been found to be normal. Furthermore, the overall rate of hydrogen ion secretion appears to be intact, as judged by studies of bicarbonate resorption and by the observation of increased rates of excretion of titratable acid, with no decrease in urinary pH, in response to infusion of neutral phosphate [52, 75, 96].

The theory in favor of an abnormality in the permeability of the distal nephron is supported mainly by the appearance of apparently classic distal RTA in patients receiving amphotericin B, a polyene antibiotic that markedly reduces pH gradients across the isolated turtle bladder [121] by increasing the permeability of cell membranes [58]. The studies of Sebastian et al. [112], which demonstrate an inability of some patients with distal RTA to conserve potassium, could also speak for leakiness of the distal nephron segment.

Studies performed during alkaline diuresis, when no secretory gradient for hydrogen ion exists, showed, however, that urinary levels of P_{CO_2} were elevated in normal subjects but not in patients with distal RTA [45]. This result is compatible with the hypothesis that in distal RTA there is a limitation in the rate of secretion of hydrogen ion rather than an increased back-diffusion of hydrogen ion in the presence of a normal secretory rate. Alternative explanations for this observation are possible, however, such as increased permeability to carbon dioxide or to carbonic acid or accelerated dehydration of carbonic acid to carbon dioxide and water. If the failure to elevate urinary P_{CO_2} above that of blood were due to a limitation in the rate of secretion of hydrogen ion, bicarbonate excretion during bicarbonate loading would be greater than in normal subjects. Conversely, if the failure to elevate urinary P_{CO_2} were due to back-diffusion of carbonic acid or its rapid conversion to carbon dioxide and water, increased urinary excretion of bicarbonate during loading would not be observed. In a study reported by Sebastian et al. [113], the latter was found to be the case.

Recently, Arruda et al. [1a] conducted studies to investigate the effect of urinary concentrating abil-ity on the generation of urinary carbon dioxide tension. In rat, dog, and man, the difference in carbon dioxide tension between blood and urine was dependent upon the urinary concentration of bicarbonate, as influenced by urinary concentrating capacity. They concluded that urinary P_{CO_2} in alkaline urine is determined by the concentration of urinary bicarbonate and does not reflect the capacity of the distal nephron to secrete hydrogen ion. Therefore, the findings of Halperin et al. [45] may reflect the impaired concentrating capacity of patients with distal RTA and have no bearing on their acidifying mechanism.

The nature of the cellular defect in distal RTA is unknown. The dominant inheritance seen in primary distal RTA is more in favor of the presence of an abnormal protein (or the absence of a normal protein) involved in membrane transport than of an enzymatic deficiency, which is generally transmitted as a recessive characteristic [44]. The nature of this protein is not known, but the association of distal RTA and elliptocytosis suggests that the renal tubule and red blood cell membranes share common characteristics. As stated by Royer and Broyer [106], the defect in distal RTA is primarily renal and represents more of a structural defect than a generalized metabolic disorder. One of their patients received two renal homotransplants without reappearance of any defect in urinary acidification in the transplanted kidneys in more than 8 years of follow-up.

The frequent association of hyperglobulinemic states and distal RTA must be considered more than coincidental. Renal tubular acidosis in such patients may be the functional expression of a generalized autoimmune disorder rather than a direct consequence of the hypergammaglobulinemia [76]. This conclusion is supported by the presence of autoantibodies to tubular antigens [17] and by the deposition of immunoglobulins and complement in the tubular cells [90, 122, 127].

DIAGNOSIS

The basic method of diagnosing distal RTA is to study urinary pH under conditions in which acidification of the urine should be maximal, such as during spontaneous or induced metabolic acidosis. In this situation values of urinary pH in patients with distal RTA are higher than those found in normal controls. The study can be done by the administration of a nonreabsorbable anion such as sulfate or more physiologically by administration of an acidifying salt such as ammonium chloride. In our hands the short test of Wrong and Davies

[131] as modified by Edelmann et al. [30] provides an adequate assessment of acidifying mechanisms, even though it does not assess ammonium adaptation during chronic acidosis. This test consists in the oral administration of an appropriate dose of ammonium chloride and the collection of urine 3 to 5 hr thereafter. Correct interpretation of the urinary response requires that the concentration of bicarbonate in blood be decreased sufficiently to ensure maximal urinary acidification, that is, to a level a few mmol below the renal bicarbonate threshold. It is obvious that any arbitrary dose of ammonium chloride may be insufficient. The dose should be calculated to decrease the concentration of plasma bicarbonate by 4 to 5 mmol per liter and to at least 20 mmol per liter in the child and 18 mmol per liter in the infant. Most patients with distal RTA present with levels of plasma bicarbonate below these figures, and it may be unnecessary to further stress the renal mechanisms of acidification. Observation of a urinary pH of 5.0 to 5.5 clearly excludes the diagnosis of distal RTA. The presence of a persistently elevated urinary pH, however, does not confirm the diagnosis of distal RTA if the level of the renal bicarbonate threshold is not known. The plotting of urine pH over a wide range of plasma bicarbonate concentrations, as discussed previously, usually will clearly differentiate distal from proximal forms of RTA.

The hydrogen ion clearance index was proposed by Elkinton and coworkers [32] in an attempt to relate the rate of excretion of hydrogen ion in the urine to hydrogen ion concentration in the blood. Although this test has had widespread application, its physiologic validity has been questioned since there is no linear correlation between the variables [30]; in our opinion, it should not be used.

TREATMENT

Treatment of distal RTA consists in the administration of alkali in adequate amounts to maintain sustained correction of the acidemia. Potassium administration is also necessary, regardless of the level of plasma potassium; in instances of severe hypokalemia, potassium should be given prior to the correction of the acidemia. The simplest maintenance therapy is the administration of sodium and potassium bicarbonate. If bicarbonate produces gastrointestinal symptoms such as bloating or belching (uncommon in our experience in infants and children), citrate can be substituted. A useful mixture is a solution of sodium and potassium citrate: 100 gm of each salt diluted in 1 liter of distilled water provides approximately 2 mEq of citrate per milliliter. The oral administration of tromethamine (THAM) has been recommended [125], but it does not seem to have any particular advantage.

The dose of alkali is about 1 to 3 mEq/kg/day, but it must be adjusted in each case according to the levels of blood pH and bicarbonate and the rate of urinary excretion of calcium. When there is associated bicarbonate wasting, as occurs frequently in infants, the requirement of alkali is larger and approximates that necessary to correct the acidemia in proximal RTA.

The principal aim of therapy, in addition to reinstitution of growth and healing of bone lesions, is the prevention of further deposition of calcium in the kidney and of progressive deterioration of renal function. The rate of urinary excretion of calcium is the most sensitive guide to therapy, and it should be kept below 2 mg/kg/day.

The administration of diuretics such as hydrochlorothiazide is not only of limited benefit but is also potentially dangerous, since it may aggravate the hypokalemia [93].

References

1. Albright, F., Burnett, C. H., Parson, W., Reifenstein, E. C., Jr., and Roos, A. Osteomalacia and late rickets. *Medicine* 25:399, 1946.
1a. Arruda, J. A. L., Nascimento, L., Mehta, P. K., Rademacher, D. R., Sehy, J. T., Westenfelder, C., and Kurtzman, N. A. The critical importance of urinary concentrating ability in the generation of urinary carbon dioxide tension. *J. Clin. Invest.* 60: 922, 1977.
2. Baehner, R. L., Gilchrist, G. S., and Anderson, E. J. Hereditary elliptocytosis and primary renal tubular acidosis in a single family. *Am. J. Dis. Child.* 115: 414, 1968.
3. Baines, G. H., Barclay, J. A., and Cooke, W. T. Nephrocalcinosis associated with hyperchloremia and low plasma bicarbonate. *Q. J. Med.* 14:113, 1945.
4. Barzel, U. S., and Hart, H. Studies in calcium absorption: Initial entry of calcium into the gastrointestinal tract in hyperparathyroidism and in a case of renal tubular acidosis. *Nephron.* 10:174, 1973.
5. Berlyne, G. M. Distal function in chronic hydronephrosis. *Q. J. Med.* 30:339, 1961.
6. Better, O. S., Goldschmid, Z., Chaimovitz, C., and Alroy, G. G. Defect in urinary acidification in cirrhosis. *Arch. Intern. Med.* 130:77, 1972.
7. Boyd, J. D., and Stearns, G. Concomitance of chronic acidosis with late rickets. *Am. J. Dis. Child.* 64:594, 1942.
8. Brenes, L. G., Brenes, J. N., and Hernandez, M. M. Familial proximal renal tubular acidosis: A distinct clinical entity. *Am. J. Med.* 63:244, 1977.
9. Brodwall, E. K., Westlie, L., and Myhre, E. The renal excretion and tubular reabsorption of citric acid in renal tubular acidosis. *Acta Med. Scand.* 192: 137, 1972.
10. Buchanan, E. U., and Komrower, G. M. The prognosis of idiopathic renal acidosis in infancy with ob-

servations on urine acidification and ammonia production in children. *Arch. Dis. Child.* 33:532, 1958.

11. Buckalew, V. M., Jr., McCurdy, D. K., Ludwig, G. D., Chaykin, L. B., and Elkinton, J. R. Incomplete renal tubular acidosis: Physiologic studies in three patients with a defect in lowering urinary pH. *Am. J. Med.* 45:32, 1968.

12. Buckalew, V. M., Jr., Purvis, M. L., Shulman, M. G., Herndon, C. N., and Rudman, D. Hereditary renal tubular acidosis: Report of a 64 member kindred with variable expression including idiopathic hypercalciuria. *Medicine* 53:229, 1974.

13. Burgess, J. L., and Birchall, R. Nephrotoxicity of amphotericin B, with emphasis on changes in tubular function. *Am. J. Med.* 53:77, 1972.

14. Butler, A. M., Wilson, J. L., and Farber, S. Dehydration and acidosis with calcification of renal tubules. *J. Pediatr.* 8:489, 1936.

15. Callis, L., Castelló, F., Fortuny, G., Vallo, A., and Ballabriga, A. Effect of hydrochlorothiazide on rickets and on renal tubular acidosis in two patients with cystinosis. *Helv. Paediatr. Acta* 25:602, 1970.

16. Carré, I. J., Wood, B. S. B., and Smallwood, W. C. Idiopathic renal acidosis in infancy. *Arch. Dis. Child.* 29:326, 1954.

17. Chanarin, I., Loewi, G., Tavill, A. S., Swain, C. P., and Tidmarsh, E. Defect of renal acidification with antibody to loop of Henle. *Lancet* 2:317, 1974.

18. Coe, F. L., and Firpo, J. J. Evidence for mild reversible hyperparathyroidism in distal renal tubular acidosis. *Arch. Intern. Med.* 135:1485, 1975.

19. Coe, F. L., Firpo, J. J., Hollandsworth, D. L., Segil, L., Canterbury, J. M., and Reiss, E. Effect of acute and chronic metabolic acidosis on serum immunoreactive parathyroid hormone in man. *Kidney Int.* 8:262, 1975.

20. Cohen, T., Brand-Auraban, A., Karshai, C., Jacob, A., Gay, I., Tsitsianov, J., Shapior, T., Jatziv, S., and Ashkenazi, A. Familial infantile renal tubular acidosis and congenital nerve deafness: An autosomal recessive syndrome. *Clin. Genet.* 4:275, 1973.

21. Cooke, R. E., Boyden, D. G., and Haller, E. The relationship of acidosis and growth retardation. *J. Pediatr.* 57:326, 1960.

22. Deck, M. D. F. Medullary sponge kidney with renal tubular acidosis: A report of 3 cases. *J. Urol.* 94:330, 1965.

23. Dedmon, R. E., and Wrong, O. The excretion of organic anion in renal tubular acidosis with particular reference to citrate. *Clin. Sci.* 22:19, 1962.

24. Donckerwolcke, R. A., Van Biervliet, J. P., Koorevaar, G., Kuijten, R. H., and Van Stekelenburg, G. J. The syndrome of renal tubular acidosis with nerve deafness. *Acta Paediatr. Scand.* 65:100, 1976.

25. Donckerwolcke, R. A., Van Stekelenburg, G. J., and Tiddens, H. A. A case of bicarbonate-losing renal tubular acidosis with defective carboanhydrase activity. *Arch. Dis. Child.* 45:759, 1970.

26. Donckerwolcke, R. A., Van Stekelenburg, G. J., and Tiddens, H. A. Therapy of bicarbonate-losing renal tubular acidosis. *Arch. Dis. Child.* 45:774, 1970.

27. Douglas, J. B., and Healy, J. K. Nephrotoxic effects of amphotericin B, including renal tubular acidosis. *Am. J. Med.* 46:154, 1969.

28. Drinkard, J. P., Lee, D. N. B., and Gonick, H. C. Parathormone (PTH) and 47 calcium kinetics changes with alkali treatment of renal tubular acidosis (RTA). In Proceedings of the Third Annual Meeting of the American Society for Nephrology, 1969. P. 17.

29. Droste, E., and Mietens, C. Diagnosis and therapy of renal tubular acidosis in infancy. *Z. Kinderheilkd.* 119:151, 1975.

30. Edelmann, C. M., Jr., Boichis, H., Rodriguez-Soriano, J., and Stark, H. The renal response of children to acute ammonium chloride acidosis. *Pediatr. Res.* 1:452, 1967.

31. Edelmann, C. M., Jr., Rodriguez-Soriano, J., Boichis, H., Gruskin, A. B., and Acosta, M. Bicarbonate reabsorption and hydrogen ion excretion in normal infants. *J. Clin. Invest.* 46:1309, 1967.

32. Elkinton, J. R., Huth, E. J., Webster, G. D., Jr., and McCance, R. A. The renal excretion of hydrogen ion in renal tubular acidosis: I. Quantitative assessment of the response to ammonium chloride as an acid load. *Am. J. Med.* 29:554, 1960.

33. Elkinton, J. R., McCurdy, D. K., Buckalew, V. M., Jr. Hydrogen Ion and the Kidney. In D. A. K. Black (ed.), *Renal Disease* (2nd ed.). Oxford, England: Blackwell, 1967. Pp. 110–135.

34. Ferris, D. O., and Odel, H. M. Electrolyte pattern of blood after bilateral ureterosigmoidostomy. *J.A.M.A.* 142:634, 1950.

35. Ferris, T., Kashgarian, M., Levitin, H., Brandt, I., and Epstein, F. H. Renal tubular acidosis and renal potassium wasting acquired as a result of hypercalcemic nephropathy. *N. Engl. J. Med.* 265:924, 1961.

36. Foss, G. L., Perry, C. B., and Wood, F. J. Y. Renal tubular acidosis. *Q. J. Med.* 25:185, 1956.

37. Fourman, P., Smith, J. W. G., and McConkey, B. Defects of water reabsorption and of hydrogen ion secretion by the renal tubules in hyperparathyroidism. *Lancet* 1:619, 1960.

38. Gill, J. R., Jr., Bell, N. H., and Bartter, F. C. Impaired conservation of sodium and potassium in renal acidosis and its correction by buffer anions. *Clin. Sci.* 33:577, 1967.

39. Goodman, A. D., Lemann, J., Jr., Lennon, E. J., and Relman, A. S. Production, excretion and net balance of fixed acid in patients with renal acidosis. *J. Clin. Invest.* 44:495, 1965.

40. Greenberg, A. J., McNamara, H., and McCrory, W. W. Metabolic balance studies in primary renal tubular acidosis: Effects of acidosis on external calcium and phosphorus balances. *J. Pediatr.* 69:610, 1966.

41. Gruskin, A. B., Patel, M. S., Linshaw, M., Ettenger, R., Huff, D., and Grover, W. Renal function studies and kidney pyruvate carboxylase in subacute necrotizing encephalomyelopathy (Leigh's syndrome). *Pediatr. Res.* 7:832, 1973.

42. Guibaud, P., Larbre, F., Freycon, M. T., and Genoud, J. Ostéopétrose et acidose tubulaire rénale: Deux cas de cette association dans une fratrie. *Arch. Fr. Pediatr.* 29:269, 1972.

43. Guignard, J. P., and Torrado, A. Proximal renal tubular acidosis in vitamin D deficiency rickets. *Acta Paediatr. Scand.* 62:543, 1973.

44. Györy, A. Z., and Edwards, K. D. G. Renal tubular acidosis. *Am. J. Med.* 45:43, 1968.

45. Halperin, M. L., Goldstein, M. B., Haig, A., Johnson, M. D., and Stinebaugh, B. J. Studies on the pathogenesis of type I (distal) renal tubular acidosis

as revealed by the urinary Pco_2 tensions. *J. Clin. Invest.* 53:669, 1974.

45a. Harrison, H. E., Chisolm, M. D., and Harrison, H. C. Congenital tubular acidosis. *Am. J. Dis. Child.* 96:588, 1958.

46. Harrison, H. E., and Harrison, H. C. The effects of acidosis upon the renal tubular reabsorption of phosphate. *Am. J. Physiol.* 134:781, 1941.

47. Huth, E. J., Mayock, R. L., and Kerr, R. M. Hyperthyroidism associated with renal tubular acidosis: Discussion of a possible relationship. *Am. J. Med.* 26:818, 1959.

48. Huth, E. J., Webster, G. D., and Elkinton, J. R. The renal excretion of hydrogen ion in renal tubular acidosis: III. An attempt to detect latent cases in a family; comments on nosology, genetics and etiology of the primary disease. *Am. J. Med.* 29:586, 1960.

49. Koningsmark, B. W. Renal tubular acidosis with progressive nerve deafness (personal communication). Cited by V. A. McKusick, *Mendelian Inheritance in Man* (2nd ed.). Baltimore: Johns Hopkins, 1968. P. 357.

50. Lamy, M., Frézal, J., Rey, J., and Larsen, C. Etude métabolique du syndrome de Lowe. *Rev. Fr. Etud. Clin. Biol.* 7:271, 1962.

51. Lathem, W. Hyperchloremic acidosis in chronic pyelonephritis. *N. Engl. J. Med.* 258:1031, 1958.

52. Latner, A. L., and Burnard, E. D. Idiopathic hyperchloremic renal acidosis in infants (nephrocalcinosis infantum): Observations on the site and nature of the lesion. *Q. J. Med.* 19:285, 1950.

53. Leaf, A. The Syndrome of Osteomalacia, Renal Glycosuria, Amino Aciduria, and Increased Phosphate Clearance (the Fanconi Syndrome). In J. B. Stanbury, J. B. Wyngaarden, and D. S. Fredrickson (eds.), *The Metabolic Basis of Inherited Disease* (2nd ed.). New York: McGraw-Hill, 1966. Pp. 1205–1220.

54. Legrain, P., Fournet, P. C., Pignard, P., and Meyer, P. Rôle joué par les anions plasmatiques dans l'excrétion rénale des ions H à la reprise de la diurèse des néphropathies tubulo-interstitielles. *J. Urol. Nephrol. (Paris)* 71:741, 1965.

54a. Lemann, J., Jr. Personal communication, 1976.

55. Lemann, J., Jr., Litzow, J. R., and Lennon, E. J. The effects of chronic acid loads in normal man: Further evidence for the participation of bone mineral in the defense against chronic metabolic acidosis. *J. Clin. Invest.* 45:1608, 1966.

56. Leumann, E. P., and Steinmann, B. Persistent and transient distal renal tubular acidosis with bicarbonate wasting. *Pediatr. Res.* 9:767, 1975.

57. Levine, A. S., and Michael, A. F., Jr. Ehlers-Danlos syndrome with renal tubular acidosis and medullary sponge kidneys. *J. Pediatr.* 71:107, 1967.

58. Lichtenstein, N. S., and Leaf, A. Effect of amphotericin B on the permeability of the toad bladder. *J. Clin. Invest.* 44:1328, 1965.

59. Lightwood, R. Calcium infarction of kidney in infants. *Arch. Dis. Child.* 10:205, 1935.

60. Lightwood, R., and Butler, N. Decline in primary infantile renal acidosis: Aetiological implications. *Br. Med. J.* 1:885, 1963.

61. Lightwood, R., Maclagan, N. F., and Williams, J. G. Persistent acidosis in an infant: Cause not yet ascertained. *Proc. R. Soc. Med.* 29:1431, 1936.

62. Lightwood, R., Payne, W. W., and Black, J. A. Infantile renal acidosis. *Pediatrics* 12:628, 1953.

63. Mason, A. M. S., McIllmurray, M. B., Golding, P. L., and Hughes, D. T. D. Fibrosing alveolitis associated with renal tubular acidosis. *Br. Med. J.* 4:596, 1970.

64. Mass, R. E., Smith, W. R., and Walsh, J. R. The association of hereditary fructose intolerance and renal tubular acidosis. *Am. J. Med. Sci.* 251:516, 1966.

65. Massry, S. G., Preuss, H. G., Maher, J. F., and Schreiner, G. E. Renal tubular acidosis after cadaver kidney transplantation: Studies on mechanism. *Am. J. Med.* 42:284, 1967.

66. Matsuda, I., Takeda, T., Sugai, M., and Matsuura, N. Oculocerebrorenal syndrome in a child with normal urinary acidification and a defect in bicarbonate reabsorption. *Am. J. Dis. Child.* 117:205, 1969.

67. McCurdy, D. K., Frederic, M., and Elkinton, J. R. Renal tubular acidosis due to amphotericin B. *N. Engl. J. Med.* 278:124, 1968.

68. McSherry, E., Sebastian, A., and Morris, R. C., Jr. Renal tubular acidosis in infants: The several kinds, including bicarbonate-wasting, classic renal tubular acidosis. *J. Clin. Invest.* 51:499, 1972.

69. Morgan, H. G., Mitchell, R. G., Stowers, J. M., and Thompson, J. Metabolic studies on two infants with idiopathic hypercalcemia. *Lancet* 1:925, 1956.

70. Morris, R. C., Jr. An experimental renal acidification defect in patients with hereditary fructose intolerance: I. Its resemblance to renal tubular acidosis. *J. Clin. Invest.* 47:1389, 1968.

71. Morris, R. C., Jr. An experimental renal acidification defect in patients with hereditary fructose intolerance: II. Its distinction from classic renal tubular acidosis, its resemblance to the renal acidification defect associated with the Fanconi syndrome of children with cystinosis. *J. Clin. Invest.* 47:1648, 1968.

72. Morris, R. C., Jr. Renal tubular acidosis: Mechanisms, classification and implications. *N. Engl. J. Med.* 281:1405, 1969.

73. Morris, R. C., Jr., McSherry, E., and Sebastian, A. Modulation of experimental renal dysfunction of hereditary fructose intolerance by circulating parathyroid hormone. *Proc. Natl. Acad. Sci. U.S.A.* 68:132, 1971.

74. Morris, R. C., Jr., McSherry, E., Sherwood, L. M., and Sebastian, A. Evidence of a pathogenetic role of hyperparathyroidism in the renal tubular dysfunction of patients with Fanconi's syndrome (abstract). *J. Clin. Invest.* 50:68a, 1970.

75. Morris, R. C., Jr., Piel, C. F., and Audioun, E. Renal tubular acidosis: Effects of sodium phosphate and sulfate on renal acidification in two patients with renal tubular acidosis. *Pediatrics* 36:899, 1965.

76. Morris, R. C., Jr., Sebastian, A., and McSherry, E. Renal acidosis. *Kidney Int.* 1:322, 1972.

77. Morris, R. C., Jr., Yamauchi, H., Palubinskas, A. J., and Howenstine, J. Medullary sponge kidney. *Am. J. Med.* 38:883, 1965.

78. Morrisey, J. F., Ochoa, M., Jr., Lotspeich, W. D., and Waterhouse, C. Citrate excretion in renal tubular acidosis. *Ann. Intern. Med.* 58:159, 1963.

79. Muldowney, F. P., Carroll, D. V., Donohoe, J. F., and Freaney, R. Correction of renal bicarbonate wastage by parathyroidectomy. *Q. J. Med.* 40:487, 1971.

80. Muldowney, F. P., Donohoe, J. F., Freaney, R., Kampff, C., and Swan, M. Parathormone-induced

renal bicarbonate wastage in intestinal malabsorption and in chronic renal failure. *Ir. J. Med. Sci.* 3: 221, 1970.

81. Mulhausen, R., Eichenholz, A., and Blumentals, A. Acid-base disturbances in patients with cirrhosis of the liver. *Medicine* 46:185, 1967.

82. Musgrave, J. E., Bennett, W. M., Campbell, R. A., and Eisenberg, C. S. Renal tubular acidosis. *Lancet* 2:1364, 1972.

83. Nance, W. E., and Sweeney, A. Evidence for autosomal recessive inheritance of the syndrome of renal tubular acidosis with deafness. *Birth Defects* 7:70, 1971.

84. Nash, M. A., Torrado, A. D., Greifer, I., Spitzer, A., and Edelmann, C. M., Jr. Renal tubular acidosis in infants and children: Clinical course, response to treatment and prognosis. *J. Pediatr.* 80:738, 1972.

85. Nordin, B. E. C., and Smith, D. A. Citric acid excretion in renal stone disease and in renal tubular acidosis. *Br. J. Urol.* 35:438, 1963.

86. Oetliker, O., Chattas, A. J., and Schultz, S. M. Characterization of renal contribution to acid-base balance in the pediatric age group. *Helv. Paediatr. Acta* 26:523, 1971.

87. Oetliker, O., and Rossi, E. The influence of extracellular fluid volume on the renal bicarbonate threshold: A study of two children with Lowe's syndrome. *Pediatr. Res.* 3:140, 1969.

88. Oetliker, O., and Zurbrügg, R. P. Renal tubular acidosis in salt-losing syndrome of congenital adrenal hyperplasia (CAH). *J. Clin. Endocrinol. Metab.* 31:447, 1970.

89. Palmer, R. H., and Cornfeld, D. Primary renal tubular acidosis recognized and treated at three days of age: A case report illustrating the value of postmortem examination. *Clin. Pediatr.* 12:140, 1973.

90. Pasternack, A., and Linder, E. Renal tubular acidosis: An immunopathological study on four patients. *Clin. Exp. Immunol.* 7:115, 1970.

91. Perez, G. O., Oster, J. R., and Vaamonde, C. A. Incomplete syndrome of renal tubular acidosis induced by lithium carbonate. *J. Lab. Clin. Med.* 86: 386, 1975.

92. Pitts, R. F., Ayer, J. L., and Schiess, W. A. The renal regulation of acid-base balance in man: III. The reabsorption and excretion of bicarbonate. *J. Clin. Invest.* 28:35, 1949.

93. Rampini, S., Fanconi, A., Illig, R., and Prader, A. Effect of hydrochlorothiazide on proximal renal tubular acidosis in a patient with idiopathic "De Toni-Debré-Fanconi syndrome." *Helv. Paediatr. Acta* 23: 13, 1968.

94. Relman, A. S. Renal acidosis and renal excretion of acid in health and disease. *Adv. Intern. Med.* 12: 295, 1964.

95. Relman, A. S. The acidosis of renal disease. *Am. J. Med.* 44:706, 1968.

96. Reynolds, T. B. Observations on the pathogenesis of renal tubular acidosis. *Am. J. Med.* 25:503, 1958.

97. Richards, P., Chamberlain, M. J., and Wrong, O. M. Treatment of osteomalacia of renal tubular acidosis by sodium bicarbonate alone. *Lancet* 2:994, 1972.

98. Richards, W., Donnell, G. N., Wilson, W. A., Stowens, D., and Perry, T. The oculocerebrorenal syndrome of Lowe. *Am. J. Dis. Child.* 109:185, 1965.

99. Richards, P., and Wrong, O. M. Dominant inheritance in a family with familial renal tubular acidosis. *Lancet* 2:998, 1972.

100. Rodriguez-Soriano, J. The renal regulation of acid-base balance and the disturbances noted in renal tubular acidosis. *Pediatr. Clin. North Am.* 18:529, 1971.

101. Rodriguez-Soriano, J., Boichis, H., and Edelmann, C. M., Jr. Bicarbonate reabsorption and hydrogen ion excretion in children with renal tubular acidosis. *J. Pediatr.* 71:802, 1967.

102. Rodriguez-Soriano, J., Boichis, H., Stark, H., and Edelmann, C. M., Jr. Proximal renal tubular acidosis: A defect in bicarbonate reabsorption with normal urinary acidification. *Pediatr. Res.* 1:81, 1967.

103. Rodriguez-Soriano, J., and Edelmann, C. M., Jr. Renal tubular acidosis. *Annu. Rev. Med.* 20:363, 1969.

104. Rodriguez-Soriano, J., Vallo, A., Chouza, M., and Castillo, G. Proximal renal tubular acidosis in tetralogy of Fallot. *Acta Paediatr. Scand.* 64:671, 1975.

105. Rodriguez-Soriano, J., Vallo, A., and Garcia-Fuentes, M. Distal renal tubular acidosis in infancy: A bicarbonate wasting state. *J. Pediatr.* 86:524, 1975.

106. Royer, P., and Broyer, M. L'acidose Rénale au Cours des Tubulopathies Congénitales. In *Actualités Néphrologiques de l'Hopital Necker*. Paris: Flammarion, 1967. P. 73.

107. Royer, P., Lestradet, H., Nordmann, R., Mathieu, H., and Rodriguez-Soriano, J. Etudes sur quatre cas d' acidose tubulaire chronique idiopathique avec hypocitraturie. *Sem. Hop. Paris (Ann. Pediatr.)* 38: 808, 1962.

108. Schloeder, F. X., and Stinebaugh, B. J. Defect of urinary acidification during fasting. *Metabolism* 15: 17, 1966.

109. Schoeneman, M., Lifshitz, F., and Diaz-Bensussen, S. The transport of bicarbonate by the small intestine of a patient with proximal renal tubular acidosis. *Pediatr. Res.* 8:735, 1974.

110. Schwartz, W. B., and Relman, A. S. Acidosis in renal disease. *N. Engl. J. Med.* 256:1184, 1957.

111. Sebastian, A., McSherry, E., and Morris, R. C., Jr. On the mechanism of renal potassium wasting in renal tubular acidosis associated with the Fanconi syndrome (type 2 RTA). *J. Clin. Invest.* 50:231, 1971.

112. Sebastian, A., McSherry, E., and Morris, R. C., Jr. Renal potassium wasting in renal tubular acidosis (RTA): Its occurrence in types 1 and 2 RTA despite sustained correction of systemic acidosis. *J. Clin. Invest.* 50:667, 1971.

113. Sebastian, A., McSherry, E., and Morris, R. C., Jr. On the mechanism of the inappropriately low urinary carbon dioxide tension in classic (type 1) renal tubular acidosis. *Clin. Res.* 22:544A, 1974.

114. Sebastian, A., McSherry, E., Ueki, I., and Morris, R. C. Jr. Renal amyloidosis, nephrotic syndrome, and impaired renal tubular reabsorption of bicarbonate. *Ann. Intern. Med.* 69:541, 1968.

115. Seedat, Y. K. Familial renal tubular acidosis. *Ann. Intern. Med.* 69:1329, 1968.

116. Seldin, D. W., and Wilson, J. D. Renal Tubular Acidosis. In J. B. Stanbury, J. B. Wyngaarden, and D. S. Fredrickson (eds.), *The Metabolic Basis of Inherited Disease* (4th ed.). New York: McGraw-Hill, 1978. Pp. 1618–1633.

117. Shapira, E., Ben-Joseph, Y., Eyal, F. G., and Rus-

sell, A. Enzymatically inactive carbonic anhydrase B in a family with renal tubular acidosis. *J. Clin. Invest.* 53:59, 1974.

118. Shear, L., Bonkowsky, H. L., and Gabuzda, G. J. Renal tubular acidosis in cirrhosis: A determinant of susceptibility to recurrent hepatic precoma. *N. Engl. J. Med.* 280:1, 1969.

119. Smith, R. Urinary acidification defect in chronic infantile malnutrition. *Lancet* 1:764, 1959.

120. Stark, H., and Geiger, R. Renal tubular dysfunction following vascular accidents of the kidneys in the newborn period. *J. Pediatr.* 83:933, 1973.

121. Steinmetz, P. R., and Lawson, L. R. Defect in urinary acidification induced in vitro by amphotericin B. *J. Clin. Invest.* 49:988, 1970.

122. Talal, N. Sjögren's syndrome, lymphoproliferation, and renal tubular acidosis (editorial). *Ann. Intern. Med.* 74:633, 1971.

123. Tannen, R. L., Falls, W. F., Jr., and Brackett, N. C., Jr. Incomplete renal tubular acidosis: Some clinical and physiologic features. *Nephron* 15:111, 1975.

124. Vainsel, M., Fondu, P., Cadranel, S., Rocmans, C., and Gepts, W. Osteopetrosis associated with proximal and distal tubular acidosis. *Acta Paediatr. Scand.* 61:429, 1972.

125. Vert, P., Marchal, C., Neimann, N., and Pierson, M.

Traitement symptomatique des acidoses renales par administration orale de citrate de tham. *Arch. Fr. Pediatr.* 25:91, 1968.

126. Vertuno, L. L., Preuss, H. G., Argy, W. P., Jr., and Schreiner, G. E. Fanconi syndrome following homotransplantation. *Arch. Intern. Med.* 133:302, 1974.

127. Vladutiu, A. O. Renal tubular acidosis: An autoimmune disease? *Lancet* 1:265, 1973.

128. Walker, W. G., Ozer, F. L., and Whelton, A. Syndrome of perceptive deafness and renal tubular acidosis. *Birth Defects* 10:163, 1974.

129. Wilson, D. R., and Siddiqui, A. A. Renal tubular acidosis after kidney transplantation: Natural history and significance. *Ann. Intern. Med.* 79:352, 1973.

130. Wrong, O. Urinary hydrogen ion excretion. *J. Clin. Pathol.* 18:520, 1965.

131. Wrong, O., and Davies, H. E. F. The excretion of acid in renal disease. *Q. J. Med.* 28:259, 1959.

132. York, S. E., and Yendt, E. F. Osteomalacia associated with renal bicarbonate loss. *Can. Med. Assoc. J.* 94:1329, 1966.

133. Young, J. D., Jr., and Martin, L. G. Urinary calculi associated with incomplete renal tubular acidosis. *J. Urol.* 107:170, 1972.

84. Clinical Syndromes Characterized by Disturbances in Phosphate Transport and Excretion

Louis V. Avioli

A systematic evaluation of inherited or acquired disorders of phosphate transport and associated skeletal abnormalities requires not only a fundamental knowledge of calcium metabolism but also an understanding of the hormonal and physical factors that regulate the absorption, excretion, and homeostatic control of inorganic phosphate. The regulation of plasma phosphate is not as readily explained as that of plasma calcium, since the circulating phosphate is not only in equilibrium with skeletal and cellular inorganic phosphate but also with a large number of organic compounds that result from cellular metabolism. The phosphate ion is essential for the metabolism of carbohydrate, lipids, and protein, as it functions as a cofactor in a multitude of enzyme systems and contributes to the metabolic potential in the form of high-energy phosphate compounds. Phosphate functions to modify acid-base equilibrium in plasma and within cells, and it plays fundamental roles in modifying the development and maturation of bone, in the renal excretion of hydrogen ions, and in modifying the effects of the B vitamins.

Phosphate Balance and Homeostatic Control
PHOSPHORUS AND BONE
Of the 11 to 14 gm of phosphorus per kilogram of fat-free tissue in the normal adult, 85 percent is in the skeleton. The remainder is distributed between tissue and membrane components of skeletal muscle, skin, nervous tissue, and other organs. Phosphorus content of bone varies slightly with age in the growing child. At term it accounts for 10.8 percent of cortical bone and reaches adult values of 11.3 percent by 5 to 9 months of age [50]. Whereas most of the phosphorus in soft tissue and cell membranes is in the form of organic esters, almost all of the phosphorus in bone is contained in the mineral phase as inorganic orthophosphate and small amounts of inorganic phosphate.

Although the sequence of events that obtain during the nucleation of bone collagen is still imperfectly understood, collagen fibrils exhibit a remarkable faculty to form covalent bonds with phosphate. As such, the phosphorylation of collagen has been considered the initiating event in the nucleation of bone [70]. In addition to this conditioning role played by phosphate in the formation of the apatitic structure, phosphate also affects bone resorption, mineralization, and collagen synthesis [75] and, as such, plays an integral role in calcium homeostasis. The available evidence is consistent with the interpretation that these effects are due to a direct effect of phosphate upon the metabolic function of osteoblasts.

PLASMA PHOSPHATE

In the human adult, plasma inorganic phosphate ranges between 2.5 and 4.4 mg per deciliter with a mean of 3.5 mg per deciliter. Dietary phosphate, stage of growth and age, time of day, hormonal interplay, and renal function all contribute to the variability of the fasting concentration of serum phosphate. Approximately 88 percent of the plasma phosphate is unfilterable, some of which is complexed with monovalent or divalent cations such as Na^+, Ca^{2+}, and Mg^{2+}. At normal blood pH, 85 percent of the ultrafilterable phosphate is in the form of $HPO_4^=$ the remainder existing mainly as $H_2PO_4^-$ [184].

The concentration of inorganic phosphate in plasma varies with age. In prepubertal children the mean value for circulating phosphate approximates 5 mg per deciliter, with an upper normal limit approaching 6 mg per deciliter. Since growth hormone decreases the phosphate Tm [29], it has been suggested that an enhanced renal response to this hormone in children might reduce phosphate excretion and contribute to the relative hyperphosphatemia [107]. Normal adult values are gradually approached by the second decade.

Total serum phosphate may fluctuate by as much as 1 to 2 mg per deciliter. These variations generally reflect abrupt shifts of inorganic phosphate between extracellular fluid and the intracellular compartments rather than a net gain or loss of phosphate from the body. In this regard, the administration of hexoses or hormones such as insulin, glucagon, or epinephrine results in a reduction in serum phosphate, presumably by stimulating the cellular utilization of glucose and accelerating the formation of intracellular phosphate esters. Systemic alkalosis is associated with a fall in circulating phosphate and has been attributed to a shift of phosphate out of the extracellular fluid compartment. The fall in plasma phosphate concentration is apparently greater in respiratory alkalosis than in comparable levels of metabolic alkalosis. Thus, the evaluation of hypophosphatemia should always include measurements of the pH and total carbon dioxide content of plasma. Whereas starvation is occasionally associated with

a decrease in plasma inorganic phosphate, acidosis and excessive catabolism of body tissue associated with starvation may lead to cellular release of phosphorus and hyperphosphatemia. Severe hypophosphatemia has also been reported in hypokalemic states and shown to be independent of the attendant metabolic alkalosis. Plasma levels of inorganic phosphorus (measured routinely as inorganic phosphate) most probably contribute to the regulation of bone turnover [75] and bioactivation of the vitamin D metabolite 25-hydroxycholecalciferol to 1,25-dihydroxycholecalciferol [45]. It is noteworthy in this regard that severe dietary phosphate deprivation results in hypophosphatemia and increased circulating 1,25-dihydroxycholecalciferol in females, whereas insignificant changes in either substance obtain in phosphate-depleted males [74].

PHOSPHATE ABSORPTION

Most if not all of the dietary phosphorus is absorbed as free phosphate. The efficiency of phosphate absorption is a function of both the dietary intake and food source [119]. On a normal intake, 60 to 70 percent of phosphate is absorbed; maximal absorption (up to 90 percent) is achieved on very low intakes [124]. Various dietary forms of organic phosphate esters, such as the phytic acid of cereals and seeds, are not readily available to humans, since the intestine is deficient in the enzyme phytase, which is essential for hydrolysis of the organic esters. Organic phosphate ester compounds may also interfere with calcium absorption, since they form insoluble calcium salts within the intestinal lumen. In animals, certain substances, e.g., unsaturated fatty acids, iron, and aluminum, interfere with intestinal phosphate absorption [42, 148, 168]. Vitamin D increases intestinal phosphate absorption in certain animal species [46]. A direct effect of vitamin D (or its biologically active metabolites) on phosphate absorption in humans is still to be adequately defined [11].

There is no known effective physiologic mechanism regulating the intestinal absorption of phosphorus in man, the control of phosphate economy being achieved primarily by a balance between variation in dietary intake and rate of renal excretion [107]. Fecal phosphorus represents both unabsorbed phosphorus and that secreted into the gastrointestinal tract. When phosphorus intakes approximate 1 to 1.50 gm per day, the endogenous secretion of phosphate into the intestinal lumen is 3 mg/kg/day [124]. Dietary phosphorus is absorbed to a greater extent than calcium, and consequently the renal excretion of phosphorus is much greater than that of calcium [107].

PHOSPHATE EXCRETION

Urinary phosphorus is largely inorganic phosphate, the amount depending primarily upon that which is absorbed from the intestinal tract. Phosphate exists in blood and in the glomerular filtrate in the form of $HPO_4^=$ and $H_2PO_4^-$ in the ratio of 4 : 1. With normal renal function, urinary phosphorus usually amounts to approximately two-thirds of the dietary phosphorus. Normally, a diurnal variation in phosphate clearance occurs with the pattern of a matitudinal increase in urinary phosphorus-creatinine ratios. This circadian rhythm is related to physical activity, with the nadir appearing a few hours after the end of sleep. The loss of diurnal variation in adrenal-insufficient states and the documented inverse correlation between phosphate excretion and plasma cortisol levels suggest that this rhythm is controlled by the adrenal glands [107].

In humans the tubular resorption of phosphate filtered by the glomeruli is normally 85 to 95 percent [107]. This process is parathyroid-hormone-dependent, age-related, and rate-limited, with a maximum tubular resorptive capacity in prepubertal children averaging 6 to 7 mg per minute. The tubular resorption of phosphate is increased by short-term cortisol therapy and growth hormone and is decreased by digoxin, estrogen, thyroid hormone, parathyroid hormone, long-term cortisol treatment, and by elevations in circulating calcium [107].

PHOSPHORUS REQUIREMENTS

The average daily phosphorus requirement of adults in the United States is estimated at 0.8 to 1.5 gm [98, 119]. The primary source of calcium in the American diet is milk, and other sources of phosphorus are poultry, fish, and meat. Nonnutritious soft drinks containing excess phosphorus in the form of phosphoric acid also serve as sources for children and adults alike. The relatively greater availability of phosphate-containing foodstuffs in Western diets has resulted in a calcium-phosphate dietary ratio much lower than that recommended to maintain the integrity of skeletal tissue. This matter is of some concern, since diets with low Ca/P ratio have led to progressive bone loss in rats [52], dogs [93, 96], and horses [6] and may stimulate secondary hyperparathyroidism in man [137].

With the exception of young infants, the recommended daily allowance of phosphorus is the same as that of calcium, although the Ca/P ratio of diets ingested throughout the world today is reportedly less than 0.75 [16, 102]. The Ca/P ratio of cow's milk of 1.3 : 1 compared with a

Ca/P ratio of 2 : 1 in breast milk [16] may contribute to the syndrome of so-called "idiopathic hypocalcemia and tetany of infants on formula feedings. Phosphorus depletion, a syndrome characterized by weakness, anorexia, malaise, and skeletal aches, can obtain during prolonged and excessive intake of nonabsorbable antacids. Specific abnormalities such as hemolytic anemia, granulocyte dysfunction, erythrocyte glycolysis, hypercalciuria, and renal calculi also result from phosphate depletion [87, 92]. The syndrome has been observed in humans and is readily reversed when the medication is discontinued and sufficient amounts of dietary phosphorus are consumed [39]. Its frequency in the very large population of individuals ingesting antacids is unknown, but it is probably rare based on the infrequency of published reports of this complication [39]. Recognition and appropriate therapy requires medical supervision, particularly when adjustments in drug therapy for peptic ulcer are involved.

Hypophosphatemia has been observed during starvation or intravenous glucose feeding and in children with early renal insufficiency, as well as in a variety of rachitic disorders resulting from vitamin D deficiency, defective bioactivation of vitamin D, or other renal phosphate transport abnormalities.

Since the kidney is capable of excreting 600 to 900 mg of phosphorus daily, hyperphosphatemia is rare in the absence of chronic renal disease (Chap. 23) and a glomerular filtration rate below 20 ml per minute [107]. Hyperphosphatemia is also characteristic of childhood disorders associated with parathyroid dysfunction, such as hypoparathyroidism, tumoral calcinosis, and pseudohypoparathyroidism, and it can be accentuated by phosphate feeding. There are no specific signs or symptoms of hyperphosphatemia per se, although the hypocalcemia often associated with the hyperphosphatemia (and exacerbated by phosphate feeding) can result in enhanced neuroexcitability, tetany, and convulsions. Chronic phosphate feeding may also result in elevations in circulating parathyroid hormone [137].

Vitamin-D-Resistant Rickets

Vitamin-D-resistant rickets (VDRR) is predominantly a familial disorder and almost always is transmitted by an X-linked dominant gene [166, 189, 191]. Sporadic instances of VDRR have also been documented in patients who are then expected to transmit the disease to their offspring in an X-linked fashion [189]. Autosomal dominant [78] and recessive [159] transmission patterns have been reported on rare occasions. In this

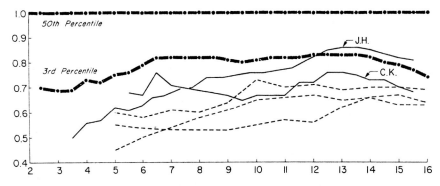

Figure 84-1. Growth rates of two girls with vitamin-D-resistant rickets (J. H. and C. K.) on combined phosphate-vitamin D therapy, compared with growth rates of three girls (broken lines) with VDRR treated with vitamin D alone. The ordinate reflects height age ÷ chronologic age, and the abcissa chronologic age in years. (From P. T. McEnery et al., J. Pediatr. 80:763, 1972.)

regard, VDRR should not be confused with so-called pseudo-vitamin-D-deficiency rickets, a separate disorder characterized by an autosomal recessive inheritance pattern (see later). Using *fasting* hypophosphatemia as a genetic determinant, the frequency of VDRR has been estimated as 1 : 25,000 [189]. Asymptomatic hypophosphatemic adult carriers (e.g., individuals with affected children but with no past history of clinical or radiographically demonstrable bone disease) are most always restricted to females. These latter VDRR individuals should be contrasted with those adults presenting with sporadic hypophosphatemia and osteomalacia, who differ from patients with the inherited form of VDRR by the onset of symptoms during adolescence or adult life, severe myopathy, and glycinuria [49, 82, 86, 155].

CLINICAL AND RADIOGRAPHIC FEATURES
Clinically VDRR is characterized by a reduced rate of growth and short stature, fractures (more often in adults), and varum and valgum deformities of the knees in growing children due to the presence of epiphyseal rachitic lesions. These changes are not specific for VDRR and may be seen in other acquired or vitamin-D-deficient forms of rickets. In untreated or poorly managed patients (i.e., those treated with vitamin D alone), the secondary deformities that present after epiphyseal closure, such as coxa vara and saber shins, may be quite severe. Trunk length is normal in children with VDRR; and leg-length shortening accounts for most of the statural defect in these patients [112]. Retardation of bone maturation is not ordinarily attended by any striking delay in bone age.

Although hypophosphatemia is the hallmark

of VDRR and supplemental phosphate administration is therapeutic, with more rapid healing and acceleration of the growth than in children treated with vitamin D alone [111] (Fig. 84-1), there is no relationship between the observed height deficits and the degree of hypophosphatemia [161]. Clinical signs of rickets, such as growth failure, genu varum, or genu valgum, are usually less obvious in affected females than in affected males despite comparable degrees of hypophosphatemia. On the average, heterozygous females manifest a mild degree of hypophosphatemia and less severe skeletal deformities. When bone disease is present, however, objective measurements such as skeletal radiograms and growth rates do not demonstrate any differences in severity between males and females.

Patients with VDRR may present initially to dental consultation because of tooth fracture or attrition. Moreover, loose, abcessed teeth with gingival fistulas, with or without gross evidence of pulpal exposure from caries, and enamel hypomineralization and hypoplasia have been observed before changes in growth rates or rachitiform deformities were apparent clinically [157]. Radiographically these changes are attended by varying degrees of facial osseous abnormalities, delayed tooth eruption, obscure lamina dura, and enlarged pulp chambers.

Radiologically, children with VDRR often present with rachitic skeletal lesions (Fig. 84-2). In severe cases diffuse skeletal osteopenia may be observed (Fig. 84-3). Defective calcification of epiphyseal cartilage is detected radiologically in the distal ends of the long tubular bones. Characteristically the space between the epiphysis and metaphysis is widened, and the metaphyseal line

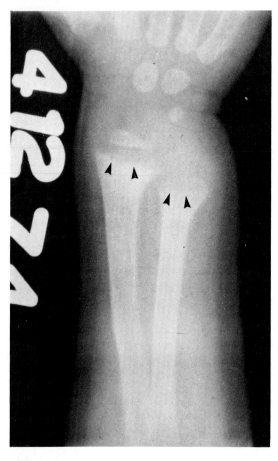

Figure 84-2. Epiphyseal changes in a child with vitamin-D-resistant rickets. Note the swollen wrists and the cup-shaped pattern of the lesions at the distal ends of the ulna and radius (arrows).

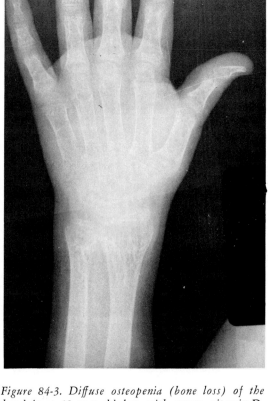

Figure 84-3. Diffuse osteopenia (bone loss) of the hand in a 12-year-old boy with severe vitamin-D-resistant rickets.

of calcification is irregular and frayed, imparting an appearance of cupping that is concave to the epiphyseal side (see Fig. 84-2).

Histologically, the skeletal lesion is generalized and is characterized by an abundance of unmineralized osteoid (collagen) and mineralization defects, specifically around the osteocytes [27]. In some skeletal areas failure of osteoclastic resorption results in osteomalacic osteosclerosis. Evidence of bone cell population dynamics in VDRR also reveals major dynamic disturbances in bone turnover, osteoprogenitor cell activity, and osteoblastic function [94, 181]. Adults with VDRR may also present with either dome-shaped or narrow and long cranial contours. These changes have been ascribed to premature closure of the cranial sutures (most commonly the sagittal suture), a phenomenon observed in one-third to one-half of children with active rickets.

CHEMICAL FINDINGS

Fasting hypophosphatemia, elevation in circulating alkaline phosphatase, phosphaturia, and hydroxyprolinuria have all been well documented in children with VDRR. Circulating levels of immunoreactive parathyroid hormone (iPTH) have been variably reported as normal [7, 63], elevated [77, 99, 138], or lower than normal [141] in VDRR, in contrast to the consistent finding of elevated values in simple vitamin-D-deficiency rickets [8]. Part of this disparity may be due to differences in the antisera used to measure the heterogeneous circulating fragments of parathyroid hormone (PTH) and the differing basal patterns of intake of phosphate and vitamin D of the patients. When a large number of untreated X-linked VDRR subjects are studied under carefully controlled conditions, their serum calciums are slightly but significantly lower and serum iPTH higher than comparable

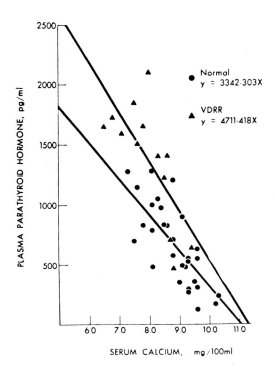

Figure 84-4. Linear regression lines (serum calcium versus immunoassayable parathyroid hormone) in normal subjects and in patients with vitamin-D-resistant rickets (VDRR) from data obtained during edetate (EDTA) infusion. Note that in VDRR a greater amount of parathyroid hormone was secreted per unit decrease in serum calcium than in normal subjects, a response attributed to hyperplastic parathyroid glands. (From R. E. Reitz and R. L. Weinstein, N. Engl. J. Med. 289:941, 1973.)

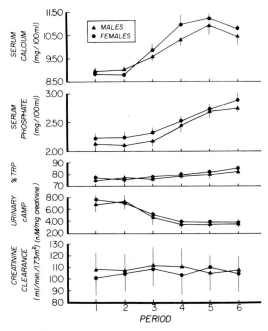

Figure 84-5. Response of patients with vitamin-D-resistant rickets to calcium infusion. Urine specimens were collected in 30-min periods with blood sampled at the midpoint of each period. Calcium, 10 mg per kilogram of ideal body weight, was infused from the end of period 2 to the end of period 4. Values represent the mean ± S.E. for 5 males and 9 females. Note the rise in serum phosphate and the increase in tubular resorption of phosphate (%TRP), which rose by 14 percent. (From T. J. Hahn et al., J. Clin. Endocrinol. Metab. 41:926, 1975.)

values in age-matched control subjects [77, 138]. Moreover, the observed above-normal iPTH response to a reduction in serum ionized calcium levels produced by infusion of edetate (EDTA) (Fig. 84-4) is also consistent with a state of increased parathyroid hormone secretion in VDRR [138]. Elevations in urinary cyclic AMP recorded in VDRR [9, 77] must be interpreted with caution and values compared with age-matched controls, since urinary cyclic AMP [182], like $TmPO_4$ [40], is age-related and is normally elevated in pediatric populations.

Although hypomagnesemia has been reported in VDRR [136], serum magnesium commonly is normal. Slight elevations in urinary amino acids, uroterpenol [68], Δ^4-3-ketosteroids [89], and glycosuria [104] also have been observed.

PATHOGENESIS

Having observed parathyroid hyperplasia in one patient with VDRR, Albright et al. originally proposed that patients with VDRR inherited either a basic defect in intestinal calcium transport or a blunted response to vitamin D [2]. They reasoned that the propensity to malabsorb calcium resulted in parathyroid overactivity, the latter leading to exaggerated phosphaturia and chronic hypophosphatemia. The skeletal lesions of rickets or osteomalacia were attributed to a persistently low Ca × P product. This hypothesis is consistent with subsequent reports of calcium malabsorption [95, 156, 164] and alterations in the morphology of the intestinal cell [125, 126], elevations in circulating iPTH [77, 138], the reversal of the phosphaturia during calcium infusion [59, 62] (Figs. 84-5, 84-6), and the development of parathyroid overactivity [138] and parathyroid adenomas [178] in patients with long-standing VDRR.

Earlier isotopic studies of vitamin D metabolism in VDRR revealed a delayed plasma disappearance of intravenously injected radioactive vitamin D_3, with decreased formation of lipid-soluble metabolites and increased formation of polar water-soluble metabolites [9, 47, 144]. These changes

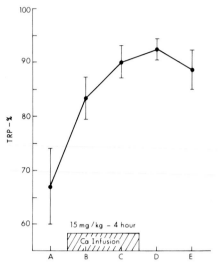

Figure 84-6. Effect of calcium infusion on the tubular resorption of phosphate (%TRP) in patients with vitamin-D-resistant rickets. Data reflect the mean ± S.E. Following a 4-hr control period (A), the percent TRP was measured for 2-hr clearance periods (B, C, D, and E); 15 mg calcium per kilogram of body weight was infused for 4 hr as indicated. (From H. M. Field and E. Reiss, J. Clin. Invest. 39:1807, 1960.)

were consistent with decreased conversion of vitamin D to one or more of its biologically active metabolites. Subsequently, it was demonstrated that circulating levels of 25-hydroxycholecalciferol (25-OHD) were normally maintained in patients with VDRR [76], with appropriate increases in 25-OHD following vitamin D administration. Recently, however, Haussler et al. have reported that serum $1,25(OH)_2D$ levels in untreated VDRR patients lie in the low normal range [80], a level inappropriate to the marked hypophosphatemia. This observation, although consistent with an abnormal 1-hydroxylase response to hypophosphatemia [80], must also be reconciled with others demonstrating paradoxical responses of 1-hydroxylase activity in normal males during phosphate deprivation when compared to females subjected to similar phosphate deprivation regimens [74]. The inappropriately low circulating $1,25(OH)_2D$ levels in patients with VDRR could result from a primary defect in the renal 1-hydroxylase enzyme system, accelerated degradation of $1,25(OH)_2D_3$, inhibition of renal 1-hydroxylase by circulating or cellular inhibitors, or derangements in renal intracellular and mitochondrial compartmentalization of calcium or phosphorus. This last possibility is presently the most intriguing, since it has been shown that mutant C57/Hyp hypophosphatemic

mice (a laboratory model for human VDRR) have normal renal cortical phosphate levels despite marked hypophosphatemia [58]. Therefore, in defense of the Albright theory [2] one could postulate that a relative deficiency (or production) of biologically active vitamin D metabolites could result in both calcium and phosphate malabsorption, secondary hyperparathyroidism, renal phosphate wasting, and hypophosphatemia. This hypothesis cannot be reconciled with other citations defining normal calcium and phosphate absorption [160] and normal circulating iPTH [7, 60] in patients with VDRR, others demonstrating a resistance to $1,25(OH)_2D$ treatment [22], nor with reports showing that the hypophosphatemia and phosphaturia persist following elective parathyroid surgery [146, 173].

In 1942 Robertson et al. proposed that the skeletal lesions and hypophosphatemia that characterize VDRR resulted from primary defects in intestinal and renal tubular phosphate transport systems [139]. Subsequently, transport defects isolated in patients with VDRR were shown to be limited to the intestine and kidney, with red cell [177] and salivary [77] phosphate transport systems apparently intact. The Robertson hypothesis is consistent with reports of defective phosphate absorption by patients with VDRR [38, 164] and by the C57/Hyp mouse model for VDRR [127], and of defective ^{32}P uptake by small-bowel mucosal biopsies obtained from hemizygous males and heterozygous females with VDRR [149]. In these latter experiments, Short et al. reported that normally two phosphate transport systems existed in the human jejunum, with either high or low affinities [149]. The high-affinity system was absent in VDRR subjects.

Consistent with the original Robertson hypothesis, Glorieux and Scriver [71] also reported that the renal tubular resorption of phosphate was mediated normally by two separate enzyme mechanisms, a PTH-sensitive system responsible for resorption of approximately two-thirds of the filtered phosphate load and a PTH-insensitive calcium-responsive system responsible for resorption of the remaining one-third. Based on observations of impaired phosphaturic response to a rapid (2-min) intravenous pulse dose of PTH in VDRR subjects, Glorieux and Scriver hypothesized that the PTH-sensitive transport system was defective [71]. This proposal is consistent with recent evidence for a PTH-independent calcium-modulated phosphate transport system along the rat nephron [5], and it may also explain earlier reports of increased tubular phosphate resorption when VDRR patients were subjected to calcium infusions [59, 62] (see Figs. 84-5, 84-6). The conclusion that phosphate excretion in VDRR is unaffected by increments in circulating PTH [71], however, must be reconciled with the observation that *prolonged* infusions of PTH in untreated patients with VDRR produces a normal to supranormal phosphaturic response in concert with a normal urinary adenosine 3′ : 5′-cyclic phosphate (cAMP) response [77, 150], even in the presence of hypercalcemia [150]. In this regard, the demonstration by Cuche et al. [43] that increments in plasma calcium actually potentiate the phosphaturic effect of PTH in the dog are worth noting.

These two apparently contradictory theories of Albright and Robertson may be reconciled if one assumes that there may be a slight initial impairment of the phosphaturic response to PTH due to impaired intracellular-transmembrane ion mobilization, to altered circulating levels of certain biologically active vitamin-D metabolites that condition or modify phosphate transport by the kidney, or to both. There may also be a defect in the PTH-independent phosphate resorptive mechanism in the proximal tubule with resultant increased phosphate delivery to the distal tubule, thereby magnifying the phosphaturic response to PTH-induced inhibition of distal tubular phosphate resorption sites. This latter hypothesis is consistent with the results of Puschett et al., who in evaluating the effects of 25-OHD_3 on urinary electrolyte excretion in VDRR concluded that proximal tubular function was faulty whereas distal transport pathways were intact [134]. It is also consistent with the observations of Cowgill et al., who showed defects in proximal and distal renal tubular phosphate transport in the mutant hypophosphatemic C57/Hyp mouse [41]. The fact that this phosphaturic, hypophosphatemic animal model for VDRR [58] also demonstrates a defect in intestinal phosphate transport [127] documented earlier in VDRR subjects [38, 164] lends additional support to this idea.

TREATMENT

The ideal response to vitamin D therapy of any rachitic or osteomalacic disorder is seen in patients with classic vitamin-D-lack rickets due to either nutritional inadequacy or poor exposure to sunlight. In treatment of simple D-lack rickets, serum calcium, phosphorus, alkaline phosphatase, and PTH return to values that are normal for the age of the patient; the skeletal lesions heal completely; and, in children, skeletal maturity and growth rate are once again normalized. This response is to be contrasted with the effect of vitamin D therapy on children with VDRR, which is characterized by healing of the rachitic lesions and a decrease in circulating alkaline phosphatase. The hypophosphatemia and growth retardation are relatively unaffected, even during long-term therapy with doses as high as 500,000 IU per day [112, 189, 191]. The dose of vitamin D required to produce increments in intestinal absorption of calcium and phosphate and ultimate healing of the skeletal lesions is usually inappropriately large [193], ranging between 50,000 and 250,000 IU per day [189, 191]. Not infrequently, the rachitic VDRR child treated only with high-dose vitamin D regimens that fail to correct the hypophosphatemia (i.e., serum phosphorus <3.0 mg per deciliter) is healed at the expense of short stature and skeletal deformities [165, 112]. The need for careful monitoring of serum and urinary calcium must be emphasized, since long-term high-dose vitamin D therapy may result in hypercalcemic crises, hypercalciuria, and nephrocalcinosis [131]. Although it has been assumed that an increase in the serum calcium level above the upper limit of normal provides a reliable sign of vitamin intoxication [131], it would be appropriate to monitor calcium excretion as well, since prolonged hypercalciuria (i.e., 24-hr urinary calcium greater than 4 mg per kilogram body weight) should be avoided. Moreover, in many instances hypercalciuria actually antedates the hypercalcemia in VDRR subjects on high-dose vitamin D regimens.

Although the ideal therapeutic dose of vitamin D is difficult to establish, the concomitant administration of oral phosphate supplements in doses of 1 to 4 gm per day results in more rapid healing of the skeletal lesions, amelioration of the hypophosphatemia, and an acceleration of growth not attainable when vitamin D is administered alone [72, 112, 114, 176, 187] (see Fig. 84-1). The recommended phosphate preparation for children with VDRR consists of dibasic sodium phosphate, 13 gm per volume; phosphoric acid (N.F. 85%), 58.5 gm per volume; and 1 liter of water. One milliliter of this solution provides 30 mg of elemental phosphorus. Treatment is usually initiated with 5-ml doses, with stepwise increments in multiples of 5 until an average intake of 15 ml every 4 hr, five times daily, is achieved [72]. When phosphate is added to the therapeutic regimen, the rachitic skeletal lesions heal with vitamin D doses of 25,000 to 75,000 IU daily, a range that rarely proves toxic [176, 187]. The main disadvantages of the phosphate therapy are the frequency (5 to 6 doses per day) with which the medication must be administered (Fig. 84-7) and the diarrhea that usually attends the first 1 to 2 weeks of therapy. These potential complications *should not preclude*

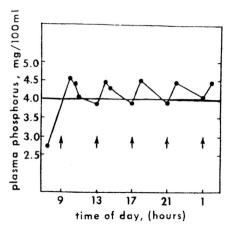

Figure 84-7. Effect of repeated oral dosing with phosphate on plasma phosphorus concentration in the patient with vitamin-D-resistant rickets. During the day 750 mg of elemental phosphorus was administered, as indicated by the arrows. (From F. Glorieux et al., N. Engl. J. Med. 287:481, 1972.)

attempts to initiate phosphate therapy in growing children with VDRR with emphasis on maintaining circulating phosphate levels >3.0 mg per deciliter (Fig. 84-7). It should be emphasized that the administration of phosphate alone cannot heal or prevent the recurrence of rickets [165], so that vitamin D therapy must be continued, albeit at lower dose schedules. During the initial stages of either vitamin D or phosphate therapy or a combination thereof, urinary total hydroxyproline and serum alkaline phosphatase increase. This seemingly paradoxical response to potentially therapeutic agents is only temporary and is actually associated with and followed by clinical, biochemical, and radiologic healing [57, 154].

Some patients with VDRR also present with mild glycosuria, a decrease in the tubular maximum resorption of glucose [15, 104], and a further decrease in the maximal tubular resorption of phosphate following oral glucose loading. High carbohydrate feeding should be avoided in these patients, since the induced phosphaturia often renders the hypophosphatemia more resistant to phosphate supplementation.

Earlier reports of potential alterations of vitamin D metabolism in VDRR have prompted a variety of short-term and long-term clinical trials with 25-OHD$_3$ and 1,25-dihydroxycholecalciferol (1,25[OH]$_2$D$_3$). Despite isolated salutary reports of skeletal healing, increased calcium absorption, decreased phosphate clearance, and reversal of the hypophosphatemia during 25-OHD$_3$ therapy in doses of 4,000 to 5,000 units per day [129, 147], it is now generally assumed that the results

of 25-OHD$_3$ do not differ qualitatively from the effects of treatment with pharmacologic doses of vitamin D$_2$ or vitamin D$_3$ [13, 35, 56]. In either instance, the hypophosphatemia rarely is corrected by 25-OHD$_3$ treatment alone. When available for routine commercial use, however, 25-OHD$_3$ may prove to be the vitamin D drug of choice, since therapeutic blood levels of 25-OHD$_3$ are not only achieved more rapidly with this substance than with the vitamin D$_3$ parent compound but they also decrease more rapidly when the drug is discontinued, as may be necessitated by marked hypercalciuria or hypercalcemia. Therapeutic attempts with 1,25(OH)$_2$D$_3$ have also resulted in less than adequate responses in VDRR patients, since despite improvements in calcium absorption, serum phosphate and phosphate clearance are unaffected [22, 143].

In the past, once the active rickets was controlled, surgery was usually considered appropriate for correction of the severe leg deformities. Operative intervention necessitating immobilization before radiographic and biochemical evidence of skeletal healing was achieved was frequently unsuccessful, and deformities recurred [174]. Moreover, spasmodic or inadequate therapy also resulted in recurrence of the deformities, although leg abnormalities that were surgically corrected in patients older than 12 years did not tend to recur [174]. Since the incidence of leg deformities and short stature should be considerably reduced if VDRR is diagnosed early in childhood and phosphate is added to vitamin D therapeutic regimens, the need for ultimate corrective surgical intervention would be minimized. If surgery necessitating strict immobilization is ultimately required, vitamin D and phosphorus supplementation should be drastically reduced until an active mobilization program is reinstituted.

Pseudovitamin-D-Deficiency Rickets

Pseudovitamin-D-deficiency rickets (PDR), also called vitamin-D-dependent rickets, hereditary pseudovitamin-D-deficiency rickets, or pseudodeficiency rickets, is often mistakenly confused with VDRR. Pseudovitamin-D-deficiency rickets, inherited as a simple autosomal recessive trait, is characterized by signs and symptoms usually appearing in the first year of life that may mimic those seen in simple nutritional vitamin D deficiency. The rachitic skeletal lesions are similar to those of VDRR, but convulsions and severe muscular weakness, notably absent in VDRR, are characteristic. Biochemically, PDR is characterized by hypocalcemia, mild hypophosphatemia (in some cases the serum phosphate is actually normal), marked elevations in alkaline phosphatase, a metabolic renal tubular acidosis, and generalized aminoaciduria [21, 66, 145, 146, 167]. Circulating levels of iPTH are usually elevated, although normal values have been reported in a pedigree with PDR and relative hypoparathyroidism [170]. Whereas controversy still exists regarding the malabsorption of calcium in VDRR, calcium malabsorption is the rule in PDR. The term *dependency* arises from the observation that the skeletal and biochemical derangements in PDR respond dramatically to vitamin D in doses that are 100 times the normal daily requirement. Unlike VDRR, in which phosphorus supplementation is mandatory for normal growth and skeletal maturation and normalization of circulating phosphate, vitamin D *alone* is therapeutic for children with PDR.

In contrast to the VDRR syndrome, which has been attributed (either directly or indirectly) to renal and intestinal phosphate transport defects independent of vitamin D, the pathogenesis of PDR has been ascribed to defective or absent 1-hydroxylation of 25-OHD to 1,25(OH)$_2$D [66, 145, 146]. This in turn supposedly results in decreased calcium absorption, hypocalcemia, and enhanced release of parathyroid hormone. The associated mild renal tubular acidosis, aminoaciduria, phosphaturia, and elevations in urinary cyclic AMP are all assumed to represent the normal renal tubular response to high circulating parathyroid hormone levels. As such, PDR may be considered a mendelian trait affecting the bioactivation of vitamin D. The fact that the requirement for vitamin D is permanently 100 times greater than normal and that patients also respond to 25-OHD$_3$ is also considered consistent with the hypothesis that PDR represents a "leaky" mutant in which high concentrations of 25-OHD$_3$ are necessary for either its uptake by the molecular enzyme complement in the renal tubule or its ultimate conversion to 1,25(OH)$_2$D$_3$ [66, 145, 146]. It should be noted, however, that levels of 25-OHD in the serum of some patients with PDR are three to seven times greater than normal and reportedly insufficient to correct the hypocalcemia and skeletal lesions [146].

Healing of the rachitic lesions and reversal of the biochemical defects of PDR have been observed with physiologic (1 μg per day) doses of 1,25(OH)$_2$D$_3$ [66] (Fig. 84-8) or the synthetic analogue 1α-hydroxycholecalciferol [135]. This therapeutic response is consistent with the hypothesis that PDR (unlike VDRR) is due to a specific inborn error of vitamin D metabolism caused by a recessively inherited defect in the renal enzyme, 25-hydroxycholecalciferol 1-hydroxylase [66, 146]. More definitive confirmation and direct evidence

of 1-hydroxylase deficiency in PDR is essential before this assumption can be accepted, however, since long-term administration of either 1,25(OH)$_2$D or 1α-hydroxyvitamin D$_3$ in doses that are therapeutic for patients with simple nutritional rickets (0.5 μg per day) have limited biologic effectiveness in patients with PDR [14]. Thus, a simple 1-hydroxylase deficiency may not account for all the biochemical and skeletal changes in PDR. Moreover, Rosen and Finberg [142], noting that some patients with PDR respond to dihydrotachysterol (a synthetic preparation that, after hydroxylation at position 25 in the liver, mimics the biologic action of 1,25(OH)$_2$D$_3$ without additional renal 1-hydroxylation), postulated that the metabolic block in PDR may be differential and variable, involving both the 25- and 1-hydroxylating enzyme systems.

Hypoparathyroidism

Hypoparathyroidism may be defined as a failure of the parathyroid glands to sustain a normal plasma ionized calcium, either naturally or when deliberate efforts are made to reduce it. Common disorders relating to parathyroid insufficiency fall into three general categories: (1) postsurgical (thyroidectomy) hypoparathyroidism; (2) idiopathic hypoparathyroidism; and (3) pseudohypoparathyroidism. Transient hypoparathyroidism may also be observed in an infant delivered by a mother with hyperparathyroidism, presumably because calcium crosses the placenta readily and suppresses fetal parathyroid activity. Despite varied etiologies for each of these syndromes, they share common abnormalities in circulating calcium and inorganic phosphorus concentrations, namely, hypocalcemia and hyperphosphatemia, and the attendant predisposition to neuromuscular irritability and tetany. The hypocalcemia and hyperphosphatemia are manifestations of the loss of parathyroid regulation of the equilibrium between extracellular and bone calcium and the tubular resorption of phosphorus. Although postsurgical and neonatal transient hypoparathyroid states still remain the most common cause of hypoparathyroidism [83, 115], this review is directed primarily to the familial or genetically determined forms of hypoparathyroidism.

DIAGNOSTIC CRITERIA

The generally accepted criteria for the diagnosis of familial or idiopathic hypoparathyroidism (IHP) are (1) a low serum calcium and high serum inorganic phosphorus; (2) absence of renal insufficiency, steatorrhea, and alkalosis; (3) no x-ray evidence of rickets or osteomalacia; (4) chronic

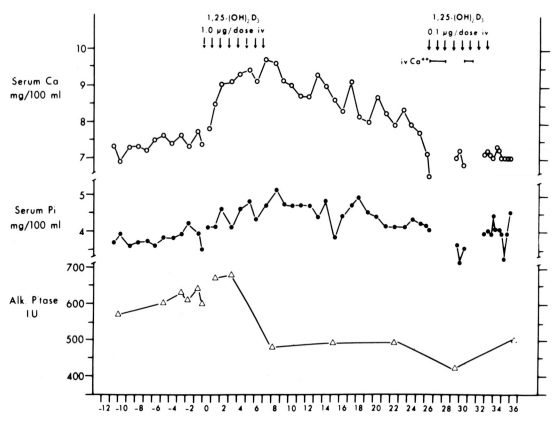

Figure 84-8. Serum calcium (Ca) and inorganic phosphorus (P$_i$) concentrations and alkaline phosphatase activity in a case of pseudo-vitamin-D-deficiency rickets (PDR) treated with 1,25(OH)$_2$D$_3$ in doses of 1.0 and 0.1 μg per day. (From D. Fraser et al., N. Engl. J. Med. *289:817, 1973.)*

tetany or its equivalent (neuromuscular irritability with paresthesias); (5) a significant phosphate diuresis following the injection of parathyroid hormone; and (6) absence of physical characteristics of pseudohypoparathyroidism, brachydactylia, dwarfing, or subcutaneous calcium deposition [163].

Infantile familial hypoparathyroidism was first reported in 1957 in three male siblings who presented with neonatal tetany [26]. Recent observations suggest that most cases of early onset IHP may be inherited as a sex-linked recessive trait [132, 163]. A distinction has been drawn between this early-onset sex-linked variety of IHP and a type of later onset that is not sex-linked. This later form is divided further clinically into familial and apparently nonfamilial varieties; each of these is again subdivided into those that are associated with Addison's disease and those that are not. The portion of the late-onset group that is genetically determined is at present uncertain. Because of the many clinical factors common to both IHP and pseudohypoparathyroidism (see later), a distinction between these syndromes on clinical and chemical [130] grounds is often impossible [19]. The association with hypoparathyroidism of moniliasis or hypoadrenalism or both favors a diagnosis of IHP, since both have been reported to complicate IHP [19] and neither has as yet been identified in patients with pseudohypoparathyroidism (Table 84-1).

In children with IHP, abnormal body growth, malformed and brittle nails, poor dentition, and thin, dry hair may often be quite striking. Roentgen examination of the skeleton in IHP is usually negative, although at times the density of bones appears increased or decreased. The serum alkaline phosphatase is characteristically normal, unlike that in children with familial hyperphosphatasia, who may also present with mental retardation and seizures [103]. Idiopathic hypoparathyroidism has also been associated with intestinal malabsorption, steatorrhea [101], and osteomalacia. The mechanism by which parathyroid deficiency might cause intestinal dysfunction and malabsorption is presently unknown. Although the relationship of gut motility to absorption is unclear, it seems conceivable that abnormalities in neuromuscular acti-

Table 84-1. Comparison of Characteristics in Idiopathic Hypoparathyroidism (IHP), Pseudohypoparathyroidism (PHP), and Pseudo-pseudohypoparathyrodism (PPHP)

Clinical Features	IHP	PHP	PPHP
Abnormalities in serum Ca and P	+	+	−
Tetany	+	+	−
Cataracts	+	+	(+)[a]
Brachydactylia	−	+	+
Round face, short stature	−	+	+
Seizures	+	+	−
Dystrophic ectopic calcification	+	+	+
Ectodermal abnormalities (skin, nails)	+	−	−
Basal ganglia calcification	+	+	−
Dental abnormalities	+	+	(+)[a]
Familial occurrence	(+)[a]	+	+
Mental retardation	+	+	+
Hypoadrenalism	(+)[a]	−	−
Gonadal dysgenesis	(−)[b]	(+)[a]	(+)[a]
Exostoses	−	+	(+)[a]
Moniliasis	+	−	−
Hypothyroidism	−	(+)[a]	(+)[a]

[a] Observed in some cases.

[b] Observed as "primary ovarian failure" in a patient without chromosomal or chromatin studies who has "irregularly spaced menstrual periods" [73].

vation of the bowel, as well as the trophic effect of chronic hypocalcemia on the gastrointestinal epithelium, could adversely affect motility and absorption.

PATHOGENESIS

The cause of IHP and its incidence as compared to pseudohypoparathyroidism are unknown. Over a third of patients with IHP have antibodies to parathyroid tissue, and 19 percent have antibodies to adrenal tissue [73, 158]. Circulating antibodies to adrenal cortex have also been demonstrated in 50 percent of patients with nontuberculous Addison's disease and parathyroid antibodies in 25 percent. These observations, combined with the more than fortuitous association of hypoadrenalism with IHP, collectively suggest that IHP represents part of a spectrum of autoimmune endocrine disorders. Since there is evidence that plasma antibodies to endocrine tissue are not cytotoxic [158], however, the role of parathyroid antibodies in the pathogenesis of IHP is still conjectural.

Pseudohypoparathyroidism

Pseudohypoparathyroidism (PHP) was originally defined as a syndrome with the chemical (hypo-calcemia and hyperphosphatemia) and clinical features of IHP, but differing from IHP by an end-organ resistance to parathyroid hormone, subcutaneous foci of ectopic calcification, and typical somatic features characterized by round facies, brachydactylia (Figs. 84-9, 84-10), and short, thick stature [105]. Subsequently, this syndrome has been identified with increasing frequency, and

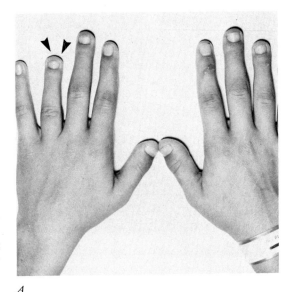

A

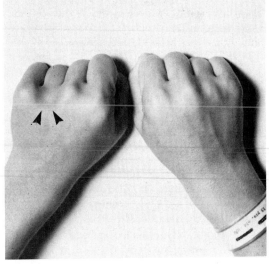

B

Figure 84-9. A. Brachydactylia (arrows) due to shortening of the left fourth metacarpal in a patient with pseudohypoparathyroidism. B. Empty knuckle sign in patient illustrated in A when fists are clenched (arrows) as a result of metacarpal shortening.

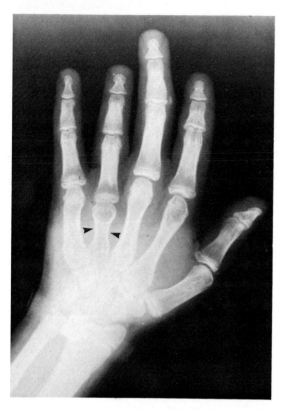

Figure 84-10. Radiographic presentation of pseudo-hypoparathyroidism. Note the shortening of the fourth metacarpal (arrows).

Table 84-2. The Ellsworth-Howard Test in Normal Subjects and in Patients with Idiopathic Hypoparathyroidism (IHP) and Pseudohypoparathyroidism (PHP)

Subjects	No. Studied	Urinary Phosphate (mg/hr)[a]		
		Control	Maximum Increment After PTE[b]	Percent Increase
Normal subjects	19	22 (4–53)	50 (19–89)	230 (90–1,150)
IHP	26	18 (5–42)	78 (23–209)	450 (120–1,320)
PHP	19	18 (3–50)	16 (2–43)	90 (20–350)

[a] Average, range in parentheses.
[b] Commercial parathyroid extract (Eli Lilly and Company).

Source: From D. Bronsky et al., *Medicine* 37:317, 1958 [25].

its variable clinical expression as well as its relationships to other genetic disorders such as pseudopseudohypoparathyroidism, Turner syndrome, basal cell nevi, and hypothyroidism have been defined [33, 116, 121, 180, 190].

PATHOGENESIS

The unresponsiveness to parathyroid hormone was initially inferred from observations which revealed that patients with PHP, unlike normal or hypoparathyroid (posthyroidectomy or IHP) subjects, failed to show a phosphorus diuresis after the parenteral administration of commercially prepared parathyroid extract (Ellsworth-Howard test) (Table 84-2) [5]. Since histologic examinations revealed either normal or hyperplastic parathyroid glands in PHP, this resistance had been alternately ascribed to alterations in the chemical structure of the hormone, rendering it biologically impotent, or to an intrinsic cellular defect leading to end-organ refractoriness.

It was noted later that the resistance to parathyroid extract need not be complete in all cases of PHP (see Table 84-2), since a twofold increase in urinary phosphorus following parathyroid hor-

mone injection was observed in some patients, while normal and hypoparathyroid subjects showed an increase of 2½ to 4 times, respectively. The Ellsworth-Howard test was the procedure most frequently used in the past to determine renal responsiveness to parathyroid extract. Results obtained with this procedure have often been misleading, due primarily to the use of nonstandardized commercial extract preparations, an inconstant variable effect of commercially prepared extract upon the glomerular filtration rate (which may affect phosphate excretion independently of tubular mechanisms), and the inconsistent response of normal individuals to potent parathyroid extract. In addition, some patients with PHP may respond initially to a single intravenous dose of parathyroid extract but demonstrate a resistance to the extract administered over a period of days. For these and related reasons, it has been suggested that the failure of the serum calcium concentration to increase following parathyroid hormone be substituted for the absence of phosphaturia in diagnosing PHP. Since elevations of serum calcium following parathyroid hormone injection are consistently noted in normal or hypoparathyroid subjects, and hypercalcemic responses to parathyroid hormone have been observed in individuals with the classic PHP syndrome, serum calcium determination is of limited value in the differentiation of IHP and PHP.

Despite these obvious limitations in tests designed to measure the phosphaturic and hypercalcemic effects of commercially prepared parathyroid extracts, reportedly normal responses to these tests in the past cast some doubt on Albright's original hypothesis that the defect in PHP is an end-organ refractoriness to parathyroid hormone. Moreover, the histologic and roentgenographic documentation of osteitis fibrosa and increased circulatory alkaline phosphatase activity in patients with PHP [18, 36, 90, 128, 151, 192] and the observed hypercalcemia following parathyroid hormone administration to some patients with PHP suggest that if an end-organ refractoriness to parathyroid hormone does in fact exist in this disorder, it may be limited to the renal tubule.

In view of these observations, alternative hypotheses have been proposed to account for the hypocalcemia and hyperphosphatemia of PHP. These include the presence of a circulating and tissue hormone-inhibitor substance and the excessive secretion of calcitonin, a potent hypocalcemia polypeptide secreted by the parafollicular cells of the thyroid gland. This latter speculation seemed to be strengthened by the demonstration that the thyroid glands of affected individuals contained 50 to 100 times the normal amount of calcitonin [3, 175] and by the temporary improvement in the serum calcium levels and the restoration of the phosphaturic effects of parathyroid hormone following thyroid ablation in a patient with PHP [109]. More recent definitive studies are more compatible with the hypothesis that elevated gland concentrations of calcitonin reflect suppression of secretion and that calcitonin is neither the cause of the hypocalcemia in PHP nor the cause of the refractoriness to parathyroid hormone [97, 172].

Parathyroid hormone, measured by radioimmunoassay in peripheral venous plasma, has been reported to be elevated in patients with PHP [97]; circulating antibodies to the C-terminal portion of the parathyroid hormone molecule have also been identified in a patient with this disorder [153]. In addition, it has been shown that purified parathyroid hormone preparations activate renal adenyl cyclase, thereby causing a marked increase in the urinary excretion of the cyclic nucleotide, $3':5'$ cAMP [30, 31, 113, 169]. Studies in normal subjects and in patients with PHP and IHP reveal that, in contrast to the gross overlap of results with measurements of phosphate clearance, parathyroid hormone induces rapid and large increments in cAMP in normal and IHP subjects, whereas the response is minimal in patients with PHP [32] (Fig. 84-11), an effect not due to a defect in parathyroid hormone metabolism [123].

These early results supported the hypothesis that the metabolic defect in PHP stemmed from a lack of or defective forms of adenylate cyclase in bone and kidney. Observations of Bell et al. [17] that dibutyryl cyclic AMP infusions increased the serum calcium, lowered the serum phosphate, and increased urinary phosphorus excretion in patients with PHP were confirmatory in this regard. The *absent adenyl cyclase* theory has been challenged, however, by at least two additional observations. In vitro adenyl cyclase studies in a kidney obtained from a patient with somatic characteristics of PHP revealed normal activation of the enzyme by parathyroid hormone and fluoride [106]. Moreover, a subgroup of patients with the somatic characteristics of PHP, hypocalcemia, and elevated levels of parathyroid hormone respond to parathyroid hormone administration with an increase in urinary cyclic AMP but no phosphaturia [53, 140]. Patients with this syndrome, or PHP *type II,* are also incapable of generating a phosphaturic response to acetazolamide (Diamox), unlike patients with the classic form of PHP, who respond to acetazolamide with a modest phosphaturia that is not mediated by cyclic AMP [152]. These observations collectively suggest that in PHP type II, the defect in phosphate excretion is located at a transport site that is unrelated to cyclic AMP generation, and they are reminiscent of the results obtained by Knox et al. in the hamster [88].

Presently, the relation between the classic form of PHP and the type II variety is still unknown. Although the hypocalcemia has been attributed to a blunted skeletal response to parathyroid hormone [20, 110], certain patients with PHP develop skeletal changes of osteitis similar to those seen in primary hyperparathyroidism [65, 90], and elevations in circulating alkaline phosphatase [36]. The skeletal response to parathyroid hormone in patients with this syndrome can also be enhanced by prior vitamin D therapy [171]. Moreover, parathyroidectomy in PHP results in a further decrease in the serum calcium [133], an observation inconsistent with complete skeletal resistance to parathyroid hormone. The hypocalcemia may result in part from decreased calcium absorption as a result of defective $1,25(OH)_2D$ synthesis [18, 122] or from a defect in renal conservation [120]. The hypothesis that invokes comparable inherited defects in renal and osseous tissue in subjects with PHP is still quite tenuous. Since it appears that a single type of interaction between parathyroid hormone and the adenyl cyclase bound to the cell membrane can account for the action of parathyroid hormones in bone as well as kidney [30, 31], PHP may represent a syndrome wherein an alteration in the responsiveness of one end-organ (kidney) to a hormone is impaired as a result of genetic or other factors without there necessarily being impaired responsiveness of another end-organ (bone) to the same

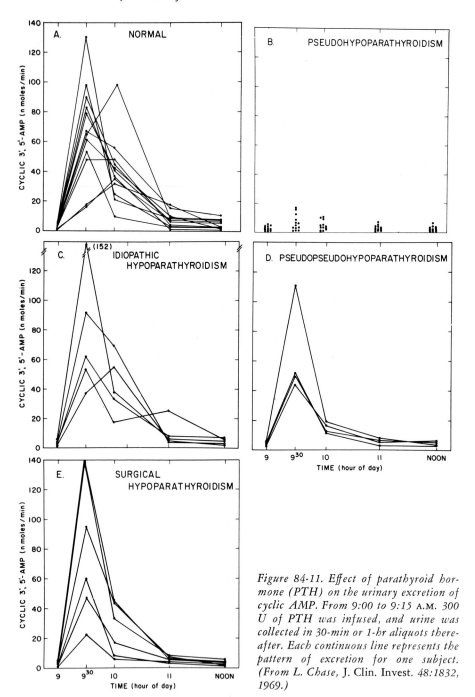

Figure 84-11. Effect of parathyroid hormone (PTH) on the urinary excretion of cyclic AMP. From 9:00 to 9:15 A.M. 300 U of PTH was infused, and urine was collected in 30-min or 1-hr aliquots thereafter. Each continuous line represents the pattern of excretion for one subject. (From L. Chase, J. Clin. Invest. 48:1832, 1969.)

hormone. Obviously, more definitive studies are needed to verify this hypothesis, including those directed toward measurements of adenyl cyclase and cAMP in the bone of PHP subjects before and after stimulation with parathyroid hormone.

DIFFERENTIAL DIAGNOSIS

As noted previously, the clinical and symptomatic features of PHP are quite similar to those of IHP

and stem from the attendant hypocalcemia and hyperphosphatemia *common* to both disorders (see Table 84-1). There are, however, specific differences that characterize these two forms of hypoparathyroidism, other than the apparent refractoriness of PHP subjects to parathyroid hormone. Idiopathic hypoparathyroidism is inherited as a sex-linked recessive trait [132], whereas X-linked dominant inheritance has been postulated for PHP

[105]. Reports of apparent male-to-male transmission suggest that an autosomal inheritance pattern may also obtain [132]. In IHP an equal distribution of the sexes is the rule, and the average age of onset is 15 to 17 years, with individual cases ranging from any age to the fifth decade [24]. In contrast, in PHP the females outnumber males 2 to 1, the average age of onset is 8 years, and the disease is invariably recognized before the second decade [19, 105]. Characteristic roentgenographic and clinical findings in PHP include disproportionate, uniform shortening of the metacarpal and metatarsal bones (brachydactylia) (see Figs. 84-9, 84-10); bilateral calcification of the basal ganglia, cerebellum, and dentate nuclei; soft-tissue (joints and extremities) calcification; cataracts, thickening of the calvarium and widening of the diploic space; osteitis fibrosa; delayed tooth eruption; and impaired dentine formation with blunting of the roots of the molar teeth [162]. Pseudohypoparathyroidism may be a difficult diagnosis to establish clinically in early childhood, since the brachydactylia is usually not evident for the first 4 to 5 years of life [118]. With the exception of the dental abnormalities, basal ganglia calcification, and cataract formation, the x-ray and clinical findings of PHP patients are rarely seen in patients with IHP, who more commonly exhibit dystrophic ectodermal changes limited to the skin, hair, and nails; alopecia; dermatitides and associated secondary *Candida* infections. Whereas hypoadrenalism is frequently seen in patients with IHP, hypothyroidism has often been noted to be associated with PHP [105, 190, 194]. The defect appears to result from a selective deficiency of thyrotropin (TSH) rather than from resistance to thyroid hormone or primary thyroid failure. It is of interest in this regard (see later) that in patients with ovarian dysgenesis (Turner syndrome), who share many features with PHP (obesity, round facies, brachydactylia, short stature, and resistance to parathyroid hormone), the incidence of hypothyroidism is also high. The somatic alterations and growth retardation seen in patients with PHP are still unexplained. Since neither growth hormone nor sulfation factor deficiency exist in PHP, the short stature has been ascribed to end-organ refractoriness to these hormones [179].

Chorea, dystonia, paralysis agitans, and transient hemisensory and hemimotor disturbances have all been reported to accompany calcification of the basal ganglia in both IHP and PHP. The calcification appears to be correlated with the duration of the hypocalcemia. The cataracts seen in both IHP and PHP are usually bilateral and lamellar, involving the subcapsular areas of the lens cortex. Cataract formation has also been attributed to the prolonged hypocalcemia characteristic of IHP and PHP. That cataract formation in PHP may be due to a genetic defect independent of the hypoparathyroid state is suggested by the presence of cataract formation in patients with pseudopseudohypoparathyroidism, despite consistently normal serum calcium levels [105].

Decreased serum calcium in both IHP and PHP also results in increased neuromuscular irritability and tetany [64]. The suppression of tetanic manifestations by concomitant hypokalemia should also always be kept in mind when evaluating hypocalcemia. Tetany associated with hypocalcemia and hypomagnesemia may not respond to calcium initially but will respond promptly to magnesium [34, 67]. Thus, hypomagnesemia should be considered as a cause of convulsions when hypocalcemic tetany fails to respond to adequate intravenous injections of calcium. Since clinical manifestations of hypomagnesemia are characterized principally by neuromuscular and CNS hyperirritability and are quite distinguishable from those of hypocalcemia, simultaneous measurements of serum calcium and magnesium should be mandatory in patients with overt tetany.

The increased neural excitability in both IHP and PHP also results in seizures and EEG abnormalities, which include a paucity of alpha rhythm, increased fast activity, sporadic spike activity, and slow waves (6 to 7 per second) with frontal preponderance [51]. In general, the abnormal EEG pattern will disappear following calcium infusions, but, since chronic hypocalcemia may also induce organic brain deterioration, calcium infusion may prove ineffective in this regard. The mechanism causing these EEG abnormalities is still unknown despite the well-known influence of relatively small variations of calcium (and magnesium) concentrations on brain function cited earlier.

The hypocalcemia of IHP and PHP is also believed to result in increased intracranial pressure. On occasion, convulsions or unilateral neurologic manifestations may be accompanied by papilledema, stimulating an expanding intracranial mass. Occasionally, patients with IHP or PHP may show cardiac arrhythmias [85], prolongation of the Q–T interval of the electrocardiogram, nausea, vomiting, and abdominal pain. The gastrointestinal symptoms may be related in part to the effect of the hypocalcemia on the symptomatic ganglia of the gastrointestinal tract, since the response to different stimuli may be increased in hypocalcemic states and the efferent discharge may be increased in the presence of a constant amount of perfusing acetylcholine. In addition, reported gustatory and olfactory abnormalities in PHP suggest an additional "sensory end-organ abnormality" [81].

In a recent review of 267 cases of hypoparathyroidism with hypocalcemia, an associated psychiatric disorder was unclassified in 54.5 percent of cases; organic brain syndrome was seen in 36.5 percent, mental subnormality in 7.1 percent, and functional psychoses in 1.9 percent [48]. Irritability, emotional lability, impairment of memory, and delusions and hallucinations have also been described, as has a specific association between depression and hypocalcemia.

The impaired mental functioning of IHP and PHP patients appears to be a combination of disordered motor coordination and memory [117]. The causal relation of the mental infirmity to repeated seizures during the development period seems inappropriate, since in patients (children) with other convulsive disorders, mental retardation, if present, is seldom a direct result of the convulsions. It cannot be excluded, however, that the mental retardation and the adverse reaction of the brain results directly from the chronic hypocalcemia and associated calcium deprivation of the central nervous system in view of the evidence that both the EEG and intellectual function in these patients may respond favorably to elevations in serum calcium [117]. Whether all the symptoms are reversible by therapy directed to elevating the serum calcium appears to depend on the age of onset. There seems to be a critical natal or neonatal period in which calcium deficiency may permanently impair brain function. If onset occurs subsequent to this crucial developmental period, the abnormal mental and neurologic effects of hypocalcemia are usually reversible.

THERAPY

Standard therapy for either IHP or PHP consists of one of the vitamin D preparations (i.e., vitamins D_2 or D_3), with or without additional calcium supplementation [10]. In the past the most commonly prescribed vitamin D preparation has been calciferol (vitamin D_2), with doses ranging from 0.225 to 19.0 mg per day. In a review of the calciferol requirements of patients with hypoparathyroidism, the mean controlling dose was 2.12 mg per day [84]. No patient was controlled (asymptomatic) on less than 1.25 mg per day, and every patient receiving doses greater than 2.50 mg per day became hypercalcemic. In these subjects the documented periods of hypercalcemia lasted 1 to 6 weeks after withdrawal of the calciferol. Recent publications have provided information on the effective dose range of another therapeutic agent, crystalline dihydrotachysterol (AT-10), with emphasis on the relative potency of this preparation in comparison to calciferol and older impotent AT-10 preparations [79].

Despite occasional reports of resistance to either calciferol or dihydrotachysterol therapy, most patients with hypoparathyroidism respond quite favorably [10]. It should be emphasized, however, that vitamin D or dihydrotachysterol may induce a significant hypercalciuria *before any reversal of the hypocalcemia is evident* [100]. Thus, one cannot rely on Sulkowitch testing for urinary calcium as a measure of serum calcium; neither can a positive result with the urinary Sulkowitch test be relied on for the early detection of overdosage with vitamin D or dihydrotachysterol. Finally, since symptomatic thresholds to hypocalcemia may vary and low blood calcium levels are tolerated quite well by some patients with chronic hypoparathyroidism, the absence of tetany or neuromuscular irritability is not a reliable indicator of the level of circulating calcium [10].

The persistent hyperphosphatemia that characterizes both IHP and PHP and the reported low circulating levels of $1,25(OH)_2D_3$ in PHP [54] have led to the suggestion that an impaired conversion of 25-OHD to $1,25(OH)_2D$ exists in both disorders [91, 152]. Isolated reports of prolactin deficiency in PHP [28] are also consistent with defective renal 1-hydroxylase activity. As a result, patients with either IHP or PHP have been successfully treated with $1,25(OH)_2D_3$ or its synthetic analogue, 1α-hydroxycholecalciferol, responding with a rise in serum calcium and an increase in calcium absorption [44, 91, 108, 122, 152, 186]. Although this form of substitution therapy may ultimately prove to be the treatment of choice, more definitive studies over prolonged intervals are necessary before it can be routinely accepted as such. Since in the human, vitamin D metabolites are not required for the renal action of parathyroid hormone [69], the phosphaturic response of patients to $1,25(OH)_2D_3$ therapy most probably stems from the correction of the hypocalcemia [122]. Recently, restoration of the renal responsiveness to parathyroid hormone has also been achieved in type II PHP by simply restoring the serum calcium to normal without benefit of vitamin D therapy [140].

Pseudo-pseudohypoparathyroidism

The term *pseudo-pseudohypoparathyroidism* (PPHP), a clinical entity unrelated to parathyroid dysfunction, was initially proposed to describe a disorder with the clinical anomalies of PHP but associated with normal serum calcium and phosphorus levels [1]. Pseudo-pseudohypoparathyroidism actually denotes a set of congenital abnormalities that bear no relationship to the parathyroid gland; in PPHP there is normal serum calcium and phosphate and a normal urinary cyclic AMP response to parathyroid hormone (see Fig. 84-11). Consequently, alternative names have been proposed for the syndrome, including Albright's hereditary osteodystrophy, dyschondroplasia with soft-tissue calcifications and ossification and normal parathyroid function, and brachymetacarpal dwarfism. In the past PPHP has also been identified with a group of disorders that includes hereditary multiple exostosis, familial brachydactylia, myositis ossificans progressiva, multiple epiphyseal dysplasia, familial calcification of the basal ganglia, and the Turner syndrome [121, 180]. The relationship between PHP and PPHP has been confusing, to say the least, since the conditions appear to comprise a spectrum of similar congenital defects, the basic etiology of which is as yet unknown (see Table 84-1). Since hypocalcemia is often a transient feature of PHP [61], some authors consider PHP and PPHP as variants of the same disease process. Reported inheritance of PHP from parents with PPHP and of PPHP from parents with PHP also supports the contention that PPHP is a forme fruste of PHP [23, 83, 116]. Mounting evidence to date seems, therefore, to indicate that PPHP is simply an incompletely expressed form of a genetically determined disorder, of which PHP and its attendant hypocalcemia represents the complete clinical syndrome. That PPHP may represent one end of the spectrum of the incompletely expressed form of PHP is suggested by the recent reports of patients without physical anomalies but with the biochemical changes of hypoparathyroidism and radiologic changes of hyperparathyroidism [4, 185]. This syndrome of hypo-hyperparathyroidism may ultimately prove to be another variant of PHP.

Despite the tendency to regard PPHP and PHP as the expression of a single genetically determined disorder, genetic confrontation to date is inconclusive. Extensive pedigree analyses reveal an autosomal dominant inheritance in which females are afflicted more frequently than males and in which male-to-male transmission is not definitely established [83]. These cases differ from "classic" forms of PPHP in the absence of feeblemindedness, ectopic calcification, or any PHP in the family. No concrete evidence or sex-linked recessive inheritance has yet been reported. The phenotypic expression of PPHP varies considerably, from individuals with shortening of the metacarpal and metatarsal bones, short stature, dental abnormalities, bossing of the frontal bone, and mental insufficiency, to individuals in whom the only anomaly may be minimal recession of the fourth metacarpal [83, 118] (see Figs. 84-9, 84-10).

Despite documented abnormal karyotypes and normal chromosome complements, the association of PPHP with gonadal dysgenesis seems more than fortuitous [121, 180]. Present evidence suggests that women with the phenotype of PPHP who are sex-chromatin negative or who have 45 (XO) chromosomes really have Turner syndrome [116]. Since the Turner syndrome is not found in every female patient with PPHP, factors other than the X-chromosome deficiency must be responsible for the phenotypic abnormalities common to both disorders. Moreover, when the Turner syndrome has been associated with the well-developed syndrome of PPHP, the sex-chromatin pattern, when reported, has been of the male type [121]. It is noteworthy in this regard that the association of PPHP and Turner syndrome recently has been reported to occur in two females, both with XO/XX mosaicism and negative sex-chromatin patterns [121]. The opinion presently prevailing is that PPHP and Turner syndrome, although phenotypically identical in many instances, represent distinct, separable genetic disorders. It has also been suggested that the characteristic changes of PPHP seen in females with Turner syndrome result from an unfavorable interuterine milieu at about the eighth or ninth week of gestation. These impressions are presently purely speculative and await confirmation or rejection by appropriate clarification of the role, if any, of the X chromosome in PPHP and the correlation of the phenotypic abnormalities of PPHP and Turner syndrome in isolated chromosomal defects.

Tumoral Calcinosis with Hyperphosphatemia

Since the original description of this syndrome by Duret in 1899 [55], over 40 well-documented cases of tumoral calcinosis have been reported. Patients with this disorder characteristically present in the first two decades of life with firm, nontender, tumorous heterotopic calcifications around the hips, elbows, and shoulders [12], although lesions have also been documented in the soft tissues surrounding smaller joints [12, 188]. The tumorous masses, which arise from fibrous tissue and fascial planes between muscles and around tendons, appear radiologically as radiopaque conglomerates in the periarticular soft tissue and contain calcium phosphate, calcium carbonate, or mixtures thereof [12]. The serum phosphate is consistently elevated in tumoral calcinosis, and glomerular filtration rates and serum calcium are normal [12, 188].

The majority of cases reported in the literature in English have been in blacks, and approximately one-third of the reported cases have been familial [12]. Since transmission from one generation to another has not been observed, an autosomal recessive inheritance pattern has been assumed for this disease. Although the hyperphosphatemia has been ascribed by some to an inherited reduction in renal tubular responsiveness to PTH [188], hyperphosphatemic subjects with tumoral calcinosis respond to PTH with a brisk phosphaturia and a decrease in serum phosphate [12]. In isolated studies, karyotype analysis of leukocyte cultures reveals a 46 XY chromosomal pattern, a normal growth hormone response to arginine infusion, normal circulating immunoassay parathyroid hormone values, and a normal parathyroid hormone response to EDTA-induced hypocalcemia [188].

Surgical excision of the tumorous masses still remains the treatment of choice in this disorder, although recurrence invariably occurs [12]. Other forms of therapy, including special diets, probenecid, corticosteroids, and radiotherapy, have been of limited value.

References

1. Albright, F.   Pseudo-pseudohypoparathyroidism. *Trans. Assoc. Am. Physicians* 65:337, 1952.
2. Albright, F., Butler, A. M., and Bloomberg, E. Rickets resistant to vitamin D therapy. *Am. J. Dis. Child.* 54:529, 1937.
3. Aliapoulis, M. A., Voelkel, E. F., and Munson, P. L. Assay of human thyroid glands for thyrocalcitonin activity. *J. Clin. Endocrinol. Metab.* 26:897, 1966.
4. Allen, E. H., Millard, F. J. C., and Nassim, J. R. Hypo-hyperparathyroidism. *Arch. Dis. Child.* 43:295, 1968.
5. Amiel, C., Kuntziger, H., Couette, S., Coreau, C., and Bergounioux, N. Evidence for a parathyroid hormone-independent calcium modulation of phosphate transport along the nephron. *J. Clin. Invest.* 57:256, 1976.
6. Argenzio, R. A., Lowe, J. E., Hintz, H. F., and Schryver, H. F. Calcium and phosphorus homeostasis in horses. *J. Nutr.* 104:18, 1974.
7. Arnaud, C. D., Glorieux, F., and Scriver, C. Serum parathyroid hormone in x-linked hypophosphatemia. *Science* 173:845, 1971.
8. Arnaud, C., Glorieux, F., and Scriver, C. R. Serum parathyroid hormone levels in acquired vitamin D deficiency of infancy. *Pediatrics* 49:837, 1972.
9. Aurbach, G. D., Marcus, R., Winickoff, R. N., Epstein, E. H., and Nigra, T. P. Urinary excretion of 3'5'-AMP in syndromes considered refractory to parathyroid hormone. *Metabolism* 19:799, 1970.
10. Avioli, L. V. The therapeutic approach to hypoparathyroidism. *Am. J. Med.* 57:34, 1974.
11. Avioli, L. V., and Birge, S. J. Controversies Regarding Intestinal Phosphate Transport and Absorption. In S. G. Massry and E. Ritz (eds.), *Phosphate Metabolism.* New York: Plenum Press, 1977. P. 507.
12. Baldursson, H., Evans, E. B., Dodge, W. F., and Jackson, W. T. Tumoral calcinosis with hyperphosphatemia: A report of a family with incidence in four siblings. *J. Bone Joint Surg. [Am.]* 51:913, 1969.
13. Balsan, S., and Garabedian, M. 25-Hydroxycholecalciferol: A comparative study in deficiency rickets and different types of resistant rickets. *J. Clin. Invest.* 51:749, 1972.
14. Balsan, S., Garabedian, M., Sorgniard, R., Holick, M. F., and DeLuca, H. F. 1,25-Hydroxyvitamin D_3 and 1,α-hydroxyvitamin D_3 in children: Biologic and therapeutic effects in nutritional rickets and different types of vitamin D resistance. *Pediatr. Res.* 9:586, 1975.
15. Barbour, B. H., Kronfield, S. J., and Pawkicki, A. M. Studies on the mechanism of phosphorus excretion in vitamin D resistant rickets. *Nephron* 3:40, 1966.
16. Beal, V. A. Calcium and phosphorus in infancy. *J. Am. Diet. Assoc.* 53:450, 1968.
17. Bell, N. H., Avery, A., Sinha, T., Clark, C., Allen, D., and Johnston, C., Jr. Effects of dibutyryl cyclic adenosine-3'5'-monophosphate and parathyroid extract on calcium and phosphorus metabolism in hypoparathyroidism and pseudohypoparathyroidism. *J. Clin. Invest.* 51:816, 1972.
18. Bell, N. H., Gerard, E. S., and Bartter, F. C. Pseudohypoparathyroidism with osteitis fibrosa cystica and impaired absorption of calcium. *J. Clin. Endocrinol. Metab.* 23:759, 1963.
19. Bergstrand, C. G., Ekengren, K., Filipsson, R., and Huggert, A. Pseudohypoparathyroidism. *Acta Endocrinol.* 29:201, 1958.
20. Birkenhager, J. C., Seldenrath, H. J., Hackeng, W. H. L., Schellekens, A. P., van der Veer, A. L., and Roelfsema, F. Calcium and phosphorus metabolism, parathyroid hormone, calcitonin and bone histology in pseudohypoparathyroidism. *Eur. J. Clin. Invest.* 3:27, 1973.
21. Birtwell, W. M., Magsamen, B. F., and Fenn, P. A. An unusual hereditary osteomalacic disease—pseudovitamin D deficiency. *J. Bone Joint Surg. [Am.]* 52:1222, 1970.
22. Brickman, A. S., Coburn, J. W., Kurokawa, K., Bethune, J. E., Harrison, H. E., and Norman, A. W. Actions of 1,25-dihydroxycholecalciferol in patients with hypophosphatemic, vitamin D-resistant rickets. *N. Engl. J. Med.* 289:495, 1973.
23. Bronsky, D. Hyperparathyroidism with Albright's osteodystrophy: Case report and a proposed new classification of parathyroid disease. *J. Clin. Endocrinol. Metab.* 31:271, 1970.
24. Bronsky, D., Kiamko, R., Waldstein, T., and Sheldon, S. Familial idiopathic hypoparathyroidism. *J. Clin. Endocrinol. Metab.* 28:61, 1968.
25. Bronsky, D., Kushner, D. S., Dubin, A., and Snapper, I. Idiopathic hypoparathyroidism and pseudohypoparathyroidism: Case reports and review of the literature. *Medicine* 37:317, 1958.
26. Buchs, S. Familiarer hypoparathyreoidismus. *Ann. Paediatr.* 188:124, 1957.
27. Buss, R. O., and Frost, H. M. The prevalence of

halo volumes in familial vitamin D-resistant rickets. *Calcif. Tissue Res.* 7:76, 1971.

28. Carlson, H. E., Brickman, A. S., and Bottazzo, G. F. Prolactin deficiency in pseudohypoparathyroidism. *N. Engl. J. Med.* 296:140, 1977.

29. Cattaneo, C. The maximum tubular reabsorption of phosphate in acromegaly. *Acta Endocrinol. (Kbn.)* 45:203, 1964.

30. Chase, L., and Aurbach, G. D. The effect of parathyroid hormone on the concentration of adenosine 3'5' monophosphate in skeletal tissue *in vitro*. *J. Biol. Chem.* 245:1520, 1970.

31. Chase, L., Fedak, S. A., and Aurbach, G. D. Activation of skeletal adenyl cyclase by parathyroid hormone *in vitro*. *Endocrinology* 84:761, 1969.

32. Chase, L., Melson, L., and Aurbach, G. D. Pseudohypoparathyroidism: Defective excretion of 3'5' AMP in response to parathyroid hormone. *J. Clin. Invest.* 48:1832, 1969.

33. Chopra, I., and Nugent, C. A. Concurrence of features of pseudohypoparathyroidism, pseudopseudohypoparathyroidism and basal-cell nevus syndrome. *Am. J. Med. Sci.* 260:171, 1970.

34. Clarke, P., and Carre, I. J. Hypocalcemic, hypomagnesemic convulsions. *J. Pediatr.* 70:806, 1967.

35. Cohanim, M., DeLuca, H. F., and Yendt, E. T. Effects of prolonged treatment with 25-hydroxycholecalciferol in hypophosphatemic (vitamin D refractory) rickets and osteomalacia. *Johns Hopkins Med. J.* 131:118, 1972.

36. Cohen, R. D., and Vince, F. P. Pseudohypoparathyroidism with raised plasma alkaline phosphatase. *Arch. Dis. Child.* 44:96, 1969.

37. Cohen, S., and Becker, G. L. Origin, diagnosis and treatment of the dental manifestations of vitamin D resistant rickets: Review of the literature and report of a case. *J. Am. Dent. Assoc.* 92:120, 1976.

38. Condon, J. R., Massim, J. R., and Rutter, A. Defective intestinal phosphate absorption in familial and non-familial hypophosphatemia. *Br. Med. J.* 3:138, 1970.

39. Cooke, N., Teitelbaum, S., and Avioli, L. V. Antacid-induced osteomalacia and nephrolithiasis. *Arch. Intern. Med.,* 138:1007, 1978.

40. Corvilain, J., and Abramow, M. Growth and renal control of plasma phosphate. *J. Clin. Endocrinol. Metab.* 34:452, 1972.

41. Cowgill, L., Goldfarb, S., Goldberg, M., Slatopolsky, E., and Agus, Z. S. Nature of the renal defect in familial hypophosphatemic rickets (FHR) (abstract). *Clin. Res.* 25:505A, 1977.

42. Cox, G. J., Dodds, M. L., Wigman, H. B., and Murphy, F. J. The effects of high doses of aluminum and iron on phosphorus metabolism. *J. Biol. Chem.* 11:92, 1931.

43. Cuche, J. L., Ott, C. E., Marchand, G. R., Diaz-Buxo, J. A., and Knox, F. G. Intrarenal calcium in phosphate handling. *Am. J. Physiol.* 230:790, 1976.

44. Davies, M., Taylor, C. M., Hill, L. F., and Stanbury, S. W. 1,25-Dihydroxycholecalciferol in hypoparathyroidism. *Lancet* 1:55, 1977.

45. DeLuca, H. F. Recent advances in our understanding of the vitamin D endocrine system. *J. Lab. Clin. Med.* 87:7, 1976.

46. DeLuca, H. F. Vitamin D: The vitamin and the hormone. *Fed. Proc.* 32:2211, 1974.

47. DeLuca, H. F., Lund, J., Rosenbloom, A., and Lobeck, C. C. Metabolism of tritiated vitamin D_3

48. Denko, J. D., and Kaelbling, R. The psychiatric aspects of hypoparathyroidism. *Acta Psychiatr. Scand.* 38 [Suppl.]:1, 1962.

49. Dent, C. E., and Stamp, T. C. B. Hypophosphatemic osteomalacia presenting in adults. *Q. J. Med.* 40:303, 1971.

50. Dickerson, J. W. T. Changes in the composition of the human femur during growth. *Biochem. J.* 82:56, 1962.

51. Dickson, L. G., Morita, Y., Gowsert, E. J., Graves, J., and Meyer, J. S. Neurological, eletcroencephalographic and heredo-familial aspects of pseudoparathyroidism and pseudo-pseudohypoparathyroidism. *J. Neurol. Neurosurg. Psychiatry* 23:33, 1960.

52. Draper, H. H., Lie, T. L., and Bergan, H. G. Osteoporosis in aging rats induced by high phosphorus diets. *J. Nutr.* 102:1133, 1972.

53. Drezner, M., Neelon, F. A., and Lebovitz, H. E. Pseudohypoparathyroidism type II: A possible defect in the reception of the cyclic AMP signal. *N. Engl. J. Med.* 289:1056, 1973.

54. Drezner, M. K., Neelon, F. A., Haussler, M., McPherson, H. T., and Lebovitz, H. E. 1,25-Dihydroxycholecalciferol deficiency: The probable cause of hypocalcemia and metabolic bone disease in pseudohypoparathyroidism. *J. Clin. Endocrinol. Metab.* 42:621, 1976.

55. Duret, H. Tumeurs multiples et singulières des bourses séreuses (endotheliomes, peut-être d'origine parasitaire). *Bull. Mem. Soc. Anat.* (Paris) 74:725, 1899.

56. Earp, H. S., Ney, R. L., Gitelman, J. H., Richman, R., and DeLuca, H. F. Effects of 25-hydroxycholecalciferol in patients with familial hypophosphatemic and vitamin D-resistant rickets. *N. Engl. J. Med.* 283:627, 1970.

57. Editorial. Vitamin D deficiency, bone turnover and urinary hydroxyproline. *Lancet* 1:1018, 1968.

58. Eicher, E. M., Southard, J. L., Scriver, C. R., and Glorieux, F. H. Hypophosphatemia: Mouse model for human familial hypophosphatemic (vitamin D resistant) rickets. *Proc. Natl. Acad. Sci. U.S.A.* 73:4667, 1976.

59. Falls, W. F., Jr., Carter, N. W., Rector, F. C., Jr., and Seldin, D. W. Familial vitamin D-resistant rickets: Study of six cases with evaluation of the pathogenetic role of secondary hypoparathyroidism. *Ann. Intern. Med.* 68:553, 1968.

60. Fanconi, A., Fischer, J. A., and Prader, A. Serum parathyroid hormone concentrations in hypophosphatemic vitamin D resistant rickets. *Helv. Paediatr. Acta* 28:187, 1974.

61. Farriaux, J. P. Pseudohypoparathyroidism. *Am. J. Dis. Child.* 130:180, 1976.

62. Field, H. M., and Reiss, E. Vitamin D-resistant rickets: The effect of calcium infusion on phosphate reabsorption. *J. Clin. Invest.* 39:1807, 1960.

63. Fischer, J. A., Binswanger, U., and Fanconi, A. Serum parathyroid hormone concentrations in vitamin D deficiency rickets of infancy: Effects of intravenous calcium and vitamin D. *Horm. Metab. Res.* 5:381, 1973.

64. Fonseca, O. A., and Calverley, J. R. Neurological manifestations of hypoparathyroidism. *Arch. Intern. Med.* 120:202, 1967.

65. Frame, B., Hanson, C. A., Frost, H. M., Block, M.,

and Arnstein, A. R.   Renal resistance to parathyroid hormone with osteitis fibrosa. *Am. J. Med.* 52:311, 1972.

66. Fraser, D., Kooh, S. W., Kind, H. P., Holick, M. F., Tanaka, Y., and DeLuca, H. F.   Pathogenesis of hereditary vitamin D-dependent rickets. *N. Engl. J. Med.* 289:817, 1973.

67. Friedman, M., Hatcher, G., and Watson, L.   Primary hypomagnesaemia with secondary hypocalcemia in an infant. *Lancet* 1:703, 1967.

68. Gellissen, K., and Duphorn, I.   Uroterpenoluria and resistant rickets. *Lancet* 1:575, 1967.

69. Gerblich, A. A., Genuth, S. M., and Haddad, J. G., Jr.   A case of idiopathic hypoparathyroidism and dietary vitamin D deficiency: The requirement for calcium and vitamin D for bone, but not renal responsiveness to PTH. *J. Clin. Endocrinol. Metab.* 44:507, 1977.

70. Glimcher, M. J., and Krane, S. M.   The Organization and Structure of Bone and the Mechanism of Calcification. In B. S. Gould (ed.), *Treatise in Collagen*. London: Academic, 1968. Vol. 2B, p. 67.

71. Glorieux, F., and Scriver, C. R.   Loss of parathyroid hormone-sensitive component of phosphate transport in x-linked hypophosphatemia. *Science* 175:997, 1972.

72. Glorieux, F., Scriver, C. R., Reade, R. N., Goldman, H., and Roseborough, A.   Use of phosphate and vitamin D to prevent dwarfism and rickets in x-linked hypophosphatemia. *N. Engl. J. Med.* 287:481, 1972.

73. Golonka, J., and Goodman, A.   Coexistence of primary ovarian insufficiency, primary adrenocortical insufficiency and idiopathic hypoparathyroidism. *J. Clin. Endocrinol. Metab.* 28:79, 1968.

74. Gray, R. W., Wilz, D. R., Caldas, A. E., and Lemann, J., Jr.   Importance of phosphate in regulating plasma 1,25(OH)$_2$ vitamin D levels in humans: Studies in healthy subjects, in calcium stone formers, and in patients with primary hyperparathyroidism. *J. Clin. Endocrinol. Metab.* 45:299, 1977.

75. Haddad, J. G., and Avioli, L. V.   Comparative effects of phosphate and thyrocalcitonin on skeletal turnover. *Endocrinology* 87:1245, 1970.

76. Haddad, J. G., Chyu, K. J., Hahn, T. J., and Stamp, T. C. B.   Serum concentrations of 25-hydroxyvitamin D in sex-linked hypophosphatemic vitamin D-resistant rickets. *J. Lab. Clin. Med.* 81:22, 1973.

77. Hahn, T. J., Scharp, C. R., Halstead, L. R., Haddad, J. G., Karl, D. M., and Avioli, L. V.   Parathyroid hormone status and renal responsiveness in familial hypophosphatemic rickets. *J. Clin. Endocrinol. Metab.* 41:926, 1975.

78. Harrison, H. E., Harrison, H. C., Lifshitz, F., and Johnson, A. D.   Growth disturbance in hereditary hypophosphatemia. *Am. J. Dis. Child.* 112:290, 1966.

79. Harrison, H. E., Lifshitz, F., and Blizzard, R. M.   Comparison between crystalline dihydrotachysterol and calciferol in patients requiring pharmacologic vitamin D therapy. *N. Engl. J. Med.* 276:894, 1967.

80. Haussler, M., Hughes, M., Baylink, D., Littledike, E. T., Cork, D., and Pitt, M.   Influence of Phosphate Depletion on the Biosynthesis and Circulating

Level of 1α, 25-Dihydroxyvitamin D. In S. G. Massry and E. Ritz (eds.), *Phosphate Metabolism*. New York: Plenum Press, 1977. P. 233.

81. Henkin, R. I.   Impairment of olfaction and of the tastes of sour and bitter in pseudohypoparathyroidism. *J. Clin. Endocrinol. Metab.* 28:624, 1968.

82. Henneman, P. H., Dempsey, E. F., Carroll, E. L., and Henneman, D. H.   Acquired vitamin D-resistant osteomalacia: A new variety characterized by hypercalcemia, low serum bicarbonate and hyperglycinuria. *Metabolism* 11:103, 1962.

83. Hermans, P. E., Gorman, C. A., Martin, W. J., and Kelly, P. J.   Pseudo-pseudohypoparathyroidism (Albright's hereditary osteodystrophy): A family study. *Mayo Clin. Proc.* 39:81, 1964.

84. Ireland, A. W., Clubb, J. S., Neale, F. C., Posen, S., and Reeve, T. S.   The calciferol requirements of patients with surgical hypoparathyroidism. *Ann. Intern. Med.* 69:81, 1968.

85. Johnson, J. D., and Jennings, R.   Hypocalcemia and cardiac arrhythmias. *Am. J. Dis. Child.* 115:373, 1968.

86. Kallmeyer, J., Dunea, G., and Schwartz, F. D.   Hypophosphatemic osteomalacia with hyperglycinuria. *Ann. Intern. Med.* 66:136, 1967.

87. Knochel, J. P.   The pathophysiology and clinical characteristics of severe hypophosphatemia. *Arch. Intern. Med.* 137:203, 1977.

88. Knox, F. G., Preiss, J., Kim, J. K., and Dousa, T. P.   Mechanism of resistance to the phosphaturic effect of the parathyroid hormone in the hamster. *J. Clin. Invest.* 59:675, 1977.

89. Kodicek, E.   Variations in Sensitivity to Vitamin D. In G. E. W. Wolstenhoeme and C. M. O'Connor (eds.), *Bone Structures and Metabolism*. Ciba Foundation Symposium. Boston: Little, Brown, 1956. P. 201.

90. Kolb, F. O., and Steinbach, H. L.   Pseudohypoparathyroidism with secondary hyperparathyroidism and osteitis fibrosa. *J. Clin. Endocrinol. Metab.* 22:59, 1962.

91. Kooh, S. W., Fraser, D., DeLuca, H. F., Holick, M. F., Belsey, R. E., Clark, M. B., and Murray, T. M.   Treatment of hypoparathyroidism and pseudo-hypoparathyroidism with metabolites of vitamin D: Evidence for impaired conversion of 25-hydroxyvitamin D to 1α,25-dihydroxyvitamin D. *N. Engl. J. Med.* 293:810, 1975.

92. Kreisberg, R. A.   Phosphorus deficiency and hypophosphatemia. *Hosp. Pract.* 12:121, 1977.

93. Krook, L., Lutwak, L., Henrikson, P., Kallfelz, F., Hirsch, C., Romanus, B., Belanger, L., Marier, J., and Sheffy, B. E.   Reversibility of nutritional osteoporosis: Physiochemical data on bones from an experimental study in dogs. *J. Nutr.* 101:233, 1971.

94. Kuhlman, R. E. and Stamp, W. F.   Biochemical biopsy evaluation of the epiphyseal mechanism in a patient with vitamin D-resistant rickets. *J. Lab. Clin. Med.* 64:14, 1964.

95. Lafferty, F. W., Herndon, C. H., and Pearson, O. H.   Pathogenesis of vitamin D-resistant rickets and the response to a high calcium intake. *J. Clin. Endocrinol. Metab.* 23:903, 1963.

96. LaFlamme, G. H., and Jowsey, J.   Bone and soft tissue changes with oral phosphate supplements. *J. Clin. Invest.* 51:2834, 1972.

97. Lee, J. B., Tashjian, A. H., Jr., Streeto, J. M., and

Frantz, A. G. Familial pseudohypoparathyroidism, role of parathyroid hormone and thyrocalcitonin. *N. Engl. J. Med.* 279:1179, 1968.

98. Leichsenring, J. M., Norris, L. M., Lamison, S. A., Wilson, E. D., and Patton, M. B. The effect of level of intake on calcium and phosphorus metabolism in college women. *J. Nutr.* 45:407, 1951.

99. Lewy, J. E., Cabana, E. C, Repetto, H. A., Canterbury, J. M., and Reiss, E. Serum parathyroid hormone in hypophosphatemic vitamin D-resistant rickets. *J. Pediatr.* 81:294, 1972.

100. Litvak, J., Moldawer, M. P., Forbes, A. P., and Henneman, P. H. Hypocalcemia and hypercalciuria during vitamin D and dihydrotachysterol therapy of hypoparathyroidism. *J. Clin. Endocrinol. Metab.* 28:246, 1958.

101. Lorenz, R., and Burr, I. M. Idiopathic hypoparathyroidism and steatorrhea: A new aid in management. *J. Pediatr.* 85:522, 1974.

102. Lutwak, L. Dietary calcium and the reversal of bone demineralization. *Nutr. News* 37:1, 1974.

103. Mabry, C. C., Bautista, A., Kirk, R. F. H., Dubilier, L. D., Braunstein, H., and Koepke, J. A. Familial hyperphosphatasia with mental retardation, seizures, and neurologic deficits. *J. Pediatr.* 77:74, 1970.

104. Magid, G. J., Maloney, J. R., Sirota, J. H., and Schwab, E. A. Familial hypophosphatemia: Studies on its pathogenesis in an affected mother and son. *Ann. Intern. Med.* 64:1009, 1966.

105. Mann, J. B., Alterman, S., and Hills, A. G. Albright's hereditary osteodystrophy comprising pseudohypoparathyroidism and pseudo-pseudohypoparathyroidism. *Ann. Intern. Med.* 56:315, 1962.

106. Marcus, R., Wilber, J. F., and Aurbach, G. D. Parathyroid hormone-sensitive adenyl cyclase from the renal cortex of a patient with pseudo-hypoparathyroidism. *J. Clin. Endocrinol. Metab.* 33:537, 1971.

107. Massry, S. G., Friedler, R. M., and Coburn, J. W. Excretion of phosphate and calcium. *Arch. Intern. Med.* 131:828, 1973.

108. Mawer, E. B., Davies, M., Taylor, C. M., Backhouse, J., and Hill, L. F. Metabolic fate of administered 1,25-dihydroxycholecalciferol in controls and in patients with hypoparathyroidism. *Lancet* 1:1203, 1976.

109. Mazzuoli, G. F., Coen, G., and Antonozzi, I. Study on calcium metabolism, thyroid calcitonin assay and effect of thyroidectomy in pseudo-hypoparathyroidism. *Isr. J. Med. Sci.* 3:627, 1967.

110. McDonald, K. M. Responsiveness of bone to parathyroid extract in siblings with pseudohypoparathyroidism. *Metabolism* 21:521, 1972.

111. McEnery, P. T., Silverman, F. N., and West, C. D. Acceleration of growth with combined vitamin D-phosphate therapy of hypophosphatemic resistant rickets. *J. Pediatr.* 80:763, 1972.

112. McNair, S. L., and Stickler, G. B. Growth in familial hypophosphatemic vitamin D-resistant rickets. *N. Engl. J. Med.* 281:511, 1969.

113. Melson, G., Chase, L., and Aurbach, G. D. Parathyroid hormone-sensitive adenyl cyclase in isolated renal tubules. *Endocrinology* 86:511, 1970.

114. Menking, M., and Sotos, J. F. Effect of administration of oral neutral phosphate in hypophosphatemic rickets. *J. Pediatr.* 75:1001, 1969.

115. Michie, W., Stowers, J. M., Frazer, S. C., and Gunn, A. Thyroidectomy and the parathyroids. *Br. J. Surg.* 52:503, 1965.

116. Miller, J. Q., Rostafinski, M. J., and Hyde, M. B. Gonadal dysgenesis and brachymetacarpal dwarfism (pseudopseudohypoparathyroidism). *Arch. Intern. Med.* 116:940, 1965.

117. Money, J., and Ehrhardt, A. Correlation of mental functioning and calcium regulation in a rare case of pseudohypoparathyroidism. *Bull. Johns Hopkins Hosp.* 123:276, 1968.

118. Monn, E., Osnes, J. B., Oye, I., and Wefring, K. W. Pseudohypoparathyroidism. *Acta Paediatr. Scand.* 65:487, 1976.

119. Moon, W., Malzer, J. L., and Clark, H. E. Phosphorus balances of adults consuming several food combinations. *J. Am. Diet. Assoc.* 64:386, 1974.

120. Moses, A. M., Breslau, N., and Coulson, R. Renal responses to PTH in patients with hormone-resistant (pseudo) hypoparathyroidism. *Am. J. Med.* 61:184, 1976.

121. Nedok, A. S., Garzicic, B. S., and Soldatovic, B. M. An association of pseudopseudohypoparathyroidism and gonadal dysgenesis with XO/XX mosaicism and negative sex chromatin pattern in two females. *J. Clin. Endocrinol. Metab.* 28:1513, 1968.

122. Neer, R. M., Holick, M. F., DeLuca, H. F., and Potts, J. T., Jr. Effects of 1α,hydroxy-vitamin D_3 and 1,25-dihydroxyvitamin D_3 on calcium and phosphorus metabolism in hypoparathyroidism. *Metabolism* 24:1403, 1975.

123. Neer, R. M., Tregear, G. W., and Potts, J. T., Jr. Renal effects of native parathyroid hormone and synthetic biologically active fragments in pseudo-hypoparathyroidism and hypoparathyroidism. *J. Clin. Endocrinol. Metab.* 38:420, 1977.

124. Nordin, B. E. C., and Smith, D. A. Phosphorus Absorption and Balance. In *Diagnostic Procedures in Disorders of Calcium Metabolism.* Boston: Little, Brown, 1965. P. 43.

125. Nordio, S., and Antener, I. The molecular conception of rickets pathogenesis: I. Clinical research. *Med. Exp.* (Basel) 18:193, 1968.

126. Nordio, S., Antener, I., Gatti, R., and Dentan, E. The molecular conception of rickets pathogenesis: II. Experimental research. *Med. Exp.* (Basel) 18:223, 1968.

127. O'Doherty, P. J., and DeLuca, H. F. Intestinal calcium and phosphate transport in genetic hypophosphatemic mice. *Biochem. Biophys. Res. Commun.* 71:617, 1976.

128. Okano, K., Fujita, T., Orimo, H., and Yoshikawa, M. A case of pseudohypoparathyroidism with increased bone turnover and demineralization. *Endocrinol. Jap.* 16:423, 1969.

129. Pak, C., DeLuca, H. F., Bartter, F. C., Henneman, D. H., Frame, B., Simopoulos, A., and Delea, C. S. Treatment of vitamin D-resistant rickets with 25-hydroxycholecalciferol. *Arch. Intern. Med.* 129:894, 1972.

130. Parfitt, A. M. The spectrum of hypoparathyroidism. *J. Clin. Endocrinol. Metab.* 34:152, 1972.

131. Paunier, L., Kooh, S. W., Conen, P. E., Gibson, A. A. M., and Fraser, D. Renal function and histology after long-term vitamin D therapy of refractory rickets. *J. Pediatr.* 73:833, 1968.

132. Peden, V. H. True idiopathic hypoparathyroidism

as a sex-linked recessive trait. *Am. J. Hum. Genet.* 12:323, 1960.

133. Potts, J. T., Jr. Pseudohypoparathyroidism. In J. B. Stanbury, J. B. Wyngaarden, and D. S. Fredrickson (eds.), *The Metabolic Basis of Inherited Disease* (3rd ed.). New York: McGraw-Hill, 1978. P. 1350.

134. Puschett, J. B., Rastegar, A., Genel, M., Anast, C., and DeLuca, H. F. Effects of 25-hydroxycholecalciferol on urinary electrolyte excretion in hypophosphatemic rickets. *Lancet* 2:920, 1974.

135. Reade, T. M., Scriver, C. R., Glorieux, F. H., Nogrady, B., Delvin, E., Poirier, R., Holick, M. F., and DeLuca, H. F. Response to crystalline 1α-hydroxyvitamin D₃ in vitamin D dependency. *Pediatr. Res.* 9:593, 1975.

136. Reddy, V., and Sivakumar, B. Magnesium-dependent vitamin D resistant rickets. *Lancet* 1:963, 1974.

137. Reiss, E., Canterbury, J. M., Bercovitz, M. A., and Kaplan, E. L. The role of phosphate in the secretion of parathyroid hormone in man. *J. Clin. Invest.* 49:2146, 1970.

138. Reitz, R. E., and Weinstein, R. L. Parathyroid hormone secretion in familial vitamin D-resistant rickets. *N. Engl. J. Med.* 289:941, 1973.

139. Robertson, B. R., Harris, R. C., and McCune, D. J. Refractory rickets: Mechanisms of therapeutic action of calciferol. *Am. J. Dis. Child.* 64:948, 1942.

140. Rodriguez, H. J., Villarreal, H., Jr., Klahr, S., and Slatopolsky, E. Pseudohypoparathyroidism type II: Restoration of normal renal responsiveness to parathyroid hormone by calcium administration. *J. Clin. Endocrinol. Metab.* 39:693, 1974.

141. Roof, B. S., Piel, C. F., and Gordon, G. S. Nature of defect responsible for familial vitamin D-resistant rickets (VDRR) based on radioimmunoassay for parathyroid hormone (PTH). *Trans. Am. Physicians* 85:172, 1972.

142. Rosen, J. F., and Finberg, L. Vitamin D-dependent rickets: Actions of parathyroid hormone and 25-hydroxycholecalciferol. *Pediatr. Res.* 6:552, 1972.

143. Russell, R. G. G., Smith, R., Preston, C., Walton, R. J., Woods, C. G., Henderson, R. G., and Norman, A. W. The effect of 1,25-dihydroxycholecalciferol on renal tubular reabsorption of phosphate, intestinal absorption of calcium and bone histology in hypophosphatemic renal tubular rickets. *Clin. Sci. Molec. Med.* 48:177, 1975.

144. Scott, K. G., Smyth, F. S., Peng, C. T., Reilly, W. A., Stevenson, E. A., and Castle, J. M. Measurement of the plasma levels of tritiated vitamin D₃ in control and patients with vitamin D-resistant rickets. *Int. J. Appl. Radiat. Isot.* 15:502, 1964.

145. Scriver, C. R. Rickets and the pathogenesis of impaired tubular transport of phosphate and other solutes. *Am. J. Med.* 57:43, 1974.

146. Scriver, C. R., Glorieux, F. H., Reade, T. M., and Tenenhouse, H. S. X-Linked Hypophosphatemia and Autosomal Recessive Vitamin D Dependency: Models for the Resolution of Vitamin D Refractory Rickets. In H. Bickel and J. Stern (eds.), *Inborn Errors of Calcium and Bone Metabolism.* Lancaster, England: MTP Press, 1976. P. 150.

147. Seely, J. R., Coussons, H., Smith, J. D., and DeLuca, H. F. Effective treatment of hypophosphatemic vitamin D resistant rickets (VDRR) with 25-hydroxycholecalciferol (25-HCC). *Pediatr. Res.* 4:451, 1970.

148. Sewell, L., Trout, E. C., Jr., Field, H., Jr., and Treadwell, C. R. Effect of dietary fat and fatty acid in fecal excretion of a calcium oleate phosphate preparation. *Proc. Soc. Exp. Biol. Med.* 92:613, 1956.

149. Short, E. M., Binder, H. J., and Rosenberg, L. E. Familial hypophosphatemic rickets: Defective transport of inorganic phosphate by intestinal mucosa. *Science* 179:700, 1973.

150. Short, E., Morriss, R. C., Jr., Sebastian, A., and Spencer, M. Exaggerated phosphaturic response to circulating parathyroid hormone in patients with familial x-linked hypophosphatemic rickets. *J. Clin. Invest.* 58:152, 1976.

151. Singleton, E. B., and Teng, C. T. Pseudohypoparathyroidism with bone changes simulating hyperparathyroidism (report of a case). *Radiology* 78:388, 1962.

152. Sinha, T. K., DeLuca, H. F., and Bell, N. H. Evidence for a defect in the formation of 1α,25-dihydroxyvitamin D in pseudohypoparathyroidism. *Metabolism* 26:731, 1977.

153. Sinha, T. K., Queener, S. F., and Bell, N. H. Acquired resistance to parathyroid hormone. *Acta Endocrinol.* 83:321, 1976.

154. Smith, R., and Dick, M. The effect of vitamin D and phosphate on urinary total hydroxyproline excretion in adult presenting "vitamin D resistant" type I renal tubular osteomalacia. *Clin. Sci.* 35:575, 1968.

155. Smith, R., Lindenbaum, R. H., and Walton, R. J. Hypophosphatemic osteomalacia and Fanconi syndrome of adult onset with dominant inheritance. *Q. J. Med.* 45:387, 1976.

156. Soergal, K. H., Mueller, K. H., Gustke, R. F., and Geenen, J. E. Jejunal calcium transport in health and metabolic bone disease: Effect of vitamin D. *Gastroenterology* 67:28, 1974.

157. Soni, N. N., and Marks, E. C. Microradiographic and polarized-light study of dental tissues in vitamin D-resistant rickets. *Oral Surg.* 23:755, 1967.

158. Spinner, M. W., Blizzard, R. M., Gibbs, J. A. H., and Childs, B. Familial distributions of organ specific antibodies in the blood of patients with Addison's disease and hypoparathyroidism and their relatives. *Clin. Exp. Immunol.* 5:461, 1969.

159. Stamp, T. C. B., and Baker, L. R. I. Recessive hypophosphatemic rickets, and possible aetiology of the "vitamin D-resistant" syndrome. *Arch. Dis. Child.* 51:360, 1976.

160. Stanbury, S. W. Intestinal Absorption of Calcium and Phosphorus in Adult Man in Health and Disease. In H. Bickel and J. Stern (eds.), *Inborn Errors of Calcium and Bone Metabolism.* Lancaster, England: MPT Press, 1976. P. 21.

161. Steendijk, R., and Latham, S. C. Hypophosphatemic vitamin D resistant rickets; an observation on height and serum inorganic phosphate in untreated cases. *Helv. Paediatr. Acta* 2:179, 1971.

162. Steinbach, H. L., and Young, D. A. The roentgen appearance of pseudohypoparathyroidism (PH) and pseudo-pseudohypoparathyroidism (PPH). *Am. J. Roentgen.* 97:49, 1966.

163. Steinberg, H., and Waldron, B. R. Idiopathic hypoparathyroidism: Analysis of 52 cases, including a report of a new case. *Medicine* 31:133, 1952.

164. Stickler, G. B. External calcium and phosphorus

balances in vitamin D-resistant rickets. *J. Pediatr.* 63:942, 1963.

165. Stickler, G. B., Hayles, A. B., and Rosevear, J. W. Familial hypophosphatemic vitamin D resistant rickets: Effect of increased oral calcium and phosphorus intake without high doses of vitamin D. *Am. J. Dis. Child.* 110:664, 1965.

166. Stickler, G. B., Beabout, J. W., and Riggs, B. L. Vitamin D-resistant rickets: Clinical experience with 41 typical familial hypophosphatemic patients and 2 atypical nonfamilial cases. *Mayo Clin. Proc.* 45:197, 1970.

167. Stoop, J. W., Schraagen, M. J. C., and Tiddens, H. A. Pseudo vitamin D deficiency rickets. *Acta Paediatr. Scand.* 56:607, 1967.

168. Street, H. R. The influence of aluminum sulfate and aluminum hydroxide upon the absorption of dietary phosphorus by the rat. *J. Nutr.* 24:111, 1942.

169. Streeto, J. M. Renal cortical adenyl cyclase: Effect of parathyroid hormone and calcium. *Metabolism* 18:968, 1969.

170. Strewler, G. J., Bernstein, D. S., and Pletka, P. Pseudo-vitamin D deficiency rickets (PDR) and relative hypoparathyroidism: A report of a family. *J. Clin. Endocrinol. Metab.* 37:220, 1973.

171. Suh, S., Fraser, D., and Kooh, S. W. Pseudohypoparathyroidism: Responsiveness to parathyroid extract induced by vitamin D_2 therapy. *J. Clin. Endocrinol. Metab.* 30:609, 1970.

172. Suh, S., Kosh, S. W., Chan, A. M., and Fraser, D. Pseudohypoparathyroidism: No improvement following total thyroidectomy. *J. Clin. Endocrinol. Metab.* 29:429, 1969.

173. Talwalkar, Y. B., Musgrave, J. E., Buist, N. R., Campbell, R. A., and Campbell, J. R. Vitamin D-resistant rickets and parathyroid adenomas: Renal transport of phosphate. *Am. J. Dis. Child.* 128:704, 1974.

174. Tapia, J., Stearns, G., and Ponseti, I. V. Vitamin D resistant rickets: A long term clinical study of eleven patients. *J. Bone Joint Surg. [Am.]* 46:935, 1964.

175. Tashjian, A. H., Jr., Frantz, A. G., and Lee, J. B. Pseudohypoparathyroidism: Assays of parathyroid hormone and thyrocalcitonin. *Proc. Natl. Acad. Sci. U.S.A.* 56:1138, 1966.

176. Teitelbaum, S. L., Rosenberg, E. M., Bates, M., and Avioli, L. V. The effects of phosphate and vitamin D therapy on osteopenia, hypophosphatemic osteomalacia of childhood. *Clin. Orthop.* 116:38, 1976.

177. Tenenhouse, H. S., and Scriver, C. R. Orthophosphate transport in the erythrocyte of normal subjects and of patients with x-linked hypophosphatemia. *J. Clin. Invest.* 55:644, 1975.

178. Thomas, W. C., Jr., and Fry, R. M. Parathyroid adenomas in chronic rickets. *Am. J. Med.* 49:404, 1970.

179. Urdanivia, E., Mataverde, A., and Cohen, M. P. Growth hormone secretion and sulfation factor activity in pseudohypoparathyroidism. *J. Lab. Clin. Med.* 86:772, 1975.

180. Van der Werfften Bosch, J. J. The syndrome of brachymetacarpal dwarfism (pseudo-pseudohypoparathyroidism) with and without gonadal dysgenesis. *Lancet* 1:69, 1959.

181. Villanueva, A. R., Ilnicki, L., Frost, H. M., and Arnstein, R. Measurement of the bone formation rate in a case of familial hypophosphatemic vitamin D resistant rickets. *J. Lab. Clin. Med.* 67:973, 1966.

182. Vitek, V., and Lang, D. J. Urinary excretion of cyclic adenosine 3'5' monophosphate in children of different ages. *J. Clin. Endocrinol. Metab.* 42:781, 1976.

183. Wade, J. S. The course of partial parathyroid insufficiency after thyroidectomy. *Br. J. Surg.* 52:497, 1965.

184. Walser, M. Protein binding of inorganic phosphate in plasma of normal subjects and patients with renal disease. *J. Clin. Invest.* 39:501, 1960.

185. Watson, L. Hypo-hyperparathyroidism. *Proc. R. Soc. Med.* 61:287, 1968.

186. Werder, E. A., Kind, H. P., Egert, F., Fischer, J. A., and Prader, A. Effective long-term treatment of pseudohypoparathyroidism with oral 1α-hydroxy- and 1,25-dihydroxycholecalciferol. *J. Pediatr.* 89: 266, 1976.

187. West, C. D., Blanton, J. C., Silverman, F. N., and Holland, N. H. Use of phosphate salts as an adjunct to vitamin D in the treatment of hypophosphatemic vitamin D refractory rickets. *J. Pediatr.* 64:469, 1964.

188. Wilber, J. F., and Slatopolsky, E. Hyperphosphatemia and tumoral calcinosis. *Ann. Intern. Med.* 64: 1044, 1968.

189. Williams, T. F., and Winters, R. W. Familial (Hereditary) Vitamin D-Resistant Rickets with Hypophosphatemia. In J. B. Stanbury, J. B. Wyngaarden, and D. S. Fredrickson (eds.), *The Metabolic Basis of Inherited Disease* (3rd ed.). New York: McGraw-Hill, 1972. P. 1465.

190. Winnacker, J. L., Becker, K. L., and Moore, C. F. Pseudohypoparathyroidism and selective deficiency of thyrotropin: An interesting association. *Metabolism* 16:644, 1967.

191. Winters, R. W., Graham, J. B., Williams, R. F., McFalls, V. W., and Burnett, C. H. A genetic study of familial hypophosphatemia and vitamin D resistant rickets with a review of the literature. *Medicine* 37:97, 1958.

192. Zampa, G. A., and Zucchelli, P. C. Pseudohypoparathyroidism and bone demineralization: Case report and metabolic studies. *J. Clin. Endocrinol. Metab.* 25:1616, 1965.

193. Zetterstrom, R., and Winberg, J. Primary vitamin D refractory rickets: II. Metabolic studies during treatment with massive doses of vitamin D. *Acta Paediatr. Scand.* 44:45, 1955.

194. Zisman, E., Lotz, M., Jenkins, M. E., and Bartter, F. C. Studies in pseudohypoparathyroidism. *Am. J. Med.* 46:464, 1969.

85. Renal Glucosuria

Johannes Brodehl

Physiologic Aspects

D-Glucose is freely filtered through the glomerular basement membrane and is almost completely reabsorbed from the tubular fluid by a combination of active and passive transport [33, 48, 109, 126, 132, 137]. In the rat more than 98 percent of filtered glucose is absorbed by the proximal tubules [48]. No net transport of glucose is found along Henle's loop and distal tubules, while in the collecting duct there is a small but definite fraction of glucose reabsorbed. Only 0.1 percent of filtered glucose appears in the final urine (for more physiologic details, see Mudge et al. [94] and Chap. 2).

BASAL GLUCOSURIA

In healthy, normoglycemic human subjects, only trace amounts of glucose can be detected in the final urine by specific, sensitive methods. The glucose concentration in noninfected urines is in the range of 2 to 30 mg per deciliter (equal to 0.1 to 1.7 mmol per liter) with a mean value of 6.5 ± 0.3 (S.E.) mg per deciliter [65]. The commonly used paper strip tests for glucose do not detect glucose below a concentration of 40 mg per deciliter. The amount of glucose excreted in the urine is about 65 mg per 24 hr (range, 32 to 93) in adults [43], or 217 ± 9 (S.E.) $\mu mol/min/1.73$ m^2 [65]. There is a slight positive correlation between glucose excretion and urine flow [65, 112], but no correlation exists with the plasma glucose levels within the physiologic range [101]. Endogenous glucose clearance averages 36.0 ± 4.3 (S.D.) $\mu l/min/1.73$m^2 [65].

Endogenous glucose excretion is independent of the maximal rate of tubular resorption of glucose and seems to be determined by the flow rate in the proximal tubules, as suggested by experiments in dogs [65]. It should be called *basal glucosuria* and is comparable to the basal aminoaciduria found in every normal subject. The existence of basal glucosuria is not included in the common definition of the renal threshold for glucose. The latter was originally defined when the laboratory methods were too insensitive to detect the trace amounts of glucose in normal urines. The appearance of glucose by those methods signals a gross increase in glucose excretion beyond the constant rate of basal glucosuria.

In newborn infants the urinary glucose concentration was found to be only slightly higher than in children or adults [10, 14]. An increase in urinary glucose concentration is observed in premature newborns [56], especially in those with gestational age below 30 weeks, in whom concentrations up to 150 mg per deciliter were observed [6]. In such very young premature infants, tubular glucose resorption was significantly lower than in older premature or full-term newborns, in whom it was found to be in the range of 99.4 percent [6].

RENAL GLUCOSE THRESHOLD

The renal threshold for glucose is the plasma glucose concentration at which frank glucosuria appears. In view of the presence of a basal glucosuria in normal subjects, as discussed above, the definition is rather imprecise. In the older literature the threshold was stated to be at plasma glucose concentrations between 140 and 190 mg per deciliter [122].

In an attempt to determine the glucose threshold more precisely, a glucose titration technique was used by Smith et al. [123] and by Reubi [102]; in these studies the plasma glucose is increased stepwise by intravenous infusion, and the urinary excretion is related to the actual amount of glucose filtered through the glomeruli. The glucose threshold is then defined by the ratio of the tubular resorption of glucose to the glomerular filtration rate (T_G/GFR) at the moment glucose appears in the urine. In view of the existence of a basal glucosuria, Elsas and Rosenberg [41] have tried to define the threshold even more precisely: A minimal threshold ($Fmin_G$) has been defined as the filtered load at which 1 mg per minute of glucose is excreted in the final urine. In seven normal adult subjects $Fmin_G$ was determined to be 224 ± 41 mg/min/1.73 m^2. No data on glucose titrations in infants and children are available in the literature. In dogs the threshold T_G/GFR was shown to increase slightly but significantly with age [7].

MAXIMAL TUBULAR GLUCOSE RESORPTION

Tubular resorption of glucose includes an active tubular process that can be saturated by increasing filtered loads of glucose and is therefore characterized by a tubular maximum (Tm_G). This was originally demonstrated in dogs by Shannon and Fisher [119] and was shown later by Smith et al. [123] to exist in man.

In the isolated perfused tubules of rabbits the transport maximum for glucose has been confirmed and was found to be independent of the perfusion rate [132]. In the isolated whole kidney of the rat, however, no Tm_G could be achieved [16]. The magnitude of Tm_G bears no direct relationship to the renal glucose threshold.

Values of Tm_G in adults, children, and infants reported in the literature [6, 19, 41, 49, 52, 76, 84, 91, 123, 125, 130, 131] are shown in Table 85-1. Variations are due mainly to different analytical methods and procedures used in determining Tm_G. There is a gradual decrease of Tm_G in older adults [90]. Children have the same values as adults when their data are corrected for surface area. The values for infants are significantly lower (Fig. 85-1); however, the lower values are not due to tubular immaturity, as suggested by Tudvad [130, 131], but rather to lower glomerular filtration rates with consequently lower filtered amounts of glucose. In our own study [19] in

infants aged $2\frac{1}{2}$ to 24 weeks, Tm_G values were found to be in the range of 147 to 318 with a mean of 213 ± 71 mg/min/1.73 m^2. Related to glomerular filtration rate (Tm_G/C_{In}; Fig. 85-2), however, Tm_G was the same in infants as in children (2.94 ± 0.74 versus 2.83 ± 0.47 mg/ml). Similar findings were reported in puppies [7] and in fetal sheep [3]. Therefore, in the handling of glucose there is no evidence for glomerulotubular imbalance in the perinatal and early postnatal period.

The Tm_G seems not to be independent from variations in the glomerular filtration rate, as was originally postulated by Shannon and Fisher [119] and later supported by other investigators [118, 128]. The early reports by Smith et al. [123] showed that Tm_G is positively correlated with the glomerular filtration rate and were subsequently confirmed by findings in man [19, 49, 136], in dogs [34, 54, 66, 72, 96, 100, 114], and in rats [16, 33, 134]. The data on infants and children demonstrate that there is a linear correlation between Tm_G and the glomerular filtration rate, as is

Table 85-1. Normal Values of Maximal Tubular Resorption of Glucose (Tm_G and Tm_G/GFR) in Adults, Children, and Infants

Authors	Tm_G (mg/min/ 1.73m^2; $X \pm$ S.D.)	Tm_G/C_{In} (mg/ml; $X \pm$ S.D.)	No. of Probands	Remarks, Method
Adults				
Smith et al. [123]	375 ± 80	2.70	24 male	Simultaneous iodopyracet
	303 ± 55	2.50	11 female	(Diodrast) loading in most cases
Letteri and Wesson [76]	306 ± 83	2.78	19	Reducing method
McPhaul and Simonaitis [84]	325 ± 36	2.34 ± 0.21	16	Glucose oxidase
Elsas and Rosenberg [41]	291 ± 27	2.38 ± 0.40	7	Glucose oxidase
Children				
Stalder [125]	304 ± 55	2.22	19 (4–16 yr)	Hagedorn Jensen
	401 ± 28	2.94	7 (4–16 yr)	Glucose oxidase
Grossmann and Zoellner [52]	254 ± 115	1.82	65 (3–15 yr)	Glucose oxidase; simultaneous para-aminohippurate loading
Brodehl et al. [19]	362 ± 96	2.83 ± 0.47	16 (1–13 yr)	Glucose oxidase
Infants				
Tudvad [130]	120–200*	—	4 (15–40 days)	Hagedorn Jensen
Gekle et al. [49]	36–288	0.90–2.38	8 (0.5–8 mo)	Hexokinase
Brodehl et al. [19]	213 ± 71	2.94 ± 0.74	8 (0.5–8 mo)	Glucose oxidase
Prematures				
Tudvad et al. [131]	59–175	2.31 (1.90–3.18)	7 (0.5–4.5 mo)	Hagedorn Jensen; simultaneous para-aminohippurate loading
Arant [6]		2.21–2.84	4 (24–28 wks gestational age)	

* Approximated values.

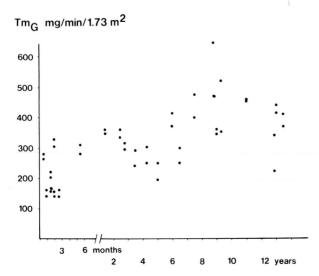

Figure 85-1. Values of maximal glucose resorption (Tm$_G$) in infants and children. Individual data are plotted against age. (Data from Brodehl et al. [18].)

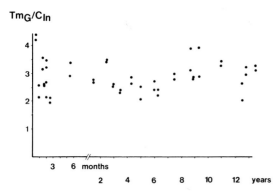

Figure 85-2. Values of Tm$_G$/C$_{In}$ in infants and children. (Data from Brodehl et al. [19].)

shown in Fig. 85-3, indicating that glomerulotubular balance in regard to glucose is maintained throughout the early period of extrauterine life [19].

THE GLUCOSE TITRATION SPLAY
Glucose titration studies reveal that the load of filtered glucose at which gross glucosuria starts, that is, at which the renal threshold is surpassed, is not identical with that which is necessary to achieve Tm$_G$, as might be expected theoretically. At renal threshold the ratio of the glucose loading to Tm$_G$ is in the range of 0.70 to 0.83; for Tm$_G$ the same ratio is 1.2 to 2.5 [76, 84, 123]. This phenomenon is designated the "splay" of the titration curve, indicating that the actual titration curve departs from the theoretical line [18, 102, 123]. The splay is interpreted as the consequence of heterogeneity in the nephron population [21,

98, 123]. Some nephrons have a relatively low capacity to reabsorb glucose, whereas others are capable of reabsorbing greater amounts and require higher glucose loads to become saturated. The whole kidney Tm$_G$ therefore, is the sum of the Tm$_G$ rates of the single nephrons. The existence of splay is also compatible with ordinary Michaelis-Menten kinetics for uptake by a single saturable system. The splay plays an important role in the recognition of renal glucosuria. It is schematically depicted in Fig. 85-4. Experimental studies have shown that splay is slightly greater in puppies than in adult dogs [7].

SOME FACTORS INFLUENCING TUBULAR
RESORPTION OF GLUCOSE AND SPLAY
There are some additional factors that influence T$_G$. Transepithelial glucose transport in the kidney is intimately related to active sodium transport [8, 9, 23, 68, 133; see 69, 70, 94, 113], as it is in the intestine [31]. It is therefore plausible that factors that change the rate of active sodium transport might also influence T$_G$. Extracellular fluid expansion lowers Tm$_G$ in the rat [11, 108, 134] and in the dog [57, 71, 114] and exaggerates the splay of the titration curve [11, 108]. Insulin in high doses reduces the Tm$_G$ [42, 90, 118], while growth hormone has the reverse effect [30, 72]. The glucoside phlorhizin exerts a competitive inhibition of T$_G$ by binding with the carrier substance on the luminal brush border [15, 24, 36, 120, 121, 135]. The binding of phlorhizin with the carrier substance is reversible and sodium dependent, as shown on isolated brush border particles [26, 45, 135]. Phlorhizin has a much higher affinity for the carrier recep-

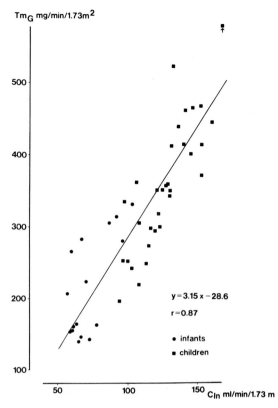

Tm$_G$ mg/min/1.73m^2

$y = 3.15 x - 28.6$

$r = 0.87$

• infants

■ children

C$_{In}$ ml/min/1.73 m

Figure 85-3. Correlation between maximal glucose resorption (Tm$_G$) *and glomerular filtration* (C$_{In}$) *in infants and children. (Data from Brodehl et al. [19].)*

tor than D-glucose [4]; it acts from the luminal side and does not penetrate into the intracellular space.

In addition to the active component of T$_G$, there is a small passive transport component; however, it plays no role in net glucose transport unless there are greatly increased transtubular concentration gradients, such as those found with a low glomerular filtration rate and high serum glucose concentrations [80]. In some experiments, especially in subjects with a low glomerular filtration rate, the Tm$_G$ was found to be related to the plasma glucose level [16, 19, 134]. There is no evidence of glucose secretion from the tubular cells to tubular urine [27]. A backflux of glucose from the periluminal to the luminal side seems to be minimal in the intact animal [12, 27]; however, it has been observed in isolated tubules [61, 132].

Clinical Aspects

DEFECTS OF TUBULAR GLUCOSE RESORPTION

Clinically, renal glucosuria can be defined as a condition characterized by constant glucosuria

without evidence of hyperglycemia, diabetes mellitus and other disturbances of carbohydrate metabolism, or renal insufficiency. The glucosuria is usually slight to moderate and rarely is severe. It can occur as a primary, isolated defect without any other tubular disturbances (primary renal glucosuria); it also may be part either of (1) a generalized tubulopathy due to metabolic diseases, intoxications, or other conditions, discussed in Chap. 81, or (2) a combined renal and intestinal defect of transepithelial glucose transport, as in the glucose-galactose malabsorption syndrome. Rarely, renal glucosuria is accompanied by other apparently primary tubular disturbances, as in glucoglycinuria or phosphate diabetes with glucosuria. Finally, slight and inconsistent renal glucosurias can be observed in various clinical conditions without recognizable pathomechanisms. These are mentioned under the term *unclassified glucosurias.*

PRIMARY RENAL GLUCOSURIA (BENIGN GLUCOSURIA)

Primary renal glucosuria is usually a benign condition that persists throughout life and needs no specific treatment. It is an inherited defect of tubular glucose resorption in which the handling of all other filtered substrates by the proximal tubules is completely normal.

Definitions of glucosuria and, consequently, the data on incidence and inheritance vary greatly in the literature. In order to avoid "an unwieldy hodgepodge of cases difficult to study" [83], stringent criteria should be used to define true renal glucosuria (see reference 69). The following criteria are based on Marble's definition [83]: (1) glucosuria should always be present; (2) the blood glucose levels should remain within normal ranges even during glucose tolerance tests; (3) the utilization of carbohydrates should be normal; (4) when ketosis develops it should be during starvation rather than following dietary excess; and (5) other types of melliturias (pentosuria, fructosuria, galactosuria, sucrosuria, maltosuria) and global renal insufficiency should be excluded. In this definition the many patients with intermittent renal glucosuria, postprandial glucosuria, starvation glucosuria, or glucosuria induced by a glucose loading test [74] are excluded. If Marble's criteria [83] are used, true renal glucosuria is not common. In the Joslin Clinic, Boston, the incidence of all melliturias was observed to be 0.17 percent [83]. Other studies report incidence rates of all melliturias ranging from 0.3 to 6.3 percent in otherwise normal populations [32, 55, 62].

There is no doubt concerning the familial incidence of primary renal glucosuria. However, the

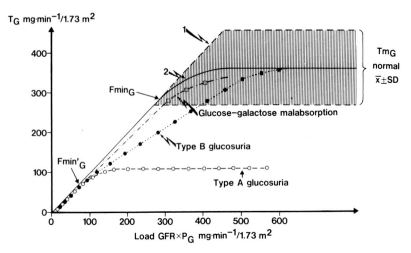

Figure 85-4. Renal tubular glucose resorption (T_G) *as a function of filtered load* (GFR × P_G). *Schematic drawing of normal and pathologic states. 1 = theoretical curve; 2 = actual curve found in normal humans;* $Fmin_G$ = *minimal renal glucose threshold in normal subjects;* $Fmin'_G$ = *minimal renal glucose threshold in renal glucosuria;* GFR = *glomerular filtration rate;* P_G = *plasma glucose concentration.*

type of inheritance is disputed. When just "glucosuria" has been used as the genetic discriminant in the affected families, a direct parent-to-offspring transmission has been observed and a dominant mode of inheritance has been postulated [20, 58, 59, 111]. This conclusion was questioned, however, by authors who used quantitative methods for evaluating the tubular defect. These investigators found that an autosomal recessive mode of transmission is the more probable type of inheritance [39, 41, 67].

In applying glucose titration methods with determination of the minimal renal glucose threshold ($Fmin_G$) and maximal capacity for glucose resorption (Tm_G), Elsas and coworkers [39] have been able to show that in type A renal glucosuria (see below) the homozygous state is accompanied by severe reduction in Tm_G leading to gross glucosuria, while in the presumed heterozygotes the defects in Tm_G and glucosuria are only mild. It remains uncertain whether type A and B renal glucosurias are really distinct genetic entities, since both types could be detected in a single family [41]. The glucose-galactose malabsorption syndrome with renal glucosuria can be separated clearly from primary renal glucosuria not accompanied by defects in intestinal glucose uptake [41]. It is probable that more than a single glucose transport site exists in the human kidney and that they may be under separate genetic control [39, 115].

Glucose titration studies in renal glucosurias reveal that two types can be differentiated on pathophysiologic grounds [17, 50, 102]; *type A*

[102] or true renal diabetes [50] is characterized by a low threshold and a low Tm_G; *type B* or pseudorenal diabetes shows a low threshold but a normal Tm_G (see Fig. 85-4). In type B, therefore, glucosuria is caused by an exaggerated splay in the titration curve. These findings may be considered analogous to in vivo enzyme saturation kinetics. Woolf and coworkers [140] derived a mathematical expression for the rate of resorption of glucose in a model nephron using Michaelis-Menten principles of enzyme kinetics. The curves closely resemble experimental results of glucose titration in normal human beings. When the expression for the number of carrier units is reduced, a curve resembling type A renal glucosuria emerges; and when the expression representing affinity is altered, a curve resembling type B renal glucosuria is found. These findings could indicate that type A renal glucosuria is the result of a reduced number of functioning glucose-binding sites, while type B is produced by an impaired affinity in the presence of a normal number of binding sites. A different, more morphologic explanation was put forward by Reubi [102], who suggested that type A renal glucosuria could be due to an overall reduction of active tubular length for glucose resorption and type B to an increased heterogeneity of the nephron population in regard to active glucose resorptive sites.

The separation of renal glucosuria into two distinct categories according to Tm_G has been questioned by other investigators [69, 93, 127]. The values of Tm_G reported in the literature in patients with renal glucosuria fail to demonstrate two clearly separable types, but rather provide a continuous distribution from lowest to highest values [69]. In our own experience with eight children with renal glucosuria from seven different families (Table 85-2), no distinct separation into the two types was observed. There may be two explanations for these conflicting findings. First, the different techniques used in various centers might not permit interpretable comparisons of the data, since type and duration of infusion and glucose loading and changes in extracellular fluid volume may interfere with tubular handling of glucose. Second, the individuals studied may be genetically heterogeneous, representing both heterozygous and homozygous states of different types of glucosurias. Therefore, quantitative studies with glucose titrations in individual families are required to clarify the genetic and pathophysiologic classification of renal glucosurias, as in the studies by Elsas and coworkers [39, 41].

A third type of renal glucosuria was postulated by Chaptal and coworkers [25]. They observed a progressive decrease in T_G in a 15-year-old girl in whom Tm_G dropped from 439 to 4.3 mg per minute during the glucose loading. Although a degree of "fatiguing" in glucose resorption was also observed by other authors (see reference 79), it was not to the severe degree reported by Chaptal et al. The postulated third type of renal glucosuria therefore remains hypothetical.

In addition to the determination of Tm_G and threshold, the splay of the glucose titration curve has to be evaluated, as demonstrated by McPhaul

Table 85-2. *Renal Handling of Glucose in Eight Children from Seven Families with Primary Renal Glucosuria*

Age (yr)	Threshold T_G/C_{In} (mg/ml)	Maximal Glucose Resorption (Tm_G) (mg/min/ 1.73 m^2)	Tm_G/C_{In} (mg/ml)
4	?	113	0.89
10	0.70	114	1.12
7	?	113	1.20
3	0.97	130	1.39
11	0.71	205	1.67
3	0.72	291	2.17
4	1.18	292	2.65
4	0.89	301	2.42

Source: author's data.
Note: T_G/C_{In} = ratio between glucose resorption and glomerular filtration rate; Tm_G/C_{In} = ratio between maximal glucose resorption and glomerular filtration rate as measured by the clearance of inulin.

and Simonaitis [84]. In their report, 6 of 14 patients with renal glucosuria had low values of Tm_G, while the remainder had normal values. However, all of them exhibited abnormally exaggerated splays in the titration curve. The splay points (T_G/Tm_G, where splay starts) in the glucosuric groups were 0.60 and 0.56, respectively, contrasted with a normal value of 0.83 ± 0.04.

The urinary glucose excretion in primary renal glucosuria is in the range of 5 to 30 gm per day and may occasionally approach 100 gm per day. There are usually no clinical signs of hypoglycemia or ketosis, however. Polyuria and polydipsia are usually absent. The patients lead a normal life and need no treatment. The only danger is that renal glucosuria may be mistaken for diabetes mellitus and the patient treated with insulin. The condition can be diagnosed as early as the first month of life [59] and seems to remain constant thereafter [83, 105]. All other kidney function tests (glomerular filtration rate, para-aminohippurate clearance, resorption of phosphate and free amino acids, urinary acidification) are normal. A high urinary lactate excretion has been reported by Anderson and Mazza [5], who suggest that the tubular resorption of lactate may be disturbed in this condition.

A few patients with renal glucosuria have subsequently developed true diabetes mellitus [2, 37]. It seems most likely, however, that these patients have had two disturbances and that no causal interrelation exists between the two conditions [83, 106]. On the other hand, true diabetes mellitus might be accompanied by a lowered renal threshold for glucose [95, 107], which has been found in as many as one third of all diabetics studied [92].

Morphologic studies of kidney specimens have failed to detect specific features of primary renal glucosuria [47, 75, 88, 103]. The finding by electron microscopy of marked changes in the proximal tubular epithelium in 2 patients with glucosuria [93] has not been confirmed by other investigators.

CONGENITAL GLUCOSE-GALACTOSE MALABSORPTION

The congenital malabsorption syndrome of glucose and galactose has been known since 1962 [73, 77, 78]. More than 20 cases have been described (see reference 51), and with one exception, all of those carefully tested have shown a mild defect in renal T_G. The disease is characterized by severe, watery diarrhea that starts directly after birth. The stools are acid and contain large amounts of glucose and galactose. The symptoms lead to severe dehydration and malnutrition unless the patients are treated by replacing all ordinary carbohydrates by fructose. The intestinal defect is due to the absence of active glucose-galactose transport systems in the jejunum [40, 86]. It is an inherited defect that is transmitted as an autosomal recessive trait [87]. The heterozygotes exhibit an intermediate defect in intestinal glucose uptake [40].

The renal defect in glucose resorption seems to be present only in homozygotes [40, 85]. It is usually mild, the daily urinary glucose excretion being in the range of 0.4 to 1.0 gm. Glucose titration studies reveal a reduced minimal threshold for glucose [40, 79]; however, Tm_G is only slightly reduced or even normal [1, 13, 40, 85]. The only exception to these findings seems to be the patient of Liu et al. [79], in whom there was a severe reduction in Tm_G accompanied by a low glomerular filtration rate and a fatigue of glucose resorption after loading. The renal defect in glucose-galactose malabsorption, therefore, resembles a mild type B renal glucosuria. Since it is associated with the severe intestinal defect, it is postulated that this syndrome might be produced by a mutation of a gene locus different from that for primary renal glucosuria [115].

COMBINED TUBULAR DEFECTS
WITH GLUCOSURIA

There are a few reports in the literature describing patients with a combination of renal glucosuria and other primary tubular defects that are not part of a generalized tubulopathy such as the Fanconi syndrome. This distinction is especially true for familial glucoglycinuria [63, 64] and for some patients with phosphate diabetes and glucosuria [35], sometimes occurring in combination with hyperglycinuria [116, author's unpublished case]. Other combinations, on the other hand, such as the glucohyperaminoacidurias [53, 81, 97], seem not to be primary tubulopathies but rather incomplete Fanconi syndromes or transitional stages of the Fanconi syndrome in which the primary mechanism may be related to disturbances in intracellular metabolism but not to defects in membrane carrier sites. Such combinations therefore will not be discussed here.

Glucoglycinuria was observed in a 9-year-old boy who suffered from cystic fibrosis with pulmonary involvement [63, 64]. His urinary glucose excretion was 2 to 4 gm per day, and the glucose titration curve revealed a low threshold for glucose (79 mg/100 ml) but a normal Tm_G (386 mg/min/1.73 m²) and Tm_G/C_{In} (2.89 mg/ml).

These findings were interpreted as characteristic of type B renal glucosuria. In addition, this patient demonstrated a constant hyperglycinuria with daily glycine excretion rates of 200 to 300 mg and occasionally up to 600 to 700 mg. The amino acid determinations were done by paper chromatography, high-voltage paper electrophoresis, and by microbiologic methods. Plasma amino acids were normal, as were the excretion of all other free amino acids and other tubular functions, including phosphate resorption. Familial studies revealed that 13 apparently normal members of 45 persons tested also exhibited glucoglycinuria. Neither of the two abnormalities occurred alone. It was concluded that this condition is probably inherited as an autosomal dominant trait. No other reports describing the same syndrome have appeared in the literature. This condition has to be differentiated from isolated hyperglycinuria, iminoglycinuria, and generalized types of hyperaminoacidurias in which glycine hyperexcretion is also a prominent feature (see Chap. 86).

The combination of renal phosphate diabetes with renal glucosuria was first mentioned as an entity by Dent [35], who reported four cases. All occurred in adults, and only one had consistent glucosuria (> 0.5 percent). The main clinical feature is osteomalacia due to decreased tubular resorption of phosphate and hypophosphatemia. Some earlier reports might have included similar cases [29, 60, 89]; however, they cannot be distinguished from idiopathic Fanconi syndromes, since exact data on amino acids are not available. In some other reports on familial and sporadic vitamin-D-resistant rickets, a mild and mostly inconsistent glycosuria has been mentioned [22, 46] (see reference 139); none of them, however, fulfills the stringent criteria of true renal glycosuria. The only case of true renal glucosuria with hypophosphatemic rickets was that reported by Magid et al. [82]. A 16-year-old boy had hypophosphatemic rickets and a renal glucosuria of 9.47 gm per day. His Tm_G was 286 mg/min/1.73 m². His mother, who also suffered from hypophosphatemia, had no glucosuria. The combination of phosphate diabetes with true renal glucosuria, therefore, seems to be a very rare entity.

Finally, a special combination of disturbed tubular resorption of phosphate, glucose, and glycine has been described by Scriver and coworkers [116]. The patient, a boy, first developed signs of rickets at the age of 9 years. Seven years later he was found to have extreme hypophosphatemia and very low tubular resorption of phosphate. The renal glucose threshold was 78 mg per deciliter then, and Tm_G was markedly decreased. Glycine clearance was in the range of 6.5 to 16.7 ml/min/1.73 m², and the percentage of tubular resorption of glycine was below 91 percent. The results of investigations of the family were negative. Recently a similar nonfamilial case with this syndrome was observed in our clinic [19a]. In early childhood the boy had developed hypophosphatemic rickets that was resistant to ordinary doses of vitamin D. At the age of 4 years glucosuria was noted that persisted until he was 17 years old. The daily amounts of glucose excreted in the urine were in the range of 10 to 40 gm. Endogenous glucose clearance was greatly increased ($C_G = 14.6$ ml/min/1.73 m²), and glucose threshold (T_G/C_{In}) was in the range of 70 mg per deciliter. The Tm_G was not determined. Except for glycine, there was no hyperaminoaciduria. Endogenous glycine clearance was 11.6 ml/min/1.73 m², and the percentage of glycine resorption was 89.4 percent. The boy received high oral phosphate substitution and vitamin D (50,000 to 100,000 U/day); he is fully active and has now reached the height of 172 cm.

UNCLASSIFIED GLUCOSURIAS

In addition to the specific types mentioned above, a nonspecific type of glucosuria is encountered rather frequently in nondiabetic subjects. These glucosurias are usually mild and are intermittent or episodic. They are often associated with several nonspecific conditions, and their pathologic mechanisms are mostly obscure. In these patients the glucosuria could result from a transient elevation of plasma glucose above the normal renal threshold, in which case it would then not be of renal origin; or it could be due to a greater inhomogeneity of the nephron population, and would then resemble a mild type B renal glucosuria. Since mechanisms and causes are so variable, this nonspecific type of glucosuria was called by Marble [83] "unclassified glucosuria." It is found in endocrine disorders such as hyperthyroidism, hyperpituitarism, and adrenal hypercorticism; in central nervous disorders such as brain tumors, injuries, or hemorrhages; in dietary alterations leading to alimentary or hunger glucosuria; in infections, toxemias, and anesthesias; in hypertension, cirrhosis of the liver, and malignant disorders; and in intoxications [83]. Patients with these findings should first be followed frequently in order not to miss the early stages of diabetes mellitus. Diagnostic procedures should include careful evaluation of the patient's history and hereditary background, quantitative examination of urinary glu-

cose before and 1 hr after a meal or a 50-gm glucose load, determination of glucose in the blood after a meal, and, in doubtful cases, a regular glucose tolerance test [83].

Finally, there are two conditions in which renal glucosuria is a rather common finding, and therefore the term *unclassified glucosuria* is not quite justified. These conditions occur during pregnancy and with severe renal insufficiency. Most pregnant women exhibit some glucosuria, mainly in the second half of pregnancy [44, 124]. This glucosuria is due to a lowered renal threshold for glucose in the presence of elevated glomerular filtration rates [28, 138]. When the glomerular filtration rate is below 15 ml/min/1.73 m² in chronic renal insufficiency, the splay of the glucose titration curve is abnormally exaggerated and is associated with intermittent glucosuria of a mild to moderate degree [84, 104, 117].

References

1. Abraham, J. M., Levin, B., Oberholzer, V. G., and Russell, A. Glucose-galactose malabsorption. *Arch. Dis. Child.* 42:592, 1967.
2. Ackerman, I. P., Fajans, S. S., and Conn, J. W. The development of diabetes mellitus in patients with non diabetic glycosuria. *Clin. Res. Proc.* 6:251, 1958.
3. Alexander, D. P., and Nixon, D. A. Reabsorption of glucose, fructose and mesoinositol by the foetal and post-natal sheep kidney. *J. Physiol.* 167:480, 1963.
4. Alvarado, F. Hypothesis for the interaction of phlorizin and phloretin with membrane carriers for sugars. *Biochim. Biophys. Acta* 135:483, 1967.
5. Anderson, J., and Mazza, R. Pyruvate and lactate excretion in patients with diabetes mellitus and benign glycosuria. *Lancet* 2:270, 1963.
6. Arant, B. S. Intrauterine and extrauterine patterns of renal functional maturation compared in the human neonate (abstract). *Pediatr. Res.* 9:373, 1975.
7. Arant, B. S., Edelmann, C. M., and Nash, M. A. The renal reabsorption of glucose in the developing canine kidney: A study of glomerulotubular balance. *Pediatr. Res.* 8:638, 1974.
8. Aronson, P. S., and Sacktor, B. Transport of D-glucose by brush border membranes isolated from the renal cortex. *Biochim. Biophys. Acta* 356:231, 1974.
9. Aronson, P. S., and Sacktor, B. The Na⁺ gradient-dependent transport of D-glucose in renal brush border membranes. *J. Biol. Chem.* 250:6032, 1975.
10. Bachmann, K.-D., and Dominick, H. C. Über die Ausscheidung von Glucose und Fructose im Harn des reifen Neugeborenen (enzymatische Bestimmungen). *Monatsschr. Kinderheilkd.* 118:290, 1970.
11. Baines, A. D. Effect of extracellular fluid volume expansion on maximum glucose reabsorption rate and glomerular tubular balance in single rat nephrons. *J. Clin. Invest.* 50:2414, 1971.
12. Banks, R. O., and Foulkes, E. C. Quantitation of urinary precession of water, potassium and other solutes. *Am. J. Physiol.* 220:1325, 1971.

13. Beauvais, P., Vaudour, G., Desjeux, J.-F., Le Balle, J.-C., Girot, J.-Y., and Brissaud, H. E. La malabsorption congénitale du glucose-galactose. *Arch. Fr. Pediatr.* 28:573, 1971.

14. Bickel, H. Mellituria, a paper chromatographic study. *J. Pediatr.* 59:641, 1961.

15. Bode, F., Baumann, K., Frasch, W., and Kinne, R. Die Bindung von Phlorrhizin an die Bürstensaumfraktion der Rattenniere. *Pfluegers Arch.* 315:53, 1970.

16. Bowman, R. H., and Maack, T. Glucose transport by the isolated rat kidney. *Am. J. Physiol.* 222:1499, 1972.

17. Bradley, S. E., Bradley, G. P., Tyson, C. J., Curry, J. J., and Blake, W. D. Renal function in renal diseases. *Am. J. Med.* 9:766, 1950.

18. Bradley, S. E., Laragh, J. H., Wheeler, H. O., MacDowell, M., and Oliver, J. Correlation of structure and function in the handling of glucose by the nephrons of the canine kidney. *J. Clin. Invest.* 40:1113, 1961.

19. Brodehl, J., Franken, A., and Gellissen, K. Maximal tubular reabsorption of glucose in infants and children. *Acta Paediatr. Scand.* 61:413, 1972.

19a. Brodehl, J., and Krohn, H. P. Unpublished data, 1977.

20. Brown, M. S., and Poleshuk, R. Familial renal glucosuria. *J. Lab. Clin. Med.* 20:605, 1935.

21. Burgen, A. S. V. A theoretical treatment of glucose reabsorption in the kidney. *Can. J. Biochem.* 34: 466, 1956.

22. Burnett, C. H., Dent, C. E., Harper, C., and Warland, B. J. Vitamin D-resistant rickets: Analysis of twenty-four pedigrees with hereditary and sporadic cases. *Am. J. Med.* 36:222, 1964.

23. Busse, D., Jahn, A., and Steinmaier, G. Carriermediated transfer of D-glucose in brush border vesicles derived from rabbit renal tubules: N+-dependent versus Na+-independent transfer. *Biochim. Biophys. Acta* 401:231, 1975.

24. Chan, S. S., and Lotspeich, W. D. Comparative effects of phlorizin and phloretin on glucose transport in the cat kidney. *Am. J. Physiol.* 203:975, 1962.

25. Chaptal, J., Benezech, C., Jean, R., Campo, C., and Dejeanne, M.-G. Étude sur le diabète rènal chez l'enfant: Exploration biologique de deux cas; Discussion nosologique. *Arch. Fr. Pediatr.* 11:273, 1954.

26. Chertok, R. J., and Lake, S. Evidence for a single kind· of D-glucose binding site on renal brush borders. *Biochim. Biophys. Acta* 339:202, 1974.

27. Chinard, F. P., Taylor, W. R., Nolan, M. F., and Enns, T. Renal handling of glucose in dogs. *Am. J. Physiol.* 196:535, 1959.

28. Christensen, P. J. Tubular reabsorption of glucose during pregnancy. *Scand. J. Clin. Lab. Invest.* 10: 364, 1958.

29. Cooke, W. T., Barclay, J. A., Govan, A. D. T., and Nagley, L. Osteoporosis associated with low serum phosphorus and renal glycosuria. *Arch. Intern. Med.* 80:147, 1947.

30. Corvilain, J., and Abramow, M. Effect of growth hormone on tubular reabsorption of glucose and phosphate. *Nature* 213:85, 1967.

31. Crane, R. K. Hypothesis for mechanism of intestinal active transport of sugars. *Fed. Proc.* 21:891, 1962.

32. Crombie, D. L. Incidence of glycosuria and diabetes. *Proc. R. Soc. Med.* 55:205, 1961.

33. Deetjen, P., and Boylan, J. W. Glucose reabsorption in the rat kidney. *Pfluegers Arch.* 299:19, 1968.

34. Dempster, W. J., Eggleton, M. G., and Shuster, S. The effect of hypertonic infusions on glomerular filtration rate and glucose reabsorption in the kidney of the dog. *J. Physiol. (Lond.).* 132:213, 1956.

35. Dent, C. E. Rickets and osteomalacia from renal tubule defects. *J. Bone Joint Surg. [Br.]* 34:266, 1952.

36. Diedrich, D. E. Glucose transport carrier in dog kidney: Its concentration and turnover number. *Am. J. Physiol.* 211:581, 1966.

37. Drucker, W. D., Fitch, R. F., and Caston, J. H. Diabetes mellitus and preexisting renal glycosuria. *Arch. Intern. Med.* 110:199, 1962.

38. Dubois, R., Loeb, H., Eggermont, E., and Mainguet, P. Etude clinique et biochimique d'un cas de malabsorption congénitale du glucose et du galactose. *Helv. Paediat. Acta* 21:577, 1966.

39. Elsas, L. J., Busse, D., and Rosenberg, L. E. Autosomal recessive inheritance of renal glycosuria. *Metabolism* 20:968, 1971.

40. Elsas, L. J., Hillman, R. E., Patterson, J. H., and Rosenberg, L. E. Renal and intestinal hexose transport in familial glucose-galactose malabsorption. *J. Clin. Invest.* 49:576, 1970.

41. Elsas, L. J., and Rosenberg, L. E. Familial renal glucosuria: A genetic reappraisal of hexose transport by kidney and intestine. *J. Clin. Invest.* 48: 1845, 1969.

42. Farber, S. J., Berger, E. Y., and Earle, D. P. Effect of diabetes and insulin on the maximum capacity of the renal tubules to reabsorb glucose. *J. Clin. Invest.* 30:125, 1951.

43. Fine, J. Glucose content of normal urine. *Br. Med. J.* 2:1209, 1965.

44. Fine, J. Glycosuria of pregnancy. *Br. Med. J.* 1: 205, 1967.

45. Frasch, W., Frohnert, P. P., Bode, F., Baumann, K., and Kinne, R. Competitive inhibition of phlorizin binding by D-glucose and the influence of sodium: A study on isolated brush border membrane of rat kidney. *Pfluegers Arch.* 320:265, 1970.

46. Freeman, S., and Dunsky, J. Resistant rickets. *Am. J. Dis. Child.* 79:409, 1950.

47. Freeman, J. A., and Roberts, K. E. A fine structural study of renal glucosuria. *Exp. Mol. Pathol.* 2:83, 1963.

48. Frohnert, P. P., Höhmann, B., Zwiebel, R., and Baumann, K. Free flow micropuncture studies of glucose transport in the rat nephron. *Pfluegers Arch.* 315:66, 1970.

49. Gekle, D., Janovsky, M., Slechtova, R., and Martinek, J. Einfluss der glomerulären Filtrationsrate auf die tubuläre Glucosereabsorption bei Kindern. *Klin. Wochenschr.* 45:416, 1967.

50. Govaerts, P. Physiopathology of glucose excretion by the human kidney. *Br. Med. J.* 2:175, 1952.

51. Gray, G. M. Intestinal Disaccharidase Deficiency and Glucose-Galactose Malabsorption. In J. B. Stanbury, J. B. Wyngaarden, and D. S. Fredrickson (eds.), *The Metabolic Basis of Inherited Disease* (4th ed.). New York: McGraw-Hill, 1978. P. 1526.

52. Grossmann, P., and Zoellner, K. Bestimmung der Funktionsfähigkeit des proximalen Tubulus mit

Hilfe von Glukose und p-Aminohippursäure bei Kindern. *Acta Biol. Med. Germ.* 20:413, 1968.

53. Halvorsen, S., and Aas, K. Renal tubular defects in fibrous dysplasia of the bones: Report of two cases. *Acta Paediatr. Scand.* 50:297, 1961.

54. Handley, C. A., Sigafoos, R. B., and La Forge, M. Proportional changes in renal tubular reabsorption of dextrose and excretion of p-aminohippurate with changes in glomerular filtration. *Am. J. Physiol.* 159:175, 1949.

55. Harkness, J. Prevalence of glycosuria and diabetes mellitus: A comprehensive survey in an urban community. *Br. Med. J.* 1:1503, 1962.

56. Haworth, J. C., and MacDonald, M. S. Reducing sugars in the urine and blood of premature babies. *Arch. Dis. Child.* 32:417, 1957.

57. Higgins, J. T., and Meinders, A. E. Quantitative relationship of renal glucose and sodium reabsorption during ECF expansion. *Am. J. Physiol.* 229:66, 1975.

58. Hjärne, V. A study of orthoglycaemic glycosuria with particular reference to its hereditability. *Acta Med. Scand.* 67:422, 1927.

59. Horowitz, L., and Schwarzer, S. Renal glycosuria: Occurrence in two siblings and a review of the literature. *J. Pediatr.* 47:634, 1955.

60. Hunter, D. Studies in calcium and phosphorus metabolism in generalized disease of bones. *Proc. R. Soc. Med.* 28:1619, 1935.

61. Imai, M., and Kokko, J. P. Effects of peritubular protein concentration on reabsorption of sodium and water in isolated perfused proximal tubules. *J. Clin. Invest.* 51:414, 1972.

62. Jackson, W. P. U., Marine, N., and Vinik, A. I. The significance of glycosuria. *Lancet* 1:933, 1968.

63. Käser, H., Cottier, P., and Antener, I. Die Glukoglycinurie, ein neues familiäre Snydrom. *Helv. Paediatr. Acta* 16:586, 1961.

64. Käser, H., Cottier, P., and Antener, I. Glucoglycinuria, a new familial syndrome. *J. Pediatr.* 61:386, 1962.

65. Keller, D. M. Glucose excretion in man and dog. *Nephron* 5:43, 1968.

66. Keyes, J. L., and Swanson, R. E. Dependence of glucose Tm on GFR and tubular volume in the dog kidney. *Am. J. Physiol.* 221:1, 1971.

67. Khachadurian, A. K., and Khachadurian, L. A. The inheritance of renal glycosuria. *Am. J. Hum. Genet.* 16:189, 1964.

68. Kleinzeller, A., Kolínská, J., and Beneš, I. Transport of glucose and galactose in kidney-cortex cells. *Biochem. J.* 104:843, 1967.

69. Krane, S. M. Renal Glycosuria. In J. B. Stanbury, J. B. Wyngaarden, and D. S. Fredrickson (eds.), *The Metabolic Basis of Inherited Disease* (3rd ed.). New York: McGraw-Hill, 1972.

70. Kurtzman, N. A., and Pillay, V. K. G. Renal reabsorption of glucose in health and disease. *Arch. Intern. Med.* 131:901, 1973.

71. Kurtzman, N. A., White, M. G., Rogers, P. W., and Flynn, J. J., III. Relationship of sodium reabsorption and glomerular filtration rate to renal glucose reabsorption. *J. Clin. Invest.* 51:127, 1972.

72. Kwong, T.-F., and Bennett, C. M. Relationship between glomerular filtration rate and maximum tubular reabsorptive rate of glucose. *Kidney Int.* 5:23, 1974.

73. Laplane, R., Polonovski, C., Etienne, M., Debray, P., Lods, J.-C., and Pissarro, B. L'intolérance aux sucres a transfert intestinal actif: Ses rapports avec l'intolérance au lactose et le syndrome coeliaque. *Arch. Fr. Pediatr.* 19:895, 1962.

74. Lawrence, R. D. Symptomless glucosuria: Differentiation by sugar tolerance tests. *Med. Clin. North Am.* 31:289, 1947.

75. Leonardi, P., Ruol, A., and Munari, R. Morphological aspects of renal glycosuria. *Am. J. Med. Sci.* 239:721, 1960.

76. Letteri, J. M., and Wesson, L. G. Glucose titration curves as an estimate of intrarenal distribution of glomerular filtrate in patients with congestive heart failure. *J. Lab. Clin. Med.* 65:387, 1965.

77. Lindquist, B., and Meeuwisse, G. W. Chronic diarrhea caused by monosaccharide malabsorption. *Acta Paediatr. Scand.* 51:674, 1962.

78. Lindquist, B., Meeuwisse, G. W., and Melin, K. Glucose-galactose malabsorption. *Lancet* 2:666, 1962.

79. Liu, H.-Y., Anderson, G. J., Tsao, M. U., Moore, B. F., and Giday, Z. Tm glucose in a case of congenital intestinal and renal malabsorption of monosaccharides. *Pediatr. Res.* 1:386, 1967.

80. Loeschke, K., Baumann, K., Renschler, H., Ullrich, K. J., and Fuchs, G. Differenzierung zwischen aktiver und passiver Komponente des D-Glucosetransports am proximalen Konvolut der Rattenniere. *Pfluegers Arch.* 305:118, 1969.

81. Luder, J., and Sheldon, W. Familial tubular absorption defect of glucose and amino acids. *Arch. Dis. Child.* 30:160, 1955.

82. Magid, G. J., Maloney, J. R., Sirota, J. H., and Schwab, E. A. Familial hypophosphatemia: Studies on its pathogenesis in an affected mother and son. *Ann. Intern. Med.* 64:1009, 1966.

83. Marble, A. Nondiabetic Melituria. In A. Marble, P. White, R. F. Bradley, and L. P. Krall (eds.), *Joslin's Diabetes Mellitus* (11th ed.). Philadelphia: Lea & Febiger, 1971.

84. McPhaul, J. J., and Simonaitis, J. J. Observations on the mechanisms of glucosuria during glucose loads in normal and nondiabetic subjects. *J. Clin. Invest.* 47:702, 1968.

85. Meeuwisse, G. W. Glucose-galactose malabsorption: Studies on renal glucosuria. *Helv. Paediatr. Acta* 25:13, 1970.

86. Meeuwisse, G. W., and Dahlqvist, A. Glucose-galactose malabsorption: A study with biopsy of the small intestinal mucosa. *Acta Paediatr. Scand.* 57:273, 1968.

87. Melin, K., and Meeuwisse, G. W. Glucose-galactose malabsorption. *Acta Paediatr. Scand.* [Suppl.] 188:19, 1969.

88. Michon, P., Larcan, A., Rauber, G., and Huriet, C. Étude biologique de 3 cas de diabète rénal étudiés par ponction-biopsie du rein. *J. Urol. Med. Chir.* 65:643, 1959.

89. Milkman, L. A. Multiple spontaneous idiopathic symmetrical fractures. *Am. J. Roentgenol.* 32:622, 1934.

90. Miller, J. H. Effect of insulin on maximal rate of renal tubular uptake of glucose in non-diabetic humans. *Proc. Soc. Exp. Biol. Med.* 84:322, 1953.

91. Miller, J. H., McDonald, R. K., and Shock, H. W. Age changes in the maximal rate of renal tubular reabsorption of glucose. *J. Gerontol.* 7:196, 1952.

92. Mohnicke, G., Lisewski, F., and Israel, J. H. Die

Eintrittsschwelle für Glukose bei Diabetes mellitus und Diabetes renalis. *Z. Gesamte. Inn. Med.* 16: 1073, 1961.

93. Monasterio, G., Olivers, J., Muiesan, G., Pardelli, G., Marinozzi, V., and MacDowell, M. Renal diabetes as a congenital tubular dysplasia. *Am. J. Med.* 37:44, 1964.

94. Mudge, G. H., Berndt, W. O., and Valtin, H. Tubular Transport of Urea, Glucose, Phosphate, Uric Acid, Sulfate, and Thiosulfate. In J. Orloff, R. W. Berliner, and S. R. Geiger (eds.), *Handbook of Physiology.* Section 8, *Renal Physiology.* Washington, D.C.: American Physiological Society, 1973.

95. Nelson, A. R., Perkoff, G. T., and Tyler, F. H. Renal glucosuria in pre-existing diabetes. *Arch. Intern. Med.* 113:649, 1964.

96. Nizet, A., Dujardin, A., Thoumsin, H., and Thoumsin-Moons, J. Excretion and tubular reabsorption of sodium, glucose and phosphate by isolated dog kidneys: Influence of blood dilution. *Pfluegers Arch.* 332:248, 1972.

97. Oetliker, O., Käser, H., Donath, A., and Rossi, E. Beitrag zur Familiarität der idiopathischen Gluko-Hyperaminoacidurie. *Helv. Paediatr. Acta* 19:556, 1964.

98. Oliver, J., and MacDowell, M. The structural and functional aspects of the handling of glucose by the nephrons and the kidney and their correlation by means of structural-functional equivalents. *J. Clin. Invest.* 40:1093, 1961.

99. Peterson, J. I. Urinary glucose measurement. *Clin. Chem.* 14:513, 1968.

100. Pitesky, J., and Last, J. H. Effects of seasonal heat stress on glomerular and tubular functions in the dog. *Am. J. Physiol.* 164:497, 1951.

101. Renschler, H. E., Weicker, H., and von Bayer, H. Die obere Normgrenze der Glukose-Konzentration im Urin Gesunder. *Dtsch. Med. Wochenschr.* 90: 3249, 1965.

102. Reubi, F. C. Glucose Titration in Renal Glycosuria. In A. A. G. Lewis and G. E. W. Wolstenholme (eds.), *The Kidney* (Ciba Foundation Symposium). Boston: Little, Brown, 1954.

103. Reubi, F. C., and Cottier, H. Un nouveau cas de diabète rénal avec controle histologique par ponction-biopsie. *J. Urol. Med. Chir.* 65:243, 1959.

104. Rieselbach, R. E., Shankel, S. W., Slatopolsky, E., Lubowitz, H., and Bricker, N. S. Glucose titration studies in patients with chronic progressive renal disease. *J. Clin. Invest.* 46:157, 1967.

105. Robbers, H., and Rümelin, K. Verlauf und Prognose des renalen Diabetes: Eine Nachuntersuchung von 60 Fällen. *Dtsch. Arch. Klin. Med.* 200:398, 1953.

106. Robbers, H., and Rümelin, K. Geht der renale Diabetes in einen echten Diabetes mellitus über? *Dtsch. Med. Wochenschr.* 78:1321, 1953.

107. Robertson, J. A., and Gray, C. H. Mechanism of lowered renal threshold for glucose in diabetes. *Lancet* 2:12, 1953.

108. Robson, A. M., Srivastava, P. L., and Bricker, N. S. The influence of saline loading on renal glucose reabsorption in the rat. *J. Clin. Invest.* 47:329, 1968.

109. Rohde, R., and Deetjen, P. Die Glucoseresorption in der Rattenniere: Mikropunktionsanalysen der tubulären Glucosekonzentration bei freiem Fluss. *Pfluegers Arch.* 302:219, 1968.

110. Schersten, B., and Fritz, H. Subnormal levels of glucose in urine. *J.A.M.A.* 20:949, 1967.

111. Schnell, A. Das Wesen der essentiellen renalen Glukosurie und ihre Beziehung zum Diabetes mellitus, unter besonderer Berücksichtigung der Erblichkeitsfrage. *Acta Med. Scand.* 92:153, 1937.

112. Schubert, G. E., Schuster, H. P., and Baum, P. Physiologische Glucosurie bei verschiedenen Diuresezuständen. *Klin. Wochenschr.* 42:619, 1964.

113. Schultz, S. G., and Curran, P. F. Coupled transport of sodium and organic solutes. *Physiol. Rev.* 50:637, 1970.

114. Schultze, R. G., and Berger, H. The influence of GFR and saline expansion on Tm_G of the dog kidney. *Kidney Int.* 3:291, 1973.

115. Scriver, C. R., Chesney, R. W., and McInnes, R. R. Genetic aspects of renal tubular transport: Diversity and topology of carriers. *Kidney Int.* 9:149, 1976.

116. Scriver, C. R., Goldbloom, R. B., and Roy, C. Hypophosphatemic rickets with renal hyperglycinuria, renal glucosuria and glycylprolinuria. *Pediatrics* 34:351, 1964.

117. Shankel, S. W., Robson, A. M., and Bricker, N. S. On the mechanism of the splay in the glucose titration curve in advanced experimental renal disease in the rat. *J. Clin. Invest.* 46:164, 1967.

118. Shannon, J. A., Farber, S., and Troast, L. The measurement of glucose Tm in the normal dog. *Am. J. Physiol.* 133:752, 1941.

119. Shannon, J. A., and Fisher, S. The renal tubular reabsorption of glucose in the normal dog. *Am. J. Physiol.* 122:765, 1938.

120. Silverman, M., Aganon, M. A., and Chinard, F. P. D-Glucose interactions with renal tubule cell surfaces. *Am. J. Physiol.* 218:735, 1970.

121. Silverman, M., and Black, J. High affinity phlorizin receptor sites and their relation to the glucose transport mechanism in the proximal tubule of dog kidney. *Biochim. Biophys. Acta* 394:10, 1975.

122. Smith, H. *The Kidney.* London: Oxford University Press, 1958.

123. Smith, H. W., Goldring, W., Chasis, H., Ranges, H. A., and Bradley, S. E. The application of saturation methods to the study of glomerular and tubular function in the human kidney. *J. Mt. Sinai Hosp.* 10:59, 1943.

124. Soler, N. G., and Malins, J. M. Prevalence of glucosuria in normal pregnancy—a quantitative study. *Lancet* 1:619, 1971.

125. Stalder, G. Funktionen des Tubulusepithels. *Mod. Probl. Paediatr.* 6:22, 1960.

126. Stolte, H., Hare, D., and Boylan, J. W. D-Glucose and fluid reabsorption in proximal surface tubule of the rat kidney. *Pfluegers Arch.* 334:193, 1972.

127. Taggart, J. V. Combined clinic on disorders of renal tubular function. *Am. J. Med.* 20:448, 1956.

128. Thompson, D. D., Barrett, M. J., and Pitts, R. F. Significance of glomerular perfusion in relation to variability of filtration rate. *Am. J. Physiol.* 167: 546, 1951.

129. Tobler, R., Prader, A., and Taiilard, W. Die familiäre primäre vitamin D-resistente Rachitis (Phosphat diabetes). *Helv. Paediatr. Acta* 11:209, 1956.

130. Tudvad, F. Sugar reabsorption in prematures and full term babies. *Scand. J. Clin. Lab. Invest.* 1:281, 1949.

131. Tudvad, F., and Vesterdal, J. The maximal tubular transfer of glucose and para-aminohippurate in premature infants. *Acta Paediatr. Scand.* 42:337, 1953.

132. Tune, B. M., and Burg, B. Glucose transport by proximal renal tubules. *Am. J. Physiol.* 221:580, 1971.

133. Ullrich, K. J., Rumrich, G., and Klöss, S. Specificity and sodium dependence of the active sugar transport in the proximal convolution of the rat kidney. *Pfluegers Arch.* 351:35, 1974.

134. Van Liew, J. B., Deetjen, P., and Boylan, J. W. Glucose reabsorption in the rat kidney: Dependence on glomerular filtration. *Pfluegers Arch.* 295:232, 1967.

135. Vick, H., Diedrich, D. F., and Baumann, K. Reevaluation of renal tubular glucose transport inhibition by phlorizin analogs. *Am. J. Physiol.* 224:552, 1973.

136. Vitelli, A., Cattaneo, C., and Martini, P. F. Maximum tubular reabsorption capacity of glucose in diabetes mellitus. *Acta Endocrinol. (Kbb.)* 50:79, 1965.

137. Walker, A. M., Bott, P. A., Oliver, J., and MacDowell, M. C. The collection and analysis of fluid from single nephrons of the mammalian kidney. *Am. J. Physiol.* 134:580, 1941.

138. Welsh, G. W., and Sims, E. A. H. Mechanisms of renal glycosuria in pregnancy. *Diabetes* 9:363, 1960.

139. Williams, T. F., and Winters, R. Familial (Hereditary) Vitamin D Resistant Rickets with Hypophosphatemia. In J. B. Stanbury, J. B. Wyngaarden, and D. S. Fredrickson (eds.), *The Metabolic Basis of Inherited Disease* (3rd ed.). New York: McGraw-Hill, 1972.

140. Woolf, L. I., Goodwin, B. L., and Phelps, C. E. Tm-limited renal tubular reabsorption and the genetics of renal glucosuria. *J. Theor. Biol.* 11:10, 1966.

86. Renal Hyperaminoaciduria

Johannes Brodehl

Physiology of Amino Acid Excretion

Amino acids are ultrafilterable and are evenly distributed in the extracellular fluid space. The only exception seems to be tryptophan, which is partially bound to protein, leaving only 10 to 40 percent of the compound dialyzable [182, 203, 316]. At the glomerulus, amino acids are filtered freely through basement membranes and are found in the same concentrations in the glomerular filtrate as in plasma water [88]. During the passage along the tubular lumen, amino acids are reabsorbed by active processes. The resorption is so effective that only 1 to 2 percent of the total amount filtered appears in the final urine, while 98 to 99 percent is recovered from renal loss by tubular transport. The resorption is active, that is, directed against an electrochemical potential difference; it is related to the sodium concentration in the extracellular fluid and depends on the intracellular supply of oxygen and energy ([64, 98, 134, 227, 228, 244, 269, 294, 303]; see reference 264). It takes place predominantly in the proximal convoluted tubule, as shown experimentally by stop-flow, micropuncture, and microperfusion studies [18, 39, 88, 108, 170, 171, 269, 270, 272].

The activity of the transport sites varies with the length of the tubules demonstrating a tubular heterogeneity [42, 43, 169–171, 252, 302, 311, 322]. There seems to be no net amino acid resorption in the distal tubule, while in the collecting ducts there is a small but definitive net resorption [88]. The small fraction of amino acids in the final urine is considered physiologic, its excretion being called aminoaciduria, while an increased loss of single or multiple amino acids is called hyperaminoaciduria.

Every amino acid detected in the blood is found in the urine; however, the pattern of the amino acids is quite different in the two fluids (Fig. 86-1), due mainly to two factors. First, individual amino acids are obviously handled specifically by the tubular cells, independent of the plasma concentration, the degree of resorption ranging from 92.2 ± 1.8 percent (for histidine) to 99.8 ± 0.1 percent (for valine). Second, some amino acids are not detectable in blood but can be found in the urine. These are mainly intermediates of amino acid metabolism that are poorly or not at all reabsorbed, thus rendering it impossible for them to accumulate in the extracellular fluid space. Several of them are involved in pathologic hyperaminoacidurias due to inborn errors of metabolism.

For most amino acids there is more than one type of active tubular transport system [18, 135, 136, 226, 255, 256]. Experimental studies and investigations in patients with inborn errors of tubular transport have demonstrated both group-specific and individual-specific transport systems. The first exhibits high capacity (high Vmax) but low

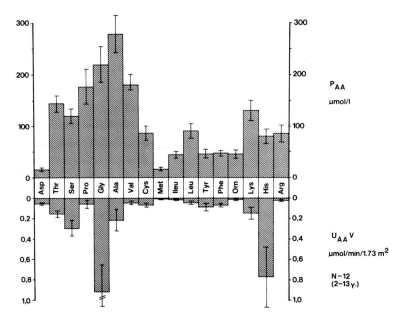

Figure 86-1. Plasma concentration P_{AA}, *μmol/l) and urinary excretion rates of free amino acids* ($U_{AA}V$, *μmol/min/1.73 m²) in normal children (N = 12). (Data from Brodehl and Gellissen [32].)*

specificity (low Km), while the latter is characterized by low capacity and high specificity (for more detail see references 236, 253, 264). The group-specific systems are listed in Table 86-1. It remains questionable whether methionine belongs in the group of neutral amino acids [17].

The nature of the transport carriers and their binding sites is still unknown. It was postulated by Meister [184–186] that amino acids are transported across the membrane by the action of membrane-bound γ-glutamyltranspeptidase, which catalyzes the binding of the transported amino acid with γ-glutamyl, which is split from glutathione (γ-glutamyl-cysteinyl-glycine). Within the cell the amino acid is released by the action of γ-glutamyl-cyclotransferase, and the γ-glutamyl is recycled to build up glutathione via the γ-glutamyl

cycle. It is still undecided whether this hypothetic transport system applies to all amino acids, and it remains questionable how the energy could be supplied for the huge amounts of amino acids involved, since their tubular transport is almost unlimited by tubular maxima.

The amounts of amino acids excreted in the urine depend on three factors: (1) the concentration of amino acids in plasma, (2) the glomerular filtration rate (GFR), and (3) the rate of tubular resorption. It is obvious that changes in the plasma amino acid concentrations are followed by proportional changes in the urinary excretion, if the fractional resorption remains unchanged. Since under physiologic conditions the largest variations of plasma amino acids are produced by dietary protein intake [207, 216, 282, 285], it is understandable that amino acid excretion depends on the nutritional state of the patient. This fact has to be considered when data in the literature are compared.

The influence of GFR on aminoaciduria is not as readily appreciated by the clinician. Pronounced lowering of GFR results in a decrease of amino acid excretion and renders a massive hyperaminoaciduria impossible, despite a decrease in tubular resorption, as occurs for instance in advanced cystinosis [31]. A large increase in GFR, on the other hand, augments aminoaciduria, as found in pregnancy [205, 306] or in vitamin-D-deficiency rickets [37]. Certainly the rate of tubular resorp-

Table 86-1. Group Specific Tubular Transport Systems

Cyclic and neutral amino acids (alanine, asparagine, citrulline, cystine, glutamine, histidine, isoleucine, leucine, methionine, phenylalanine, serine, threonine, tryptophan, tyrosine, valine)

Dibasic amino acids (arginine, lysine, ornithine) and cystine

Imino acids (proline, hydroxyproline) and glycine

Dicarboxylic amino acids (aspartic, glutamic)

Beta-amino acids (β-alanine, β-amino isobutyric, taurine)

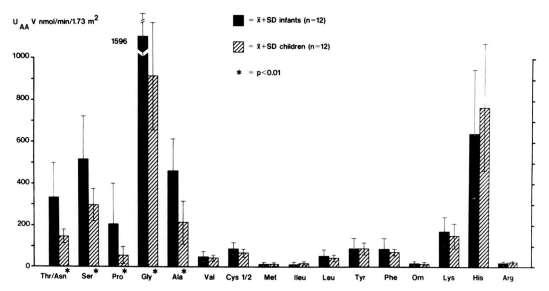

Figure 86-2. Endogenous urinary excretion rates of free amino acids in infants (16 days to 4 months) and children (2 to 13 years). (Data from Brodehl and Gellissen [32].)

tion exerts the strongest effect on the degree of hyperaminoaciduria: a decrease in the resorption of only 1 to 2 percent produces hyperaminoaciduria with a twofold increase in amino acid excretion.

Developmental Aspects

In early infancy the rate of urinary excretion of amino acids is increased as compared with that in later life. This phenomenon has been known for a long time and has been called physiologic hyperaminoaciduria of infancy [44, 82, 112, 278]. It is certainly not due to increased plasma amino acid levels, since those are identical in children and infants after the newborn period [32, 77, 78, 109, 168]. Particularly since GFR is relatively low in early infancy, less complete tubular resorption is considered to be responsible for the physiologic hyperaminoaciduria.

The extent of hyperaminoaciduria reported in the literature depends on the methods of determination and on the standards for comparing infants with adults. As long as the total amounts of amino acids or amino nitrogen were measured and their values were related to the creatinine or total nitrogen excretion rates (both very low in infancy), all free amino acids were considered to be excreted in higher amounts in infancy than in later childhood. By comparing, however, the net excretion rates of individual amino acids corrected for surface area of adults, it has become evident that only some of the free amino acids are involved in the physiologic hyperaminoaciduria [32]. These amino

acids are threonine, serine, proline, glycine, alanine, and hydroxyproline (Fig. 86-2). Excretion of the other amino acids does not exhibit significant differences when the mean values of a group of infants in the first few months of life are compared with those of older children. This, however, is not quite correct, since in the early months of life, the rates of excretion and resorption are changing rapidly and the infants are not homogeneous groups. Therefore, aminoaciduria has to be studied longitudinally. This has been tried in a recent study by Brodehl [30], in which the number of probands could be increased considerably over those of the former report [32]. The data for cystine and valine are depicted in Figs. 86-3 and 86-4, respectively. Although both amino acids belonged to those that did not exhibit significant differences in the mean excretion rates in infancy in the earlier study (see Fig. 86-2), their rates in the longitudinal plotting are obviously increased in the very young age period. The large variation in the values reflects variation in the individual maturation of GFR and tubular activity. The clearance rates behave similarly. It is obvious that the rates of urinary excretion in the early periods of life are determined by both the degree of development in glomerular filtration and the degree of tubular resorption. A low GFR may mask the decreased rates of tubular resorption, thus resulting in normal rates of urinary excretion.

The most sensitive measure of renal amino acid handling is tubular resorption related to GFR, especially the percentage of tubular resorption

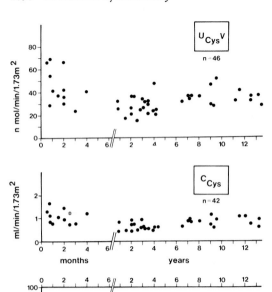

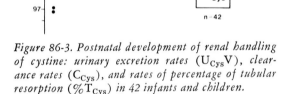

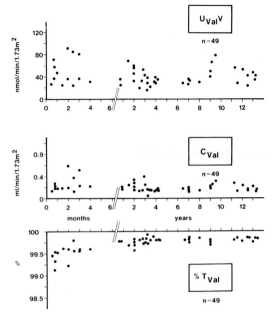

Figure 86-3. Postnatal development of renal handling of cystine: urinary excretion rates (U$_{Cys}$V), clearance rates (C$_{Cys}$), and rates of percentage of tubular resorption (%T$_{Cys}$) in 42 infants and children.

Figure 86-4. Postnatal development of renal handling of valine: urinary excretion rates (U$_{Val}$V), clearance rates (C$_{Val}$), and rates of percentage of tubular resorption (% T$_{Val}$) in 49 infants and children.

(%T$_{AA}$ = 100 × (1 − C$_{AA}$/GFR), where C$_{AA}$ = clearance of amino acids). The latter is reduced for all amino acids in early infancy, as shown in Fig. 86-5), indicating that the tubular resorption is less complete in early infancy for all amino acids studied. A greater degree of glomerulotubular imbalance in this period of life was considered to be responsible for the hyperaminoaciduria, although this could not explain why the contribution of individual amino acids to the hyperaminoaciduria was so variable. It seems more probable that different tubular transport systems mature at different stages of development, as suggested by Segal and coworkers [261–263] and Scriver and coworkers [13, 14, 253] in their studies of dibasic amino acids and glycine and imino acid excretion, respectively.

The basal aminoaciduria of infants is not related to the maximal capacity of tubular resorption of amino acids. Even in early infancy the maximal tubular resorption seems to be immeasurably high, as shown for phenylalanine in untreated phenylketonuric infants [33] and for methionine in infants with homocystinuria [author's unpublished data]. It is tempting to speculate that the "leakage" of amino acids into the tubular lumen might be due to increased permeability of the tubular cell membrane or to higher intracellular amino acid concentrations, permitting a greater fraction of amino acids to leak out of the cell rather than to decreased resorption.

Experimental in vivo studies in developing rats [13, 309] and in chick embryos [52] have generally confirmed the findings in the human species. Although in the chick embryo the clearance rates for glycine, tyrosine, and lysine were significantly lower than in hatched chickens, the percentages of filtered loads excreted were greater (at least for glycine and tyrosine) and the resorption rates expressed per gram of kidney tissue increased markedly after hatching. In vitro studies of cellular uptake of amino acids in kidney cortex slices did not give unequivocal results. Baerlocher et al. [13, 14] described a less efficient uptake of proline and glycine by the newborn rat and the absence of the low K$_m$ system for both amino acids. Segal and coworkers [220, 261–263], however, found an enhanced uptake of lysine and glycine in immature rat kidney slices that could be due to a decreased rate of efflux from the cell, while cystine was not taken up in the first neonatal period. These data indicate that various amino acid transport systems may begin functioning at different developmental ages, following a general phenomenon of developmental biology [47].

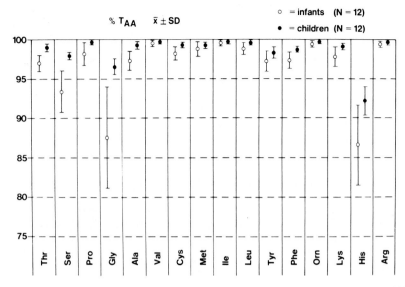

Figure 86-5. The tubular resorption of free amino acids in infancy and childhood: comparison of percentage of tubular resorption (% T_{AA}). All differences between the two groups are statistically significant (p < 0.02) with the exception of methionine, isoleucine, leucine, and tyrosine. (From Brodehl and Gellissen [32].)

Diagnosis and Normal Values

The first step in evaluating the renal handling of amino acids is the measurement of free amino acids in the urine by screening or semiquantitative methods ([21, 87, 137, 143, 163, 281, 299, 315]; for reviews see references 140, 253, 279). The amounts of amino acids are most often related to the rate of excretion of creatinine, which, unfortunately, exhibits great variation [3, 19, 55, 84, 212, 326]. Therefore experience is necessary in the evaluation of semiquantitative methods in order to avoid misinterpretations, and attention has to be paid to exogenously administered substances such as ampicillin or N-acetylcysteine [86, 166, 210, 211, 267, 284]. If hyperaminoaciduria is suspected, a timed collection of urine should be examined, first with the same methods, and, if the result is the same, by more accurate methods such as column chromatography or gas chromatography. The amounts excreted should be calculated in relation to time and body size. Normal values for urinary free amino acids in infants, children, and adults are listed in Table 86-2 (see references 32, 41, 213, 216, 248, 283, 323).

The urinary excretion rates do not reveal the mechanism by which amino acid excretion is altered. The next step in elucidating a hyperaminoaciduria, therefore, is the determination of the clearance of amino acids, which relates their excretion rates to their concentrations in plasma. The urinary collection periods should not be too long, since plasma amino acid concentrations show diurnal and nutritional variations. Normal amino acid clearance values are listed in Table 86-3 (see references 4, 31, 65, 110, 248). High clearance rates are suggestive of *renal* hyperaminoaciduria, while low clearance rates in the presence of high excretion rates are indicative of *prerenal* hyperaminoaciduria.

The final step in evaluating patients with hyperaminoaciduria is the simultaneous measurement of GFR and amino acid clearance in order to determine the net tubular resorption,

$$T_{AA} = (GFR \times P_{AA}) - U_{AA}V$$

where P_{AA} = plasma concentrations of amino acids
$U_{AA}V$ = urinary amino acid excretion rate

and the percentage of tubular resorption:

$$\% T_{AA} = 100 \, (1 - C_{AA}/GFR)$$

The last measurement is the most sensitive in determining the completeness of tubular amino acid resorption, since it is almost independent of the tubular load. Normal values for percent of T_{AA} are given in Table 86-4 (see references 31, 248, 323). Tubular maxima for amino acid resorption (Tm_{AA}) are practically never approached in human beings, with the exception of proline and hydroxyproline [251]. The determination of Tm_{AA} is therefore of no use in clinical nephrology.

Table 86-2. Urinary Excretion Rates of Free Amino Acids in Infants, Children, and Adults

Amino Acid	Prematures (Przyrembel et al. [216]*; N = 11; 10 days) 24-hr urine; μmol/24 hr — Mean	Range	Infants (Brodehl and Gellissen [32]; N = 12; 16 days–4 mo) Short-term clearance; nmol/min/1.73 m² — Mean	± S.D.	Children (Brodehl and Gellissen [32]; N = 12; 2–13 yr) Short-term clearance; nmol/min/1.73 m² — Mean	± S.D.	Children (Scriver and Davies [248]; N = 9; 3–10 yr) Short-term clearance; nmol/min/1.73 m² — Mean	Range	Adults (Soupart [283]; N = 15) 24-hr urine; μmol/24 hr — Mean	Range	Adults (Yü et al. [323]; N = 13) 24-hr urine; nmol/min — Mean	± S.D.
Alanine (Ala)	38.2	17–95	459	164	214	104	189	44–352	257	60–500	198	28
β-Alanine (β-Ala)	1.4	0.6–2.7	—	—	—	—	—	—	47	20–120	—	—
α-amino-n-butyric acid (Abu)	—	—	—	—	—	—	—	tr–62	—	—	—	—
Arginine (Arg)	3.7	0.9–6.5	22	7	23	6	20	8–44	26	10–80	21	5
Aspartic acid (Asp)	3.3	0.4–9.2	—	—	55	5	23	tr–71	41	10–222	21	—
Citrulline (Cit)	—	—	—	—	—	—	—	tr–22	—	—	—	—
Cystine (Cys)$_2$	26.9	5–82	89	31	68	17	—	tr–79	82	30–280	44	18
Glutamine (Gln)	—	—	—	—	—	—	364 (+Asn)	40–752	515	290–770	440	78
Glutamic acid (Glu)	—	—	—	—	—	—	61	13–132	—	—	27	6
Glycine (Gly)	201.1	79–400	1596	790	912	258	769	331–1541	1687	710–4160	785	355
Histidine (His)	20.3	7–58	642	314	768	294	471	109–995	790	130–1370	717	162
Hydroxyproline (Hypro)	67.2	36–133	—	—	—	—	—	—	—	—	—	—
Isoleucine (Ile)	3.5	0.4–6.2	10	8	15	5	25	7–67	94	40–180	32	17
Leucine (Leu)	5.0	2.2–11	54	30	43	14	36	18–107	74	10–150	45	9
Lysine (Lys)	36.8	13–85	172	70	152	61	113	41–211	44	0–120	591	237
Methionine (Met)	3.0	0.8–7.6	9	7	10	6	26	6–37	36	20–80	25	7
1-Methylhistidine (1Me-his)	4.0	1.8–9.7	—	—	—	—	—	—	433	130–930	—	—
3-Methylhistidine (3Me-his)	4.5	2.6–7.2	—	—	—	—	—	—	323	180–520	—	—
Ornithine (Orn)	7.0	1.9–18	19	8	18	8	20	12–27	11	0–80	—	—
Phenylalanine (Phe)	2.3	1.1–5.8	87	48	71	15	49	14–105	80	40–250	58	14
Proline (Pro)	58.4	11–186	205	202	57	39	—	0–38	—	—	—	—
Serine (Ser)	51.9	14–124	517	207	296	75	233	93–335	374	210–620	260	35
Taurine (Tau)	2.5	0.7–4.7	—	—	—	—	1145	764–1912	812	220–1850	710	336
Threonine (Thr)	55.0	12–153	330 (+Asn)	165	146 (+Asn)	33	105	36–174	168	20–300	134	45
Tyrosine (Tyr)	4.7	2.3–9.8	90	46	92	34	85	34–125	94	40–150	98	25
Valine (Val)	2.5	0.4–10	48	20	42	15	45	tr–85	72	0–260	33	12

* Mean values calculated from published data of low protein diet group.

Note: N = number of subjects; S.D. = standard deviation; +Asn = includes asparagine; tr = trace.

Table 86-3. Clearance Rates of Free Amino Acids in Infants, Children, and Adults (ml/min/1.73 m²)

Amino Acids	Prematures (O'Brien and Butterfield [201]; N = 4; 36–53 days) Short-term Clearance Range	Infants (Brodehl and Gellissen [32]; N = 12; 16 days to 4 mo) Short-term Clearance Mean	± S.D.	Infants (Ghisolfi et al. [110]; N = 7; 10 days to 1 mo) 24-hr Urine Mean	Range	Children (Brodehl and Gellissen [32]; N = 12; 2 to 13 yr) Short-term Clearance Mean	± S.D.	Children (Scriver and Davies [248]; N = 9; 3 to 10 yr) Short-term Clearance Mean	Range	Adults (Ghisolfi et al. [110]; N = 9) 24-hr Urine Mean	Range
Alanine	1.5–3.7	1.7	0.8	2.4	1.0–4.9	0.8	0.4	0.8	0.2–1.3	1.3	0.3–2.6
Arginine	—	0.4	0.1	0.8	0.2–1.6	0.3	0.1	0.5	0.2–1.2	0.3	0.1–0.3
Aspartic acid	4.2	—	—	—	—	3.6	0.9	2.8	tr–8.8	—	—
Citrulline	0.6–2.5	—	—	—	0–2.2	—	—	—	0.6	—	0–3.2
Cystine	3.6–8.8	1.1	0.3	1.8	0.6–4.0	0.8	0.2	—	1.0–1.4	0.8	0.6–1.2
Glutamine	1.2–3.6 (+Asn)	—	—	0.9	0.3–1.5	—	—	1.3 (+Asn)	0.1–2.3	0.8	0.4–1.3
Glutamic	0.2–1.5	—	—	0.4	0.1–0.8	—	—	0.8	0.1–2.4	0.8	0.3–2.1
Glycine	12–26	7.4	3.2	10.6	6.6–16.0	4.2	1.4	4.4	1.2–8.6	4.3	2.2–6.8
Histidine	7.1–19	8.5	4.5	7.9	4.3–13.7	9.5	2.6	9.2	1.9–21.8	7.5	2.1–14.5
Hydroxyproline	16–34	—	—	24.8	3.1–117.8	—	—	—	—	0	0
Isoleucine	0.4–1.0	0.3	0.2	0.4	0.2–0.9	0.3	0.1	0.5	0.2–1.1	0.5	0.2–1.1
Leucine	0.4–1.3	0.8	0.5	0.6	0.2–1.3	0.5	0.2	0.5	0.2–0.9	0.3	0.1–0.6
Lysine	1.6–5.2	1.3	0.4	1.6	0.8–3.6	1.2	0.4	1.1	0.3–2.4	1.4	0.3–2.9
Methionine	2.3–5.8	0.8	0.6	1.6	0.3–2.4	1.2	0.3	1.9	1.0–3.4	1.1	0.4–2.1
Ornithine	0.9–1.0	0.4	0.1	0.8	0.2–2.7	0.4	0.1	0.5	0.2–0.8	0.5	0.1–1.0
Phenylalanine	1.2–2.2	1.7	0.9	1.2	0.9–1.5	1.5	0.3	1.2	0.3–2.3	0.9	0.4–1.3
Proline	2.1–13	1.0	0.7	1.6	0.7–3.6	0.4	0.2	—	0–0.3	—	0–0.2
Serine	4.6–13	4.1	1.9	5.0	1.8–8.0	2.4	0.5	2.4	1.2–3.4	2.3	1.4–3.5
Taurine	0.6–1.3	—	—	1.6	0.7–3.7	—	—	13.7	9.9–26.2	12.9	1.7–33.1
Threonine	3.0–8.2	2.0 (+Asn)	1.4	2.9	1.2–5.1	1.0 (+Asn)	0.2	1.4	0.5–2.5	0.9	0.5–1.3
Tryptophan	—	—	—	1.1	0.5–2.0	—	—	—	—	1.1	0.1–2.7
Tyrosine	0.6–2.6	1.8	0.4	1.6	0.5–2.8	2.0	0.8	2.0	0.8–3.3	1.3	0.5–2.9
Valine	0.2–0.6	0.3	0.1	0.3	0.1–0.7	0.2	0.1	0.2	0.2–0.3	0.2	0–0.4

Note: N = number of subjects; S.D. = standard deviation; +Asn = includes asparagine.

Table 86-4. *Values of Percentage of Tubular Resorption of Free Amino Acids in Infants, Children, and Adults*

	Premature	Infants		Children				Adults	
	(O'Brien and Butterfield [201]; N = 4; 36–53 days) Short-term Clearance	(Brodehl and Gellissen [32]; N = 12; 16 days–4 mo) Short-term Clearance		(Brodehl and Gellissen [32]; N = 12; 2–13 yr) Short-term Clearance		(Scriver and Davies [248]; N = 9; 3–10 yr) Short-term Clearance		(Yü et al. [323]*; N = 13) Short-term Clearance	
Amino Acid	Ranges	Mean	± S.D.	Mean	± S.D.	Mean	Range	Mean	± S.D.
Alanine	87–95	97.3	1.1	99.3	0.4	99.5	99.1–99.9	99.5	0.1
Arginine	—	99.4	0.2	99.8	0.2	99.6	99.0–99.9	99.8	0.1
Aspartic acid	85	—	—	96.8	1.1	97.1	92.4–99.2	—	—
Citrulline	92–98	—	—	—	—	—	—	—	—
Cystine	68–89	98.2	0.8	99.3	0.2	—	—	99.3	0.3
Glutamine	89–96 (+Asn)	—	—	—	—	99.0	98.1–99.9	99.3	0.1
Glutamic	95–99	—	—	—	—	99.0	98.5–99.8	99.5	0.2
Glycine	15–63	87.6	6.4	96.5	0.9	97.0	92.9–99.0	97.5	1.0
Histidine	31–78	86.6	5.1	92.2	1.8	95.2	90.3–98.4	94.2	1.7
Hydroxyproline	15–51	—	—	—	—	—	—	—	—
Isoleucine	96–99	99.5	0.3	99.7	0.1	99.5	99.2–99.9	99.6	0.2
Leucine	97–99	98.8	0.7	99.6	0.2	99.7	99.6–99.9	99.7	0.1
Lysine	81–95	97.8	1.1	99.0	0.3	99.4	98.5–99.8	97.8	1.0
Methionine	85–93	98.8	0.9	99.3	0.3	98.8	98.3–99.7	99.2	0.3
Ornithine	96–98	99.4	0.3	99.7	0.2	99.6	99.5–99.8	—	—
Phenylalanine	94–96	97.4	1.0	98.8	0.3	99.2	98.8–99.7	99.2	0.2
Proline	53–94	98.3	1.4	99.7	0.2	—	98.8–100	—	—
Serine	54–86	93.4	2.7	98.0	0.3	98.4	97.3–99.1	98.1	0.4
Taurine	96–98	—	—	—	—	93.0	83.1–95.3	85.8	7.4
Threonine	71–91	97.0 (+Asn)	1.1	99.1 (+Asn)	0.3	98.2	92.4–99.6	99.2	0.3
Tyrosine	93–98	97.2	1.1	98.3	0.6	98.7	98.2–99.3	98.7	0.3
Valine	98–99	99.5	0.4	99.8	0.1	99.8	99.7–99.9	99.9	0.1

* Recalculated.

Note: N = number of subjects; S.D. = standard deviation; +Asn = includes asparagine.

Table 86-5. Classification of Hyperaminoaciduria

I. Renal hyperaminoaciduria
   A. Specific tubular hyperaminoaciduria
      1. Defective individual-specific transport system
         a. Isolated hypercystinuria
         b. Hyperglycinuria
      2. Defective group-specific transport systems
         a. Classic cystinuria
         b. Hyperdibasic aminoaciduria
         c. Iminoglycinuria
         d. Hyperdicarboxylic aminoaciduria
         e. Hartnup disease
   B. Generalized tubular hyperaminoaciduria
      1. Caused by inborn errors of metabolism (Chap. 81)
         a. Cystinosis
         b. Glycogenosis with Fanconi syndrome
         c. Lowe's syndrome
         d. Galactosemia
         e. Fructose intolerance
         f. Tyrosinemia
         g. Wilson's disease
         h. Hyperammonemia [206]
      2. Caused by acquired diseases
         a. Multiple myeloma (Chap. 67)
         b. Nephrotic syndrome (Chap. 52)
         c. Transplanted kidney (Chap. 36)
      3. Caused by deficiency diseases
         a. Vitamin D deficiency [37, 101, 148]
      4. Caused by intoxications
         a. Heavy metals (mercury, uranium, lead, cadmium) (Chap. 79)
         b. Organic toxins (maleic acid, Lysol)
         c. Drugs (outdated tetracycline, methyl-3-drome) (Chap. 81)
      5. Of unknown cause
         a. Idiopathic renal Fanconi syndrome (Chap. 81)

II. Prerenal hyperaminoaciduria
   A. With hyperaminoacidemia, but without tubular competition ("overflow" hyperaminoaciduria)
      1. Phenylketonuria
      2. Tyrosinosis
      3. Histidinemia
      4. Maple syrup urine disease (branched-chain ketonuria)
      5. Hypervalinemia
      6. Hyperglycinemia
      7. Hypermethioninemia
      8. Citrullinemia
      9. Hypersarcosinemia
      10. Homocystinuria
      11. Hypophosphatasia with phosphorethanol-aminuria
      12. Hydroxylysinemia
   B. With hyperaminoacidemia and tubular competition ("competitive" hyperaminoaciduria)
      1. Hyperprolinemia
      2. Hyperhydroxyprolinemia
      3. Hyperlysinemia
      4. Hyperargininemia
      5. Hyperornithinemia
      6. Hyper-β-alaninemia

   C. With no or low tubular resorption ("non-threshold" hyperaminoaciduria)
      1. Cystathioninuria
      2. Argininosuccinicaciduria
      3. β-Amino-iso-butyric aciduria

Types of Hyperaminoaciduria

The mechanisms that lead to hyperaminoaciduria are easily deduced from the physiologic facts of renal amino acid handling. Either tubular resorption is impaired while the filtered amounts are normal, or amino acids are filtered in excess due to an overproduction or defective catabolism in the organism. Both situations result in hyperexcretion of single or multiple amino acids. In the first type, the defect is located in the kidney, the resulting hyperaminoaciduria being of renal origin; it is termed *renal hyperaminoaciduria,* as originally proposed by Dent and Walshe [74] in 1954. In the second type of hyperaminoaciduria, the defect is located outside the kidney, reflecting a systemic metabolic derangement; the resulting hyperaminoaciduria is of *prerenal* origin.

Renal hyperaminoaciduria can be subdivided into two groups, depending on the mechanism of impairment (Table 86-5). The first group is characterized by defects in specific tubular transport systems that are located in the tubular membranes. The defects may involve either an individual-specific transport carrier or a group-specific transport system. The specific tubular hyperaminoaciduria is characterized by a constant and distinct pattern of amino acids in the urine, which in most cases renders the diagnosis easy. The excretion of other amino acids not involved in the specific defect remains completely normal. The concentrations in blood of the involved amino acids are normal or slightly lowered, the clearance rates are increased, and the tubular resorption rates are diminished. The defects are genetically determined and demonstrate the typical features of Garrod's inborn errors of metabolism [107].

The second group of renal hyperaminoacidurias is caused by systemic metabolic disturbances, intoxications, or deficiencies that secondarily affect tubular cell metabolism and usually lead to multiple nonspecific tubular defects, including the resorption of all amino acids and of other substances such as glucose, phosphate, and bicarbonate. The hyperaminoaciduria is of a generalized type. In its full expression it is described as the renal Fanconi syndrome (see Chap. 81).

Prerenal hyperaminoaciduria is caused by an increased metabolic production of a single or multiple amino acids. Depending on the mechanism of tubular transport of the involved amino acid, three different types of hyperaminoacidurias (see Table 86-5) can be separated in this prerenal group: (1) a pure "overflow" hyperaminoaciduria without any additional tubular competition for resorptive sites; (2) an overflow hyperaminoaciduria with additional competition in the resorption of related amino acids ("competitive" hyperaminoaciduria); and (3) a "nonthreshold" hyperaminoaciduria of amino acids with poor or no tubular resorption and absence of elevated plasma levels. These prerenal hyperaminoacidurias are not renal diseases and will therefore be mentioned only briefly in the following section. The known types are listed in Table 86-5, which is not intended to be complete.

Renal Hyperaminoacidurias
ISOLATED HYPERCYSTINURIA
In 1966 a new type of cystinuria was described in two siblings (a girl with idiopathic hypoparathyroidism and her brother) who showed high urinary excretion rates for cystine but normal excretions of lysine, ornithine, and arginine [34, 35]. This tubular defect seems to be very rare, since no further cases have been reported. In order to distinguish it from classic cystinuria it was called isolated hypercystinuria. The rates of amino acid clearance and tubular resorption in both children and their unaffected sister are given in Table 86-6. Cystine clearance is elevated up to thirty times normal, and the tubular resorption is decreased to 72 to 80 percent. The tubular defect, therefore, is much less pronounced than in classic cystinuria, and it has remained constant during a 4-year follow-up period. Loading with L-lysine produced an increase in the clearance both of cystine and of the dibasic amino acids (see reference 31). None of the children has developed nephrolithiasis so far, which is consistent with the fact that the highest urinary cystine concentrations measured were 260 mg per liter. The plasma levels for cystine were low normal. Oral loading tests with L-cystine, L-cystine hydrochloride, L-cysteine, and L-lysine failed to show an additional defect in intestinal absorption, in contrast to classic cystinuria. The parents showed normal urinary amino acid excretion.

Although isolated hypercystinuria has only minimal clinical importance, it has strongly influenced the theory of tubular transport systems for dibasic amino acids and cystine, which had long been considered to be ruled by a common carrier, as originally postulated by Dent and Rose [71] in 1951. The finding of isolated hypercystinuria was supplemented 2 years later by the description of hy-

Table 86-6. Isolated Hypercystinuria: Amino Acid Values in One Unaffected and Two Affected Siblings

Amino Acid Value	Unaffected M. K. (F, 9 yr)	Affected K. K. (F, 4 yr)	Affected H. K. (M, 1 yr)
P_{AA} (μmol/L)			
Half-cystine	74.1	50.8	57.4
Lysine	123.1	97.8	140.9
Ornithine	43.1	35.6	41.6
Arginine	118.8	72.3	63.7
$U_{AA}V$ (nmol/ min/1.73 m^2)			
Half-cystine	80	1534	1776
Lysine	83	64	114
Ornithine	17	7	7
Arginine	19	14	27
C_{AA} (ml/min/ 1.73 m^2)			
Cystine	1.1	30.2	30.9
Lysine	0.5	0.7	0.8
Ornithine	0.2	0.2	0.2
Arginine	0.1	0.2	0.4
Percent T_{AA}			
Cystine	99.0	78.0	74.6
Lysine	99.5	99.5	99.3
Ornithine	99.8	99.8	99.8
Arginine	99.9	99.8	99.7

Note: P_{AA} = plasma amino acids; $U_{AA}V$ = urinary excretion rates of amino acids; C_{AA} = amino acid clearance; T_{AA} = amino acid tubular resorption.

perdibasic aminoaciduria without cystinuria in a French-Canadian family [314]. Both observations and the recognition of isolated cystinuria in dogs [25, 139] are strong evidence against the hypothesis of a common carrier as the only tubular transport system for those amino acids, which is supported by the in vitro studies of the groups of Scriver, Segal, and Rosenberg (see Classic Cystinuria. The Tubular Defect).

HYPERGLYCINURIA
The isolated defect of tubular glycine resorption seems to be a very rare transport defect also, described so far only in two Jewish families, the first by DeVries et al. [76] in 1957 and the second by Greene et al. [115] in 1973. Hyperglycinuria is characterized by excessive excretion of glycine in the presence of normal plasma glycine levels, while all other amino acids, including proline and hydroxyproline, are excreted in normal amounts; other tubular defects have not been detected. In both families the inheritance was autosomal dom-

inant. It is still uncertain, however, whether this type of hyperglycinuria is (1) a homozygous state of a distinct entity; (2) the heterozygous state of iminoglycinuria, as suggested by Scriver [246, 247]; or (3) a distinct form of iminoglycinuria (type II) that has to be separated from the more common type I, as suggested by Greene et al. [115]. The tubular defect may be associated with an increased tendency to develop urinary calculi, which cannot be explained, however, by the hyperexcretion of glycine alone. Otherwise there seem to be no further symptoms.

In hyperglycinuria the urinary glycine excretion is in the range of 10 to 16 mmol per day [76, 115]. The endogenous clearance rates for glycine (C_{Gly}) are between 33 and 60 ml per minute (for adults), with the exception of one patient reported by Green in whom the C_{Gly} was only 12 ml per minute. The percentage of glycine resorption is in the range of 60 percent. According to DeVries and Alexander [75], intravenous glycine loading decreased the percentage of tubular glycine resorption further [115]. Proline loading, on the other hand, had no influence on glycine resorption, as was reported to occur in iminoglycinuria [246]. The endogenous tubular resorption of proline was almost complete, and, under intravenous loading with proline, an exaggerated splay in the titration curve was noted by Scriver et al. [249]. A normal tubular maximum for proline (Tm_{Pro}), however, was approached when filtered loads were increased to 45 mg per minute [115]. Hydroxyproline excretion was slightly increased in one member of the family reported by Greene and, as in normal subjects [249], it did increase greatly during proline loading. The intestinal absorption of glycine seems not to be impaired as suggested by oral glycine loading [115].

In experimental studies with isolated proximal tubules of rabbits it has been shown that glycine resorption is mediated by at least three distinct transport systems [135]: one is shared by proline and hydroxyproline; a second by alanine and possibly other neutral amino acids; and a third seems to be specific for glycine [193]. Studies with rat kidney slices confirmed these findings, while microperfusions in rats showed, in addition, that a certain fraction of glycine is reabsorbed also by passive diffusion [269]. It remains debatable whether these animal data could be transferred directly to human tubules, and if so, which one of those transport systems would most likely be disturbed in the different types of glycinuria and iminoglycinuria.

Specific tubular hyperglycinuria is also observed in association with other tubular defects, as in glucoglycinuria, a dominantly transmitted trait [152], and in certain types of familial and nonfamilial hypophosphatemic vitamin-D-resistant rickets [70, 132, 250]. Nonspecific hyperglycinuria (i.e., hyperglycinuria in combination with other amino acids) is, in addition, a prominent finding in all forms of generalized hyperaminoaciduria and can be found in prerenal hyperaminoaciduria, such as in ketotic and nonketotic hyperglycinemia and in hyperprolinemia.

CLASSIC CYSTINURIA

Cystinuria is one of the oldest recognized metabolic disorders. It was first described by Wollaston [318] in 1810 and discussed as one of four examples of inborn errors of metabolism by Garrod in 1908 [107]. After many years of unsuccessful trials by various investigators to elucidate the metabolic block in cystinuria, Dent and Rose [71] in 1951 were able to identify the defect as an inborn error of tubular transport concerning the "common transport system" of dibasic amino acids and cystine. An associated intestinal defect in the absorption of dibasic amino acids was recognized 10 years later by Milne et al. [189]. Thus, cystinuria is regarded as an inherited defect in specific transepithelial transport mechanisms of dibasic amino acids and cystine, including both the tubular and the intestinal cells (for more details on the history see references 62, 159, 236, 253, 296).

Cystinuria is characterized by excessive urinary excretion of cystine and the three dibasic amino acids, lysine, ornithine, and arginine (see Fig. 86-6). Due to poor solubility, cystine crystallizes in the urine, leading to the development of calculi in the urinary tract with the potential for obstruction, infection, and ultimately renal insufficiency. The urinary loss of dibasic amino acids and the intestinal defect are of no clinical significance. Cystinuria is inherited as an autosomal recessive trait with at least three different alleles and a variable expression in the heterozygotes. In order to avoid confusion with isolated hypercystinuria and other types of cystine-lysinuria, cystinuria should be called classic cystinuria. Cystinuria has long been confused with cystinosis, which, however, is a completely different metabolic disease (see Chap. 81).

The Tubular Defect

The most prominent finding in cystinuria to which all clinical symptoms can be attributed is the hyperexcretion of cystine, which persists throughout life. In homozygous adult carriers cystine excretion is in the range of 0.5 to 1.8 gm per day [4, 51, 73, 103, 123, 195], with mean values of 0.98 ± 0.38 gm per day [51], 99 ± 24 mg/kg/day

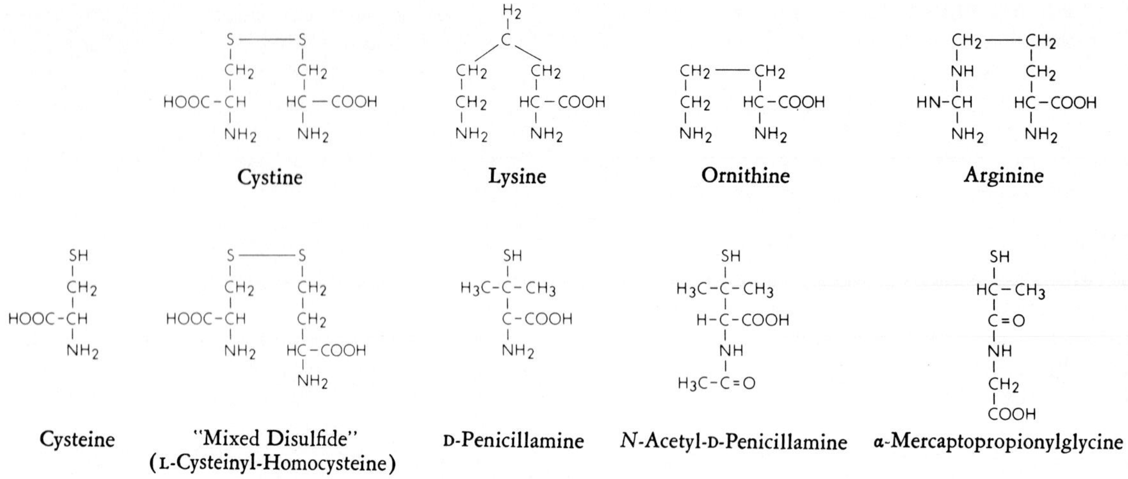

Figure 86-6. Molecular structures of cystine and dibasic amino acids and related compounds.

[195], 630 ± 64 mg per gram of creatinine [123], respectively. In short-term clearance examinations performed in children and adults, the urinary excretion rates are between 2,750 and 4,370 nmol/min/1.73 m² (author's unpublished data). The excretion rates are variable and depend on both the rate of glomerular filtration and the plasma cystine levels, which are related to the ingestion of metabolic precursors of cystine, mainly methionine and cysteine. It is still unknown whether the degree of the tubular defect in cystine resorption is fixed or whether it could be influenced by factors such as plasma levels or filtered loads of lysine, methionine, or other amino acids.

The concentration of cystine in the urine is very variable, depending mostly on the urinary flow rate. Water diuresis does not increase net urinary cystine excretion per se [165]. The plasma levels of cystine are normal or below the normal range [4, 29, 58, 106, 173]. Cystine clearance rates, therefore, are extremely high. In short-term clearance studies it could be shown in several homozygous patients that the clearance of cystine can exceed the glomerular filtration rate, up to a ratio of 2 [31, 58, 106]. This indicates that net tubular secretion of cystine takes place in these patients. Loading with lysine is able to increase the cystine clearance even further, as is shown in Fig. 86-7 [31]. This finding seems to be in contrast to an earlier negative report by Robson and Rose [221]; however, they did not achieve such high plasma levels for lysine. It was confirmed recently by Lester and Cusworth [165] in 3 out of 4 homozygous patients. Therefore, the tubular defect in classic cystinuria cannot be explained solely by the absence of a transport carrier in the tubular membrane, but rather seems to involve cystine or cysteine metabolism or transfer within the tubular cells.

The tubular defect in the resorption of lysine and the other two dibasic amino acids is usually not as severe as it is for cystine. The net amount of urinary lysine excretion, however, is higher than cystine, due to higher blood levels of lysine; they are in the range of 0.4 to 2.6 gm per day [4, 51, 106, 123, 195]. The clearance rates of lysine almost never exceed the glomerular filtration rate, the percentage rate of tubular resorption being in the range of 10 to 40 percent [4, 58, 106, 195]. Arginine excretion is in the range of lysine, while ornithine excretion is usually least severely involved.

In addition to these four amino acids, other metabolites and derivatives are excreted in classic cystinuria. Frimpter [102] identified the "mixed disulfide" of L-cysteine and L-homocysteine (see Fig. 86-6) in all cystinuric patients studied [103], but it was not found in the urine of healthy controls. It is excreted in amounts of 14 to 225 mg per day; its excretion rates are not correlated with those of cystine but rather to the intake of methionine. Homoarginine seems to be excreted constantly in cystinuria [54], and citrullinuria is observed frequently [191]. The excretion of cystathionine has not been reported to be increased [105], with the exception of one patient in whom cystinuria was associated with cystathioniuria [104]. Glycine resorption was found to be decreased in a few patients with cystinuria [58, 106, 304], while increased excretion of methionine and

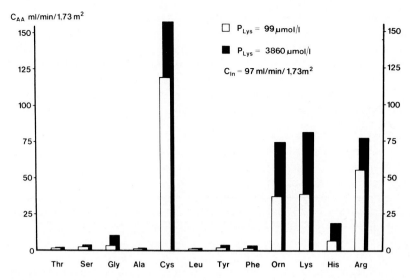

C_{AA} ml/min/1,73 m²

P_{Lys} = 99 µmol/l
P_{Lys} = 3860 µmol/l
C_{In} = 97 ml/min/ 1,73m²

Figure 86-7. Clearance rates of free amino acids (C_{AA}) *in a 5-year-old boy with classic cystinuria. Intravenous loading with* L-*lysine produces a gross increase in the clearance of cystine and the dibasic amino acids, while other amino acids are only slightly increased.*

uric acid [158, 304] was considered to be of extrarenal origin.

Cysteine, the reduced form of cystine, is not found in the urine [97] even after oral loading with cystine. The determination of cysteine, however, remains a difficult procedure due to spontaneous oxidation of cysteine to cystine, which could already occur in the urine during passage along the urinary tract. In the plasma, cysteine is found to be lower in cystinuria than in control subjects (8 ±2 versus 16 ± 6 µmol/L) [97]. After oral loading with cysteine, plasma levels of cystine increase as high as in the controls. It is of interest that cystine did not decline more rapidly than it does in normal subjects, which could have been expected since the urinary cystine excretion was massively augmented by this loading procedure [97]. Cysteine was reported to show a higher rate of renal extraction in cystinuria [103], while cystine and other amino acids are only minimally extracted. This finding could indicate a special role of cysteine in the mechanism of cystine hyperexcretion; however, it could not be confirmed by Rosenberg et al. [233].

Experimental studies have demonstrated the cellular defect of the tubules in the uptake of lysine, ornithine, and arginine; however, so far the defect in cystine uptake has not been revealed. Kidney slices from the renal cortex of rats [231] and human subjects [99] are able to accumulate the dibasic amino acids against a concentration gradient and are competitive inhibitors of each

other. Cystine, however, does not share this pathway; it does not competitively inhibit, nor is it inhibited, by the three dibasic amino acids. Slices from cystinuric patients demonstrate a defect in the ability to transport lysine and arginine, but cystine uptake is unimpaired, both at low and high initial cystine concentrations [99]. Lysine and cystine demonstrate different biochemical characteristics in their transport mechanisms ([242–244, 260]; for more details see references 264, 296) and in their ontogenetic development, both in rats [262] and, in vivo, in human infants [30].

The in vitro uptake of cysteine is not defective in kidney slices of cystinuric patients, and there is no interaction of dibasic amino acids with the cysteine influx mechanism [260]. Only the incubation of cysteine with lysine produced a higher intracellular accumulation of the sulfur amino acid, which is possibly explained by an inhibition of cysteine efflux by lysine [242, 243]. Kinetic and ontogenic studies have indicated further that the renal cystine and cysteine transport systems are different [260, 263]. Recent studies in rats have shown that the in vivo uptake of ^{14}C lysine [11] and ^{35}S cystine [116] is more rapid than in vitro. Additional loading with arginine enhances the cellular uptake of lysine, although lysine clearance is considerably increased; similarly, loading with lysine enhances the uptake of cystine, although cystine clearance is also increased. These findings are interpreted as evidence for a dissociation between cellular accumulation and transepithelial transport. They could explain the paradoxical findings in cystinuria, in which there appears to be a luminal transport defect for cystine but no defect for the cellular accumulation of cystine from the peritubular side.

Microperfusion studies in rats have shown that dibasic amino acids are reabsorbed by active and saturable transport systems and that there is no evidence for passive diffusion [270, 271]. Tubular resorption of arginine is strongly inhibited by lysine and ornithine and also by agmatine, homoarginine, and canavanine, but not by cysteine or citrulline [272]. The effect of cystine on arginine resorption could not be tested due to low solubility of cystine. In the same microperfusion experiments, however, the resorption of cystine was strongly inhibited by the dibasic amino acids and also by cysteine, but not by glycine, agmatine, and 2,6-diaminopimelic acid [271]. From these experiments it was postulated that two systems are responsible for the resorption of the dibasic amino acids and cystine/cysteine [268, 271].

Cystinuria is found in species other than man. Datta and Harris [66] described excessive "cystine" excretion in the Kenya blotched genet, which was not accompanied by increased excretion of dibasic amino acids and not followed by cystine stone formation [90]. Later, however, it was shown that the genet excretes not cystine but the far more soluble amino acid, S-sulfo-L-cysteine [61]. There is no abnormality of cystine transport in this species. In 1956 a male mink was described with large numbers of stones that consisted of pure cystine [202].

The oldest known and best studied type of nonhuman cystinuria, however, is canine cystinuria [26, 196]. There seem to be various types of cystinuria that so far have been observed only in male dogs: isolated hypercystinuria, cystine-lysinuria, and the classic type of cystinuria [25, 56, 139]. An intestinal defect for lysine also has been postulated [301], which, however, could not be confirmed in in vitro studies [139]. Recently hypermethioninemia was found in most of the cystinuric dogs, and there was a positive correlation between plasma methionine and fractional cystine resorption, suggesting a metabolic disease manifesting itself as abnormal tubular resorption [25].

The Intestinal Defect

Some reports in the older literature indicated intestinal absorption defects in cystinuria. These are the reports by Von Udransky and Baumann [305], who in 1889 observed increased amounts of putrescine and cadaverine, diamines derived from arginine and lysine, respectively, in the urine of patients with cystinuria; this finding was later confirmed by other investigators [172, 293]. High protein diets are followed by increased excretion of diamines in the urine [293]; high lysine intake especially leads to increased excretion of cadaverine, while arginine leads to putrescine excretion [172]. Reexamination more than 50 years later confirmed the old findings [28, 189]. Oral loading with lysine produces massive increase in fecal lysine and cadaverine in cystinuric patients; this has not been observed in control subjects. Comparable results are obtained after arginine loading [10]. Treatment with neomycin abolishes the fecal conversion to putrescine. Cystine loading in cystinuric patients is not followed by a normal rise in plasma cystine when compared with control subjects [173]. Cysteine, on the other hand, is absorbed completely as in normal subjects [173]. In vitro studies demonstrated that jejunal tissues from patients with cystinuria failed to accumulate ^{14}C-labeled lysine, ornithine, arginine, and cystine, while tissues from controls maintained a high concentration gradient [180, 295, 297]. Further studies revealed that the ability of intestinal mucosa to accumulate these four amino acids was different in different groups of patients. Some cystinuric patients demonstrated a total impairment for all four amino acids, others had a small but detectable cystine transport but no dibasic amino acid transport, and still another group showed normal cystine transport and only slightly impaired uptake of lysine and arginine [230]. Cysteine uptake was not at all impaired [229]. In normal individuals a common intestinal transport system for the three dibasic amino acids could be demonstrated, which, in contrast to the kidney, is shared by cystine also, but not by cysteine. Recently an intestinal perfusion technique was used in order to study the intestinal absorption of amino acids in vivo. Loading with cysteine and cystine [274] and with dibasic amino acids [130, 273] confirmed the former results elegantly.

All these findings demonstrate that there is in classic cystinuria an intestinal as well as a renal tubular transport defect; this combination is comparable to that in the Hartnup syndrome and some cases of iminoglycinuria. It has to be pointed out, however, that the transport characteristics are not at all identical; instead, marked discrepancies exist between the recognized transport systems in the kidney and intestine, especially in those for cystine.

Despite the poor intestinal absorption of four amino acids, although one of these (lysine) definitely is essential and another (arginine) is essential at least in infants, cystinuric patients do not suffer from detectable nutritional defects except for a slight reduction in total height [51]. This paradox can be explained by findings that demonstrate that lysine and arginine are well absorbed by the intestinal tract in the form of their oligopeptides, as L-lysylglycine and L-arginyl-L-aspartate and others, thus avoiding malabsorption syndromes [57–9, 131]. Even in normal persons intestinal absorption of amino acids is faster in the form of their oligopeptides than as free amino acids. Those findings are interpreted as evidence for the existence of dipeptide transport systems in the intestinal mucosa that are independent of those for free amino acids [131].

Clinical Signs
The only relevant clinical sign of classic cystinuria is nephrolithiasis [23]. The renal loss of the four amino acids and the defect in intestinal amino acid absorption is of negligible nutritional significance, at least in adult patients. It could be of some importance in infants, however, since in a study of 44 patients with stone-forming cystinuria it was found that their mean height was 2.5 cm less than that of normal subjects, possibly related to a mild nutritional disadvantage during the growth period [51]. Otherwise the daily protein intake provides enough amino acids, especially lysine and arginine, to cope for the renal loss. The intestinal defect is of no great importance due to the fact that oligopeptides can be absorbed undisturbed. Scriver and coworkers [254] have reported that the incidence of cystinuria in a population with mental illness is ten times higher than in the normal population. The significance of this observation awaits further elucidation.

Renal calculi are the consequence of poor solubility of cystine, which depends on urinary pH and is about 300 mg per liter in acid solutions [72]. The solubility changes very little between pH 4.5 and 7.0 but increases to about 500 mg per liter at pH 7.5 and above. It is higher in urine than in water, and most cystinuric patients will dissolve 150 mg per liter more cystine than theoretically expected [188]. Therefore, heterozygotes of cystinuria are unlikely to form stones, since they usually excrete less than 300 mg of cystine per day. In homozygous carriers, however, the urine is liable to become oversaturated with cystine, especially during the night when urine tends to be more concentrated and more acid than during the daytime [72].

The majority of homozygous carriers develop renal calculi during their lifetime. Their clinical symptoms are related exclusively to this consequence, as described in a large series of patients by Niemann [199], Reander [219], and Boström and Hambraeus [23] and in a smaller pediatric series by Pruzanski [215]. Calculi are mainly formed in the third and fourth decade, but they occur also in early childhood: 7 to 10 percent of the cystine stones appear before the age of 10 years [23] and 25 percent before the age of 20 years [197]. In one series [215], 8 of 15 children with cystinuria already had renal calculi when they were diagnosed. Cystine stones account for 1 to 2 percent of renal calculi in adults [280]; the percentage in children is considerably higher [188].

Cystine stones are radiopaque, even if they are of pure cystine, due to their sulfur content [125, 219]. Sometimes they are coated with calcium phosphate, especially the large ones and those in infected urine. The roentgenologic density is less than that of most other renal stones. As a result, small cystine stones may be undetected by radiographic examination in about 10 percent of patients [188].

The clinical symptoms of cystine urolithiasis are the same as those produced by other types of calculi. Colic may be associated with obstruction of the urinary tract; subsequent hydronephrosis, infection, pyelonephritis, and eventual loss of renal function may occur. Males are usually more severely affected than females. Life expectancy is significantly reduced; in about 46 percent of patients in the Swedish series who died [23], the cause of death was related to kidney involvement. The diagnosis of cystinuria should be suspected in any patient with urinary calculi. It can be tested easily by microscopic examination of the urinary sediment, preferably of a morning specimen, which should be acidified with a few drops of acetic acid. In homozygous untreated patients the typical hexagonal, flat, birefringent crystals should appear in polarized light.

As a biochemical screening method the cyanide nitroprusside test for disulfides originally described by Lewis [167] in 1932 or similar tests are widely used ([122, 222, 224]; see reference 253). The lower limit of sensitivity is in the range of 60 mg cystine per liter or 80 mg per gram of creatinine, respectively; therefore the reaction (magenta-red color complex) permits an easy detection of homozygous cystinuria. This test may be positive in some patients with heterozygous cystinuria with increased cystine excretion, in homocystinuria, in cysteine-β-mercapto-lactate disulfiduria, and in severe types of generalized hyperaminoacidurias.

Acetone and drugs with disulfide groups can give false-positive results. In patients with positive microscopic or screening tests, the urine should be examined for the characteristic amino acid pattern by more quantitative methods.

Genetics and Incidence

The genetic basis of classic cystinuria was already observed by the earliest reports of the disease [107, 199]. In 1908 Garrod pointed out that cystinuria is rarely found in two successive generations, and that consanguinity was frequently observed in families with affected offspring, suggesting an autosomal recessive inheritance. After methods for quantitative determinations of amino acids in the urine had become available, a homozygous state could be defined more accurately by quantification of urinary metabolites. By this means Harris and his coworkers [126–128] were able to survey 27 families and analyze their data by statistical means. They concluded that there must be two genetic types of cystinuria. In one type, the genetic defect was expressed exclusively in the affected generation, while the obligate heterozygotes showed normal amino acid excretion (complete autosomal recessive type); in the other type, heterozygotes demonstrated increased urinary cystine and lysine excretion (incomplete autosomal recessive), while the homozygotes did not behave differently from the first type.

The elucidation of the intestinal defect in cystinuric patients led to the recognition of an even greater genetic heterogeneity of classic cystinuria. By surveying 13 families, Rosenberg and coworkers [225, 230] were able to define three genetically distinct types of cystinuria (Table 86-7). Type I cystinuria, which corresponds with the complete recessive type of Harris, is characterized by the absence of active transport of cystine, lysine, or arginine in gut mucosa in the affected subjects and by normal urinary excretion rates for the four amino acids in the heterozygotes. In type II cystinuria the active transport of cystine, but not of lysine, is retained in the intestinal mucosa of affected subjects, while the heterozygotes excrete distinctly increased amounts of cystine and lysine; it is comparable to the incompletely recessive type of Harris. In type III cystinuria the intestinal transport of cystine, lysine, and arginine is reduced but not absent in the affected subjects, while the heterozygotes excrete also increased amounts of dibasic amino acids; it again corresponds with the incomplete recessive type of Harris. The study of more families with obviously double heterozygotes led to the conclusion that the genetic heterogeneity is probably due to multiple allelic mutations [195, 225].

The incidence of cystinuria depends on the methods used for screening the population and the definition of cystinuria. Therefore, the figures given in the literature show great variation. Lewis [167] found a positive nitroprusside test in 1 : 600 of 10,534 asymptomatic students. This test, however, cannot distinguish between homozygotes, some heterozygotes of classic cystinuria, and other defects with increased disulfide excretion. Among 7,793 schoolchildren in Sweden, 3 had classic cystinuria identified by screening plus quantitative methods [24]. The calculated incidence of 1 in 2,600, however, is in contrast to the actual observed cases of cystinuria in Sweden, that is, 98 cases in the 92 years from 1870–1962 [23]. In 8,203 schoolchildren in Zurich, Switzerland, 32 had a strong positive nitroprusside test and 29 a slight or questionable reaction [183]. On repeated examination with high-voltage electrophoresis, 18 of the 61 children were found to be normal and 37 could be considered to be heterozygotes for type II and type III cystinuria; 6 had other types of hyperaminoaciduria. From these data a frequency of 1 in 17,000 for homozygous or double heterozygous cystinuria was calculated, which corresponds fairly well with the figure of 1 in 16,000 given by the Massachusetts Screening Program [179].

Treatment

Treatment of classic cystinuria is directed toward prevention of urinary tract calculi and dissolution of stones that have already been formed. Complications of nephrolithiasis are treated as in other forms of urolithiasis. Heterozygous carriers of cystinuria usually do not require prophylactic procedures, since their urinary cystine content remains below 250 mg per liter or 200 mg per gram of creatinine. All homozygous carriers of cystinuria should be treated, however, whether stones are already formed or not.

Table 86-7. The Three Genetic Types of Classic Cystinuria

Type	Active Intestinal Transport in Homozygotes			Excretion of Dibasic Amino Acids and Cystine by Heterozygotes
	Cystine	Lysine	Arginine	
I	Absent	Absent	Absent	Normal
II	Present	Absent	Not determined	2+ Increased
III	Present	Present	Present	1+ Increased

Source: L. E. Rosenberg et al. [230].

Since crystallization of cystine depends mainly on its concentration in the urine, the most important aspect of treatment is the maintenance of a high urinary output by a large fluid intake [69, 72]. This is especially important during nighttime, when the urine tends to be concentrated and acid. The urinary volume should be continuously not less than 2 ml/min/1.73 m², which in adults is 3 liters per day. The fluid intake has to be adjusted, especially during periods of excessive extrarenal fluid losses. Special attention has to be paid to be sure that the patients take their fluid before retiring and at least once during the night in order to prevent nighttime oliguria. This continuous fluid therapy is rewarded with complete success, if it is strictly followed; for many patients, however, especially children, it often is not acceptable. Only two-thirds of an adult group treated by Dent and coworkers [69] complied. Those who did comply did not develop new concretions, and stones already present could be dissolved [69].

Cystine solubility can be enhanced by providing an alkaline urine with a pH value of at least 7.5 [72]. Although this high urinary pH can be achieved by the continuous administration of sodium bicarbonate or citrate, the very large amounts of alkali required make the treatment difficult to follow. The urinary pH should be checked in the morning specimen and should be greater than 7.4. Successful prevention of stone formation with this consequent treatment has been reported in children by Bickel [22]. It should never be the only regimen, however, but must always be combined with fluid therapy.

The effect of dietary treatment, especially of a low methionine [280] diet, has been questioned [324], although there are reports in which continuous low methionine therapy has resulted not only in stone dissolution [161] but even in disappearance of cystinuria while the dibasic aminoaciduria remained unchanged [160]. Experiments in pediatric patients with cystinuria have not been reported, since a low protein and methionine diet in children has its own hazards.

In spite of all the prophylactic efforts mentioned above, cystine stone formation cannot be prevented in all cases. In patients with recurrent urinary calculi, often requiring surgery for relief of urinary tract obstruction, treatment with D-penicillamine or its analogues has offered a great advantage. This treatment was introduced by Crawhall et al. [59] in 1963, and since then many reports have appeared in the literature [57, 60, 174, 177, 181].

D-Penicillamine is a dimethylcysteine (see Fig. 86-6) that reacts with cysteine to form a soluble mixed disulfide. Its application dramatically reduces cystine excretion, thus preventing the formation of stones and promoting the dissolution of calculi. It is given daily in a divided dosage of 30 mg per kilogram. Under this regimen the urinary cystine concentration should be kept below 150 mg per liter.

D-Penicillamine has many undesirable side effects, including fever and rash [63, 177], proteinuria and nephrotic syndrome [63, 145, 176, 218, 234], systemic lupus erythematosus [217], pancytopenia [53], thrombocytosis [95], and loss of taste [153]. In addition, penicillamine is a potent vitamin B_6 antagonist [144], and patients on long-term therapy should receive supplements of pyridoxine. The use of penicillamine, therefore, should be restricted to those patients in whom the fluid and alkali therapy has failed or is not manageable or in whom special indications exist; it is not the first choice of treatment. Whether the use of analogues of penicillamine, such as N-acetyl-D-penicillamine [287, 288] or α-mercaptopropionyl glycine [157], offers any advantage, especially in the pediatric age group, has to await further clarification. Cystine crystallization is also said to be reduced by administration of chlordiazepoxide [93].

Atypical Cystinuria (Cystine-lysinuria)
Atypical cases of cystinuria have been described in which only the tubular resorption of cystine and lysine is disturbed, while the resorption of arginine and ornithine is fully retained. Such cases have occurred either as sporadic or as familial cases and are often accompanied by various other abnormalities that intiated the urinary investigations. Since in none of them could a direct relationship to classic cystinuria be established, the question remains open whether these cases represent distinct entities as variants of cystinuria, or whether they are just heterozygotes of type II and type III classic cystinuria.

Gross and coworkers [117, 118] described cystine-lysinuria in a kindred with hereditary pancreatitis. Both defects are transmitted as an autosomal dominant trait, but they are not linked obligately. The tubular lysine resorption is in the range of 90 percent; exact data for cystine are not available. Bremer [27] mentioned 3 of 8 siblings who suffered from protein-losing enteropathy and had cystine-lysinuria. Their tubular defect (percent T_{AA}) for cystine was 93 to 97 percent, and for lysine it was 90 to 96 percent (author's unpublished data). See et al. [258] reported on a 20-month old girl with severe muscular hypotonicity, skeletal deformities, chromosomal aberration, and mental retardation who also had definitive cystine-lysinuria, and Hurwitz and coworkers [141] observed two brothers in a family with muscular dystrophy who showed lysinuria with ornithinuria. In our clinic a girl of 8 years was observed who showed mental retardation and brachytelephalangia and whose cystine and lysine resorption was in the range of 90 percent, while arginine and ornithine were completely reabsorbed (author's unpublished data).

In other patients with cystinuria associated with various abnormalities, the genetic relationship to classic cystinuria or the urinary amino acid pattern is so well established that the patients can be considered as heterozygotes or homozygotes for classic cystinuria; these include patients with dermatomyositis [94], celiac disease [124], osteogenesis imperfecta and mental retardation [20], muscular hypotonicity and dwarfism [48], and mental retardation with neurologic abnormalities [298].

HYPERDIBASIC AMINOACIDURIA

The isolated disturbance of the tubular resorption of the dibasic amino acids lysine, ornithine, and arginine without increased excretion of cystine was first recognized as a distinct tubular entity by Whelan and Scriver [314] in 1968, although similar cases had been described previously [96, 154, 209]. Since then several more cases have appeared in the literature [12, 38, 156, 178, 204, 277], most of them with intestinal defects in the absorption of dibasic amino acids leading to protein or lysine intolerance with periods of diarrhea, severe malnutrition, failure of growth, hyperammonemia, and often mental retardation. Hyperdibasic aminoaciduria, or lysinuric protein intolerance, as it is often referred to, is a genetic entity that is clearly distinguished clinically and chemically from classic cystinuria. It represents an intestinal and tubular defect in the transport of dibasic amino acids, but not of cystine; in addition, it is characterized by protein intolerance leading to hyperammonemia and slow urea production after protein loads. The slow urea production could be caused by a defective hepatic transport of dibasic amino acids, especially ornithine, as suggested by Simell [276]. This transport defect could deprive hepatic cells of ornithine, which is necessary for urea production via the Krebs-Henseleit cycle.

Lysinuria is the most prominent renal feature in hyperdibasic aminoaciduria. Urinary excretion rates for lysine are in the range of 1 to 7 mmol/24 hr/ 1.73 m² [277]; 0.3 to 1.5 μmol/min/1.73 m² [12, 314]; or 0.9 to 1.6 mg per milligram of creatinine [156, 204]. The clearance rates for lysine

are between 5 and 68 ml per minute [12, 155, 209, 277, 314]. The defect in arginine and ornithine resorption is less severe, the clearance rates of arginine being in the range of 0.5 to 22 ml per minute, and those of ornithine between 0.8 and 8 ml per minute [276]. In addition, the urinary excretion rates of homocitrulline were found elevated ten to fifteen times normal [204]. Values of dibasic amino acids in plasma usually are lower than normal.

Special renal function studies in seven patients with lysinuric protein intolerance were performed by Simell and Perheentupa [276]. Glomerular filtration rates were found to be in the lower range of normal. Although under endogenous conditions the tubular load is extremely low, only 37 percent of filtered lysine, on the average, is reabsorbed by the tubules. Tubular lysine secretion, however, could not be demonstrated unequivocally. The endogenous resorption of arginine and ornithine are also diminished (76 percent and 87 percent, respectively). After stepwise infusion with arginine and ornithine, the fractional resorption of both amino acids and of lysine diminished; however, under very high loads the resorption capacity approached approximately the same level as the controls.

The genetic pattern of hyperdibasic aminoaciduria is questionable. The Finnish pedigrees are interpreted as an autosomal recessive trait [200], while in the French Canadian pedigree an autosomal dominant inheritance was reported [314]. Scriver and Rosenberg [253] suggested that isolated hyperdibasic aminoaciduria may represent the heterozygous manifestation, while those with the severe biochemical and clinical disturbances may represent the homozygous state. Simell and coworkers [277] claim that there are two types of hyperdibasic aminoaciduria: In the first, diamino acid transport is defective only in renal tubules and in the intestine; in the second, the same defect is shared by the hepatic cells.

Treatment of hyperdibasic aminoaciduria consists of a low protein diet. Supplementation with arginine, ornithine, or citrulline abolishes the hyperammonemic response after protein loading and has been used successfully [12, 154].

IMINOGLYCINURIA

The tubular resorption of glycine and the imino acids proline and hydroxyproline is disturbed in familial iminoglycinuria, first described in 1958 by Joseph et al. [150] in France and 7 years later by Tada et al. [290] in Japan. Several cases and families have been described [15, 100, 113, 194, 232, 291, 313]. The levels of proline in plasma are normal, in contrast to hyperprolinemia, which can mimic the urinary amino acid pattern [246, 253]. It is postulated that the group-specific tubular transport system for glycine and imino acids is disturbed in this defect, which in some cases is accompanied also by a defect in intestinal absorption of proline [113, 194]. Associated neurologic and mental disturbances [100, 232, 290, 291] are questionably related to the tubular defect, since many cases are otherwise completely undisturbed. Iminoglycinuria is inherited as an autosomal recessive trait in which the heterozygotes may reveal hyperglycinuria without hyperprolinuria.

The tubular resorption of glycine and the imino acids was extensively studied in humans and in animal models (see references 247, 253). Titration studies with L-proline loading in man demonstrated that net tubular absorption undergoes saturation and that a tubular maximum for proline can be achieved [249]. The Tm_{Pro} is in the range of 170 to 260 μmol per minute, or 1.25 to 1.86 μmol per milliliter of glomerular filtrate, respectively. Similar studies have been performed with hydroxyproline [251]. Infusion with one imino acid increases urinary excretion of the other and of glycine, while glycine infusion does not increase the rate of excretion of the imino acids [249, 251]. Patients with familial hyperprolinemia demonstrate iminoglycinuria [80, 239]. In rat kidney cortex slices, the uptake of glycine and imino acids can be saturated and follows Michaelis-Menten kinetics [193, 255]. In human kidney cortex slices, the uptake of L-proline is intimately related to the extent of intracellular proline metabolism [138]. Intracellular proline is rapidly metabolized, mainly to glutamic acid. Kinetic analysis of the entry process in human kidney slices suggested the existence of two saturable transport systems: one with a low capacity operating at low physiologic concentrations of proline, but shared with some neutral amino acids, and the other operating at higher proline concentration with an affinity value ten times less, but with a high capacity [138]. Studies in isolated tubules have shown that both L-proline and glycine are transported by more than one system [135, 136].

Patients with homozygous iminoglycinuria show urinary excretion rates for glycine in the range of 4 to 12.8 mmol per day [232, 291], 1.7 to 17 μmol/kg/day [290], or 4.8 to 7.0 μmol/min/1.73 m^2 [291], respectively. The clearance values for glycine are in the range of 12 to 39 ml/min/1.73 m^2 [15, 232, 290, 291], while glycine resorption ranges between 61 and 78.6 percent [15, 100, 232, 291]. The urinary excretion rates for proline are in the range of 0.3 to 3.0 mmol per day [15, 232], 28 to 45 μmol/kg/day [290], or 0.3 to 2.2 μmol/min/1.73 m^2 [291], respectively. The proline clearances are between 1.7 and 32 ml/min/1.73 m^2 [15, 232], while the percentage of tubular resorption varies between 61 and 98 percent [15, 100, 232]. The defect in hydroxyproline resorption is less severe. The urinary excretion rates of all other free amino acids and the levels of all amino acids in plasma are within the normal range.

The maximum rates of tubular resorption of L-proline and L-hydroxyproline are significantly lowered in homozygous patients with iminoglycinuria. Their imino acid transport is already saturated at normal concentrations in plasma [232, 246]; however, some transport capacity is retained, which explains the fact that prolinuria may disappear when plasma proline levels are very low [247]. The Tm values in heterozygotes are between those of homozygotes and normal subjects. In the heterozygotes the urinary excretion rates of glycine are either increased or normal, while the excretion rates of proline and hydroxyproline are always within the normal range. The "hyperglycinuric" heterozygotes of iminoglycinuria have glycine clearance rates between 8.6 and 26.2 ml/min/1.73 m^2 [246], and their percentage of tubular resorption is in the range of 82 to 95 percent, which means that glycine resorption is better retained by them than in patients with isolated hyperglycinuria (see Hyperglycinuria).

Normal intestinal transport of L-proline has been demonstrated in several patients with iminoglycinuria [15, 232, 246, 290, 291], while others have revealed impaired L-proline absorption as shown by delayed increase in plasma levels and augmentation of fecal amino acids [113, 194]. Obviously familial iminoglycinuria is also a heterogenous genetic entity with various defects in epithelial transport. Treatment is neither necessary nor possible.

Hematuria, renal malformations, and hereditary nephritis have been found in some patients with type I hyperprolinemia, due to a defect in proline oxidase [85, 114, 162, 192, 223, 239]. These patients sometimes demonstrate lowered tubular thresholds for proline, thus presenting a kind of renal prolinuria that probably is due to a general impairment of kidney function [114]. Similar findings have been reported in endemic Balkan nephropathy [81]. The demonstration of increased plasma proline levels, however, distinguishes the latter patients from patients with renal iminoglycinuria. A thorough investigation of inheritance patterns has revealed that hyperprolinemia and familial renal disease represent different genetic traits, one being transmitted by recessive and the other by dominant traits [253]. It has to be added that some patients with advanced renal insufficiency may show modestly increased plasma levels of proline per se [253].

HYPERDICARBOXYLIC AMINOACIDURIA

Recently this new type of tubular disturbance was described by Teijema and coworkers [292] in a 2-year-old girl with congenital athyreosis who demonstrated mental retardation and growth failure in spite of adequate thyroid substitution. She was found to have low plasma bicarbonate levels, attacks of hypoglycemia, hyperprolinemia (0.4 to 0.9 mmol/L), and a gross increase in the urinary excretion of glutamic acid and aspartic acid. The patient excreted 50 to 250 times more glutamic acid (6.2 to 12.7 μmol/min/1.73 m^2) than normal controls (61 $\pm$ 26 nmol/min/1.73 m^2) and 100 to 200 times more aspartic acid (0.8 to 1.23 μmol/min/1.73 m^2) than controls (8 $\pm$ 5 nmol/min/1.73 m^2). The levels of both amino acids in plasma were in the normal range (P$_{Glu}$ = 44 $\pm$ 8, normal = 30 $\pm$ 10 μmol/L; P$_{Asp}$ = 3.3 $\pm$ 1.4, normal = 2.9 $\pm$ 1.1 μmol/L). The clearance of glutamic acid was in the range of 275 to 310 ml/min/1.73 m^2 and that of aspartic acid between 150 and 600 ml/min/1.73 m^2, demonstrating a net tubular secretion for both amino acids. Neutral and basic amino acids were excreted in normal amounts except for proline and glycine, which were increased whenever proline in plasma exceeded 1 mmol per liter. The excretion rates for asparagine (0.03 to 0.06 μmol/min/1.73 m^2) and glutamine (0.2 to 0.5 μmol/min/1.73 m^2) were within the normal range. The intestinal absorption of L-glutamate seemed to be impaired also. The authors discuss the possibility that the defect might be another example of tubular overproduction, as in pyroglutamic aciduria [89], or a total tubular defect in the resorption of the dicarboxylic acids resulting in a net tubular secretion, as for cystine in classic cystinuria. Treatment was tried with oral glutamine supplementation, which succeeded in preventing hypoglycemic attacks when given continuously both day and night.

A similar type of hyperdicarboxylic aminoaciduria was described by Melançon and coworkers [187] in 4 unrelated French Canadian children. Two of them demonstrated tubular secretion of glutamic and aspartic acid, while the other two had no net secretion. All patients had normal levels of the dicarboxylic amino acids in plasma and cerebrospinal fluid.

Several years ago it was postulated from animal studies that the dicarboxylic amino acids are reabsorbed by a common transport system, since infusion of one dicarboxylic amino acid produced a steep increase in the excretion of the other dicarboxylic amino acid [151, 307, 308]. The finding of hyperdicarboxylic aminoaciduria in the human species is a fine confirmation of this early postulate.

HARTNUP DISEASE

This complex disturbance in the epithelial transport of neutral amino acids was first recognized in four siblings of an English family with the surname of Hartnup [16]; they later consented to lend their name to this syndrome [146], which although very rare, has been reported to occur in almost all parts of the world (for a complete list of published cases see reference 146). Hartnup syndrome is characterized by a tubular and intestinal defect in the (re)absorption of monocarboxylic-monoamino acids (cyclic and neutral amino acids) leading to a characteristic hyperaminoaciduria and to intestinal malabsorption with secondary decomposition of amino acids in the stool. The malabsorption, especially the defective tryptophan absorption, is responsible for the clinical signs, including pellagra-like photosensitive rash, attacks of cerebellar ataxia, and other central nervous system symptoms; these usually appear in successions of exacerbations and remissions and become less severe in adolescence. Hartnup disease is transmitted as an autosomal recessive trait.

The hyperaminoaciduria present in all Hartnup disease patients is remarkably constant, usually massive, and correlates neither with the severity of clinical signs nor with the therapeutic response to agents such as nicotinamide or antibiotics. Urinary excretion rates of amino acid nitrogen are in the range of 1 gm per day. The urinary pattern of amino acids is unique, indicating that the disturbance is located in the transport system for the neutral amino acids. It includes all cyclic and neutral amino acids: alanine, serine, threonine, asparagine, glutamine, valine, leucine, isoleucine, phenylalanine, tyrosine, tryptophan, histidine and citrulline; those of the iminoglycine, dicarboxylic, and dibasic transport systems usually are excluded or less severely involved. Methionine also is often found not to be increased, which implicates a specific and independent tubular transport system for this amino acid. The levels of the involved amino acids in plasma are often slightly reduced or in the lower normal range.

The clearance rates of the involved amino acids are highly increased [2, 65, 121, 289, 320], as shown on Fig. 86-8, which is taken from the data given by Antener and coworkers [2]. Some clear-

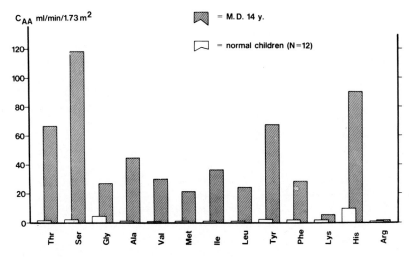

Figure 86-8. Clearance rates of free amino acids (C_{AA}) *in a 14-year-old girl with Hartnup disease. (Data from Antener et al. [2].)*

ance values, especially those of histidine and threonine, approach the glomerular filtration rate, which indicates the severity of the defect in tubular resorption. The values for the percentage of tubular resorption are correspondingly low. All other tubular functions are well retained; morphologic alterations are not found [67]. The hyperaminoaciduria of Hartnup disease is of little clinical importance; it has not been shown to result in any nutritional disturbance. The urine contains increased quantities of indoles also, but this is secondary to the intestinal defect and does not appear to reflect an additional tubular disturbance.

The intestinal defect in Hartnup disease was first demonstrated to exist for tryptophan. Milne and coworkers [190] performed oral tryptophan loading tests and showed that increased amounts of tryptophan can be found in the feces, that the plasma tryptophan levels exhibit a delayed response, and that patients excrete abnormally large amounts of products derived from tryptophan by bacterial decomposition in the intestinal lumen, especially indican, indolyl-3-acetic acid and indolyl-acetylglutamine [6]. The latter can be diminished by pretreatment with antibiotics. Fecal amino acids were found to be highly increased [245], especially after loading with tryptophan [2, 68, 320], although the stool amino acids show great variation. Intestinal malabsorption could be demonstrated also for tyrosine, lysine, and phenylalanine [198, 214, 257], while histidine was not found to be involved [121, 257]. Shih and coworkers [266] reported reduced in vitro uptake of tryptophan and methionine by intestinal mucosa of patients with Hartnup disease. Oligopeptides containing

tryptophan, phenylalanine, and histidine, however, are absorbed normally [5, 198]. The intestinal defect, therefore, seems to be specific for free amino acids, and nutritional disturbances are unlikely to arise from those defects.

The bacterial decomposition of tryptophan leads to intermediary products, which may then be absorbed and appear in the urine; indican, indolyl-acetic acid and indolyl-acetylglutamine are often excreted in the urine on normal diets and always after a tryptophan load [2, 6, 312, 319, 320]. Furthermore, the patients have a lowered ability to convert tryptophan to kynurenine and nicotinamide, probably due to the reduced tryptophan absorption in the intestine [190, 320]. Deficiency of endogenous nicotinamide formation has been considered to be the possible cause of skin rash and ataxia, since the symptoms are improved by nicotinamide, as in pellagra.

Treatment of Hartnup disease with nicotinamide (40 to 200 mg/day) is usually followed by marked improvement of the dermatitis and neurologic picture [2, 68, 120, 319], although such improvement also occurs spontaneously. An undue exposure to sunlight should be avoided, and temporary sterilization of the colon with neomycin may reduce the bacterial decarboxylation of unabsorbed dietary amino acids and thereby decrease the absorption of indoles and other amines [188].

GENERALIZED HYPERAMINOACIDURIA
The second group of renal hyperaminoacidurias does not demonstrate specific patterns of urinary amino acid excretion pathognomonic for the dis-

eases involved; the patterns are nonspecific regardless of the various causes leading to this syndrome. Usually all free amino acids are involved. The extent of involvement, however, is characteristic of each individual amino acid and mimics the degree to which amino acids are excreted in normal conditions. This nonspecific pattern is an exaggeration of the physiologic pattern and is called generalized hyperaminoaciduria. Generalized hyperaminoaciduria may exist as a singular tubular defect but is mostly accompanied by other disturbances of tubular or general kidney function. It is probably always acquired in the sense that it is secondary to some underlying disease. Therefore it always has to be considered as a symptom of tubular injury requiring further investigation, rather than a diagnostic entity per se.

Generalized hyperaminoaciduria is of renal origin. Its degree varies widely and depends on the severity and nature of the underlying disease. The plasma amino acids are normal or slightly decreased unless there is, in addition, a systemic metabolic derangement, especially of the liver, as in hyperammonemia or in intoxications accompanied by hyperaminoacidemias.

The pattern of generalized hyperaminoaciduria is shown in Figs. 86-9 and 86-10, in which the mean values of seven children with generalized hyperaminoaciduria due to various causes are compared with those of age-matched controls. In Fig. 86-9 the clearance values (C_{AA}) are depicted; individual values used to derive these data are shown in Fig. 81-3 in Chap. 81, since all of the patients suffered from complex tubular syndromes. Although the individual data exhibit great variation, the mean values reveal the typical pattern of generalized hyperaminoaciduria: those amino acids that under normal conditions are excreted in higher amounts (i.e., glycine and histidine) are most severely involved, while those amino acids that normally show only minimal excretion rates (i.e., proline, valine, isoleucine, ornithine, and arginine) are least involved.

Figure 86-10 shows the corresponding data for the percentage of tubular resorption; again the mean values of hyperaminoaciduric children are compared with normal values. The generalized pattern is obvious: there are low tubular resorption rates of those amino acids that show physiologically the lowest resorption rates and still rather high resorption rates in those amino acids normally almost completely reabsorbed. Methionine seems to be the only exception; it has, however, the lowest value in plasma so that analytical errors cannot be excluded. Net tubular secretion of amino acids, as seen in classic cystinuria or hyperdicarboxylic aminoaciduria, was never encountered in our own patients with generalized hyperaminoaciduria, indicating again a basic difference in the pathologic mechanisms.

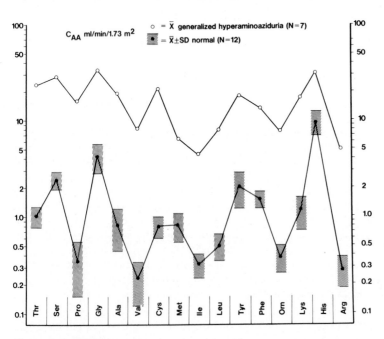

Figure 86-9. Clearance rates of free amino acids (C_{AA}) in patients with generalized hyperaminoaciduria (mean values of 7 children) as compared with normal values of age-matched controls. (Mean ± S.D. from Brodehl and Gellissen [32].)

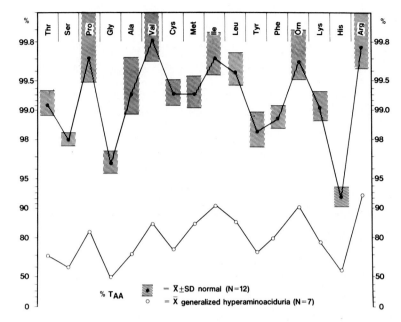

Figure 86-10. Percentage of tubular resorption (% T_{AA}) in generalized hyperaminoaciduria (mean values of 7 children) as compared with normal values. (Mean ± S.D. from Brodehl and Gellissen [32].)

Generalized hyperaminoacidurias are probably produced by defective energy metabolism in the tubular cells, as discussed in Chap. 81; however, molecular disturbances that lead to generalized hyperaminoaciduria are not understood. It is especially mysterious why the degrees and combinations of tubular defects could be so different for particular noxious substances or metabolic disturbances. In a few instances amino acid transport seems to be exclusively afflicted, as in patients with hyperammonemia due to enzymatic deficiencies in the urea cycle [206, author's unpublished observation] or in healing vitamin-D-deficiency rickets, when the defective phosphate resorption is already completely normalized [37]. In other cases typical combinations of tubular dysfunctions are present; thus in vitamin D deficiency phosphate resorption and amino acid resorption are most severely disturbed [37, 45, 101, 148], while bicarbonate resorption is only slightly affected [317] and glucose resorption is affected not at all by the metabolic disturbance, which includes the effect of hyperparathyroidism [101]. In the Fanconi syndrome of glycogenosis (Chap. 81), glucose resorption is most severely involved, while in galactosemia and fructose intolerance glucose resorption is only minimally disturbed, although all three conditions may exhibit severe generalized hyperaminoaciduria. Thus the molecular pathomechanism and the derangement in enzymatic activities are not known for the various types of these complex tubular dysfunctions. It is therefore mandatory to perform exact and quantitative measurements of tubular functions in these patients in order to get a better understanding of the underlying mechanisms that lead to tubular defects.

There are more than thirty different causes described that lead to generalized hyperaminoaciduria (see references 40, 164, 188, 253, 321). Most of them are listed in Table 86-5. Several are described under the heading of the Fanconi syndrome (Chap. 81) and will therefore not be discussed here. A critical analysis of the reports in the literature seems to be necessary, however, since it is obvious that some of the alleged causes of hyperaminoaciduria can no longer be incriminated, for the following reasons: (1) the underlying disease has been recognized as belonging to another entity, (2) hyperaminoaciduria could not be confirmed by later investigators using more precise methods, (3) the type of hyperaminoaciduria reported is not concordant with generalized hyperaminoaciduria, or (4) the influence of elevated plasma amino acids was not fully appreciated in the earlier studies. For instance, the Luder-Sheldon syndrome [175] turned out to be a familial type of idiopathic Fanconi syndrome [265, 321], the hyperaminoaciduria after thermal burns [83] is due mainly to peptide hydroxyproline excretion [91, 142], and the hyperaminoaciduria of kwashiorkor [240] is much influenced by elevated blood amino acid levels [238, 241]. Furthermore, the type of hyperaminoaciduria reported in patients with growth retardation and cor pulmonale [236, 237] is so unusual for a generalized form that it remains questionable whether this is not another tubular transport defect; this possibility is supported by the fact that no other tubular dysfunction could be detected in these cases. The same could apply for the patients with osteogenesis imperfecta [46]. Vitamin C deficiency was reported to be accompanied by renal hyperaminoaciduria [147, 149]. Since in short-term clearance studies with exact measurement of tubular amino acid resorption no defect could be found in three infants with scurvy [36], this cause is also eliminated from the list of hyperaminoacidurias. Finally, several reports have appeared in the literature describing different types of hyperaminoacidurias that are often accompanied by other abnormalities, which, however, cannot be classified properly as long as they are not confirmed by further investigation; these include patients with hyperaminoaciduria and xeroderma pigmentosum [50, 129], fibrous dysplasia of the bones [119], Blackfan-Diamond anemia [92], progeria [286], various dermatologic alterations [1, 49, 133, 208], steroid treatment [325], and vitamin B_{12} deficiency [300].

Prerenal Hyperaminoaciduria

In prerenal hyperaminoaciduria the urinary excretion rates of amino acids reflect the response of the kidney to increased loads of endogenously produced amino acids. These are therefore not renal disorders but are, from the renal point of view, experiments of nature by which the normal response of the kidney can be studied. Dipeptides and oligopeptides deriving from disturbed metabolism should also be included in the prerenal hyperaminoaciduria; however, they are not listed in Table 86-5.

The urinary pattern of amino acids in prerenal hyperaminoaciduria depends on the type of amino acid involved (see Table 86-5).

1. Amino acids with high specific resorption (mainly the cyclic and neutral amino acids) will "overflow" and not influence the resorption of related amino acids competitively. The mechanism of overflow could be either saturation of the tubular transport system by exceeding the maximal tubular resorptive capacity or a proportional increase in the net amount that escapes complete resorption without exceeding the tubular maximum. The first mechanism seems to be valid for the hyperexcretion of phosphoethanolamine in hypophosphatasia [217]. With the second mechanism, the percent of filtered amino acids to be reabsorbed is

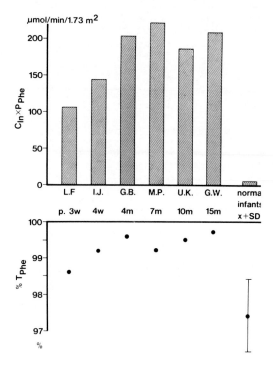

Figure 86-11. Filtered loads of phenylalanine ($C_{In} \times P_{Phe}$) and percentage of tubular resorption of phenylalanine (% T_{Phe}) in 6 untreated infants with phenylketonuria (p = prematures; w = week, m = month). (Normal values from Brodehl and Gellissen [32].)

either decreased, producing an exaggerated "splay" of the titration curve, as in hypersarcosinemia [111]; or the percentage of tubular resorption remains unchanged, as in phenylketonuria [33, 79]. The latter is shown on Fig. 86-11, in which the response of six untreated infants with phenylketonuria is depicted in comparison to the normal state. In spite of the increase in the tubular load ($C_{In} \times P_{Phe}$) up to forty times normal, the percentage of tubular resorption (% T_{Phe}) is not at all diminished; it even seems to be higher than found normally in age-matched controls [33]. Furthermore, there is no influence on the tubular resorption of all the other amino acids. Comparable results have been obtained for methionine in infants with homocystinuria [author's unpublished data] and could be assumed to exist in many of the inborn errors of metabolism listed in Table 86-5 under overflow hyperaminoaciduria; exact data in these latter conditions are not available from the literature. This type of hyperaminoaciduria, therefore, is strictly limited to the amino acid that is involved in the metabolic error.

2. Amino acids that share a group-specific transport system compete for tubular resorptive

sites with related amino acids when their load is increased. This effect can be found in metabolic errors of amino acids related to the iminoglycine, dibasic, and β-amino transport system. The competitive hyperaminoaciduria then reflects both the amino acid involved metabolically and its influence on the tubular resorption of other related amino acids.

3. The rate of excretion of amino acids with very low tubular resorption increases to the same extent as the metabolic production is increased. Usually there will be no accompanying change in the rate of excretion of other amino acids by a renal mechanism. This nonthreshold hyperaminoaciduria is specific for the amino acid involved in the metabolic error. The plasma amino acid levels depend on the rate of metabolic production; mostly they are very low or not measurable in comparison with those in the other two types of prerenal hyperaminoaciduria. The diagnosis of the underlying metabolic error therefore is primarily performed by urinary investigation.

References

1. Adler, R. C., and Nyhan, W. L. An oculocerebral syndrome with aminoaciduria and keratosis follicularis. *J. Pediatr.* 75:436, 1969.

2. Antener, I., Bartelheimer, H. K., Grüttner, R., and Rybak, C. Das Hartnup-Syndrom: II. Untersuchungen zur selektiven Aminosäuren-Malabsorption, zum Tryptophanmetabolismus und zur selektiven Hyperaminoaciduriе unter oraler Belastung mit L-Tryptophan. *Monatsschr. Kinderheilkd.* 121:571, 1973.

3. Applegarth, D. A., Hardwick, D. F., and Ross, P. M. Creatinine excretion in children and the usefulness of creatinine equivalents in amino acid chromatography. *Clin. Chim. Acta* 22:131, 1968.

4. Arrow, V. K., and Westall, R. G. Amino acid clearances in cystinuria. *J. Physiol.* 142:141, 1958.

5. Asatoor, A. M., Bandon, J. K., Lant, A. F., Milne, M. D., and Navab, F. Intestinal absorption of carnosine and its constituent amino acids in man. *Gut* 11:250, 1970.

6. Asatoor, A. M., Craske, J., London, D. R., and Milne, M. D. Indole production in Hartnup disease. *Lancet* 1:126, 1963.

7. Asatoor, A. M., Crouchman, M. R., Harrison, A. R., Light, F. W., Loughridge, L. W., Milne, M. D., and Richards, A. R. Intestinal absorption of oligopeptides in cystinuria. *Clin. Sci.* 41:23, 1971.

8. Asatoor, A. M., Freedman, P. S., Gabriel, J. R. T., Milne, M. D., Prussser, D. I., Roberts, J. T., and Willoughby, C. P. Amino acid imbalance in cystinuria. *J. Clin. Pathol.* 27:500, 1974.

9. Asatoor, A. M., Harrison, B. D. W., Milne, M. D., and Prosser, D. I. Intestinal absorption of an arginine-containing peptide in cystinuria. *Gut* 13: 95, 1972.

10. Asatoor, A. M., Lacey, B. W., London, D. R., and Milne, M. D. Amino acid metabolism in cystinuria. *Clin. Sci.* 23:304, 1962.

11. Ausiello, D. A., Segal, S., and Thier, S. O. Cellu-

lar accummulation of L-lysine in rat kidney cortex in vivo. *Am. J. Physiol.* 222:1473, 1972.

12. Awrich, A. E., Stackhouse, W. J., Cantrell, J. E., Patterson, J. H., and Rudman, D. Hyperdibasic aminoaciduria, hyperammonemia and growth retardation: Treatment with arginine, lysine, and citrulline. *J. Pediatr.* 87:731, 1975.

13. Baerlocher, K. E., Scriver, C. R., and Mohyuddin, F. The ontogeny of amino acid transport in rat kidney: 1. Effect on distribution ratios and intracellular metabolism of proline and glycine. *Biochim. Biophys. Acta* 249:353, 1971.

14. Baerlocher, K. E., Scriver, C. R., and Mohyuddin, F. The ontogeny of amino acid transport in rat kidney: 2. Kinetics of uptake and effect of anoxia. *Biochim. Biophys. Acta* 249:364, 1971.

15. Bank, H., Crispin, M., Ehrlich, D., and Szeinberg, A. Iminoglycinuria: A defect of renal tubular transport. *Isr. J. Med. Sci.* 8:606, 1972.

16. Baron, D. N., Dent, C. E., Harris, H., Hart, E. W., and Jepson, J. B. Hereditary pellagra-like skin rash with temporary cerebellar ataxia, constant renal amino-aciduria and other bizarre biochemical features. *Lancet* 2:421, 1956.

17. Bartsocas, C. S., Thier, S. O., and Crawford, J. D. Transport of L-methionine in rat intestine and kidney. *Pediatr. Res.* 8:673, 1974.

18. Bergeron, M., and Morel, F. Amino acid transport in rat renal tubules. *Am. J. Physiol.* 216:1139, 1969.

19. Bergstedt, J., O'Brien, D., and Lubschenco, L. O. Interrelationships in the urinary excretion of creatine, creatinine, free alpha amino acid nitrogen, and total nitrogen in premature infants. *J. Pediatr.* 56:635, 1960.

20. Berry, H. K. Cystinuria in mentally retarded siblings with atypical osteogenesis imperfecta. *Am. J. Dis. Child.* 97:196, 1959.

21. Berry, H. K., Leonard, C., Peters, H., Granger, M., and Chunekamra, N. Detection of metabolic disorders: Chromatographic procedures and interpretation of results. *Clin. Chem.* 14:1033, 1968.

22. Bickel, H. Harnsteinprophylaxe bei Cystinurie. *Urologe* 1:288, 1962.

23. Boström, H., and Hambraeus, L. Cystinuria in Sweden: VII. Clinical, histo-pathological, and medico-social aspects of the disease. *Acta Med. Scand.* [Suppl.] 411:1, 1964.

24. Boström, H., and Tottie, K. Cystinuria in Sweden: II. The incidence of homozygous cystinuria in Swedish schoolchildren. *Acta Paediatr. Scand.* 48:345, 1959.

25. Bovee, K. C., Thier, S. O., Rea, C., and Segal, S. Renal clearance of amino acids in canine cystinuria. *Metabolism* 23:51, 1974.

26. Brand, E., Cahill, G. F., and Kassell, B. Canine cystinuria: V. Family history of two cystinuric Irish terriers and cystine determinations in dog urine. *J. Biol. Chem.* 133:431, 1940.

27. Bremer, H. J. Die Cystinurie, Typen, Diagnostik und Behandlung. *Monatsschr. Kinderheilkd.* 117:1, 1964.

28. Bremer, H. J., Kohne, E., and Enders, W. The excretion of diamines in human urine: II. Cadaverine, putrescine, 1,3-diaminopropane, 2,2-dithiobis-(ethylamine) and spermidine in urine of patients with cystinuria and cystinlysinuria. *Clin. Chim. Acta* 32:407, 1971.

29. Brigham, M. P., Stein, W. H., and Moore, S. The

concentration of cysteine and cystine in human blood plasma. *J. Clin. Invest.* 39:1633, 1960.

30. Brodehl, J. Postnatal Development of Tubular Amino Acid Reabsorption. In S. Silbernagl, F. Lang, and R. Greger (eds.), *Amino Acid Transport and Uric Acid Transport.* Stuttgart: Thieme, 1976.

31. Brodehl, J., and Bickel, H. Aminoaciduria and hyperaminoaciduria in childhood. *Clin. Nephrol.* 1: 149, 1973.

32. Brodehl, J., and Gellissen, K. Endogenous renal transport of free amino acids in infancy and childhood. *Pediatrics* 42:395, 1968.

33. Brodehl, J., Gellissen, K., and Kaas, W. P. The renal transport of amino acids in untreated infants with phenylketonuria. *Acta Paediatr. Scand.* 59:241, 1970.

34. Brodehl, J., Gellissen, K., and Kowalewski, S. Isolated Cystinuria (without Lysine-Ornithine- and Argininuria) in a Family with Hypocalcemic Tetany. In *Abstracts of the 3rd International Congress of Nephrology, Washington, 1966.* P. 165.

35. Brodehl, J., Gellissen, K., and Kowalewski, S. Isolierter Defekt der tubulären Cystin-Rückresorption in einer Familie mit idiopathischem Hypoparathyroidismus. *Klin. Wochenschr.* 45:38, 1967.

36. Brodehl, J., and Kaas, W. P. The tubular reabsorption of free amino acids in infants with scurvy. *Clin. Chim. Acta* 28:409, 1970.

37. Brodehl, J., Kaas, W. P., and Weber, H.-P. Vitamin D deficiency rickets: Renal handling of phosphate and free amino acids. *Pediatr. Res.* 5:591, 1971.

38. Brown, J. H., Fabre, L. F., Fabrell, G. L., and Adams, E. D. Hyperlysinuria with hyperammonemia. *Am. J. Dis. Child.* 124:127, 1972.

39. Brown, J. L., Samiy, A. H., and Pitts, R. F. Localization of amino-nitrogen reabsorption in the nephron of the dog. *Am. J. Physiol.* 200:370, 1961.

40. Calcagno, P. L., and Hollerman, C. E. Hereditary Renal Disease and Certain Renal Tubular Disorders. In M. I. Rubin and T. M. Barratt (eds.), *Pediatric Nephrology.* Baltimore: Williams & Wilkins, 1975. Pp. 668–728.

41. Carver, M. J., and Paska, R. Ion exchange chromatography of urinary amino acids: I. Normal children. *Clin. Chim. Acta* 6:721, 1961.

42. Chan, A. W. K., Burch, H. B., Alvey, T. R., and Lowry, O. H. A quantitative histochemical approach to renal transport: I. Aspartate and glutamate. *Am. J. Physiol.* 229:1034, 1975.

43. Chan, Y.-L., and Huang, K. C. Microperfusion studies on renal tubular transport of tryptophan derivatives in rats. *Am. J. Physiol.* 221:575, 1971.

44. Childs, B. Urinary excretion of free alpha-amino acid nitrogen by normal infants and children. *Proc. Soc. Exp. Biol. Med.* 81:225, 1952.

45. Chisolm, J. J., and Harrison, H. E. Aminoaciduria in vitamin D deficiency states in premature infants and older infants with rickets. *J. Pediatr.* 60:206, 1962.

46. Chowers, I., Czaczkes, J. W., Ehrenfeld, E. N., and Landau, S. Familial aminoaciduria in osteogenesis imperfecta. *J.A.M.A.* 181:771, 1962.

47. Christensen, H. N. On the development of amino acid transport systems. *Fed. Proc.* 32:19, 1973.

48. Clara, R., and Lowenthal, A. Aminoacidurie tubulaire congénitale et familiale avec nanisme grave et hypotonie musculaire à évolution favorable chez quatre enfants d'une même fratrie. *Acta Neurol. Belg.* 65:911, 1965.

49. Clodi, P. H., Deutsch, E., and Niebauer, G. Hyperaminoacidurie bei Lichtdermatosen. *Wien. Klin. Wochenschr.* 76:623, 1964.

50. Clodi, P. H., Wewalka, F., and Zweymüller, E. Xeroderma pigmentosum mit körperlichem sowie geistigem Entwicklungsrückstand und intermittierender Aminoacidurie: Ein neues Syndrom? *Z. Kinderheilkd.* 93:223, 1965.

51. Colliss, J. E., Levi, A. J., and Milne, M. D. Stature and nutrition in cystinuria and Hartnup disease. *Br. Med. J.* 1:590, 1963.

52. Cooke, H., and Young, J. A. Amino acid transport in the developing chicken kidney. *Aust. J. Exper. Biol. Med. Sci.* 51:199, 1973.

53. Corcos, J. M., Soler-Bechera, J., Mayer, K., Freyberg, R. H., Goldstein, R., and Jaffé, I. Neutrophilic agranulocytosis during administration of penicillamine. *J.A.M.A.* 189:265, 1964.

54. Cox, B. D., and Cameron, J. S. Homoarginine in cystinuria. *Clin. Sci. Molec. Med.* 46:173, 1974.

55. Cramér, K., Cramér, H., and Selander, S. A comparative analysis between variation in 24-hour urinary creatinine output and 24-hour urinary volume. *Clin. Chim. Acta* 15:331, 1967.

56. Crane, C. W., and Turner, A. W. Amino acid pattern of urine and blood plasma in a Labrador dog. *Nature (Lond.)* 177:237, 1956.

57. Crawhall, J. C., Scowen, E. F., Thompson, C. J., and Watts, R. W. E. Dissolution of cystine stones during D-penicillamine treatment of a pregnant patient with cystinuria. *Br. Med. J.* 1:216, 1967.

58. Crawhall, J. C., Scowen, E. F., Thompson, C. J., and Watts, R. W. E. The renal clearance of amino acid in cystinuria. *J. Clin. Invest.* 46:1162, 1967.

59. Crawhall, J. C., Scowen, E. F., and Watts, R. W. E. Effect of penicillamine on cystinuria. *Br. Med. J.* 1:588, 1963.

60. Crawhall, J. C., Scowen, E. F., and Watts, R. W. E. Further observations on use of D-penicillamine in cystinuria. *Br. Med. J.* 1:1411, 1964.

61. Crawhall, J. C., and Segal, S. Sulphocysteine in the urine of the blotched Kenya genet. *Nature (Lond.)* 208:1320, 1965.

62. Crawhall, J. C., and Watts, R. W. E. Cystinuria. *Am. J. Med.* 45:736, 1968.

63. Crawhall, J. C., and Watts, R. W. E. Some complications observed in the treatment of cystinuria with D-penicillamine and N-acetyl-D-penicillamine. *Postgrad. Med. J.* 44:8, 1968.

64. Curran, P. F. Active transport of amino acids and sugars. *Arch. Intern. Med.* 129:258, 1972.

65. Cusworth, D. C., and Dent, C. E. Renal clearances of amino acids in normal adults and in patients with aminoaciduria. *Biochem. J.* 74:550, 1960.

66. Datta, S. P., and Harris, H. Urinary amino acid patterns of some mammals. *Ann. Eugen. (Lond.)* 18:107, 1953.

67. Daute, K. H., Dietel, K., and Ebert, W. Das Hartnup Syndrom: Bericht über einen tödlichen Krankheitsverlauf. *Z. Kinderheilkd.* 95:103, 1966.

68. De Laey, P., Hooft, C., Timmermans, J., and Shoeck, J. Biochemical aspects of the Hartnup disease: I. Results of intravenous and oral tryptophan loading tests in a case of Hartnup disease. *Ann. Paediatr. (Basel)* 202:145, 1964.

69. Dent, C. E., Friedman, M., Green, H., and Watson,

L. C. A. Treatment of cystinuria. *Br. Med. J.* 1: 403, 1965.

70. Dent, C. E., and Harris, H. Hereditary forms of rickets and osteomalacia. *J. Bone Joint Surg. [Br.]* 38:204, 1956.

71. Dent, C. E., and Rose, G. A. Amino acid metabolism in cystinuria. *Q. J. Med.* 20:205, 1951.

72. Dent, C. E., and Senior, B. Studies on the treatment of cystinuria. *Br. J. Urol.* 27:317, 1955.

73. Dent, C. E., Senior, B., and Walshe, J. M. The pathogenesis of cystinuria: II. Polarographic studies of the metabolism of sulphur containing amino acids. *J. Clin. Invest.* 33:1216, 1954.

74. Dent, C. E., and Walshe, J. M. Amino acid metabolism. *Br. Med. Bull.* 10:247, 1954.

75. DeVries, A., and Alexander, B. Studies on amino acid metabolism: II. Blood glycine and total amino acids in various pathological conditions with observations on the effects of intravenously administered glycine. *J. Clin. Invest.* 27:655, 1958.

76. DeVries, A., Kochwa, S., Lazebnik, J., Frank, M., and Djaldetti, M. Glycinuria, a hereditary disorder associated with nephrolithiasis. *Am. J. Med.* 23:408, 1957.

77. Dickinson, J. C., Rosenblum, H., and Hamilton, P. B. Ion exchange chromatography of the free amino acids in the plasma of the newborn infant. *Pediatrics* 36:2, 1965.

78. Dickinson, J. C., Rosenblum, H., and Hamilton, P. B. Ion exchange chromatography of the free amino acids in the plasma of infants under 2500 gm at birth. *Pediatrics* 45:606, 1970.

79. Dodinval, P., Heusden, A., Willems, C., and Dodinval-Versie, J. Clearance rénale et réabsorption tubulaire de la phénylalanine chez l'enfant phénylcétonurique. *Rev. Fr. Etud. Clin. Biol.* 10: 1064, 1965.

80. Dodinval, P., Willems, C., Heusden, A. M., Hainaut, H., and Gottschalk, C. Clearance rénale des acides aminés chez un enfant hyperprolinémique. *J. Genet. Hum.* 17:297, 1969.

81. Dotchev, D., Hungerland, H., Liappis, N., and Oyanagi, K. Hyperiminoazidurie und Dysaminoazidurie bei der Endemischen (Balkan-) Nephropathie. *Munch. Med. Wochenschr.* 116:363, 1974.

82. Dustin, J. P., Moore, S., and Bigwood, E. J. Chromatographic studies on the excretion of amino acids in early infancy. *Metabolism* 4:75, 1955.

83. Eades, C. H., Pollack, R. L., and Hardy, J. D. Thermal burns in man: IX. Urinary amino acid patterns. *J. Clin. Invest.* 34:1756, 1955.

84. Edwards, O. M., Bayliss, R. I. S., and Millen, S. Urinary creatinine excretion as an index of the completeness of 24-hour urine collections. *Lancet* 2: 1165, 1969.

85. Efron, M. L. Familial hyperprolinemia: Report of a second case, associated with congenital renal malformations, hereditary hematuria and mild mental retardation, with demonstration of an enzyme defect. *N. Engl. J. Med.* 272:1243, 1965.

86. Efron, M. L., McPherson, T. C., Shih, V. E., Welsh, C. F., and MacCready, R. A. D-Methioninuria due to DL-methionine ingestion. *Am. J. Dis. Child.* 117: 104, 1969.

87. Efron, M. L., Young, D., Moser, H. W., and MacCready, R. A. A simple chromatographic screening test for the detection of disorders of amino acid metabolism. *N. Engl. J. Med.* 270:1378, 1964.

88. Eisenbach, G. M., Weise, M., and Stolte, H. Amino acid reabsorption in the rat nephron. Free flow micropuncture study. *Pfluegers Arch.* 357:63, 1975.

89. Eldjarn, L., Jellum, E., and Stokke, O. Pyroglutamic aciduria: Studies on the enzymic block and on the metabolic origin of pyroglutamic acid. *Clin. Chim. Acta* 40:461, 1972.

90. Elliot, J. S., Ribeiro, M. E., and Eusebio, E. Cystinuria in the blotched genet. *Invest. Urol.* 5:568, 1968.

91. Estes, F. L., and Wetzel, R. L. The recovery of amino acids from acid hydrolysates of whole urine from patients with thermal burns. *Clin. Chim. Acta* 15:421, 1967.

92. Falter, M. L., and Robinson, M. G. Autosomal dominant inheritance and amino aciduria in Blackfan-Diamond anaemia. *J. Med. Genet.* 9:64, 1972.

93. Fariss, B. L., and Kolb, F. O. Factors involved in crystal formation in cystinuria. *J.A.M.A.* 205:846, 1968.

94. Fawcett, N. P., and Nyhan, W. L. Cystinuria and dermatomyositis. *Clin. Pediatr.* 9:727, 1970.

95. Fawcett, N. P., Nyhan, W. L., and Anderson, W. W. Thrombocytosis during treatment of cystinuria with penicillamine. *J. Pediatr.* 69:976, 1966.

96. Fleming, W. H., Avery, G. B., Morgan, R. I., and Cone, T. E. Gastrointestinal malabsorption associated with cystinuria: Report of a case in a Negro. *Pediatrics* 32:358, 1963.

97. Foley, T. H., and London, D. R. Cysteine metabolism in cystinuria. *Clin. Sci.* 29:549, 1965.

98. Fox, M., Thier, S., Rosenberg, L. E., and Segal, S. Ionic requirements for amino acid transport in rat kidney cortex slices: I. Influence of extracellular ions. *Biochim. Biophys. Acta* 79:167, 1964.

99. Fox, M., Thier, S., Rosenberg, L. E., Kiser, W., and Segal, S. Evidence against a single renal transport defect in cystinuria. *N. Engl. J. Med.* 270:556, 1964.

100. Fraser, G. R., Friedman, A. I., Ratton, V. M., Wade, D. N., and Woolf, L. I. Imino glycinuria—a "harmless" inborn error of metabolism. *Humangenetik* 6:362, 1968.

101. Fraser, D., Kooh, S. W., and Scriver, C. R. Hyperparathyroidism as the cause of hyperaminoaciduria and phosphaturia in human vitamin D deficiency. *Pediatr. Res.* 1:425, 1967.

102. Frimpter, G. W. The disulfide of L-cysteine and L-homocysteine in urine of patients with cystinuria. *J. Biol. Chem.* 236:51, 1961.

103. Frimpter, G. W. Cystinuria: Metabolism of the disulfide of cysteine and homocysteine. *J. Clin. Invest.* 42:1956, 1963.

104. Frimpter, G. W. Cystathioninuria in a patient with cystinuria. *Am. J. Med.* 46:832, 1969.

105. Frimpter, G. W., and Greenberg, A. J. Renal clearance of cystathionine in homozygous and heterozygous cystathioninuria, cystinuria and the normal state. *J. Clin. Invest.* 46:975, 1967.

106. Frimpter, G. W., Horwith, M., Furth, E., Fellows, R. E., and Thompson, D. D. Inulin and endogenous amino acid renal clearances in cystinuria: Evidence for tubular secretion. *J. Clin. Invest.* 41:281, 1962.

107. Garrod, A. E. *Inborn Errors of Metabolism* (1909). Reprint. London: Oxford University Press, 1963.

108. Gayer, J., and Gerok, W. Die Lokalisierung der

L-Aminosäure-Rückresorption in der Niere durch Stop-flow-Analysen. *Klin. Wochenschr.* 39:1054, 1961.

109. Ghadimi, H., and Pecora, P. Plasma amino acids after birth. *Pediatrics* 34:182, 1964.

110. Ghisolfi, J., Angier, D., Dalous, A., and Regnier, C. Les clearances renales endogenes des acides amines. Etude des variations en fonction de l'age. *Arch. Fr. Pediatr.* 30:131, 1973.

111. Glorieux, F. H., Scriver, R., Delvin, E., and Mohyuddin, F. Transport and metabolism of sarcosine in hypersarcosinemic and normal phenotypes. *J. Clin. Invest.* 50:2313, 1971.

112. Goebel, F. Über die Aminosäurenfraktion im Säuglingsharn. *Z. Kinderheilkd.* 34:94, 1923.

113. Goodman, S. I., McIntyre, C. A., and O'Brien, D. Impaired intestinal transport of proline in a patient with familial iminoaciduria. *J. Pediatr.* 71:246, 1967.

114. Goyer, R. A., Reynolds, J., Burke, J., and Burkholder, P. Hereditary renal disease with neurosensory hearing loss, prolinuria and ichthyosis. *J. Med. Sci.* 256:166, 1968.

115. Greene, M. L., Lietman, P. S., Rosenberg, L. E., and Seegmiller, J. E. Familial hyperglycinuria: New defect in renal tubular transport of glycine and imino acids. *Am. J. Med.* 54:265, 1973.

116. Greth, W. E., Thier, S. O., and Segal, S. Cellular accumulation of L-cystine in rat kidney cortex in vivo. *J. Clin. Invest.* 52:454, 1973.

117. Gross, J. B., Ulrich, J. A., and Jones, J. D. Urinary excretion of amino acids in a kindred with hereditary pancreatitis and aminoaciduria. *Gastroenterology* 47:41, 1964.

118. Gross, J. B., Ulrich, J. A., Jones, J. D., and Maher, F. T. Endogenous renal clearances of 12 individual amino acids in four apparently healthy subjects and in four aminoaciduric persons of a kindred with hereditary pancreatitis. *J. Lab. Clin. Med.* 63:933, 1964.

119. Halvorsen, S., and Aas, K. Renal tubular defects in fibrous dysplasia of the bones: Report of two cases. *Acta Paediatr. Scand.* 50:297, 1961.

120. Halvorsen, K., and Halvorsen, S. Hartnup disease. *Pediatrics* 31:29, 1963.

121. Halvorsen, S., Hygstedt, O., Jagenburg, R., and Sjaastad, O. Cellular transport of L-histidine in Hartnup disease. *J. Clin. Invest.* 48:1552, 1964.

122. Hambraeus, L. Comparative studies of the value of two cyanide-nitroprusside methods in the diagnosis of cystinuria. *Scand. J. Clin. Lab. Invest.* 15:657, 1963.

123. Hambraeus, L. Cystinuria in Sweden: X. Quantitative studies of the urinary amino acid excretion in cystinuria. *Acta Soc. Med. Ups.* 69:1, 1964.

124. Hambraeus, L., and De Hevesy, G. Cystinuria in Sweden: VIII. A case of coeliac disease associated with cystine-lysinuria. *Acta Paediatr.* 53:213, 1964.

125. Hambraeus, L., and Lagergren, C. Cystinuria in Sweden: VI. Biophysical and roentgenological studies of urinary calculi from cystinurias. *J. Urol.* 88:826, 1962.

126. Harris, H., Mittwoch, U., Robson, E. B., and Warren, F. L. Phenotypes and genotypes in cystinuria. *Ann. Hum. Genet.* 20:57, 1955.

127. Harris, H., Mittwoch, U., Robson, E. B., and Warren, F. L. The pattern of amino acid excretion in cystinuria. *Ann. Hum. Genet.* 19:196, 1955.

128. Harris, H., and Warren, F. L. Quantitative studies on the urinary cystine in patients with cystine stone formation and in their relatives. *Ann. Eugen. (Lond.)* 18:125, 1953.

129. Hatano, H., Ohkido, M., Arai, J., and Mamiya, G. Aminoaciduria in xeroderma pigmentosum. *Acta Derm. Venereol. (Stockh.)* 48:571, 1968.

130. Hellier, M. D., Holdsworth, C. D., and Perrett, D. Dibasic amino acid absorption in man. *Gastroenterology* 65:613, 1973.

131. Hellier, M. D., Holdsworth, C. D., Perrett, D., and Thirumalai, C. Intestinal dipeptide transport in normal and cystinuric subjects. *Clin. Sci.* 43:659, 1972.

132. Henneman, P. H., Dempsey, E. F., Caroll, E. L., and Henneman, D. H. Acquired vitamin D resistant osteomalacia: A new variety characterized by hypercalcemia, low serum bicarbonate and hyperglycinuria. *Metabolism* 11:103, 1962.

133. Hermans, P. E., Ulrich, J. A., and Markowitz, H. Chronic mucocutaneous candidiasis as a surface expression of deep-seated abnormalities: Report of a syndrome of superficial candidiasis, absence of delayed hypersensitivity and aminoaciduria. *Am. J. Med.* 47:503, 1969.

134. Hewitt, J., Pillon, D., and Leibach, F. H. Inhibition of amino acid accumulation in slices of rat kidney cortex by diamide. *Biochim. Biophys. Acta* 363:267, 1974.

135. Hillman, R. E., Albrecht, I., and Rosenberg, L. E. Identification and analysis of multiple glycine transport systems in isolated mammalian renal tubules. *J. Biol. Chem.* 243:5566, 1968.

136. Hillman, R. E., and Rosenberg, L. E. Amino acid transport by isolated mammalian renal tubules: II. Transport systems for L-proline. *J. Biol. Chem.* 244:4494, 1969.

137. Holmgren, G., Jeppson, J. O., and Samuelson, G. High-voltage electrophoresis in urinary amino acid screening. *Scand. J. Clin. Lab. Invest.* 26:313, 1970.

138. Holtzapple, P., Genel, M., Rea, C., and Segal, S. Metabolism and uptake of L-proline by human kidney cortex. *Pediatr. Res.* 7:818, 1973.

139. Holtzapple, P., Rea, C., Bovee, K., and Segal, S. Characteristics of cystine and lysine transport in renal and jejunal tissue from cystinuric dogs. *Metabolism* 20:1016, 1971.

140. Hsia, D. Y.-Y., and Inouye, T. *Inborn Errors of Metabolism.* Part 2. Laboratory Methods. Chicago: Year Book, 1966.

141. Hurwitz, L. J., Carson, N. A. J., Allen, I. V., Fannin, T. F., Lyttle, J. A., and Neill, D. W. Clinical, biochemical, and histopathological findings in a family with muscular dystrophy. *Brain* 90:799, 1967.

142. Jackson, S. H., and Elliott, T. G. The origin of the urinary peptide hydroxyproline in burns. *Clin. Chim. Acta* 23:97, 1969.

143. Jackson, S. H., Sardharwalla, J. B., and Ebers, G. C. Two systems of amino acid chromatography suitable for mass screening. *Clin. Biochem.* 2:163, 1968.

144. Jaffe, I. A., Altman, K., and Merryman, P. The antipyridoxine effect of penicillamine in man. *J. Clin. Invest.* 43:1869, 1964.

145. Jaffe, I. A., Treser, G., Suzuki, Y., and Ehrenreich, T. Nephropathy induced by D-penicillamine. *Ann. Intern. Med.* 69:549, 1968.

146. Jepson, J. B. Hartnup Disease. In J. B. Stanbury,

J. B. Wyngaarden, and D. S. Fredrickson (eds.), *The Metabolic Basis of Inherited Disease* (4th ed.). New York: McGraw-Hill, 1978. P. 1563.

147. Jonxis, J. H. P., and Huisman, T. H. J. Aminoaciduria and ascorbic deficiency. *Pediatrics* 14:238, 1954.
148. Jonxis, J. H. P., Smith, P. A., and Huisman, T. H. J. Rickets and amino-aciduria. *Lancet* 2:1015, 1952.
149. Jonxis, J. H. P., and Van Lukk, W. H. J. Tubular reabsorption of amino acids in vitamin C deficiency. *Arch. Dis. Child.* 48:402, 1973.
150. Joseph, R., Ribierre, M., Job, J.-C., and Girault, M. Maladie familiale associante des convulsions à début très précoce une hyperalbuminorachie et une hyperaminoacidurie. *Arch. Fr. Pediatr.* 15:374, 1958.
151. Kamin, H., and Handler, P. Effect of infusion of single amino acids upon excretion of other amino acids. *Am. J. Physiol.* 164:654, 1951.
152. Käser, H., Cottier, P., and Antener, I. Glucoglycinuria, a new familial syndrome. *J. Pediatr.* 61:386, 1962.
153. Keiser, H. R., Henkin, R. I., Bartter, F. C., and Sjoerdsma, A. Loss of taste during therapy with penicillamine. *J.A.M.A.* 203:381, 1968.
154. Kekomäki, M., Toivakka, E., Häkkinen V., and Salapuro, M. Familial protein intolerance with deficient transport of basic amino acids. *Acta Med. Scand.* 183:357, 1968.
155. Kekomäki, M., Visakorpi, J. K., Perheentupa, J., and Saxén, L. Familial protein intolerance with deficient transport of basic amino acids: An analysis of 10 patients. *Acta Paediatr. Scand.* 56:617, 1967.
156. Kihara, H., Valente, M., Porter, M. T., and Fluharty, A. L. Hyperdibasic aminoaciduria in a mentally retarded homozygote with a peculiar response to phenothiazines. *Pediatrics* 51:223, 1973.
157. King, J. S. Treatment of cystinuria with α-mercaptopropionylglycine: A preliminary report with some notes on column chromatography of mercaptans. *Proc. Soc. Exp. Biol. Med.* 129:927, 1968.
158. King, J. S., and Wainer, A. Cystinuria with hyperuricemia and methioninuria: Biochemical study of a case. *Am. J. Med.* 43:125, 1967.
159. Knox, W. E. Sir Archibald Garrod's "inborn errors of metabolism": I. Cystinuria. *Am. J. Hum. Genet.* 10:13, 1958.
160. Kolb, F. O., Earll, J. M., and Harper, H. A. Disappearance of cystinuria in a patient treated with prolonged low methionine diet. *Metabolism* 16:378, 1967.
161. Kolb, F. O., and Harper, H. A. Disappearance of cystine stones on low methionine diets. *Clin. Res.* 8:141, 1960.
162. Kopelman, H., Asatoor, A. M., and Milne, M. D. Hyperprolinaemia and hereditary nephritis. *Lancet* 2:1075, 1964.
163. Kraffczyk, F., Helger, R., Lang, H., and Bremer, H. J. Thin layer chromatographic screening test for amino acid anomalies in urine without desalting using internal standards. *Clin. Chim. Acta* 35:345, 1971.
164. Leaf, A. The Syndrome of Osteomalacia, Renal Glucosuria, Aminoaciduria, and Increased Phosphate Clearance (the Fanconi Syndrome). In J. B. Stanbury, J. B. Wyngaarden, and D. S. Fredrickson (eds.), *The Metabolic Basis of Inherited Disease* (2nd ed.). New York: McGraw-Hill, 1966. P. 1205.

165. Lester, F. T., and Cusworth, D. C. Lysine infusion in cystinuria: Theoretical renal thresholds for lysine. *Clin. Sci.* 44:99, 1973.
166. Levy, H. L., Madigan, P. M., and Lum, A. Fecal contamination in urine amino acid screening: Artifactual cause of hyperaminoaciduria. *J. Clin. Pathol.* 51:765, 1969.
167. Lewis, H. B. The occurrence of cystinuria in healthy young men and women. *Ann. Intern. Med.* 6:183, 1932.
168. Lindblad, B. S., and Baldesten, A. Time studies on free amino acid levels of venous plasma during the neonatal period. *Acta Paediatr. Scand.* 58:252, 1969.
169. Lingard, J. M., Györy, A. Z., and Young, J. A. Microperfusion study of the kinetics of reabsorption of cycloleucine in early and late segments of the proximal convolution of the rat nephron. *Pfluegers Arch.* 357:51, 1975.
170. Lingard, J., Rumrich, G., and Young, J. A. Reabsorption of L-glutamine and L-histidine from various regions of the rat proximal convolution studied by stationary microperfusion: Evidence that the proximal convolution is not homogeneous. *Pfluegers Arch.* 342:1, 1973.
171. Lingard, J., Rumrich, G., and Young, J. A. Kinetics of L-histidine transport in the proximal convolution of the rat nephron studied using the stationary microperfusion technique. *Pfluegers Arch.* 342:13, 1973.
172. Loewy, A., and Neuberg, C. Zur Kenntnis der Diamine. *Z. Physiol. Chem.* 43:355, 1904.
173. London, D. R., and Foley, T. H. Cystine metabolism in cystinuria. *Clin. Sci.* 29:129, 1965.
174. Lotz, M., and Bartter, M. C. Stone dissolution with D-penicillamine in cystinuria. *Br. Med. J.* 2:1408, 1965.
175. Luder, J., and Sheldon, W. A familial tubular absorption defect of glucose and amino acids. *Arch. Dis. Child.* 30:160, 1955.
176. Luke, R. G., Briggs, J. D., Fell, G. S., and Kennedy, A. C. Proteinuria associated with D-penicillamine therapy of cystinuria. *J. Urol.* 99:207, 1968.
177. MacDonald, W. B., and Fellers, F. X. Penicillamine in the treatment of patients with cystinuria. *J.A.M.A.* 197:396, 1966.
178. Malmquist, J., Jagenburg, R., and Lindstedt, G. Familial protein intolerance—possible nature of enzyme defect. *N. Engl. J. Med.* 284:997, 1971.
179. Massachusetts Department of Public Health. Newborn screening for metabolic disorders. *N. Engl. J. Med.* 288:1299, 1973.
180. McCarthy, C. F., Borland, J. L., Lynch, H. J., Owen, E. E., and Tyor, M. P. Defective uptake of basic amino acids and L-cystine by intestinal mucosa of patients with cystinuria. *J. Clin. Invest.* 43:1518, 1964.
181. McDonald, J. E., and Henneman, P. H. Stone dissolution in vivo and control of cystinuria with D-penicillamine. *N. Engl. J. Med.* 273:578, 1965.
182. McMenamy, R. H., Lund, C. C., and Oncley, J. L. Unbound amino acid concentration in human blood plasmas. *J. Clin. Invest.* 36:1672, 1957.
183. Meier, P., Rampini, S., Baerlocher, K., and Prader, A. Über die Häufigkeit vermehrter Zystinausscheidung bei Zürcher Schulkindern. *Helv. Paediatr. Acta* 29:237, 1974.
184. Meister, A. On the enzymology of amino acid transport. *Science* 180:33, 1972.

185. Meister, A. The γ-glutamyl cycle: Disease associated with specific enzyme deficiencies. Ann. Intern. Med. 81:247, 1974.

186. Meister, A. Glutathione: Metabolism and function via the γ-glutamyl cycle. Life Sci. 15:177, 1974.

187. Melançon, S. B., Dallaire, L., Lemieux, B., Robitaille, P., and Portier, M. Dicarboxylic aminoaciduria: A new inborn error of glutamic and aspartic acid transport with genetic heterogeneity. Pediatr. Res. 9:377, 1975.

188. Milne, M. D. Renal Tubular Dysfunction. In M. B. Strauss and L. G. Welt (eds.), Diseases of the Kidney (2nd ed.). Boston: Little, Brown, 1971. P. 1071.

189. Milne, M. D., Asatoor, A. M., Edwards, K. D. G., and Loughridge, L. W. The intestinal absorption defect in cystinuria. Gut 2:323, 1961.

190. Milne, M. D., Crawford, M. A., Girao, C. B., and Loughridge, L. W. The metabolic disorder in Hartnup disease. Q. J. Med. 29:407, 1960.

191. Milne, M. D., London, D. R., and Asatoor, A. M. Citrullinuria in cases of cystinuria (letter to the editor). Lancet 2:49, 1962.

192. Minder, F. C., Dubach, U. C., and Antener, I. Hereditäre Nephropathie und Schwerhörigkeit (mit Aminosäuren- und Fettstoffwechselstörungen in einer Familie in der Schweiz). Z. Klin. Med. 158: 601, 1965.

193. Mohyuddin, F., and Scriver, C. R. Amino acid transport in mammalian kidney: Multiple systems for imino acids and glycine in rat kidney. Am. J. Physiol. 219:1, 1970.

194. Morikawa, T., Tada, K., Ando, T., Yoshida, T., Yokoyama, Y., and Arakawa, T. Prolinuria: Defect in intestinal absorption of imino acids and glycine. Tohoku J. Exp. Med. 90:105, 1966.

195. Morin, C. L., Thompson, M. W., Jackson, S. H., and Sass-Kortsak, A. Biochemical and genetic studies in cystinuria: Observations on double heterozygotes of genotype I/II. J. Clin. Invest. 50:1961, 1971.

196. Morris, M. L., Green, D. F., Dinkel, J. H., and Brand, E. Canine cystinuria. North Am. Vet. 16: 16, 1935.

197. Morrison, H. R. A roentgenological study of cystine urinary calculs. Am. J. Roentgenol. 44:537, 1940.

198. Navab, F., and Asatoor, A. M. Studies on intestinal absorption of amino acids and a dipeptide in a case of Hartnup disease. Gut 11:373, 1970.

199. Niemann, A. Beitrag zur Lehre von Cystinurie beim Menschen. Dtsch. Arch. Klin. Med. 18:232, 1876.

200. Norio, R., Perheentupa, J., Kekomäki, M., and Visakorpi, J. K. Lysinuric protein intolerance, an autosomal recessive disease; a genetic study of 10 Finnish families. Clin. Genet. 2:214, 1971.

201. O'Brien, D., and Butterfield, L. J. Further studies on renal tubular conservation of free amino acids in early infancy. Arch. Dis. Child. 38:437, 1963.

202. Oldfield, J. E., Allen, P. H., and Adair, J. Identification of cystine calculi in mink. Proc. Soc. Exp. Biol. Med. 91:560, 1956.

203. Opienska-Blauth, J., Charezinski, M., and Brzusziewicz, H. Tryptophan in human plasma. Clin. Chim. Acta 8:260, 1963.

204. Oyanagi, K., Miura, R., and Yamanouchi, T. Congenital lysinuria: A new inherited transport disorder of dibasic amino acids. J. Pediatr. 77:259, 1970.

205. Page, E. W., Glendening, M. B., Dignam, W., and Harper, H. A. The cause of histidinuria in normal pregnancy. Am. J. Obstet. Gynecol. 68:110, 1954.

206. Palmer, T., Oberholzer, V. G., and Levin, B. Amino acid levels in patients with hyperammonemia and argininosuccinic aciduria. Clin. Chim. Acta 52: 335, 1974.

207. Palmer, T., Rossiter, M. A., Levin, B., and Oberholzer, V. G. The effect of protein loads on plasma amino acid levels. Clin. Sci. Molec. Med. 45: 827, 1973.

208. Passwell, J., Zipperkorski, L., Katznelson, D., Szeinberg, A., Crispin, M., Pollak, S., Goodman, R., Bat-Miriam, M., and Cohen, B. E. A syndrome characterized by congenital ichthyosis with atrophy, mental retardation, dwarfism, and generalized aminoaciduria. J. Pediatr. 82:466, 1973.

209. Perheentupa, J., and Visakorpi, J. K. Protein intolerance with deficient transport of basic amino acids: Another inborn error of metabolism. Lancet 2:813, 1965.

210. Perrett, D. Ampicillin and amino acid analysis. Clin. Chim. Acta 64:343, 1975.

211. Perry, T. L. Iatrogenic urinary amino-acid derived from penicillin. Nature (Lond.) 206:895, 1965.

212. Peters, W.-H. A study of the possible usefulness of the α-amino nitrogen/creatinine ratio in urine. Clin. Chim. Acta 45:387, 1973.

213. Peters, J. H., Lin, S. C., Berridge, B. J., Cummings, J. G., and Chao, W. R. Amino acids, including asparagine and glutamine, in plasma and urine of normal human subjects. Proc. Soc. Exp. Biol. Med. 131:281, 1969.

214. Pomeroy, J., Efron, M. L., Dayman, J., and Hoefnagel, D. The Hartnup disorder in a New England family. N. Engl. J. Med. 278:1214, 1968.

215. Pruzanski, W. Cystinuria and cystine urolithiasis in childhood. Acta Paediatr. Scand. 55:97, 1966.

216. Przyrembel, H., Leupold, D., Tosberg, P., and Bremer, H. J. Amino acid excretion of premature infants receiving different amounts of protein. Clin. Chim. Acta 49:27, 1973.

217. Rasmussen, K. Phosphorylethanolamine and hypophosphatasia. Dan. Med. Bull. 15:1, 1968.

218. Rasmussen, K. Observations during treatment of cystinuria with D-penicillamine. Acta Med. Scand. 189:367, 1971.

219. Reander, A. The roentgen density of the cystine calculus; a roentgenographic and experimental study including a comparison with more common uroliths. Acta Radiol. (Diagn.) (Stockh.) [Suppl.] 41:1, 1941.

220. Reynolds, R., Rea, C., and Segal, S. Regulation of amino acid transport in kidney cortex of newborn rats. Science 184:68, 1974.

221. Robson, E. B., and Rose, G. A. The effect of intravenous lysine on the renal clearances of cystine, arginine and ornithine in normal subjects, in patients with cystinuria and Fanconi syndrome and their relatives. Clin. Sci. 16:75, 1957.

222. Roesel, R. A., and Coryell, M. E. Determination of cystine excretion by the nitroprusside method during drug therapy of cystinuria. Clin. Chim. Acta 52:343, 1974.

223. Rokkones, T., and Løken, A. C. Congenital renal dysplasia, retinal dysplasia and mental retardation associated with hyperprolinuria and hyper-OH-prolinuria. *Acta Paediatr. Scand.* 57:225, 1968.

224. Rootwelt, K. Quantitative determination of thiols and disulphides in urine by means of Ellman's reagent and thiolated sephadex and its application in cystinuria. *Scand. J. Clin. Lab. Invest.* 19:325, 1967.

225. Rosenberg, L. E. Cystinuria: Genetic heterogeneity and allelism. *Science* 154:1341, 1966.

226. Rosenberg, L. E., Albrecht, I., and Segal, S. Lysine transport in human kidney: Evidence for two systems. *Science* 155:1426, 1967.

227. Rosenberg, L. E., Berman, M., and Segal, S. Studies of the kinetics of amino acid transport, incorporation into proteins and oxidation in kidney-cortex slices. *Biochim. Biophys. Acta* 71:664, 1963.

228. Rosenberg, L. E., Blair, A., and Segal, S. Transport of amino acids by slices of rat-kidney cortex. *Biochim. Biophys. Acta* 54:479, 1961.

229. Rosenberg, L. E., Crawhall, J. C., and Segal, S. Intestinal transport of cystine and cysteine in man: Evidence for separate mechanisms. *J. Clin. Invest.* 46:30, 1967.

230. Rosenberg, L. E., Downing, S., Durant, J. L., and Segal, S. Cystinuria: Biochemical evidence for three genetically distinct diseases. *J. Clin. Invest.* 45:365, 1966.

231. Rosenberg, L. E., Downing, S. J., and Segal, S. Competitive inhibition of dibasic amino acid transport in rat kidney. *J. Biol. Chem.* 237:2265, 1962.

232. Rosenberg, L. E., Durant, J. L., and Elsas, L. J. Familial iminoglycinuria: An inborn error of renal tubular transport. *N. Engl. J. Med.* 278:1407, 1968.

233. Rosenberg, L. E., Durant, J. L., and Holland, J. M. Intestinal absorption and renal extraction of cystine and cysteine in cystinuria. *N. Engl. J. Med.* 273:1239, 1965.

234. Rosenberg, L. E., and Hayslett, J. P. Nephrotoxic effects of penicillamine in cystinuria. *J.A.M.A.* 201:698, 1967.

235. Rosenberg, L. E., Mueller, P. S., and Watkin, D. M. A new syndrome: Familial growth retardation, renal amino aciduria and cor pulmonale: II. Investigation of renal function, amino acid metabolism and genetic transmission. *Am. J. Med.* 31:205, 1961.

236. Rosenberg, L. E., and Scriver, C. R. Disorders of Amino Acid Metabolism. In P. K. Bondy (ed.), *Duncan's Diseases of Metabolism* (6th ed.). Philadelphia: Saunders, 1969. P. 366.

237. Rowley, P. T., Mueller, P. S., Watkin, D. M., and Rosenberg, L. E. Familial growth retardation, renal aminoaciduria and cor pulmonale: I. Description of a new syndrome, with case report. *Am. J. Med.* 31:187, 1961.

238. Saunders, S. J., Barbezat, G. O., Wittmann, W., and Hansen, J. D. L. Aminoaciduria of kwashiorkor. *Am. J. Clin. Nutr.* 20:760, 1967.

239. Schafer, I. A., Scriver, C. R., and Efron, M. L. Familial hyperprolinemia, cerebral dysfunction and renal anomalies occurring in a family with hereditary nephropathy and deafness. *N. Engl. J. Med.* 267:51, 1962.

240. Schendel, H. E., Antonis, A., and Hansen, J. D. L. Increased aminoaciduria in infants with kwashiorkor fed natural and synthetic diets. *Pediatrics* 23:662, 1959.

241. Schendel, H. E., and Hansen, J. D. L. Study of factors responsible for the increased aminoaciduria of kwashiorkor. *J. Pediatr.* 60:290, 1962.

242. Schwartzman, L., Blair, A., and Segal, S. A common renal transport system for lysine, ornithine, arginine and cysteine. *Biochem. Biophys. Res. Commun.* 23:220, 1966.

243. Schwartzman, L., Blair, A., and Segal, S. Exchange diffusion of dibasic amino acids in rat-kidney cortex slices. *Biochim. Biophys. Acta* 135:120, 1967.

244. Schwartzman, L., Blair, A., and Segal, S. Effect of transport inhibitors on dibasic amino acid exchange diffusion in rat-kidney cortex. *Biochim. Biophys. Acta* 135:136, 1967.

245. Scriver, C. R. Hartnup disease: A genetic modification of intestinal and renal transport of certain neutral alpha amino acids. *N. Engl. J. Med.* 273:530, 1965.

246. Scriver, C. R. Renal tubular transport of proline, hydroxyproline, and glycine: III. Genetic basis for more than one mode of transport in human kidney. *J. Clin. Invest.* 47:823, 1968.

247. Scriver, C. R. Familial Iminoglycinuria. In J. B. Stanbury, J. B. Wyngaarden, and D. S. Fredrickson (eds.), *The Metabolic Basis of Inherited Disease* (4th ed.). New York: McGraw-Hill, 1978. P. 1593.

248. Scriver, C. R., and Davies, E. Endogenous renal clearance rates of free amino acids in pre-pubertal children. *Pediatrics* 36:592, 1965.

249. Scriver, C. R., Efron, M. L., and Schafer, I. A. Renal tubular transport of proline, hydroxyproline, and glycine in health and in familial hyperprolinemia. *J. Clin. Invest.* 43:374, 1964.

250. Scriver, C. R., Goldbloom, R. B., and Roy, C. Hypophosphatemic rickets with renal hyperglycinuria, renal glucosuria and glycylprolinuria. *Pediatrics* 34:357, 1964.

251. Scriver, C. R., and Goldman, H. Renal tubular transport of proline, hydroxyproline, and glycine: II. Hydroxy-L-proline as substrate and as inhibitor in vivo. *J. Clin. Invest.* 45:1357, 1966.

252. Scriver, C. R., and Mohyuddin, F. Amino acid transport in kidney: Heterogeneity of α-amino iso butyric uptake. *J. Biol. Chem.* 243:3207, 1968.

253. Scriver, C. R., and Rosenberg, L. E. Amino Acid Metabolism and Its Disorders. In A. L. Schaffer (ed.), *Major Problems in Clinical Pediatrics*. Philadelphia: Saunders, 1973. Vol. 10.

254. Scriver, C. R., Whelan, D. T., Clow, C. L., and Dallaire, L. Cystinuria: Increased prevalence in patients with mental disease. *N. Engl. J. Med.* 283:783, 1970.

255. Scriver, C. R., and Wilson, O. H. Possible locations for a common gene product in membrane transport of imino acids and glycine. *Nature (Lond.)* 202:92, 1964.

256. Scriver, C. R., and Wilson, O. H. Amino acid transport: Evidence for genetic control of two types in human kidney. *Science* 155:1428, 1967.

257. Seakins, J. W. T., and Ersser, R. S. Effect of amino acid load on a healthy infant with the biochemical features of Hartnup disease. *Arch. Dis. Child.* 42:682, 1967.

258. See, G., Lejeune, J., Dayras, J.-C., and Raoul, M. Cystinurie-lysinurie avec nanisme, dysmorphie faciale, hypoplasie musculaire et retard psycho-motor. *Ann. Pediatr. (Paris)* 17:846, 1970.

259. Segal, S., and Crawhall, J. C. Transport of cysteine by human kidney cortex in vitro. *Biochem. Med.* 1:141, 1968.

260. Segal, S., and Crawhall, J. C. Characteristics of cystine and cysteine transport in the rat kidney cortex slices. *Proc. Natl. Acad. Sci. U.S.A.* 59:231, 1968.

261. Segal, S., Rea, C., and Smith, I. Separate transport systems for sugars and amino acids in developing rat kidney cortex. *Proc. Natl. Acad. Sci. U.S.A.* 68:372, 1971.

262. Segal, S., and Smith, I. Delineation of separate transport systems in rat kidney cortex for L-lysine and L-cystine by developmental patterns. *Biochem. Biophys. Res. Commun.* 35:771, 1969.

263. Segal, S., and Smith, I. Delineation of cystine and cysteine transport systems in rat kidney cortex by developmental patterns. *Proc. Natl. Acad. Sci. U.S.A.* 63:926, 1969.

264. Segal, S., and Thier, S. O. Renal Handling of Amino Acids. In J. Orloff and R. W. Berliner (eds.), *Handbook of Physiology.* Section 8: *Renal Physiology.* Washington, D.C.: American Physiological Society, 1973.

265. Sheldon, W., Luder, J., and Webb, B. A familial tubular absorption defect of glucose and amino acids. *Arch. Dis. Child.* 36:90, 1961.

266. Shih, V. E., Bixby, E. M., Alpers, D. H., Bartsocas, C. S., and Thier, S. O. Studies of intestinal transport defect in Hartnup disease. *Gastroenterology* 61:445, 1971.

267. Shih, V. E., and Schulman, J. D. N-acetylcysteine-cysteine disulfide excretion in the urine following N-acetylcysteine administration. *J. Pediatr.* 74:129, 1969.

268. Silbernagl, S. Renal handling of amino acids: Recent results of tubular microperfusion. *Clin. Nephrol.* 5:1, 1976.

269. Silbernagl, S., and Deetjen, P. Glycine reabsorption in rat proximal tubules. *Pfluegers Arch.* 323:342, 1971.

270. Silbernagl, S., and Deetjen, P. L-arginine transport in rat proximal tubules. *Pfluegers Arch.* 336:79, 1972.

271. Silbernagl, S., and Deetjen, P. The tubular reabsorption of L-cystine and L-cysteine: A common transport system with L-arginine or not? *Pfluegers Arch.* 337:277, 1972.

272. Silbernagl, S., and Deetjen, P. Molecular specificity of the L-arginine reabsorption mechanism: Microperfusion studies in the proximal tubule of rat kidney. *Pfluegers Arch.* 340:325, 1973.

273. Silk, D. B. A., Perrett, D., and Clark, M. L. Jejunal and ileal absorption of dibasic amino acids and an arginine containing dipeptide in cystinuria. *Gastroenterology* 68:1426, 1975.

274. Silk, D. B. A., Perrett, D., Stephens, A. D., Clark, M. L., and Scowen, E. F. Intestinal absorption of cystine and cysteine in normal human subjects and patients with cystinuria. *Clin. Sci. Mol. Med.* 47:393, 1974.

275. Simell, O. Diamino acid transport into granulocytes and liver slices of patients with lysinuric protein intolerance. *Pediatr. Res.* 9:504, 1975.

276. Simell, O., and Perheentupa, J. Renal handling of diamino acids in lysinuric protein intolerance. *J. Clin. Invest.* 54:9, 1974.

277. Simell, O., Perheentupa, J., Rapola, J., Visakorpi, J. K., and Eskelin, L. E. Lysinuric protein intolerance. *Am. J. Med.* 59:229, 1975.

278. Simon, S. Zur Stickstoffverteilung im Urin des Neugeborenen. *Z. Kinderheilkd.* 2:1, 1911.

279. Smith, I. (ed.). *Chromatographic and Electrophoretic Techniques.* Vol. I, *Chromatography* (3rd ed.), 1969; Vol. II, *Electrophoresis* (2nd ed.), 1968. London: Heinemann.

280. Smith, D. R., Kolb, F. O., and Harper, H. A. The management of cystinuria and cystine-stone disease. *J. Urol.* 81:61, 1959.

281. Snyderman, S. E. Diagnosis of metabolic disease. *Pediatr. Clin. North Am.* 18:199, 1971.

282. Snyderman, S. E., Holt, L. E., Jr., Norton, P. M., Roitman, E., and Phansalkar, S. V. The plasma aminogram: I. Influence of the level of protein intake and a comparison of whole protein and amino acid diets. *Pediatr. Res.* 2:131, 1968.

283. Soupart, P. Urinary excretion of free amino acids in normal adult men and women. *Clin. Chim. Acta* 4:265, 1959.

284. Steginck, L., Boaz, D. P., VonBehren, P., and Mueller, S. Ampicillin and amino acid chromatography. *J. Pediatr* 81:1214, 1972.

285. Stein, W. H., and Moore, S. The free amino acids of human blood plasma. *J. Biol. Chem.* 211:915, 1954.

286. Steinberg, A. H., Szeinberg, A., and Cohen, B. E. Aminoaciduria and hypermetabolism in progeria. *Arch. Dis. Child.* 32:401, 1957.

287. Stephens, A. D., and Watts, R. W. E. The treatment of cystinuria with N-acetyl-D-penicillamine, a comparison with the results of D-penicillamine treatment. *Q. J. Med.* 40:355, 1971.

288. Stokes, G. S., Potts, J. T., Lotz, M., and Bartter, F. C. New agent in the treatment of cystinuria, N-acetyl-D-penicillamine. *Br. Med. J.* 1:284, 1968.

289. Tada, K., Hirono, H., and Arakawa, T. Endogenous renal clearance rates of free amino acids in prolinuric and Hartnup patients. *Tohoku J. Exp. Med.* 93:57, 1967.

290. Tada, K., Morikawa, T., Ando, T., Yoshida, T., and Minagawa, A. Prolinuria: A new renal tubular defect in transport of proline and glycine. *Tohoku J. Exp. Med.* 87:133, 1965.

291. Tancredi, F., Guazzi, G., and Auricchio, S. Renal iminoglycinuria without intestinal malabsorption of glycine and imino acids. *J. Pediatr.* 76:386, 1970.

292. Teijema, H. L., VanGelderen, H. H., Giesberts, M. A. H., and Laurent De Angulo, M. S. L. Dicarboxylic amino aciduria: An inborn error of glutamate and aspartate transport with metabolic implications, in combination with hyperprolinemia. *Metabolism* 23:115, 1974.

293. Thiele, F. H. Concerning cystinuria and diamines. *J. Physiol. (Lond.)* 36:68, 1907.

294. Thier, S. O., Blair, A., Fox, M., and Segal, S. The effect of extracellular sodium concentration on the kinetics of α-aminosiobutyric acid transport in the rat kidney cortex slices. *Biochim. Biophys. Acta* 135:300, 1967.

295. Thier, S. O., Fox, M., Segal, S., and Rosenberg, L. E. Cystinuria: In vitro demonstration of an intestinal transport defect. *Science* 143:482, 1964.

296. Thier, S. O., and Segal, S. Cystinuria. In J. B. Stanbury, J. B. Wyngaarden, and D. S. Fredrickson (eds.), *The Metabolic Basis of Inherited Dis-*

ease (4th ed.). New York: McGraw-Hill, 1978. P. 1578.

297. Thier, S. O., Segal, S., Fox, M., Blair, A., and Rosenberg, L. E. Cystinuria: Defective intestinal transport of dibasic amino acids and cystine. *J. Clin. Invest.* 44:442, 1965.

298. Thiriar, M. J., Seliwowski, H. B., and Vis, H. L. Cystin-lysinurie associée chez deux frères à une arriération mentale et à des anomalies morphologiques et neurologiques. *Acta Neurol. Psychiatr. Belg.* 68:216, 1968.

299. Tocci, P. M. The Biochemical Diagnosis of Metabolic Disorders by Urinalysis and Paper Chromatography. In W. L. Nyhan (ed.), *Amino Acid Metabolism and Genetic Variation*. New York: McGraw-Hill, 1967. P. 461.

300. Todd, D. Observations on the amino-aciduria in megaloblastic anemia. *J. Clin. Pathol.* 12:238, 1959.

301. Treacher, R. J. Intestinal absorption of lysine in cystinuric dogs. *J. Comp. Pathol.* 75:309, 1965.

302. Ullrich, K. J., Fasold, H., Klöss, S., Rumrich, G., Salzer, M., Sato, K., Simon, B., and DeVries, J. X. Effect of SH- NH$_2$-, and COOH-site group reagents on the transport processes in the proximal convolution of the rat kidney. *Pfluegers Arch.* 334:51, 1973.

303. Ullrich, K. J., Rumrich, G., and Klöss, S. Sodium dependence of the amino acid transport in the proximal convolution of the rat kidney. *Pfluegers Arch.* 351:49, 1974.

304. Vergis, J. G., and Walker, B. R. Cystinuria, hyperuricemia and uric acid nephrolithiasis—case report. *Nephron* 7:577, 1970.

305. Von Udransky, L., and Baumann, E. Über das Vorkommen von Diaminen, sogenannten Ptomaine, bei Cystinurie. *Z. Physiol. Chem.* 13:562, 1889.

306. Wallraff, E. B., Brodie, E. C., and Borden, A. L. Urinary excretion of amino acids in pregnancy. *J. Clin. Invest.* 29:1542, 1950.

307. Webber, W. A. Interactions of neutral and acidic amino acids in renal tubular transport. *Am. J. Physiol.* 202:577, 1962.

308. Webber, W. A. Characteristics of acidic amino acid transport in mammalian kidney. *Can. J. Biochem. Physiol.* 41:131, 1963.

309. Webber, W. A. Amino acid excretion patterns in developing rats. *Can. J. Physiol. Pharmacol.* 45:867, 1967.

310. Webber, W. A., Brown, J. L., and Pitts, R. F. Interaction of amino acids in renal tubular transport. *Am. J. Physiol.* 200:380, 1961.

311. Wedeen, R. P., and Thier, S. O. Intrarenal distribution of nonmetabolized amino acids in vivo. *Am. J. Physiol.* 220:507, 1971.

312. Weyers, H., and Bickel, H. Photodermatose mit Aminoacidurie, Indolaceturie und cerebraler Manifestation (Hartnup-Syndrom). *Klin. Wochenschr.* 36:893, 1958.

313. Whelan, D. T., and Scriver, C. R. Cystathioninuria and renal iminoglycinuria in a pedigree. *N. Engl. J. Med.* 278:924, 1968.

314. Whelan, D. T., and Scriver, C. R. Hyperdibasic-aminoaciduria: An inherited disorder of amino acid transport. *Pediatr. Res.* 2:525, 1968.

315. White, H. H. Separation of amino acids in physiological fluids by two-dimensional thin-layer chromatography. *Clin. Chim. Acta* 21:297, 1968.

316. Williams, W. M., and Huang, K. C. In vitro and in vivo transport of tryptophan derivatives. *Am. J. Physiol.* 219:1468, 1970.

317. Winberg, J., and Bergström, T. Renal acidification defect in infants with mild deficiency rickets. *Acta Paediatr. Scand.* 54:139, 1965.

318. Wollaston, W. H. On cystic oxide: A new species of urinary calculus. *Phil. Trans. R. Soc.* 100:223, 1810.

319. Wong, P. W. K., Lambert, A. M., Pillai, P. M., and Jones, P. M. Observations on nicotinic acid therapy in Hartnup disease. *Arch. Dis. Child.* 42:642, 1967.

320. Wong, P. W. K., and Pillai, P. M. Clinical and biochemical observations in two cases of Hartnup disease. *Arch. Dis. Child.* 41:383, 1966.

321. Woolf, L. I. *Renal Tubular Dysfunction*. Springfield, Ill.: Thomas, 1966.

322. Wright, L. A., and Nicholson, T. F. The proximal tubular handling of amino acids and other ninhydrin positive substances. *Can. J. Physiol. Pharmacol.* 44:183, 1966.

323. Yü, T.-F., Adler, M., Bobrow, E., and Gutman, A. B. Plasma and urinary amino acids in primary gout, with special references to glutamine. *J. Clin. Invest.* 48:885, 1969.

324. Zinneman, H. H., and Jones, J. E. Dietary methionine and its influence on cystine excretion in cystinuric patients. *Metabolism* 15:915, 1966.

325. Zischka, R., Orti, E., and Castells, S. Effect of short-term administration of dexamethasone on urinary and plasma free amino acids in children. *J. Clin. Endocrinol.* 31:95, 1970.

326. Zorab, P. A. Normal creatinine and hydroxyproline excretion in young persons. *Lancet* 2:1164, 1969.

87. Disorders of Renal Transport of Sodium, Potassium, and Magnesium

George J. Schwartz and Adrian Spitzer

Disorders of Sodium Transport

Renal tubular disorders of sodium, potassium, and magnesium transport are uncommon in childhood in the absence of glomerular damage. They may occur singly or be part of a constellation of tubular dysfunctions, such as in the Fanconi syndrome. Even when isolated, these defects may severely stress the body's homeostatic mechanisms, since sodium is the predominant extracellular cation and potassium and magnesium are the first and the second most common intracellular cations, respectively. The tubular disorders to be discussed in this chapter include the salt-losing syndrome of pseudohypoaldosteronism, the potassium-losing conditions of pseudohyperaldosteronism (the Liddle syndrome), hyperplasia of the juxtaglomerular complex with secondary aldosteronism without hypertension (the Bartter syndrome); a potassium-retaining disorder associated with hyperkalemia and acidosis (the Spitzer-Weinstein syndrome), and, finally, two disorders of magnesium transport leading to hypomagnesemia.

PSEUDOHYPOALDOSTERONISM

Synonyms for pseudohypoaldosteronism include pseudohypoadrenalocorticism [6], pseudohypoadrenocorticalism [15], and congenital renal salt-losing syndrome [1].

In 1958 Cheek and Perry [3] described a salt-wasting syndrome in a 3-month-old male infant who failed to thrive and was unable to maintain water balance. He was found to have renal sodium wasting, and this defect could not be corrected by the administration of deoxycorticosterone acetate (DOCA). Renal function, as estimated from blood urea nitrogen, appeared to be normal. Urinary excretion of 17-ketosteroids and 11-oxysteroids were within the expected range for age, and the adrenal gland responded adequately to corticotropin stimulation. An appropriately low concentration of sodium in sweat suggested adequate production of mineralocorticoids. The transitory nature of this disease became apparent at the age of 8 months, when salt supplementation was no longer required.

Epidemiology. Twenty-two cases of pseudohypoaldosteronism have been reported [1, 3, 4, 6, 9–16, 18, 20, 21, 22, 26], with a slight preponderance of males. A genetic transmission is suggested by detection in sibships [1, 15], in offspring of consanguineous parents [16, 20], and in the mother of an affected infant [10]. On the basis of its appearance in two sisters, Bierich and Schmidt considered the disease to have an autosomal recessive mode of inheritance [1].

Clinical Features. Pseudohypoaldosteronism typically is recognized in the second week of life following an apparently normal prenatal course and delivery. The baby is noted to be feeding poorly, to vomit, to fail to gain weight, and to be moderately dehydrated. Urine output is usually normal even during acute episodes of dehydration.

Laboratory Findings. Isotonic or hyponatremic dehydration with hyperkalemia is usually present in pseudohypoaldosteronism. Hypochloremia may accompany hyponatremia. Prerenal azotemia is common. Acidosis is seldom encountered. Despite

hyponatremia and dehydration, the infant excretes inappropriately large amounts of sodium in the urine. There are no other urinary abnormalities, no evidence of distortion of the kidneys or urinary tract on intravenous urogram, and the renal biopsy is usually normal, although a case with juxtaglomerular hyperplasia and elevated plasma renin levels has been reported [1].

As already mentioned, plasma cortisol levels and urinary 17-hydroxycorticosteroids, 17-ketosteroids, and pregnanetriol are within normal limits. Urinary aldosterone excretion and aldosterone secretion rates are elevated; plasma aldosterone concentration and plasma renin activity are high. Treatment with salt supplements tends to reduce these levels, but not into the range appropriate to the level of sodium intake. Administration of exogenous aldosterone, DOCA, or 9α-fluorohydrocortisone has no effect on sodium balance or the clinical condition. The aldosterone antagonist spironolactone, however, aggravates the sodium loss [20]. The cases described by Rosler et al. may represent a variant of the classic disorder, since both DOCA and 9α-fluorohydrocortisone decreased the salt wastage [16].

Pathophysiology. The association of renal salt loss with elevated levels of renin and aldosterone in the absence of any other renal abnormality has suggested an end-organ unresponsiveness similar to that observed in pseudohypoparathyroidism or nephrogenic diabetes insipidus. The fact that spironolactone exacerbates the salt loss, however, suggests that the renal tubule is not totally unresponsive to aldosterone [20]. Moreover, the presence of low maximal tubular resorption of glucose (Tm_G) [12, 13] and a normal response of the colon [12, 13] and the sweat glands [3, 4, 15, 20] to aldosterone indicate that at least some of the salt wasting might reflect impaired resorption in the proximal tubule [13, 14]. Supporting this conclusion are the recent findings of Bierich and Schmidt [1] that Na^+-K^+-ATPase activity in microdissected tubules from a kidney biopsy of an affected patient was minimal in the ascending limb of Henle's loop and absent in the proximal and distal convoluted tubules.

Differential Diagnosis. Once a diagnosis of salt wasting is made in an infant, it is necessary to investigate steroid metabolism. A defect in 21-hydroxylase or β-1-dehydrogenase is present in congenital virilizing adrenal hyperplasia, whereas a defect in 20,22-cholesterol desmolase is found in nonvirilizing adrenal hyperplasia (congenital lipoid adrenal hyperplasia) [2, 22]. A generalized failure to increase steroid production in response to corticotropin (ACTH) is apparent in adrenal insufficiency [11]. Salt wasting may also occur in congenital hypoaldosteronism, which may result from a defect in the biosynthetic pathway between corticosterone and aldosterone and possibly from a defect in 18-hydroxylation or in 18-dehydrogenation [20]. In such cases aldosterone secretion rates are very low, but corticosterone production increases with age, leading to spontaneous remission [11, 19]. Unlike classic pseudohypoaldosteronism, the salt wasting of hypoaldosteronism can be controlled with DOCA.

Salt loss may occur in complex tubulopathies such as the Fanconi syndrome and renal tubular acidosis. In occasional cases of renal insufficiency, the magnitude of salt wasting is greater than anticipated and is termed *salt-losing nephritis* [7, 25]. These patients may present with what initially appears to be adrenocortical insufficiency [25] but then are found to have renal abnormalities such as dysgenesis, hereditary polycystic disease, oligomeganephronia, juvenile nephronophthisis, chronic pyelonephritis, or interstitial nephritis [18].

Finally, a similar constellation of electrolyte abnormalities has been documented in low birth weight infants [5, 8, 17, 24] in whom hyponatremia, hyperkalemia, and inadequate renal conservation of sodium appear in the second or third week of life associated with a few nonspecific symptoms. Spontaneous resolution usually occurs by 6 weeks of age. Although systematic studies of aldosterone metabolism have not been done, it has been suggested that the immature renal tubules respond poorly to aldosterone [8]. Animal experiments suggest, however, that the high levels of aldosterone encountered in these infants are not the consequence of relative tubular unresponsiveness to the hormone but represent a compensatory response to the tendency toward sodium loss resulting from the rapid increase in the filtration rate of the superficial nephrons, not attended by a concomitant and proportional rise in sodium resorption at the level of the proximal tubules [23].

Treatment. Salt supplements of 3 to 6 gm daily (50 to 100 mEq/day) have proved sufficient to restore plasma electrolytes to normal and reduce the production of renin and aldosterone in pseudohypoaldosteronism [5, 17].

Course. Untreated patients with pseudohypoaldosteronism may die of dehydration, vascular collapse, or hyperkalemia. Treated patients usually outgrow their need for salt within the first 2 to 4 years of life. Subsequently they exhibit some catch-up growth, although most of them remain two standard deviations below the mean height and weight, at least over the limited periods of observation available so far. Despite clinical improvement, the elevation of the plasma renin activity may persist [13], justifying the need for long-term follow-up of such patients.

Potassium-Retaining Disorders
THE SPITZER-WEINSTEIN SYNDROME

Occurrence. Hyperkalemia associated with inappropriately reduced urinary potassium excretion and systemic acidosis in the absence of reduction in the glomerular filtration rate (GFR) has been reported in 4 children. There have been no reports of affected sibs, parents, or relatives.

Clinical Features. Three of the four patients with the Spitzer-Weinstein syndrome presented with short stature [28, 31, 33]. Hypertension was found in 2 patients, each of whom gave a history of recurrent attacks of weakness [27, 28, 30, 32]. Three patients had associated findings: absent [30] or hypoplastic [28] upper incisors or a history of urinary tract infection and a calcium oxalate stone [33].

Laboratory Findings. Each patient with Spitzer-Weinstein syndrome exhibited persistent hyperkalemia and metabolic acidosis. Urinalysis was normal, and GFR was within an appropriate range for age. Testing of renal tubular function revealed an inability of the kidneys to excrete adequate amounts of potassium, some reduction in the excretion of phenolsulfonphthalein despite normal maximal tubular resorption of para-aminohippurate (Tm_{PAH}) and normal clearance of PAH (C_{PAH}), slightly reduced excretion of ammonium and total acid [27], and reduced threshold for resorption of bicarbonate [31, 33]. No defect was found in conservation of sodium while the patients were on a restricted intake of salt. Correction of acidemia did not affect plasma potassium values [28, 31, 33], suggesting that the metabolic acidosis was not the cause of the hyperkalemia.

The 2 patients with hypertension had low plasma renin activities, and one was found to have an increased plasma volume, although edema was not evident [28]. Plasma renin and urinary aldosterone values rose, but they remained below normal following salt restriction. On the other hand, correction of the hyperkalemia was associated with an increase in plasma renin levels to normal and elevation of aldosterone production [32]. The two normotensive patients had no gross abnormalities of aldosterone metabolism [31, 33].

Pathophysiology. Since none of the patients with Spitzer-Weinstein syndrome was insensitive to aldosterone, none showed abnormalities in renal handling of sodium, and all had normal levels of GFR, it was suggested that the primary abnormality is a defect in renal secretion of potassium

[31]. The resulting hyperkalemia was thought to impair proximal resorption of bicarbonate, as found in the cases reported by Spitzer et al. [31] and Weinstein et al. [33]; both cases had reduced renal thresholds for resorption of bicarbonate. It was postulated [31] that the loss of base in the urine along with the failure to excrete sufficient potassium led to hyperkalemic acidosis. The acidosis in turn would further interfere with potassium secretion, exaggerating the hyperkalemia and possibly causing stunting in growth. This hypothesis was supported by the finding that these children had a low potassium excretion for a given amount of bicarbonate delivered into the distal tubule [31].

The two patients with hypertension [27, 28, 30, 32] might have had a different abnormality [28], such as a primary renal tubular avidity for sodium leading to extracellular volume expansion and subsequent proximal tubular sodium "escape." The volume expansion would suppress renin and aldosterone secretion, leading to hyperkalemia and acidosis. In favor of this hypothesis is the fact that sodium restriction corrected hyperkalemia, acidosis, and hypertension. The dental anomalies found in the hypertensive patients represent another feature that distinguishes them from the patients described by Spitzer [31] and Weinstein [33].

Differential Diagnosis. Hyperkalemia and acidosis with normal adrenocorticoid levels may result from failure of aldosterone production; however, salt wasting is also present. Familial periodic paralysis may occur with hyperkalemia, but serum potassium levels are usually normal between attacks [28].

Treatment. Chlorothiazide, 4 to 10 mg/kg/day, usually corrects hyperkalemia and acidosis within 1 or 2 weeks, presumably by enhancing delivery of sodium to the distal tubule, which in turn facilitates the secretion of potassium; or by affecting directly the transport of these ions at the level of the distal tubule [29]. Bicarbonate administration may be required to correct persistent acidosis. Hypertension responded to the administration of sodium polystyrene sulfonate in one case [27]. As already mentioned, Gordon et al. found sodium restriction alone to be adequate to correct hyperkalemia, acidosis, and hypertension [28].

Course. Correction of electrolyte abnormalities has resulted in improved growth [28, 31], although long-term follow-up has not been reported in Spitzer-Weinstein syndrome.

Potassium-Losing Disorders
LIDDLE'S SYNDROME
Synonyms for the Liddle syndrome include pseudohyperaldosteronism and pseudoaldosteronism.

In 1964 Liddle et al. [38] described a familial disorder characterized by hypertension, hypokalemic alkalosis, and failure of the kidneys to conserve potassium; aldosterone secretion was low. A similar constellation of findings had been noted by Ross 4 years earlier [40] in an asymptomatic 13-year-old boy.

Occurrence. The Liddle syndrome has been diagnosed as early as 10 months of age [37]. Its appearance in siblings of both sexes and in successive generations suggests an autosomal dominant mode of inheritance.

Clinical Features. Symptoms of the Liddle syndrome, when present, have included headaches, paresthesias, epigastric cramping pain, occasionally tetany [38], and acute paralysis [34]. Weakness, polyuria, and polydipsia usually accompany hypokalemia. Short stature has been noted once [40]. Hypertension is constantly present and is usually associated with retinopathy.

Laboratory Findings. The Liddle syndrome is characterized by hypokalemic metabolic alkalosis found in association with failure of the kidneys to conserve potassium; the GFR is normal. Plasma renin activity and aldosterone secretion and excretion rates are low. Correction of hypokalemia elevates aldosterone secretion, but to levels lower than those appropriate for the sodium intake [34, 35, 38, 39]. Sodium restriction has a similar effect on aldosterone and results in a slightly negative sodium balance. Administration of physiologic doses of aldosterone to these patients enables them to return to a balanced state [38].

Neither inhibition of aldosterone synthesis nor blockage by spironolactone affects either electrolyte excretion or hypokalemia, probably because of the low endogenous aldosterone level [38, 39]. On the other hand, triamterene, a diuretic that inhibits distal tubular ion transport independently of aldosterone, causes a marked rise in sodium excretion and a concomitant fall in potassium excretion, resulting in normalization of plasma potassium concentration [34, 37, 38].

Pathophysiology. On the basis of their studies, Liddle et al. [38, 39] concluded that the kidneys have an unusual tendency to conserve sodium and to excrete potassium, even in the virtual absence of mineralocorticoids. Hypertension follows from excessive sodium retention. Bravo et al. [35] noted that sodium restriction caused an appropriate rise in corticosterone secretion rate, whereas it remained subnormal for aldosterone. They suggested a possible block in corticosterone-to-aldosterone synthesis, with overproduction of the former hormone contributing to the electrolyte abnormalities. Liddle et al., on the other hand, found high concentration ratios of sodium to potassium in saliva and sweat and normal amounts of urinary corticosterone metabolites, and they concluded that production of mineralocorticoids was not excessive [38, 39].

It is possible that the Liddle syndrome reflects a generalized abnormality of sodium transport. Helbock and Reynolds [37] studied the erythrocytes from a patient with the Liddle syndrome and observed an increased sodium influx and a high intracellular sodium concentration. They postulated that the same applies to the renal tubular cells and that the high intracellular sodium concentration stimulates the sodium-potassium exchange in the distal tubule leading to retention of sodium and enhanced excretion of potassium. Treatment of their patient with triamterene and salt restriction resulted in a decrease in red cell sodium uptake and intracellular concentration of sodium. Gardner and coworkers found that both fractional efflux and influx of sodium were increased in the erythrocytes of two sisters with the Liddle syndrome, although the intracellular concentration of sodium was normal. Incubation of the red cells in plasma containing normal concentrations of potassium, renin, and aldosterone did not alter the results [36].

Differential Diagnosis. Patients with primary aldosteronism exhibit a similar picture to that in the Liddle syndrome except they have high aldosterone secretory rates and their electrolyte excretion is affected by both aldosterone synthesis inhibitors and spironolactone; their sweat and salivary sodium-potassium ratios are low [39].

Patients with the Bartter syndrome (see under The Bartter Syndrome) are normotensive and usually have hyperreninemia with secondary hyperaldosteronism.

Treatment. The combination of sodium restriction, potassium supplementation, and administration of triamterene, 8 to 10 mg/kg/day, has corrected the serum and urinary electrolyte abnormalities and the hypertension.

Course. Reports of long-term follow-up of the few patients described have not been published. It is not known if patients on long-term therapy maintain normal concentrations of potassium in plasma and eventually achieve normal rates of aldosterone secretion.

Renal Wasting of Magnesium

Idiopathic hypomagnesemia secondary to renal magnesium wasting has been described in two familial forms as an isolated tubular defect [41–43, 49] or associated with hypokalemia and renal potassium wasting [44–46, 48, 50]. In all cases the GFR and blood pressure have been normal.

Occurrence. Both forms of hypomagnesemia have occurred in successive generations (such as mother and son [43, 50]), in sisters [44, 45], and in a sister and brother [48], suggesting autosomal recessive inheritance. It is not clear whether hypomagnesemia may occur as an acquired defect.

Clinical Features. In subjects experimentally depleted of magnesium, symptoms and signs of tetany include a positive Trousseau sign, tremor, fasciculation, and carpopedal spasm. The presence of these signs seems to depend on the combination of low concentration in serum of magnesium, potassium, and calcium [51, 52]. Personality changes, such as irritability, apathy, weakness, poor appetite, and nausea, were noted by Shils and others [51, 52]. Some patients present with seizures in the newborn period [42, 43] that typically fail to respond to calcium therapy despite concomitant hypocalcemia [42].

Growth retardation has been noted in one hypomagnesemic patient who was subsequently found to have generalized aminoacidemia, aminoaciduria, and glycosuria [41]. Since failure to thrive did not occur in other patients with renal magnesium wasting, it is likely that one of the other abnormalities was responsible for this finding. Finally, a chronic nonspecific dermatitis with thickening of the skin and purple-red hues has been described by Gitelman et al. and linked in appearance to the erythematous rash of magnesium-depleted rats [44, 45].

Laboratory Findings. Hypomagnesemia is usually associated with urinary magnesium excretion rates that are appropriate for subjects with normal magnesium levels, indicating failure of renal conservation. The three patients studied by Gitelman et al. were placed on severe magnesium restriction, 1 mEq per day, yet they excreted three to five times more magnesium than control subjects and showed marked decreases in their previously low serum values [44, 45].

Since about half of the total body magnesium is found in bone [52], it is not surprising to note two cases of osteochondrosis associated with renal magnesium wasting. Miller reported a 6-year-old boy with Legg-Calvé-Perthes disease, a newborn history of tetany and tremors, a recent history of carpopedal spasm, and hypomagnesemia that responded to oral magnesium supplementation [49]. Although further studies were not reported except for normal serum electrolytes and calcium, it it likely that this boy had a congenital renal tubular defect in magnesium resorption. An additional case reported by Klingberg was in an otherwise asymptomatic 5-year-old boy who presented with carpopedal spasm and was found to have hypomagnesemia and hypokalemia along with "mild osteochondrosis of shoulders, knees, and hips (Legg-Perthes-like)" [46]. Despite hypomagnesemia, the child excreted 5 to 9 mEq per day of magnesium (0.2–0.45 mEq/kg/day in the urine) and required 2 mEq/kg/day of magnesium acetate to achieve positive magnesium balance. After 6 months of therapy, the bony lesions had reverted almost to normal. In both of these patients tetany recurred when magnesium therapy was discontinued.

Patients with hypomagnesemia and hypokalemia have a mild metabolic alkalosis and may show abnormalities in urinary concentration tests, possibly attributable to hypokalemia rather than hypomagnesemia. No other defects in glomerular or in tubular function have been reported.

The increased plasma renin activity found in patients with both hypomagnesemia and hypokalemia probably reflects stimulation by potassium depletion [47]. The normal aldosterone levels are probably the result of the well-known inhibitory effect of hypokalemia on aldosterone production [47]. It would be anticipated, although it has not been demonstrated, that both plasma renin activity and aldosterone production would be normal in isolated renal magnesium wasting.

Differential Diagnosis. Malabsorptive and hormonal disorders such as hyperaldosteronism, hyperparathyroidism, and hyperthyroidism must be considered in the differential diagnosis of hypomagnesemia. Failure of renal conservation of magnesium during magnesium dietary restriction, especially in the presence of normal blood pressure, together with hypomagnesemia and possibly hypokalemia, provide the diagnosis and exclude the other conditions.

Bartter syndrome with hypokalemia and occasional hypomagnesemia is differentiated by early growth retardation, severe urinary concentrating defect, very high plasma renin activity and aldosterone excretion rate, possibly insensitivity to angiotensin II, and marked hypertrophy of the juxtaglomerular apparatus [48].

Treatment. Supplementation of the diet with magnesium gluconate, magnesium acetate, or magnesium oxide to provide 1 to 2 mEq/kg/day in three or four divided doses usually causes improvement in symptomatology and partial to full correction of the hypomagnesemia. Potassium chloride may be required for patients with the combined disorder: 4 to 6 mEq/kg/day has corrected the serum levels to normal [48].

Course and Prognosis. Withdrawal of magnesium supplementation has resulted in recurrence of symptoms and severe hypomagnesemia. It is not clear whether treatment can ever be discontinued.

The Bartter Syndrome

The *Bartter syndrome,* first defined in 1962, is characterized by hypertrophy and hyperplasia of the renal juxtaglomerular apparatus, hyperaldosteronism, hyperreninemia with diminished blood pressure response to infused angiotensin II, and hypokalemic metabolic alkalosis [57]. Although symptoms such as polyuria, polydipsia, constipation, poor feeding, and vomiting usually occur during infancy, the diagnosis may be delayed for years until failure to thrive, weakness, salt craving, or episodes of dehydration lead to more thorough investigation. The Bartter syndrome affects family members of both sexes and may be transmitted as an autosomal recessive disorder.

It is likely that the constellation of signs and symptoms that comprise the Bartter syndrome occurs in association with disorders having diverse etiologies and pathophysiologic mechanisms. For the present it is useful to dichotomize patients into those who can conserve salt and those who are salt wasters [55].

In this chapter the clinical characteristics of 80 patients reported in 63 papers are reviewed, including nine cases with presumed Bartter syndrome occurring prior to 1962 [53, 54, 57, 58, 61, 63–68, 70–76, 78, 87, 90, 92, 93, 95–97, 101–104, 106, 107, 111, 112, 114–119, 121, 122, 124–133, 135–137, 139, 140]. These latter nine cases have been reported under names such as congenital hypokalemia, chronic hypokalemia, congenital alkalosis, low potassium syndrome, and congenital renal tubular alkalosis.

Occurrence

The Bartter syndrome has occurred in both sexes, with a slight male predominance (58 percent); 30 percent of cases were in blacks. There was a positive family history in 17 cases in siblings [53, 76, 86, 93, 116, 127, 131, 137, 139], cousins [67], and in offspring of incestuous relationships [62, 115, 123, 127, 132]. In addition, biochemical features have been demonstrated in otherwise asymptomatic relatives: abnormal erythrocyte sodium transport [88], hyperlipidemia in a mother [72], increased aldosterone secretion on a low sodium diet in a normokalemic sister [92], tubular proteinuria in a brother, maternal grandfather, and two maternal great uncles [117].

Clinical Manifestations

In three-fourths of the cases symptoms were noted in infancy (first 2 years of life), although the diagnosis of Bartter syndrome was often made much later. Thirteen of twenty-one patients whose onset of symptoms occurred after the second year of life were 14 years of age or older.

Clinical manifestations have included salt craving, weakness, constipation, anorexia, vomiting, nocturia, enuresis, paresthesias, seizures, failure to grow, and poor school performance. The constellation of polyuria, polydipsia, and a tendency toward dehydration was noted in over 80 percent of the cases; more than one-half of those without these symptoms presented at 14 years of age or older.

Physical examination is notable for the universal absence of hypertension and edema. Failure to thrive or failure to attain the third percentile in height or weight has been noted in 75 percent of cases but in less than 33 percent of adults (19 years of age and older). It has been suggested that normal height may be attained sometime after the seventeenth year, following a belated adolescent growth spurt [120].

Other physical findings include weakness, tetany, and carpopedal spasm, all generally unresponsive to calcium therapy. Gouty arthritis was reported in three adult patients [105, 106].

James et al. have described two infants with the Bartter syndrome who had a characteristic facial appearance: a large head with respect to the body, and a prominent forehead with a triangular facies having protruding pinnae, large eyes, and a pouting expression caused by drooping corners of the mouth [96].

Mental function was normal in almost two-thirds of the patients evaluated.

Laboratory Findings

Routine biochemical findings in the Bartter syndrome include marked hypokalemia with metabolic alkalosis, often accompanied by low or low normal concentrations of sodium and chloride in serum. Glomerular filtration rate was normal in 80 percent of patients and below 70 ml/min/ 1.73 m² in 17 percent; the two brothers described by Arant et al. [53] were severely azotemic. Serum calcium levels are usually normal, although one episode or more of hypercalcemia (>5.7 mEq/L) was apparent in 22 percent of cases. Hypercalciuria above 4 mg/kg/day (or 2 mEq/kg/ day) was present in nine patients [80, 103, 104, 115, 116]. Uric acid in nonazotemic subjects was above 7 mg per deciliter in 50 percent of the patients in whom it was measured [74, 103, 105, 106]. Serum magnesium values, although not necessarily reflecting total body magnesium stores, were below 1.5 mEq per liter in 33 percent of those investigated, while serum phosphorus levels were below 3.5 mg per deciliter (2.2 mEq/L) in 32 percent of cases on at least one occasion. Hy-

perlipidemia, or elevated serum cholesterol, was noted in 8 cases. Plasma volumes have been reported as normal in 3 patients [63, 90, 128], increased in 4 [58, 96, 97] and decreased in 2 [82, 106]. One hypovolemic patient had been hypervolemic 10 years earlier [82].

Examination of the urine is remarkable for its alkaline pH and hypotonicity, and a 30 percent incidence of proteinuria. Maximal urinary concentration is usually subnormal even after severe water deprivation, administration of vasopressin, and potassium repletion. Less than 15 percent of patients can achieve urinary osmolalities above 850 mOsm per liter or specific gravities above 1.019. In one 4-year-old girl, an infusion of cyclic AMP reduced urine volume although vasopressin did not [110].

Urinary acid excretion following acid loading is generally inadequate, with the vast majority of hydrogen ion being excreted as ammonium, even following potassium repletion. Urine pH minima were abnormal in three-fourths of the patients who were subjected to acid loading tests; only 28 percent attained urine pH of 5.4 or less, and almost one-third failed to reach pH 6. White found increased bicarbonate resorption in his two patients [139].

Water loading studies demonstrated normal diluting capacity in 5 patients, as assessed by urinary specific gravity. However, 3 of 6 other patients studied more extensively were found to have a normal C_{H_2O} per 100 ml GFR, whereas the fraction of glomerular filtrate delivered distally (determined as $C_{H_2O} + C_{Na}/100$ ml GFR) ranged from 22 to 35 percent as compared to a normal range of 7 to 17 percent [56, 71]. Furthermore, the fraction of distal fluid converted to free water ($C_{H_2O}/C_{H_2O} + C_{Na}$) was below 60 percent in five of the subjects studied, with the normal range being 71 to 89 percent. It appears, therefore, that sodium transport at the diluting segment is impaired [70] and that normal free water clearances are found only when massive amounts of filtrate are delivered to the distal nephron [56].

Sodium conservation under conditions of severe salt restriction was abnormal in half of the patients studied. In several patients sodium was present in the urine for a number of days after sodium intake was reduced below 10 mEq per day, whereas in normal individuals subjected to a similar stress, urine sodium falls rapidly to near zero. Ultimately maximal salt conservation occurs in patients with the classic features of the syndrome and hypovolemia is avoided; in contrast, salt wasters develop hyponatremia and hypovolemia.

Irrespective of their ability to conserve sodium,

more than 50 percent of all patients with the Bartter syndrome had high serum potassium levels under conditions of sodium restriction. Conversely, sodium loading caused exacerbations of hypokalemia in nearly 90 percent of cases. Potassium loading usually resulted in quantitative increases in urinary potassium excretion, reaching 125 to 180 percent of the filtered load. Hypokalemia, accordingly, was substantially corrected by potassium loading in less than 50 percent of cases.

Plasma renin activity (PRA) is elevated, usually markedly, in all patients with the Bartter syndrome. Volume expansion with isotonic saline or hyperoncotic albumin solution resulted in reductions of PRA in 8 of the 13 patients studied, of whom only 3 returned to normal [122, 139]. In 5 patients [68, 103, 104, 119] volume expansion failed to suppress or led to elevations in PRA. These results could not be correlated with sodium intake, the presence or absence of salt wasting, or with the state of potassium balance.

Angiotensin II infusions were performed in 36 patients according to the procedure of Kaplan and Silah [99]; a mean pressor dose of 7.4 ± 1.3 ng/kg/min causes a 20 mm Hg rise in diastolic blood pressure in normal subjects. A fourfold increase in dose was required for an equivalent rise in pressure in patients with secondary hyperaldosteronism due to nephrotic syndrome, congestive heart failure, or cirrhosis [98]. In patients with the Bartter syndrome the mean minimal dose required was greater than 200 ng/kg/min. Volume expansion restored vascular sensitivity to normal in 3 of 9 patients [90, 139] while partially correcting sensitivity in 3 others. Indomethacin therapy alone (vide infra) restored vascular sensitivity in a tenth patient [133]. Finally, Sasaki et al. [118] reported a study in a patient showing marked insensitivity to angiotensin II (750 to 825 ng/kg/min). An infusion of the analogue, 1-Sar, 8-Ile-angiotensin II, caused a marked hypotensive response, revealing the presence of some vascular reactivity to this compound.

Aldosterone production or excretion was increased in 74 percent of patients. Those with normal levels usually increased production following potassium supplementation.

Intravenous urograms disclose normal configuration of the kidneys, although reduced concentration of dye is frequently noted and attributed to high rates of urine flow. Mild dilatation of collecting system, ureters, and bladder has been ascribed to the high rate of urine flow as well as to the effect of potassium depletion on ureteral peristalsis and bladder contractility [74]. Nephrocalcinosis was noted in 9 patients [53, 54, 80, 86, 103, 104]. Renal angiography of 1 patient showed medullary hypertrophy with a corticomedullary ratio of 1 : 6 [69].

Hematologic abnormalities in the Bartter syndrome are uncommon; three cases of polycythemia not attributable to hemoconcentration have been reported [79, 97, 128]. The patients of Jepson et al. [97] and Erkelens et al. [79] showed mild reticulocytosis and increased erythropoietic activity as measured on bioassay. Platelet counts have been reported to be elevated above 500,000 mm³ in 3 patients [80, 116].

Adrenal function generally is normal. Skeletal survey usually shows retarded bone age; osteoporosis has been noted in 6 nonazotemic patients [102, 104, 116, 117, 131].

Studies of various tissues have shown that transport defects in the Bartter syndrome may involve organ systems other than the kidneys. The magnesium content of muscle has been reported to be reduced by 40 percent despite a normal level in serum [101]. Similarly, the potassium content of muscle is below normal [57, 86, 93] in association with a reduced ratio of sodium- and potassium-activated to magnesium-activated ATPases [93]. The sodium content of the erythrocytes has usually been found to be elevated [79, 87, 88], while potassium was low prior to supplementation [79, 86, 133]. Gardner et al. found that 6 of 8 patients with the Bartter syndrome showed both increased erythrocyte sodium concentrations and reduced fractional sodium efflux [88]. Gall et al. reported the red cells of one patient to have increased concentration of sodium with increased fractional efflux and influx [87]. The results of these studies are consistent with the concept of abnormal membrane cation transport or permeability.

In a study of parotid salivary secretion in a patient with the Bartter syndrome, Heidland et al. [94] found potassium secretion to be more than twice normal. Along with a slight decrease in sodium resorption, there was increased secretion of calcium, magnesium, bicarbonate, and phosphorus. In contrast, 2 patients with primary aldosteronism showed a marked increase in sodium resorption [94].

Finally, the measurement of prostaglandins using radioimmunoassay and gas chromatography-mass spectrometry has enabled investigators to document elevated prostaglandin A_2 levels in the plasma of one male [82] and elevated urinary prostaglandin E_2 in 5 females [89] with the Bartter syndrome. The latter group has reported preliminary studies in 6 patients with the Bartter syndrome showing elevated levels of plasma bradykinin and urinary kallikrein in parallel with elevated urinary prostaglandin E_2 and plasma renin activity [134].

Pathology

The classic finding in the Bartter syndrome is hypertrophy and hyperplasia of the juxtaglomerular complex of many but not all glomeruli [55]. The hyperplasia involves all elements of the complex, including the macula densa. There is a variable degree of hyalinization and glomerular atrophy. Proliferative changes were reported in 25 percent of the cases, adhesions or crescents in 14 percent, and arteriolar thickening in 11 percent. Tubular atrophy or vacuolization was seen in nearly half the cases. The adrenal gland zona glomerulosa is often hypertrophic and infiltrated by lipid material.

An explanation for the increased distal delivery of sodium may be found in the biopsies of several patients [55, 60], in whom a loss of continuity of glomerular basement membrane, with adherence of capillary tufts to the wall of Bowman's capsule, has been found. This lesion, possibly an old glomerulitis, theoretically might permit an ultrafiltrate of plasma to drain into an adjacent distal tubule.

There have been few examinations of the renal medullary tissue because so little is obtained with the needle biopsy technique. However, hyperplasia of medullary interstitial cells has been reported [79, 86] and subsequently suggested to be of pathophysiologic importance [133]. These authors found a proliferation of polyhedral or fusiform renomedullary interstitial cells with histochemical staining characteristics identifying them to be similar to cells known to produce renal prostaglandins (see under Pathophysiology).

Pathophysiology

The pathophysiology of the Bartter syndrome is subject to much controversy. Since it is possible that more than one disorder may result in what is now called the Bartter syndrome, the hypotheses are not necessarily mutually exclusive. Of the 40 authors suggesting a mechanism for the disorder, 21 have invoked a tubular defect in sodium handling, especially in the proximal tubule; while others have leaned toward primary vascular insensitivity to angiotensin II or have suggested a membrane transport defect, primary potassium wasting, hormone-mediated or prostaglandin-induced sodium wasting, abnormal macula densa feedback, abnormal volume regulation, or adrenal hyporesponsiveness to angiotensin II.

Bartter originally suggested vascular resistance to angiotensin with limited feedback control of re-

nin mediated by blood pressure [87]. Excess renin production would lead in turn to an increase in aldosterone production and hypokalemic alkalosis. In support of this theory is the finding that 10 to 100 times the usual dose of angiotensin II is required for a pressor response, and vascular reactivity is restored to normal following volume expansion in only one-third of patients. The fact that renin is partially suppressible in two-thirds of cases tends to rule out a completely autonomous renin-angiotensin system. However, the failure of adrenalectomy and inhibitors or antagonists of aldosterone to correct hypokalemia fully (see under Treatment) suggests that this mechanism alone is insufficient to explain the pathophysiology. Moreover, tachyphylaxis arising from continued high levels of angiotensin is unlikely, since patients with renin-secreting tumors continue to have hypertension and metabolic alkalosis [113].

In patients who are obligatory salt wasters, the resulting hypovolemia leads to overproduction of renin and aldosterone and reduced vascular sensitivity to infused angiotensin II [68]. As noted above, however, sodium depletion with secondary hyperaldosteronism does not usually lead to a tenfold to hundredfold reduction in vascular reactivity. Furthermore, most patients studied had normal or high plasma volumes. Most of them also had increased distal delivery of water and salt, with a reduced fraction converted to free water; this is consistent with a defect in chloride transport in the cortical diluting segment of the ascending limb of the loop of Henle, as well as with an impairment in the proximal tubular resorption of sodium. Such defects would be expected in patients having shunt lesions between the glomeruli and the distal tubules or perhaps early acquired forms of glomerulitis.

The abnormalities in electrolyte concentration observed in the erythrocytes and parotid secretion lend support to a generalized defect in membrane ion transport or permeability. This would contribute to increased distal delivery of sodium and would lead to increased distal sodium-potassium exchange and renal potassium wasting.

The recent findings of renomedullary cell hyperplasia and elevated levels of urinary prostaglandin E_2 and plasma prostaglandin A_2 are consistent with a role of these hormones in mediating the hyperreninemia of patients with the Bartter syndrome. Indomethacin, a prostaglandin synthetase inhibitor, caused marked reductions in prostaglandins to subnormal levels, with concomitant reductions in plasma renin activity and aldosterone production and restoration of vascular sensitivity to exogenous angiotensin II [77, 82, 89, 133]. It has been postulated from these data that overproduction of prostaglandins by the hyperplastic renomedullary cells (due to some unknown factor) leads to decreased sodium resorption, decreased effective arteriolar volume, and angiotensin insensitivity, resulting in increased plasma renin activity and secondary hperaldosteronism [133]. An alternative hypothesis suggested by Gill et al. [89] refers to the primary vascular insensitivity to angiotensin leading to elevated renin and angiotensin levels, which evoke excessive release of prostaglandins. These potent vasodilators then cause subnormal arteriolar constriction resulting in further increases in renin production and secondary hyperaldosteronism. The role of the other potent vasodepressor system, kallikrein and kinin, is highly speculative.

Differential Diagnosis

The Liddle syndrome and the disorder of potassium and magnesium wasting described by Gitelman et al. [44, 45] are discussed in earlier sections of this chapter. Multiple tubular disorders such as the Fanconi syndrome and renal tubular acidosis are discussed in Chapters 81 and 83.

Primary aldosteronism is differentiated from the Bartter syndrome on the basis of its association with hypertension and very low plasma renin levels, plus the excellent response of hypokalemia to salt restriction. A similar clinical picture occurs with renin-secreting renal tumors, in which hypertension and hypokalemic alkalosis, as well as symptoms of polyuria and polydipsia, have been described [100, 113]. One finds increased production of renin and aldosterone attributable to a localized hemangiopericytoma arising from the juxtaglomerular apparatus. The Bartter syndrome may be mimicked by chronic licorice intake because of the aldosterone-like effects of the glycyrrhizic acid contained in licorice [103].

The pseudo-Bartter syndrome is manifested by secondary hyperaldosteronism with hypokalemic alkalosis, hyperreninemia, and even juxtaglomerular cell hyperplasia and vascular resistance to angiotensin infusion. Chronic volume and electrolyte depletion appear to be consistent findings, since pseudo-Bartter syndromes have been described in familial chloride diarrhea [109] and in psychiatric disturbances associated with ulcerative colitis [108], surreptitious vomiting [138], and self-administration of laxatives [84, 141] and diuretics [59]. The angiotensin resistance in one patient was not corrected by volume expansion with saline [84]. Most abnormalities would be expected to disappear following elimination of the cause.

Finally, a presentation of hypokalemic metabolic alkalosis with failure to thrive has been described in infants subsequently diagnosed as having cystic fibrosis [91, 119a]. The cause is probably related to excessive loss of salt in sweat leading to volume contraction, excessive resorption of bicarbonate, and resulting metabolic alkalosis with hypokalemia.

Treatment

Treatment of the Bartter syndrome until recently has been symptomatic and generally unsuccessful in fully correcting the electrolyte disturbances or reducing plasma renin levels to normal. Potassium chloride supplements in excess of 10 mEq/kg/day have improved the general condition and symptomatology. The addition of spironolactone, up to 15 mg/kg/day, may further increase serum potassium, but it usually causes hyponatremia requiring sodium supplementation of 5 to 10 mEq/kg/day. However, of those patients whose serum potassium levels were raised following spironolactone, nearly 75 percent became resistant to therapy after several weeks, usually receiving progressively larger doses without significant effect. Triamterene possibly may be more effective; however, experience with this drug is limited. Propranolol in combination with potassium-retaining diuretics has been reported to be ineffective [124], partially effective [82, 106, 119], and successful [122] or only temporarily effective in correcting hypokalemia because of the escape phenomenon [119]. Suppression of renin activity by methyldopa appears to be transient [125]. Weekly or semiweekly infusions of albumin combined with supplemental potassium may be helpful [76, 120]. The data on sodium restriction have been conflicting. Magnesium supplementation may be advantageous [101]. Suppression of aldosterone synthesis [90], subtotal adrenalectomy [57, 65, 128], and total adrenalectomy [131] have failed to correct hypokalemia.

Recent success with prostaglandin inhibition has been reported [77, 82, 89, 133]. A follow-up of 8 months demonstrated normokalemia and no escape from indomethacin therapy [133]. There is no experience with the use of this drug in patients under 14 years of age; one child was successfully treated with aspirin [107].

Course

The course of the Bartter syndrome is chronic and may be especially severe if the onset of disease occurs in infancy. Of the 11 deaths reported, 10 occurred in children whose age at onset was less than 1 year. Death may be the consequence of dehydration and vascular collapse, acute electrolyte imbalance, or intercurrent infection. It is likely that progressive renal insufficiency develops in some cases over a period of years [115].

Growth is usually impaired in children with the Bartter syndrome and fails to improve following therapy in two-thirds of cases. Simopoulos and Bartter [120], however, have reported that 2 patients reached an appropriate adult height following a delayed adolescent growth spurt. Indeed, follow-up has been insufficient for one to speculate further on the long-term course in this condition.

References

Disorders of Sodium Transport

1. Bierich, J. R., and Schmidt, U. Tubular Na$^+$-K$^+$-ATPase deficiency, the cause of the congenital renal salt-losing syndrome. *Eur. J. Pediatr.* 121:81, 1976.
2. Bongiovanni, A. M. Action and Metabolism of Adrenocortical Hormones. In H. L. Barnett and A. H. Einhorn (eds.), *Pediatrics*. New York: Appleton-Century-Crofts, 1972. Pp. 1093–1102.
3. Cheek, D. B., and Perry, J. W. A salt-wasting syndrome in infancy. *Arch. Dis. Child.* 33:252, 1958.
4. Corbeel, L. Diabète salin du nourrison sans insuffisance surrénaliene. *Pédiatrie* 18:557, 1963.
5. Day, G. M., Radde, I. C., Balfe, J. W., and Chance, G. W. Electrolyte abnormalities in very low birth weight infants. *Pediatr. Res.* 10:522, 1972.
6. Donnell, G. N., Litman, N., and Roldan, M. Pseudohypo-adrenalocorticism: Renal sodium loss, hyponatremia, hyperkalemia due to renal tubular insensitivity to mineralocorticoids. *Am. J. Dis. Child.* 97:813, 1959.
7. Gonick, H. C., Maxwell, M. H., Rubini, M. E., and Kleeman, C. R. Functional impairment in chronic renal disease: I. Studies of sodium-conserving ability. *Nephron* 3:137, 1966.
8. Honour, J. W., Shackleton, C. H. L., and Valman, H. B. Sodium homeostasis in preterm infants (letter). *Lancet* 2:1147, 1974.
9. Jeune, M., Lamit, J., Loras, B., Do, F., and Forest, M. Pseudo-hypoaldostéronisme (abstract). *Arch. Fr. Pédiatr.* 27:714, 1967.
10. Lelong, M., Alagille, D., Philippe, A., Gentil, C., Gabilan, J. C. Diabète salin par insensibilité congénitale du tubule à l'aldostérone: "Pseudo-hypo-adrénocorticisme." *Rev. Fr. Etud. Clin. Biol.* 5:558, 1960.
11. Polonovski, C., Zittoun, R., and Mary, F. Hypocorticisme global, hypoaldostéronisme, et pseudo-hypoaldostéronisme du nourisson: Trois observations. *Arch. Fr. Pédiatr.* 22:1061, 1965.
12. Postel-Vinay, M. C. Sodium balance, aldosterone excretion and secretion rates: Study of colon receptors to aldosterone in a 9-year-old boy known as a case of pseudohypoadrenocorticism (abstract). *Acta Paediatr. Scand.* 61:261, 1971.
13. Postel-Vinay, M. C., Alberti, G. M., Ricour, C., Limal, J. M., Rappaport, R., and Royer, P. Pseudohypoaldosteronism: Persistence of hyperaldosteronism and evidence for renal tubular and intestinal responsiveness to endogenous aldosterone. *J. Clin. Endocrinol. Metab.* 39:1038, 1974.
14. Proesmans, W., Geussens, H., Corbeel, L., and Eeckels, R. Pseudohypoaldosteronism. *Am. J. Dis. Child.* 126:510, 1973.
15. Raine, D. N., and Roy, J. A salt-losing syndrome in infancy: Pseudohypoadrenocorticalism. *Arch. Dis. Child.* 37:548, 1962.
16. Rosler, A., Theodor, R., Gazit, E., Boichis, H., and Rabinowitz, D. Salt-wastage, raised plasma-renin activity, and normal or high plasma-aldosterone: A form of pseudohypoaldosteronism. *Lancet* 1:959, 1973.
17. Roy, R. N., Chance, G. W., Radde, I. C., Hill, D. E., Willis, D. M., and Sheepers, J. Late hyponatremia in very low birth weight infants (<1.3 kilograms). *Pediatr. Res.* 10:526, 1976.
18. Royer, P. The Hereditary Tubular Diseases. In P. Royer, R. Habib, H. Mathieu, and M. Broyer (eds.), *Pediatric Nephrology*. Philadelphia: Saunders, 1974. Pp. 56–98.
19. Royer, P. L'hypoaldostéronisme congénital. *Rev. Fr. Etud. Clin. Biol.* 12:111, 1963.
20. Royer, P., Bonnette, J., Mathieu, H., Gabilan, J. C., Klutchko, G., and Zittoun, R. Pseudo-hypoaldostéronisme. *Ann. Pediatr.* 39:2612, 1963.
21. Savitt, M., Molitch, M., Kawoaka, E., and Leake, R. Pseudohypoaldosteronism (abstract). *Clin. Res.* 23:165A, 1975.
22. Shakleton, C. H. L., and Snodgrass, G. H. A. I. Steroid excretion by an infant with an unusual salt-losing syndrome: A gas-chromatographic-mass spectrometric study. *Ann. Clin. Biochem.* 11:91, 1974.
23. Spitzer, A., and Schoeneman, M. The role of the kidney in sodium homeostasis during maturation. In preparation.
24. Sulyok, E. The relationship between electrolytes and acid-base balance in the premature infant during early postnatal life. *Biol. Neonate* 17:227, 1971.
25. Thorn, G. W., Keopf, G. F., and Clinton, M., Jr. Renal failure simulating adrenocortical insufficiency. *N. Engl. J. Med.* 231:76, 1944.
26. Trung, P. H., Piussan, C., Rodary, C., Legrand, S., Attal, C., and Mozziconacci, P. Etude du taux de secretion de l'aldostérone et de l'activité de la rénine plasmatique. *Arch. Fr. Pédiatr.* 27:603, 1970.

Potassium-retaining Disorders

27. Arnold, J. E., and Healy, J. K. Hyperkalemia, hypertension and systemic acidosis without renal failure associated with a tubular defect in potassium excretion. *Am. J. Med.* 47:461, 1969.
28. Gordon, R. D., Geddes, R. A., Pawsey, C. G. K., and O'Halloran, M. W. Hypertension and severe hyperkalemia associated with suppression of renin and aldosterone and completely reversed by dietary sodium restriction. *Aust. Ann. Med.* 4:287, 1970.
29. Kunau, R. T., Jr., Weller, D. R., and Webb, H. L. Clarification of the site of action of chlorothiazide in the rat nephron. *J. Clin. Invest.* 56:401, 1975.
30. Paver, W. K. A., and Pauline, G. J. Hypertension and hyperpotassaemia without renal disease in young male. *Med. J. Aust.* 2:305, 1964.
31. Spitzer, A., Edelmann, C. M., Jr., Goldberg, L. D., and Henneman, P. H. Short stature, hyperkalemia and acidosis: A defect in renal transport of potassium. *Kidney Int.* 3:251, 1973.
32. Stokes, G. S., Gentle, J. L., Edwards, K. D. G., Stewart, J. H., Scroggins, B. A., and Coghland, J. P. Syndrome of idiopathic hyperkalaemia and

hypertension with decreased plasma renin activity: Effects of plasma renin and aldosterone on reducing the serum potassium level. *Med. J. Aust.* 2:1050, 1968.

33. Weinstein, S. F., Allan, D. M. E., and Mendoza, S. A. Hyperkalemia, acidosis, and short stature associated with a defect in renal potassium excretion. *J. Pediatr.* 85:355, 1974.

Potassium-losing Disorders

34. Aarshog, D., Stoa, K. F., Thorsen, T., and Wefring, K. W. Hypertension and hypokalemic alkalosis associated with underproduction of aldosterone. *Pediatrics* 39:884, 1970.

35. Bravo, E. L., Smith, H. C., Retan, W. C., and Bartter, R. C. Hypertension, Decreased Aldosterone Secretion Rate, Suppressed Plasma Renin Activity. In Proceedings of the 52nd Meeting of the Endocrine Society, St. Louis, Mo., 1970. P. 66.

36. Gardner, J. D., Lapey, A., Simopoulos, A. P., and Bravo, E. L. Abnormal membrane sodium transport in Liddle's syndrome. *J. Clin. Invest.* 50:2253, 1971.

37. Helbock, H. J., and Reynolds, J. W. Pseudoaldosteronism (Liddle's syndrome): Evidence for increased cell membrane permeability to Na$^+$ (abstract). *Pediatr. Res.* 4:455, 1970.

38. Liddle, G. W., Bledsoe, T., and Coppage, W. S., Jr. A familial disorder simulating primary aldosteronism but with negligible aldosterone secretion. *Trans. Assoc. Am. Physicians* 76:199, 1963.

39. Liddle, G. W., Bledsoe, T., and Coppage, W. S., Jr. A Familial Disorder Simulating Primary Aldosteronism but with Negligible Aldosterone Secretion. In E. E. Baulieu and P. Robel (eds.), *Aldosterone.* Oxford, England: Blackwell, 1964. Pp. 353–368.

40. Ross, E. J. Hypertension and hypokalemia associated with hypoaldosteronism (abstract). *Proc. R. Soc. Med.* 52:1056, 1959.

Renal Wasting of Magnesium

41. Booth, B. E., and Johanson, A. Hypomagnesemia due to renal tubular defect in reabsorption of magnesium. *J. Pediatr.* 84:350, 1974.

42. Dooling, E. C., and Stern, L. Hypomagnesemia with convulsions in a newborn infant: Report of a case associated with maternal hypophosphatemia. *Can. Med. Assoc. J.* 97:827, 1967.

43. Freeman, R. M., and Pearson, E. Hypomagnesemia of unknown etiology. *Am. J. Med.* 41:645, 1966.

44. Gitelman, H. J., Graham, J. B., and Welt, L. G. A new familial disorder characterized by hypokalemia and hypomagnesemia. *Trans. Assoc. Am. Physicians* 79:221, 1966.

45. Gitelman, H. J., Graham, J. B., and Welt, L. G. A new familial disorder characterized by hypokalemia and hypomagnesemia. *Ann. N.Y. Acad. Sci.* 162:856, 1969.

46. Klingberg, W. G. Idiopathic hypomagnesemia and osteochondritis (abstract). *Pediatr. Res.* 4:452, 1970.

47. Laragh, J. H., and Sealy, J. E. The Renin-Angiotensin-Aldosterone Hormonal System and Regulation of Sodium, Potassium and Blood Pressure Homeostasis. In J. Orloff and R. W. Berliner (eds.), *Handbook of Physiology.* Section 8: *Renal Physiology.* Washington, D.C.: American Physiological Society, 1973. Pp. 831–908.

48. McCredie, D. A., Blair-West, J. R., Scroggins, B. A., and Shipman, R. Potassium-causing nephropathy of childhood. *Med. J. Aust.* 1:129, 1971.

49. Miller, J. G. Tetany due to deficiency in magnesium: Its occurrence in a child of six years with associated osteochondrosis of capital epiphysis of femur (Legg-Perthes disease). *Am. J. Dis. Child.* 67:117, 1944.

50. Paunier, L., and Sizonenko, P. C. Asymptomatic chronic hypomagnesemia and hypokalemia in a child: Cell membrane disease. *J. Pediatr.* 88:51, 1976.

51. Shils, M. E. Experimental human magnesium depletion. *Medicine* 48:61, 1969.

52. Wacker, W. E. C., and Parisi, A. F. Magnesium metabolism. *N. Engl. J. Med.* 278:658, 712, 772, 1968.

Bartter Syndrome

53. Arant, B. S., Brackett, N. C., Jr., Young, R. B., and Still, W. J. S. Case studies of siblings with juxtaglomerular hyperplasia and secondary aldosteronism associated with severe azotemia and renal rickets— Bartter's syndrome or disease? *Pediatrics* 46:344, 1970.

54. Barjon, P., Fourcade, J., Mimran, A., Philippot, J., and de Costecaude Saint-Victor, A. Reconsidération du syndrome de Bartter: A propos d'une nouvelle observation. *Sem. Hop. Paris* 50:1715, 1974.

55. Bartter, F. C. The syndrome of juxtaglomerular hyperplasia with aldosteronism, hypokalemic alkalosis and normal blood pressure. *Birth Defects* 10:104, 1974.

56. Bartter, F. C., Delea, C. S., Kawasaki, T., and Gill, J. R., Jr. The adrenal cortex and the kidney. *Kidney Int.* 6:272, 1974.

57. Bartter, F. C., Pronove, P., Gill, J. R., Jr., and MacCardle, R. C. Hyperplasia of the juxtaglomerular complex with hyperaldosteronism and hypokalemic alkalosis: A new syndrome. *Am. J. Med.* 33:811, 1962.

58. Beilin, L. J., Schiffman, N., Crane, M., and Nelson, D. H. Hypokalaemic alkalosis and hyperplasia of the juxtaglomerular apparatus without hypertension or edema. *Br. Med. J.* 4:327, 1967.

59. Ben-Ishay, D., Levy, M., and Birnbaum, D. Self-induced secondary hyperaldosteronism simulating Bartter's syndrome. *Isr. J. Med. Sci.* 8:1835, 1972.

60. Biava, C., Desjardins, R., Bravo, E., and Bartter, F. Glomerular changes with glomerulo-distal tubular shunts in patients with Bartter's syndrome (abstract). *Lab. Invest.* 20:575, 1969.

61. Borst, J. R., and Smith, P. A. Chronic hypopotassaemia, refractory to potassium treatment, and tetany, in a girl aged 14 years. *Acta Med. Scand.* 161:207, 1958.

62. Bos, C. Discussion of A. H. F. Van Olphen, P. J. J. Van Munster, and J. P. Slooff, Chronic Hypokalemia, Hypochloremia and Alkalosis of Probably Renal Origin. In J. deGraeff and B. Leijnse (eds.), *Water and Electrolyte Metabolism II.* Amsterdam: Elsevier, 1964. P. 147.

63. Brackett, N. C., Jr., Koppel, M., Randall, R. E., Jr., and Nixon, W. P. Hyperplasia of the juxtaglomerular complex with secondary aldosteronism with-

out hypertension (Bartter's syndrome). *Am. J. Med.* 44:803, 1968.

64. Bravo, E., and Bartter, F. C. The syndrome of juxtaglomerular hyperplasia and hyperaldosteronism without hypertension: Studies on pathophysiological mechanisms (abstract). *Clin. Res.* 16:263, 1968.

65. Bryan, G. T., MacCardle, R. C., and Bartter, F. C. Hyperaldosteronism, hyperplasia of the juxtaglomerular complex, normal blood pressure, and dwarfism: Report of a case. *Pediatrics* 37:43, 1966.

66. Calcagno, P. L., Rubin, M. I., Esperanca, M. J., and Mattimore, J. M. Congenital renal tubular alkalosis (abstract). *Am. J. Dis. Child.* 102:726, 1961.

67. Camacho, A. M., and Blizzard, R. M. Congenital hypokalemia of probable renal origin. *Am. J. Dis. Child.* 103:43, 1962.

68. Cannon, P. J., Leeming, J. M., Sommers, S. C., Winters, R. W., and Laragh, J. H. Juxtaglomerular cell hyperplasia and secondary hyperaldosteronism (Bartter's syndrome): A reevaluation of the pathophysiology. *Medicine* 47:107, 1968.

69. Cha, E. M., and Ramanathan, K. Bartter's syndrome: With angiographic evaluation. *Radiology* 113:703, 1974.

70. Chaimovitz, C., Levi, J., Better, O. S., Oslander, L., and Benderli, A. Studies on the site of renal salt loss in a patient with Bartter's syndrome. *Pediatr. Res.* 7:89, 1973.

71. Chan, J. C. M., Malekzadeh, M. H., and Anand, S. K. Defect in renal tubular sodium reabsorption in a patient with Bartter's syndrome. *Clin. Proc. Child. Hosp. Natl. Med. Cent.* 31:67, 1975.

72. Cheek, D. B., Robinson, M. J., and Collins, F. D. The investigation of a patient with hyperlipidemia, hypokalemia and tetany. *J. Pediatr.* 59:200, 1961.

73. Codaccioni, J. L., Boyer, J., Jubelin, J., Conte-Devolx, B., and Habreard, J. Alcalose hypokaliémique avec hyperplasie de l'appareil juxtaglomérulaire: Syndrome de Bartter? *Ann. Endocrinol. (Paris)* 33:281, 1972.

74. Dehart, H. S., Bath, N. M., Glenn, J. F., and Gunnells, J. C. Urologic considerations in Bartter's syndrome. *J. Urol.* 111:420, 1974.

75. Desmit, E. M. Hypokalemic Alkalosis. In J. deGraeff and B. Leijnse (eds.), *Water and Electrolyte Metabolism II.* Amsterdam: Elsevier, 1964. Pp. 125–133.

76. Desmit, E. M., Cost, W. B., Brown, J. J., Fraser, R., Lever, A. F., and Robertson, J. I. S. An unusual type of hypokalaemic alkalosis with a disturbance of renin and aldosterone. *Acta Endocrinol. (Kbh.)* 64:75, 1970.

77. Donker, A. J. M., deJong, P. E., Van Eps, L. W. S., Brentjens, J. R., Bakker, K., and Doorenbos, H. A study on the treatment of Bartter's syndrome with indomethacin (abstract). *Kidney Int.* 9:449, 1976.

78. Earle, D. P., Sherry, S., Eichna, L. W., and Conan, N. J. Low potassium syndrome due to defective renal tubular mechanisms for handling potassium. *Am. J. Med.* 11:283, 1951.

79. Erkelens, D. W., and Van Eps, L. W. S. Bartter's syndrome and erythrocytosis. *Am. J. Med.* 55:711, 1973.

80. Fanconi, A., Schackenmann, G., Nussli, R., and Prader, A. Chronic hypokalaemia with growth retardation, normotensive hyperrenin-hyperaldosteronism ("Bartter's syndrome"), and hypercalciuria: Report of two cases with emphasis on natural history and on catch-up growth during treatment. *Helv. Paediatr. Acta* 26:144, 1971.

81. Fashena, G. J., and Martin, P. J. Congenital alkalosis of renal origin (abstract). *Am. J. Dis. Child.* 79:1127, 1950.

82. Fichman, M. P., Telfer, N., Zia, P., Speckart, P., Golub, M., and Rude, R. Role of prostaglandins in the pathogenesis of Bartter's syndrome. *Am. J. Med.* 60:785, 1976.

83. Fisher, C. E., Olambinwanu, O., Frasier, S. E., and Horton, R. Renin-aldosterone dynamics in Bartter's syndrome (abstract). *Clin. Res.* 21:282, 1973.

84. Fleischer, N., Brown, H., Graham, D. Y., and Delena, S. Chronic laxative-induced hyperaldosteronism and hypokalemia simulating Bartter's syndrome. *Ann. Intern. Med.* 70:791, 1969.

85. Fleisher, D. S. Prolonged hypokalemic alkalosis: A specific disorder associated with dwarfism and elevated serum levels of unidentified anions (abstract). *Am. J. Dis. Child.* 102:705, 1961.

86. France, R., Stone, W. J., Michelakis, A. M., Island, D. P., Merrill, J. M., and Tolleson, W. J. Renal potassium-wasting of unknown cause in a clinical setting of chronic potassium depletion: Report of a case. *South. Med. J.* 66:115, 1973.

87. Gall, G., Vaitukaitis, J., Haddow, J. E., and Klein, R. Erythrocyte Na flux in a patient with Bartter's syndrome. *J. Clin. Endocrinol.* 32:562, 1971.

88. Gardner, J. D., Simopoulos, A. P., Lapey, A., and Shibolet, S. Altered membrane sodium transport in Bartter's syndrome. *J. Clin. Invest.* 51:1565, 1972.

89. Gill, J. R., Jr., Frolich, J. C., Bowden, R. E., Taylor, A. A., Keiser, H. R., Seyberth, H. W., Oates, J. A., and Bartter, F. C. Bartter's syndrome: A disorder characterized by high urinary prostaglandins and a dependence of hyperreninemia on prostaglandin synthesis. *Am. J. Med.* 61:43, 1976.

90. Goodman, A. D., Vagnucci, A. H., and Hartroft, P. M. Pathogenesis of Bartter's syndrome. *N. Engl. J. Med.* 281:1435, 1969.

91. Gottlieb, R. P. Metabolic alkalosis in cystic fibrosis. *J. Pediatr.* 79:930, 1971.

92. Greenberg, A. J., Arboit, J. M., New, M. I., and Worthen, H. G. Normotensive secondary hyperaldosteronism. *J. Pediatr.* 69:719, 1966.

93. Haljamae, H., Enger, E., and Sigstrom, L. Cellular potassium transport and ATPase activity in Bartter's syndrome. *Scand. J. Clin. Lab. Invest.* 35:53, 1975.

94. Heidland, A., Kreusser, W., Hennemann, H., Knauf, H., and Wigand, M. E. Excretion of the mono- and divalent ions in relation to flow rate in Bartter's and pseudo-Bartter's syndromes in parotid saliva: Comparative studies to the syndrome of Conn. *Klin. Wochenschr.* 50:959, 1972.

95. Imai, M., Yabuta, K., Murata, H., Takita, S., Ohbe, Y., and Sokabe, H. A case of Bartter's syndrome with abnormal renin response to salt load. *J. Pediatr.* 74:738, 1969.

96. James, T., Holland, N. H., and Preston, D. Bartter's syndrome: Typical facies and normal plasma volume. *Am. J. Dis. Child.* 129:1205, 1975.

97. Jepson, J., and McGarry, E. E. Polycythemia and increased erythropoietin production in a patient with hypertrophy of the juxta-glomerular apparatus. *Blood* 32:370, 1968.

98. Johnston, C. I., and Jose, A. D. Reduced vascular

response to angiotensin II in secondary hyperaldo-steronism. *J. Clin. Invest.* 42:1411, 1963.

99. Kaplan, N. M., and Silah, J. G. The effect of angiotensin II on the blood pressure in humans with hypertensive disease. *J. Clin. Invest.* 43:659, 1964.

100. Kihara, I., Kitamura, S., Hoshino, T., Seida, H., and Watanabe, T. A hitherto unreported vascular tumor of the kidney: A proposal of "juxtaglomerular cell tumor." *Acta Pathol. Jpn.* 18:197, 1968.

101. Mace, J. W., Hambidge, K. M., Gotlin, R. W., Dubois, R. S., Solomons, C. S., and Katz, F. H. Magnesium supplementation in Bartter's syndrome. *Arch. Dis. Child.* 48:485, 1973.

102. Mathieu, H., Habib, R., Lestradet, H., Recher, P., and Royer, P. Nephropathie chronique avec perte de potassium: Lésions rénales insolites et surcharge lipidique cortico-surrénale chez un enfant. *Arch. Fr. Pédiatr.* 17:1161, 1960.

103. McCredie, D. A., Blair-West, J. R., Scroggins, B. A., and Shipman, R. Potassium-losing nephropathy. *Med. J. Aust.* 1:129, 1971.

104. McCredie, D. A., Rotenburg, E., and Williams, A. L. Hypercalciuria in potassium-losing nephropathy: A variant of Bartter's syndrome. *Aust. Paediatr. J.* 10:286, 1974.

105. Meyer, W. J., III, Gill, J. R., Jr., and Bartter, F. C. Gout as a complication of Bartter's syndrome: A possible role for alkalosis in the decreased clearance of uric acid. *Ann. Intern. Med.* 83:56, 1975.

106. Modlinger, R. S., Nicolis, G. L., Krakoff, L. R., and Gabrilove, J. L. Some observations on the pathogenesis of Bartter's syndrome. *N. Engl. J. Med.* 289:1022, 1973.

107. Norby, L. H., Lentz, R., Flamenbaum, W., and Ramwell, P. Prostaglandins and aspirin therapy in Bartter's syndrome. *Lancet* 2:604, 1976.

108. Pasternack, A. Anorexia nervosa, secondary aldosteronism and angiopathy. *Acta Med. Scand.* 187:139, 1970.

109. Pasternack, A., Perheentupa, J., Launiala, K., and Hallman, N. Kidney biopsy findings in familial chloride diarrhoea. *Acta Endocrinol. (Kbh.)* 55:1, 1967.

110. Proesmans, W., Eggermont, E., and Eechels, R. Antidiuretic therapy in Bartter syndrome (letter). *J. Pediatr.* 82:538, 1973.

111. Pronove, P., MacCardle, R. C., and Bartter, F. C. Aldosteronism, hypokalemia, and a unique renal lesion in a five year old boy (abstract). *Acta Endocrinol.* [Suppl.] (Kbh.) 51:167, 1960.

112. Ramanathan, K., Gantt, C., and Grossman, A. Six-year follow-up of a child with Bartter syndrome. *Am. J. Dis. Child.* 126:230, 1973.

113. Robertson, P. W., Klidjian, A., Harding, L. K., Walters, G., Lee, M. R., and Robb-Smith, A. H. T. Hypertension due to a renin-secreting renal tumor. *Am. J. Med.* 43:963, 1967.

114. Rosenbaum, P., and Hughes, M. Persistent, probably congenital hypokalemic metabolic alkalosis with hyaline degeneration of renal tubules and normal urinary aldosterone (abstract). *Am. J. Dis. Child.* 94:560, 1957.

115. Royer, P. The Hereditary Tubular Diseases. In P. Royer, R. Habib, H. Mathieu, and M. Broyer, (eds.), *Pediatric Nephrology.* Philadelphia: Saunders, 1974. Pp. 56–98.

116. Royer, P., Delaitre, R., Mathieu, H., Gabilan, J. C., Raynaud, C., Pasqualini, J. R., Debris, P., Gerbeaux,

S., and Habib, R. L'Hypokaliémie chronique idiopathique avec hyperkaliurie de l'enfant. *Rev. Fr. Etud. Clin. Biol.* 9:61, 1964.

117. Sann, L., Moreu, P., Longin, B., Sassard, J., and François, R. Un syndrome de Bartter associant un hypercortisolisme, d'un diabète phosphoré et magnesien et d'une tubulopathie d'origine familiale. *Arch. Fr. Pédiatr.* 32:350, 1975.

118. Sasaki, H., Okumura, M., Ideda, M., Kawasaki, T., and Fukiyama, K. Hypotensive response to angiotensin II analogue in Bartter's syndrome (letter). *N. Engl. J. Med.* 294:611, 1976.

119. Schwartz, G. J., and Cornfeld, D. Bartter's syndrome: Clinical study of its treatment with salt loading and propranolol. *Clin. Nephrol.* 4:45, 1974.

119a. Schwartz, G. J., and Cornfeld, D. Unpublished observation, 1973.

120. Simopoulos, A. P., and Bartter, F. C. Growth characteristics and factors influencing growth in Bartter's syndrome. *J. Pediatr.* 81:56, 1972.

121. Slater, R. J., Azzopardi, P., Stater, P. E., and Chute, A. L. An unusual case of chronic hypokalemia associated with renal tubular degeneration (abstract). *Am. J. Dis. Child.* 96:469, 1958.

122. Solomon, R. J., and Brown, R. S. Bartter's syndrome: New insights into pathogenesis and treatment. *Am. J. Med.* 59:575, 1975.

123. Stanbury, J. Discussion of A. H. F. Van Olphen, P. J. J. Van Munster, and J. P. Slooff, Chronic Hypokalemia, Hypochloremia and Alkalosis of Probable Renal Origin. In J. deGraeff and D. Leijnse (eds.), *Water and Electrolyte Metabolism II.* Amsterdam: Elsevier, 1964. Pp. 146–147.

124. Stokes, G. S., Andrews, B. S., Hagon, E., Thornell, I. R., Palmer, A. A., and Posen, S. Bartter's syndrome presenting during pregnancy: Results of amiloride therapy. *Med. J. Aust.* 2:360, 1974.

125. Strauss, R. G. Failure of methyldopa therapy in Bartter's syndrome. *J. Pediatr.* 85:101, 1974.

126. Strauss, R. G., Mohammed, S., Loggie, J. M. H., Schubert, W. K., Fasola, A. F., and Gaffney, T. E. The effect of methyldopa on plasma renin activity in a child with Bartter's syndrome. *J. Pediatr.* 77:1071, 1970.

127. Sutherland, L. E., Hartroft, P., Balis, J. U., Bailey, J. D., and Lynch, M. J. Bartter's syndrome: A report of four cases, including three in one sibship, with comparative histologic evaluation of the juxtaglomerular apparatuses and glomeruli. *Acta Paediatr. Scand.* [Suppl.] 201:1, 1970.

128. Takayasu, H., Aso, Y., Nakauchi, K., and Kawabe, K. A case of Bartter's syndrome with surgical treatment followed for four years. *J. Clin. Endocrinol.* 32:842, 1971.

129. Tarm, F., Juncos, L. L., Anderson, C. F., and Donadio, J. V., Jr. Bartter's syndrome: An unusual presentation. *Mayo Clin. Proc.* 48:280, 1973.

130. Tomko, D. J., Yeh, B. P. Y., and Falls, W. F., Jr. Bartter's syndrome: Study of a 52-year-old man with evidence for a defect in proximal tubular sodium reabsorption and comments on therapy. *Am. J. Med.* 61:111, 1976.

131. Trygstad, C. W., Mangos, J. A., Bloodworth, J. M. B., Jr., and Lobeck, C. C. A sibship with Bartter's syndrome: Failure of total adrenalectomy to correct the potassium wasting. *Pediatrics* 44:234, 1969.

132. Van Olphen, A. H. F., Van Munster, P. J. J., and

Slooff, J. P. Chronic Hypokalemia, Hypochloremia, and Alkalosis of Probably Renal Origin. In J. de-Graeff and B. Leijnse (eds.), *Water and Electrolyte Metabolism II.* Amsterdam: Elsevier, 1964. Pp. 134–142.

133. Verberckmoes, R., Van Damme, B., Clement, J., Amery, A., and Michielsen, P. Bartter's syndrome with hyperplasia of renomedullary cells: Successful treatment with indomethacin. *Kidney Int.* 9:302, 1976.

134. Vinci, J. M., Telles, D. A., Bowden, R. E., Izzo, J. L., Jr., Keiser, H. R., Radfar, N., Taylor, A. A., Gill, J. R., Jr., and Bartter, F. C. The kallikrein-kinin system in Bartter's syndrome and its response to prostaglandin synthetase inhibition (abstract). *Clin. Res.* 24:414A, 1976.

135. Visser, H. K. A., Degenhart, H. J., Desmit, E., and Cost, W. S. Mineralocorticoid excess in two brothers with dwarfism, hypokalaemic alkalosis and normal blood pressure. *Acta Endocrinol. (Kbh.)* 55: 661, 1967.

136. Wald, M. K., Perrin, E. V., and Bolande, R. P. Bartter's syndrome in infancy: Physiologic, light and electron miscroscopic observations. *Pediatrics* 47: 254, 1971.

137. Walker, S. H. Severe Bartter syndrome in blacks (letter). *N. Engl. J. Med.* 285:1150, 1971.

138. Wallace, M., Richards, P., Chesser, E., and Wrong, O. Persistent alkalosis and hypokalaemia caused by surreptitious vomiting. *Q. J. Med.* 37:577, 1968.

139. White, M. G. Bartter's syndrome: A manifestation of renal tubular defects. *Arch. Intern. Med.* 129:41, 1972.

140. Williams, G. H., Handwerger, S., Hickler, R. B., and Crigler, J. R., Jr. Primary renal potassium wasting in a patient with juxtaglomerular hyperplasia (Bartter's syndrome) (abstract). *J. Clin. Invest.* 49:103a, 1970.

141. Wolff, H. P., Vecsei, P., Kruck, F., Roscher, S., Brown, J. J., Dusterdieck, G. O., Lever, A. F., and Robertson, J. I. S. Psychiatric disturbance leading to potassium depletion, sodium depletion, raised plasma-renin concentration, and secondary hyperaldosteronism. *Lancet* 1:257, 1968.

Section Seven. Circulatory Disorders

88. Renal Arterial Disease and Renovascular Hypertension

Gunnar B. Stickler

A number of conditions decrease flow in the renal artery and are associated with hypertension. These conditions can be diagnosed with the help of selective aortography and the determination of renal vein renin levels. Operative techniques to revascularize the kidney have been developed and refined, and these have improved considerably the prognosis for patients with these obstructive lesions.

The differential diagnosis of hypertension is discussed in Chap. 9. The pathogenesis of renovascular hypertension is discussed in Chap. 18. Some patients not only have hyperreninemia, but also secondary hyperaldosteronism with hypokalemia and polyuria [26, 37]. Review of the extensive literature leaves one with the impression that renal arterial lesions are still underdiagnosed, particularly in the newborn period and after trauma.

In the past, the term *renal artery stenosis* was used to describe intrinsic obstructions. During the past 15 years, *fibromuscular dysplasia* has been considered the most frequent cause in children for the narrowing of the lumen of the renal artery

and its branches. In the adult population, atheromatous lesions are the most frequent cause. In 1967 Favre [11] reviewed the case reports of 42 children who had hypertension due to an obstructive process of the renal artery. Of these children, 20 had renal artery stenosis or fibromuscular dysplasia, 9 had aneurysms, 1 had an arteriovenous fistula, 2 had external compression of the renal artery by a ganglioneuroma, and 10 had various other lesions. In 1971 Cukier and associates [7] summarized the reports of 61 pediatric patients with renal artery obstruction; the majority had fibromuscular dysplasia.

Fibromuscular Dysplasia of the Renal Artery

Harrison and McCormack [17] use the term *dysplasia of the renal artery* to indicate a morphologic alteration of the renovascular conduit without etiologic implication. The term is applied to disruptive or hyperplastic processes that predominantly involve the tunica media and result in stenosis of the artery, with or without an associated

The critical review and constructive criticisms by Drs. Philip E. Bernatz and James C. Hunt were deeply appreciated.

aneurysm. These authors proposed a unified histologic classification according to the layer of the artery that is predominantly involved: intimal fibroplasia; periarterial fibroplasia; and the condition most commonly found, fibromuscular dysplasia (when the tunica media is involved). These lesions are found almost exclusively in patients with hypertension, although they may be incidental findings.

The first patient with fibromuscular dysplasia of the renal artery was described by Leadbetter and Burkland [24]. This 5½-year-old boy obtained relief of hypertension when the affected kidney was removed. The histologic changes in the renal artery later were called fibromuscular hyperplasia [28]. Further historic contributions have been summarized by Hunt and coworkers [19].

The pathogenesis of fibromuscular dysplasia is unknown. A familial aggregation has been noted in some instances [1]. The disease occurs with equal frequency in boys and girls.

There have been a number of reports of fibromuscular dysplasia in infants. Ljungqvist and Wallgren [27] described a 10-day-old boy with stenosis of the left renal artery who died of a cerebral hemorrhage. Schmidt and Rambo [34] reported a 7-week-old infant with hypertension who died of congestive failure; the child had severe intimal hyperplasia of the renal arteries and the abdominal aorta. A 10-month-old boy with involvement of the renal artery and coronary arteries was described by Dawson and Nabarro [10].

In the series of Fry and coworkers [15], almost half of the 22 patients had hypertension diagnosed during the course of a routine physical examination. Others in the series were brought to medical attention because of symptoms such as headache, dizziness, irritability, and loss of weight. Seizures may occur in as many as 25 percent of children with severe hypertension [38]. In young infants the symptoms include vomiting, failure to thrive, and cardiac failure.

In addition to the positive funduscopic findings and elevated blood pressure, bruits may be revealed by auscultation of the central areas of the abdomen and the renal region.

When other causes of hypertension, predominantly parenchymal renal disease, are ruled out (see Chap. 18), rapid sequence urography may give a clue to the diagnosis, such as discrepancy in size of the kidney and delayed excretion of contrast material (Fig. 88-1A). Isotope renograms and renal scans in children are considered unreliable by Fry and associates [15]. However, Bernatz [3] believes that isotope renograms provide the surgeon with a reliable noninvasive method for following function, particularly during the postoperative period. In order to arrive at a definitive diagnosis, selective aortography (Fig. 88-1B) is the method of choice, combined with determination of renin levels in both renal veins.

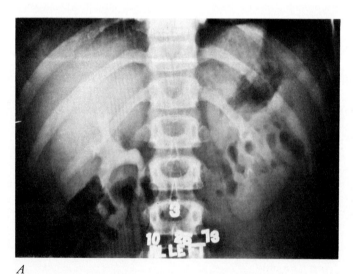

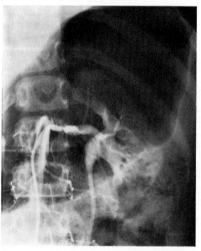

A   B

Figure 88-1. A. Excretory urogram in 9-year-old girl with hypertension due to fibromuscular disease of the left renal artery is compatible with delay in excretion of contrast material. B. Aortogram reveals stenosis of the left renal artery due to fibromuscular dysplasia.

This technique has generally replaced the split renal function test. Renal vein determinations have a lateralizing value when the ratio of the affected to the nonaffected side is greater than 1.5 : 1.

In the decision regarding treatment, the age of the child has to be considered. Definite guidelines have not been developed, but if medical control of the hypertension in the very young infant fails and only one renal artery is involved, nephrectomy probably is the best approach. Fry and associates [15] successfully revascularized the kidney in a 21-month-old boy and in two 3-year-old boys by using a saphenous vein bypass procedure. Occasionally revascularization has been accomplished by anastomosing the splenic artery to the renal artery distal to the lesion, but this is not considered to be the therapy of choice. Kaufman and coworkers [21] have used the interposition of the right hypogastric artery to revascularize the kidney. Serrallach-Mila and coworkers [35] were the first to utilize renal autotransplantation, and Fay and colleagues [12, 13] have applied this technique to children.

The prognosis for children with fibromuscular hyperplasia is uncertain. There has been a high failure rate in children because of thrombosis in the bypass, and eventually nephrectomy has been required. In follow-up of 5 children after surgical treatment, Foster and associates [14] found that 2 developed contralateral renal artery disease.

Aneurysms of the Renal Artery

Hock and Jones [18] described a child with hypertension who had an aneurysm with thrombosis within the lesion. Nephrectomy corrected the hypertension. Cummings and associates [8] studied the association of renal aneurysm and hypertension and found that in 13 patients, including 1 child, the aneurysm alone did not cause hypertension. Nephrectomy or operation to accomplish revascularization is indicated only if the aneurysm is associated with narrowing of the renal artery. Fibromuscular dysplasia may be associated with the aneurysm. These authors recommend revascularization procedures in patients with aneurysms only if lateralization is confirmed by renin studies.

Disease of the Renal Artery in Neurofibromatosis

Tilford and Kelsch [39] reported their experience with 4 patients who had neurofibromatosis and stenosis of the renal artery and reviewed all the reported cases, bringing the total, mostly pe-

diatric patients, to 30. They noted that renal arterial disease in neurofibromatosis was more frequent in males than in females (21 : 9). Mena and associates have also reviewed the subject [29].

In the pediatric age group, neurofibromatosis with renovascular hypertension is more frequent than neurofibromatosis and hypertension due to pheochromocytoma. Only three patients with the latter combination have been reported below the age of 18 years.

Tilford and Kelsch [39] noted that both renal arteries were narrowed in 40 percent of their patients, and 53 percent had aneurysmal or poststenotic dilatations of the involved vessel. Of the patients with neurofibromatosis and renal arterial disease, 23 percent had narrowing of the abdominal aorta.

Mena and coworkers [29] emphasized that renal artery stenosis in neurofibromatosis is usually seen within 1 cm of the origin from the aorta, while in fibromuscular disease, the involvement usually begins in the middle or the distal segments of the main renal artery.

Microscopically, the lesions in the artery represent hyperplasia of the intima and media. Mena and associates [29] mentioned that the histologic appearance was difficult to distinguish from that of fibromuscular dysplasia. Revascularization operations were their treatment of choice, with aortorenal vein grafts being their preferred method.

Arteritis of the Aorta With Stenosis of the Renal Artery

Patients have been reported from various countries in Asia with a nonspecific aortic arteritis that is indistinguishable from Takayasu's arteritis (synonyms are pulseless disease, middle aortic syndrome, atypical coarctation of the aorta, and aortic arch syndrome characterized by aortitis). The nonspecific aortic arteritis occurs predominantly in young adults. The aortic arch is affected primarily, but the renal artery also may be involved. Inoue et al. [20] summarized their experience in 1972. Danaraj and Ong [9] described two children in whom this condition affected the renal arteries and caused hypertension. An 8½-year-old boy seen by Sinaiko and coworkers [36] had involvement of the abdominal aorta and both renal arteries with a surrounding severe fibrotic reaction; however, the authors believed that the patient's condition was fibromuscular dysplasia. Following failure of a saphenous vein bypass, the hypertension was corrected after a renal autotransplantation.

Thrombosis of the Renal Artery in the Newborn

In a review of arterial occlusions in infants, Gross [16] noted 47 patients 2 to 3 weeks of age with lesions at various arterial sites. Four of the 47 infants had thrombosis of the renal artery. He suggested that causes of arterial embolism and thrombosis were sepsis, "immaturity of peripheral circulation," and congenital heart disease, particularly patent ductus arteriosus.

Zuelzer et al. [43] found four instances of thrombosis of the renal artery among 2,058 autopsies, all in newborns. This condition probably was recognized only at postmortem examination until Woodard and associates [42] diagnosed it in a newborn who had hypertension and evidence of congestive heart failure. The child had proteinuria, hematuria, and azotemia; no mass was felt. Nephrectomy was followed by a decrease in blood pressure, and the patient recovered.

Renal vein thrombosis is a well-known entity in the newborn period, but if the newborn, particularly one with impaired circulation due to congenital heart disease, presents with hypertension, azotemia, proteinuria, and hematuria in the absence of renal enlargement, more frequent use of an aortogram may allow early diagnosis of an arterial lesion; prompt treatment with nephrectomy may be carried out if arterial thrombosis is found. The relatively high incidence in the series by Zuelzer et al. [43] may lead one to speculate that partial arterial occlusion of the renal artery may be more common than previously assumed.

Thrombosis of the Renal Artery Due to Trauma

Von Recklinghausen [40] described the first patient with posttraumatic thrombosis of the renal artery in 1861. In 1972 Morton and Crawford [30] found reports of only 9 such patients in the literature, and they added an additional case; 3 of the 10 were children.

It has been postulated that trauma causes stretching of the renal vascular pedicle and rupture of the arterial intima, with subsequent dissection and hematoma and thrombus formation. During the last few years, a large number of case reports have been published. The availability and more frequent use of selective aortograms, particularly in patients with abdominal trauma and nonfunction of one or both kidneys, may allow the diagnosis to be made more often. Cornell et al. [6] saw 5 patients with renal artery thrombosis due to trauma during a 3-year period; 3 were children. Two patients presented with hypertension, one patient 3 months and the other 10 years after the abdominal injury. Ready and coworkers [33] summarized the reports of 4 patients with bilateral traumatic renal artery thrombosis, including one of their own. All 4 patients were teenagers who were involved in automobile or motorcycle accidents. Excretory urography failed to demonstrate excretion of dye from either kidney, and aortography demonstrated bilateral renal artery obstruction in all four. Two of the four patients died. Their own patient had irreversible renal failure and had to undergo transplantation.

The patient reported by Morton and Crawford [30] was operated on 18 hr after an accident, and revascularization was accomplished. He had partial return of renal function, his serum creatinine level remained elevated at 1.7 mg per deciliter, and he continued to be hypertensive.

In 1974 Fay and coworkers [12] noted reports of 38 patients who had posttraumatic renal artery thrombosis. These authors also were the first to use renal autotransplantation for this condition in one patient, with a good result. Another four teenagers with posttraumatic thrombosis of the renal artery were observed by Caponegro and Leadbetter [4].

With the increasing use of motorcycles by children and teenagers, more posttraumatic renal artery thrombosis probably will be observed. Prompt revascularization procedures within hours after the injury may save a kidney and may be lifesaving if there is bilateral thrombosis.

Intrarenal Arteriovenous Fistula

Palmer and Connolly [31] reviewed 45 cases of arteriovenous fistula in 1966 and included an additional case of their own. Of these, 25 cases were congenital. Trauma was presumed to be the cause in 14 patients; 5 of the 14 had arteriovenous fistula after a needle biopsy and 3 after surgery. Six fistulas were found in patients with renal carcinoma; the authors, however, did not indicate the age distribution of the patients reviewed. The most common presenting symptom was hematuria. Thirteen patients had hypertension, and eleven were in congestive failure. Bernatz [3] has seen several asymptomatic patients with arteriovenous fistulas. The presence of an abdominal bruit or murmur is helpful in the diagnosis of intrarenal arteriovenous fistula, but for precise delineation, selective aortograms and renin studies (when there is associated hypertension) are indicated. The treatment for these fistulas is surgical, with nephrectomy being done frequently. Partial nephrectomy or selective hypothermia with removal of the lesion has been done successfully in a few instances. There have been no reports of renal autotransplantation for this condition, but this may be a procedure in the future.

Miscellaneous Causes of Renovascular Hypertension

Other conditions infrequently cause renovascular hypertension in children. Obstruction from the external compression of the renal artery by tumors such as ganglioneuromas [11], Wilms' tumor [22], or scar tissue [41] has been reported. Periarteritis nodosa has been mentioned as a cause for narrowing of the renal artery and subsequent hypertension [5]. Clayman and Bookstein [5] mentioned renovascular hypertension in a patient with homocystinuria. Lefèbvre and associates [25] stated that renal artery disease has been found in patients with the Marfan syndrome. They [25] also reported renovascular hypertension associated with severe idiopathic hypercalcemia and the Williams triad (see Chap. 74), proved by selective aortography.

Renal artery stenosis was found in a boy with a solitary hydronephrotic kidney on the basis of ureteropelvic obstruction [32]; this patient also had a patent ductus arteriosus. During the first year of life, severe hypertension was noted in identical twins who had persistent medial hypertrophy of the renal arterioles [2] as well as interstitial fibrosis and tubular atrophy. Recently Krawczynski and coworkers [23] described their experience doing aortograms in patients with Turner's syndrome. Of 28 patients, 25 had one or more additional renal arteries on one or both sides, but none had hypertension.

References

1. Assendelft, P. M. van, Kooiker, C. J., Mees, E. J., and Hameleers, A. J. Renovascular hypertension in three children from one family. *J. Clin. Pathol.* 26:359, 1973.
2. Bergstein, J. M., Fangman, J., Fish, A. J., Herdman, R., and Good, R. A. Severe hypertension in identical twin infants. *Am. J. Dis. Child.* 122:348, 1971.
3. Bernatz, P. E. Personal communication, 1975.
4. Caponegro, P. J., and Leadbetter, G. W., Jr. Traumatic renal artery thrombosis. *J. Urol.* 109:769, 1973.
5. Clayman, A. S., and Bookstein, J. J. The role of renal arteriography in pediatric hypertension. *Radiology* 108:107, 1973.
6. Cornell, S. H., Reasa, D. A., and Culp, D. A. Occlusion of the renal artery secondary to acute or remote trauma. *J.A.M.A.* 219:1754, 1972.
7. Cukier, J., Perelman, D., Beurton, D., Vacant, J., Ott, R., and Marie, J. Sténoses multiples d'une artère rénale responsables d'une hypertension artérielle chez l'enfant: Guérison par pontage aorto-rénal. *Ann. Pediatr.* 18:741, 1971.
8. Cummings, K. B., Lecky, J. W., and Kaufman, J. J. Renal artery aneurysms and hypertension. *J. Urol.* 109:144, 1973.
9. Danaraj, T. J., and Ong, W. H. Primary arteritis of abdominal aorta in children causing bilateral stenosis of renal arteries and hypertension. *Circulation* 20:856, 1959.
10. Dawson, I. M. P., and Nabarro, S. A case of intimal hyperplasia of arteries with hypertension in a male infant. *J. Pathol. Bacteriol.* 66:493, 1953.
11. Favre, R. Hypertension artérielle rénale et son traitement chirurgical chez l'enfant. *Helv. Paediatr. Acta* 22:54, 1967.
12. Fay, R., Brosman, S., Lindstrom, R., and Cohen, A. Renal artery thrombosis: A successful revascularization by autotransplantation. *J. Urol.* 111:572, 1974.
13. Fay, R., and Kaufman, J. J. Renal hypertension in children. *Urology* 3:148, 1974.
14. Foster, J. H., Oates, J. A., Rhamy, R. K., Klatte, E. C., Burko, H. C., and Michelakis, A. M. Hypertension and fibromuscular dysplasia of the renal arteries. *Surgery* 65:157, 1969.
15. Fry, W. J., Ernst, C. B., Stanley, J. C., and Brink, B. Renovascular hypertension in the pediatric patient. *Arch. Surg.* 107:692, 1973.
16. Gross, R. E. Arterial embolism and thrombosis in infancy. *Am. J. Dis. Child.* 70:61, 1945.
17. Harrison, E. G., Jr., and McCormack, L. J. Pathologic classification of renal arterial disease in renovascular hypertension. *Mayo Clin. Proc.* 46:161, 1971.
18. Hock, E. F., and Jones, E. M. Aneurysm of the renal artery causing hypertension. *Am. J. Dis. Child.* 89:606, 1955.
19. Hunt, J. C., Harrison, E. G., Jr., Kincaid, O. W., Bernatz, P. E., and Davis, G. D. Idiopathic fibrosis and fibromuscular stenoses of the renal arteries associated with hypertension. *Proc. Staff Meet. Mayo Clin.* 37:181, 1962.
20. Inoue, T., Kawada, K., Takeuchi, S., Sohma, Y., Koyanagi, H., Hosoda, Y., and Hata, J. Surgical considerations of the aortic and arterial lesions due to nonspecific aorta-arteritis. *J. Thorac. Cardiovasc. Surg.* 63:599, 1972.
21. Kaufman, J. J., Goodwin, W. E., Waisman, J., and Gyepes, M. T. Renovascular hypertension in children: Report of seven cases treated surgically including two cases of renal autotransplantation. *Am. J. Surg.* 124:149, 1972.
22. Koons, K. M., and Ruch, M. K. Hypertension in a 7-year-old girl with Wilms' tumor relieved by nephrectomy. *J.A.M.A.* 115:1097, 1940.
23. Krawczynski, M., Maciejewski, J., Grzybkowska, B., and Bartkowiak, K. Les anomalies de la vascularisation du système urogénital dans le syndrome de Turner. *Pediatrie* 29:413, 1974.
24. Leadbetter, W. F., and Burkland, C. E. Hypertension in unilateral renal disease. *J. Urol.* 39:611, 1938.
25. Lefèbvre, J., Labrune, M., and Benacerraf, R. Renovascular hypertension in childhood. *Progr. Pediatr. Radiol.* 3:252, 1970.
26. Leumann, E. P., Bauer, R. P., Slaton, P. E., Biglieri, E. G., and Holliday, M. A. Renovascular hypertension in children. *Pediatrics* 46:362, 1970.
27. Ljungqvist, A., and Wallgren, G. Unilateral renal artery stenosis and fatal arterial hypertension in a newborn infant. *Acta Paediatr. (Stockh.)* 51:575, 1962.
28. McCormack, L. J., Hazard, J. B., and Poutasse, E. F. Obstructive lesions of the renal artery associated with remediable hypertension (abstract). *Am. J. Pathol.* 34:582, 1958.

29. Mena, E., Bookstein, J. J., Holt, J. F., and Fry, W. J. Neurofibromatosis and renovascular hypertension in children. *Am. J. Roentgenol. Radium Ther. Nucl. Med.* 118:39, 1973.

30. Morton, J. R., and Crawford, E. S. Bilateral traumatic renal artery thrombosis. *Ann. Surg.* 176:62, 1972.

31. Palmer, J. M., and Connolly, J. E. Intrarenal arteriovenous fistula: Surgical excision under selective renal hypothermia with kidney survival. *J. Urol.* 96:599, 1966.

32. Presto, A. J., III, and Middleton, R. G. Cure of hypertension in a child with renal artery stenosis and hydronephrosis in a solitary kidney. *J. Urol.* 109:98, 1973.

33. Ready, L. B., Wright, C., and Baltzan, R. B. Bilateral traumatic renal artery thrombosis. *Can. Med. Assoc. J.* 109:885, 1973.

34. Schmidt, D. M., and Rambo, O. N., Jr. Segmental intimal hyperplasia of the abdominal aorta and renal arteries producing hypertension in an infant. *Am. J. Clin. Pathol.* 44:546, 1965.

35. Serrallach-Mila, N., Paravisini, J., Mayol-Valls, P., Alberti, J., Casellas, A., and Nolla-Panadés, J. Renal autotransplantation (letter to the editor). *Lancet* 2:1130, 1965.

36. Sinaiko, A., Najarian, J., Michael, A. F., and Mirkin, B. L. Renal autotransplantation in the treatment of bilateral renal artery stenosis: Relief of hypertension in an 8-year-old boy. *J. Pediatr.* 83:409, 1973.

37. Stefan, H., Helge, H., Merker, H. J., and Bachmann, D. Nierenarterienstenose, renale Hypertonie und sekundärer Hyperaldosteronismus bei einem 8 Jahre alten Knaben. *Helv. Paediatr. Acta* 23:509, 1968.

38. Still, J. L., and Cottom, D. Severe hypertension in childhood. *Arch. Dis. Child.* 42:34, 1967.

39. Tilford, D. L., and Kelsch, R. C. Renal artery stenosis in childhood neurofibromatosis. *Am. J. Dis. Child.* 126:665, 1973.

40. Von Recklinghausen, F. Hämorrhagische Niereninfarkte. *Virchows Arch. Pathol. Anat. Physiol.* 20:205, 1861.

41. Wilk, F. Der renovaskuläre Hochdruck beim Kind. *Arch. Kinderheilkd.* 183:327, 1971.

42. Woodard, J. R., Patterson, J. H., and Brinsfield, D. Renal artery thrombosis in newborn infants. *Am. J. Dis. Child.* 114:191, 1967.

43. Zuelzer, W. W., Kurnetz, R., and Newton, W. A., Jr. Circulatory diseases of the kidneys in infancy and childhood: IV. Occlusion of the renal artery. *Am. J. Dis. Child.* 81:21, 1951.

89. Renal Venous Obstruction

Gavin Cranston Arneil

Definition. Renal venous obstruction may be caused by intraluminal, luminal, or extraluminal interference with the normal flow pattern of venous channels in the kidney. In practice the overwhelming majority of cases observed and reported relate to intraluminal renal venous thrombosis. Luminal obstruction or extraluminal obstruction due to a neoplasm or other mass is exceedingly rare in the child.

Renal Venous Thrombosis. Renal venous thrombosis (RVT) is the preferred term applied to a clotting process, whether progressing forward from venous radicles toward the main renal vein or more rarely in the reverse direction. The use of the phrase "renal *vein* thrombosis" is usually incorrect and is almost always misleading in relation to the pathogenesis of the condition in the child.

Historical Aspects
The original description of RVT is usually attributed to Rayer in 1840 [23]. There were few reports during the nineteenth century, although in fact the incidence at that time was not low, at least in Europe [5]. A number of accounts now available in the literature [1, 3, 10, 16, 20, 21, 24] shed light on progress in recognizing and treating the disease while suggesting that many cases remain unrecognized even today. Several large series have been published relating to as many as 36 [20], 45 [10], 96 [16], and 165 [3] children, respectively.

The surgical approach to the problem of RVT in the past has consisted in attempts to improve prognosis by heroic procedures such as immediate nephrectomy [10] and thrombectomy [17]. Today neither procedure is considered to have a useful role in the vast majority of affected children.

Familial Incidence and Genetics
Familial occurrence of RVT is rare, and there are not enough examples to permit analysis of a potential hereditary factor. The best recorded familial record is that noted by Dundon [14], published here for the first time as a personal communication [13].

A 26-year-old woman whose first child had been stillborn was delivered of her second child, a male with a birth weight of 4.1 kg, after 36 weeks' gestation. At the age of 5 weeks the infant was admitted and treated for left RVT, which was confirmed on later nephrectomy. One year later the third child, a male with a birth weight of 4.5 kg, was admitted at the age of 12 days with right RVT, which was confirmed on later nephrectomy. Nine days following the birth of her fifth child this unfortunate lady died of pulmonary embolism. Transient abnormal glucose tolerance curves were noted during each of her five pregnancies, but this curve returned to within normal limits (but abnormal on glucocorticosteroid stress) between pregnancies.

There may be a link between the prediabetic pattern of the mother and the occurrence of RVT in two of her newborn offspring.

Epidemiology
Neither the incidence nor the prevalence of RVT has been properly defined in a sufficiently large population over a long enough period of time to give reliable data. Where interest has been aroused and where *routine* postmortem studies with histologic examination of renal tissue from all infants and children dying has been instituted, the condition of RVT has been found to be much commoner than anticipated. Routine questions asked concerning every ill baby should include:

1. Is water and electrolyte disequilibrium causing a hyperosmolar state?
2. Is thrombocytopenia, burr cells, or other evidence of intravascular coagulation present?

If the answer to either of the above questions is yes, then the question, "Is RVT present?" follows naturally. A high index of suspicion leads to more frequent recognition and definition of the lesser degrees of RVT. Estimations of frequency are based on review of postmortem material and, since the disease is dominantly one of the newborn, the estimations must be influenced by the relative proportion of neonatal and other deaths in any series. Figures quoted range from 0.4 to 0.7 percent of childhood deaths [9, 20]. In one series from this hospital [6] the overall incidence in childhood postmortems was 0.4 percent, and in the newborn deaths it was 2.7 percent (these were newborns admitted to a children's hospital and not newborns dying in a maternity hospital). Another report recorded an incidence of 1.9 percent for RVT in 800 routine neonatal postmortem examinations [12].

Age Distribution. It has always been clear that the majority of cases of RVT occur during the early weeks of life. The results from various studies are difficult to compare, since the compilation of statistics for areas over a sufficient period has not yet been possible. In the largest European sur-

vey of 115 cases [3], 35 were diagnosed during the first week of life, 49 between 1 week and 1 month, and 23 between 1 month and 1 year. The comparable figures for the other large British report of 36 cases [20] were 20 during the first month and 15 during the remainder of the first year of life.

Sex Distribution. In the European group of RVT cases there were 71 boys and 44 girls (1.6 : 1) [3] and in a British series there were 21 boys and 15 girls (1.4 : 1) [20]. The male preponderance is common to all major series, but this could be due to vulnerability of the male to a primary and contributory disorder rather than to RVT directly. In the European series [3] the sex ratio in the patients aged less than a month was 2 : 1, but for those aged more than 1 month it was 1 : 1, suggesting specific factors operative in male newborn infants. There does not seem to be any difference between the incidence of right-sided, left-sided, and bilateral RVT in males and females [20].

Other Factors. The majority of reports of RVT, particularly of large series, have come from Europe. Whether this indicates a higher incidence, a higher awareness, or more thorough postmortem histologic study of newborns is not clear. The condition does not seem to be confined to any specific socioeconomic group, and there is no obvious seasonal incidence. The frequent history of preceding diarrhea in the children aged 1 to 12 months (55 percent) does suggest an association, but this has not been proved causal. A secondary link in this chain may be a hyperosmolar state. The occurrence of RVT following angiocardiography for congenital heart lesions is certainly suggestive [20] and may provide a clear link between hyperosmolar states, coagulopathy, and RVT [22]. The reported association between maternal diabetes and RVT in the offspring is difficult to interpret [4, 17]. Dramatic incidents such as recorded by Dundon [13] make a big impression, but in the 115 European children there was no *recognized* incidence of maternal diabetes or prediabetes [3].

Pathology
Renal venous thrombosis most commonly starts in the smaller veins such as the interlobular or ascending vasa recta and the arcuate veins, which anastomose with each other sparingly [3] (Fig. 89-1). Backward spread to the smaller venous tributaries may occur. Thrombosis may occur over a wide range of comparable arcuate veins or it may progress along the interlobar and hilar veins to the main renal vein and occasionally to the inferior

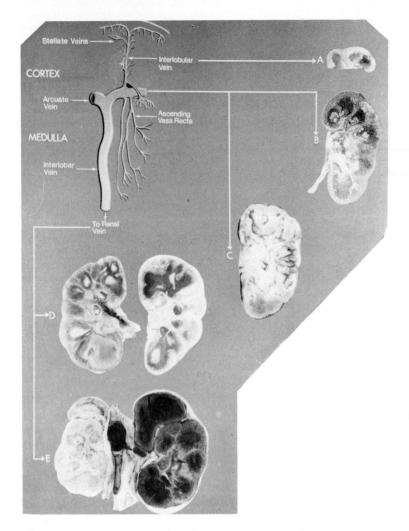

Figure 89-1. Renal venous thrombosis. Severity depends upon extent of vascular involvement. A. Interlobular vein, little damage. B. Arcuate veins, extensive lesion. C. Arcuate veins, marked parenchymal death. D. Hilar and renal veins involved. E. Renal vein, inferior vena cava, and adrenal gland involved.

vena cava and adrenal veins. Such thrombotic episodes may be unilateral or bilateral, and if bilateral they may be symmetrical or asymmetrical. Very rarely in children, but commonly in adults, the initial mechanism is thrombosis of the main renal vein with spread to the venous tributaries [8].

The morbid anatomy of the kidneys varies widely, depending on the degree of venous involvement, the duration of the thrombosis, and the age of the patient. Small areas related to interlobular, vasa recta, or even arcuate venous thrombosis may be missed if only a longitudinal section of kidney is made. Diffuse involvement of many smaller veins is not always obvious on gross inspection but is revealed on histology. On the other hand, involvement of interlobar, hilar, or

main renal vein produces gross obvious changes. The later stage, with gross lobulation, scarring, and contraction is often mistaken for dysplastic kidneys or chronic pyelonephritis. When the lesion has begun prenatally, calcification is the rule.

The marked tendency to intravascular coagulation in the newborn frequently produces focal microthrombi before, during, or after birth [7]. In the Glasgow series [3] three perinatal examples were reported in which one kidney was affected prenatally (with calcification following) and the other postnatally. It seems likely that the slow double capillary circulation in the kidney is particularly vulnerable to thrombosis under circumstances of hemoconcentration, dehydration, hyperosmolality, and hypercoagulability, particularly in the perinatal period. Histologically the appearance is that of a thrombus which initially consists almost entirely of platelets but which later organizes. This thrombus fibroses and may eventually recanalize to a greater or lesser extent. If local anastomosis is not adequate, then massive infarction with hemorrhage into adjacent tissues occurs, leading to death of cortical or medullary cells or both. Pigmentation from alteration of hemoglobin and then progressive sclerosis occurs rapidly.

Clinical Findings
SIGNS AND SYMPTOMS

Three out of four patients with RVT are less than 1 month of age. The infant with RVT may fail to thrive, with anorexia and oliguria. In 64 percent of infants and 49 percent of older children hematuria is noted [3]. Occasionally there is a history of maternal diabetes or prediabetes. Contributory factors in the newborn are asphyxia and cyanotic congenital heart disease, and angiocardiography in such infants is a frequent precipitating factor. Palpable, enlarged kidney(s) are a positive sign in only 60 percent of infants and children. Diarrhea, vomiting, and shock are present in only 10 to 20 percent of the very young children (0 to 7 days) but are noted in 40 to 60 percent of the older infants [3]. Metabolic acidosis may be observed in 50 percent of the children.

Blood pressure is variable in the early stages of RVT and is more likely to be lowered than raised, although hypertension is encountered. Signs and symptoms of an underlying primary disorder may be obvious. The most likely pattern is that of the hyperosmolar syndrome with primary failure of water intake either absolutely or in relation to solute load.

Clinical manifestations of RVT vary from relatively mild, with minimal to gross hematuria, to rapidly progressive renal failure with azotemia, uremia, hyperosmolality, anuria, and death. The patient may present with tachypnea, shock, and pallor, and only the detection of a firm, palpable kidney or kidneys may lead to an appreciation of the underlying lesion. The condition of the patient may deteriorate rapidly if thrombosis spreads. Hemoperitoneum has been reported in association with RVT, and a nephrotic syndrome sometimes occurs, more often in adults than in children.

HEMATOLOGIC FINDINGS

Significant anemia is found in one-third of young infants and two-thirds of older children [3] with RVT. The most significant, simple, and reliable test is that for progressing thrombocytopenia, which is found in 90 percent of cases.

Microangiopathic hemolytic anemia with falling hemoglobin level, red cell fragmentation (burr cells) on the blood film, and thrombocytopenia have been found in the majority of RVT cases studied recently at the Royal Hospital for Sick Children in Glasgow. These changes were frequently accompanied by elevated serum fibrin degradation products (>10 μg/ml) and low plasma fibrinogen levels (<200 mg/100 ml). In half the cases plasma factor V and plasminogen levels were also low [17]. These findings reflect the consumption of platelets and coagulation factors within the renal venous system and perhaps, in some of the severe cases, in other sites also, such as the brain or liver. Serial observations may be more informative than single tests, both in regard to evidence of progressive intravascular consumption and as an index of response to therapy.

Although this pattern of hematologic change in ill infants should strongly alert one to the possibility of RVT, the same picture can also be seen in septicemia [11] and even to a lesser extent in hypertonic dehydration without overt renal venous thrombosis [22].

Serum Nitrogen and Electrolyte Levels. Azotemia and uremia are the rule in RVT and may be severe (urea >100 mg/dl in 55 percent) [3]. Metabolic acidosis is frequent but not invariable. The level of serum sodium is highly variable, being less than 130 mEq per liter in 26 percent and greater than 150 mEq per liter in 28 percent. The serum chloride level is equally variable, but serum potassium levels tend to be normal or raised (35 percent >6 mEq/L) [3]. There is confusion as to whether hypertonic, hypernatremic, hyperosmolar states follow or (more probably) precede the occurrence of some cases of RVT. Serial study of electrolyte concentrations is desirable, but it must not be forgotten that electrolytes are measured per unit volume of extracellular fluid, and attention should be paid to the possible existence of overhydration, underhydration, or disparity between hydration of intracellular and extracellular compartments.

RADIOLOGIC FINDINGS

Radiology has been of great value in improving the diagnosis of RVT [3], particularly in the azotemic, anuric, and potentially anephric neonate. The questions posed to the radiologist are

1. Are both kidneys present and normal?
2. Are both kidneys functioning and functioning normally?
3. Is there a change in these findings on repeat study?

The first step is a plain radiograph of the abdomen and then intravenous urography, including a nephrogram and tomography if indicated. Abdominal films are taken in the supine and lateral position and aim at demonstrating the existence, location, and size of the kidney and the presence of intrarenal or adrenal calcification. In the shocked infant, bowel gas shadows are often reduced and enlarged kidneys are usually demonstrable.

Prior to intravenous urography attention must be paid to the general state of the patient and in particular to the osmolality of the plasma. Unless the baby is oliguric there must be *no* fluid restriction; it is not only unnecessary but may prove detrimental to the precarious circulatory state of the infant. A relatively high dose of contrast material is used, such as 3 to 5 ml of sodium diatrizoate (Hypaque) per kilogram of body weight.

The 5-min supine film should show a nephrogram and a faint, partial, or complete pyelogram if some areas are functioning well in contrast to infarcted areas. Subsequent films designed to improve demonstration of the renal areas involved may include (1) a posteroanterior view; (2) high-speed tomography to blur gas shadows; or (3) a long-exposure film that blurs out bowel gas shadows by respiratory movement and may be more effective than low-speed tomography [3]. Further films may be required, but the examination should not exceed 1 hr in duration unless obstructive uropathy is suspected.

In the European series [3] 41 of 45 children (91 percent) examined were found to have radiologic abnormalities on intravenous urography. These tended to be severe cases, a nonfunctioning kidney or kidneys being present in 34 of the 41 children. Interpretation of the lesser degrees of involvement with patchy distribution and altered function of some kidney segments requires considerable radiologic expertise. Selective angiography and in particular venography may be helpful on rare occasions.

Repeat examination by intravenous urography is indicated to study the recovery from the acute stages of RVT, to watch for calcification in infarcted tissue, and to observe restoration of function. A nonfunctioning kidney should be reassessed after 6 weeks.

The usefulness of pulsed diagnostic sonar in kidney disorders has dramatically increased in the past few years [3, 18, 19]. It is now well established as an alternative or complement to radiologic investigation. This noninvasive technique is particularly helpful in RVT when the infant is too ill to tolerate intravenous urography or when no nephrogram is visible (see Chap. 11).

Differential Diagnosis

In hyperosmolar states in young infants with or without RVT, oliguria, azotemia, metabolic acidosis, and electrolyte disequilibrium are present; the infant is often moderately dehydrated, and diarrhea or vomiting may occur. The presence of palpable kidney(s) is a strong indication of gross RVT, as is hematuria.

Circulating burr cells, thrombocytopenia, and altered fibrin degradation products may be present in either RVT or in other hyperosmolar states. Radiologic studies are invaluable. Palpable kidney(s) with or without hematuria raise the possibility of hydronephrosis, nephroblastoma, neuroblastoma, or cystic disease of the kidney; radiologic and ultrasonic investigation will help differentiate these. Renal venous thrombosis should be suspected in any acutely ill baby whose condition has no obvious cause; and it should be especially suspected in the newborn in whom dehydration, asphyxia, maternal prediabetes or diabetes, or cyanotic congenital heart disease has been a feature.

Treatment

Treatment of RVT, which should be initiated once it is suspected or established, falls into four general phases: maintaining homeostasis; minimizing further thrombosis; correcting uremia; and treating or preventing hypertension. The age of the patient may range from a few days to several years, but the basic problems are the same, modified by any primary illness or complicating feature such as cyanotic congenital heart disease. Treatment may conveniently be considered under the following headings: general measures, treatment of water and electrolyte disturbances, management of azotemia and uremia, anticoagulant therapy, surgery, and prevention.

GENERAL MEASURES

A newborn infant affected with RVT may be very ill with shock, hypotension, and cyanosis. Warmth, oxygen therapy (preferably in an incubator to permit easy inspection), and gentle handling are required. The infant preferably is nursed in the lateral position. Thought and skill are required both in timing investigations and in ensuring that they do not cause chilling or hypoxia. Children older than 1 week often present with diarrhea. If bacterial infection is seriously considered or proved, then antimicrobial treatment is indicated on the "best guess" principle [2], taking into account the extra hazards of antimicrobial therapy in the newborn who has poor renal function.

TREATMENT OF WATER AND ELECTROLYTE DISTURBANCES

The first problem in the treatment of RVT is to decide the appropriate water and electrolyte intake. Extracellular dehydration is easily assessed, but intracellular hydration is more intangible. In RVT the problem of overhydration may be present. A critical factor is the volume of urine being voided. This may vary from a considerable output of normal urine, when one kidney functions well and the other is obliterated, to oliguria with hematuria or virtual anuria. Since the output is unpredictable, it is necessary to avoid overhydrating the patient. Hyperosmolality with hypernatremia and hyperchloremia are best dealt with by dialysis. Diuretics are of very dubious value. Metabolic acidosis may be corrected to some extent by intravenous sodium bicarbonate. Clearly the risk of aggravating hypernatremia is real, and dialysis may be a better answer.

MANAGEMENT OF AZOTEMIA AND UREMIA

Azotemia is common in infants with RVT, particularly in geographic areas where high-solute milk feeding is the rule [15]. In young infants, relatively mild water loss or lack of water intake leads to a marked rise in the level of serum urea nitrogen and serum creatinine as compared to older children or adults. The loss of function in one kidney or in parts of one or both kidneys greatly increases the vulnerability of the infant to this biochemical change. The degree of azotemia must therefore be viewed with caution, and levels of blood urea nitrogen up to 40 mg per deciliter may not be of great significance. In the well-established case, azotemia is much more pronounced. The degree of hyperphosphatemia, metabolic acidosis, overhydration, hyperosmolality, and the general state of the kidney are all relevant to the decision as to whether or not to dialyze [3]. With experience it has become the practice to dialyze *early* rather than *late*.

ANTICOAGULANT THERAPY

If there is evidence of continuing intravascular coagulation, such as thrombocytopenia, a fall in factor V level, a fall in fibrinogen level, or an increase in fibrin degradation products, heparin therapy may be indicated in the treatment of RVT. Although the lesions are often if not always bilateral, they are usually asymmetric and may be asynchronous; a good case can be made, therefore, for heparin treatment of all children with RVT.

Heparin is administered initially intravenously in a dosage of 100 units per kilogram of body weight followed by continuous intravenous infusion at 25 units/kg/hr. The dosage level is subsequently adjusted by monitoring the capillary clotting time, which should be perceptibly raised above the normal value (120 to 165 sec) to a level of 240 to 300 sec [3]. The capillary clotting time is simple, easy to read, and well suited to young infants. Heparin is continued for 5 days or longer until the platelet count returns to normal or there is significant improvement in renal function and other indicators of coagulopathy. After stopping heparin, the platelet count and clotting factors should continue to be monitored; and heparin should be restarted if thrombocytopenia reappears. During such heparin therapy and with thrombocytopenia intramuscular injections *must* be avoided.

SURGERY

In the past surgery was undertaken during the acute phase of RVT, involving either thrombectomy or nephrectomy. However, because the thrombosis usually begins deep within the kidney and spreads to the larger veins, thrombectomy is rarely of value [17]. During the acute phase, when the baby is ill and in water and electrolyte disequilibrium with a disturbed acid-base state, in a hypercoagulable state with thrombocytopenia, and is in shock and is oliguric, surgery in any form carries a great risk. For this reason, nephrectomy during the acute stage is not only unnecessary and of no proved value but is potentially dangerous and increases mortality [3]. Surgery during the acute phase thus is contraindicated.

Fibrosis of the kidney with malignant hypertension may ensue rapidly within a few months of RVT. If following RVT a kidney is functionless for 2 months, an elective nephrectomy should be carried out when the baby is 4 to 6 months old. At this age the baby is large enough to be easily operable and small enough for maternal separation to be relatively less important. If malignant hypertension occurs, it must be controlled by antihypertensive therapy (Chap. 32) either preoperatively, or, if the lesion is bilateral, then indefinitely or until bilateral nephrectomy, dialysis, and transplantation are undertaken.

PREVENTION

Since RVT is uncommon and its occurrence is largely unpredictable, prevention is not easy. However, some infants at increased risk may be identified and preventive measures taken. If a pregnant woman is known to be prediabetic or diabetic, her infant should be monitored for early signs of RVT. If cyanotic congenital heart disease is present, care must be exercised in the use of hypertonic fluids in angiocardiography. The practice in some countries of giving high-solute milk formulas to newborn infants should be discouraged, as recommended in the United Kingdom [15], in order to reduce the osmolal, nitrogen, and phosphorus load. It is essential that mothers of young infants be aware that a baby who fails to ingest its milk feeds must take in an equal daily volume of water and that failure to take fluids for 24 hr requires urgent medical attention. There should be an increased index of suspicion of RVT among the medical staff, particularly when faced with newborn infants or babies with diarrhea or hyperosmolal states.

PROGNOSIS

In the European investigation, mortality was 66 percent in the 113 children diagnosed as having RVT. This survey was retrospective, and it can confidently be predicted that with modern therapy controlling homeostasis and with the use of peritoneal dialysis, heparin therapy, and elective surgery, the prognosis now is much better, even for asymmetric bilateral RVT. Mortality was particularly high in male children with congenital heart defects and in those subjected to early nephrectomy as opposed to late nephrectomy (25 percent mortality compared to 7 percent) [3]. The extent of kidney involvement often seems worse on first radiologic examination, possibly because areas close to the actual infarction cease to function well temporarily but with appropriate therapy are rapidly restored.

References

1. Abeshouse, B. S. Thrombosis and thrombophlebitis of the renal vein. *Urol. Cutan. Rev.* 49:661, 1945.
2. Arneil, G. C., and McAllister, T. A. *Textbook of Paediatrics.* Edinburgh: Churchill Livingstone, 1973. Chap. 32.
3. Arneil, G. C., MacDonald, A. M., Murphy, A. V., and Sweet, E. M. Renal venous thrombosis. *Clin. Nephrol.* 1:119, 1973.
4. Avery, M. E., Oppenheimer, E. H., and Gordon, H. H. Renal vein thrombosis in infants of diabetic mothers. *N. Engl. J. Med.* 256:1134, 1957.
5. Barenberg, L. H., Greenstein, N. M., Levy, W., and Rosenbluth, S. B. Renal thrombosis with infarction complicating diarrhea of the newborn. *Am. J. Dis. Child.* 62:362, 1941.
6. Bassett, W. Personal communication, 1967.
7. Boyd, J. F. Thrombo-embolism among stillbirths and neonatal deaths. *J. Pathol. Bacteriol.* 90:53, 1965.
8. Bruns, W. T. Ascending thrombosis involving inferior vena cava and renal veins. *Am. J. Dis. Child.* 99:276, 1960.
9. Campbell, M. F. *Pediatric Urology.* New York: Macmillan, 1937.
10. Campbell, M. F., and Matthews, W. F. Renal thrombosis in infancy. *J. Pediatr.* 20:614, 1942.
11. Corrigan, J. J., Ray, W., and May, N. Changes in the blood coagulation system associated with septicaemia. *N. Engl. J. Med.* 279:851, 1968.
12. Cruickshanks, J. N. Causes of 800 Neonatal Deaths. *Special Report Series Medical Research Council, No. 145,* 1930.
13. Dundon, S. Renal venous thrombosis in siblings. Personal communication, 1974.
14. Dundon, S., O'Donnell, B., and Doyle, C. Renal vein thrombosis in the newborn. *J. Ir. Med. Assoc.* 60:99, 1967.
15. Her Majesty's Stationery Office. *Present-Day Practice in Infant Feeding.* Edinburgh, 1974.
16. Kaufmann, H. J. Renal vein thrombosis. *Am. J. Dis. Child.* 95:377, 1958.
17. Lowry, M. F., Mann, J. R., Abrams, L. D., and Chance, G. W. Thrombectomy for renal venous thrombosis in infant of diabetic mother. *Br. Med. J.* 3:687, 1970.
18. Lyons, E. A., Arneil, G. C., and Murphy, A. V. Sonar and its use in kidney disease in children. *Arch. Dis. Child.* 47:777, 1972.
19. Lyons, E. A., Fleming, J. E. E., Arneil, G. C., Murphy, A. V., Sweet, E. M., and Donald, I. Nephrosonography in infants and children: A new technique. *Br. Med. J.* 2:689, 1972.
20. McFarland, J. B. Renal venous thrombosis in children. *Q. J. Med.* 34:269, 1965.
21. Morison, J. E. Renal venous thrombosis and infarction in the newborn. *Arch. Dis. Child.* 20:129, 1945.
22. Murphy, A. V., and Willoughby, M. L. N. Unpublished data, 1974.
23. Rayer, P. F. O. *Traité des Maladies des Reins et des Alterations de la Secretion Urinaire.* Paris, 1840.
24. Sandblom, P. Renal thrombosis with infarction in newborn. *Acta Paediatr. Scand.* 35:160, 1948.

90. Renal Cortical and Medullary Necrosis *Jay Bernstein*

Renal cortical necrosis and renal medullary necrosis [19, 20], which are relatively uncommon conditions in childhood, occur as primary renal lesions and also as secondary lesions in several well-recognized associations, for example, in the hemolytic-uremic syndrome and in neonatal venous thrombosis. Cortical necrosis and medullary necrosis are defined as ischemic, sometimes hemorrhagic, bland, coagulative lesions involving the cortex and medulla, either alone or in combination and without evidence of major vascular thrombosis. The definition, stated in these broad terms, leaves room for ischemic medullary necrosis as a complication of hydronephrosis and of infection and for cortical necrosis as a consequence of disseminated intravascular coagulation (DIC) with glomerular and arteriolar thrombosis.

Pathogenesis

The cause of cortical and medullary necrosis is renal ischemia secondary to diminished blood flow and parenchymal perfusion. The two abnormalities that have been implicated in the pathogenesis of renal ischemia are vasoconstriction and intravascular coagulation. The former is thought to be mediated by shock, by hypovolemia, and possibly by nephrotoxic factors. The latter has been ascribed to sepsis, toxins, and the factors that trigger the clotting mechanism. Differentiating these two mechanisms and defining their roles have been the subject of considerable experimental study, but the pathogenesis of the lesion encountered in clinical practice remains far from clear. It would be appropriate to say that several factors, some of them still undefined, probably play roles [10]. Experimental studies on induced interruption of renal blood flow show that vasospasm persists following release of prolonged occlusion [18], that parenchymal necrosis ensues, and that the occurrence of cortical or medullary necrosis may be related to the duration of vascular occlusion [5]; moreover, the lesion is complicated by secondary vascular thrombosis within the kidney. Other experimental studies have demonstrated that the Shwartzman reaction induced by endotoxin is associated with intravascular coagulation, glomerular capillary thrombosis, and cortical necrosis [17]. These relationships to DIC are invoked to account for the observed association of renal cortical necrosis with bacterial sepsis. A number of difficulties

arise, however, in the interpretation of clinical material, because (1) fibrin deposits in the intrarenal vasculature are an inconstant finding in renal necrosis, and (2) renal necrosis is only sometimes associated with clinically demonstrated DIC. The relationship of cortical necrosis to DIC is therefore a tenuous one, and morphologic evaluation for the presence or absence of intravascular fibrin precipitates may or may not be a reliable criterion, because on the one hand local coagulation can be a consequence of necrosis and on the other hand fibrinolysis ordinarily removes clots very rapidly. The clinical demonstration of depleted clotting factors and of increased fibrin split-products suffers from the same uncertainty for the same reasons.

Epidemiologic Factors

Frequency data concerning cortical and medullary necrosis are not available; these lesions are uncommon in childhood. They may occur at any age, although several age-related peaks may be identified. A small peak occurs in the newborn period, when renal necrosis develops in association with asphyxial and anemic shock (Chap. 5). A pathogenetically and morphologically different sort of medullary necrosis occurs also in newborns with severe hyperbilirubinemia as a direct consequence of high concentrations of unconjugated bilirubin within the renal medulla. Cortical necrosis in later infancy and in childhood may be an expression of microangiopathy, and it is one of the morphologic features of the hemolytic-uremic syndrome (Chap. 56). Renal medullary necrosis as a complication of sickle cell disease (Chap. 60) occurs occasionally in childhood but more often in young adults. Another age-related peak beyond the pediatric age group is in young women, in whom toxemia of pregnancy accounts for approximately one-half of all cases of renal cortical necrosis. A third age-related peak is in the elderly, in whom diabetes mellitus, urinary tract obstruction, and renal infection form the background of papillary and medullary necrosis. Medullary necrosis is also part of the spectrum of analgesic nephropathy, which is rare in childhood.

Clinical Manifestations

Renal cortical and medullary necrosis both occur in early infancy, apart from the specific associations mentioned above, as complications of gastroenteritis, diarrhea, and dehydration. The patient, who is usually under 1 year of age, experiences a relatively acute onset of dehydration followed by anuria or severe oliguria. Cortical necrosis is the more common lesion following generalized sepsis [10], and medullary necrosis has been seen following the administration of angiographic media [7, 9]. The kidneys are usually enlarged to palpation, and the urine, even though scanty, is sometimes grossly bloody. Mild proteinuria may also be present. Laboratory data include elevated serum electrolytes as a consequence of dehydration, and the serum concentration of potassium is often disproportionately elevated. Clinical differentiation between cortical and medullary necrosis may be impossible, partly because of common clinical findings and partly because the two abnormalities frequently coexist.

The initial oliguria in medullary necrosis is followed by impaired ability to concentrate urine and impaired ability to conserve sodium. The oliguric phase may, however, be exceedingly short, with a rapid onset of diuresis [11]. The urinary findings of elevated sodium concentration, reduced osmolality, and reduced urea concentration have been attributed to renal tubular damage [1], which is present in both the medulla and the cortex. The concentrating defect can become permanent because of a loss of medullary tissue. Functional studies in a child who survived cortical necrosis, on the other hand, have shown a relative preservation of tubular function in relation to glomerular filtration rate, a finding attributed to the relative sparing of the juxtamedullary nephrons [8]. Clinical management of children who survive the acute episode is concerned, therefore, with maintenance of fluid and electrolyte balance. Other clinical problems are the management of hypertension and chronic renal failure.

Radiographic studies early in the course of disease often show poor renal visualization. A prolonged nephrogram with dense opacification of the pyramids is characteristic of medullary necrosis [3, 4]. The necrotic tissue in renal cortical necrosis rapidly undergoes calcification and is visualized radiographically as a peripheral radiopaque shell or rim [14]. Later x-rays show the effects of renal atrophy and scarring. Medullary necrosis with loss of tissue is followed by pyelocalyceal deformity [11, 15, 16].

Renal Pathology

Cortical and medullary necrosis may be diffuse or patchy. The lesions of cortical necrosis are usually bilateral, though not necessarily symmetrical. Medullary necrosis is less often bilateral because of its occasional relationship to urinary obstruction and infection. Gross and histopathologic examination in cortical necrosis shows a lesion resembling patchy infarction. The involved tissue may be pale and have a coagulated appearance. At other times necrosis is accompanied by hemorrhage. Microscopic examination discloses ischemic necrosis, with irregular extravasation of blood and with irregularly distributed thrombosis of arterioles, glomerular capillaries, and cortical venules [2, 13]. The frequency of thrombosis is unclear; it has been as high as 30 percent in some series and has been negligible in others. The lesion in medullary necrosis is also bland and coagulative, with variable hemorrhage [6].

Calcification of necrotic cortical tissue occurs rapidly. The necrotic tissue undergoes resorption, and the areas of cortical and medullary damage are the sites of tubular atrophy, glomerular involution, interstitial fibrosis, vascular thickening, and the general features of scarring (Fig. 90-1). The affected segment of kidney in cases of segmental necrosis may appear to be severely hypoplastic because of atrophy and because subsequent growth is impaired. Medullary necrosis is followed by sequestration and loss of involved tissue, with blunting of pyramids and calyceal enlargement.

Differential Diagnosis

The differential diagnosis of renal medullary and cortical necrosis includes acute renal failure (with or without tubular necrosis), renal vein thrombosis, and renal arterial embolism. Radiographic identification of medullary necrosis may be made on the presence of a prolonged, dense nephrogram with medullary opacification [3, 4]. Renal vein thrombosis in dehydrated children may be impossible to differentiate from cortical and medullary necrosis on clinical grounds; radiographic features of venous thrombosis include demonstration of large thrombi by venography and the demonstration of intrarenal phleboliths after the acute episode. Renal infarction due to arterial embolism, which occurs in newborns, is extremely rare in infancy and childhood.

Treatment and Prognosis

The treatment is supportive and in the recovery phase involves maintaining salt and water balance. The efficacy of anticoagulation therapy has not been demonstrated, although infusions of heparin and urokinase may be of value [12].

The ultimate outcome depends upon the degree

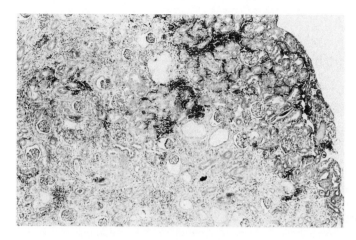

Figure 90-1. Renal cortical atrophy in an infant with erythroblastosis and severe neonatal distress. He had oliguria, gross hematuria, and azotemia. At 4 weeks of age he had persistent azotemia and hypertension. A renal biopsy showed severe changes in the inner cortex, with tubular atrophy, glomerular sclerosis, and parenchymal loss consistent with resolving cortical necrosis. Note the sparing of the peripheral subcapsular cortex. (Specimen generously provided by Drs. Geoffrey Altshuler and James Wenzl, Children's Memorial Hospital, Oklahoma City, OK.) (H&E, ×40.)

of damage and loss of parenchyma. Permanently impaired concentrating ability and relative glomerular insufficiency may precede the eventual development of chronic renal failure. The development of hypertension is another factor that affects prognosis. Finally, renal injury in early infancy may, in addition to damaging existing renal tissue, impair the subsequent growth and development of the kidney, causing high-grade hypoplasia.

References

1. Banister, A., and Hatcher, G. W. Renal tubular and papillary necrosis after dehydration in infancy. *Arch. Dis. Child.* 48:36, 1973.
2. Bouissou, H., Familiades, J., Fabre, J., Regnier, C., and Hamousin-Metregiste, R. La glomérulo-nécrose, lésion initiale de la nécrose corticale symétrique des reins. *Sem. Hop. Paris* 39:282, 1963.
3. Chrispin, A. R., Hull, D., Lillie, J. G., and Risdon, R. A. Renal tubular necrosis and papillary necrosis after gastroenteritis in infants. *Br. Med. J.* 1:140, 1970.
4. Chrispin, A. R., and Lillie, J. G. Acute kidney damage with tubular necrosis and papillary necrosis in young infants. *Ann. Radiol.* 14:199, 1971.
5. Davies, D. J. The patterns of renal infarction caused by different types of temporary ischaemia. *J. Pathol.* 102:151, 1970.
6. Davies, D. J., Kennedy, A., and Roberts, C. Renal medullary necrosis in infancy and childhood. *J. Pathol.* 99:125, 1969.
7. Gilbert, E. F., Khoury, G. H., Hogan, G. R., and Jones, B. Hemorrhagic renal necrosis in infancy: Relationship to radiopaque compounds. *J. Pediatr.* 76:49, 1970.
8. Groshong, T. D., Taylor, A. A., Nolph, K. D., Esterly, J., and Maher, J. F. Renal function following cortical necrosis in childhood. *J. Pediatr.* 78:267, 1971.
9. Gruskin, A. B., Oetliker, O. H., Wolfish, N. M., Gootman, N. L., Bernstein, J., and Edelmann, C. M., Jr. Effects of angiography on renal function and histology in infants and piglets. *J. Pediatr.* 76:41, 1970.
10. Heptinstall, R. M. *Pathology of the Kidney* (2nd ed.). Boston: Little, Brown, 1974. Chap. 6.
11. Husband, P., and Howlett, K. A. Renal papillary necrosis in infancy. *Arch. Dis. Child.* 48:116, 1973.
12. Jones, F. E., Black, P. J., Cameron, J. S., Chantler, C., Gill, D., Maisey, M. N., Ogg, C. S., and Saxton, H. Local infusion of urokinase and heparin into renal arteries in impending renal cortical necrosis. *Br. Med. J.* 4:547, 1975.
13. Koffler, D., and Paronetto, F. Fibrinogen deposition in acute renal failure. *Am. J. Pathol.* 49:383, 1966.
14. Leonidas, J. C., Berdon, W. E., and Gribetz, D. Bilateral renal cortical necrosis in the newborn infant: Roentgenographic diagnosis. *J. Pediatr.* 79:623, 1971.
15. Malpuech, G., Godeneche, P., Meyer, M., and Raynaud, E. M.-J. Nécrose papillaire des reins chez un nourrisson. *Arch. Fr. Pediatr.* 32:433, 1975.
16. Mauer, S. M., and Nogrady, M. B. Renal papillary and cortical necrosis in a newborn infant: Report of a survivor with roentgenologic documentation. *J. Pediatr.* 74:750, 1969.
17. McKay, D. G. *Disseminated Intravascular Coagulation: An Intermediary Mechanism of Disease.* New York: Harper & Row, 1965.
18. Sheehan, H. L., and Davis, J. C. Renal ischaemia with failed reflow. *J. Pathol.* 78:105, 1959.
19. Stirling, G. A. Renal papillary necrosis in childhood. *J. Clin. Pathol.* 11:296, 1958.
20. Zuelzer, W. W., Charles, S., Kurnetz, R., Newton, W. A., Jr., and Fallon, R. Circulatory diseases of the kidneys in infancy and childhood. *Am. J. Dis. Child.* 81:1, 1951.

91. Clinical Aspects of Acute Renal Failure (Vasomotor Nephropathy)

Donald E. Oken

Used in its literal sense, the term *acute renal failure* denotes any abrupt, severe deterioration of renal function, regardless of cause. Various parenchymal renal diseases that produce this syndrome (see Table 91-1) are considered in detail elsewhere. The major topic of discussion in this chapter is the form of acute renal failure that results from shock, trauma, sepsis, hemolytic reactions, depletion of the blood volume, tissue ischemia, anoxia, or poisoning. It has several characteristic features, follows a well-delineated course, and, although potentially reversible, it constitutes a serious threat to life.

The acute renal failure syndrome has been graced with many titles. The term *lower nephron nephrosis* achieved popularity in the 1940s until it was generally recognized that tubular necrosis, when present, was more a feature of the proximal than the distal tubule. Bull and coworkers [15] introduced the name acute tubular necrosis in the belief that tubular injury was the essential renal abnormality. Finckh and others [32, 81] soon pointed out, however, that frank necrosis of the renal tubular epithelium is relatively uncommon and that distinct tubular abnormalities may be found at autopsy of patients who have been neither azotemic nor oliguric before death. Although cellular injury undoubtedly affects the transport capacity of the kidney, most authorities no longer believe that tubular necrosis is the immediate cause of renal failure (see Chap. 7) and have adopted the term *acute renal failure* to avoid the morphologic connotations implicit in the term *acute tubular necrosis*. This choice also is less than ideal, however, since it is so nonspecific.

The renal cortical blood flow of patients with acute renal failure due to shock, trauma, poisoning, or hemorrhage characteristically is reduced by 50 to 70 percent [14, 45, 56]. That degree of ischemia appears to be due to preglomerular vascular constriction. Renal angiograms performed in such subjects, indeed, have shown marked attenuation of the arcuate and interlobular vessels [45]. This preglomerular constriction, possibly coupled with efferent arteriolar dilatation, can lower glomerular capillary pressure below the level necessary to sustain glomerular filtration. A vascular basis for renal insufficiency in man thus seems well established, the hemodynamic alterations being essentially the same regardless of the underlying cause [43]. Hence the term *vasomotor nephropathy* [70] has been proposed and will be used throughout this chapter.

Incidence

Perhaps as a result of the recognition and treatment of factors that predispose to its development, the syndrome of vasomotor nephropathy has become relatively uncommon in many parts of the world. Excluding antibiotic-induced acute renal failure, we saw fewer than two dozen adult patients with this syndrome per year on the Renal Service of the Peter Bent Brigham Hospital between 1963 and 1974. Only 1 in every 600 severely injured combat casualties in Vietnam developed renal failure [93], and, reviewing 1,659 cases of lower aortic surgery performed in ten centers, Kountz and coworkers found the overall incidence of vasomotor nephropathy to be only 3.8 percent [53]. Powers et al. [76] estimated that the syndrome occurs in 0.1 percent of adult patients undergoing major surgery. The precise incidence in adults is unknown, and reliable figures are even more difficult to obtain for the pediatric population. It is clear, however, that vasomotor nephropathy is not a common cause of acute renal failure in childhood. Wiggelinkhuizen and Pokroy, for example, reported the existence of "acute tubular necrosis" in only 12 of 132 infants and children with acute renal failure [94]. Our own experience is similar; we found the syndrome occurring predominantly in traumatized older children and in severely dehydrated infants. Indeed, Gordillo and associates found that of 100 infants under the age of 2 years who had developed vasomotor nephropathy, 55 had done so on the basis of infectious diarrhea [39]. Extreme trauma in severely ill infants also carries a distinct risk. Chesney and coworkers, for example, reported that 8 percent of infants undergoing cardiac surgery developed renal failure with characteristics compatible with vasomotor nephropathy. Thirteen of these 20 babies died [20]. Regardless of its incidence, the high mortality rate of children with this form

Supported by U.S. Public Health Service grant HL-AM 19463. This paper focuses on the clinical presentation of vasomotor nephropathy. Pathogenesis and treatment are detailed in Chaps. 7 and 33.

of acute renal failure makes it of serious importance.

Pathology

Starting 1 or 2 days after the onset of renal failure, the kidneys become large, firm, and edematous; kidney weight ultimately may exceed one and one-half times normal. The swelling is predominantly interstitial and seems best explained by altered capillary permeability [61]. The renal capsule is smooth, glistening, and nonadherent. The cortical parenchyma is pale, a reflection not only of interstitial edema but also of cortical ischemia [45]. In stark contrast, the medulla is often deep burgundy in color, a hue imparted by engorgement of the vasa recta and, at times, by the presence of heme pigments in Henle's loop and collecting ducts. Tubules no longer lie in immediate proximity to one another, as is normal, but are separated by a distinct interstitial space, evidencing edema. Small patches of leukocytes are often present in the interstitium and at times are widespread. The lymphocyte is the predominant cell in this infiltrate, with occasional plasma cells and polymorphonuclear and eosinophilic leukocytes often intermixed.

Glomeruli are entirely normal, whether examined by light or electron microscopy [23, 73], although capillary constriction has been noted in some experimental models [22a, 86a]. The endothelial cells, epithelial cells, mesangium, and basement membranes show no characteristic alterations. At times, tubular epithelial cells are found free in Bowman's space, a phenomenon termed *infraglomerular reflux* [41]. The same abnormality can be produced in experimental animals by the injection of serotonin and other materials [91], perhaps due to increased intrarenal pressure. The blood vessels also appear normal on both light and electron microscopy. Much has been made of the presence of islands of cells in the vasa recta. These islands are believed by some to represent intravascular hematopoiesis, but their true significance remains to be determined.

Tubular injury, variable in degree from subject to subject and patchy in distribution within a given kidney, is frequently most notable at the corticomedullary junction. One often sees little or no change in cellular architecture on light microscopy [32, 81]. At the other extreme, there may be frank tubular necrosis with nuclear pyknosis, cellular disruption, and shedding of masses of epithelium into tubular lumens. Even when the tubules appear normal on light microscopy, electron microscopic examination reveals degeneration of cellular nuclei, swelling of mitochondria with distortion of

their cristae, and disintegration of outer mitochondrial membranes [23]. Such changes may explain the grossly depressed transport capacity of the nephron in vasomotor nephropathy. There is, however, no correlation between the severity of the histologic lesions and the clinical status of the patient [32].

Regardless of the degree of renal injury found at postmortem examination, the tubular lumens typically are not collapsed as in other autopsy material, a feature considered to be of diagnostic importance by Bohle [13]. Luminal "casts" of proteinaceous material, heme pigments, or cellular debris vary in amount from patient to patient. Many authors have assumed that these materials cause tubular obstruction and hence serve as an important factor in the pathogenesis of acute renal failure; however, the absence of luminal casts in many patients tends to contradict that belief [32, 81]. It seems likely that such casts more often are the result rather than the cause of impaired filtration (Chap. 7).

After several days, nuclear mitoses become evident in increasing numbers of tubular cells and herald the repair of parenchymal injury prior to the onset of functional recovery. Interstitial edema persists into the early recovery phase, resolving slowly thereafter. The renal architecture may then become entirely normal, or islands of tubular atrophy and interstitial fibrosis can persist indefinitely. Very rarely, the healing process is associated with progressive parenchymal atrophy [58].

Differential Diagnosis of Renal Failure— Acute Versus Chronic Nephropathy

When faced with a child just noted to be azotemic and oliguric, one must decide whether the problem is acute or represents a covert, chronic process. A careful history, physical examination, and evaluation of appropriate laboratory data are of great help in distinguishing between these possibilities. The *family history*, for example, may suggest medullary cystic or polycystic kidney disease, Alport's syndrome, oxalosis, cystinuria, cystinosis, or other heritable diseases. A *history* of polyuria and polydipsia, enuresis beyond age 5 or 6, failure to thrive in infancy, or impaired growth in later childhood suggests that renal disease has been present for some time. The previous excision of a sacrococcygeal tumor or an abdominoperineal surgical procedure signals the possibility of a neurogenic bladder. Previously documented urinary tract anomalies, a history of hesitancy, gross hematuria, pain (or crying) on urination, or a poor urinary stream suggest the possibility of obstructive uropathy. Infants noted to have a single umbilical artery have an especially high incidence of congenital anomalies of the urinary tract [31], as do infants with other extrarenal birth defects [31]. Recurrent pyelonephritis, abdominal radiation, chronic suppurative diseases, long-standing diabetes, or other systemic afflictions that might affect the kidneys all point to the likelihood of chronic nephropathy. Similarly, chronic renal failure may be strongly suspected when proteinuria, an abnormal urinary sediment, hypertension, or even minimal elevation of the blood urea concentration has been found at any time in the past.

On *physical examination,* the peculiar, sallow coloration of long-standing azotemia; hypertensive retinopathy; cardiomegaly; small stature; polycystic nephromegaly; clearly old, pruritic excoriations of the skin; rickets; and dystrophic fingernails bespeak the chronicity of the process. The characteristic skin lesions of Fabry's disease and the gingival "lead line" of lead or bismuth poisoning are readily recognizable. Stigmata of juvenile rheumatoid arthritis, old decubiti, and osteomyelitis, coupled (or not) with macroglossia and other stigmata of amyloidosis, are worthy of note. Spina bifida or a meningomyelocele associated with a lax anal sphincter and perianal anesthesia connote that a neurogenic bladder and urinary dysfunction are likely to have been present since birth.

Laboratory procedures may be of great help in separating chronic from acute disease. Chronic renal failure typically progresses at a slow rate with a negligible rise in serum creatinine concentration from day to day. Accordingly, an appreciable, progressive increase in serum creatinine strongly suggests that renal disease is of recent origin or that, if chronic, an additional acute problem has been superimposed.

The finding of small kidneys, renal asymmetry, or staghorn calculi on abdominal x-rays points strongly to a chronic problem. Nephrocalcinosis may reflect long-standing renal tubular acidosis, undetected partial cortical necrosis of infancy, hyperparathyroidism, or vitamin D intoxication with progressive renal failure. Particularly large renal outlines may be indicative of cystic kidney disease, hydronephrosis, or bilateral tumors, any of which may have produced renal failure over a protracted period of time. The osseous manifestations of osteitis fibrosa or rickets are classic signs of chronic rather than acute renal disease.

Differential Diagnosis of Acute Renal Failure

The majority of cases of actue renal failure in childhood stem from the glomerular abnormalities listed in Table 91-1. The hemolytic-uremic syndrome is seen with remarkable frequency in spo-

Table 91-1. Causes of Acute Renal Failure in Pediatric Practice

1. *Glomerulonephritis (especially necrotizing, proliferative, membranoproliferative, rapidly progressive):* Streptococcus* and other bacteria, viruses, lupus erythematosus, Wegener's granulomatosis, eclampsia
2. *Vascular and thrombotic disease:* Malignant hypertension, Wegener's granulomatosis, hypersensitivity angiitis, periarteritis nodosa, thrombotic thrombocytopenic purpura, hemolytic-uremic syndrome,* Shwartzman reaction (cortical necrosis),* collagenosis, scleroderma, acute allograft rejection, fat embolism, renal venous*-vena caval thrombosis, posttraumatic arterial thrombosis or avulsion, aortic coarctation with arterial thrombosis, renal artery dysplasia
3. *Interstitial disease:* Allergic, postinfectious, and idiosyncratic interstitial nephritis, fulminating pyelonephritis, papillary necrosis
4. *Functional renal failure ("prerenal" renal failure):* Severe volume depletion,* shock,* sepsis,* trauma,* heart failure
5. *Vasomotor nephropathy (acute tubular necrosis, acute renal failure):* All causes of functional renal failure (e.g., nephrotic syndrome, hemorrhage, vomiting, diarrhea, hypotension) if not adequately treated*; blunt trauma, burns, surgery, fractures, intravascular hemolysis, heat-stroke, malaria, snake bite, electric shock, dissecting aneurysm (e.g., Marfan's, homocystinuria), septicemia, rhabdomyolysis; poisons,* especially antibiotics (see text), mercury, bismuth, phosphorus, lead, carbon tetrachloride, ethylene, glycol, methanol, mushrooms, Lysol, methoxyflurane (see reference 79), other poisons are rare
6. *Hepatorenal syndrome*
7. *Urinary obstruction:* Ureter, bladder, or urethra, including inflammation stone, blood clot, urate crystallization, tumor, retroperitoneal mass or fibrosis

* Common cases in children.

radic outbreaks in various parts of the world [38] and in some series constitutes the most common single cause of infantile acute renal failure [59]. Scleroderma and polyarteritis occur so infrequently in early childhood that the pediatrician is unlikely to see acute renal failure secondary to either affliction. Lupus erythematosus is a well-established cause of acute renal failure in early adolescence [22, 47, 62]. Acute pyelonephritis rarely, if ever, causes renal failure in older children and adults unless it is associated with papillary necrosis, but it may do so in young children [19]. The hepatorenal syndrome, multiple myeloma, and spontaneous renal artery occlusion also are distinctly rare in childhood. Posttraumatic renal artery occlusion occurs at any age, however, and no age group is exempt from interstitial nephritis and hypersensitivity angiitis. The latter, usually a manifestation of an idiosyncratic or hypersensitivity drug reaction [69], may relate to virtually any medication, but particularly to methicillin, phenylbutazone, sulfonamides, and the thiazide diuretics [69]. Renal vein thrombosis is by no means a rare cause of acute renal failure in dehydrated infants [59]. Acute urinary tract obstruction may be intrinsic or the result of nephrolithiasis or urate crystallization.

Vasomotor nephropathy has the same underlying basic causes in childhood as in adult life: dehydration, hemorrhage, shock, hemolytic reactions, anoxia, burns, trauma, sepsis, and poisons. The widespread and sometimes indiscriminate use of the aminoglycoside antibiotics in excessive dosage has become another major cause. Ninety percent of all cases of poisoning involve children, three-quarters of whom are less than 5 years old [3]. The concomitant appearance of acute hepatic disease and renal shutdown in a previously well child strongly suggests the possibility of poisoning, most particularly with mushrooms, carbon tetrachloride, phosphorus, iron or arsenic [3].

Functional or so-called prerenal renal failure in small children is most often the result of a massive loss of fluid from vomiting or diarrhea, or the sequestration of extracellular fluid in third-spaces in the presence of burns, paralytic ileus, or the nephrotic syndrome. Cardiovascular instability or frank shock of any etiology may produce similar reductions in cardiac output, renal perfusion, and glomerular filtration.

The oliguria and progressive azotemia of functional failure are rapidly and totally reversible with the restoration of normal cardiac output, unless vasomotor nephropathy or renal cortical necrosis has already supervened. As judged from response to therapy, over two-thirds of the small children we have seen with acute oliguria and azotemia had a functional rather than an organic basis for their renal failure. Wiggelinkhuizen and Pokroy [94] attributed 28 percent of their cases of childhood acute renal failure to prerenal causes, and Doxiadis found an organic cause for renal insufficiency in only 4 of 47 infants [26].

Fortunately it is rarely difficult to distinguish between functional renal insufficiency and established vasomotor nephropathy in childhood. Volume depletion is usually apparent on physical examination, and a history of an illness leading to volume depletion is easy to elicit. Except when due to covert poisoning, vasomotor nephropathy will almost universally be preceded by major trauma or other equally evident catastrophic events. Acute renal failure appearing de novo is, then, highly unlikely to be due to this cause. In infancy, however, the same circumstances of shock, dehydration, sep-

sis, and fever may produce either functional renal failure, vasomotor nephropathy, or renal cortical necrosis. In addition, systemic diseases such as the hemolytic-uremic syndrome, the Schönlein-Henoch syndrome, or lupus erythematosus may cause severe gastrointestinal symptoms, dehydration, and intrinsic renal disease concomitantly and thus produce considerable diagnostic uncertainty.

Urinalysis

Examination of the urine often provides essential clues to the type of abnormality responsible for acute renal failure. Erythrocytes and erythrocyte casts are the hallmark of glomerular disease. Little can be made of erythrocyturia alone, since red cells can be shed anywhere in the genitourinary tract for a multitude of reasons. Erythrocyte casts, on the other hand, always are of renal origin, reflect some element of glomerular injury, and when diligently searched for almost invariably are found in the presence of acute glomerular disease. They are not pathognomonic of primary glomerular disease, however, and one sometimes sees large numbers of erythrocytes and scattered erythrocyte casts early in the course of vasomotor nephropathy. Fortunately for the diagnostician, proteinuria usually is not notable in this syndrome, except at times in small children [20]. The continued excretion of erythrocyte casts and large amounts of protein argues against the presence of vasomotor nephropathy and in favor of established glomerular or vascular disease, particularly when associated with diastolic hypertension. By contrast, masses of tubular epithelial cells or casts of whole tubule segments are often present in the urine of patients with vasomotor nephropathy and strongly suggest that diagnosis.

The presence of pigment-stained casts or pink, red, or brown urine after erythrocytes have been sedimented by centrifugation most often reflects hemoglobinuria or myoglobinuria, both likely determinants of vasomotor nephropathy. The so-called broad cast, formerly believed to be indicative of the syndrome, is seen in any oliguric state regardless of cause and is merely a manifestation of slowed flow through collecting tubules in a diseased kidney. Pyelonephritis, allergic interstitial nephritis, and other disorders of the renal interstitium manifest leukocyturia and leukocyte casts as the predominant abnormality of the sediment; in such patients proteinuria usually is not marked. The cells appearing in the urine originate from, and are therefore identical with, those infiltrating the renal interstitium. It is often of diagnostic value, therefore, to examine the urine sediment with modified Wright's stain to aid in the identification of the predominant cell type. Eosinophils found in large numbers strongly suggest the diagnosis of allergic interstitial nephritis. Masses of polymorphonuclear leukocytes, especially within casts, are indicative of an acute inflammatory process and suggest fulminating pyelonephritis or papillary necrosis.

Patients with obstructive uropathy may manifest all the urinary findings of pyelonephritis, secondary infection being a frequent concomitant. Microscopic or gross hematuria also may be found as a result of calculi or acute dilatation of the renal pelvis, but proteinuria typically is scant and erythrocyte casts rarely, if ever, are seen. Masses of uric acid, oxalate, or cystine crystals in the urine warn of the possibility that accretion of these materials may have produced urinary tract obstruction and renal failure; however, uricosuria is expected following intravenous pyelography and should not be given undue consideration under that circumstance. Additionally, the excretion of masses of oxalate crystals may indicate the presence of vasomotor nephropathy due to ethylene glycol poisoning [37] or methoxyflurane anesthesia [66].

Functional acute renal failure associated with severe volume depletion produces neither an abnormal urinary sediment nor significant proteinuria. Congestive heart failure, by contrast, may cause marked proteinuria and frequently is associated with the excretion of numbers of hyaline and finely granular casts. Erythrocytes occasionally are excreted in excess numbers, but erythrocyte casts are distinctly uncommon. The presence of erythrocyte casts thus is helpful in the differential diagnosis of the patient with acute renal failure and volume overload leading to heart failure.

Since the urine sediment is apt to be normal and proteinuria scant in both vasomotor nephropathy and functional acute renal failure due to volume depletion, examination of the sediment is usually of little help in distinguishing between these two diagnoses. Two physiologic responses that are retained by patients with functional renal failure do aid in this differentiation. The increase in aldosterone secretion in functional renal failure causes maximal conservation of sodium. The concentration of sodium in urine, therefore, is predictably less than 10 to 20 mEq per liter and usually is less than 5 mEq per liter. As a result of antidiuretic hormone release, the urine osmolality is at least 50 mOsm per kilogram higher than that of plasma. The capacity to conserve sodium to this degree and the retained ability to concentrate the urine indicate integrity of the tubule transport system, a situation which contrasts sharply with that in vaso-

motor nephropathy, in which the transport capacity of the tubule is significantly impaired. As a result, the urinary sodium concentration in vasomotor nephropathy lies between 30 and 90 mEq per liter (most commonly 40 to 60 mEq/L), and the urinary osmolality is always nearly identical with that of plasma, regardless of the patient's fluid and electrolyte status [15, 85]. It must be stressed, however, that whereas a low urinary sodium concentration and high osmolality effectively rule out the diagnosis of vasomotor nephropathy, the opposite findings do not necessarily denote that vasomotor nephropathy is present. Similar results are observed in renal cortical necrosis, obstructive uropathy, fulminating interstitial nephritis, and, at times, in glomerular diseases.

One must be cautious in interpreting urinary findings in the first voiding after the onset of vasomotor nephropathy, however, since this urine may have been formed in the incipient phase of renal failure, when urinary sodium concentration was low and the osmolality high. In the presence of functional renal failure, on the other hand, pharmacologic diuretics or an osmotic diuresis induced with glucose, mannitol, or radiographic contrast material will interfere with the kidney's capacity to conserve sodium, even in the most dehydrated patient, and will falsely suggest other causes of renal failure.

Over the years, various other laboratory examinations have been proposed as diagnostic indexes of acute renal failure (Table 91-2). Foremost among these are the urine-plasma concentration ratios of urea and creatinine [33, 75] and the so-called renal failure ratio [42], that is, the product of the urinary sodium concentration and the plasma-urine creatinine concentration ratio. Obviously, urine that is isosmotic with plasma and contains 40 mEq per liter or more of sodium, along with potassium and the attendant anions, cannot have a very high concentration of either urea or creatinine. The measurement of urinary sodium and osmolality, therefore, generally will suffice, and I have found no advantage in using the other factors to differentiate vasomotor nephropathy from functional acute renal failure.

It must be stressed that examination of urinary sodium and osmolality will not distinguish between vasomotor nephropathy and obstructive uropathy. Vasomotor nephropathy, however, is characterized by a relatively constant daily urine volume until the onset of recovery leads to a progressive, continuous rise in output. Random changes in daily urine volume of more than 20 or 25 percent should lead the physician to question the diagnosis

*Table 91-2. Urine Characteristics in Oliguric Renal Failure**

Etiology	Urine-Plasma Concentration Ratio			Urinary		Sediment and Protein
	Urea Nitrogen	Creatinine	Osmolality	Na (mEq/L)	K	
Functional (volume depletion, low cardiac output)	>20	>40	>1.15	<30 (usually <10)	Any	Benign proteinuria with heart failure
Vasomotor nephropathy	<10 (usually 2–5)	<15 (usually 3–8)	~1.1	30–90 (usually 40–60)	Any	May be myoglobinuria, hemoglobinuria, or casts; RBC, RBC casts may be seen early; scant proteinuria
Obstructive uropathy	Urine identical to that in vasomotor nephropathy, but urine volume may fluctuate spontaneously and in response to fluid administration—an important difference				Any	Typically benign—may show RBC/WBC if due to stone or stricture
Glomerular-vascular diseases	May resemble either functional renal failure or vasomotor nephropathy, depending on degree of tubular involvement				Any	RBC, RBC casts, marked proteinuria

* The values given are representative of each form of acute renal failure. Values intermediate between those typical of "functional" and vasomotor nephropathy may be seen occasionally; the true cause may be discovered only after the normalization of cardiac output.
Note: RBC = red blood cells; WBC = white blood cells.

of vasomotor nephropathy; it may be the only clue to the existence of incomplete urinary tract obstruction.

Functional Abnormalities and Complications of Vasomotor Nephropathy

Glomerular Filtration Rate. The glomerular filtration rate of subjects with vasomotor nephropathy typically is 1 to 5 percent of normal. Nitrogenous wastes are retained, and the ability of the kidney to maintain fluid, electrolyte, and hydrogen ion homeostasis is lost. Urine production usually is below 200 ml/m²/day, a volume that nevertheless represents up to 30 percent of the glomerular filtrate. Rarely, there is total anuria; conversely, perhaps one-tenth of patients are not oliguric [51] but excrete urine volumes up to 1 liter/m²/day or more. The latter patients, classified as having "high output" or nonoliguric renal failure, often have a somewhat better maintained (but still grossly reduced) glomerular filtration rate and experience a shorter period of renal shutdown [87]. The extravagant use of the nephrotoxic aminoglycoside antibiotics appears to account for a significant proportion of such cases in recent years. Regardless of the volume excreted, however, the urine is isosmotic with plasma until recovery of glomerular function is well underway, and the concentration of sodium almost invariably ranges between 30 and 90 mEq per liter.

Blood Urea Nitrogen. In nonoliguric renal failure the rate at which the blood urea nitrogen concentration rises is more a function of the patient's catabolic rate than the degree of renal impairment. Patients with burns, severe traumatic injuries, or heat stroke, or whose renal failure is complicated by sepsis, fever, blood sequestered in extravascular sites, or tissue necrosis may experience a daily rise in blood urea nitrogen concentration of 50 to 60 mg per deciliter, whereas in less severely ill patients with equivalent depressions in the glomerular filtration rate, such as follows simple transfusion reactions or uncomplicated hypotension, the blood urea nitrogen concentration increases by less than 10 mg/dl/day.

Tetracycline antibiotics (except doxycycline) and corticosteroids also accelerate the rate of increase in blood urea nitrogen, the former by inhibiting protein anabolism [83] and the latter by promoting more rapid catabolism [16]. The use of these agents in patients with acute renal failure of any form, therefore, should be entertained only when essential. Unlike blood urea nitrogen, the serum creatinine concentration is not greatly influenced by the catabolic state of the patient. It thus reflects the degree of renal failure quite faithfully (except, perhaps, in certain patients with myoglobinuric acute renal failure [40]). Since, however, the clinical manifestations of uremia correlate well with the degree of blood urea nitrogen elevation, it is well to follow the changes in both values.

Acidosis. The rate at which severe metabolic acidosis develops tends to correlate with the catabolic state of the patient. The ability to acidify the urine is at least partially retained, as the urinary pH of subjects with vasomotor nephropathy ranges between 5.5 and 6.5 [24]. Nevertheless, with grossly reduced rates of glomerular filtration, parsimonious delivery of buffer to the acidifying segment of the nephron, and impaired ammonia production, the total amount of hydrogen ion excreted does not equal that produced. Hydrogen ion retention thus is inevitable unless the impaired renal excretion is matched by the loss of acid through pernicious vomiting or gastric suction. Moreover, severe metabolic acidosis may be present at the onset of renal failure because of diabetic ketosis; lactic acidosis; severe diarrhea; or poisoning with salicylates, methanol, or ethylene glycol.

Hyperkalemia. Hyperkalemia may develop very soon after the onset of vasomotor nephropathy. Neonates, who may be fed a diet rich in potassium, are particularly at risk unless renal failure is recognized and an artificial formula is substituted. Several other factors contribute to the development of this complication in patients of all ages. Potassium derived from the diet, as well as that released from catabolized muscle, necrotic tissue, and hemolyzed erythrocytes, cannot be excreted quantitatively by the kidney, although patients with renal failure do display remarkable variability in their urinary potassium concentration. Medications in the form of the potassium salt (e.g., potassium penicillin) and blood transfusions are frequently overlooked exogenous sources of potassium. Most importantly, metabolic acidosis results in the movement of potassium from cell water to the extracellular fluid compartment [49]. On the other hand, extrarenal potassium losses in vomitus and diarrheal stool can be quite large and may offset the development of hyperkalemia. Finally, some patients, in the absence of vomiting and diarrhea, show little tendency toward hyperkalemia, for reasons that are entirely unclear.

Modest degrees of hyperkalemia produce no symptoms, and in the severely ill child the manifestations of severe hyperkalemia may be mistakenly attributed to uremia or to other causes. Hypoactive or absent tendon reflexes, ileus, weakness of the extremities (particularly if asymmetric), a tingling sensation of the mouth, tongue, or distal extremities, and bradycardia with or without cardiac arrhythmias all may be signs of severe potassium intoxication. If left untreated, the patient with such a degree of hyperkalemia may die suddenly. Close monitoring of the electrocardiogram is mandatory (see Chap. 33).

Other Electrolytes. For reasons that are unclear, hypocalcemia is an almost constant and early finding in vasomotor nephropathy, despite increased secretion of parathormone [54]. Concentrations of calcium in serum generally range between 7 and 8.5 mg per deciliter, but we have seen values below 6 mg per deciliter. Clinical manifestations of even severe degrees of hypocalcemia are not commonly encountered, however, perhaps due in part to the attendant metabolic acidosis and the tendency to hyperkalemia. Except in young children, the Trousseau and Chvostek signs rarely can be elicited, and the transient correction of hypocalcemia during hemodialysis usually has little effect on the neuromuscular irritability to which the acutely uremic child is prone (see under Neurologic Findings).

Hypermagnesemia is an almost universal concomitant of vasomotor nephropathy [88]; it is mild and very unlikely to produce serious effects unless magnesium salts have been (ill-advisedly) administered to control convulsions or as an osmotic cathartic to remove residual gastrointestinal blood. The increase in magnesium is reported to parallel that of potassium [88] and presumably is derived from the intracellular pool.

A slow and modest rise in serum phosphate concentration is to be expected but is not invariably seen. It bears no relationship to the patient's serum calcium concentration, which often falls before significant hyperphosphatemia has occurred. Instead, the progressive elevation in serum phosphate concentration relates primarily to reduction in the amount filtered. Gastrointestinal excretion of phosphate, of course, remains intact.

Sodium and potassium are excreted in scant amounts during the oliguric phase of vasomotor nephropathy. In the face of already impaired tubular transport capacity, even the potent loop diuretics (furosemide and ethacrynic acid) are incapable of modifying the urine volume and composition [29].

Medications that are primarily excreted by the kidney may reach toxic levels when renal function is seriously impaired. Each medicine given, therefore, should be considered in the light of its normal route of excretion and its potential toxicity [11, 44].

Anemia and Bleeding Tendencies. Normocytic, normochromic anemia is an expected complication in any form of acute renal failure, even in the absence of overhydration and demonstrable blood loss [85]. Poikilocytosis, spherocytosis, and distorted burr and helmet cells are present to a variable but modest degree [80]. The bone marrow generally is hypocellular [57, 74] but may be normal [55].

The severity of anemia correlates well with the duration and severity of azotemia [84]. Reticulocytosis varies from subject to subject, but generally is depressed [84]. The anemia has been attributed to "maturational arrest" [8], depressed erythropoietin production [2], ineffective erythropoiesis [30], impaired utilization of iron [25], and impaired erythrocyte survival.

Bruising and abnormal bleeding are frequently encountered in severe uremia and are late complications of vasomotor nephropathy. Significant thrombocytopenia occurs in a minority of acutely uremic subjects [50, 84]. Probably of more significance is the marked deficiency of platelet factor 3, which results in altered platelet aggregation and activity [18]. Defective platelet function can be induced experimentally with high concentrations of urea [27] guanidinosuccinic acid [21], and phenol compounds [77].

Infection. Infection is among the most serious complications of vasomotor nephropathy, constituting a leading cause of death in both the oliguric and the recovery phase [85]. Trauma, burns, and major surgery, which are frequent causes of renal failure, predispose to serious infection, even in children with normal renal function. Coma and immobilization do likewise. Central venous catheters inserted for measurement of pressure or for hyperalimentation [1] provide portals of entry for invading organisms. Infection introduced by an indwelling bladder catheter is reprehensible, since such catheters are rarely necessary for the care of oliguric patients. Arteriovenous shunts and performance of peritoneal dialysis provide further routes of infection.

It is generally agreed that the prophylactic use of antibiotics in renal failure is ill-advised [92]. Immune processes in acute uremia have been reported to be normal [7] or depressed [65], but no means of improving phagocytosis and antibody formation is known. Most centers now utilize early and vigorous regimens of dialysis in hopes of improving the patient's overall clinical status, alertness, and resistance to infection. Although some authors suggest that such treatment is effective [52], firm proof is still lacking. Perhaps equally valuable is the awareness of potential causes of sepsis, prompt and vigorous therapy of established infection, and the use of reverse isolation precautions [89].

Gastrointestinal Symptoms. Gastrointestinal abnormalities are extremely common in children with vasomotor nephropathy. Anorexia, nausea, vomiting, and ileus are particularly notable early in the course of illness. Parotitis [12] and monilial glossitis [64] are largely preventable by appropriate oral hygiene and occur less frequently than in the distant past. Gastrointestinal bleeding due to stress ulcers [48], nonspecific gastritis [82], bleeding diathesis (see above), or enterocolitis [60] is a common and dreaded complication, only the two latter causes being predictably preventable by dialysis. Hemodialysis, in turn, may initiate gastrointestinal bleeding because of the need for administration of heparin.

Cardiovascular Findings. Hypertension, other than that due to gross volume overload, is an unusual concomitant of vasomotor nephropathy. Heart failure generally is an entirely preventable complication of injudicious hydration, but it may be seen following open heart surgery [20] or blunt trauma to the chest. Immobilization, severe dehydration, and tissue injury predispose to pulmonary embolization.

Uremic pericarditis, usually a manifestation of severe uremia, has occurred less frequently since the advent of early dialysis. Since it is totally reversible with dialysis, it presumably is the result of retention by the failing kidney of one or more unidentified low molecular weight products. In contrast to chronic renal failure [10], significant pericardial effusion is relatively uncommon, although even cardiac tamponade has been reported [46].

Neurologic Findings. The neurologic manifestations of acute uremia are poorly understood and often difficult to separate from those related to severe illness. A bewildering array of symptoms occur, many suggesting fixed organic lesions of the brain; they reverse promptly as renal function is restored. Abnormalities of affect, attitude, and mentation are the earliest clinical signs of uremia. The concentration span is short, and the child is apt to be sullen, withdrawn, and dull. Occasionally he is hyperactive, aggressive, and demanding, only to become disoriented and progressively lethargic before slipping into coma. Asterixis of the outstretched hand, muscular twitching, myoclonic jerks, and hyperreflexia are common manifestations and portend the need for vigorous dialysis before the more serious signs of uremia become evident. A stiff neck or positive Kernig's sign occurs in some uremic children, particularly (in my experience) those with myotonia and hyperreflexia. Although spinal fluid pressure and protein may be slightly elevated [86], the absence of pleocytosis and normal cerebrospinal fluid sugar concentrations differentiate such patients from those with meningitis.

The electroencephalogram of acutely uremic subjects shows a variety of abnormalities. Diffuse slowing or intermittent paroxysms of slow activity and focal changes are seen most commonly [17]. Their cause is very poorly understood. The older concept that acute uremic encephalopathy relates to cerebral edema is now open to question [4, 5] except in recently dialyzed patients [5]. The anatomic alterations of brain that have been described are probably nonspecific and of doubtful pathogenic significance [72]. The reversal of the cerebral manifestations by dialysis underscores that fact. Recently, a 47 to 66 percent increase in calcium and a lesser change in magnesium content has been demonstrated in the brains of acutely uremic dogs [4]. This change, related to increased parathormone secretion, could be prevented by parathyroidectomy and was independent of the animals' acid-base status. Nonetheless, brain calcium fell significantly with hemodialysis.

The Prevention of Vasomotor Nephropathy

There is little doubt that depletion of the plasma volume is an important factor in the development of vasomotor nephropathy. Furthermore, there appears to be a phase of incipient renal failure [28] in which vasomotor nephropathy is imminent, yet still reversible, as long as plasma volume, blood pressure, and cardiac output are returned promptly to normal. Mannitol has been claimed to be of particular value in reversing this "incipient" phase of vasomotor nephropathy [6, 9, 28], although volume expansion in response to saline is effective in many instances. The renal vasodilator effect of mannitol has been suggested as an additional, important mechanism of action, over and above volume expansion. However, experimental data supporting a specific prophylactic role of mannitol, summarized elsewhere [71], is meager. The early belief that furosemide might prevent vasomotor nephropathy [67] has not been supported subsequently [68]. In the absence of the proved value of either mannitol or furosemide, the use of these drugs in patients at risk of renal failure is not universally recommended. Either will produce a diuretic response, even in severely dehydrated subjects, as long as renal failure is not yet established. This favorable response tends to reassure the attending physician and may result in failure to restore fluid volume deficits and to normalize the cardiac output and blood pressure.

Recovery from Vasomotor Nephropathy

The oliguric phase of vasomotor nephropathy usually lasts 10 to 12 days, with a range of 3 days to over 3 weeks. Then, while fluid intake remains unchanged, there is a stepwise although variable increase in urine volume. The first day or so of recovery may witness a 10 to 20 percent rise in urine

output. Thereafter the increment may amount to 20 to 50 percent a day until normal or above normal volumes of urine are excreted.

The urinary concentration of sodium and potassium and the urinary osmolality remain unchanged throughout the early phase of recovery. The concentrations of urea and creatinine in plasma visually continue to rise for the first 2 to 4 days of recovery, plateau for a further 2 to 4 days, and then fall progressively toward normal. Except when renal failure has been particularly protracted, the total time required to achieve a normal blood urea nitrogen and serum creatinine usually is about equal to the duration of the oliguric period. Thus, except for an improved ability to excrete water, the patient remains azotemic, unable to excrete medications normally, and at risk of severe acidosis and hyperkalemia for several days after increased urine output heralds recovery. Infection continues to be a life-threatening complication throughout the recovery period; one-half of all deaths due to this cause occur after renal recovery has begun.

At times a massive diuresis ensues, and it then becomes necessary to closely monitor the urine volume and its electrolyte content to prevent serious hypokalemia, dehydration, and sodium imbalance. Anemia improves slowly and may not be fully repaired for weeks after the serum creatinine concentration has normalized [63]. Gastrointestinal and neurologic manifestations usually improve as the child's total condition improves, although convulsions occasionally occur in the face of rapid amelioration of renal function [86]. A degree of general debilitation may last for several weeks after the serum creatinine concentration has returned to normal and is attributable in part to the severity of the illness that produced renal failure.

Detailed studies of residual renal function following recovery from vasomotor nephropathy have not yet been performed in children. In adults, however, creatinine clearances are often mildly depressed 6 months or more after recovery [34]. The urinary sediment and excretion of protein are normal, and deterioration in renal function is extremely rare [36]. Hypertension is not an expected sequel. Slight defects in maximum concentrating capacity may persist [90] but are not of major clinical importance.

References

1. Abel, R. M., Beck, C. H., Jr., Abbott, W. M., Ryan, J. A., Jr., Barnett, G. O., and Fischer, J. E. Improved survival from acute renal failure after treatment with intravenous essential L-amino acids and glucose. Results of a prospective, double-blind study. *N. Engl. J. Med.* 288:695, 1973.

2. Adamson, J. W., Eschbach, J., and Finch, C. A. The kidney and erythropoiesis. *Am. J. Med.* 44:785, 1968.

3. Arena, J. M. *Poisoning* (2nd ed.). Springfield, Ill.: Thomas, 1970.

4. Arieff, A. I., and Massry, S. G. Calcium metabolism of brain in acute renal failure: Effects of uremia, hemodialysis, and parathyroid hormone. *J. Clin. Invest.* 53:387, 1974.

5. Arieff, A. I., Massry, S. G., Barrientos, A., and Kleeman, C. R. Brain water and electrolyte metabolism in uremia: Effects of slow and rapid hemodialysis. *Kidney Int.* 4:177, 1973.

6. Augur, R., Dayton, D., Harrison, C. E., Tucker, R. M., and Anderson, C. F. Use of ethacrynic acid in mannitol-resistant oliguric renal failure. *J.A.M.A.* 206:891, 1968.

7. Balch, H. H. The effect of severe battle injury and of post-traumatic renal failure on resistance to infection. *Ann. Surg.* 142:145, 1955.

8. Baldini, M., and Pannaciull, I. The maturation rate of reticulocytes. *Blood* 15:614, 1960.

9. Barry, K. G., Mazze, R. I., and Schwartz, F. D. Prevention of surgical oliguria and renal-hemodynamic suppression by sustained hydration. *N. Engl. J. Med.* 270:1371, 1964.

10. Beaudry, C., Nakamoto, S., and Kolff, W. J. Uremic pericarditis and cardiac tamponade in chronic renal failure. *Ann. Intern. Med.* 64:990, 1966.

11. Bennett, W. M., Singer, I., and Coggins, C. J. A guide to drug therapy in renal failure. *J.A.M.A.* 230:1544, 1974.

12. Bluemle, L. W., Jr., Webster, G. D., and Elkinton, J. R. Acute tubular necrosis: Analysis of one hundred cases with respect to mortality, complications and treatment with and without dialysis. *A.M.A. Arch. Intern. Med.* 104:180, 1959.

13. Bohle, A. Pathologische anatomie des akuten Nierenversagens. *Verh. Dtsch. Ges. Pathol.* 49:56, 1965.

14. Brun, C., Crone, C., Davidsen, H. G., Fabricius, J., Tybjaerg-Hansen, A., Lassen, N. A., and Munck, O. Renal blood flow in anuric human subject determined by use of radioactive krypton 85. *Proc. Soc. Exp. Biol. Med.* 89:687, 1955.

15. Bull, G. M., Joekes, A. M., and Lowe, K. G. Renal function studies in acute tubular necrosis. *Clin. Sci.* 9:379, 1950.

16. Bush, I. E. Chemical and biological factors in the activity of adrenocortical steroids. *Pharmacol. Rev.* 14:317, 1962.

17. Cadilhac, J., Ribstein, M., and Jean, R. The EEG and metabolic disorders. *Electroencephalogr. Clin. Neurophysiol.* 10:755, 1958.

18. Castaldi, P. A., Rozenberg, M. C., and Stewart, J. H. The bleeding disorder of uraemia: A qualitative platelet defect. *Lancet* 2:66, 1966.

19. Chan, J. C. M. Acute renal failure in children: Principles of management. *Clin. Pediatr.* 13:686, 1974.

20. Chesney, R. W., Kaplan, B. S., Freedom, R. M., Haller, J. A., and Drummond, K. N. Acute renal failure: An important complication of cardiac surgery in infants. *J. Pediatr.* 87:381, 1975.

21. Cohen, B. D. Guanidinosuccinic acid in uremia. *Arch. Intern. Med.* 126:846, 1970.

22. Cook, C. D., Wedgewood, R. J. P., Craig, J. M., Hartmann, J. R., and Janeway, C. A. Systemic lupus erythematosus: Description of 37 cases in children and a discussion of endrocrine therapy in 32 of the cases. *Pediatrics* 26:570, 1960.

23. Dalgaard, O. Z., and Pedersen, K. J. Renal tubular degeneration: Electron microscopy in ischaemic anuria. *Lancet* 2:484, 1959.

24. DeLuna, M. B., Metcalfe-Gibson, A., and Wrong, O. Urinary excretion of hydrogen-ion in acute oliguric renal failure. *Nephron* 1:3, 1964.

25. Desforges, J. F., and Dawson, J. P. The anemia of renal failure. *Arch. Intern. Med.* 101:326, 1958.

26. Doxiadis, S. A. Azotaemia in infancy. *Arch. Dis. Child.* 23:50, 1948.

27. Eknoyan, G., Wacksman, S. J., Glueck, H. I., and Will, J. J. Platelet function in renal failure. *N. Engl. J. Med.* 280:677, 1969.

28. Elliahou, H. E. Mannitol therapy in oliguria of acute onset. *Br. Med. J.* 1:807, 1964.

29. Epstein, M., Schneider, N. S., and Befeler, B. Effect of intrarenal furosemide on renal function and intrarenal hemodynamics in acute renal failure. *Am. J. Med.* 58:510, 1975.

30. Eschbach, J. W., Adamson, J. W., and Cook, J. D. Disorders of red blood cell production in uremia. *Arch. Intern. Med.* 126:812, 1970.

31. Feingold, M., Fine, R. N., and Ingall, D. Intravenous pyelography in infants with single umbilical artery. *N. Engl. J. Med.* 270:1178, 1964.

32. Finckh, E. S., Jeremy, D., and Whyte, H. M. Structural renal damage and its relation to clinical features in acute oliguric renal failure. *Q. J. Med.* 31:429, 1962.

33. Fine, L. G., and Elliahou, H. E. Acute oliguric intrinsic renal failure: Diagnostic criteria and clinical features in 61 patients. *Isr. J. Med. Sci.* 5:1024, 1969.

34. Finkenstaedt, J. T., and Merrill, J. P. Renal function studies in acute tubular necrosis. *Clin. Sci.* 9:379, 1950.

35. Fishman, R. A., and Raskin, N. H. Experimental uremic encephalopathy: Permeability and electrolyte metabolism of brain and other tissues. *Arch. Neurol.* 17:10, 1967.

36. Fox, M. Progressive renal fibrosis following acute tubular necrosis: An experimental study. *J. Urol.* 97:196, 1967.

37. Friedman, E. A., Greenberg, J. B., Merrill, J. P., and Dammin, G. J. Consequences of ethylene glycol poisoning. *Am. J. Med.* 32:891, 1962.

38. Gianantonio, C. A., Vitacco, M., Mendilaharzu, F., Rutty, A., and Mendilaharzu, J. The hemolytic-uremic syndrome. *J. Pediatr.* 64:478, 1964.

39. Gordillo, G., Ledezna, J. P., and Pertuz, C. M. Acute renal failure in infants: Observations on 100 cases. *Bol. Med. Hosp. Inf. (Mexico)* 3:203, 1962.

40. Grossman, R. A., Hamilton, R. W., Morse, B. M., Penn, A. S., and Goldberg, M. Nontraumatic rhabdomyolysis and acute renal failure. *N. Engl. J. Med.* 291:807, 1974.

41. Handa, S. P. Glomerular lesions in acute tubular necrosis. *Postgrad. Med. J.* 46:79, 1970.

42. Handa, S. P., and Moran, P. A. F. Diagnostic indices in acute renal failure. *Can. Med. Assoc. J.* 96:78, 1967.

43. Hollenberg, N. K., Adams, D. F., Oken, D. E., Abrams, H. L., and Merrill, J. P. Acute renal failure due to nephrotoxins. *N. Engl. J. Med.* 282:1329, 1970.

44. Hollenberg, N. K., and Epstein, M. The use of

drugs in the patient with uremia. In J. P. Merrill (ed.), Treatment of acute renal failure. *Mod. Treat.* 6:1011, 1969.

45. Hollenberg, N. K., Epstein, M., Rosen, S. M., Basch, R. I., Oken, D. E., and Merrill, J. P. Acute oliguric renal failure in man: Evidence for preferential renal cortical ischemia. *Medicine* 47:455, 1968.

46. Hutt, M. P., and Holmes, J. H. Pericardial effusion complicating acute tubular necrosis. *Arch. Intern. Med.* 108:226, 1961.

47. Jacobs, J. C. Systemic lupus erythematosus in childhood: Report of 35 cases. *Pediatrics* 32:257, 1963.

48. Jungers, P., Maillard, J.-N., Bienayme, J., Glaser, P., and Mery, J. P. Hemorrhagies digestives par ulcerations gastro-duodenales au cours de l'insuffisance renale aiguë: A propos de cinq cas opérés et gueris. *Proc. Eur. Dialysis Transplant Assoc.* 4:301, 1967.

49. Keating, R. E., Weicheslbaum, T. E., Alanis, M., Margraf, H. W., and Elman, R. The movement of potassium during experimental acidosis and alkalosis in the nephrectomized dog. *Surg. Gynecol. Obstet.* 96:323, 1953.

50. Kendall, A. G., Lowenstein, L., and Morgen, R. O. The hemorrhagic diathesis in renal disease (with special reference to acute uremia). *Can. Med. Assoc. J.* 85:405, 1961.

51. Kerr, D. N. S., Rabindranath, G., and Elliot, R. W. The treatment of acute renal failure. In O. Wrong (ed.), *Fourth Symposium on Advanced Medicine.* London: Pitman, 1968. P. 74.

52. Kleinknecht, D., Jungers, P., Chanard, J., Barbanel, C., and Ganeval, D. Uremic and non-uremic complications in acute renal failure: Evaluation of early and frequent dialysis on prognosis. *Kidney Int.* 1:190, 1972.

53. Kountz, S. L., Tuttle, K. L., Cohn, L. H., Eschelman, L. T., and Cohn, R. Factors responsible for acute tubular necrosis following lower aortic surgery. *J.A.M.A.* 183:447, 1963.

54. Kovithavongs, T., Becker, F. O., and Ing, T. S. Parathyroid hyperfunction in acute renal failure: Serial studies in man. *Nephron* 9:349, 1972.

55. Kuroyanagi, T. Anemia associated with chronic renal failure, with special reference to kinetics of the erythron. *Acta Haematol. Jpn.* 24:156, 1961.

56. Ladefoged, J., and Winkler, K. Hemodynamics in acute renal failure: The effect of hypotension induced by dihydralazine on renal blood flow, mean circulation time for plasma, and renal vascular volume in patients with acute oliguric renal failure. *Scand. J. Clin. Lab. Invest.* 26:83, 1970.

57. Leitner, S. J. *Bone Marrow Biopsy.* New York: Grune & Stratton, 1949. P. 127.

58. Levin, M. L., Simon, N. M., Herdson, P. B., and Greco, F. Acute renal failure followed by protracted, slowly resolving chronic uremia. *J. Chronic Dis.* 25:645, 1972.

59. Lieberman, E. Management of acute renal failure in infants and children. *Nephron* 11:193, 1973.

60. Mason, E. E. Gastrointestinal lesions occurring in uremia. *Ann. Intern. Med.* 37:96, 1952.

61. McLachlan, M. S. F., Davies, R. L., and Leach, K. G. Diatrizoate levels in the kidney and lymph nodes in acute renal failure in the rat. *Nephron* 13:443, 1974.

62. Meislin, A. G., and Rothfield, N. Systemic lupus erythematosus in childhood: Analysis of 42 cases, with comparative data on 200 adult cases followed concurrently. *Pediatrics* 42:37, 1968.

63. Merrill, J. P. *The Treatment of Renal Failure* (2nd ed.). New York: Grune & Stratton, 1965. P. 167.

64. Merrill, J. P. *The Treatment of Renal Failure* (2nd ed.). New York: Grune & Stratton, 1965. P. 172.

65. Montgomerie, J. Z., Kalmanson, G. M., and Guze, L. B. Renal failure and infection. *Medicine (Baltimore)* 47:1, 1968.

66. Mostert, J. W., Kim, U., and Woodruff, M. W. Hepatorenal failure with renal oxalosis after methoxyflurane anesthesia. *N.Y. State J. Med.* 71:2676, 1971.

67. Muth, R. G. Furosemide in severe renal insufficiency. *Postgrad. Med. J.* 47:21, 1971.

68. Muth, R. G. Furosemide in Acute Renal Failure. In E. A. Friedman and H. E. Eliahou (eds.), *Proceedings of a Conference on Acute Renal Failure* (DHEW Publication [NIH] 74–608). Washington, D.C.: U.S. Govt. Printing Office, 1973.

69. Oken, D. E. Drug-induced renal disease. *Practitioner* 201:461, 1968.

70. Oken, D. E. Nosologic considerations in the nomenclature of acute renal failure. *Nephron* 8:505, 1971.

71. Oken, D. E. Mannitol and the Prevention of Vasomotor Nephropathy. In S. Giovannetti, V. Bonomini, and G. D'Amico (eds.), *Proceedings of the 6th International Congress of Nephrology, 1975.* Basel: Karger, 1976. Pp. 578–583.

72. Olsen, S. The brain in uremia. *Acta Psychiatr. Scand.* [Suppl. 156] 36:1, 1961.

73. Olsen, T. S., and Skjoldborg, H. The fine structure of the renal glomerulus in acute anuria. *Acta Pathol. Microbiol. Scand.* [8] 70:205, 1967.

74. Pasternack, A., and Wahlberg, P. Bone marrow in acute renal failure. *Acta Med. Scand.* 181:505, 1967.

75. Perlmutter, M., Grossman, S. L., Rottenberg, S., and Dobkin, G. Urine-serum urea nitrogen ratio. *J.A.M.A.* 170:1533, 1959.

76. Powers, S. R., Jr., Boba, A., Hostnik, W., and Stein, A. Prevention of post-operative acute renal failure with mannitol in 100 cases. *Surgery* 55:15, 1964.

77. Rabiner, S. F., and Molinas, F. Cited by H. I. Horowitz, The role of phenol and phenolic acids on the thrombocytopathy and defective platelet aggregation of patients with renal failure. *Arch. Intern. Med.* 126:823, 1970.

78. Rubenstein, M., Meyer, R., and Bernstein, J. Congenital abnormalities of the urinary system. *J. Pediatr.* 58:356, 1961.

79. Schreiner, G. E., and Maher, J. F. Toxic nephropathy. *Am. J. Med.* 38:409, 1965.

80. Schwartz, S. O., and Motto, S. A. Diagnostic significance of "Burr" red blood cells. *Am. J. Med. Sci.* 218:563, 1949.

81. Sevitt, S. Pathogenesis of traumatic uremia: A revised concept. *Lancet* 2:135, 1959.

82. Shackman, R., and Perkash, I. Gastro-intestinal bleeding in acute renal failure. *Proc. Eur. Dialysis Transplant Assoc.* 1:15, 1964.

83. Shils, M. E. Renal disease and the metabolic effects of tetracycline. *Ann. Intern. Med.* 58:389, 1963.

84. Stewart, J. H. Haemolytic anaemia in acute and chronic renal failure. *Q. J. Med.* 36:85, 1967.

85. Swann, R. C., and Merrill, J. P. The clinical course of acute renal failure. *Medicine* 32:215, 1953.

86. Tyler, H. R. Neurological Complications of Acute and Chronic Renal Failure. In J. P. Merrill (ed.), *The Treatment of Renal Failure* (2nd ed.). New York: Grune & Stratton, 1965. P. 332.

87. Vertel, R. M., and Knochel, J. P. Non-oliguric acute renal failure. *J.A.M.A.* 200:598, 1967.

88. Wacker, W. E. C., and Vallee, B. L. A study of magnesium metabolism in acute renal failure employing a multichannel flame spectrometer. *N. Engl. J. Med.* 257:1254, 1957.

89. Walter, C. W. Isolation Technic for Containment or Exclusion of Bacteria for the Prevention of Cross Infection in Hospitals. In J. P. Merrill (ed.), *The Treatment of Renal Failure* (2nd ed.). New York: Grune & Stratton, 1965. P. 306.

90. Ward, E. E., Richard, P., and Wrong, O. M. Urine concentration after acute renal failure. *Nephron* 3: 289, 1966.

91. Waugh, D., and Beschal, H. Infra-glomerular epithelial reflux in the evolution of serotonin nephropathy in rats. *Am. J. Pathol.* 39:547, 1961.

92. Weinstein, L., Goldfield, M., and Chan, T. W. Infections occurring during chemotherapy: A study of their frequency, type and predisposing factors. *N. Engl. J. Med.* 251:247, 1954.

93. Whelton, A., and Donadio, J. V., Jr. Post-traumatic acute renal failure in Vietnam: A comparison with the Korean War experience. *Johns Hopkins Med. J.* 124:95, 1969.

94. Wiggelinkhuizen, J., and Pokroy, M. V. Acute renal failure in infancy and childhood. *S. Afr. Med. J.* 48:2129, 1974.

III. Diseases of the Urinary Tract

92. Urinary Tract Infections in Infants and Children

Jan Winberg

Urinary tract infection (UTI) is one of the major bacterial diseases of childhood. The risk of a newborn girl having symptomatic UTI during childhood is at least 3 percent and for a boy about 1 percent. The prevalence of asymptomatic bacteriuria in girls of preschool and school age is about 1 percent. One-half of the patients with symptomatic infections (about 80 percent of those with asymptomatic bacteriuria) will develop one or several recurrences. About 5 to 10 percent of patients with symptomatic infections will develop a renal scar; a few of them will become hypertensive or uremic.

The possibility of surgically correctable lesions calls for radiologic examination in most of these patients. They all receive antibiotics for shorter or longer periods of time, and some need to be followed systematically for their entire life. Thus, UTI is a common disease that causes suffering and inconvenience to many patients; it results in huge costs for the family or society and requires a great deal of the pediatrician's time.

Definition

The general term *urinary tract infection* describes a group of conditions that have one feature in common: the presence of significant numbers of bacteria in the urine. These conditions differ in pathogenesis and consequently in course and prognosis. They can be classified with regard to pathogenesis, localization, and therapeutic implications.

CLASSIFICATION WITH REGARD TO PATHOGENESIS

A classification based on pathogenesis facilitates understanding of the disease process and also has clinical implications. The major categories are distinguished on the basis of whether or not obstruction is present. Obstruction may be structural or functional, as with neurogenic bladders. Infections associated with obstructive lesions represent only a small minority of all UTI in childhood (1 to 2 percent in girls; 5 to 10 percent in boys);

however, they are qualitatively important, since irreversible renal damage may occur rapidly. Bacteriuria detected through screening ("asymptomatic"; symptomless; covert; latent) is revealed by examination of healthy populations, and it occurs mainly in girls. A special host-aggressor relationship present under these circumstances may justify classifying it separately, although the pathogenetic mechanism may be the same as in uncomplicated symptomatic infections.

CLASSIFICATION WITH REGARD TO LOCALIZATION

Urethritis. This infection is limited to the urethra; it remains to be proved that a true bacterial urethritis exists.

Cystitis. This infection is limited to the bladder. The symptoms vary from frequency and severe pain and burning on micturition to only occasional dull pain over the bladder. Patients are usually afebrile. These symptoms can also be present in association with infection of the renal parenchyma; thus the term *cystitis* should not be used until proof exists that the kidneys are not affected (see Acute Pyelonephritis, below).

Pyelitis. This term has been used especially in the past to designate a febrile condition allegedly caused by an infection of the renal pelvis and leading to local inflammation and loin pain. It is impossible, however, to demonstrate that the infection is confined to the pelvis; consequently there is no reason to continue to use this term, and it should be dropped.

Acute Pyelonephritis. This is an acute bacterial infection of the renal parenchyma. The symptoms vary from fever, chills, severe malaise, vomiting, loin pain, and dysuria to no symptoms at all. Temporary impairment of the renal concentrating capacity and a transitory increase of serum antibody titer are considered evidence of renal involvement. When these findings are lacking, the infection may be localized by (1) an increased C-reactive protein [45]; (2) demonstration of ureteral bacteriuria by

Aided by the Swedish Medical Research Council, Project No. 19X-765.

one of the washout methods [25, 100]; (3) finding in the urine bacteria coated with antibody [44, 104]; or (4) an increased urinary excretion of lactic dehydrogenase [18].

Chronic Pyelonephritis. This confusing term is used variously to describe (1) certain histologic lesions of the renal parenchyma; (2) renal parenchymal abnormalities visible on radiographs, consisting usually of papillary shrinking and a defect of the corresponding part of the renal outline ("scarring"); and (3) a clinical condition characterized by continuous excretion of bacteria or by frequent recurrences of infection. These multiple definitions clearly are misleading.

Cystourethral Syndrome (Cystourethritis; Abacterial Cystitis; Urethritis). This designation is often used to describe a condition manifested by the classic symptoms of "cystitis" but lacking demonstrable bacteriuria. Pyuria, suggesting inflammation, may be present. Vulvitis and balanitis should be ruled out by inspection. The etiology is unknown; on endoscopy some patients show evidence of inflammation of the bladder, especially the area of the trigone. In some a low bacterial count may be due to frequent voiding. The condition is not uncommon in girls before puberty.

CLASSIFICATION WITH REGARD TO MANAGEMENT

There has long been a need for a new classification of urinary infection that can serve as a guide for management with antimicrobial therapy. Stamey [95] has suggested four simple categories: (1) first infection; (2) unresolved bacteriuria during therapy (failure to sterilize the urine); (3) bacterial persistence (in a locus not amenable to antibiotics); and (4) reinfection. Note that a distinction is made between failure to sterilize the urine (unresolved bacteriuria) and failure to sterilize a certain site within the urinary tract (bacterial persistence). In the latter instance voided urine temporarily may be sterile.

First (Onset) Infection. Bacteria causing initial infection in infants and children are, with few exceptions, sensitive to most antimicrobial agents. Sulfonamides will cure almost 100 percent of these patients. In infants and toddlers the first infection usually is associated with fever and involves the renal parenchyma. Demonstration of the presence or absence of gross reflux is essential in regard to follow-up and prophylaxis in these patients.

Unresolved Bacteriuria During Therapy. The clinician often fails to recognize this condition either because cultures of the urine are not obtained during treatment, or, if they are obtained,

he misinterprets bacterial counts of $< 10^5$ per milliliter as contaminants. Clearly, if any bacteria of the infecting strain are present in a midstream specimen of urine, one cannot be certain that the bacteriuria has been eradicated. According to Stamey [95], the causes of unresolved bacteriuria, in descending order of importance, are as follows:

1. Bacterial resistance to the drug selected for therapy. If a patient has received therapy in the recent past, there is a considerable chance that resistant organisms may be responsible for the current bacteriuria. Resistant mutants may also be selected from an initially sensitive bacterial population in the urinary tract.
2. The occurrence of two different bacterial species simultaneously in the bladder that have mutually exclusive antimicrobial sensitivities. Initial therapy unmasks the presence of a second species.
3. Azotemia. Unresolved bacteriuria may continue with sensitive bacteria solely because renal failure prevents attainment of the urinary concentration of antibiotic required to kill the organism.
4. Giant staghorn calculi associated with a "critical mass" of sensitive bacteria too great for antimicrobial inhibition. The role of stagnant urine in therapeutic failure has been emphasized [73].

The first two of these causes for failure to sterilize the urine can be resolved by in vitro antimicrobial sensitivity testing.

Bacterial Persistence. Once the urine is sterile, recurrence with the same organism from a site within the urinary tract can occur in two circumstances—in the presence of infected stones (struvite), and with chronic bacterial prostatitis. The existence of prostatitis in children is questionable. A structural abnormality such as a nonfunctioning duplication, urachal cyst, or a nonrefluxing ureteral stump may represent a third but less common cause of bacterial persistence.

Reinfections. All other infections can be classified as reinfections, including rapid reinfection occurring within 24 to 48 hours after cessation of therapy. Some 95 to 99 percent of recurrences seem to be reinfections [113].

Diagnostic Procedures

Demonstration of a "significant" number of bacteria in the urine is the only valid criterion for the diagnosis of a UTI. Other commonly used methods test only secondary phenomena and therefore can give only supportive evidence.

DEMONSTRATION OF BACTERIA

Kass's definition of significant bacteriuria is statistically based [48]. He examined urine (not midstream specimens) obtained from apparently healthy adult women. The following criteria were suggested by the Kass study: $<10^4$ bacteria per milliliter of urine probably represents contamination; 10^4 to 10^5 bacteria per milliliter of urine probably represents infection. These criteria usually are regarded as valid for infants and children, but further investigation to substantiate this is required.

Office Methods for Demonstration of Bacteriuria

Microscopy. 1 bacterium per high power field corresponds to 5×10^4 to 10^5 bacteria per milliliter when uncentrifuged urine is examined.

Dipslide[1] Culture. This is an easy and inexpensive method for demonstration of significant bacteriuria. The accuracy is higher than that of the standard loop method routinely used for quantitative cultures [4]. Dipslide culture represents a major advance in the diagnosis of UTI, and its use is encouraged. The set consists of a glass slide covered with blood agar on one side and clear agar on the other; the latter inhibits the growth of gram-positive organisms. The slide is dipped into the urine or, still better, is placed in the urinary stream; the excess urine is allowed to run off onto a scrap of filter paper. The slide, fitted in a plastic tube, is best incubated at 37°C, but room temperature also gives accurate results. The growth is compared to a visual scale that corresponds to the number of bacteria per milliliter.

Accurate diagnosis requires careful attention to the following: (1) method of collection of urine, (2) storage of urine, (3) discontinuation of antibiotic treatment before collecting a urine specimen for culture.

Collection of Urine

Four methods are available for the collection of urine: clean catch of midstream urine; collection by plastic bag; catheterization; and bladder puncture.

Clean Catch. This should be the routine procedure, collecting, if possible, a midstream urine. The preputial folds of noncircumcised boys may contain large numbers of bacteria even after cleaning and must be irrigated before a urine culture is taken.

Collection by Plastic Bag. With meticulous washing of the genital region (renewed if the

[1] Manufactured under the name Uricult.

patient has not voided within 3 hr), detachment of the bag within 15 to 20 min after voiding, and immediate culture or chilling to +4°C, reliable results can be obtained when urine is collected by plastic bag. Nevertheless, the risk of false-positive results is great.

Catheterization. When bladder puncture is not convenient, chiefly in patients above the age of 1 year, catheterization may be performed. The risk of infecting previously healthy patients is small; it may be considerable, however, in patients with a history of recurring infections [63].

Bladder Puncture. This is used mainly during the first year of life. The procedure has been described in detail [69]. The use of a Vacutainer facilitates the procedure. Complications are rare. Urine obtained in this way from normal subjects is supposed to be sterile, but data on this point are lacking.

The indications for bladder puncture include (1) persistent bacteriuria of doubtful significance, (2) seriously ill patients in whom rapid and accurate diagnosis is essential prior to initiation of therapy, (3) obstruction of bladder outflow or of the urethra, (4) uncircumcised boys with a non-retractable prepuce when the urine contains $>10^4$ bacteria per milliliter (it is probably unnecessary, though, to confirm such a questionable culture when it is combined with massive pyuria), and (5) fever of unknown origin before beginning antibiotic therapy as a therapeutic test.

Transportation and Storage

Bacterial multiplication starts rapidly in vitro. After 24 hr at room temperature urines have similar bacterial numbers irrespective of the number present at voiding (Fig. 92-1). It is mandatory

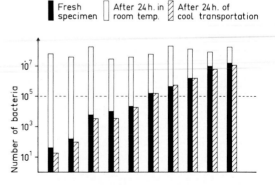

Figure 92-1. The concentration of bacteria in urine specimens before and after 24 hr at room temperature and after 24 hr at +4°C. Dotted line represents the limit for significant bacteriuria [47].

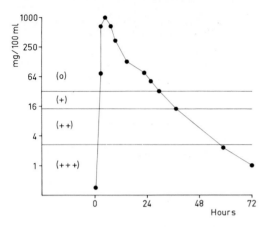

Figure 92-2. Concentration of sulfonamide in the urine after single dose of 50 mg per kilogram of a short-acting sulfisoxazole (Gantrisin). Levels defining the degree of sensitivity are indicated. (Courtesy of Dr. K. Lincoln.)

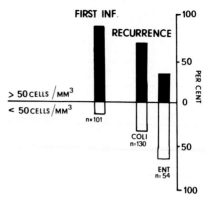

Figure 92-3. Occurrence of pyuria in girls with urinary tract infections. A count below 50 cells per cubic millimeter in the uncentrifuged urine is common, especially in recurrent infection due either to E. coli (COLI) or enterococci (ENT). N = number of cases.

that urine be kept cold from the moment of voiding until the seeding on plates. At 0 to 4°C, the bacterial count remains unchanged for at least 48 hr.

Influence of Antibiotics Present in the Urine

Even at low concentrations in blood, most antibiotics appear in active form in high concentrations in the urine and influence bacterial multiplication. Figure 92-2 shows that 48 hr after one single dose of 50 mg per kilogram of body weight of a short-acting sulfonamide compound (sulfisoxazole) the concentration in urine was sufficient to inhibit bacterial growth. The implication of this is that therapy should be discontinued for at least 72 hr before culture to permit complete excretion of the antibiotic. Another cause of falsely negative urine is perineal washing with antiseptic solutions.

DEMONSTRATION OF PHENOMENA SECONDARY TO INFECTION

White Cell Count

Pyuria is only a sign of inflammation of the genital region or urinary tract; it may be either bacterial or nonbacterial, and it cannot replace cultures in the diagnosis of bacterial UTI. Conversely, a normal white cell count in the urine does not exclude a UTI. In consecutive urine specimens white cells may vary between none and gross pyuria [28]. It is more common to find a normal concentration of white cells in recurrent infections than in apparent first infections (Fig. 92-3). Counting of urinary white cells is best done by placing the uncentrifuged urine in a counting

chamber[2] [43]. In voided specimens boys should have less than 10 cells per cubic millimeter; girls usually also have few cells, but counts between 50 and 100 may be found without demonstrable disease.

White cell counting is of help in three situations: (1) in making a tentative diagnosis in acutely ill patients before the results of culture are available; (2) in support of the diagnosis (a) in patients with low bacterial counts due to frequency; (b) in patients with symptoms of doubtful significance or with asymptomatic bacteriuria; (c) in all boys below the age of 3 to 4 years, where the preputial bacteria may contaminate urine heavily; and (3) in suggesting renal involvement by the presence of white cell casts. Testing for proteinuria is of no help in the diagnosis of UTI. Hematuria is not uncommon, especially in infections in neonates and in males.

Determination of Antibody Titer

Agglutinating and hemagglutinating antibodies to the O antigen of the infecting *Escherichia coli* can be demonstrated regularly in the serum of patients with pyelonephritis but not in those with cystitis [75, 112]. The antibodies are highly specific and can be used diagnostically to verify that the isolated bacteria are the cause of the infection.

Renal Function

In actue infection of a previously healthy kidney,

---

[2] For example, the four-chamber Fuchs-Rosenthal leukocyte counting chamber, which is obtainable from Hawksley and Sons, Lancing, Sussex, England.

renal concentrating capacity is transiently reduced. In uncomplicated infections it improves rapidly, but it may not be completely restored to normal until after 8 to 12 weeks. If concentrating capacity does not return to normal, the possibility of obstruction of the urine flow, renal scarring, or persistent infection should be considered.

Increase in the concentration of urea or creatinine in blood is uncommon in uncomplicated acute UTI. When present, it suggests either bilateral obstruction or marked parenchymal reduction. During the newborn period an increase in blood urea nitrogen may occur, even in the absence of obstruction [10]. A decrease in renal plasma flow during and after acute infection also has been described [17].

In scarred kidneys all types of functional defects may be seen, including reduced ability to excrete a sodium chloride load [3] and a lowering of the renal threshold for resorption of sodium bicarbonate [8]. The latter may be the earliest functional defect to become manifest.

RADIOGRAPHIC DIAGNOSTIC PROCEDURES

Excretory pyelography (IVP) and micturition cystourethrography (MCU) are discussed in detail elsewhere (Chap. 10). The three main aims of these examinations are (1) to detect factors predisposing to or encouraging infection, that is, congenital or acquired obstruction of the urinary flow, calculus, gross vesicoureteral reflux, and intrarenal reflux; (2) to detect and outline renal tissue narrowing and calyceal dilatation, which may be early signs of renal scarring; (3) to check the rate of growth of the kidney, which may be a valuable aid in assessing the effect of treatment [38].

Reports of the frequency of positive findings on radiographic procedures in children with UTI vary widely, from as high as 25 to 50 percent in some urologic centers to as low as 5 to 10 percent in boys and 1 to 2 percent in girls in many pediatric practices [111]. The variations are probably due chiefly to differences in patient selection and in criteria for diagnosing abnormalities.

Indications for Radiologic Investigation
1. Apparent first infection
   a. All infants and toddlers with symptomatic infections
   b. All boys with symptomatic infections, irrespective of age
   c. All patients with bacteriuria detected on screening
   d. When a mass is seen or palpated over the symphysis after micturition, indicating incomplete bladder emptying
   e. Palpation of a mass in the upper part of the abdomen, suggesting the possibility of hydonephrosis
   f. Increased blood urea or serum creatinine or persistently reduced concentrating capacity
   g. Increased blood pressure
   h. When infection fails to resolve in spite of administration of an adequate antibiotic
2. Recurrent infections: patients of all ages and both sexes should have an IVP and MCU.

When Should Radiologic Investigations Be Repeated?
In patients with recurrent infections but without obstruction, we check renal growth and calyceal appearance at intervals of 6 months during the first year of life, at the end of the second year of life, and thereafter at intervals of 2 to 3 years. Radiologic follow-up of patients with reflux is controversial. Since UTIs occurring in children without obstruction result so rarely in renal damage, many believe that frequent follow-up examinations that involve exposure to x-rays are not indicated. Since preservation of renal tissue is the aim of the therapy, however, I prefer to evaluate treatment by checking the growth of the kidneys by IVP.

LOCALIZATION STUDIES
Localizing the site of infection is required when it is important to know whether or not an infection involves the renal parenchyma and when persistent unilateral infection is suspected. The washout technique of Stamey et al. [100] with ureteral catheterization and the Fairley method [25] using only bladder catheterization are used most commonly. The results of these so-called direct techniques must be interpreted with caution. The discharge of bacteria may be intermittent, and results may indicate bladder infection when in fact there is renal infection. The opposite misinterpretation is also possible if bacteria are carried up from the bladder, either by the catheter or by reflux. Even minimal amounts of the bladder disinfectant left behind after saline irrigation may inhibit bacterial growth and erroneously suggest lower UTI. The only truly direct method for demonstrating renal infection is renal biopsy, which for obvious reasons can be performed only in very selected cases. Even here, cultures of the biopsy material may be negative in the presence of other strong evidence of renal infection.

A transitory decrease in renal concentrating capacity or an increase in serum antibody titer against the O antigen of infecting bacteria (as determined by direct agglutination) is widely used to indicate renal involvement. These tests appear to be valuable in defining groups of patients with renal infection; however, they may be difficult to interpret in an individual patient [45, 56]. Both a low concentrating capacity and a high antibody titer may have explanations other than a renal infection. The correlation between concentrating capacity, antibody titer, and sedimentation rate in patients with an apparent first symptomatic infection is better than that in patients with frequent recurrences or asymptomatic bacteriuria. In these instances the infection is often caused by bacteria with a deficient cell wall. When such bacteria are used as sources of antigen, the measured antibody titer may be low, whereas it is high when a laboratory strain with a more complete antigenic structure is used [56]. Unfortunately, it is in patients with frequent recurrences or asymptomatic bacteriuria that localization of infection is most essential.

Demonstration of antibody-coated bacteria in the urine has recently been suggested as a means of separating renal from bladder infection [104]. Since there is considerable local antibody production in the bladder in patients with repeated infections [44], it is unlikely that this method can differentiate between upper and lower tract infections. In recent studies [45, 56] it was suggested that C-reactive protein may be the most reliable method for discriminating between renal and nonrenal infections.

Carvajal et al. [18] measured urinary concentrations of lactic dehydrogenase isoenzymes in children with urinary infection. Isoenzyme 5 ranged from 0 to 11.4 mU per milliliter in 22 children with bladder infections (mean 3.1 mU/ml), in contrast to values of 5.9 to 640 mU per milliliter in 16 children with renal infection (mean 120 mU/ml). Only 1 child with renal infection had a urinary value within the bladder infection range, suggesting that measurement of this isoenzyme might provide an accurate method of differentiating upper and lower infection.

Epidemiology
SYMPTOMATIC INFECTIONS
The age and sex distribution of 596 consecutive patients with presumed first (onset) infections appearing within a defined population during a defined period of time are shown in Fig. 92-4 [111]. The age and sex distribution is discussed under Pathogenesis and Predisposing Factors. From these data the risk of a child developing a symptomatic UTI before age 11 years has been

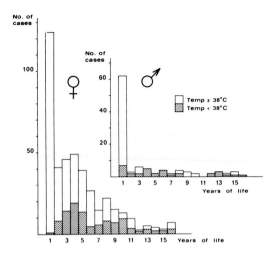

Figure 92-4. *Apparently primary onset of symptomatic UTI in 419 girls and 104 boys between second month and 16 years. The proportion of nonfebrile infections was very small during the first year of life, but it increased with age. Not included are 52 boys and 21 girls with neonatal infections (0 to 30 days). (From Winberg et al. [111].)*

calculated to be 1.1 percent for boys and 3.0 percent for girls. Most of the infants and small children with acute symptomatic infections do not continue to have repeated infections, although a small proportion will. This explains the fact that although first infections have their peak incidence during the first year of life, girls of school age dominate the patients with UTI seen by pediatricians.

SCREENING BACTERIURIA (ASYMPTOMATIC, COVERT, LATENT, SYMPTOMLESS BACTERIURIA)
Screening bacteriuria is defined here as infection diagnosed by surveys of so-called healthy populations. The designation *asymptomatic* may not be accurate, since some of these patients show improvement in their general state after eradication of bacteriuria, although this effect is difficult to document. In apparently healthy girls between 4 and 16 years the prevalence of bacteriuria is between 0.7 and 2 percent; there is no definite increase with age, although a yearly acquisition rate of 0.32 percent has been observed [51]. In boys the frequency is very low beyond the newborn period [51, 67], when asymptomatic bacteriuria associated with a heavy pyuria may be seen in 1 to 3 percent [110]; the significance is unknown. The significance of asymptomatic bacteriuria in various populations is discussed under Screening Bacteriuria at the end of this chapter.

Table 92-1. Bacterial Etiology in 596 Apparent First Nonobstructive Urinary Tract Infections in Relation to Sex and Age

Bacteria	Percent of Neonates of Both Sexes (N = 73)	Percent of Girls		Percent of Boys	
		1 mo–10 yr[a] (N = 389)	10–16 yr (N = 30)	1 mo–1 yr (N = 62)	1–16 yr[a] (N = 42)
E. coli	75[b]	83	60	85	33
Klebsiella	11	<1	0	2	2
Proteus	0	3	0	5	33
Enterococci	3	2	0	0	2
Staphylococcus albus	1	<1	30	0	12[c]
Other bacteria	4	<1	0	3	2
Mixed etiology	4	1	3	2	5
Unknown	1	9	7	3	10

[a] No differences between girls 1 month to 1 year and 1 to 10 years. No differences between boys 1 to 10 and 10 to 16 years except for *S. albus;* see footnote b.
[b] In girls, 57 percent; in boys, 83 percent; $\chi^2 : p = 0.016$.
[c] Four of the five patients were above 11 years of age.

Bacterial Etiology and Pattern of Resistance

Escherichia coli causes the majority of urinary tract infections in patients without complicating disorders of the urinary system such as calculus, obstruction, and neurogenic bladder. Other organisms are not uncommon, however, especially under certain circumstances, such as *Proteus* in older boys, coagulase-negative *Staphylococcus* at puberty in either sex, and *Klebsiella* in the newborn period (Table 92-1). Of about 150 known *E. coli* serotypes, some 8 to 10 O groups, including O_1, O_2, O_4, O_6, O_7, O_{18}, and O_{75}, cause about two-thirds of all *E. coli* UTI. These same subgroups are usually also the dominant ones in the fecal flora of the community [33]. *Escherichia coli* isolated in the urine are usually of the same serogroup as those dominating the fecal flora of an individual (see reference 33). Such observations suggest that UTI usually is not caused by special uropathogenic bacteria. *Staphylococcus* and *Proteus* do not infect the special groups mentioned above because of fecal dominance, however; it is possible, therefore, that they may have special pathogenicity.

A vast majority of infecting bacteria are sensitive to most of the antimicrobials commonly used, including sulfonamides. There are several exceptions to this general rule, however. A recurrence during the first few months after a course of sulfonamide is often due to resistant organisms. This sequence is due to antibiotic-induced changes in the sensitivity of the organisms in the intestinal flora (see under Chemotherapy, Fecal Flora, and Transmissible Chemoresistance). The same evolution occurs after ampicillin and tetracycline therapy, but not during treatment with nitrofurantoin;

consequently, recurrences are rarely due to nitrofurantoin-resistant organisms.

In patients with complications, *E. coli* is common, but other species, such as *Proteus, Pseudomonas, Alcaligenes faecalis, Klebsiella, Enterobacter,* white and yellow staphylococci, enterococci (fecal streptococci), and *Candida,* are frequently found. The pattern of resistance of these organisms is often impossible to predict.

Pathogenesis and Predisposing Factors

Bacteria are supposed to enter the urinary tract mainly by one of two routes; hematogenous or ascending. It is generally assumed, but not proved, that most infections are ascending except for those appearing during the newborn period, which are blood-borne.

Gram-negative bacteremia associated with UTI during the neonatal period is usually of obscure origin, but sometimes the site of entry may be identified (intrauterine manipulations, tracheal tubes, umbilical catheters, omphalitis).

Presumed ascending infections seem to affect 3 to 5 percent of all girls. The risk of these girls developing a symptomatic UTI may be 50 times greater than that of a previously healthy girl [111]. Moreover, the risk of reinfection seems to increase with the number of previous infections (Fig. 92-5). The female population can thus be divided into those *prone* and those *not prone* to UTI. During the first year of life the same holds true for the male population. The causes of the difference between susceptible and nonsusceptible groups have been a matter of much speculation but are still unknown.

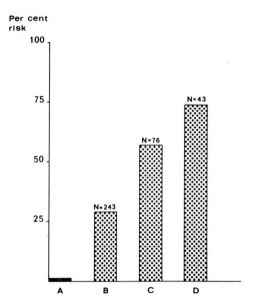

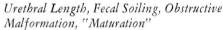

Figure 92-5. Recurrence rate of symptomatic UTI in girls within 1 year of a preceding infection related to the number of earlier infections. (A) Approximate risk of a 30-day-old healthy girl having an infection before 11 years of age. (B) Observed risk in 243 girls with one earlier infection. (C) Observed risk in 76 patients with two earlier infections. (D) Observed risk in 43 patients with three earlier infections. (From Winberg et al. [111].)

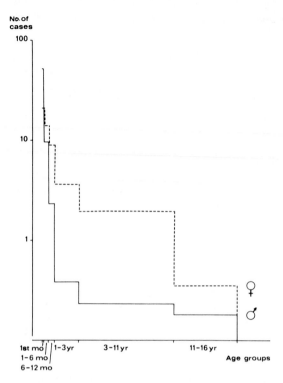

Figure 92-6. Mean number of new cases per month in different age groups and in 104 boys and 419 girls with UTI. Calculated from data shown in Fig. 92-4.

Urethral Length, Fecal Soiling, Obstructive Malformation, "Maturation"

The typical age and sex distribution in onset infections (see Fig. 92-4) helps to define possible pathogenetic mechanisms. The mean number of new cases per month of life in different age periods was calculated from this population (Fig. 92-6). More than 50 boys fell ill during the first month of life; during the following 5 months there were about 10 new cases per month; and during the next 6 months there were between 1 and 2 new cases per month. Thus UTI in boys is largely a disease of infancy. The decline in morbidity in girls is similar but slower.

Several possibilities must be considered to explain the slope of the curves in Fig. 92-6. First, demonstrable obstructive malformations cannot account for the age distribution, since such patients were excluded. Second, pathogenetic factors operating in very early infections may be different from those in infections occurring later on. For example, the early peak incidence may be due to gram-negative septicemia, which occurs much less frequently after the first month of life. Asymptomatic bacteriuria associated with pyuria, a condition that is more probably due to ascending than hema-

togenous infection, appears in about 1 to 3 percent of newborn boys (see Neonatal Asymptomatic Bacteriuria, at the end of this chapter), suggesting a decreased local defense at this age. Third, fecal soiling, proposed as a predisposing factor, can hardly be of decisive importance, since the rapid decrease in frequency begins during the first few months of life.

Female preponderance in UTI is usually attributed to the short female urethra. The successive change of the sex ratio with age demonstrated in Table 92-2 is hardly compatible with this view. It is more suggestive of a successive functional maturation of some defense mechanism or disappear-

Table 92-2. Sex Ratio at Time of First Nonobstructive Urinary Tract Infection in Different Age Groups

Age Group	Female-Male Ratio
First mo	0.4
2–6 mo	1.5
7–12 mo	4
2–3 yr	10
4–11 yr	9

ance of a predisposing factor developing at different rates in the two sexes.

Meatal Stenosis, Bladder Neck Obstruction,
Incomplete Bladder Emptying,
Vesicoureteral Reflux

So-called bladder neck obstruction and urethral meatal stenosis have often been mentioned as major causes of recurrent infections. Critical evaluation suggests that these conditions play little, if any, role [49]. Incomplete emptying of the urinary system [72, 73] may encourage infection in some patients, especially in those with posterior urethral valves, ureterocele, bladder diverticula, neurogenic disorders, and calculus. This group is very small.

Vesicoureteral reflux has also been incriminated as a factor facilitating infection of the bladder. With the possible exception of gross reflux, evidence seems to be more against than for this hypothesis [31, 49]. The role of *reflux* in pyelonephritis is dealt with under that heading.

Cooling, Hygiene, Social Conditions,
and Genetic Factors

Although it is well known that cooling may provoke urgency, there is no evidence that it predisposes to infection. General hygienic and socioeconomic conditions do not appear to play a role [102]. Acute respiratory infections have been reported to precede UTI in 13 percent of cases [102]. Black girls may be more resistant to infection than white girls [50], which suggests that a genetic factor may be operating.

Immune Response and Bacterial Adhesion to the
Epithelial Surface of the Urogenital Sphere

Since simple anatomic and hygienic explanations for repeated reinfections have been largely abandoned, more biologic pathogenetic explanations have been sought.

Immune Response. A gram-negative infection of the urinary tract elicits both a general and a local immune response. The humoral response has been extensively studied, whereas little is known about the cell-mediated response. So far no immune defects have been demonstrated in patients with increased susceptibility to infections. Immunodiffusion studies have shown that, in addition to the O, K, and H antigens, at least some 20 antigens from an *E. coli* strain may elicit antibody synthesis. These antibodies might differ with regard to immune globulin class and avidity, which will explain why, for example, indirect hemagglutination and direct agglutination methods sometimes give different results. The antibody synthesis induced by gram-negative bacteria is not only IgM,

but also IgG. The latter occurs especially after several infections. The commonly used agglutination methods favor IgM antibodies and underestimate IgG; therefore, direct measurement of antibodies yields more accurate information about the distribution of Ig classes.

IgM antibodies against the O antigen may be protective, as judged from experimental studies. IgG antibodies may form antigen-antibody complexes, which may fix complement and, at least theoretically, cause renal damage. Antibodies against K_1 capsular antigen are of interest, since they may induce host tolerance to the infecting organism.

Urine from normal humans contains antibodies. Patients with repeated infections have an augmented excretion. These antibodies are of the IgG and IgA class and are probably synthesized locally. In recurrent infection of the renal parenchyma, antibody-producing cells are demonstrable. It thus seems as if a defect in local antibody response cannot explain increased liability to recurrent infections. Local antibodies may play a clinical role by inhibiting bacterial adhesion to epithelial surfaces and contributing to selection of less virulent strains.

Determination of serum antibody response is a good method for localizing the infection, but it is of limited value in the management of individual patients. Although persistently high titers are sometimes seen in patients with severe renal damage [2], their significance is unknown. The presence of antibody-coated bacteria in the urinary sediment has been demonstrated and claimed to indicate a renal infection. An extensive review of the present knowledge of immune response in urinary tract infections has been published [34, 37].

Periurethral Flora. Because the proximity of the anal and urethral openings would favor ascending infections, a highly efficient local defense mechanism has been assumed, and a first line of defense may be located in the periurethral area. Dense colonization of gram-negative bacteria is only exceptionally found in this area in healthy boys and girls over 4 to 5 years of age [14] and also in adult females [101]. The mechanism by which this area clears bacteria is unknown. By contrast, in UTI-prone girls there is often a high density of gram-negative bacteria, often several species at one time in the periurethral area, even between infections. Infections typically are preceded by periurethral colonization with the infecting organism. When proneness to infection eventually disappears, as it does in many patients, the liability to periurethral colonization seems to vanish as well [15]. These observations would suggest that proneness to urinary infection runs parallel to a defect of some unknown mechanism that normally clears the periurethral region of gram-negative bacteria. The typical age and sex distribution in Figs. 92-4 and 92-6 might be explained by the maturation of such a factor.

Bacterial characteristics may also play a role in colonization by encouraging adherence to the epithelial lining [23, 60, 90]. There is, in fact, a specificity of the ability of different bacterial species to adhere to the cell surfaces; for example, *E. coli* adheres better to urinary than to oral epithelium [23].

Clinical Features

GENERAL ASPECTS

The clinical features of UTI are influenced by several factors, including the age and sex of the patient, the presence of anatomic disorders of the urinary tract, the localization of the infection, the number of earlier infections, and the time interval since the last infection. A febrile infection almost always indicates a renal infection, which may be present, however, in the absence of any symptoms.

The more infections a patient has had earlier, or the closer a recurrence follows upon an earlier infection, the less the symptoms seem to be. These relationships may be due to tolerance to endotoxin [61, 62] or to the effect of antibodies to lipid A [37]. Another explanation might be that recurrent infections are often caused by bacteria with a deficient cell wall rendering them [56] less virulent [79] (see Table 92-7). Bacteria such as enterococci, *Proteus, Pseudomonas,* and staphylococci often cause fewer symptoms than infections caused by *E. coli.*

Increased blood urea nitrogen or arterial hypertension in patients above the age of 2 months almost always indicates the existence of bilateral hydronephrosis or advanced renal parenchymal reduction.

In the cystourethral syndrome or urethritis in children with symptoms of urgency, burning, and pain on micturition or daytime enuresis, the urine may be sterile in spite of the presence of pyuria. If tuberculosis can be disregarded, this finding suggests an inflammation of the urinary or genital tract, but not a bacterial UTI. Such patients should not be classified as having UTI only on the basis of symptomatology and pyuria.

SYMPTOMATOLOGY IN RELATION TO SEX, AGE, AND PRESENCE OF OBSTRUCTION

Neonatal Infections (1 to 30 Days)
It is generally thought, but by no means proved, that symptomatic neonatal UTI is a manifestation of a generalized septicemia. The symptomatology is varied [10] (Table 92-3). Some symptoms may precede positive urinary findings by several days. Classic symptoms such as sluggishness, feeding difficulties, irritability, and tenderness upon touching may be noted. A change of an initially normal weight curve may often be noted before any other symptoms and can focus early attention on the possibility of a urinary infection. An abnormally slow weight gain may be noted for several weeks after successful treatment. The central nervous system symptoms (see Table 92-5) consist of generalized convulsions with loss of consciousness, marked hypotonicity or irritability, respiratory inadequacy, and absent or barely elicitable primitive reflexes. Pleocytosis of the spinal fluid without demonstrable bacterial meningitis was found in one-third of those who had a spinal tap. In this series bacteremia was found in 50 percent of those investigated; blood urea was increased in 20 percent. There may be marked oliguria and a transient increase in renal size.

Girls and Boys from About 1 Month to 3 Years of Age, with or without Obstruction
In infants 1 to 3 months old, acute symptomatic infections, especially the first, often appear with fever. Meningisms, irritability, and hypersensitivity of the skin to touch are common symptoms, as are abdominal pains, vomiting, a certain pale or even gray color of the skin, and malodorous diapers. A few patients have macroscopic hematuria; otherwise, symptoms or findings pointing to the urinary tract are usually lacking. Failure to thrive (feeding difficulties, sluggishness, poor weight

Table 92-3. Prominent Symptoms in Neonatal (0–30 Days) Nonobstructive Urinary Tract Infection

Symptom	Percent (N = 75)
Weight loss*	76
Fever	49
Cyanosis or gray color	40
Distended abdomen	16
Central nervous system symptoms (purulent meningitis not included)	23
History of generalized convulsions	7
Purulent meningitis	8
Jaundice (conjugated bilirubin increased)	7
Other	16

* Registered only for 46 patients falling ill on days 0–10. Weight loss was not explained by vomiting, diarrhea, or refusal to eat.

gain, abdominal discomfort) is a leading feature of UTI during the first few years of life.

Older Girls without Obstruction

With increasing age, urinary tract symptoms in girls, including enuresis, become more frequent during UTI, as does abdominal discomfort. Pains over the loins appear later during childhood, but tenderness on palpation over the loins may be noted at a rather young age.

Older Boys without Obstruction

Boys above the age of 1 to 2 years often have still fewer general symptoms of UTI. Fever is seen in half or less of the patients, even if they have an apparent first infection. When present, fever is often moderate. Macroscopic or microscopic hematuria is common [9]. Pain on micturition or urgency may be present. Coliform bacteria do not dominate etiologically to the same extent as in girls. *Proteus* and other atypical bacteria are relatively frequent invaders. An apparent late onset infection in older boys usually represents a recurrence [9].

Infections Complicated by Obstruction

When complicated by a congenital malformation causing bilateral hydronephrosis, infection usually starts during the first few months of life. In patients with acquired obstruction, the onset of infection may be at any age. The presenting features are those of infantile infections. On physical examination, a distended bladder or a mass in the loin may be found. When an acute UTI is associated with arterial hypertension, dehydration, a high blood urea, or electrolyte disturbances (including acidosis), an obstructive complication should be suspected [24, 64]. Straining at micturition, dribbling, or a poor urinary stream that is often voided intermittently, characterize urethral obstruction; however, the symptoms may be absent even if obstruction is marked.

Reflux

Vesicoureteral reflux is a pathologic phenomenon, except possibly during the first few weeks of life, when studies of healthy subjects are few. Reflux may be congenital or acquired; in some instances, it may possibly be genetically determined [22]. Any evaluation of the importance of reflux must consider its grade. Smellie et al. recognized four grades, taking into account whether reflux takes place only during micturition or also at other times (free) [91]. A classification not accounting for whether reflux is free or not is proposed in Fig. 92-7. Grades I and II seem to be of little or no importance. Grade IV (gross reflux) bears a risk of renal damage. With lesser dilatation (grade III) the risk seems to diminish [83]. The demarcation between grade III and grade IV is indefinite. Scott [88] therefore distinguishes only between two grades, that is, reflux with and without dilatation.

Two effects have been ascribed to reflux, namely that it may facilitate recurrent infections by preventing complete emptying of the bladder, and that it predisposes to renal scarring by effectively transporting bacteria from the bladder up into the kidney tissue. Evidence supporting the first effect is weaker [31, 49] than that for the latter, which is well established. Whether gross reflux itself damages the kidney is debatable; however, when associated with infection, the risk is considerable [26, 92, 94]. The exact significance of reflux in the pathogenesis of renal scarring remains unsettled, however. Children with severely scarred kidneys often have gross reflux [26, 40]. On the other hand, children with reflux and infection only occasionally develop scarring when followed prospectively, the risk of renal damage increasing

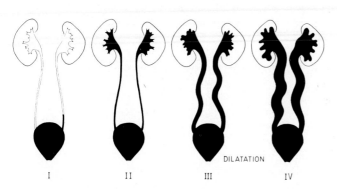

Figure 92-7. Grades of reflux, not taking into account whether reflux is free or not. (From Winberg et al. [115].)

with the grade of reflux [13, 26, 115]. This sequence suggests that in addition to infection and gross vesicoureteral reflux, another factor must be operative to cause renal damage.

Williams [109] was the first to suggest that in children with reflux the difference between kidneys with and without focal scars might be a difference in local defense at the level of the papillae. Hodson et al. [39, 41] showed that intrarenal reflux could occur in the multipapillary kidney of the pig and cause a renal scar. Rolleston et al. [82] found that in infants gross vesicoureteral reflux associated with intrarenal reflux and infection was predictive of future renal damage in the area with intrarenal reflux. Ransley and Risdon [76–78] have explored the anatomic basis of intrarenal reflux and found that in pigs as well as in humans, the collecting ducts open at the renal papillae with either slitlike orifices or round ones. The slitlike openings appear on the cone-shaped single papillae, while the circular openings are found in the center of the area cribrosa of the conglomerate or fused papillae. When pressure in the renal pelvis and calyces was increased in the experimental animal, the slitlike orifices tended to become occluded, while the gaping orifices of the compound papillae in the flat or even concave area cribrosa tended to remain open and contrast was forced into the renal parenchyma. This mechanism seems very simple and would explain why gross reflux is not invariably associated with renal damage, since conglomerate papillae with gaping orifices are not always present; it also would explain why the highest frequency of scarring is in the upper pole, less in the lower, and least in the midzone of the kidney. These frequencies of scars follow the distribution of conglomerate papillae in human kidneys.

If congenital anatomic variants were the only prerequisite for scarring, however, one would expect similar frequencies of scarring in various series of patients, which seems not to be the case. Ten percent were reported to have focal scars in one series with abacteriuric girls [55], some 25 percent in others [66, 86], and only 4.5 percent among girls followed after a symptomatic infection, which in most instances was febrile [111].

It is probable that renal scarring has multifactorial causes, with intrarenal reflux being one important factor (see Renal Focal Scar—"Chronic Pyelonephritis").

Management of vesicoureteral reflux is still controversial, and to quote Scott [89], "decisions still tend to be based on personal experience rather than applied scientific knowledge." There is general agreement on the importance of early diagno-

sis, control of infection, assessment of renal status, and surgery in selected patients, mainly in those with progressive dilatation of the pelvis and minor calyces. Our approach is to follow patients closely and to carry out frequent assessment of morphologic and functional states of the kidneys. If reflux is massive, renal growth is impaired, concentrating capacity is persistently low, or infection cannot be controlled, consideration is given to surgical intervention. There is a great tendency for reflux to disappear spontaneously [92]. Surgery should therefore not be too readily attempted. Excellent brief position papers on vesicoureteral reflux have recently been published [29, 94, 107].

Renal Focal Scar—"Chronic Pyelonephritis"
DIAGNOSTIC CRITERIA AND PATHOGENESIS
Infections may cause retardation of renal growth, focal scars, or both. Such changes may also have causes other than infection. A scar is wedge-shaped, with the tip in the papilla and a distinct demarcation from healthy renal tissue [35]. The cause of this is uncertain; the distribution of intrarenal reflux, as well as vascular or immunologic barriers, have been incriminated. In any case the distribution clearly suggests the ascending nature of the infection.

Radiologic criteria for the diagnosis of pyelonephritis have been defined by Hodson and Wilson [42] and consist of a papillary lesion, in the most advanced cases with "clubbing," and a corresponding defect of the renal outline. It may take up to 24 months for a scar to become visible radiographically [26]. Differentiation from congenital renal dysplasia may be difficult, and the diagnosis should rest on strictly defined histologic criteria [12].

The growing human kidney seems to be much more vulnerable to focal scarring than that of the adult. This has also been shown in the experimental animal [5]. Particularly vulnerable are kidneys of small children with gross reflux [26, 92].

Scars may already be present on the first radiographic examination. Smellie and Normand [94] rightly point out that in such instances the damage is either congenital or that the first infection, initiating the damage, went unrecognized. The last possibility is strongly favored, since scarring and renal growth retardation [113] are less commonly seen on the first radiograph in infantile infections than when the first recognized infection occurs at an older age (Table 92-4).

The pathogenesis of scar formation is obscure. Most onset infections in infants and small children are febrile and seem to involve the renal paren-

Table 92-4. Renal Lesion Seen on the First X-ray in 38 Patients with Focal Scar at Follow-up

First Recognized Infection	With Scar at First X-ray
Before 1 yr (N = 16)	3
After 1 yr (N = 22)	12

chyma. Yet, in one study of 20 patients in only 1 was a scar visible radiographically [111], and other studies have reported 1 in 5 [58]. Boys may run a much greater risk than girls [111]. Thus factors other than infection of the renal parenchyma seem to be decisive. Massive intrarenal reflux seems to be one important scar-promoting factor (see under Reflux), but age of onset of infection, sex, presence of obstruction, pattern of immune response, early diagnosis, and adequate antibiotic treatment and checkup may be equally important. As a matter of fact, scarring developed four times more often and progressed more rapidly when the first pyelonephritis attack was not properly diagnosed and treated than when it was handled properly [113]. This view is supported by other studies [31, 92].

Other factors that have been incriminated as inducing renal damage are persistence of bacterial antigen; formation of immune complexes with complement fixation; cross-reactions between kidney and certain *E. coli* antigens with formation of autoantibodies; infections with especially invasive strains rich in K_1 antigen [30, 46]; and a direct toxic effect of lipid A [108]. The possible role of such mechanisms in the pathogenesis of renal scar formation has been reviewed recently [34, 37].

Although there is often a correlation between the number of pyelonephritic attacks and the risk of scarring, it is also striking how silently even severe renal destruction may develop [2, 66]. In such cases there may have been a very early acute attack of pyelonephritis that was unrecognized or not remembered [2].

Diagnosis, Therapy, and Follow-up
GENERAL MANAGEMENT
The goal of management of UTI is to prevent progressive renal disease. The physician's first concern should be to look for evidence of obstruction of the urinary flow. The genital organs and the abdomen, especially the suprapubic area, must be examined thoroughly. A distended bladder, a mass in the loin, arterial hypertension, a high blood urea nitrogen or creatinine, or electrolyte disturbances (including acidosis) should evoke suspicion of an obstruction [24]. The main key to differentiation between obstructed and nonobstructed infections is the response to treatment. If the temperature is not normalized after 2 to 3 days of therapy and the urinary sediment is not cleared after 4 to 5 days, it is highly likely either that the bacteria are resistant to the antibiotic given or that there is an obstruction. The same is true if the renal concentrating capacity does not return toward normal within 3 weeks. Such patients should have a full radiologic investigation as soon as possible.

If a urethral obstruction is suspected on physical examination, the patient should have a retention catheter until expert evaluation can be performed. If urethral obstruction is confirmed, the catheter should be left in place until a free urinary flow is established surgically. Direct drainage of a unilaterally obstructed renal pelvis may sometimes be necessary. It should be remembered that infection in itself may cause moderate dilatation of ureters and pelves [81, 103] due to damage to muscles or interference with the transmission of neural impulses.

If the patient is severely ill or dehydrated, an intravenous drip should be set up and treatment begun at once. Appropriate antimicrobials should be given parenterally as soon as urine culture has been collected.

GENERAL POINTS ON ANTIBIOTIC THERAPY
A 10-day course of a suitable antibiotic will eradicate infection in close to 100 percent of cases, provided that the bacteria are sensitive. The high rate of recurrence after a short course of antibiotic treatment used to be interpreted as due to recrudescence of incompletely healed infections. This was the original basis of "long-term treatment," the idea being that bacteria in the renal tissue could be eradicated only after therapy for weeks or months. This reason for long-term treatment is rarely, if ever, relevant, since most recurrences are reinfections; that is, therapy of the foregoing infection has been effective, but new bacteria have invaded [11]. Even when recurrences appear within 2 to 3 days after discontinuation of therapy, they are usually due to reinfection. The current approach, therefore, is to try to eradicate the infection by a short course of an antimicrobial agent, and, in selected cases, to continue with small dosages of antibiotics to prevent reinfection. Some authors prefer to put all patients on long-term prophylaxis [71]; others select for such a regimen only those who have had repeated infections at very short intervals [50, 114]. Infants and toddlers with a grade IV reflux, however, possibly should be given prophylaxis even before they

have demonstrated a liability to recurrence (see under Reflux).

Although the majority of recurrences are reinfections, a few are not. These represent either an unresolved bacteriuria or persistence of bacteria in a focus unamenable to antibiotics (see Bacterial Persistence, above). A change of drug or dosage helps in most instances of unresolved bacteriuria, whereas surgical treatment is required in most instances of obstruction. Whether or not bacteria may persist in the renal parenchyma is debatable. If so, bactericidal drugs in high doses for long periods may be tried [16].

INITIAL TREATMENT OF ACUTE INFECTIONS

The choice of antimicrobial drug and duration of treatment should be considered in relation to the individual patient, with attention to whether there have been single episodes with long intervals or frequently repeated infections; whether the patient is severely dehydrated and vomiting; whether he has a neurogenic bladder or renal insufficiency; or whether the patient is a newborn. With all drugs, 10 days of therapy seems to be enough to eradicate infection, irrespective of whether there is renal involvement or not. Shorter courses may work as well, but this has not been established in properly performed studies. Nighttime doses requiring awakening of the child are not needed.

Single Episodes of Symptomatic Infections Separated by Long Intervals

Sulfonamide still holds its position as a good first choice in patients with single episodes of UTI, whether they have pyelonephritis or so-called cystitis. In vivo sulfonamide resistance is uncommon in these patients, as contrasted to those with frequently recurring infections, but local differences may exist. Cure of the infection will follow a 10-day course in close to 100 percent of cases [113]. In addition to effectiveness, solubility, frequency of side reactions, and costs should guide the choice of the sulfonamide compound. Preparations with a short excretion time, such as sulfisoxazole (Gantrisin) and sulfasomidine (Elkosin), have a high solubility in urine, and allergic reactions are infrequent. Garrod and O'Grady [27] recommend these two drugs in urinary infections. These authors point out that sulfamethazine (Sulfamezathine), which is widely used in some centers, may have a lower potency than other rapidly excreted sulfonamide compounds. Sulfonamide preparations with long or half-long excretion times do not seem to hold any advantages. Even with rapidly excreted drugs the antibacterial activity of urine remains

high for 12 to 24 hr or even 46 hr following a single dose, as was shown in Fig. 92-2 [105]. There is also some evidence that the concentration of antibiotics in urine is more important than the concentration in blood [99, 100]. Considering these circumstances, it is possible that dose intervals can be considerably prolonged. Studies to test this possibility have not been performed.

In addition to sulfonamide, other suitable drugs for treating UTI are nitrofurantoin, nalidixic acid, trimethoprim sulfamethoxazole, and ampicillin and related penicillin substances. Indications, doses, and complications for all these agents are listed in Table 92-5. Nitrofurantoin is a very suitable drug, especially in regard to its limited ecologic effects (see Bacterial Etiology and Pattern of Resistance). There are, however, no controlled studies on its efficiency in treating acute febrile pyelonephritis. Gastrointestinal side effects will be few with a recommended dose of 3 mg/kg/24 hr. Allergic pulmonary reactions and pulmonary fibrosis have been reported with increasing frequency. These reactions, however, are rare in children. Nitrofurantoin is ineffective when the glomerular filtration rate is reduced to 50 percent or less of normal. The rapid development of resistance to nalidixic acid in a previously sensitive bacterial population [84] seems to occur mainly with underdosage [96]. The combination of trimethoprim with a sulfonamide (Septra, Bactrim) has become widely used during recent years. Both compounds interfere with bacterial folate metabolism but on different levels, and they have a synergistic effect in vitro. This effect, if it occurs in vivo, may be of benefit in treating infections resistant to sulfonamides. The value of these drugs seems now to be well established. Doses of 5 to 7 mg per kilogram of body weight of trimethoprim and 25 to 35 mg per kilogram of body weight of sulfamethoxazole twice daily for 8 to 12 days have been used. The pharmacokinetics of this new drug in infants and small children have not been sufficiently investigated.

Trimethoprim, unlike other antimicrobial substances, seems to concentrate by nonionic diffusion across vaginal as well as prostatic epithelium. This property of the drug may play a major role in treatment and especially in prevention of certain urinary infections [97, 98].

Checkup After Therapy

The first checkup should be done when therapy has been discontinued for 2 to 3 days; the second should be carried out 2 to 3 weeks later. The third, fourth, and fifth checkups are spread over the first year after the infection. If possible, the patients

Table 92-5. Drugs of Choice in Management of Urinary Tract Infection

Drug	Dose (mg/kg body weight/24 hr*)	No. of Doses/Day	Duration of Therapy (days)	Remarks
Short-acting sulfonamide:				
Sulfisoxazole	100–200	4	10	Not to be used as long as neonatal jaundice persists
Sulfasomidin	100	4	10	
Nitrofurantoin	3	4	10	Not to be used first month of life; not effective when GFR 50 percent of normal or less; pulmonary side reactions reported with increasing frequency; seems so far to be rare in children. Limited ecologic side effects
Nalidixic acid	60	3–4	10	Not to be used in newborns. Dose at 1–4 mo of age 30 mg/kg/24 hr. Rise in intracranial pressure described in infants and children
Trimethoprim sulfamethoxazole	6 30	3–4	10	Not to be used before 6 weeks of life. Experience with this drug limited in infants and toddlers. Diffuses into prostate and vagina
Ampicillin Pivampicillin Amoxicillin	50–100 25–50 25–50	3–4	10	Neonatal infections often caused by *Klebsiella,* resistant to ampicillin. Gastrointestinal complications very common with ampicillin

* First dose upon awakening, last dose at bedtime, one or two doses in between; night doses are not necessary.
Note: GFR = glomerular filtration rate.

should be followed for several years thereafter. Note that whenever chemotherapy has been given, the drug should be omitted for 2 to 3 days before each checkup; otherwise, evaluation of negative or doubtfully positive cultures will be difficult.

MANAGEMENT OF RECURRENT INFECTIONS

The etiology and resistance pattern in recurrent infections is more variable than in single infections. If the patient's condition permits, therapy should be postponed until the resistance of the bacteria has been determined. If immediate therapy is imperative, a different drug is used than that in the preceding infection. Prophylaxis is carried through after treatment in patients with frequent reinfections. Nitrofurantoin is the drug of choice for this purpose because of its insignificant effect on the gastrointestinal flora [114]. Dosage is 1 mg/kg/24 hr, divided into one morning and one evening dose. An alternative drug is nalidixic acid, 20 mg/kg/24 hr. Trimethoprim-sulfamethoxazole may be a good alternative, since it may keep the vestibular area clean [98].

With regard to duration of prophylaxis, a trial-and-error approach is suggested. Treatment is started for a period of 2 to 4 months. If a recurrence occurs shortly after stopping prophylaxis, a new therapeutic course is given for 10 days, and this is followed by prophylaxis for half a year. Prophylaxis is then discontinued, and the patient

is followed with repeated cultures and other examinations. Some patients need prophylaxis for several years.

Checkups are done 2 to 3 days after each therapeutic course and at each or every second or third month during prophylaxis, depending on the liability to recurrence. The use of dipslide cultures [4] facilitates checkups for both patients and doctor.

MANAGEMENT OF INFECTIONS IN PATIENTS WITH NEUROGENIC BLADDERS, SPECIFICALLY WITH MYELOMENINGOCELE

Organic obstructive changes may complicate disorders such as neurogenic bladder, and the urinary problems therefore should be managed by pediatricians and urologists in close cooperation. The etiology and the type of infecting bacteria and their patterns of resistance are unpredictable. In nonacute infections, therapy is best postponed until the results of culture and sensitivity tests are available. Antimicrobial therapy should be given to patients who have urinary symptoms, a high sedimentation rate, or nonspecific symptoms such as fatigue or anorexia without other obvious explanations. Antimicrobial treatment of asymptomatic infections in these patients is probably of little value. Recurrences, which usually are reinfections, are almost impossible to prevent by prophylaxis. Application of an antiseptic ointment over the urethral orifice has been tried unsuccessfully. Continence training of children with neurogenic bladder dysfunction using pharmacologic agents to increase bladder volume, relax the external sphincter, and stimulate detrusor contraction may prove to be helpful [70].

MANAGEMENT OF INFECTIONS IN NEWBORNS

Urinary tract infections in newborns are sometimes part of a generalized septicemia. A combination of gentamicin and ampicillin is then a good choice for treatment. The glomerular filtration rate is often severely reduced by infection, so the concentration in serum of any potentially toxic drug should be followed. If renal infection is the only manifestation, ampicillin in a dosage of 100 to 200 mg per kilogram of body weight may be sufficient. If response is not prompt, therapy should be changed, since *Klebsiella* and Enterobacteriaceae organisms are common pathogens in this age group. When diagnosed early, neonatal *E. coli* pyelonephritis has a good prognosis [10]. Infections at this age are often caused by *E. coli* with a K_1 antigen that seems to be a virulence factor [80]. Recommendations regarding the use of gentamicin are given by Nelson and McCracken [68].

MANAGEMENT OF PATIENTS WITH RENAL INSUFFICIENCY AND URINARY INFECTION

The ideal qualities of an antimicrobial agent for patients with urinary infection and renal insufficiency can be summarized as follows: (1) rapid renal excretion, (2) low toxicity, even in high serum concentrations, (3) slow metabolism by the liver, (4) no alternative pathways of excretion. Ampicillin is a suitable drug if therapy must be started before antibiotic sensitivity results are obtained. Sulfonamides with short half-lives are preferable to those with a long half-life. Nitrofurantoin should not be used. Gentamicin can be used with great caution if dosage is guided by determination of concentrations in serum.

CHEMOTHERAPY, FECAL FLORA, AND TRANSMISSIBLE CHEMORESISTANCE (R-FACTORS)

The management of UTI is seriously hampered by the increasing frequency of infections caused by organisms with resistance mediated by R factor. Urinary infections caused by such strains are *preceded* by their appearance in feces and in the periurethral flora [114]. Selective antibiotic usage has been shown to favor intestinal colonization with resistant mutants present in the environment. This is seen with sulfonamide [114], tetracycline [19],

ampicillin [20], and probably with most other antibiotics, with one, nitrofurantoin, being the one proved exception [114]. The influence of environment on bacterial selection has also been suggested. The difference in the effects of these various antibiotics on physiologic bacterial reservoirs explains the common failure of long-term prophylaxis with sulfonamide and the good effect of nitrofurantoin [59, 74, 114]. The influence on the periurethral flora [114] may be especially relevant, since bacterial colonization of this area may be a predecessor to bladder infection [15, 101]. Since enteric bacilli other than *E. coli* are often resistant to nitrofurantoin, nitrofurantoin may be less suitable for prophylaxis in heavily contaminated hospital wards.

Recurrences following nitrofurantoin treatment are often caused by the same strain as that causing the preceding infection. Such cases used to be considered relapses of persisting renal infection, but the identity of organisms in two consecutive infections separated by treatment with nitrofurantoin is probably explained better by reinfection from an unchanged fecal and periurethral reservoir.

The problem of resistant urinary infections should be considered in the light of the influence of therapy on the intestinal and periurethral flora. The evaluation of any drug used for treatment of UTI should be done with regard to its effect on the physiologic bacterial reservoirs. Progress is not bound to come from the introduction of more and more potent drugs. It is more apt to come from the use of drugs with limited ecologic effects. Since resistance to nitrofurantoin, nalidixic acid [96], and trimethoprim [32] rarely is mediated by R factor, these drugs may offer some advantages for prophylaxis. Possibly there will also be a renaissance in the use of agents such as methenamine mandelate [36].

Course and Prognosis

The course and prognosis of UTI are influenced by age at onset, sex, earlier history, and the presence or absence of reflux and obstruction. The prognosis can be evaluated at three levels: the risk of recurrence, the risk of scarring, and the risk for development of hypertension and uremia. The statistics given below are from a prospective study in which the patients were diagnosed, treated, and checked at the apparent first infection [111, 113]. Prognosis may be worse where initial infection has not been recognized.

INFECTIONS COMPLICATED BY OBSTRUCTION

The nature of the obstruction, the success of surgical intervention, and the time lapse between onset of infection and establishment of adequate drainage are the main factors determining the degree of permanent renal damage. If such damage occurs and is bilateral, it may manifest itself clinically as sodium-losing nephropathy, acidosis necessitating treatment with sodium bicarbonate, or uremia.

Repeated infections occur in some patients although the obstruction is removed. In these patients, as in others with frequent recurrences, absence of either symptoms or pyuria never excludes infection. Checking these patients only by history or examination of urinary sediment is inadequate (see Chap. 96).

GIRLS WITHOUT OBSTRUCTION FALLING ILL BEYOND THE NEWBORN PERIOD

Recurrence Rate

The most characteristic feature of girls with UTI beyond the newborn period is their liability to develop recurrent UTI, which often continues for many years, sometimes for decades [58]. In such cases it is not the infection but the inclination to acquire repeated infection that is chronic. This distinction is essential with regard to therapy.

The risk of recurrence is about 30 percent within 1 year and is probably somewhat below 50 percent within the first 5 years after onset of infection. An unexplained feature is that reinfections tend to accumulate soon after the preceding infection. The risk of recurrence seems to increase with the number of preceding infections, up to 75 percent (see Fig. 92-5). This suggests that the postulated defect of the defense mechanism varies in degree of severity.

In patients whose disease is detected by screening, the risk of recurrence was 80 percent, irrespective of the number of preceding periods of treatment [51], and thus was about the same as in patients with several symptomatic infections. These figures fit the hypothesis that girls with asymptomatic bacteriuria represent a selected group with a great liability to asymptomatic infection following early symptomatic ones.

There seems to be no obvious correlation between age, localization of infection, presence or absence of reflux, and liability to recurrence. A possible exception, though, is patients with gross reflux. In patients with asymptomatic bacteriuria there was a positive correlation between residual urine volume, even if small, and liability to infection [54].

Scarring

A young girl falling ill with her first acute, symptomatic urinary tract infection may run a risk of

Table 92-6. Radiologic Scarring in Girls with Symptomatic and Asymptomatic Bacteriuria

	Percent with Scarring	
Bacteriuria	England	Sweden
Symptomatic	13[a, b] (N = 281)	4.5[c, d] (N = 440)
Asymptomatic	26[e] (N = 296)	10[f] (N = 119)

[a] Referred with a history of recurrent infection.
[b] Recalculated from J. M. Smellie and I. C. S. Normand, Experience of Follow-up of Children with Urinary Tract Infection. In F. O'Grady and W. Brumfitt (eds.), *Urinary Tract Infection,* London: Oxford University Press, 1968. P. 123.
[c] Followed introspectively from first symptomatic infection.
[d] From J. Winberg, H. J. Andersen, T. Bergström, B. Jacobsson, H. Larson, and K. Lincoln, Epidemiology of symptomatic urinary tract infection in childhood. *Acta Paediatr. Scand.* [Suppl. 252] 63:1, 1974.
[e] From D. C. L. Savage, M. I. Wilson, M. McHardy, D. A. E. Dewar, and W. M. Fee, Covert bacteriuria of childhood: A clinical and epidemiological study. *Arch. Dis. Child.* 48:8, 1973.
[f] From U. Lindberg, I. Claesson, L. Å. Hanson, and U. Jodal, Asymptomatic bacteriuria in schoolgirls. I. Clinical and laboratory findings. *Acta Paediatr. Scand.* 64:425, 1975a.

some 5 percent of developing a scar (Table 92-6) (the risk for a boy ranges from 10 to 15 percent). These figures are for children in whom the infection is diagnosed, treated, and checked [111]. However, scars are often present already at the first examination, especially in boys (see Renal Focal Scar); in clinical reports of patients not selected during apparent first infections, the frequency of scarring is considerably greater [58, 93]. A 25 percent frequency of scarring in asymptomatic bacteriuric girls, probably representing a selection of girls with an early unrecognized symptomatic infection, may estimate approximately the risk in untreated patients.

Clinically Severe Complications

It is unknown how often patients with recurrent infections will develop hypertension, uremia, tubular disorders, and obstructing stones. In the absence of obstruction, the risk for renal insufficiency and hypertension seems to be remote. However, since UTI is a common disease, the number of patients with renal insufficiency and hypertension due to renal infections is considerable. It is probable that patients with these complications are recruited from those with early childhood scarring. Complications of pregnancy, such as intrauterine fetal death and delivery of babies prematurely or small for gestational age, are another and probably more common consequence of childhood infection and renal damage.

NEONATAL INFECTIONS

Early Prognosis. Neonatal UTI infections seem to be part of a generalized bacteremia, the course of which will determine the early prognosis.

Recurrence Rate. Early recurrences during the months following the first UTI infection appear in about one-quarter of neonatal patients [10]. Recurrences after more than 1 year seem to be rare. This feature clearly distinguishes the infections appearing during the newborn period from those of older girls.

Scarring. The frequency of scarring following neonatal UTI infection is unknown. In the study mentioned above, it was seen in 2 of 75 patients.

BOYS FALLING ILL DURING FIRST YEAR OF LIFE (NEONATES EXCLUDED)

Early recurrences appear in these baby boys as they do in girls, but infant boys, like neonates, seem to grow out of their susceptibility to infection. It is thus rare to see a recurrence more than 1 year after the onset of infection [113]. Scarring may be more common than in girls.

OLDER BOYS (1 TO 16 YEARS) WITHOUT OBSTRUCTION

There seems to be no systematic observation of UTI in boys aged 1 to 16. Early recurrences do occur after onset infection, as in girls; late recurrences, however, are less common [9]. Focal renal scarring, sometimes extensive, is a common finding, even at the so-called first infection [9]. Whether such defects are congenital or acquired is unknown, but it is an attractive hypothesis that they are consequences of earlier unrecognized infections. In boys iterated reinfections are less common than in girls, and therefore they do not alert the physician.

The pathogenesis of the kind of UTI seen in girls and women without obstruction is unknown; however, more and more clearly the picture unfolds as a disease that (1) begins during the first or one of the first years of life; (2) in which the tendency to acquire UTI often remains for many years, perhaps for life; and (3) in which the prognosis to a great extent will be determined by the way the patient is cared for during infancy or childhood. Against this background, both increased knowledge of the clinical manifestations of the disease in infancy and improved, inexpensive diagnostic methods that are practical and usable by practitioners are very important.

Screening Bacteriuria (Asymptomatic, Covert, Symptomless)

GIRLS OF PRESCHOOL AND SCHOOL AGE

The definition of asymptomatic bacteriuria and the epidemiology in girls of this age are discussed under Epidemiology.

Clinical Findings

About one-third of the patients with asymptomatic bacteriuria have a past history of symptoms referable to the urinary tract; pyuria often is absent. Reflux is seen in 20 to 35 percent and focal renal scars in 10 to 25 percent [1, 51, 55, 66, 67] without any increase in frequency or progression between the ages of 4 and 16 years [66]. These findings suggest that asymptomatic bacteriuria does not cause appreciable damage, at least not after the age of 4 years.

The reason why infection is asymptomatic in some patients is not well understood. One possibility is an acquired endotoxin tolerance [61, 62], another that the cell wall lipopolysaccharides of the infecting bacteria have a deficient polysaccharide moiety [57] that may render the bacteria less virulent [79].

Bacteriology

There are prominent differences in *E. coli* isolated from patients with symptomatic pyelonephritis or cystitis and bacteria from those with asymptomatic bacteriuria (Table 92-7). Some of the differences may be due to selection of polysaccharide-deficient mutants as an adaptation to the infection or the

Table 92-7. Characteristics of E. coli *Strains Isolated from Patients with Pyelonephritis and Asymptomatic Bacteriuria*[a]

Characteristics of Urinary *E. coli*	Pyelonephritis (N = 119) (percent)	Asymptomatic Bacteriuria (N = 115) (percent)
O serogroups: O$_1$, O$_2$, O$_4$, O$_6$, O$_7$, O$_{16}$, O$_{18}$, O$_{75}$	80	31
Spontaneous agglutination	2	45
Serum bactericidal sensitivity		
Strains highly[b] resistant	69	12
Strains highly[c] sensitive	4	70

[a] From Lindberg et al. [57].
[b] Less than 50 percent of bacteria killed.
[c] More than 99 percent of bacteria killed.

local immune response of the host [34, 57]. After elimination of these mutants by therapy, the urinary tract may be invaded by intact bacteria from the fecal reservoir, which may explain why therapy in asymptomatic bacteriuria sometimes is followed by symptomatic recurrences [7, 53].

Localization of the actual infection is difficult. C-reactive protein may be more reliable than washout tests, sedimentation rate, concentrating capacity, or antibody determinations [56]. It is still uncertain how often the infection involves the renal parenchyma.

Therapy

A 7- to 10-day course of antibiotics eliminates infection in some 90 percent of girls with asymptomatic bacteriuria, but only 20 to 25 percent remain uninfected 1 to 2 years later [51, 53, 85, 106]. Spontaneous "cures" persisting for 1 year occur in about 10 percent [6, 106]. Treatment is followed by an increase of renal concentrating capacity in patients with scars or reflux [53] and growth of the healthy kidney when one is damaged [85]. The growth of the damaged kidney, however, seems to be the same whether or not treatment is given. Sometimes patients feel better after treatment, although they have not complained of any symptoms. On the other hand, restriction of chemotherapy may be indicated since, as mentioned above, pyelonephritis not infrequently follows elimination of an asymptomatic infection [7, 53]. Thus it is still controversial whether or not asymptomatic bacteriuria should be treated. At present it would seem reasonable to treat and follow patients with symptoms, even if slight, as well as patients with foul urine or gross reflux.

Course

The crucial question is whether asymptomatic bacteriuria is a forerunner of renal damage or whether it is a consequence of earlier symptomatic infections. Since renal scarring in asymptomatic bacteriuria patients is similar at 4 years and at 16 [66], the latter hypothesis seems more probable. Table 92-6 compared the frequency of renal scarring found in girls with symptomatic infections with that seen in girls with asymptomatic bacteriuria. Two interpretations for the lower incidence of scarring in symptomatic infections are possible. Either asymptomatic bacteriuria is a more serious disease than symptomatic infection, or patients with symptomatic infections have been diagnosed, treated, and checked, while the asymptomatic bacteriuria patients represent a group whose initial symptomatic infections have not been cared for. If so, performing screening programs may be a kind of medical archeology registering events that happened long ago. If screening programs are performed, patients should be submitted to complete radiologic examination until ongoing research has clarified the significance of asymptomatic bacteriuria. If resources are restricted, it seems more urgent to screen infants and small children with fever for urinary infections rather than to spend money on school screening programs. A similar position is also taken by Schwartz and Edelmann [87].

NEONATAL ASYMPTOMATIC BACTERIURIA

Several investigations (see reference 110) have shown that true but asymptomatic bacterial excretion in the urine may be seen in 1 to 3 percent of newborns, mainly boys. The significance of this finding is unknown. In some patients the bacteriuria may persist if untreated and may eventually cause overt symptoms after 1 to 2 months or more [52].

Neonatal asymptomatic bacteriuria, as well as symptomatic UTI, rarely occurs before day four or five after delivery, which may explain why some studies have revealed very few if any neonatal infections [21]. So far there is no clinical indication for screening healthy neonates, however, except possibly premature infants [21].

References

1. Anders, D., Anders, I., and Sitzmann, F. C. Feldstudie zur Epidemiologie inapparenter Harnweginfektionen bei Mädchen im Vorschulalter. *Med. Klin.* 69:1850, 1974.
2. Andersen, H. J., Jacobsson, B., Larson, H., and Winberg, J. Hypertension, asymmetric renal parenchymal defect, sterile urine and high *E. coli* antibody titre. *Br. Med. J.* 3:14, 1973.
3. Aperia, A., Berg, U., and Broberger, D. Control of sodium homeostasis in children with recurrent infections and reduced glomerular filtration rates. *Acta Paediatr. Scand.* 60:695, 1971.
4. Arneil, G. C., McAllister, T. A., and Kay, P. Measurement of bacteriuria by plane dipslide culture. *Lancet* 1:94, 1973.
5. Asscher, A. W., and Chick, S. Increased susceptibility of the kidney to ascending *Escherichia coli* infection following unilateral nephrectomy. *Br. J. Urol.* 44:202, 1972.
6. Asscher, A. W., McLachlan, M. S. F., Verrier-Jones, R., Meller, S., Sussman, M., and Harrison, S. Screening for asymptomatic urinary-tract infection in schoolgirls. *Lancet* 2:1, 1973.
7. Asscher, A. W., Sussman, M., Waters, W. E., Evans, J. A. S., Campbell, H., Evans, K. T., and Edmund, J. Asymptomatic bacteriuria in the non-pregnant woman: II. Response to treatment and follow-up. *Br. Med. J.* 1:804, 1969.
8. Berg, U., Aperia, A., and Broberger, O. Subclinical defects in renal regulation of acid base balance in children with recurrent urinary tract infections. *Acta Paediatr. Scand.* 60:521, 1971.

9. Bergström, T.   Sex differences in childhood: Urinary tract infection. *Arch. Dis. Child.* 47:227, 1972.

10. Bergström, T., Larson, H., Lincoln, K., and Winberg, J.   Studies of urinary tract infections in infancy and childhood: XII. Eighty consecutive patients with neonatal infection. *J. Pediatr.* 80:858, 1972.

11. Bergström, T., Lincoln, K., Ørskov, F., Ørskov, I., and Winberg, J.   Studies of urinary tract infections in infancy and childhood: VIII. Reinfection vs relapse. *J. Pediatr.* 71:13, 1967.

12. Bernstein, J.   Developmental Abnormalities of the Renal Parenchyma: Renal Hypoplasia and Dysplasia. In S. C. Sommers (ed.), *Pathology Annual 1968.* New York: Appleton-Century-Crofts, 1969.

13. Blank, E., and Girdany, B. R.   Prognosis with vesicoureteral reflux. *Pediatrics* 48:782, 1971.

14. Bollgren, I., and Winberg, J.   The periurethral aerobic bacterial flora in healthy boys and girls. *Acta Paediatr. Scand.* 65:74, 1976.

15. Bollgren, I., and Winberg, J.   The periurethral aerobic flora in girls highly susceptible to urinary infections. *Acta Paediatr. Scand.* 65:81, 1976.

16. Brumfitt, W., and Percival, A.   Laboratory control of antibiotic therapy in urinary tract infection. *Ann. N.Y. Acad. Sci.* 145:329, 1967.

17. Calcagno, P. L., D'Albora, J. B., Tina, L. U., Papadopoulou, Z. L., Deasy, P. F., and Hollerman, C. E.   Alterations in renal cortical blood flow in infants and children with urinary tract infections. *Pediatr. Res.* 2:332, 1968.

18. Carvajal, H. F., Passey, R. B., Berger, M., Travis, L. B., and Lorentz, W. B.   Urinary lactic dehydrogenase isoenzyme 5 in the differential diagnosis of kidney and bladder infections. *Kidney Int.* 8:176, 1975.

19. Daikos, G. K., Kontomichalou, P., Bilalis, D., and Pimenidou, L.   Intestinal flora ecology after oral use of antibiotics: Terramycin, chloramphenicol, ampicillin, neomycin, paromomycin, aminodidin. *Chemotherapia* 13:146, 1968.

20. Datta, N., Faiers, M. C., Reeves, D. S., Brumfitt, W., Ørskov, F., and Ørskov, I.   R-factors in *Escherichia coli* in faeces after oral chemotherapy in general practice. *Lancet* 1:312, 1971.

21. Edelmann, C. M., Jr., Ogwo, J. E., Fine, B. P., and Martinez, A. B.   The prevalence of bacteriuria in full-term and premature newborn infants. *J. Pediatr.* 82:125, 1973.

22. Editorial.   Vesicoureteral reflux and its familial distribution. *Br. Med. J.* 4:726, 1975.

23. Ellen, R. P., and Gibbons, R. J.   Parameters affecting the adherence and tissue tropisms of streptococcus pyogenes. *Infect. Immunol.* 9:85, 1974.

24. Ericsson, N. O., Winberg, J., and Zetterström, R.   Renal function in infantile obstructive uropathy. *Acta Paediatr.* 44:444, 1955.

25. Fairley, K. F., Carson, N. E., Gutch, R. C., Leighton, P., Grounds, A. D., Laird, E. C., McCallum, P. H. G., Sleeman, R. L., and O'Keefe, C. M.   Site of infection in acute urinary tract infection in general practice. *Lancet* 2:615, 1971.

26. Filly, R., Friedland, G. W., Govan, D. E., and Fair, W. R.   Development and progression of clubbing and scarring in children with recurrent urinary tract infections. *Radiology* 113:145, 1974.

27. Garrod, L. P., and O'Grady, F.   *Antibiotic and Chemotherapy.* Edinburgh: Livingstone, 1968.

28. Geisinger, J. F.   Intermittency of pyuria at the level of the renal papillae. *J. Urol.* 25:649, 1931.

29. Girdany, B. R., and Price, S. E.   Vesicoureteral reflux and renal scarring. *J. Pediatr.* 86:998, 1975.

30. Glynn, A. A., Brumfitt, W., and Howard, C. J.   K-antigens of *Escherichia coli* and renal involvement in urinary tract infections. *Lancet* 1:514, 1971.

31. Govan, D. E., Fair, W. R., Friedland, G. W., and Filly, R. A.   Urinary tract infections in children: III. Treatment of ureterovesical reflux. *Western Med. J.* 121:382, 1974.

32. Gruneberg, R. N., Leakey, A., Bendall, M. J., and Smellie, J. M.   Bowel flora in urinary tract infection: Effect of chemotherapy with special reference to cotrimoxazole. *Kidney Int.* 8:122, 1975.

33. Gruneberg, R. N., Leight, D. A., and Brumfitt, W.   *Escherichia coli* Serotypes in Urinary Tract Infection: Studies in Domiciliary, Antenatal and Hospital Practice. In F. O'Grady and W. Brumfitt (eds.), *Urinary Tract Infection.* London: Oxford University Press, 1968. P. 68.

34. Hanson, L. A., Ahlstedt, S., Jodal, U., Kaijser, B., Larsson, P., Lidin-Janson, G., Lincoln, K., Lindberg, U., Mattsby, I., Olling, S., Peterson, H., and Sohl, A.   The host-parasite relationship in urinary tract infections. *Kidney Int.* 8:28, 1975.

35. Heptinstall, R. H.   *Pathology of the Kidney.* Boston: Little, Brown, 1966. P. 421.

36. Holland, N. H., and West, C. D.   Prevention of recurrent urinary tract infections in girls. *Am. J. Dis. Child.* 105:560, 1963.

37. Holmgren, J., and Smith, J. W.   Immunological aspects of urinary tract infections. *Progr. Allergy* 18:289, 1975.

38. Hodson, C. J.   The kidneys in urinary infection. *Proc. R. Soc. Med.* 59:416, 1966.

39. Hodson, C. J.   Abstract 598. In *Proceedings of the 5th International Congress for Nephrology, 1972.*

40. Hodson, C. J., and Edwards, D.   Chronic pyelonephritis and vesicoureteric reflux. *Clin. Radiol.* 11:219, 1960.

41. Hodson, C. J., Maling, T. M. J., McManamon, P. J., and Lewis, M. G.   The pathogenesis of reflux nephropathy (chronic atrophic pyelonephritis). *Br. J. Radiol.* [Suppl. 13] 48:1, 1975.

42. Hodson, C. J., and Wilson, S.   Natural history of chronic pyelonephritic scarring. *Br. Med. J.* 2:191, 1965.

43. Houston, I. B.   Pus cell and bacterial counts in the diagnosis of urinary tract infections in childhood. *Arch. Dis. Child.* 38:600, 1963.

44. Jodal, U., Ahlstedt, S., Carlsson, B., Hanson, L. A., Lindberg, U., and Sohl, A.   Local antibodies in childhood urinary tract infection: A. Preliminary study. *Int. Arch. Allergy Appl. Immunol.* 117:537, 1974.

45. Jodal, U., Lindberg, U., and Lincoln, K.   Level diagnosis of symptomatic urinary tract infections in childhood. *Acta Paediatr. Scand.* 64:201, 1975.

46. Kaijser, B.   Immunology of *E. coli* strains with special reference to K-antigen and its relation to urinary tract infection. *J. Infect. Dis.* 127:670, 1973.

47. Kallings, L. O.   Medicinsk behandling av urinvägsinfektioner (1). Bakteriologisk översikt. *Sven. Lakartidningen* [Suppl. III] 65:30, 1968.

48. Kass, E. H.   Asymptomatic infection of the urinary tract. *Trans. Assoc. Am. Physicians* 69:56, 1956.

49. Kendall, A. R., and Karafin, L.   Urinary tract infec-

tion in children: Fact and fantasy. *J. Urol.* 107:1068, 1972.

50. Kunin, C. M. Pattern of Recurrent Urinary Tract Infections in Girls. In *Symposium on Pyelonephritis.* Edinburgh: Livingstone, 1966. P. 1.

51. Kunin, C. M., Deutscher, R., and Paquin, A. Urinary tract infection in school children: An epidemiologic, clinical and laboratory study. *Medicine* 43:91, 1964.

52. Lincoln, K., and Winberg, J. Studies of urinary tract infections in infancy and childhood: II. Quantitative estimation of bacteriuria in unselected neonates with special reference to the occurrence of asymptomatic infections. *Acta Paediatr. Scand.* 53: 307, 1964.

53. Lindberg, U. Asymptomatic bacteriuria in schoolgirls: V. The clinical course and response to treatment. *Acta Paediatr. Scand.* 64:718, 1975.

54. Lindberg, U., Bjure, J., Haugstvedt, S., and Jodal, U. Asymptomatic bacteriuria in schoolgirls: III. Relation between residual urine volume and recurrence. *Acta Paediatr. Scand.* 64:437, 1975.

55. Lindberg, U., Claesson, I., Hanson, L. Å., and Jodal, U. Asymptomatic bacteriuria in schoolgirls: I. Clinical and laboratory findings. *Acta Paediatr. Scand.* 64:425, 1975a.

56. Lindberg, U., Jodal, U., Hanson, L. Å., and Kaijser, B. Asymptomatic bacteriuria in schoolgirls: IV. Difficulties of level diagnosis and the possible relation to the character of infecting bacteria. *Acta Paediatr. Scand.* 64:574, 1975.

57. Lindberg, U., Hanson, L. Å., Jodal, U., Lidin-Janson, G., Lincoln, K., and Olling, S. Asymptomatic bacteriuria in schoolgirls: II. Differences in *Escherichia coli* causing asymptomatic and symptomatic bacteriuria. *Acta Paediatr. Scand.* 64:432, 1975.

58. Lindblad, B. S., and Ekengren, K. The long-term prognosis of nonobstructive urinary tract infection in infancy and childhood after the advent of sulphonamide. *Acta Paediatr. Scand.* 58:25, 1969.

59. Lippman, R. W., Wrobel, C. J., Rees, R., and Hoyt, R. A. Theory concerning recurrence of urinary infection. *J. Urol.* 80:77, 1958.

60. Mackintosh, I. P., Watson, B. W., and O'Grady, F. Theory of hydrokinetic clearance of bacteria from the urinary bladder. *Invest. Urol.* 12:473, 1975.

61. McCabe, W. R. Endotoxin tolerance: II. Its occurrence in patients with pyelonephritis. *J. Clin. Invest.* 42:618, 1963.

62. McCabe, W. R., and Anderson, V. Endotoxin tolerance: I. Its induction by experimental pyelonephritis. *J. Clin. Invest.* 42:610, 1963.

63. McCabe, W. R., and Jackson, G. Treatment of pyelonephritis: Bacterial, drug and host factors in success or failure among 252 patients. *N. Engl. J. Med.* 272:1037, 1965.

64. McCrory, W. W., Shibuya, M., Leuman, E., and Karp, R. Studies of renal function in children with chronic hydronephrosis. *Pediatr. Clin. North Am.* 18:445, 1971.

65. McGregor, M. Pyelonephritis lenta: Consideration of childhood urinary infection as a forerunner of renal insufficiency in later life. *Arch. Dis. Child.* 45: 159, 1970.

66. McLachlan, M. S. F., Meller, S. T., Verrier-Jones, E. R., Asscher, A. W., Fletcher, E. W. L., Mayon-White, R. T., Ledingham, J. G. G., Smith, J. C., and Johnston, H. H. Urinary tract in schoolgirls with covert bacteriuria. *Arch. Dis. Child.* 50:253, 1975.

67. Meadow, W. R., White, R. H. R., and Johnston, N. M. Prevalence of symptomless urinary tract disease in Birmingham school children: I. Pyuria and bacteriuria. *Br. Med. J.* 3:81, 1969.

68. Nelson, J. D., and McCracken, G. H. The current status of gentamicin for the neonate and young infant. *Am. J. Dis. Child.* 124:13, 1972.

69. Nelson, J. D., and Peters, P. C. Suprapubic aspiration of urine in premature and term infants. *Pediatrics* 36:132, 1965.

70. Nergårdh, A., von Hedenberg, C., Hellström, B., and Ericsson, N. O. Continence training of children with neurogenic bladder dysfunction. *Dev. Med. Child. Neurol.* 16:47, 1974.

71. Normand, I. C. S., and Smellie, J. M. Prolonged maintenance chemotherapy in the management of urinary infection in childhood. *Br. Med. J.* 1:1023, 1965.

72. O'Grady, F., and Cattell, W. R. Kinetics of urinary tract infection: II. The bladder. *Br. J. Urol.* 38:156, 1966b.

73. O'Grady, F., Mackintosh, I. P., Greenwood, D., and Watson, B. W. Treatment of "bacterial cystitis" in fully automatic mechanical models simulating conditions of bacterial growth in the urinary bladder. *Br. J. Exp. Pathol.* 54:283, 1973.

74. Olbing, H., Reischauer, H. C., and Kovacs, I. Prospektiver Vergleich von Nitrofurantoin und Sulfamethoxydiazin bei der Langzeittherapie von Kindern mit schwerer chronischrezidivierender pyelonephritis. *Dtsch. Med. Wochenschr.* 95:2469, 1970.

75. Percival, A., Brumfitt, W., and de Louvois, J. Serum-antibody levels as an indication of clinically inapparent pyelonephritis. *Lancet* 2:1027, 1964.

76. Ransley, P. G., and Risdon, R. A. Renal papillae and intrarenal reflux in the pig. *Lancet* 2:1114, 1974.

77. Ransley, P. G., and Risdon, R. A. Renal papillary morphology and intrarenal reflux in the young pig. *Urol. Res.* 3:105, 1975.

78. Ransley, P. G., and Risdon, R. A. Renal papillary morphology in infants and young children. *Urol. Res.* 3:111, 1975.

79. Roantree, R. J. The Relationship of Lipopolysaccharide Structure to Bacterial Virulence. In S. Kadis, G. Weinbaus, and S. Ajl (eds.), *Microbial Toxins.* V. Bacterial Endotoxins. New York: Academic, 1971. P. 1.

80. Robbins, J. B., McCracken, G. H., Gotschlich, E. C., Ørskov, F., Ørskov, I., and Hanson, L. Å. *Escherichia coli* K_1 capsular polysaccharide associated with neonatal meningitis. *N. Engl. J. Med.* 290:1216, 1974.

81. Roberts, J. A. Experimental pyelonephritis in the monkey: III. Pathophysiology of ureteral malfunction induced by bacteria. *Invest. Urol.* 13:117, 1975.

82. Rolleston, G. L., Maling, T. M. J., and Hodson, C. J. Intrarenal reflux and the scarred kidney. *Arch. Dis. Child.* 49:531, 1974.

83. Rolleston, G. L., Shannon, F. T., and Utley, W. L. Follow-up of vesico-ureteric reflux in the newborn. *Kidney Int.* 8:59, 1975.

84. Ronald, A. R., Truck, M., and Petersdorf, R. G. A critical evaluation of nalidixic acid in urinary tract infections. *N. Engl. J. Med.* 275:1081, 1966.

85. Savage, D. C. L. Natural history of covert bacteriuria in schoolgirls. *Kidney Int.* 8:90, 1975.

86. Savage, D. C. L., Wilson, M. I., McHardy, M., Dewar, D. A. E., and Fee, W. M. Covert bacteriuria of childhood, a clinical and epidemiological study. *Arch. Dis. Child.* 48:8, 1973.

87. Schwartz, G. J., and Edelmann, C. M., Jr. Screening for bacteriuria in children. *Kidney* 8:1, 1975.

88. Scott, J. E. S. A Critical Appraisal of the Management of Ureteric Reflux. In J. H. Johnston and R. J. Scholtmeijer (eds.), *Problems in Pediatric Urology.* Amsterdam: Excerpta Medica, 1972. P. 271.

89. Scott, J. E. S. The role of surgery in the management of vesico-ureteric reflux. *Kidney Int.* 8:73, 1975.

90. Silverblatt, F. J. Host-parasite interaction in the rat renal pelvis: A possible role for pili in the pathogenesis of pyelonephritis. *J. Exp. Med.* 140:1696, 1974.

91. Smellie, J. M. Medical aspects of urinary infection in children. *J. R. Coll. Physicians Lond.* 1:189, 1967.

92. Smellie, J. M., Edwards, D., Hunter, N., Normand, I. C. S., and Prescod, N. Vesico-ureteric reflux and renal scarring. *Kidney Int.* 8:65, 1975.

93. Smellie, J. M., and Normand, I. C. S. Experience of Follow-up of Children with Urinary Tract Infection. In F. O'Grady and W. Brumfitt (eds.), *Urinary Tract Infection.* London: Oxford University Press, 1968. P. 123.

94. Smellie, J. M., and Normand, I. C. S. Bacteriuria, reflux and renal scarring. *Arch. Dis. Child.* 50:581, 1975.

95. Stamey, T. A. A clinical classification of urinary tract infections based upon origin. *South Med. J.* 68:934, 1975.

96. Stamey, T. A., and Bragonje, J. Resistance to nalidixic acid: A misconception due to underdosage. *J.A.M.A.* 236:1857, 1976.

97. Stamey, T. A., Bushby, S. R. M., and Bragonje, J. The concentration of trimethoprim in prostatic fluid: Nonionic diffusion or active transport? *J. Infect. Dis.* [Suppl.] 128:S686, 1973.

98. Stamey, T. A., and Condy, M. The diffusion and concentration of trimethoprim in human vaginal fluid. *J. Infect. Dis.* 131:261, 1975.

99. Stamey, T. A., Fair, W. R., Timothy, M. M., Millar, M. A., Mihara, G., and Lowery, Y. C. Serum versus urinary antimicrobial concentrations in cure of urinary tract infections. *N. Engl. J. Med.* 291:1159, 1974.

100. Stamey, T. A., Govan, D. E., and Palmer, J. M. The localization and treatment of urinary tract infections: The role of bactericidal urine levels as opposed to serum levels. *Medicine (Baltimore)* 44:1, 1965.

101. Stamey, T. A., Timothy, M., Millar, M., and Mihara, G. Recurrent urinary infections in adult women: The role of introital enterobacteria. *Calif. Med.* 115:1, 1971.

102. Stansfeld, J. M. Clinical observations relating to incidence and aetiology of urinary tract infections in children. *Br. Med. J.* 1:631, 1966.

103. Teague, W., and Boyarsky, S. The effect of coliform bacteria upon ureteral peristalsis. *Invest. Urol.* 5:423, 1968.

104. Thomas, V., Shelokov, A., and Forland, M. Antibody-coated bacteria in the urine and the site of urinary tract infection. *N. Engl. J. Med.* 290:588, 1974.

105. Tschudi Madsen, S. Antibacterial effect of urine after single oral doses of sulphonamide. *Chemotherapia* 13:16, 1968.

106. Verrier-Jones, E. R., Meller, S. T., McLachlan, M. S. F., Sussman, M., Asscher, A. W., Mayon-White, R. T., Ledingham, J. G. G., Smith, J. C., Fletcher, E. W. L., Smith, E. H., Johnston, H. H., and Sleight, G. Treatment of bacteriuria in schoolgirls. *Kidney Int.* 8:85, 1975.

107. VUR + IRR = CPN? (lead article). *Lancet* 2:1120, 1974.

108. Westenfelder, M., Galanos, C., and Madsen, P. O. Experimental lipid A induced nephritis in the dog. *Invest. Urol.* 12:337, 1975.

109. Williams, D. I. The ureter, the urologist, and the paediatrician. *Proc. R. Soc. Med.* 63:595, 1970.

110. Winberg, J. Screening in the Newborn Period. In *Colloquium on Pyelonephritis, 14th International Congress of Pediatrics, 1974.*

111. Winberg, J., Andersen, H. J., Bergström, T., Jacobsson, B., Larson, H., and Lincoln, K. Epidemiology of symptomatic urinary tract infection in childhood. *Acta Paediatr. Scand.* [Suppl. 252] 63:1, 1974.

112. Winberg, J., Andersen, H. J., Hanson, L. Å., and Lincoln, K. Studies of urinary tract infections in infancy and childhood. *Br. Med. J.* 2:524, 1963.

113. Winberg, J., Bergström, T., and Jacobsson, B. Morbidity, age and sex distribution, recurrences and renal scarring in symptomatic urinary tract infection in childhood. *Kidney Int.* 8:101, 1975.

114. Winberg, J., Bergström, T., Lidin-Janson, G., and Lincoln, K. Treatment trials in urinary tract infection (UTI) with special reference to the effect of antimicrobials on the fecal and periurethral flora. *Clin. Nephrol.* 1:142, 1973.

115. Winberg, J., Larson, H., and Bergström, T. Comparison of the Natural History of Urinary Infection in Children with and without Vesico-ureteric Reflux. In P. Kincaid-Smith and K. Fairley (eds.), *Renal Infection and Renal Scarring.* Melbourne: Mercedes, 1971. P. 293.

93. Urologic Trauma in Childhood

Selwyn B. Levitt

Serious trauma has reached epidemic proportions in our complex, urban, mechanized society. Accidents are the leading cause of mortality in children, accounting for 40 percent of childhood deaths in the United States. In addition to the 13,000 children killed annually, an estimated 100,000 are permanently disabled. Abdominal injuries rank third among causes of accidental death in children, with burns and head injuries heading the list. The alarming rise in automobile accidents, which steadily increase each year, has resulted in greater numbers of children with blunt abdominal trauma and urologic injury.

Kidney

The slow but significant rise in the incidence of renal trauma is reflected in figures related to pediatric hospital admissions. Campbell [14] in 1941 reported an incidence of 1 renal injury in 2,000 pediatric admissions at Bellevue Hospital. Charron and Brault [17] noted 1 per 1,000 pediatric admissions in a report from Montreal in 1963. More recently, Smith et al. [100], in a review of pediatric hospital admissions at Englewood Hospital, New Jersey, found 1 renal injury in 860 children admitted.

Blunt abdominal trauma is more likely to result in renal injury in children than in adults. Osgood and Campbell [119] noted that 20 to 25 percent of all patients with renal trauma are children and that the kidney is injured more often than any other urinary organ in the young. Hood and Smyth [43] reported a 32 percent incidence of renal injury in a recent review of 130 children who had sustained blunt abdominal trauma; indeed, in this series the kidney was involved more frequently than any other intraabdominal organ. Richardson et al. [91] noted a 10 percent incidence in their 80 children with blunt abdominal injuries. Comparable adult series of patients with blunt abdominal trauma report urologic injuries in only 2.5 percent of patients, with the kidney being the involved organ in one-half of these cases (i.e., 1.2 percent) [112, 115]. There are certain anatomic features peculiar to children that might account for their predisposition to renal trauma:

1. The size of the kidneys in children is relatively greater than in the adult.
2. Lobulation often persists until puberty, and the contiguous portions of lobules seem to represent areas of weakness.
3. The perirenal fat and Gerota's (fascia) do not become fully developed until puberty.
4. The secondary ossification centers for the eleventh and twelfth ribs do not close until the twenty-fifth year.
5. The kidneys during childhood tend to be somewhat lower in position and consequently are less protected by the rib cage and vertebral musculature.
6. The incidence of renal anomalies is higher; the abnormal kidney is particularly prone to rupture from relatively minor trauma.

INCIDENCE

The peak incidence of renal trauma occurs in the 10- to 14-year age group. A collation of three recent reports showed that 141 (61 percent) of 231 children were between 10 and 14 years of age. Renal trauma is least common in the first quinquennium in all published series.

Boys predominate in all reports, with the average male-female ratio being 3 : 1. This figure is supported by a compilation of five series of renal trauma in which there were 379 children (291 boys and 88 girls [30, 46, 70, 84, 100]). Mertz et al. [70] noted that among the children less than 10 years old, 22 of 34 were boys (2 : 1), whereas 29 of 36 children more than 10 years old were boys (4 : 1). Forsythe [30] observed the same trend of greater male involvement in children more than 10 years old. This probably reflects the more rugged types of play that older boys indulge in.

Right and left kidneys are about equally involved. In the combined series of Mertz et al. [70], Javadpour and Bush [46], and Morse et al. [79] comprising 260 renal injuries, 127 involved the right kidney and 115 the left; 14 were bilateral. In 4 children the side of the injury was not recorded. It should be noted that this relatively high incidence of bilateral involvement is misleading, since of Javadpour's 110 children 34 suffered from stabs and gunshot wounds (31 percent), whereas most publications list these etiologies in less than 1 percent of cases. A more accurate estimate of bilateral involvement would be in the order of 2 to 3 percent.

Hood and Smyth [43] reported a preponderance

of right renal injuries when the child was involved as a pedestrian in an automobile accident. This seems to be the pattern in Great Britain, where automobiles are driven on the left side of the road. The authors suggested that the child who runs into the roadway is more likely to be struck by an automobile coming toward him on his right. His right side would receive the impact directly and would be more likely to be injured. The converse would be anticipated when traffic is driven on the right. Arcari's figures [2] suggest that injury in Detroit, Michigan, is more common on the left side of the abdomen, lending support to Hood and Smyth's theory.

ETIOLOGY

Renal injury may result from direct or indirect trauma. Direct trauma may be blunt or penetrating in nature, although in children blunt trauma is more common. Consideration must be given to contributing or predisposing factors, as well as to the types of injury inflicted. Spontaneous injuries occur with underlying disease. Spontaneous subcapsular hemorrhage or bleeding into the perirenal spaces should arouse suspicion of an underlying neoplasm such as a ruptured Wilms' tumor. Minor trauma, which ordinarily would go unnoticed, can result in major renal injury in hydronephrotic kidneys. Ravich and Schell [88] reported a newborn with hematuria and a flank mass that required urgent exploration and nephrectomy. The specimen showed a grossly hydronephrotic kidney secondary to ureteropelvic junction obstruction, with a laceration of the renal pelvis. A retroperitoneal perirenal hematoma was evacuated at the time of surgery. They postulated an intrauterine rupture secondary to increased intrauterine pressure, which, with uterine contractions during labor, can reach as high as 250 mm Hg. Alternatively, the injury could have resulted from passage of the baby through the birth canal or from obstetric manipulation during delivery.

I recently encountered a newborn with peripelvic bleeding around a hydronephrotic kidney secondary to a ureteropelvic junction obstruction. A dismembered pyeloplasty with excision of the redundant pelvis and ureter resulted in salvage of the kidney. Histopathologic examination disclosed a stricture of the pelviureteric junction with fibrosis and an organizing hematoma in the pelvic wall [59a].

Spontaneous urinary extravasation in the newborn is a well-recognized complication of posterior urethral valves [33] and has also been described with urethral stricture [74], bladder neck obstruction [5], an anomalous [120] or edematous ure-terovesical junction [38], and pelvic neuroblastoma [114]. Urinary extravasation may present as ascites, presumably from spontaneous rupture of a calyceal fornix.

Rarely, ingested foreign bodies perforate through the posterior wall of the second part of the duodenum and then gain entry to the kidney. All of the reported cases of ingested foreign bodies in children have involved the right kidney and a metallic foreign body (usually a bobby pin). Broomstraws have been implicated in two children in whom perforation into the left kidney resulted in hematuria. The portal of entry was presumed to be the urethra, with ascent up the left ureter by retrograde peristalsis [73]. No case of a bullet or shell fragment entering the skin and then migrating through to the kidney has been reported in a child.

Iatrogenic injury to the kidney occasionally occurs during the course of abdominal or retroperitoneal surgery. Retrograde pyelographic procedures may result in perforation or extravasation of contrast material. Injuries result from overdistention of the renal pelvis with contrast material or from injection under too high a pressure, with resultant rupture of the calyceal fornices (Fig. 93-1*A*). This allows contrast material to extravasate intrarenally or directly into the tubules, lymphatics, or venous channels. Pyelotubular, pyelolymphatic, and pyelovenous backflow results, as well as subcapsular accumulation of dye. The other mode of injury during retrograde pyelography is forceful advancement of the ureteral catheter with perforation through a papilla into the renal substance (Fig. 93-1*B*). These injuries almost all heal spontaneously and only rarely require operative intervention.

The most common iatrogenic injury occurs as a result of diagnostic percutaneous renal biopsy. Renal injuries occurring during liver biopsies are also on record. The incidence of postbiopsy complication is dependent to a large extent on the definition of significant bleeding. Almost all subjects have transitory microscopic hematuria or experience temporary flank or abdominal pain. Intrarenal or perirenal bleeding is by far the most common postbiopsy complication. Serious bleeding manifested by prolonged gross hematuria (with or without colic from clots), hypotension, or a fall in hematocrit occurs in less than 5 percent of children [60, 61]. Approximately 1 percent require transfusion and 0.3 percent require surgical intervention, at times resulting in nephrectomy. The mortality is reportedly slightly less than 0.1 percent. Arteriovenous fistulas are the second most frequent postbiopsy complication [23, 26, 27, 58].

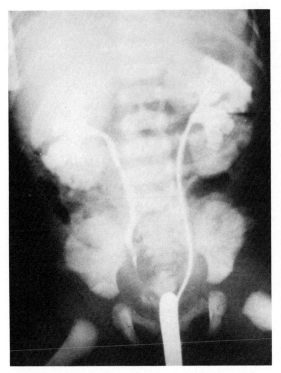 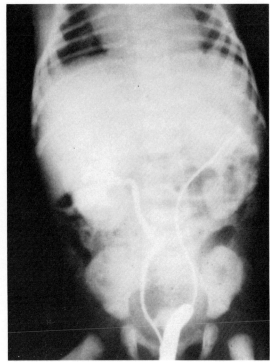

A   B

Figure 93-1. Extravasated contrast material after bilateral retrograde ureteropyelograms for suspected obstruction were performed in a newborn with anuria and a prolonged nephrogram on an intravenous pyelogram. A. On the right there is overdistention with forniceal rupture and subcapsular extravasation of Hypaque. B. On the left the ureteral catheter has perforated through the papilla into the parenchyma to a subcapsular position.

Most fistulas are small and disappear spontaneously. Severe renal lacerations and pedicle injuries are unusual when the biopsy is performed by an experienced nephrologist under x-ray or scanning control.

The majority of renal injuries in children result from blunt abdominal trauma. Falls with the trunk athwart an object, against a paling fence or the edge of a trampoline, onto a diving board, onto the branch of a tree, and from a bicycle against a sidewalk or onto a fence are the most common mode of injury. Of 494 children reviewed [30, 46, 61, 70, 84, 89, 100], 172 (34 percent) were injured in this manner. A higher proportion of children sustain renal injuries with falls than do adults, in whom falls account for approximately 16 percent of renal injuries. Noteworthy is the fact that children who fall generally sustain more severe types of injury than adults. Reid [89] noted that half of his children with complete fractures or type IV parenchymal lacerations were injured by falls.

Vehicular accidents accounted for 151 renal injuries in the series cited above (30 percent of the total group of 494 children) and were the second most common cause of renal injury. (Vehicular injuries were even more common in the 1- to 5-year-old age group in Reid's [89] series, with falls being the predominant mode of injury in the older age groups.) Kicks, blows to the abdomen, athletic accidents, and contrecoup or decelerating injuries (Fig. 93-2B) consequent to falling from a height and landing on the feet or buttock accounted for most of the remainder. Penetrating injuries from stabs and gunshot wounds were sustained by 37 of the 494 injured children (7 percent). As mentioned above, however, the Chicago experience reported by Javadpour and Bush [46] was most unusual in that 34 of their 110 children were injured by stabs or gunshot wounds. In other reports, gunshot and stab wounds account for only 1 to 2 percent of all renal injuries in children.

TYPES OF INJURY
Management of renal injuries requires clear definition of the pathologic anatomic changes that have resulted from the traumatic episode. Any classification must take into account the four essential

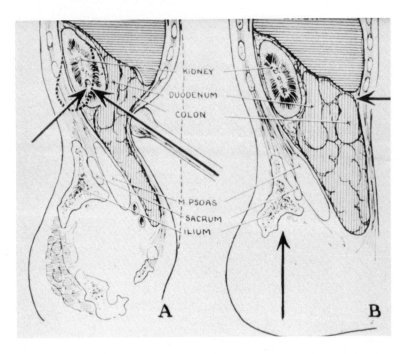

Figure 93-2. A. Mechanism of direct renal injury. B. Contrecoup or decleration injury. The body suddenly decelerates on impact with the ground. The kidney continues its downward descent because of its loose attachments, causing shearing stress on the pedicle and resulting in intimal tears and subsequent thrombosis of the artery or complete vessel avulsion. (From A. J. Scholl and E. F. Nation, Injury of the Kidney. In M. F. Campbell and J. H. Harrison [eds.], Urology *[3rd ed.]. Philadelphia: Saunders, 1970. Vol. I, p. 786.)*

anatomic elements of kidney structure: parenchyma, capsule, collecting system, and blood supply. Many classifications have been proposed, but all recognize the need to correlate clinical and radiologic features as a means of differentiating mild from severe injuries.

There is little argument as to what constitutes a mild injury or contusion, but there is a great deal of confusion in the literature when it comes to differentiating the various types of severe injuries or lacerations. This differentiation is important if one is to assess the claims of one or another modality of therapy. The more recent publications on renal trauma have recognized this problem and have attempted to provide a more precise classification of the injury based upon better visualization of the kidney, either by high-dose or infusion urography. Nunn's classification [80] (Fig. 93-3), presented here, correlates the clinical and radiologic features with the pathology.

Type I Injury—Contusion
Children with simple renal contusions present with a history and sometimes clinical evidence of trauma to the renal area. This might take the form of pain, tenderness, contusions, or abrasions in the flank region. Gross or microscopic hematuria is a constant feature. No flank mass is palpable. The psoas and renal outlines are intact on plain roentgenograms. The excretory urogram shows a normal nephrogram, with little or no evidence of depressed renal function. The pelvocalyceal system is intact, although the amount of contrast material seen in the collecting system is usually less on the injured side (Fig. 93-4A). After a few hours, the parenchyma may swell and compress the collecting system, limiting the amount of contrast material in the collecting system and giving the appearance of markedly impaired or even absent excretory function. These effects subside after a day or two (Fig. 93-4B). No extravasation of dye occurs. In children in whom parenchymal swelling is severe enough to markedly diminish or totally prevent visualization of the kidney, classification as a type I injury cannot be made until further radiologic studies are performed.

Type II—Cortical Lacerations (Incomplete Parenchymal Tears)
The renal capsule provides a great deal of support for the parenchyma. In type II renal injuries the capsule is disrupted, and the underlying paren-

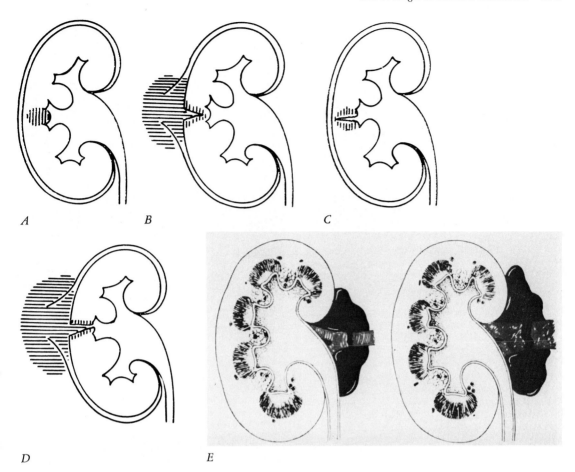

Figure 93-3. Types of renal injury according to I. N. Nunn's classification. A. Type I: contusion. The capsule and pelvocalyceal system are left intact. This is the most common type of injury (approximately 60 percent of all injuries). B. Type II: cortical laceration (incomplete parenchymal tear). The capsule ruptures, but the pelvocalyceal system is left intact and there is extravasation of blood only. The adjacent injured parenchyma does not secrete urine. C. Type III: Calyceal laceration (incomplete parenchymal tear). The capsule is intact, but the pelvocalyceal system is ruptured and there is intrarenal urinary and bloody intravasation. D. Type IV: Complete parenchymal tear. The hallmark of this injury is urinary extravasation; there is extravasation of blood as well. Type IV accounts for approximately 20 percent of all renal injuries. E. Addition to the Nunn classification—Type V. This is a pedicle injury in which the main component of injury is vessel damage. Type V injuries are the least common; they account for approximately 6 percent of renal injuries. (From I. N. Nunn, Aust. N.Z. J. Surg. 31:263, 1962.)

chymal injury is apt to be severe. Clinical evidence of trauma to the renal area is likely to be more manifest than in type I injuries. Extrarenal bleeding from the lacerated parenchymal margins accumulates in the perirenal space and often produces a palpable mass. A soft tissue shadow and loss of the renal and psoas outlines are often apparent on the plain film. On excretory urography, the nephrogram is normal or less intense than usual due to parenchymal swelling and bleeding. The collecting system is intact. The injured nephrons along the edge of the parenchymal laceration do not produce

significant amounts of urine, and thus no extravasation of urine is evident.

Type III—Calyceal Lacerations (Incomplete Parenchymal Laceration with an Intact Capsule but Lacerated Calyx or Calyces)

Clinical evidence of loin injury is evident in type III renal injuries, and marked hematuria is characteristic. There is no flank mass. Urography shows distortion of the pelvocalyceal system but no disruption of the renal outline. Intrarenal intravasa-

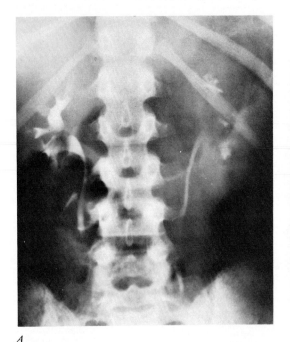 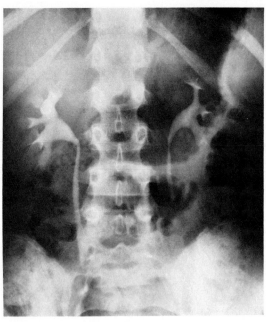

A   B

Figure 93-4. A. An intravenous pyelogram shows decreased excretion on the left in a 7-year-old girl following trauma. Left flank tenderness and hematuria were evident. B. Normal equal excretion is seen 3 weeks later. No treatment other than observation was necessary.

tion of dye and blood clot in the pelvocalyceal system may appear as a space-occupying lesion.

Type IV—Complete Tears—Injuries Involving the Capsule, Parenchyma, and Collecting System

Here the clinical and radiologic evidence of injury combines the features of type II and III renal injuries. The capsule and renal pelvis provide support for the friable parenchyma. When both of these supporting structures are disrupted, the intervening parenchyma is always severely injured. Complete separation of the renal parenchyma from the pelvis or calyces to the capsule is evident. The hallmark of this injury is extravasation of urine beyond the confines of the kidney. The injury is usually sharply localized in children; most of the kidney tissue remains intact.

The addition of a fifth category to Nunn's classification seems warranted for those lesions that primarily involve the renal vessels. The renal artery may sustain the brunt of the trauma, resulting in an intimal tear, as in contrecoup injuries, or complete avulsion. The urine may be devoid of red blood cells if it all comes from the uninjured kidney. The child with an avulsion injury presents in shock with an expanding flank mass. The excretory urogram shows no function on the affected side. Arteriography and selective renal angiogra-

phy will elucidate the lesion. The bleeding may be unremitting, requiring immediate surgery. Were a retrograde pyelogram to be done in such a situation, it would appear normal.

Renal injuries in childhood most commonly are type I (renal contusions). Four recent reports revealed 166 such injuries among a total of 260 patients (64 percent) [61, 79, 84, 89]. Type II injuries are least common, followed by type III. Type IV lesions account for 12 to 22 percent, and they occur most commonly in road accidents in which the child is a pedestrian. Isolated pedicle injuries are the rarest form of renal injury in children, although Reid [89] reported 5 such injuries among 78 children (6.4 percent).

CLINICAL FEATURES

Symptoms and signs of renal trauma are related both to the severity of renal injury as well as to the presence of associated injuries. The cardinal features of renal trauma are *hematuria, pain, tenderness,* and *abdominal rigidity.* Hematuria, either gross or microscopic, is almost always present. It is the most dramatic indicator of renal injury, although the degree is not a good index of the extent of injury. Isolated pedicle injury is the classic example of serious renal trauma in which hematuria is absent; blood clot with ureteral obstruction and pelvic rupture or complete avulsion of the ureter from the pelvis are other examples. Hematuria usually occurs shortly after injury, but its appearance may be delayed by hypotension severe enough to cause a drop in urinary output. Colic is sometimes prominent and results from clots obstructing the renal pelvis and ureter. Passage of elongated clots from the bladder confirms the presence of upper urinary tract bleeding. Urinary retention may result from accumulation of blood clots in the bladder.

The extravasation of blood or urine into the perirenal tissues leads to the development of a mass in the loin. Often the degree of local muscular rigidity renders accurate palpation of the renal area impossible; however, large perirenal collections can usually be felt or even seen through the rigid abdominal musculature. Diffuse abdominal distention commonly occurs as a result of reflex paralytic ileus secondary to retroperitoneal extravasation. Pain and tenderness are most commonly confined to the injured flank but on occasion may be primarily abdominal. Fever often develops later because of the absorption of blood or urine, and it is important to note that its occurrence does not necessarily indicate infection. Shock, which may be delayed in onset in the young, is reported frequently in some series [89].

ASSOCIATED INJURY

Many authors have stressed the association of renal injuries with multiple injuries to other organ systems. Four recent publications on renal trauma in the pediatric age group, with a cumulative experience of 297 children, reported the incidence of associated injuries to range from 25 to 40 percent [46, 61, 70, 79]. The most frequent extraurinary tract injuries are skeletal fractures, usually involving either the ribs or extremities. Morse et al. [79] recorded splenic ruptures in 8 of 32 left-sided renal injuries. In general, the more severe the renal injury, the greater the likelihood of multiorgan injury. The mode of injury is also important in determining the degree of associated injuries. Vehicular accidents and, to a lesser extent, gunshot and stab wounds, are much more likely to involve multiple organ systems. However, it should be emphasized that most kidney trauma occurs as an isolated injury.

UNDERLYING ANOMALIES

Seemingly minor renal injuries in children must be carefully evaluated with intravenous urography, since the incidence of underlying urologic anomalies is significant. Among nine reports, 87 of 697 children with renal trauma had underlying anomalies (13 percent), with a range from 3.9 percent [46] to 23 percent [84]. Obstructive uropathy accounted for the majority of cases, with pelviureteric junction obstructions being most common, followed by megaloureter. Ectopic and solitary kidneys were frequent. A few instances of hypoplasia and an occasional cystic kidney were detected. Wilms' tumor was found in 6 of the 87 children.

DIAGNOSTIC RADIOLOGY

Adequate visualization of the kidneys is the key to classification of the extent and the type of renal injury. Intravenous urography is mandatory, even if the injury appears slight or is only suspected. Hypotension is not a contraindication to excretory urography.

Infusion or high-dose urography is recommended as the first and most useful radiologic investigation. The procedure has been adapted from that described for use in adults by Harris and Harris [36] and by Schencker [96], who observed that most unsatisfactory pyelograms result from insufficient filling of the collecting system rather than from inadequate concentration of the contrast material. Infusion pyelography produces a diuresis that distends the collecting system to its physiologic maximum and supplies contrast material in sufficient quantity so that the copious supply of urine is densely opacified. Exposures are made in the anteroposterior projection at 3, 10, 20, and 30 min after the start of the infusion. A lateral exposure is made at 20 or 30 min. Finally, an oblique exposure is made with the child voiding.

Morse et al. [79] have advised early radiologic study within a few hours of injury so that optimal visualization can be obtained before parenchymal swelling interferes. Orkin [81] found that routine intravenous pyelograms were diagnostic in less than half of his adult patients and concluded that the only real value of the study was to show the presence of a normal contralateral kidney. Kazmin et al. [51], however, found that 48 of 54 high-dose studies were adequate for diagnosis, compared with 32 of 56 low-dose urograms. Mahoney and Persky [64] reported that urograms were diagnostic in 93 percent of patients studied with high-dose infusion pyelograms; they used nephrotomography as an adjunct. Moreover, Morrow and Mendez [76] stated that the results of infusion urography correlated with those of selective renal angiography in 87 percent of 48 patients.

Cystoscopy and retrograde pyelography have been used less frequently in the evaluation of renal injuries since the advent of high-dose urography and scintigraphic studies. I agree with Water-

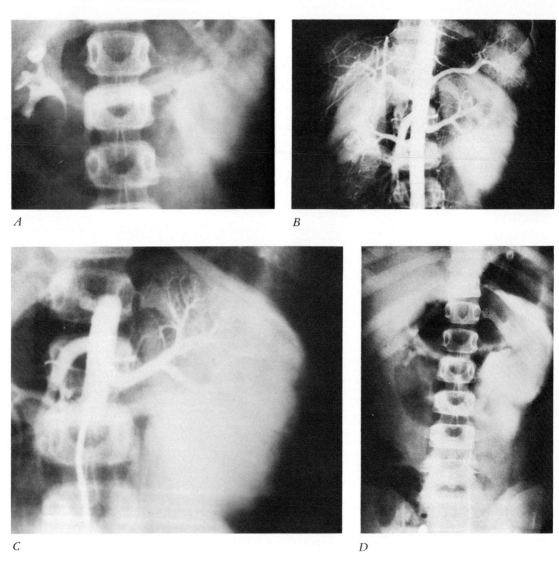

Figure 93-5. Studies of a 6-year-old girl injured in an auto accident in 1972. A. An intravenous pyelogram shows left hilar extravasation. The upper calyces are filled. B. The aortogram shows decreased filling of the left lower pole renal arteries. No gross parenchymal separation is visualized. C. A left selective renal arteriogram shows diminished filling of lower pole arterial branches. No arterial extravasation is evident. D. A retrograde ureteropyelogram shows gross urinary extravasation. The retrograde pyelogram rather than the IVP and arteriogram indicates that the main pathology involves the collecting system. At surgery a small parenchymal laceration was noted with a large tear in the renal pelvis. (Courtesy of C. H. Meng.)

house and Gross [112a] that, generally, arteriography rather than retrograde pyelography is the procedure of choice if the infusion urogram is not diagnostic. Definite indications do remain for cystoscopy and retrograde pyelography, however, such as when the excretory pyelogram and arteriograms do not adequately visualize the collecting system (Fig. 93-5). Scholl and Nation [98] allude to the possible hazards of retrograde pyelography, which include infection, exacerbation of hemorrhage, or worsening of the patient's condition during positioning for the study. They continue to recommend early use of cystoscopy and retrograde pyelography, however, if the procedure seems indicated. An added hazard in children is the need for anesthesia. However, these children generally require operative exploration, so that the cystoscopy and retrograde pyelogram can be done just prior to that procedure, utilizing the same anesthetic.

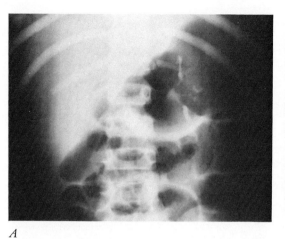
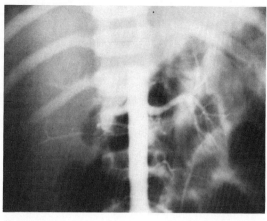

A   *B*

Figure 93-6. Studies of a 5-year-old boy who was hit by a truck, sustaining multiple fractures in addition to hematuria. A. An intravenous pyelogram done 8 hr after injury—a 40-min film—shows nonvisualization of the right kidney. B. An aortogram done 12 hr after injury shows complete occlusion of the right renal artery. There is definite thrombosis of the renal artery as opposed to agenesis, hypoplasia, or poor renal artery perfusion, as is frequently seen with severe parenchymal swelling. (Courtesy of C. H. Meng.)

Arteriography is the only direct method of clearly delineating the vascular architecture of the kidney. A nonvisualizing kidney on urography or radionuclide scintiscan is strong circumstantial evidence for vascular disruption or thrombosis, but it does not define the pathologic anatomy. Congenital absence or severe hypoplasia of a kidney will appear as nonvisualization on urography and scintiscan, whereas the angiogram will clearly separate these entities from disruption or thrombosis of the renal artery or its branches (Fig. 93-6).

Differentiating renal artery thrombosis or disruption from congenital renal hypoplasia or agenesis is not generally a problem since the contralateral normal kidney shows compensatory hypertrophy; however, on occasion the compensatory hypertrophy is not so marked as to convince the clinician or radiologist of the exact pathology. Moreover, in the case of vascular obstruction or avulsion as well as in complete parenchymal lacerations or major injuries that may require surgical intervention, accurate definition by angiography of the arterial architecture is extremely valuable information for the surgeon (Fig. 93-7). Selective celiac angiograms done at the same time may also be helpful in delineating injuries to the spleen and liver.

Bronklaus et al. [7], McDonald and Hiller [68] and Nebesar et al. [79a] have reported performance of renal angiography in children with few complications. Temporary spasm of the femoral artery was the most common complication. Small hematomas are the next most frequent complica-tion. Femoral artery thrombosis is the most serious hazard and occurs in approximately 2 percent of children undergoing angiography. Small diameter catheters, percutaneous rather than open surgical placement of the femoral artery catheter, and heparinization reduce this incidence. Most of the reported cases of femoral artery thrombosis have occurred in children younger than age 5 years. Almost all children can be studied under sedation and local anesthesia.

The renal scan with [197]Hg-labeled chlormerodrin has been demonstrated to be a simple, highly accurate, and rapid study that is totally free of complications and has none of the allergic problems that may result from the use of organic iodides [31, 53a, 94, 97]. Its prime use is as a screening procedure for children who are allergic to Hypaque. Its sensitivity and accuracy have been amply demonstrated [31, 94] (Fig. 93-8). This, as well as its ease of performance and the lower radiation doses of the newer technetium agents make the renal scan an ideal study for long-term, serial follow-up of patients with renal injuries. It should be performed as part of the early work-up of patients in whom the need for further studies is anticipated.

MANAGEMENT

Treatment of the injured child must first be directed to maintenance of an adequate airway and to the correction of hypovolemia. Mannitol has not been shown to be protective or to reduce the traumatic effect on injured parenchyma in the experi-

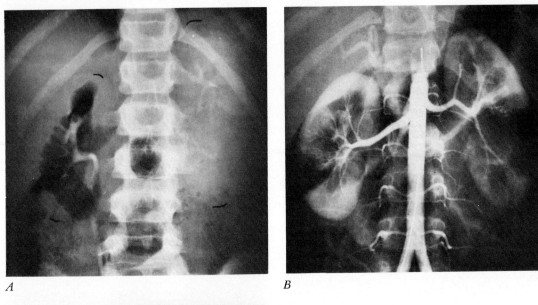

A

B

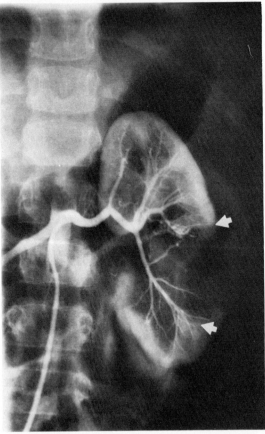

C

Figure 93-7. *A. An intravenous pyelogram shows decreased visualization of the left kidney with poor delineation of the pelvocalyceal system. B. An aortogram shows single renal arteries bilaterally. The lacerated left kidney has a good vascular supply to the separated parenchymal segments. C. A selective renal angiogram shows perfect definition of the intrarenal arterial tree. The lack of secondary and tertiary branches at the junction of the middle and lower pole parenchymal segments (arrows) is secondary to thrombosis.*

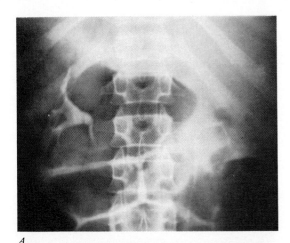

A

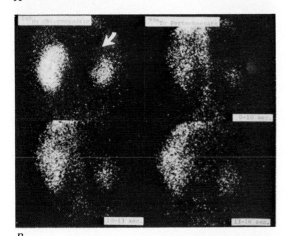

B

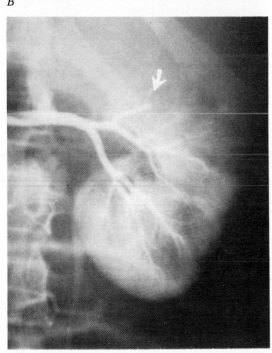

C

mental animal [45a]. Hemorrhage from a renal injury is retained within and tamponaded by the renal capsule of Gerota and therefore is rarely an immediate threat to life. Even when the kidney is completely avulsed from its vascular pedicle, the bleeding may be restrained sufficiently to prevent hypovolemia [52].

In nearly all cases of closed renal injury, an initial conservative regimen is indicated. Careful monitoring of blood pressure and pulse and frequent abdominal examinations to discover whether a loin swelling is appearing or increasing in size will allow time for adequate excretory urography and assessment of the degree of injury. In the unusual case in which emergency lifesaving surgery is needed for persistent hemorrhage, a transperitoneal approach through a long midline abdominal incision is indicated in order to permit immediate control of the renal pedicle before the restraining renal fascia is opened. Once this has been accomplished and the bleeding has been controlled, stabilization of the child's vital signs will be possible by blood transfusion. If a preoperative urogram was not possible, an infusion urogram should be obtained on the operating room table in order to establish the normality of the contralateral kidney before any definitive treatment of the injured kidney is undertaken. When an unsuspected renal injury is detected during emergency exploration for other intraabdominal catastrophies, it is wise to refrain from entering the tamponaded retroperitoneal hemorrhage unless it is expanding, is very tense, or has resulted from a penetrating wound. In these instances a urogram on the table is mandatory in order to establish the presence of a contralateral normal kidney.

The very common Nunn type I injury (renal contusion) can be treated conservatively with bed rest and observation with the expectation of complete recovery without sequelae. The very uncommon, *totally* fragmented shattered kidney or the

Figure 93-8. A. An inadequate intravenous pyelogram (IVP) with poor nephrographic delineation of the right parenchymal margins (posteroanterior orientation of the IVP corresponds with scan). B. Renal scan with [197]Hg-labeled chlormerodrin demonstrates absence of activity in the upper pole of the right kidney (arrow). Poor perfusion of the kidney with no uptake in the upper pole is obtained with rapid sequential ^{99m}Tc-labeled pertechnetate scintigraphy. C. A right selective renal angiogram shows a fracture of the right kidney with thrombosis of the artery to the upper pole (arrow). (From M. Koenigsberg, M. D. Blaufox, and L. M. Freeman, Traumatic injuries of the renal vasculature and parenchyma. Semin. Nucl. Med. 4:117–132, 1974. By permission.)

kidney avulsed from its renal pedicle should be removed. Most type II and III injuries, that is, incomplete parenchymal tears without perirenal urinary extravasation, can be managed conservatively.

Controversy exists concerning the management of the 15 to 20 percent of patients with extravasation of urine from a kidney with at least partial preservation of its architecture. There are those who advocate absolute conservatism with surgical exploration only for clinical deterioration, such as an expanding flank mass from continuing severe hemorrhage or from increasing urinary extravasation [6, 67, 86, 95, 109]. McCague [67] has summarized the nonoperative view: "While recognizing the necessity for prompt and radical surgery in a small group, we believe that if the majority of traumatic renal lesions are submitted to *immediate* surgery, many of these kidneys will be sacrificed that might have been salvaged if treated in a conservative manner" [italics added]. Hodges et al. [42] and McKay et al. [69] advocated aggressive treatment with early exploration before the sequelae of hemorrhage and extravasation of urine become manifest and to avoid protracted convalescent periods following injury. Orkin [81] endorsed the surgical approach to renal rupture but felt that the operation was best done at a propitious time after injury rather than on an emergency basis. He emphasized the importance of a shortened hospital stay and salvage of kidneys that might otherwise have come to nephrectomy. However, as Morse and associates [79] note, he did not define the key phrase "the propitious time."

Morse et al. [79], adopting a middle course, have recently demonstrated optimum results with conservative surgery for Nunn type IV renal injuries (with perinephric urinary extravasation). Since most renal injuries in children are localized to a small portion of the kidney, appropriate surgery can salvage major portions of healthy renal tissue. Morse and associates [79] found the propitious time to be 2 to 7 days after injury. Ischemic segments of the kidney by that time have become clearly demarcated, hemorrhage is relatively easy to control, and perirenal infection has not usually supervened. All seven of their patients who were handled in this manner had functioning kidneys. Prolonged infection, progressive hydronephrosis, and hypertension did not occur. One child required a secondary operation to relieve obstruction caused by scar tissue. In both instances of immediate exploration within the first 24 hr using the flank approach, the surgeon induced uncontrollable hemorrhage that necessitated immediate nephrectomy of a presumably salvageable kidney. At the other extreme, three children with obvious extrarenal extravasation were treated nonoperatively for more than 1 week, and two developed perinephric abscesses requiring nephrectomies.

I endorse the Morse approach in any type IV injury with more than just minor degrees of urinary extravasation, but I use aortography and selective renal angiography preoperatively in order to define the blood supply to the injured segments. Prior knowledge of the number of renal arteries supplying the injured kidney is extremely useful for gaining control of the renal pedicle before mobilization of the kidney. A transperitoneal rather than an extraperitoneal operation is used unless obvious infection has already supervened.

Those children in whom the injured kidney cannot be visualized on infusion urography should undergo investigation with aortography and selective renal angiography without delay. Kidneys deteriorate rapidly at body temperature; expeditious diagnostic workup and prompt surgery are mandatory in patients with intimal tears and thrombosis of the renal artery. Observation, repeat intravenous urograms, and retrograde studies merely delay the diagnosis and work against possible conservative surgery. The literature in traumatic renal artery thromboses consists almost entirely of cases that were diagnosed too late for reparative surgery [19, 29, 47]. In the more common event of intimal disruption and subsequent thrombosis of the renal artery, a period of time may elapse prior to the development of complete occlusion. This period may allow for the development of enough collateral circulation to at least partially satisfy the metabolic needs of the kidney [63]. Sullivan and Stables described a patient with bilateral artery occlusion who recovered useful renal function despite a 10-hour delay before surgical correction [105].

SEQUELAE

Mortality was reported in 19 of 574 children with renal trauma [30, 46, 61, 70, 79, 89, 100] (3.3 percent). Only 2 of the 19 deaths, however, could be attributed directly to the renal injury. Perinephric hematomas, particularly when associated with urinary extravasation, are apt to become infected and result in perinephric abscesses. Some authors have suggested using prophylactic antibiotics in order to prevent this dreaded complication. Urinary leaks may persist and become walled off, forming pararenal pseudohydronephroses or urinomas. The perirenal urinoma communicates with the pelvocalyceal system, and its persistence is due to an obstruction to pelvic emptying that may have preceded the trauma, be consequent to it, or result from the distortion caused by the cyst itself. The cyst wall later may become hyalinized or calcified intrarenal extravasation and an intact capsule developed scarring, whereas 6 of 7 children with extrarenal extravasation on the initial urogram developed scars. Hutchison and Nogrady further noted that the growth of a recognizably damaged kidney is abnormal. The greatest reduction in kidney size occurred within the first year following injury. In general, the atrophied kidney subsequently increases in size, but at a slower rate than the normal one, which may undergo compensatory hypertrophy. When focal hypertrophy is excessive, it may simulate a neoplasm. The degree of permanent renal damage is likely to be established within 1 year following trauma.

Hypertension subsequent to renal trauma is a well-known complication, although its incidence is unknown. Massumi et al. [66], in a report on renal hypertension in a 16-year-old boy, quoted four cases from the literature (age 4 to 7 years) who developed arterial hypertension subsequent to trauma. Grant et al. [34] reported two cases of hypertension 12 and 16 years after injury. Hypertension secondary to renal trauma rarely develops at the age when patients attend pediatric hospitals; therefore, children with known posttraumatic radiologic renal scarring should continue to be observed for the possibility of hypertension after leaving the pediatric center.

Obstructive uropathy secondary to scarring, if it is going to occur, will generally do so in the first year following injury. Urinary tract infection was absent in all 111 patients followed by Hutchison and Nogrady [45], and in no patient did calculi form.

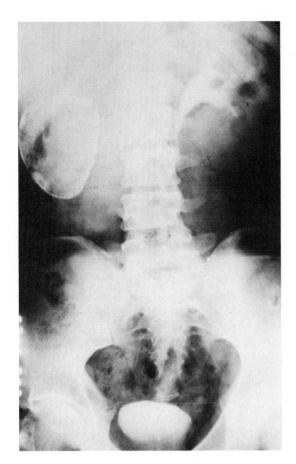

Figure 93-9. Calcified right pseudohydronephrosis or urinoma secondary to renal trauma with nonvisualization on the intravenous pyelogram.

(Fig. 93-9). Urothorax has been reported as an unusual complication of multiple injuries, with urinary extravasation tracking into the pleural cavity [44].

Delayed hemorrhage may occur following conservative treatment, reparative surgery, or partial nephrectomy. It usually occurs between 10 days and 4 weeks after the injury.

The true incidence of long-term complications is unknown because of inadequate follow-up of asymptomatic patients. Patients with Nunn type I injuries without urographic abnormalities do not develop late sequelae [82]. Hutchison and Nogrady [45], however, reported follow-up studies in 59 children with renal trauma in whom delayed or decreased visualization or definite distortion of the calyceal pattern had been observed on their initial urogram. Eleven of 47 children without extravasation were observed to have posttraumatic scarring. The more severe the injury, the higher the rate of scarring. Three of the 5 children with

Ureteral Injuries

Injuries of the ureter are rare in childhood. The position of the ureter deep in the retroperitoneum, protected by the full thickness of the abdomen, the rigid bony spine, and the heavy paraspinal muscle complex, poses a formidable barrier to injury. Operative trauma during pelvic dissection, the most common mechanism in adult ureteral injury, is readily avoidable in children, since the lack of extraperitoneal fat allows the course of the ureter to be easily visualized. Penetrating external injuries from stabs and gunshots rarely involve children. Blunt abdominal trauma, the most common mode of abdominal injury both in children and adults, only rarely results in ureteral injury.

INCIDENCE

There are only 21 case reports of ureteral injury secondary to blunt abdominal trauma in the literature. Patient age is listed in 17 cases; 8 are children

[21, 32, 35, 49, 99, 101, 121], including 5 boys and 2 girls. All of the childhood injuries were avulsions of the ureter at or just below the ureteropelvic junction. Seven cases were unilateral; the right side was involved in 5 and the left in 2. The one bilateral avulsion occurred in a 3-year-old girl [49]. All injuries resulted from severe and violent blows caused by moving vehicles. All but 2 children had fractures of the pelvis, ribs, lumbar vertebrae, or skull. Other intraabdominal injuries were frequent.

MECHANISM OF INJURY

The mechanism of injury in cases of ureteral avulsion has been the subject of speculation and investigation. Küster [56] thought the injury resulted from compression of the kidney and pelvis against the lower ribs or upper transverse processes, together with stretching of the ureter by lateral flexion of the trunk. Wilenius [116] thought that wheels rolling across the abdomen produced ureteral crushing and tears at the level of the second, third, and fifth lumbar vertebrae. Ainsworth et al. [1] stated that their case of bilateral involvement in an adult ruled out lateral flexion as an important etiologic factor. Simultaneous direct compression of both ureters also seemed highly unlikely, since the fact that one ureteral end was buried within the vertebral column could not be explained by either of these mechanisms. The vertebral fracture site or intervertebral space must have been widely open anteriorly at the instant of ureteral separation, suggesting extreme hyperextension of the lumbar spine at the moment of impact. They postulated that this hyperextension plus the additional force due to sudden acceleration imposed enough tension on the ureters to result in avulsion.

SYMPTOMS AND SIGNS

Early diagnosis of ureteral injury is difficult. Examination of the first urine voided is critical, as it will almost always show gross or microscopic hematuria. Subsequent urines may be entirely free of blood, as was reported by Halverstadt and Fraley [35]. In unsuspected injury urine will accumulate in the retroperitoneum and result in a palpable flank mass or urinary fistula that may not present for several days or weeks. Secondary infection of the urinary cyst may intervene. Johnston [49a] suggested that in those children in whom the diagnosis is made only after several days or even weeks after injury the ureter might not have been ruptured immediately; rather, it suffered vascular trauma which led to its subsequent necrosis and separation.

DIAGNOSIS

High-dose intravenous urography should be done during the initial evaluation of the child with multiple trauma. If there is ureteral injury, dye will extravasate in the region of the ureteropelvic junction (Fig. 93-10). Rotation and upward displacement of the kidney may be apparent. If a ureteral injury is suspected on urography and if the general condition of the patient allows, a retrograde ureteropyelogram under anesthesia should be made in order to confirm the diagnosis and localize precisely the area of injury. The retrograde pyelogram will also differentiate partial from complete severance of the ureter. The ureteral catheter should be left in place to facilitate location of the avulsed distal ureter, and exploration should follow immediately upon completion of the study.

TREATMENT

Treatment ideally consists in early retroperitoneal exploration, if no intraabdominal injury is suspected, and adequate mobilization of the kidney to allow for its maximal descent as a means of reducing tension on the ureteral anastomosis. If it is impossible to achieve approximation of the ureteral ends despite thorough mobilization of the kidney and ureter, anastomosis of the distal ureteral segment to the most inferior portion of the renal calyceal system can be performed or autotransplantation can be considered.

Delayed exploration and repair are fraught with technical difficulty because of extensive fibrosis at the site of injury, distortion of normal anatomic relationships, and the presence of infection. Nevertheless, Seright [99] reported salvaging a kidney with good function despite some hydronephrosis 10 weeks after complete avulsion.

RESULTS AND SEQUELAE

Two of the seven patients with unilateral ureteral injury reported in the literature underwent nephrectomy. Five underwent successful repair. Three have normal pyelograms, and two have residual hydronephrosis but good visualization. One required reoperation at 3 months because of a ureteropelvic junction stricture before a satisfactory result was attained. In the only bilateral ureteral avulsion reported [49], primary repair was successful on one side. These results suggest that every effort should be made to achieve primary reconstruction, with nephrectomy reserved for those patients in whom reconstruction has failed.

Injuries of the Bladder

There are no published reports that specifically analyze bladder injuries in children. The available

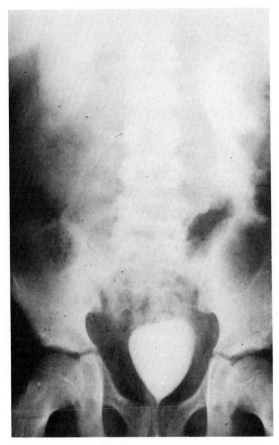

A

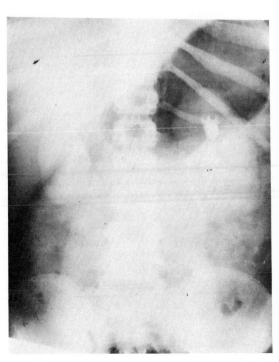

B

information regarding the mode of presentation of such injuries, the best method of treatment, and the related morbidity and mortality have all been garnered from isolated case reports and by extrapolation from experience in adults.

The child's bladder is an abdominal rather than a pelvic organ. According to Campbell [11, 12] the bladder does not attain its adult pelvic position until about the twentieth year; thus the proportionate area of the bladder covered by peritoneum is considerably greater. Consequently it has been stated that the child's bladder, when full, is more susceptible to injury of the closed or penetrating type [119]. Despite the apparent vulnerability of the bladder, however, the literature contains only isolated case reports of bladder injury in children.

Levitt and Zuckerman [59b] reviewed the records of all children admitted to the Bronx Municipal Hospital Center in New York City from July, 1966, through July, 1974, with the diagnosis of pelvic fracture or rupture of the bladder. Fifty children had fractures of the pubis alone, while sixteen others additionally had iliac bone fractures. Forty-six had hematuria. All but 2 were evaluated by intravenous urography, and many had cystography. Perivesical or pelvic hematomas were evident in 33, but *only* 2 children had *lacerations* of the bladder. In 1 of these all four pubic rami were fractured, and in the other there were no pelvic fractures at all, although the patient did have hematuria and difficulty voiding.

TYPES OF INJURY

Bladder injuries are classified into two types, contusions and ruptures. Ruptures are further subdivided according to whether they are intraperitoneal or extraperitoneal.

Contusions

Contusions refer to nonperforating injuries of the bladder wall. The effect may be evident only on

Figure 93-10. Studies of an 11-year-old boy who was struck by an automobile. A. An intravenous urogram shows prompt excretion bilaterally with marked extravasation of contrast material from the left ureter. Both calyceal systems appear normal. B. Excretory urogram 3 months postoperatively following end-to-end ureteroureterostomy of the avulsed ureter 1 cm below the ureteropelvic junction and temporary nephrostomy. Prompt excretion is noted bilaterally. There is slight narrowing at the site of anastomosis but no calicectasis. (From B. Fruchtman and H. Newman, Upper ureteral avulsion secondary to nonpenetrating injury, J. Urol. 93:452. Copyright © 1965, The Williams & Wilkins, Co., Baltimore.)

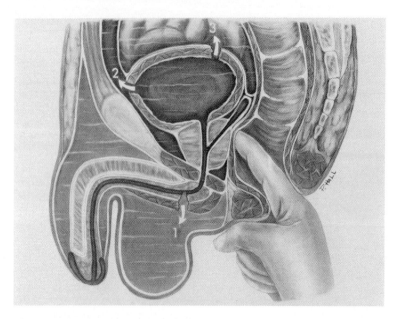

Figure 93-11. Anatomy of the bladder and male urethra showing difference between intraperitoneal and extraperitoneal bladder rupture. 1. Bulbomembranous urethral rupture. 2. Extraperitoneal rupture of bladder. 3. Usual site of intraperitoneal bladder rupture. (From S. S. Clark and R. F. Prudencio, Surg. Clin. North Am. 52:183, 1972.)

the mucous membrane, or the muscle layer and serosa may be involved as well. The wall of the bladder remains intact, however, and no urine escapes.

Catheterization and endoscopic procedures often result in mucosal ecchymosis. Surgery on organs adjacent to the bladder may be followed by contusions of the bladder wall. Fractures of the bony pelvis that do not cause rupture of the bladder nearly always produce sufficient trauma to cause contusion. Symptoms are irritative in nature, with dysuria and frequency predominating. Hematuria may be gross, microscopic, or absent. Usually no treatment is required, and spontaneous healing can be expected. When the contusion has resulted from instrumentation, an antibiotic generally is prescribed for 5 to 7 days.

Ruptures

Intraperitoneal Rupture. This denotes a complete break in the continuity of the bladder wall with communication into the peritoneal cavity. It most commonly follows blunt trauma to the lower abdomen or crush injuries when the bladder is distended. The ample mobility, elasticity, and lack of attachment of the bladder to the symphysis pubis prevents it from being injured more frequently by direct pelvic trauma. Distention is the critical factor that renders it more vulnerable to injury, since mobility and compressibility are decreased and surface area is increased. Since the distal and

lateral aspects of the bladder wall are supported by bony or muscular structures, the peritoneal surface is the weakest point and is most susceptible to rupture. The perforation generally occurs in the fundus or posterior aspect of the dome (Fig. 93-11).

The adult bladder is classically injured by bony spicules from pelvic fractures piercing the bladder wall extraperitoneally. This occurs less frequently in children because the bladder is intraperitoneal and the compression effect exerted at the time of impact more commonly results in an intraperitoneal rupture [18].

Kroll et al. [54] and Miller et al. [71] reported intraperitoneal bladder rupture in neonates. Presumably compression of the distended bladder occurred during birth, either from uterine contractions, compression during passage through the birth canal, or from obstetric manipulation. "Spontaneous" intraperitoneal perforations have also been reported in children with underlying bladder pathology. Sullivan et al. [104] reported a 1-year-old boy with spontaneous intraperitoneal rupture of a paraureteric diverticulum. No bladder outlet obstruction could be detected. Urinary ascites has also been reported in the newborn secondary to posterior urethral valves. One of the mechanisms that might allow for this to occur is spontaneous perforation of a small bladder saccule [74].

Extravasation of sterile urine intraperitoneally

initially evokes little peritoneal reaction. Watson and Cunningham [113] quoted Tuffier's experimental studies, which showed that slow injection of sterile urine or allowing sufficient time between larger injections does not produce peritonitis. The continued flow of urine in moderate or larger quantities, however, does produce peritoneal irritation. The omentum or adjacent bowel becomes adherent and seals the rupture if it is small, but the plugging effect is not adequate with larger rents. In those cases in which the diagnosis is not suspected early and in which there is persistent extravasation of sterile urine into the peritoneal cavity, a condition of peritoneal autodialysis occurs [53]. Equilibration between the plasma and intraperitoneal fluid results in a fall in serum sodium and chloride content and a rise in urea and potassium, accompanied by acidosis. These metabolic changes are manifested as convulsions, stupor, and, finally, coma. Unsuspected bladder ruptures have also been reported to cause serum blood urea nitrogen-creatinine disproportion. Measurement of ammonia levels in peritoneal fluid has been found to be helpful in identifying urinary extravasation in patients with possible "spontaneous" intraperitoneal bladder ruptures. Levels greater than 3 μg per milliliter are significant. Mansberger and Young [65] reported a case of unsuspected intraperitoneal urinary extravasation in which the cystogram was interpreted as normal and urinary output seemed adequate; the diagnosis was suggested only by a high ammonia level in intraperitoneal fluid. Laparotomy revealed a posterior bladder wall perforation. Urea content might also aid in identifying the fluid as urine; however, the difference in urea concentration between plasma and urine may not be sufficient to be diagnostic.

Extraperitoneal Rupture. This term denotes a break in the continuity of the bladder wall in an area that is not covered by peritoneum. Almost all extraperitoneal injuries of the bladder occur on the anterolateral bladder wall, close to the vesical neck. Extraperitoneal bladder rupture is most commonly seen in association with fractures of the bony pelvis, particularly when the pubic symphysis and rami are involved. The bladder is either torn by traction on its attachments or is penetrated by bony spicules. An empty bladder is not immune to extraperitoneal rupture.

Prather and Kaiser [85] reported a 10 percent incidence of rupture of the bladder in 1,798 cases of pelvic fracture in adults. When the rupture occurred in conjunction with the pelvic fraction, 82 percent were of the extraperitoneal type. As noted earlier, however, in my unpublished review of 66 children with pelvic fractures there was only 1

case of bladder rupture, and this was of the intraperitoneal type [59b].

The posterior aspect of the bladder may be injured when a child falls on a spike that enters the anus and penetrates the rectum and bladder (Fig. 93-12). A similar posterior injury may occur in an infant if a thermometer breaks in the rectum. Urine extravasates into the perivesical tissues, and if left undrained, it will extend along fascial planes to the anterior abdominal wall or perinephric areas through the inguinal canals to the scrotum, via the sciatic foramina to the buttocks, or through the obturator foramen into the thigh. In addition to urinary extravasation, extraperitoneal hemorrhage generally is severe, particularly when associated with a pelvic fracture. Bleeding from the pubic branch of the inferior epigastric and obturator arteries, which anastomose on the posterior surface of the pubis, and from the internal pudendal vessels and their branches coursing through the urogenital diaphragm, as well as from the vesical vessels and muscle bleeders, leads to large hematomas.

CLINICAL PRESENTATION

The diagnosis of rupture of the bladder is usually suspected from a history of trauma. An extreme desire to void, with inability to do so, is frequently present. Lower abdominal or suprapubic pain is usually present. The abdomen becomes distended. Suprapubic tenderness without muscular rigidity or absent bowel sounds is common. If untreated, infection occurs in about 60 percent [13, 41, 43, 71] of those with intraperitoneal rupture, leading to peritonitis with abdominal rigidity and ileus. Medial compression of the iliac crests or pressure over the symphysis pubis is apt to result in severe pain in those with associated fractures. When a fractured pelvis is present, the signs of bladder injury are often obscured by the bony trauma. In extraperitoneal rupture the lower abdomen is full and is often accompanied by scrotal hematomas in the male. Diffuse pelvic swelling may be evident on rectal examination.

DIAGNOSIS

The diagnosis of vesical perforation is best made by retrograde cystography [14, 39, 93] using an 8F polyethylene pediatric feeding tube for urethral catheterization. Intraperitoneal contrast medium gravitates to the dependent paracolic gutters and may be visible radiologically between coils of small intestine (Fig. 93-13). A large rupture may produce a sunburst appearance. Several investigators have reported negative cystographic findings in the presence of bladder ruptures, despite ade-

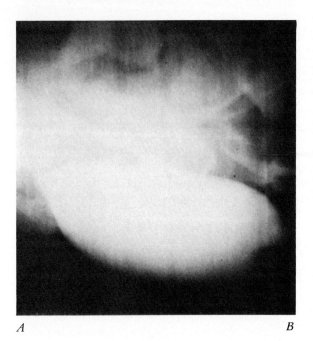
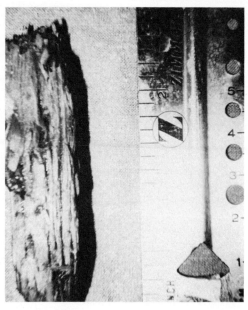

A   B

Figure 93-12. A foreign body was removed at exploration from a 10-year-old boy who sustained a posterior extraperitoneal bladder rupture in association with an anterior rectal tear. The boy fell onto a splintered wooden broomstick that perforated his rectum and posterior bladder wall, resulting in a rectovesical fistula. A. Cystogram with foreign body in situ demonstrating vesicorectal communication. B. Foreign body removed at surgery.

quate distention and good radiographic technique [13, 90, 92]. In doubtful cases cystoscopy [118] may be diagnostic. It is particularly useful in diagnosing suspected puncture wounds, in which cystographic findings are negative.

In extraperitoneal hemorrhage, contrast medium is visible in the perivesical tissues. Often the bladder is circumferentially compressed by accumulation of blood and urine so that it assumes a long, narrow ovoid shape—the so-called teardrop bladder.

The formerly recommended diagnostic technique of comparing the volumes of injected and recovered fluid is unreliable [14, 90, 118]. Fallacies arise if the catheter becomes blocked by blood clot or if the catheter traverses the rupture and fluid is aspirated from the peritoneal cavity.

TREATMENT
When the diagnosis of bladder rupture is established and the child's general condition has been stabilized, urgent surgery is performed. The peritoneal cavity is opened through a midline subumbilical incision. Extravasated urine and blood are aspirated. The vesical rupture is closed with absorbable sutures. It is important to establish effective bladder drainage postoperatively, and in the

male a large-bore catheter is brought out suprapubically from the anterior extraperitoneal portion of the bladder. Urethral catheterization will allow equally good urinary drainage in the female. The catheter should be connected to a closed catheter drainage system so as to lessen the likelihood of bacteriuria [55].

COMPLICATIONS AND SEQUELAE
Mortality rates in unsuspected or untreated bladder injuries are very high [10, 20, 22, 87]. Electrolyte disturbances secondary to peritoneal autodialysis, peritonitis, and perivesical necrosis from concentrated urine with superimposed infection almost always prove fatal unless adequate bladder drainage is established. With prompt recognition of bladder injuries and early adequate bladder drainage, the outlook for complete recovery is excellent.

Urethral Injuries
Urethral injuries can involve the anterior or posterior urethral segments (Fig. 93-14). They result from external violence or are secondary to instrumentation. The iatrogenic injuries resulting from instrumentation usually damage the anterior urethra. External violence more commonly injures the

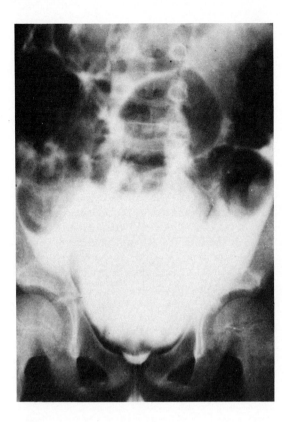

Figure 93-13. Cystogram showing intraperitoneal extravasation of contrast outlining coils of intestine and gravitating into the paracolic gutters.

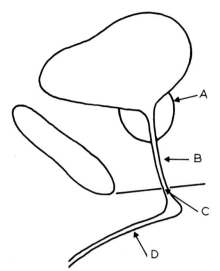

Figure 93-14. Sites of urethral injuries.
A. Bladder neck urethral disruptions—very rare
B. Supramembranous urethral rupture
C. Membranous urethral rupture
D. Anterior urethral injury
} *Posterior Urethral Injuries*

(From J. P. Mitchell, Br. J. Urol. 40:649, 1968; by permission of E. & S. Livingstone.)

posterior urethra, in association with pelvic fractures or dislocations.

INTRAPELVIC URETHRAL RUPTURE (RUPTURE OF THE POSTERIOR URETHRA)
Urethral ruptures above the urogenital diaphragm occur as a complication of fracture dislocations of the pelvis.

Incidence
A review of 2,419 [59, 117] cases of fractured pelves in both adults and children showed a 14.5 percent incidence of urinary injuries. In one compilation of 427 lower urinary tract injuries [18], 58.3 percent involved the urethra alone, 9.4 percent involved both urethra and bladder, and in only 32.3 percent was the bladder the sole structure injured.

Harrison [37] and Uhle and Erb [108] reported crush injuries compressing the pelvis in the transverse plane as the commonest cause of posterior urethral ruptures. During childhood the injury is usually consequent to an automobile accident in which the child is run over. Younger children are more commonly affected. Almost all reported cases have been in males, although Mitchell [72] reported rupture of the posterior urethra in two females, one an adult and the other a child.

Mechanism of Injury
The location of the posterior urethra within the angle of the pubic arch and its lack of mobility renders it particularly vulnerable to direct as well as indirect injury when the pelvis is fractured. The radiologic severity of the pubic arch fracture generally correlates with the degree of lower urinary tract injury [18, 40]. In patients with unilateral fractures of the pubic rami, the incidence of posterior urethral rupture was 15.5 percent; in bilateral fractures of the pubic rami, the incidence was 40.8 percent [40, 83]. The "sprung" or exploded pelvis is an exception to this rule. It occurs most commonly in children and often demonstrates few radiologic findings; yet the degree of trauma to the soft tissues and the urinary tract is great. Such injuries are frequently caused by a heavy vehicle passing over the child's pelvis. With the application of the force, the pelvis becomes disrupted at both the symphysis pubis and sacroiliac joints. After the force is removed, the pelvis springs back into a relatively normal position while the soft tissues are compressed and rapidly decompressed, resulting in total disruption of the rectum and urinary tract.

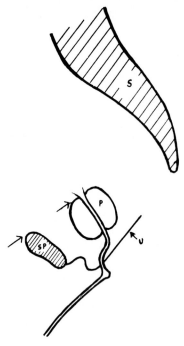

The shearing effect of a dislocation of the symphysis pubis (SP), which drives the prostate (P) backward in relation to the urogenital diaphragm (U). Sacrum (S).

Figure 93-15. Crush injury with disruption of pubo-prostatic ligaments and posterior dislocation of prostatic urethra on fixed membranous portion. (From J. P. Mitchell, Br. J. Urol. 40:649, 1968; by permission of E. & S. Livingstone.)

Crush injuries in the transverse plane produce sudden shortening in the transverse pelvic diameter with an increase in the anteroposterior diameter. The sudden, severe, shearing strain in the sagittal plane ruptures the puboprostatic ligaments, allowing the prostatic urethra greater mobility. The fixed supramembranous segment of urethra stretches acutely, leading to a simple contusion of the urethral wall and partial laceration or total disruption of the supramembranous urethra, shearing it from the membranous urethra (Fig. 93-15). The disruption may in addition be at the level of the vesical neck, leading to a free-floating prostate gland. In Mitchell's series [72] the only ruptures occurring above the lower border of the prostate were in children. Presumably the still undeveloped state of the prostate had something to do with this phenomenon. Associated with this unfortunate occurrence is the disruption of the periprostatic venous plexus, resulting in large hematomas that displace the prostate cephalad and posteriorly.

When bivalve separation of the symphysis pubis has occurred, the urethra is prone to injury by a different mechanism. In this instance the puboprostatic ligament on one side and the urogenital diaphragm on the other side are severed as the pubic arch separates, disrupting the membranous urethra (Fig. 93-16).

Diagnosis
The child with posterior urethral rupture is usually in severe shock and has sustained multiple injuries. Perivesical hemorrhage leads to a tender, palpable swelling in the lower abdomen and pelvis. On occasion blood will track from the perivesical tissue into the scrotum, perineum, thighs, and into the buttocks along tissue planes. Inability to urinate combined with a desire to do so is a common complaint. Blood at the external meatus is nearly always seen, but Mitchell noted its absence in two children with ruptured urethras. Rectal examination may reveal a free-floating prostate, although a large pelvic hematoma often will make adequate palpation of the prostate impossible. A high index of suspicion is necessary in the child with a pelvic fracture. A palpable bladder is a useful sign for distinguishing partial from complete rupture. In the latter, spasm of the bladder neck prevents extravasation into the retropubic space.

The diagnosis, when suspected, is best established by retrograde urethrography (Fig. 93-17). Blind passage of a urethral catheter carries the risk of making a false diagnosis. The catheter may pass with ease and curl up under the trigone or track perivesically, giving one a false impression that it is within the bladder. Recovery of bloody urine may be from the perivesical space in combined injuries of the bladder and urethra. Partial urethral ruptures may be missed. Incomplete urethral ruptures may be converted into complete disruptions by repeated efforts at instrumentation. Similarly, sterile perivesical hematomas, free of extravasated urine, may become infected by vigorous attempts at catheterization. Mitchell [72] advocated making the diagnosis of urethral injury solely on clinical grounds and avoiding all forms of urethral manipulation. As soon as the patient is in satisfactory condition, he performs a simple suprapubic cystostomy. Definitive diagnostic tests are performed electively at a later time. Cystoscopic examination is absolutely contraindicated.

TREATMENT AND COMPLICATIONS
The most urgent requirement in most cases of pelvic fracture with posterior urethral injury is resuscitation of the child with blood transfusions.

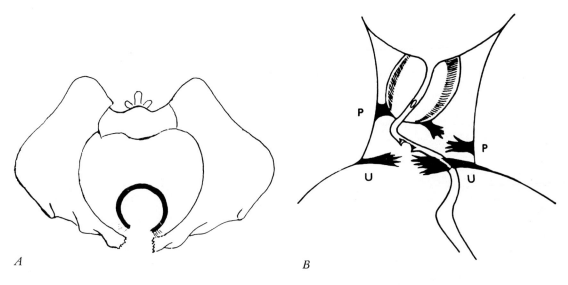

Figure 93-16. Mechanism of urethral injury in bivalve separation of symphysis pubis. A. Symphyseal separation (bivalve). B. Rupture of the puboprostatic ligament (P) on one side and urogenital diaphragm (U) on the other. (From J. P. Mitchell, Br. J. Urol. 40:649,1968; by permission of E. & S. Livingstone.)

Attempts at surgical control of bleeding are not feasible [83]. Early immobilization of the pelvis using a pelvic sling is often helpful, since every breath, cough, or movement of the unstabilized fracture fragments promotes further bleeding. A careful rectal examination in the child with a "sprung" pelvis is necessary to diagnose an associated rectal laceration and resultant fecal contamination. A diverting transverse colostomy is mandatory in such cases.

Radiologic differentiation of complete from partial rupture is often very difficult. When the diagnosis is made of a partial rupture without separation of the posterior urethral fragment, however, a simple diversion by suprapubic cystostomy tube drainage through the bladder dome is sufficient. No attempt is made to evacuate perivesical hematomas. The hematomas will absorb if left undisturbed, and the urethra will heal, often without stricture, allowing removal of the cystostomy tube in 10 days to 2 weeks.

There is no doubt that any complete transection of the urethra will ultimately lead to stricture formation. There is considerable controversy regarding the best program of management. Johanson [48], Morehouse et al. [75], Clark and Prudencio [18], as well as Mitchell [72] advocate initial simple suprapubic cystostomy drainage without any form of urethral stent. They maintain that urethral injuries are usually incomplete, with continuity being maintained at least by a bridge of intact urethra in most cases. Urethral instrumentation tends

to destroy this bridge and the normal alignment of bladder and urethra. They argue that with time the perivesical hematoma will subside, leaving a short stricture between the lacerated urethral segments that is relatively simple to treat by a later primary urethroplasty. Wilkinson [117], on the other hand, reported excellent results in 6 patients treated by suprapubic drainage together with "railroading" of the urethra in order to reestablish continuity. Apposition was maintained by constant traction on a Foley urethral catheter for 10 days. He treated a further 6 patients in the same fashion, but no traction was applied to the urethral catheter, which was left indwelling merely as a stent. A much poorer result was obtained. Malek et al. [64a] recently reported excellent results in 7 boys with partial or complete rupture of the posterior urethra. All were managed with the time-honored technique of early suprapubic cystostomy and concomitant primary realignment of the urethra over a catheter. Gentle traction was maintained for 4 to 7 days; thereafter the urethral stent was left indwelling for 4 to 6 weeks. Of the 4 children who had a functionally significant urethral stricture, 3 were cured within a few months by one or two simple urethral dilatations and 1 by subsequent transperineal lysis of the angulated urethra from its surrounding fibrous tissue. Follow-up data for 8 to 22 years (mean of 14 years) indicate that all 7 patients void with an excellent stream and are continent, free from infection, and potent. In fact, 3 of the 4 married and have fathered chil-

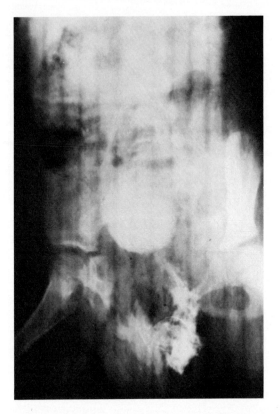

Figure 93-17. Retrograde urethrogram following intravenous pyelogram. It demonstrates complete rupture of the membranous urethra with no communication between the urethra and bladder. Extravasation of contrast into the perineum distal to the urogenital diaphragm is evident. Note the high-riding bladder (filled during IVP) and fractured pubis.

dren. Johnston [49a] advocates aligning the ruptured urethral ends and maintaining them in apposition using traction via a perineal urethrostomy. Turner-Warwick's [107] method of maintaining alignment and opposition using a nylon stitch through the prostate with elastic band traction on the emerging ends in the perineum seems particularly applicable in children.

Complications

The complications of rupture of the posterior urethra as well as of its treatment are significant. As noted by Devereux and Williams [25], strictures develop within weeks of injury. In their experience complications of treatment resulting from improper urethral stenting were frequent. Upper tract changes ranging from mild dilatation of the lower ureters to severe hydronephrosis were already present in 6 of 14 boys with posterior urethral strictures within a few months of injury. Urinary tract infection was present in more than half

the children. One patient had a vesical diverticulum, and another had a bladder calculus.

Long-term urethral dilatations are generally unsatisfactory for managing urethral strictures in children. However, scrotal inlay urethroplasties of the Turner-Warwick type [107] or other methods such as the Leadbetter [57] and Johanson [48] operations, as well as the Badenoch [4] pull-through procedure, are eminently successful in achieving an unobstructed urethra with continence in most cases. More recently, Waterhouse and Gross [112a] achieved excellent results using a transpubic approach with direct anastamosis of the normal anterior urethra to the anterior wall of the prostatic urethra, proximal to the stricture. A minority of children have injuries that cannot be reconstructed and require urinary diversion. Impotence may be a late sequel resulting from interruption of vascular and neural connections to the penile erectile tissue.

ANTERIOR URETHRAL INJURIES

Iatrogenic injuries consequent to urethral instrumentation most frequently involve the anterior urethra. The penoscrotal junction is the most vulnerable portion. Endoscopy and urethral catheter drainage are the main causes. Forcible insertion of large sounds and cystoscopes can rupture the urethra, leading to urinary extravasation, a periurethral phlegmon, and subsequent stricture formation. Devereux and Williams [25] noted 17 iatrogenic strictures among 26 anterior urethral strictures in boys aged 2 to 11 years. Seven were the result of complications related to transurethral posterior valve resections. The remainder occurred from indwelling urethral catheters.

Strictures developing secondary to injury are recognized by symptoms of obstruction. Dilation as a definitive method of treatment is advisable only for mild strictures that are cured by a few infrequent dilations. The treatment of choice for short penile urethral strictures is resection with end-to-end anastomosis of healthy proximal and distal segments. Longer strictures require primary marsupialization [48] with subsequent urethroplasty [8, 28, 106].

Bulbar urethral injuries result from straddle injuries or are secondary to blows in the perineum that compress the urethra against the pubic arch. A hematoma will develop in the perineum and scrotum. Bleeding occurs from the urethral meatus. These injuries may result in urethral contusion or partial and complete tears. The children often are unable to void. Retrograde urethrography confirms the diagnosis. Simple contusion may require an indwelling urethral catheter for several days to allow for perineal swelling and pain to subside and for spontaneous urination to recommence. Lacerations are best treated by suprapubic cystostomy tube diversion. Total rupture results in stricture formation that will require subsequent urethroplasty.

References

1. Ainsworth, T., Weems, W. L., and Merrel, W. H., Jr. Bilateral ureteral injury due to non penetrating external trauma. *J. Urol.* 96:439, 1966.
2. Arcari, F. A. Blunt abdominal trauma in infants and children. *J. Mich. Med. Soc.* 61:335, 1962.
3. Bacon, S. K. Rupture of the urinary bladder: Clinical analysis of 147 cases in the past 10 years. *J. Urol.* 49:432, 1943.
4. Badenoch, A. W. Pull-through operation for impassible traumatic stricture of urethra. *Br. J. Urol.* 22:404, 1950.
5. Baghdassarian, O. M., Koehler, R. P., and Schultze, G. M. Neonatal ascites. *Radiology* 76:586, 1961.
6. Bailey, H. Injuries to the kidney and ureter. *Br. J. Surg.* 11:609, 1924.
7. Bronklaus, M., Riley, R. R., and Girdany, B. R. Pediatric arteriography in abdominal and extremity lesions. *Radiology* 92:1241, 1969.
8. Brown, D. An operation for hypospadias. *Proc. R. Soc. Med.* 42:466, 1949.
9. Butt, A. J., and Perry, J. Q. Ureteral injury complicating fracture of the bony pelvis. *South. Surg.* 16:1139, 1950.
10. Cahill, G. F. Rupture of the bladder and urethra. *Am. J. Surg.* 36:653, 1937.
11. Campbell, M. F. Rupture of the bladder. *Surg. Gynecol. Obstet.* 49:540, 1929.
12. Campbell, M. F. *Pediatric Urology.* New York: Macmillan, 1937. Vol. 2, p. 172.
13. Campbell, M. F. *Clinical Pediatric Urology.* Philadelphia: Saunders, 1951. P. 617.
14. Campbell, M. F. Injuries of the kidneys. *Surg. Clin. North Am.* 21:443, 1941.
15. Campbell, M. F. and Harrison, J. H. *Urology* (3rd ed.). Philadelphia: Saunders, 1970. Vol. 1, chap. 22.
16. Carvajal, H. F., Travis, L. B., Srivastaua, R. N., DeBeukelaer, M. M., Dodge, W. F., and Dupree, E. Percutaneous renal biopsy in children: An analysis of complications in 890 consecutive biopsies. *Texas Rep. Biol. Med.* 29:3, 1971.
17. Charron, J. W., and Brault, J. P. Recognition and early management of injuries to the urinary tract. *J. Trauma* 4:702, 1964.
18. Clark, S. S., and Prudencio, R. F. Lower urinary tract injuries associated with pelvic fracture. *Surg. Clin. North Am.* 52:183, 1972.
19. Cornell, S., Reasa, D. A., and Culp, D. A. Occlusion of the renal artery secondary to acute or remote trauma. *J.A.M.A.* 219:1754, 1972.
20. Crane, J. J., and Schenck, G. F. Rupture of the urinary bladder. *Urol. Cutan. Rev.* 36:614, 1932.
21. Crosby, D. L. An unusual case of renal trauma. *Br. J. Urol.* 31:159, 1959.
22. Culp, O. S. Treatment of ruptured bladder and urethra. *J. Urol.* 48:266, 1942.
23. DeBeukelaer, M. M., Schreiber, M. H., Dodge, W. F., and Travis, L. B. Intrarenal arteriovenous fistulas following needle biopsy of the kidney. *J. Pediatr.* 78:266, 1971.
24. Del Villar, R. G., Ireland, G. W., and Cass, A. S. Ureteral injury owing to external trauma. *J. Urol.* 107:29, 1972.
25. Devereux, M. H., and Williams, D. I. The treatment of urethral stricture in boys. *J. Urol.* 108:489, 1972.
26. Dowse, J. L., and Kihn, R. B. Renal injuries: Diagnosis, management and sequelae in 67 cases. *Br. J. Surg.* 50:353, 1963.
27. Dumitresco, D. A case of traumatic rupture of the ureter, with remarks on the diagnosis of such ruptures in general. *Med. Press Circ.* 99:494, 1915.
28. Duplay, S. Perineoscrotal hypospadias and its repair. *Arch. Gen. Med. Paris* 1:513, 1874.
29. Evans, J., and Mogg, R. A. Renal artery thrombosis due to closed trauma. *J. Urol.* 105:330, 1971.
30. Forsythe, W. E. Renal trauma in children. *Hosp. Med.* 68, 1969.
31. Freeman, L. M., Kay, C. J., and Meng, C. H. The contribution of renal scanning in the evaluation of renal trauma. *Radiology* 86:1021, 1966.
32. Fruchtman, B., and Newman, H. Upper ureteral avulsion secondary to non-penetrating injury. *J. Urol.* 93:452, 1965.
33. Garrett, R. A., and Franken, E. A., Jr. Neonatal ascites: Perirenal urinary extravasation with bladder outlet obstruction. *J. Urol.* 102:627, 1969.
34. Grant, R. P., Jr., Gifford, R. W., Pudvan, W. R., Meaney, W. F., Straffon, R. A., and McCormack, L. J. Renal trauma and hypertension. *Am. J. Cardiol.* 27:173, 1971.
35. Halverstadt, D. B., and Fraley, E. E. Avulsion of the upper ureter secondary to blunt trauma. *Br. J. Urol.* 39:588, 1967.
36. Harris, J. H., and Harris, J. H., Jr. Infusion pyelography. *Am. J. Roentgenol.* 92:1391, 1964.
37. Harrison, J. H. The treatment of rupture of the urethra, especially when accompanying fractures of the pelvic bones. *Surg. Gynecol. Obstet.* 72:622, 1941.
38. Harrow, B. R. Unusual renal peripelvic extravasation requiring operative drainage. *J. Urol.* 102:564, 1969.
39. Hartley, B. Traumatic intraperitoneal rupture of the urinary bladder. *Aust. N.Z. J. Surg.* 28:233, 1959.
40. Hartmann, K. Blasen—Und Harnrohrenverletzungen Becken Bruchen. *Arch. Klin. Chir.* 282:943, 1955.
41. Hershman, H., and Allen, H. L. Spontaneous rupture of the normal urinary bladder. *Surgery* 35:805, 1954.
42. Hodges, C. V., Gilbert, D. R., and Scott, W. W. Renal trauma: A study of 71 cases. *J. Urol.* 66:627, 1951.
43. Hood, J. M., and Smyth, B. T. Non-penetrating intraabdominal injuries in children. *J. Pediatr. Surg.* 9:69, 1974.
44. Hume, H. A., Stevens, L. W., and Erb, W. H. Urothorax: An unusual complication of multiple traumatic injuries. *N. Engl. J. Med.* 267:289, 1962.
45. Hutchison, R. J., and Nogrady, M. B. Late sequelae of renal trauma in the pediatric age group. *J. Can. Assoc. Radiol.* 24:3, 1973.
45a. Jaffe, J. W., Persky, L., and Downs, T. D. Parenteral therapy in the management of mechanical renal trauma. *J. Urol.* 100:133, 1968.

46. Javadpour, G. P., and Bush, I. M.   Renal trauma in children. *Surg. Gynecol. Obstet.* 136:237, 1973.

47. Jevtich, M. J., and Montero, G.   Injuries to renal vessels by blunt trauma in children. *J. Urol.* 102:493, 1969.

48. Johanson, B.   Reconstruction of the Male Urethra in Strictures. In E. W. Riches (ed.), *Modern Trends in Urology.* London: Butterworth, 1953. P. 344.

49. Johnson, J. M., Chernov, M. S., Cloud, D. T., Linkner, L. M., Dorman, G. W., and Trump, D. S.   Bilateral ureteral avulsion. *J. Pediatr. Surg.* 7:723, 1972.

49a. Johnston, J. H.   *Paediatric Urology* (3rd ed.). London: Butterworth, 1968. Pp. 356, 360.

50. Kaiser, T. F., and Franklin, F. C.   Injury to the bladder and prostatomembranous urethra associated with fracture of the bony pelvis. *Surg. Gynecol. Obstet.* 120:99, 1965.

51. Kazmin, M. H., Brosman, S. A., and Cockett, A. T. K.   Diagnosis and early management of renal trauma: A study of 120 patients. *J. Urol.* 101:783, 1969.

52. Knappenberger, S. T., Akes, R. E., and Galuszka, A. A.   Complete avulsion of the renal pedicle by non-penetrating trauma with survival. *J. Urol.* 89:316, 1963.

53. Ko-Kwang, W., Judson, R., and Fellers, F. X.   Peritoneal self dialysis following traumatic rupture of the bladder. *J. Urol.* 91:343, 1964.

53a. Koenigsberg, M., Blaufox, M. D., and Freeman, L. M.   Traumatic injuries of the renal vasculature and parenchyma. *Semin. Nucl. Med.* 4:117, 1974.

54. Kroll, V., Dickman, F., and Chalstrom, H.   Rupture of the urinary bladder in the neonatal period with report of a case. *La. State Med. Soc. J.* 108:58, 1956.

55. Kunin, C. M., and McCormack, R. C.   Prevention of catheter-induced urinary tract infections by sterile closed drainage. *N. Engl. J. Med.* 274:1155, 1966.

56. Küster, E.   *Dtsch. Chir.* 52B, 1896. Cited by W. Seright, Traumatic closed rupture of the ureter. *Br. J. Surg.* 46:511, 1959.

57. Leadbetter, G. W., Jr.   A simplified urethroplasty for strictures of the bulbous urethra. *J. Urol.* 83:54, 1960.

58. Leiter, E., Gribetz, D., and Cohen, S.   Arteriovenous fistula after percutaneous needle biopsy—surgical repair with preservation of renal function. *N. Engl. J. Med.* 287:971, 1972.

59. Levine, J. I., and Crampton, R. A.   Major abdominal injuries associated with pelvic fractures. *Surg. Gynecol. Obstet.* 116:223, 1963.

59a. Levitt, S. B., and Lutzker, L. G.   Urine extravasation secondary to upper urinary tract obstruction. *J. Pediatr. Surg.* 11:575, 1976.

59b. Levitt, S. B., and Zuckerman, H.   A review of children with pelvic fractures, urethral and bladder injuries. Unpublished data, 1973.

60. Lindeman, R. D.   Percutaneous renal biopsy. *Kidney* 7:1, 1974.

61. Linke, C. A., Frank, I. N., Young, L. W., and Cockett, A. T.   Renal trauma in children. *N.Y. State J. Med.* 72:2414, 1972.

62. Lloyd, F. A.   Historical notes on the Twelfth General Hospital (U.S.)—war injuries of the ureter. *Q. Bull. Northwest. Univ. Med. Sch.* 30:74, 1956.

63. Love, L., and Bush, I. M.   Early demonstration of renal collateral arterial supply. *Am. J. Roentgenol. Nucl. Radium. Ther.* 104:296, 1968.

64. Mahoney, S. A., and Persky, L.   Intravenous drip nephrotomography as an adjunct in the evaluation of renal injury. *J. Urol.* 99:513, 1968.

64a. Malek, R. S., O'Dea, M. J., and Kelalis, P. P.   Management of ruptured posterior urethra in childhood. *J. Urol.* 117:105, 1977.

65. Mansberger, A. R., Jr., and Young, J. D., Jr.   The value of ammonia levels as an aid in the diagnosis of urinary extravasation. *J. Urol.* 94:125, 1965.

66. Massumi, R. A., Andrade, A., and Kramer, N.   Arterial hypertension in traumatic subcapsular perineal haematuria (Page kidney). *Am. J. Med.* 46:635, 1969.

67. McCague, E. J.   Renal trauma—conservative management. *J. Urol.* 63:773, 1950.

68. McDonald, P., and Hiller, H. G.   Angiography in abdominal tumours in childhood with particular reference to neuroblastoma and Wilms tumour. *Clin. Radiol.* 19:1, 1968.

69. McKay, H. W., Baird, H. H., and Lynch, K. M., Jr.   Management of the injured kidney. *J.A.M.A.* 141:575, 1949.

70. Mertz, J. H., Wishard, W. N., Jr., Nourse, M. H., and Mertz, H. O.   Injury of the kidney in children. *J.A.M.A.* 183:730, 1963.

71. Miller, A. L., Jr., Sharp, L., Anderson, E. V., and Emlet, J. R.   Rupture of the bladder in the newborn. 83:630, 1960.

72. Mitchell, J. P.   Injuries to the urethra. *Br. J. Urol.* 40:649, 1968.

73. Mitnik, M., Weill, W. B., Wolfson, S. L., and Drummond, C. D., Jr.   Renal foreign bodies—unusual cause of hematuria and pyuria. *Clin. Pediatr.* 8:281, 1969.

74. Moncada, R., Wang, W. J., Love, L., and Busch, I.   Neonatal ascites associated with urinary outlet obstruction (urine ascites). *Radiology* 90:1165, 1968.

75. Morehouse, D. D., Belitsky, P., and MacKinnow, K.   Rupture of the posterior urethra. *J. Urol.* 107:255, 1972.

76. Morrow, J. W., and Mendez, R.   Renal trauma. *J. Urol.* 104:649, 1970.

77. Morse, T. S.   Infusion pyelography in the evaluation of renal injuries in children. *J. Trauma* 6:693, 1966.

78. Morse, T. S.   Trauma: A call to action. Presented at the American Pediatric Surgical Association Trauma Workshop, Hot Springs, Va., April 12, 1972.

79. Morse, T. S., Smith, J. P., Howard, W. H. R., and Howe, M. I.   Kidney injuries in children. *J. Urol.* 98:693, 1967.

79a. Nebesar, R. A., Fleischli, D. J., Pollard, J., and Griscom, N. T.   Arteriography in infants and children. *Radiology* 94:476, 1970.

80. Nunn, I. N.   The management of closed renal injury. *Aust. N.Z. J. Surg.* 31:263, 1962.

81. Orkin, L. A.   Evaluation of the merits of cystoscopy and retrograde pyelography in the management of renal trauma. *J. Urol.* 63:9, 1950.

82. Palavatara, C., Graham, S. R., and Silverman, F. N.   Delayed sequels to renal injury in childhood. *Am. J. Roentgenol.* 91:659, 1964.

83. Peltier, L. F.   Complications associated with frac-

tures of the pelvis. *J. Bone Joint Surg.* 47:1060, 1965.

84. Persky, L., and Forsythe, W. E. Renal trauma in childhood. *J.A.M.A.* 182:709, 1962.

85. Prather, G. C., and Kaiser, T. F. The bladder in fracture of the bony pelvis; significance of "tear drop bladder." *J. Urol.* 63:1019, 1950.

86. Priestley, J. T. Renal trauma. *Surg. Clin. North Am.* 19:1033, 1939.

87. Quain, E. P. Rupture of the bladder associated with fracture of pelvis. *Surg. Gynecol. Obstet.* 23:55, 1916.

88. Ravich, L., and Schell, N. B. Rupture of the kidney in the newborn infant. *N.Y. State J. Med.* 61:2822, 1961.

89. Reid, I. S. Renal trauma in children: A ten-year review. *Aust. N.Z. J. Surg.* 42:260, 1973.

90. Reid, R. E., and Herman, J. R. Rupture of the bladder and urethra: Diagnosis and treatment. *N.Y. State J. Med.* 65:2685, 1965.

91. Richardson, D., Belin, R. P., and Griffen, W., Jr. Blunt abdominal trauma in children. *Ann. Surg.* 176:213, 1972.

92. Rieser, C., and Nicholas, E. Rupture of the bladder—unusual features. *J. Urol.* 90:53, 1963.

93. Robertson, J. P., and Headstream, J. W. The use of cystogram and urethrogram in the diagnosis and management of rupture of the urethra and bladder. *South. Med. J.* 44:895, 1951.

94. Samuels, L. D., and Smith, J. P. Kidney scanning in pediatric renal trauma. *J. Trauma* 8:583, 1968.

95. Sargent, J. C., and Marquardt, C. R. Renal injuries. *J. Urol.* 63:1, 1950.

96. Schencker, B. Drip infusion pyelography: Indications and applications in urologic roentgen diagnosis. *Radiology* 83:12, 1964.

97. Schiller, M., Harris, B. H., Samuels, L. D., Clatworthy, W. H., Jr., and Morse, T. A. Diagnosis of experimental renal trauma. *J. Pediatr. Surg.* 7:2, 1972.

98. Scholl, A. J., and Nation, E. J. Injuries of the Kidney. In M. F. Campbell and J. H. Harrison (eds.), *Urology* (3rd ed.). Philadelphia: Saunders, 1970. Vol. 1, pp. 800–801.

99. Seright, W. Traumatic closed rupture of the upper ureter. *Br. J. Surg.* 46:511, 1969.

100. Smith, M. J. V., Seidel, R. F., and Bonacarti, A. F. Accident trauma to the kidneys in children. *J. Urol.* 96:845, 1966.

101. Smith, M. J. V., Wanson, E. M., and Campbell, J. M. An unusual case of closed rupture of the ureter. *J. Urol.* 83:277, 1960.

102. Stickel, D. L., and Howse, R. M. Injuries of the ureter due to external violence—a review of the litera-

ture and report of two cases. *Am. Surg.* 154:137, 1961.

103. Stone, H., and Quillian, J. Penetrating and nonpenetrating injuries to the ureter. *Surg. Gynecol. Obstet.* 114:52, 1962.

104. Sullivan, M. J., Lackner, L. H., and Banowsky, L. H. Intraperitoneal extravasation of urine: BUN/serum creatinine disproportion. *J.A.M.A.* 221:491, 1972.

105. Sullivan, M. J., and Stables, D. P. Renal arterial occlusion from trauma—letter to the editor. *J.A.M.A.* 221:1282, 1972.

106. Thiersch, C. On the origin and operative treatment of epispadias. *Arch. Heilk.* 10:20, 1869.

107. Turner-Warwick, R. T. Urethral structures in relation to the sphincters. *Br. J. Urol.* 40:677, 1968.

108. Uhle, C. A. W., and Erb, H. E. Reconstruction of the membranous urethra: Case reports. *J. Urol.* 52:42, 1944.

109. Vermillion, C. D., McLaughlin, A. P., III, and Pfister, R. C. Management of blunt renal trauma. *J. Urol.* 106:478, 1971.

110. Vital Statistics of the United States. *Mortality.* Volume II, part A, 1960–1967. Washington, D.C.: U.S. Department of Health, Education, and Welfare.

111. Walker, J. A. Injuries of the ureter due to external violence. *J. Urol.* 102:410, 1969.

112. Waterhouse, K. The surgical repair of membranous urethral strictures in children. *Trans. Am. Assoc. Genitourin. Surg.* 67:81, 1975.

112a. Waterhouse, K., and Gross, M. Trauma to the genito-urinary tract: A five-year experience with 251 cases. *J. Urol.* 101:241, 1969.

113. Watson, F. S., and Cunningham, J. A. *Diseases and Surgery of the Genitourinary System.* Philadelphia: Lea & Febiger, 1908. Pp. 447–456.

114. Weller, M. H., and Miller, K. Unusual aspects of urine ascites. *Radiology* 109:665, 1973.

115. Wellers, S. P., and Kellner, G. *Urologische Begleitverletzumgen bei Unfallheilkd.* 71:409, 1968.

116. Wilenius, R. Subcutaneous rupture of the ureter. *Ann. Chir. Gynaec. Fenn.* 39:1, 1950.

117. Wilkinson, F. O. W. Rupture of the posterior urethra—with a review of twelve cases. *Lancet* 1:1125, 1961.

118. Williams, D. I. *Paediatric Urology.* London: Butterworth, 1968. P. 358.

119. Young, J. D., Jr. *Urology.* New York: Harper & Row, 1973. Volume 2, chap. 3, p. 2.

120. Zaidi-Zafar, H. Spontaneous intraperitoneal rupture of pyelonephrotic kidney in infancy. *J. Pediatr.* 55:78, 1959.

121. Zufall, R. Traumatic avulsion of the upper ureter. *J. Urol.* 85:246, 1961.

The presence of stones in the urinary tract has fascinated medical scientists for centuries. Perhaps it is the preposterous idea that the human body should manufacture something so foreign and mundane as a stone that has caused the subject to be viewed more with humorous fascination than scientific erudition. In recent years, however, serious investigations have been conducted in the area of urolithiasis, clarifying some of the pathogenetic mechanisms involved in stone production.

As opposed to their occurrence in adults, urinary stones are relatively infrequent in childhood, at least in the United States. In several other areas of the world, however, the condition is frequent enough to pose a major health problem. For example, a survey of two hospitals in New Delhi over a period of 2 years disclosed stones in 600 children [1]; 60 percent of these were bladder calculi. Similarly, surveys in Canton, China, and in Thailand revealed that 25 and 22 percent, respectively, of stones in children were bladder stones [31]. In addition, about 90 percent of these endemic vesical stones occur in boys and are most often composed of uric acid [8, 18]. This very high frequency of boys, of localization in the bladder, and of uric acid composition, together with the frequency of occurrence, strongly suggest that stone disease is etiologically different in these endemic areas than in other areas of the world. In the United States, for example, bladder stones are distinctly uncommon in the absence of a foreign body or neurogenic bladder. Various dietary deficiencies related to low socioeconomic levels have been investigated as possible etiologic factors, but a specific deficiency has not been found to have etiologic significance.

Urinary stone disease occurs more frequently in males, although this sex preponderance is not present in all surveys. The large experience of Williams and Eckstein [32] suggests that the majority of stones in children occur under 4 years of age, with a peak during the second and third years.

Composition of Calculi

Urinary stones are composed of a crystalline fraction imbedded in a mucoid matrix. This matrix material, which has been extensively investigated by Boyce [3], is about two-thirds protein, the remainder being various mixtures of simple and complex sugars. The matrix comprises 2.5 to 10 percent of stone weight. Although this material is undoubtedly important in calculus formation, it does not appear to be the inciting agent.

The recent application of the tools of crystallography and mineralogy to the crystalline composition of urinary stones has demonstrated a far greater complexity of chemical composition than was heretofore suspected [26]. Whereas analysis by chemical techniques identifies ions such as Ca^{2+}, $PO_4^{\equiv}$, and Mg^{2+}, x-ray diffraction and polarizing microscopy reveal such complex structures as brushite, hydroxyapatite, struvite, or weddelite. The vast majority of stones (65 percent) are composed of combinations of calcium phosphate and calcium oxalate. Magnesium ammonium phosphate, usually associated with urinary tract infections, comprises about 15 percent of stones, the remaining 20 percent being uric acid, cystine, and xanthine.

Pathogenesis of Stone Formation

Theories of the pathogenesis of stone formation have focused on either matrix formation or crystal precipitation as primary inciting events. While the matrix material probably acts as an adhesive and influences stone growth, it appears unlikely that these proteins are of primary etiologic importance.

The precipitation of crystals from solution seems to be primary in most instances of stone formation. A useful approach to the etiology of crystal formation in urine is to examine the behavior of urine as an aqueous solvent. It can be shown that far greater amounts of calcium, phosphate, oxalate, and uric acid can be held in solution in urine than in water [29, 30]. The factors that determine the capacity of an aqueous solvent are almost sufficient to account for the superiority of urine to water. Theoretically, any or all of these factors could be important in the pathogenesis of stone formation, and, to the extent they can be manipulated in a favorable direction, important in the therapy of recurrent stones. These implications are discussed below.

QUANTITY OF SOLVENT

Given a fixed quantity of solute for excretion, it is obvious that the greater the quantity of solvent, the more dilute the solution and the lesser the probability of precipitation. Decreased quantity of urine, however, is not often the primary etiologic factor in stone formation. It has been implicated in the increased incidence of stones seen in British soldiers stationed in desert areas and in endemic stone formation in children in areas where gastroenteritis is prevalent and access to water is restricted. Although a decreased quantity of solvent may not often be of etiologic importance, the therapeutic significance of increasing urine volume to prevent recurrent precipitation is obvious. Thus an increased fluid intake is a hallmark of treatment in all patients with recurrent urolithiasis. Since the longest period of fluid deprivation usually is during sleep, it is advisable to wake the patient at least once during the sleeping period to drink. The results of this therapy can be evaluated by measuring the osmolality of the first voided morning urine and the concentration of the substance of concern. For example, cystine is soluble in urine up to a concentration of about 300 μg per milliliter.

QUANTITY OF SOLUTE

Whether or not precipitation occurs is related, not to the total amount of solute, but to its concentration, assuming the volume of solvent is not fixed. In reality it is not the *concentration* of ions, but their *activity,* which determines their interaction in complex solutions. This reflects the concept that the likelihood of two ions in solution coming together is decreased by the presence of other particles. The considerable influence of the presence of other ions on the solubility of calcium salts has been shown in Vermuelen's studies creating an artificial urine [14, 30]. These investigations have begun with water; ions normally present in urine are progressively added, and their effect on the solubility of calcium salts is measured.

Utilizing the activities of ions rather than their concentrations, precipitation should occur when the product of the ionic activities of the salt in question exceeds the formation constant. Pak has utilized these concepts to measure the degree of saturation for brushite in urine by examining the ratio of the activity product to the formation product for that particular urine [20]. Precipitation occurs when this ratio exceeds 1 [11].

Thus increases in the activity product or decreases in the formation product theoretically could have pathogenic significance for urolithiasis. Such alterations could be caused by an increase in the quantity of precipitable solute for excretion without a concomitant increase in urine volume or ionic strength. Such changes in excretory load appear to have primary import in the calculus diseases in which calcium excretion is increased,

including hyperparathyroidism, vitamin D intoxication, distal renal tubular acidosis, immobilization, thyrotoxicosis, and sarcoidosis. Hypercalciuria and urolithiasis have been associated with total parenteral alimentation [1]. Uric acid excretion is augmented in the Lesch-Nyhan syndrome, in the leukemias when treated with cytotoxic drugs, and in some forms of gout. Oxalate excretion is increased in the inborn errors of metabolism called type I and II hyperoxaluria [33] as well as in pyridoxine deficiency [14], ethylene glycol poisoning, methoxyflurane anesthesia [10], ileal diseases [4], and following large doses of ascorbic acid. There is a marked increase in cystine excretion in the inborn error of metabolism known as cystinuria. Xanthine excretion is increased in the metabolic disorder xanthinuria and in patients treated with the xanthine oxidase inhibitor allopurinol. A complete deficiency of the enzyme adenine phosphoribosyltransferase has been associated with urinary stones composed of 2,8-dihydroxyadenine [7a, 28a]. This is due to increased oxidation of adenine to this substance through the pathway catalyzed by xanthine oxidase, a situation exactly comparable to the increased uric acid production in the Lesch-Nyhan syndrome, in which there is deficiency of hypoxanthine guanine phosporibosyltransferase. In addition, a considerable number of both children and adults with recurrent stone formation are found to have hypercalciuria without an identifiable cause.

Therapy directed toward abnormalities in solute excretion should either lower the activity product or increase the formation product [11]. Decreases in activity product can be accomplished by limiting gastrointestinal absorption through dietary restrictions of calcium, purines (uric acid), or sulfoproteins (cystine). The oral administration of cellulose phosphate will inhibit intestinal calcium absorption [21]. Other approaches to lowering the activity product include decreasing the formation of uric acid or 2,8-dihydroxyadenine by inhibiting the enzyme xanthine oxidase with allopurinol and converting cystine into a more soluble disulfide by the administration of penicillamine. Thiazide therapy will decrease calcium excretion by increasing renal resorption. The formation product can be increased by augmenting the excretion of substances having a particular solubilizing action greater than that attributable to their contribution to total ionic strength (see below).

pH

Solubility may vary markedly with alterations in urinary pH. Thus calcium phosphate (apatite) and magnesium ammonium phosphate are more soluble at a pH less than 6, and uric acid is more soluble at a pH greater than 6. Cystine demonstrates little change in solubility up to pH 7.0, but there is a marked increase in solubility at higher pH levels. Calcium oxalate shows little variation in solubility in vitro with changes in pH.

Several pieces of evidence suggest that disturbances in urinary acidification may play a primary etiologic role in calculus disease. The majority of patients with uric acid stones, for example, have neither hyperuricemia nor hyperuricosuria. It has been shown, however, that as a group these patients have (1) a lower mean urinary pH than controls, and (2) lower ammonium excretion at comparable levels of urinary pH [12]. Magnesium ammonium phosphate stones are limited almost exclusively to two types of patients: those with long-standing urinary tract infections with urea-splitting organisms, and thus a persistently alkaline urine, and those receiving long-term alkali therapy. Patients with distal renal tubular acidosis have a persistently alkaline urine and also form calcium stones, suggesting that the two may be related; other urinary alterations contributing to stone formation in renal tubular acidosis will be discussed below.

Therapy directed at alteration of urine pH would seem beneficial in patients with recurrent calcium phosphate, magnesium ammonium phosphate, or uric acid stones. Such therapy would not be effective in patients with cystine stones unless urinary pH is maintained at 7.5 or greater. Although calcium oxalate solubility is affected little by pH in vitro, in experimental animals with hyperoxaluria stone formation is increased in acid urines and decreased in alkaline urines [2]. These relationships were thought to be due to an absolute decrease in calcium excretion with alkalinization coupled with an increase in citrate excretion (see below). It should be noted that an initiating stone nucleus may be, for example, uric acid. Due to secondary infection, this uric acid nucleus might grow by deposition of magnesium ammonium phosphate. Failure to recognize the etiologic importance of the uric acid nucleus would lead to misdirected attempts to acidify the urine, aggravating further the primary disorder, the formation of uric acid stones.

Alkalinization may be accomplished with the use of oral sodium bicarbonate or citrate, and acidification may be established with ammonium chloride, ascorbic acid, or methionine. Obviously urinary acidification cannot be achieved in distal renal tubular acidosis, but correction of the systemic acidosis will decrease calcium excretion [19].

PRESENCE OF SUBSTANCES HAVING A PARTICULAR SOLUBILIZING ACTION

Vermuelen's artificial urine experiments suggested that magnesium ions had a much greater effect on calcium phosphate solubility than could be accounted for by their contributions to total ionic strength [30]. Other studies using hyperoxaluric rats have shown the protective effect of magnesium [2], and a similar solubilizing effect is seen in experiments with rachitic rat cartilage [17]. Several studies have reported decreased frequency of stone formation in patients with recurrent calculus disease treated with magnesium [16].

Urinary citrate has a profound effect on the solubility of calcium salts, probably due to the formation of calcium citrate complexes, which decrease the activity of ionized calcium. Citrate excretion is increased in alkaline urines. The low urinary citrate excretion in patients with distal renal tubular acidosis may explain, along with hypercalciuria, their propensity to stone formation.

The artificial urine experiments have shown that the effects of total ionic strength, and of magnesium and citrate can explain fully the greater solubility of calcium oxalate in urine than in water; these effects are not sufficient to explain the solubility of calcium phosphate, however [30]. Other studies have shown that for any degree of oversaturation of urine with calcium oxalate, normal subjects excrete crystals of smaller size than do recurrent stone formers [27a]. This suggests the presence of substances that inhibit crystal aggregation and growth. One of these substances is pyrophosphate, which accounts for about 15 percent of this inhibition [27b]. A second substance appears to be an acid mucopolysaccharide that is responsible for the majority of the inhibitory activity [27b].

Therapy directed at increasing the excretion of substances having particular solubilizing activity could include oral magnesium therapy. Although several reports have indicated a decrease in stone formation in patients with recurrent calculus disease treated with magnesium, such therapy has not found wide use, nor has it been extensively investigated. Urinary pyrophosphate can be increased by the oral administration of phosphates or thiazides [9, 22], which do seem to be effective in preventing stone formation. Diphosphonates, which are synthetic analogues of pyrophosphate, inhibit nucleation and growth of calcium salts in vitro. Since they are resistant to pyrophosphatase, they can be administered orally and will be excreted in urine in amounts sufficient to inhibit nucleation and growth of stones in vivo. However, side effects of diphosphonate therapy have so far prohibited general clinical use [27c].

TIME

One need only note the precipitate formed in urine allowed to stagnate in a collection bottle to realize that time has an adverse effect on solubility. Time may be important in situations of urinary stasis, such as ureteropelvic obstruction and megaureter, both of which are associated with stone formation. Stones are not seen frequently in patients with obstructed bladder, however, such as those with posterior urethral valves. Immobilization, as in paraplegia or osteomyelitis, may lead to calculi due to a combination of stasis and hypercalciuria. Stone formation following repair of bladder exstrophy probably represents a combination of stasis and abnormal bladder mucosa. Treatment in these cases consists in relief of obstruction and establishment of adequate drainage.

PRESENCE OF NIDUS

Much as encrustations may form on a rock projecting from a stream, so the presence of a foreign or irregular particle in the urinary tract may stimulate precipitation. Such a particle may take the form of an indwelling catheter, a postoperative or self-introduced foreign body, blood clots, desquamated cells, or debris associated with infection; treatment consists in removal of the nidus through surgery or antibiotics.

The Special Problem of Idiopathic Hypercalciuria

Calcium stones are the most common variety encountered; after extensive evaluation most of these patients are found to have either (1) no identifiable cause for their calcium urolithiasis or (2) hypercalciuria with no definable etiology, that is, idiopathic hypercalciuria. Among those with apparent normocalciuria, studies have suggested that either hypercalciuria is present but intermittent [27] or relative hypercalciuria is present when examined as a ratio of calcium excretion to urinary osmolality [5].

There is considerable overlap in the rate of calcium excretion and the activity product of calcium oxalate between normal controls and patients with recurrent stone formation. Robertson et al. [28] have suggested that this overlap might be resolved by evaluating simultaneously the activity product of calcium oxalate and the ability of the urine to inhibit crystal formation. When the log of the ratio between the activity product of calcium oxalate and its solubility product was plotted against the

percent inhibitory activity of the urine, a line of discrimination could be calculated that separated stone-forming patients from control subjects. The distance from this discriminant line for a given urine provided a relative measure of the propensity to stone formation. These investigators called this value the saturation-inhibition index. This index, if its value is confirmed, could be used to define the risk for recurrent stone formation in a given patient. Of even greater theoretical importance would be the ability to quantify the effects of various therapies designed to decrease this risk.

Among those patients with idiopathic hypercalciuria, the underlying mechanism must be increased gastrointestinal absorption of dietary calcium, increased endogenous production of calcium (bone resorption), or a renal tubular defect in calcium resorption. All three theoretical causes have been described in patients with idiopathic hypercalciuria, although their relative frequency is not clear. Several studies have suggested the primacy of gastrointestinal hyperabsorption in these patients [24, 25]; however, calcium excretion in patients fasting or on a usual diet may be normal, the defect becoming apparent only with a calcium load. There is a suggestion that the urinary excretion of calcium may be dependent in part on gastrointestinal glucose load [13].

Increased bone resorption as a cause of idiopathic hypercalciuria is generally associated with primary hyperparathyroidism and identified by the presence of hypercalcemia, elevated urinary cyclic adenosine monophosphate, increased serum parathyroid hormone, and radiologic evidence of bone disease. Although normocalcemic hyperparathyroidism is theoretically possible, its actual occurrence is rare.

Finally, a primary defect in the renal tubular resorption of calcium has been demonstrated in a few patients with idiopathic hypercalciuria in the series reported by Pak et al. [24] and in half the patients of Coe et al. [6]. In this condition serum parathyroid hormone is elevated; however, the elevation is secondary, as shown by its suppression when calcium excretion is normalized by the administration of thiazides [6].

Since therapy is different in these three forms of idiopathic hypercalciuria, it is important to separate them as described in the protocol proposed by Pak et al. [24]. Therapy in the hyperabsorptive form entails dietary restriction of calcium and inhibition of absorption with cellulose phosphate [23]. The effects of such treatment on the urinary excretion of calcium and oxalate should be monitored, since at times dietary restriction of calcium and not of oxalate may increase oxalate excretion and actually elevate the activity product [15]. The mechanism of this increase in oxalate excretion is presumably greater gastrointestinal resorption of oxalate secondary to decreased binding with calcium in the intestinal tract. This monitoring precaution is of greater concern in those patients with borderline hypercalciuria or normocalciuria, where the resultant decrease in calcium excretion is small, than it is in those with frank hypercalciuria, where any increase in oxalate excretion is more than offset by greater decreases in calcium excretion. As noted above, covert, normocalcemic hyperparathyroidism is rare, but if clearly documented, the therapy is parathyroidectomy. Finally, a primary renal defect in calcium resorption may be treated with thiazides to decrease calcium excretion, the presumed mechanism being this stimulation of sodium and calcium resorption by mild extracellular volume contraction.

An intriguing observation, shown repeatedly, is that hyperuricemia and hyperuricosuria are more frequent in those who form calcium stones than in control subjects. There is evidence to suggest that crystals of sodium urate may form the nucleus upon which crystals of calcium oxalate grow [24a]. Other investigations have demonstrated that urate inhibits the activity of the acid mucopolysaccharide inhibitor of crystal aggregation [27b]. Of therapeutic interest is the demonstration that treatment of these patients with allopurinol may reduce markedly the recurrence of calcium stones [7].

Diagnosis

The majority of stones in children are discovered incidentally or during evaluation of urinary tract infection. Those that become symptomatic present with flank or inguinal pain, hematuria, fever, or recurrent urinary tract infections.

The diagnosis of urolithiasis should be entertained in any child with the above symptomatology. Confirmation is through the urinary passage of gravel-like material or a stone or through visualization of a calculus on a plain abdominal radiograph or intravenous urogram. Uric acid and xanthine stones are radiolucent, if pure, but they often contain enough calcium to render them radiopaque.

Exploring the etiology of urolithiasis is based more profitably on a consideration of the factors discussed above that affect the ability of urine to hold salts in solution rather than on the perfunctory elimination of named diseases. Once the underlying urinary abnormality is revealed, the specific pathogenic mechanisms producing the ab-

Table 94-1. Factors Contributing to Stone Formation

Composition of Stone	Contributory Factors

Calcium phosphate	Hypercalciuria
	    Hyperparathyroidism
	    Vitamin D intoxication
	    Distal renal tubular acidosis
	    Immobilization
	    Thyrotoxicosis
	    Sarcoidosis
	    Idiopathic
	    High calcium diet (in susceptible individuals) (?)
	Alkaline urinary pH
	Decreased urinary pyrophosphate (?)
	Decreased urinary Mg^{++}/Ca^{++} ratio (?)
	Foreign body
	Urinary stasis

Calcium oxalate	All of the above except pH
	Hyperoxaluria
	    Types I and II hyperoxaluria
	    Ethylene glycol poisoning
	    Pyridoxine deficiency
	    Methoxyflurane anesthesia
	    Ileal disease
	    Massive doses of ascorbic acid
	Hyperglycinuria
	Hyperuricosuria

Magnesium ammonium phosphate	Infection with urea-splitting organism Alkaline urine Foreign body Urinary stasis

Uric acid	Hyperuricosuria
	    Gout
	    Lesch-Nyhan syndrome
	    Hematologic malignances
	    High-purine diet
	Acid urine

Xanthine	Xanthinuria Acid urine Allopurinol therapy
Cystine	Cystinuria Acid urine

Table 94-2. Normal Excretion Rates for Substances Important in Calculus Formation

Calculus Component	Normal Excretion Rate
Calcium	$\leq$2–4 mg/kg/24 hr $\leq$300 mg/24 hr on normal diet in adults
Oxalate*	<50 mg/1.73 m²/24 hr
Cystine	<70 mg per gram of creatinine
Uric acid	$\leq$500 mg/m²/24 hr

* Normal values for oxalate vary with the analytical method used. Values for an individual patient should be compared to normal values for the laboratory performing the particular analysis.

normality may be investigated. These mechanisms are summarized in Table 94-1.

The evaluation should include a search for a family history of stones or metabolic diseases, urine culture, and radiographic examination of the urinary tract. If spontaneous urines with pH 5.0 or less are not obtained, the ability to acidify urine may be tested by the administration of ammonium chloride. If a calculus is obtained, it should be analyzed, preferably using crystallographic techniques. Multiple 24-hr urine specimens should be analyzed for calcium, oxalate, cystine,* and uric acid. Normal values for these substances are listed in Table 94-2. Serum should be analyzed for urea nitrogen, creatinine, calcium, phosphorus, alkaline phosphatase, electrolytes, uric acid, and acid-base profile. A creatinine clearance is helpful as an estimate of renal damage and as a basis for later evaluation of renal function.

Treatment

The treatment of stones too large to pass spontaneously is surgical removal. Prophylaxis to prevent recurrence involves alteration of urine composition by one or (usually) more of the techniques discussed above. Early institution of prophylactic therapy with careful monitoring of the urinary response, together with prompt detection and treatment of infection and obstruction, will help prevent irreversible renal damage.

References

1. Adelman, R. D., Abern, S. B., Merten, D., and Halsted, C. H. Hypercalciuria with nephrolithiasis: A complication of total parenteral nutrition. *Pediatrics* 59:473, 1977.
1a. Aurora, A. L., Taneja, O. P., and Gupta, D. N. Bladder stone disease of childhood. *Acta Paediatr. Scand.* 59:177, 1971.
2. Borden, T. A., and Lyon, E. S. Effects of magnesium and pH on experimental calcium oxalate stone disease. *Invest. Urol.* 6:412, 1969.
3. Boyce, W. H. Organic matrix of human urinary concretions. *Am. J. Med.* 45:673, 1968.
4. Chadwick, V. S., Modha, K., and Dowling, R. H. Mechanism for hypoxaluria in patients with ileal dysfunction. *N. Engl. J. Med.* 289:172, 1973.
5. Chambers, R. M., and Dormandy, T. L. Hypercalciuria—Relative and Absolute. In A. Hodgkinson and B. E. C. Nordin (eds.), *Renal Stone Research Symposium.* London: Churchill, 1969. P. 233.
6. Coe, F. L., Canterbury, J. M., Firpo, J. J., and Reiss, E. Evidence for secondary hyperparathyroidism in idiopathic hypercalciuria. *J. Clin. Invest.* 52:134, 1973.
7. Coe, F. L., and Paisen, L. Allopurinol treatment of uric-acid disorders in calcium-stone formers. *Lancet* 1:129, 1973.
7a. Debray, H., Cartier, P., Temstet, A., and Cedron, J. Child's urinary lithiasis revealing a complete deficit in adenine phosphoribosyltransferase. *Pediatr. Res.* 10:762, 1976.
8. Eckstein, H. B. Harnstein in Kindersalter. *Z. Kinderchir.* 2:451, 1965.
9. Ettinger, B., and Kalb, F. O. Inorganic phosphate treatment of nephrolithiasis. *Am. J. Med.* 55:32, 1973.
10. Frascino, J. A., Parker, V., and Rosen, P. P. Renal oxalosis and azotemia after methoxyflurane anesthesia. *N. Engl. J. Med.* 283:676, 1970.
11. Halzbach, R. T., and Pak, C. Y. C. Metastable supersaturation: Physicochemical studies provide new insights into formation of renal and biliary tract stones. *Am. J. Med.* 56:141, 1974.
12. Henneman, P. H., Wallach, S., and Dempsey, E. P. The metabolic defect responsible for uric acid stone formation. *J. Clin. Invest.* 41:537, 1962.
13. Lemann, J., Jr., Piering, W. F., and Lennan, E. J. Possible role of carbohydrate-induced calciuria in calcium oxalate kidney-stone formation. *N. Engl. J. Med.* 280:232, 1969.
14. Lyon, E. S., Borden, T. A., Ellis, J. E., and Vermuelen, C. W. Calcium oxalate lithiasis produced by pyridoxine deficiency and inhibition with high magnesium diets. *Invest. Urol.* 4:133, 1966.
15. Marshall, R. W., Cochran, M., and Hodgkinson, A. Relationships between calcium and oxalic acid intake in the diet and their excretion in the urine of normal and renal-stone-forming subjects. *Clin. Sci.* 43:91, 1972.
16. Moore, C. A., and Bunce, G. E. Reduction in frequency of renal calculus formation by oral magnesium administration. *Invest. Urol.* 2:7, 1964.
17. Mukai, T., and Howard, J. E. Some observations on the calcification of rachitic cartilage by urine. *Bull. Johns Hopkins Hosp.* 112:279, 1963.
18. Myers, N. A. A. Urolithiasis in childhood. *Arch. Dis. Child.* 32:48, 1957.
19. Nash, M. A., Torrado, A. D., Greifer, I., Spitzer, A., Edelmann, C. M., Jr. Renal tubular acidosis in infants and children. *J. Pediatr.* 80:738, 1972.
20. Pak, C. Y. C. Physicochemical basis for formation of renal stones of calcium phosphate origin: Calculation of the degree of saturation of urine with respect to brushite. *J. Clin. Invest.* 48:1914, 1969.
21. Pak, C. Y. C. Effects of cellulose phosphate and sodium phosphate on formation product and activity product of brushite in urine. *Metabolism* 21:447, 1972.
22. Pak, C. Y. C. Hydrochlorothiazide therapy in nephrolithiasis: Effect on urinary activity product and formation product of brushite. *Clin. Pharmacol. Therap.* 14:209, 1973.
23. Pak, C. Y. C., Delea, C. S., and Bartter, F. C. Successful treatment of recurrent nephrolithiasis (calcium stones) with cellulose phosphate. *N. Engl. J. Med.* 290:175, 1974.
24. Pak, C. Y. C., Masahire, O., Lawrence, E. C., and

---

* The nitroprusside test on a random urine specimen will give an adequate indication of markedly increased cystine concentration. A few drops of ammonium hydroxide and 2 ml of fresh 5% NaCN are added to 5 ml of urine. After 10 min for equilibration, a few drops of 5% sodium nitroprusside are added. A deep purple color indicates a positive reaction. False-positive results occur from ketonuria.

Snyder, W. The hypercalciurias: Causes, parathyroid functions, and diagnostic criteria. *J. Clin. Invest.* 54:387, 1974.

24a. Pak, C. Y. C., Waters, O., Arnold, L., Holt, K., Cox, C., and Barilla, D. Mechanism for calcium urolithiasis among patients with hyperuricosuria: Supersaturation of urine with respect to monosodium urate. *J. Clin. Invest.* 59:426, 1977.

25. Peacock, M., and Nordin, B. E. C. The Hypercalciuria of Renal Stone Disease. In A. Hodgkinson and B. E. C. Nordin (eds.), *Renal Stone Research Symposium.* London: Churchill, 1969. P. 253.

26. Prien, E. L., and Prien, E. L., Jr. Composition and structure of urinary stone. *Am. J. Med.* 45:654, 1968.

27. Revisova, V. Dynamics of Hypercalciuria in Children with Urolithiasis. In A. Hodgkinson and B. E. C. Nordin (eds.), *Renal Stone Research Symposium.* London: Churchill, 1969. P. 245.

27a. Robertson, W. G. Physical Chemical Aspects of Calcium Stone-formation in the Urinary Tract. In H. Fleisch, W. G. Robertson, L. H. Smith, and W. Vahlensieck (eds.), *Urolithiasis Research.* New York: Plenum, 1976. P. 25.

27b. Robertson, W. G., Knowles, F., and Peacock, M. Urinary Acid Mucopolysaccharide Inhibitors of Calcium Oxalate Crystallisation. In H. Fleisch, W. G. Robertson, L. H. Smith, and W. Vahlensieck (eds.), *Urolithiasis Research.* New York: Plenum, 1976. P. 331.

27c. Robertson, W. G., Peacock, M., Marshall, R. W., and Knowles, F. The effect of ethane-1 hydroxy-1,1-diphosphonate (EHDP) on calcium oxalate crystalluria in recurrent renal stone-formers. *Clin. Sci. Mol. Med.* 47:13, 1974.

28. Robertson, W. G., Peacock, M., Marshall, R. W., Marshall, D. H., and Nordin, B. E. C. Saturation-inhibition index as a measure of the risk of calcium oxalate stone formation in the urinary tract. *N. Engl. J. Med.* 294:249, 1975.

28a. Van Acker, K. J., Simmonds, A., Potter, C., and Cameron, J. S. Complete deficiency of adenine phosphoribosyltransferase: Report of a family. *N. Engl. J. Med.* 297:127, 1977.

29. Vermeulen, C. W., Lyon, E. S., and Fried, F. A. On the nature of the stone forming process. *J. Urol.* 94: 176, 1965.

30. Vermeulen, C. W., Lyon, E. S., and Miller, G. H. Calcium phosphate solubility in urine as measured by a precipitation test: Experimental urolithiasis. XIII. *J. Urol.* 79:596, 1958.

31. Waller, J. I., and Adney, F. Vesical calculi in young female children. *Am. J. Dis. Child.* 79:684, 1950.

32. Williams, D. I., and Eckstein, H. B. Urinary Lithiasis. In D. I. Williams (ed.), *Pediatric Urology.* London: Butterworth, 1968. P. 323.

33. Williams, H. E., and Smith, L. H. L-Glyceric aciduria. *N. Engl. J. Med.* 278:233, 1968.

95. Enuresis

S. Roy Meadow

The term *enuresis* is given to the inappropriate voiding of urine in a child who has reached an age at which bladder control is expected. In normal children this ranges from 1 to 5 years. The usual stages for the development of bladder control are as follows. At 1½ years the child passes urine at regular intervals and can defer micturition for a reasonable period. At 2 years the child exclaims while voiding. At 2½ years 90 percent of girls and 80 percent of boys make known their need to micturate [26]. From this stage the child begins to hold his urine even though aware of the need to micturate. If he can walk to an approved place and remove his pants, he will be able to control the situation most of the time. At 3 years most children go to the lavatory themselves, proudly announcing the fact to everyone. Sometimes they hold on too long, especially if preoccupied with play. The child will void between 8 and 14 times per 24 hr.

At 4 years the child is a connoisseur of water closets and reports with great interest on the various features of different lavatories. This passion lasts less than a year. At 5 years the child voids seven or eight times per 24 hr and may refuse to void unless in private. By this age he is usually able to initiate emptying of the bladder at any degree of fullness, a skill limited to dogs and man.

Thus, by the age of 2½ most children, with the help of a sympathetic adult, can be dry during the day. Night control is most commonly achieved a little later, between the ages of 2½ and 3½. At the age of 3½ years, 75 percent of children are dry at night.

The emergence of dryness is not dependent on training (any more than it is in lions or pigs, neither of which foul their sleeping quarters). Early toilet training has not been shown to increase the chance of dryness ultimately and most methods have been shown to increase the chance of enuresis [30]. However, when adverse social factors can be removed and when it is practicable for mothers to delay potty and toilet awareness until 2½ to 3 years of age, long-lasting dryness is more likely to be achieved. When this delayed approach is combined with efforts to reduce the child's anxiety about his family's expectations of dryness, then 98.5 percent of several hundreds of children have become reliably dry by the age of 5 years [5, 30].

Nocturnal Enuresis

Bed-wetting is a common and troublesome condition for children and their parents. *Primary enuresis* describes the situation in which the child has never been reliably dry. *Secondary* (acquired or onset) *enuresis* refers to wetting that occurs in someone who has been reliably dry for at least 1 year. It is much less common than primary enuresis. Approximately 10 percent of children with nocturnal enuresis also have some diurnal (daytime) enuresis.

EPIDEMIOLOGY

There is a variation in the prevalence of enuresis in different countries. Australia and the United States have a higher prevalence than Scandinavian countries [24]. Most of the larger surveys have originated from Europe and North America. The figures below are representative values for the many different surveys.

At the age of 5 years between 10 and 15 percent of children wet their beds at least once a month. Most of them wet their beds several times a week. At 10 years 7 percent wet, and at 15 years 1 percent.

Bed-wetting is commoner in first-born children, in the lower social classes, and in children who have suffered a social or psychological handicap in the first 4 years of life [12, 13a]. Up to the age of 11 years it is nearly twice as common in boys as in girls [8]. After that age the sex incidence is equal or weighted toward females [18]. Eighty percent of nocturnal enuresis is primary; 20 percent is secondary.

ETIOLOGY

Enuresis is a symptom, and its origins may be multiple.

Genetic Factors. Nocturnal enuresis is a familial disorder occurring with high frequency in the parents and siblings of bed wetters. The frequency in other members of the family is directly related to the closeness of the genetic relationship. Monozygotic twins are concordant for enuresis twice as frequently as dizygotic twins [3, 17]; 74 percent of boys and 58 percent of girls have one or both parents with a history of enuresis [11a].

Bladder Function. Frequency of micturition is often associated with both nocturnal and diurnal enuresis. The enuretic child has a smaller functional bladder capacity [13]. The bladder is functionally but not structurally smaller [28]. Children with combined day and night wetting usually have considerable urgency of micturition by day. Urodynamic studies show abnormal physiologic responses compared with night-wetters. They are unable to suppress voluntary bladder contraction [29a].

Psychological Stress. Stress and anxiety certainly may result from enuresis; moreover, they may cause it. A variety of stressful events in early childhood have been shown to be associated with enuresis later on. The chance of enuresis is proportional to both the severity of the stress and the number of stressful events, particularly those occurring in the third and fourth year of life [12]. Separation from mother, prolonged hospital admission, and broken homes are all associated with an increased incidence of enuresis in later life. It is as if stress during the sensitive developmental period for night bladder control—$2\frac{1}{2}$ to $3\frac{1}{2}$ years—interferes with the emergence of dryness. The optimal stage for developing dryness passes, and though the stress may be transient, the symptom of enuresis may persist [19]. If it persists long enough, it may generate enough anxiety itself to convert the family and home situation into one in which it is most difficult for the child to acquire bladder control; the symptom persists though the cause has changed.

Psychiatric Illness. Most children who wet the bed are psychiatrically normal. However, there is consistent evidence from controlled studies on unselected populations of a relationship at all ages between emotional disorder and enuresis. Children with combined diurnal and nocturnal enuresis have a greater frequency of psychiatric disturbance than children with nocturnal enuresis alone, neurotic disorders being common in the girls and antisocial disorders, including fecal soiling, in the boys [3a]. It is difficult to differentiate between psychiatric illness that causes enuresis and psychiatric illness that results from enuresis.

Depth of Sleep. Despite the common claim by parents that their enuretic child is a very deep sleeper, there is conflicting evidence on the rousability of bed wetters. Wetting can occur during any phase of sleep except in stage one, when rapid eye movement is occurring [25]. It is most common during stages 3 and 4.

In summary, it is clear that the necessary anatomic and physiologic relationships between the brain and bladder become developed and mature enough for dryness at varying ages up to the age of 5 years. Genetic factors are responsible for some of this variation. Environmental factors ranging from stress experiences to social handicap and coercive toilet training may adversely affect the emergence and retention of dryness.

ORGANIC CAUSES OF ENURESIS

Infection. There is a strong association between urinary tract infection and enuresis. Enuresis is the presenting symptom in 15 percent of children with urine infection [29]. It is also common in school children with asymptomatic bacteriuria [22]. Conversely, children with enuresis have a higher incidence of urine infection than those without enuresis. A girl over 5 years of age who wets the bed has a 5 to 10 percent chance of having a urine infection [11, 21a]. It is uncertain whether the infection causes the enuresis, for it can be suggested that the wet perineum of the enuretic child might predispose to ascending infection. The latter theory is supported by the fact that the incidence of radiological abnormality is unusually low in enuretic children who also have urinary tract infection [21a]. When enuresis is associated with urine infection, successful treatment of that infection cures the enuresis in about one-third of the children. Children with combined nocturnal and diurnal enuresis have a particularly high incidence of urinary infection; in one series 50 percent of such children had significant bacteriuria [3a].

Polyuria. Any condition causing polyuria makes enuresis more likely, particularly if the polyuria develops in a child with a previously normal urine output. Thus the polyuria of diabetes mellitus or acquired renal insufficiency may cause the child to present to the doctor with enuresis. It is worth noting that extreme polyuria does not necessarily cause nocturnal enuresis, even in the very young (one of my patients is a $3\frac{1}{2}$-year-old boy with nephrogenic diabetes insipidus who voids every hour during the night, uses a bucket, and does not wet the bed).

Urinary Tract Abnormalities. A large number of minor abnormalities of the bladder neck and urethra have been alleged to cause primary enuresis. None have withstood the tests of time or a controlled study. A variety of surgical assaults have been perpetrated on the genitalia and urinary tracts of enuretic children. No controlled trials have proved their value.

Secondary enuresis is more likely to be associated with an organic cause or severe psychological stress than is primary enuresis. After the age of 10, secondary enuresis is rare and is invariably associated with either an organic or psychiatric illness [23].

THE NATURAL HISTORY OF UNTREATED ENURESIS

Long-term studies of children with nocturnal enuresis who have not been treated with the buzzer alarm show that the spontaneous remission rate rises with age. The annual spontaneous cure rate between 5 and 9 years is 14 percent and between 10 and 19 years is 16 percent [14].

MANAGEMENT

Nocturnal enuresis is a challenging and rewarding condition to treat. There are few conditions which cause so much family turmoil for so long and yet which have an appreciable spontaneous cure rate and an even higher cure rate with enthusiastic management.

Most children presenting with enuresis will have neither an organic nor a psychiatric illness; however, the history and examination should exclude these. A full history and examination have an important therapeutic effect on the child and family. The history may yield positive clues as to the causes of the wetting—for instance, a family history of wetting, slowness at achieving all skills, poor social conditions with no inside toilet, or stressful events in early life. It is important to get a clear story about the wetting, including what is the longest period of dryness (careful questioning usually reveals that the child who is "always" wet is in fact very occasionally dry for a night, which means that dryness is possible and that there is no "leak in the plumbing").

Frequency, dysuria, or a poor stream of urine may indicate urinary tract abnormalities. Neurologic causes of incontinence are likely to disturb bowel function also and to cause other neurologic symptoms. It is important to find out exactly what happens when the child wets: Who gets up, who moves beds, who gets cross or upset, and who takes either a punitive or lackadaisical attitude. One needs to know just why the parents have come for help at that particular moment: Do they fear a particular disease, or does the child need to be dry quickly because of an important event such as going to camp? Physical examination is highly unlikely to reveal an abnormality, particularly if the history is unexceptional. But the examination is therapeutic and reassuring to all parties.

The only obligatory laboratory investigation is examination of the urine for infection and testing for albumin, sugar, and blood. Spinal x-ray is not helpful unless there are neurologic symptoms or signs. In general, intravenous urograms and micturating cystograms are not indicated, although they are recommended by some authors. Since secondary enuresis over the age of 10 is rare, more detailed examination and investigation is likely to be needed than in other types of enuresis.

Therapy comprises a number of general and specific measures. The most important of the *general measures* is a sympathetic and helpful doctor. The physician needs to show concern and involvement and may have to quiet a disastrously tense home situation and then calmly promise cure.

Parent and child will need to be interviewed separately to achieve the necessary opportunity for ventilation of worries, explanation, and reassurance. Thereafter the therapeutic regimen will vary according to the child, the family, and the beliefs of the doctor. All regimens should aim to involve the child directly in the therapy so that he cures himself; the doctor helps. It is best to embark on a few months of energetic therapy rather than on years of desultory and sporadic management.

The following maneuvers are widely used:

1. Chart and stars: These records kept by the child have a dual purpose. They are a useful record of progress for the doctor, and they involve the child actively. Most young children enjoy sticking colored stars on diary cards; older children can keep a progress record in a notebook. It is usually possible to praise their neatness if not their dryness. After one initial interview with the doctor and the issuing of a record chart, up to 10 percent of children stop wetting. Some physicians call this the placebo effect, and others call it good doctoring.
2. Fluid restriction: Apart from advising against excess fluid in the evening, fluid restriction is unnecessary and unhelpful.
3. Interval training: Interval training is often used and may be successful, particularly for young children with daytime frequency. The mother is instructed to take the child to the toilet and ensure voiding every half hour on the first day. The interval is increased by half an hour per day until the child can manage intervals of 3 or 4 hr. At this stage some children stop wetting the bed.
4. Lifting and waking: Lifting the child on to a pot when the parents go to bed does not train the child to be dry. Few of the children fully awaken; they virtually void in their sleep. But it may diminish the number of nights of sheet changing and days of sheet washing for the mother.
5. Rewards and punishments: These must be used cautiously. The child has to want to be dry and should know that the parents want him to be dry. But too much tension makes dryness difficult to acquire. It is best if the child can feel

secure in the knowledge that the doctor and the parents are quietly and encouragingly confident that the child will soon be dry, without mention of punishment or reward.

The two main *specific measures* in the treatment of enuresis are drugs and the enuresis alarm. A great many drugs ranging from stimulants to sedatives have been used for nocturnal enuresis [4]. The only drugs shown to be superior to placebo in adequately conducted trials are the tricyclic antidepressants. Their mode of action in enuresis is uncertain. Benefit occurs in up to 50 percent of children, usually within the first week of treatment. A favorable response is more likely in girls and in those with severe enuresis [4]. On stopping the drug the relapse rate is high. Permanent cure with drugs occurs in less than 25 percent of those who become dry during drug therapy, limiting the usefulness of such treatment [21]. My personal practice is to use drug therapy for children who are unsuitable for or have failed to respond to other therapeutic measures and in whom there is an urgent need to achieve dryness because of an important social or family happening. The dose required and tolerated varies considerably. Children who wet before midnight should be given the drug at 5:00 P.M. rather than bedtime [1]. The initial dose of imipramine hydrochloride is 25 mg for a young child or 50 mg for one over 8 years. The dose can be increased in 25-mg stages, according to tolerance, up to a maximum of 100 mg. The commonest reason for having to stop the drug is the onset of mood or sleep disturbance as the dose is increased.

Enuresis alarms are a deservedly popular form of treatment. They work. They are known by many titles: "bell and pad," "buzzer alarm," "bed buzzer," "conditioning therapy." The aim of the treatment is to awaken the child as soon as micturition occurs. The child sleeps on some form of detector mechanism such as mesh or foil pads that are connected to an alarm buzzer. The mechanism is triggered by voided urine completing the electrical circuit. At first the child awakens after wetting, but within a few weeks he either awakens before wetting or does not need to void at all. The alarm is most successful for children over the age of 7 years. With the help of an enthusiastic doctor or instructor, 75 percent will become dry. Up to 20 percent of these may relapse, but they usually respond quickly to a second course with the alarm. The technique of overlearning, in which the child is deliberately given excess fluid at night just as he is becoming dry with the alarm, results in fewer relapses [31]. The enuresis alarm is an important method of treatment. To be used successfully, great attention must be paid to instructing the child and family in the practical details of its use. Any person loaning or advising the use of a buzzer alarm should study the detailed guidance available [10].

Diurnal Enuresis

Isolated daytime enuresis unaccompanied by nocturnal enuresis is uncommon; however, it is not as uncommon as its scanty literature might suggest. In a large series of children with enuresis, Hallgren reported that 10 percent had diurnal enuresis without nocturnal enuresis [15]. Frequency of micturition and urgency are commonly associated [3a]. The epidemiology of diurnal enuresis differs in two major ways from that of nocturnal enuresis. It is more common in girls, and there is a greater likelihood of psychiatric disturbance [16, 27]. If the child wets only in the daytime, and then only when the mother is bound to notice, referral to a child psychiatrist is usually indicated.

Slight dampening of the pants is very common, particularly in girls, throughout the school years. It should not be confused with diurnal enuresis, in which the child voids inappropriately leaving a puddle of urine on the chair or on the floor.

Urgency Syndrome

One of the normal stages in the achievement of bladder control is that stage in which the toddler has awareness of bladder fullness, but perceives it suddenly and at the last moment. In order to keep dry he has to micturate almost at once. This is normal in a child of 2 or 3 years of age [19].

When this sudden, unpredictable urge to micturate is present after the age of 4, it is called the urgency syndrome. It is somewhat analogous to the irritable bladder syndrome or the urethral syndrome of adults [6].

Urgency syndrome is much more common in girls than boys. Generally it occurs in girls who have had a normal pattern of micturition at an earlier stage, though it certainly may persist from the age of 2 or 3 years without a normal intervening period. It is often associated with frequency and a tendency to dampen the pants (mild urge incontinence rather than overt enuresis). The etiology is uncertain. There is a familial predisposition [9]. Conditions such as urinary tract infection may precipitate the syndrome, but most children with urgency syndrome have neither infection nor any identifiable organic lesion causing bladder irritability. The urge to micturate comes on suddenly, and many of the children then suppress micturition by a combination of pelvic floor muscle contraction and external compression of the perineum. They may adopt a variety of characteristic postures: crouching with the heel of one foot pressed into the perineum, forced adduction of the thighs, or sitting on the extreme corner of a hard seat.

The syndrome usually subsides by the age of 10 years [8]. A variety of different treatments have been used without conclusive proof of their benefit. When there is an associated urinary tract infection, treatment of that infection may produce cure. For the rest, that is, the majority who have no infection, sympathetic explanation and a commonsense approach for both child and parent are needed. For them it is a troublesome (and smelly) condition; too much reproach or punishment will only aggravate the situation.

Pollakiuria (Extreme Frequency)

The sudden onset of extreme frequency of micturition in a child should prompt a search for a urinary tract infection or some organic condition that might irritate the urinary tract. A few children are found to have no organic cause for their urinary frequency. The child is healthy but suddenly starts voiding 30 or more times a day. She will use the pot in the doctor's office several times during the visit and will be in and out of bed throughout the night, often falling asleep on the pot or toilet. The episodes are usually triggered by an identifiable stress situation. The symptom may persist several weeks. Therapy is aimed at either relieving the stress or helping the child cope with the situation [2].

Giggle Micturition

This is a rare syndrome characterized by sudden, involuntary, uncontrollable and complete emptying of the bladder on giggling in a person who is otherwise fully continent. It is not comparable to stress incontinence in an adult, for the child empties the bladder completely, and once micturition has started, the child cannot stop even though the giggling or laughter may have stopped. Other situations and physical exertion do not cause voiding. It is twice as common in girls as boys [19]. It usually begins in the early school years and sometimes but not always ceases during adolescence [19]. There is no effective cure. Since it is an embarrassing and socially disastrous syndrome, practical advice should be given. Frequent micturition will reduce the amount of wetting when it does occur. Boys can be advised to wear a penile sheath urine collecting bag and girls to wear a sanitary napkin on special social occasions.

References

1. Alderton, H. R. Imipramine in childhood enuresis: Further studies on the relationships of time of administration to effect. *Can. Med. Assoc. J.* 102:1179, 1970.
2. Asnes, R. S., and Mones, R. L. Pollakiuria. *Pediatrics* 52:615, 1973.
3. Bakwin, H. Enuresis in twins. *Am. J. Dis. Child.* 121:222, 1971.
3a. Berg, I., Fielding, D., and Meadow, R. Psychiatric disturbance, urgency, and bacteriuria in children with day and night wetting. *Arch. Dis. Child.* 52:651, 1977.
4. Blackwell, B., and Currah, J. The Psychopharmacology of Nocturnal Enuresis. In I. Kolvin, R. C. MacKeith, and S. R. Meadow (eds.), *Bladder Control and Enuresis* (Clinics in Developmental Medicine Nos. 48/49). Philadelphia: Lippincott, 1973. P. 231.
5. Brazelton, T. B. A child-oriented approach to toilet training. *Pediatrics* 29:121, 1962.
6. Brooks, D., and Maudar, A. Pathogenesis of the urethral syndrome in women and its diagnosis in general practice. *Lancet* 2:893, 1972.
7. Cooper, C. E. Giggle Micturition. In I. Kolvin, R. C. MacKeith, and S. R. Meadow (eds.), *Bladder Control and Enuresis* (Clinics in Developmental Medicine Nos. 48/49). Philadelphia: Lippincott, 1973. P. 61.
8. DeJonge, G. A. Epidemiology of Enuresis: A Survey of the Literature. In I. Kolvin, R. C. MacKeith, and S. R. Meadow (eds.), *Bladder Control and Enuresis* (Clinics in Developmental Medicine Nos. 48/49). Philadelphia: Lippincott, 1973. P. 39.
9. DeJonge, G. A. The Urge Syndrome. In I. Kolvin, R. C. MacKeith, and S. R. Meadow (eds.), *Bladder Control and Enuresis* (Clinics in Developmental Medicine Nos. 48/49). Philadelphia: Lippincott, 1973. P. 66.
10. Dische, S. Treatment of Enuresis with an Enuresis Alarm. In I. Kolvin, R. C. MacKeith, and S. R. Meadow (eds.), *Bladder Control and Enuresis* (Clinics in Developmental Medicine Nos. 48/49). Philadelphia: Lippincott, 1973. P. 211.
11. Dodge, W. F., West, E. F., Bridgforth, E. B., and Travis, L. B. Nocturnal enuresis in 6- to 10-year-old children: Correlation with bacteriuria, proteinuria, and dysuria. *Am. J. Dis. Child.* 120:32, 1970.
11a. Dorfmuller, M. Enuresis. Zur Frage der Hereditaren Disposition. *Med. Klin.* 69:637, 1974.
12. Douglas, J. W. B. Early Disturbing Events and Later Enuresis. In I. Kolvin, R. C. MacKeith, and S. R. Meadow (eds.), *Bladder Control and Enuresis* (Clinics in Developmental Medicine Nos. 48/49). Philadelphia: Lippincott, 1973. P. 109.
13. Esperanca, M., and Gerrard, J. W. Nocturnal enuresis: Studies in bladder function in normal children and enuretics. *Can. Med. Assoc. J.* 101:324, 1969.
13a. Essen, J., and Peckham, C. Nocturnal enuresis in childhood. *Dev. Med. Child Neurol.* 18:577, 1976.
14. Forsythe, W. I., and Redmond, A. Enuresis and spontaneous cure rate. *Arch. Dis. Child.* 49:259, 1974.
15. Hallgren, B. Enuresis. *Acta Psychiatr. Neurol. Scand.* 31:379, 1956.
16. Hallgren, B. Enuresis. *Acta Psychiatr. Neurol. Scand.* 31:405, 1956.
17. Hallgren, B. Nocturnal enuresis in twins. *Acta Psychiatr. Neurol. Scand.* 35:73, 1960.
18. Hawkins, D. N. Enuresis: A survey. *Med. J. Aust.* 1:979, 1962.
19. MacKeith, R. C. Micturition induced by giggling. *Guys Hosp. Rep.* 113:250, 1964.
20. MacKeith, R. C., Meadow, S. R., and Turner, R. K. How Children Become Dry. In I. Kolvin, R. C. MacKeith, and S. R. Meadow (eds.), *Bladder Control and Enuresis* (Clinics in Developmental Medicine Nos. 48/49). Philadelphia: Lippincott, 1973. P. 3.
21. Meadow, S. R. Drugs for bed-wetting. *Arch. Dis. Child.* 49:257, 1974.
21a. Meadow, R., Berg, I., and Fielding, D. Enuresis and urinary tract infection—cause or effect. *Arch. Dis. Child.* 52:808, 1977.
22. Meadow, S. R., White, R. H. R., and Johnston, N. M. Prevalence of symptomless urinary tract disease in Birmingham school children: I. Pyuria and bacteriuria. *Br. Med. J.* 3:81, 1969.
23. Miller, F. J. W. Children Who Wet the Bed. In I. Kolvin, R. C. MacKeith, and S. R. Meadow (eds.), *Bladder Control and Enuresis* (Clinics in Developmental Medicine Nos. 48/49). Philadelphia: Lippincott, 1973. P. 47.
24. Oppel, W. C., Weiner, G., Harper, P. A., and Rider, R. V. The age of attaining bladder control. *Pediatrics* 42:614, 1968.
25. Ritvo, E. R., Gottlieb, F., Poussaint, A. F., Maron, B. T., Ditman, K. S., Blinn, K. A., and Ornitz, E. M. Arousal and non-arousal enuretic events. *Am. J. Psychiatry* 126:77, 1969.
26. Roberts, K. E., and Shoellkopf, J. A. Eating, sleeping, and elimination practices of a group of two-and-one-half-year-old children. *Am. J. Dis. Child.* 82:121, 1951.
27. Rutter, M., Yule, W., and Graham, P. Enuresis and Behavioural Deviance: Some Epidemiological Considerations. In I. Kolvin, R. C. MacKeith, and S. R. Meadow (eds.), *Bladder Control and Enuresis* (Clinics in Developmental Medicine Nos. 48/49). Philadelphia: Lippincott, 1973. P. 137.
28. Starfield, B. Functional bladder capacity in enuretic and non-enuretic children. *J. Pediatr.* 70:777, 1967.
29. Stansfeld, J. M. Enuresis and Urinary Tract Infection. In I. Kolvin, R. C. MacKeith, and S. R. Meadow (eds.), *Bladder Control and Enuresis* (Clinics in Developmental Medicine Nos. 48/49). Philadelphia: Lippincott, 1973. P. 102.
29a. Whiteside, C. G., and Arnold, E. P. Persistent primary enuresis: A urodynamic assessment. *Br. Med. J.* 1:364, 1975.
30. Young, G. C. The relationship of "potting" to enuresis. *J. R. Inst. Public Health Hyg.* 27:23, 1964.
31. Young, G. C., and Morgan, R. T. T. Overlearning in the conditioning treatment of enuresis. *Behav. Res. Ther.* 10:147, 1972.

96. Congenital Urogenital Pathology: General Considerations

Alan B. Retik

In the following chapters various congenital abnormalities, obstructive disorders, and tumors of the genitourinary tract will be discussed. Some of the disorders, such as exstrophy of the bladder and various penile abnormalities, are easily diagnosed by inspection. Most of them, however, require a thorough history, physical examination, and special diagnostic procedures.

Congenital abnormalities of the urinary tract may be single or multiple. They may be simple and of no functional importance, or they may be severe and cause irreversible renal damage. Renal duplication, horseshoe kidney, and congenital solitary kidney are usually asymptomatic and most often go undetected. The majority of children with congenital posterior urethral valves, on the other hand, present in early infancy with signs and symptoms of severe obstructive uropathy and renal insufficiency. Due to their common embryologic derivation, abnormalities of the genitalia are often associated with urinary tract anomalies.

Ureteral duplications, vesicoureteral reflux, and hypospadias are familial disorders and may be genetically transmitted. Little is known concerning their genetic pattern, however, making it difficult to offer recommendations regarding screening of family members.

Urogenital malformations often are multiple, necessitating complete urologic examination for adequate evaluation. For example, genitourinary anomalies are associated with imperforate anus, tracheoesophageal fistula, and various cardiac anomalies. Renal anomalies, notably horseshoe kidney, are commonly seen in the child with the Turner syndrome. Tumors of the urinary tract also may be associated with abnormalities of other organ systems, for example, Wilms' tumor in children with congenital hemihypertrophy or aniridia.

The presence of oligohydramnios suggests renal agenesis, hypoplasia, or obstructive disease. The infant who exhibits the Potter facies, with a flat nose, recession of the chin, a prominent fold running downward and outward from the inner canthus, and flattened, aberrantly folded ears, may have renal agenesis. Infants with congenital hypo-plasia of the abdominal musculature always have associated urinary tract abnormalities.

Clinical Manifestations of Obstructive Uropathy

Abnormalities of the urinary sediment, symptoms and signs of urinary tract infection, and manifestations of renal insufficiency may indicate congenital urologic abnormalities as well as many other types of disorders. These are dealt with in other chapters. In this chapter emphasis will be placed on urinary retention and anuria, urinary incontinence, and abdominal masses as prima facie evidence of urologic disease.

Acute urinary retention in the newborn is rare and must be distinguished from *anuria*. The normal infant may not void for 24 to 48 hr after birth. If voiding has not occurred after this period of time, anuria due to renal agenesis, severe dysplasia, or obstructive uropathy must be considered. Urinary retention in the newborn most often is due to occlusion of the urethral meatus with epithelial debris, particularly in infants with coronal hypospadias. Complete obliteration of the membranous urethra is sometimes seen in children with hypoplasia of the abdominal musculature. Vaginal distention in the neonate with hydrometrocolpos may cause compression of the urethra and is another important cause of urinary retention.

Acute urinary retention in the older infant or child is not common and may be due to transitory causes, such as meatal ulceration or constipation. Retention may also be caused by congenital anomalies or tumors causing intrinsic or extrinsic obstruction of the urethra or the bladder neck. Bladder diverticula presenting posteriorly may fill with urine and obstruct the bladder neck and the prostatic urethra. Calculi impacted in the urethra may also be obstructive. Congenital diverticula and valves of the anterior urethra, prolapsing ectopic ureteroceles, urethral strictures, and lymphomatous infiltration of the bladder neck protruding into the urethra on occasion are responsible for acute urinary retention.

Urinary incontinence is one of the more prominent presenting symptoms in children with disorders of the urinary tract. One of the most common types of incontinence is urge incontinence, usually associated with urinary tract infection. These children are usually incontinent day and night, but they are not wet continuously, as in the child with dribbling incontinence, which is usually due to an organic disorder such as a vaginal ectopic ureter. On physical examination of the child with dribbling incontinence one may see a constant drip of urine from the vagina. A bifid clitoris in the girl who is wet most of the time is indicative of subsymphyseal epispadias with a deficiency of the urethral sphincter mechanism. Dribbling incontinence may also be seen in patients with an obstructed bladder and overflow or in patients with neurogenic bladder dysfunction. A worthwhile bedside maneuver to differentiate the latter two forms of incontinence is to attempt to express urine from the bladder manually (as in the Credé method). A normally innervated obstructed bladder cannot be emptied in this way except in the newborn. In addition, children with neurogenic bladder dysfunction may have an easily palpable spinal defect or a prominent dimple or hairy nevus in the lower back or sacrum.

Nocturnal enuresis without daytime wetting is usually not indicative of an organic abnormality (Chap. 95). Stress incontinence is not common in children, but it may occur with a well-compensated organic abnormality such as epispadias or neurogenic bladder dysfunction.

The kidney of the normal infant is palpable during the first several months of life. Nevertheless, a significantly high percentage of *abdominal masses* in the infant and child are related to the urinary tract. Most renal masses are palpated by the pediatrician during a routine examination and are asymptomatic. In a roentgenographic study [1] of abdominal masses in 117 newborns, 63 of the masses were renal, 39 being discovered during the first 2 days of life and 24 in the first 4 weeks. Twenty-five of the masses were multicystic kidneys, and twenty represented hydronephrosis. These last two conditions constituted almost 40 percent of the abdominal masses in the newborn.

Multicystic kidneys are almost always unilateral, have a lobulated surface, and can be transilluminated. Hydronephrosis due to ureteropelvic obstruction usually presents as a unilateral tense, cystic mass that may on occasion change size due to the intermittency of the obstruction. In the male infant with severe lower urinary tract obstruction, usually secondary to posterior urethral valves, it may be possible to palpate ureters, kidneys, and bladder. The diameter of these ureters is often much larger than that of the intestine; such ureters feel like diffuse, cystic structures on both sides of the abdomen.

Infantile polycystic disease often is detectable at birth, presenting as bilateral smooth masses that encompass the entire abdomen.

Adrenal hematoma and renal vein thrombosis are encountered most commonly during the first 2 to 3 weeks of life in a very sick infant. Adrenal hematoma is usually unilateral and is seen either in a large infant who has suffered birth trauma or in the premature child with hypoxia. Renal vein thrombosis classically is seen in a markedly dehydrated infant, often with a maternal history of diabetes.

Wilms' tumor and neuroblastoma are very uncommonly palpated in the newborn and are more likely to be detected between the ages of 6 months and 4 years. Wilms' tumors are large, hard, painless tumors usually projecting anteriorly into the abdomen. Adrenal neuroblastomas are very hard and immovable tumors projecting deeper into the abdomen, often extending across the midline. Metastases often are present at the time this tumor is detected.

Renal carbuncle and perinephric abscess are rare lesions that are usually secondary to hematogenous staphylococcal infections. They occur in children who have been sick for several weeks and who have had a preexisting staphylococcal infection in another area of the body. The renal carbuncle is a hard mass that is usually tender.

It may be possible in the infant to palpate a number of lesions on rectal examination. The markedly dilated prostatic urethra in the boy with posterior urethral valves is a good example. Sarcomas of the bladder, prostate, and female genital organs are firm, rubbery, lobulated masses. The various retrorectal tumors, such as teratoma, sacral neuroblastoma, and sacrococcygeal tumors, are easily palpable on rectal examination.

Diagnostic Procedures

As mentioned above, urinary tract infection is a common presenting symptom of many infants and children with congenital anomalies of the urinary system. Appropriate studies to document the presence of infection are mandatory, as discussed in Chap. 92. The two basic studies in the evaluation of a child with urinary tract infection are the excretory urogram and the voiding cystourethrogram.

Cystourethroscopy may be indicated in the evaluation of children with a number of congenital anomalies and recurrent urinary infections. This procedure is always done under general anesthesia. Excellent visualization of the urethra and bladder is obtained with the newer fiberoptic instruments. Cystoscopy will help to confirm anatomic abnormalities of the bladder and urethra visualized radiologically and will clearly define the anatomy of the trigone and ureteral orifices in the child with vesicoureteral reflux. It is also useful in girls with many recurrent urinary tract infections in whom minor anatomic abnormalities not apparent by x-ray may be detailed. It can also define the nature and extent of an inflammatory disorder, for example, cystitis cystica, which may dictate the type and duration of antibiotic therapy.

Retrograde pyelography is not often necessary in children. Performed as a dynamic study with the use of image amplification, it can be helpful in delineating an obstructive ureteral or ureteropelvic lesion. Ureteral peristalsis also may be studied.

Radioisotopic and sonographic methods are extremely useful in the evaluation of patients with obstructive uropathy (Chap. 11). Radioisotope cystograms have been employed in the follow-up of children with vesicoureteral reflux to determine whether or not the reflux has subsided. Radiation dosage is appreciably less than with conventional voiding cystourethrography.

Renal angiography is used frequently in infants and children in the evaluation of renal and retroperitoneal tumors, hypertension, and certain instances of renal trauma (Chap. 10). Arteriography may be performed in the newborn through the umbilical artery. This procedure recently delineated a renal artery stenosis in a 2-day-old girl on our service with severe hypertension and congestive heart failure.

PHYSIOLOGIC STUDIES OF BLADDER FUNCTION

In order to gain further insight into disorders of micturition, certain physiologic studies may be of value. These include cystometry, uroflowmetry, sphincter electromyography, and measurement of intraurethral resistance during voiding. These studies are difficult to perform and interpret in the young uncooperative child and therefore are most applicable in children over the age of 4 or 5 years. Physiologic studies of bladder function may be helpful in (1) neurogenic vesical dysfunction; (2) urinary incontinence, retention, or diurnal and nocturnal enuresis of undetermined etiology; and (3) repeated urinary tract infections without an obvious anatomic abnormality.

Cystometry is done by asking the child to void, following which a small catheter is passed through the urethra into the bladder and left in place. The volume of residual urine is measured. Water is instilled into the bladder at a flow rate of approximately 1 ml per second. Proprioception is determined by ascertaining from the child when the first desire to urinate occurs and when capacity is reached. Intravesical pressures (in cm H_2O) are recorded with each 50-ml increment of bladder filling. In the older, more cooperative child, exteroceptive sensation may be tested by instillation of cold and then warm water. The advantage of the commercially available water and air cystometers is their ability to record intravesical pressure graphically. A continuous pressure recording is therefore available, allowing for evaluation and identification of uninhibited bladder contractions.

The bethanechol chloride (Urecholine) supersensitivity test advocated by Lapides et al. [2] is an extremely helpful adjunct in cystometry and should be employed whenever possible. After filling the bladder with 100 ml of H_2O, the intravesical pressure is recorded and the flow of fluid is stopped. Urecholine is then given subcutaneously, and the cystometrogram is repeated 20 to 30 min later. A denervated (supersensitive) bladder may show a hyperactive response, suggesting a neurogenic component.

The normal child has a residual urine of less than 20 ml and is able to perceive hot and cold sensation. The first urge to void and bladder capacity vary with age. During the initial bladder filling, intravesical pressure rises sharply to between 5 and 25 cm H_2O. The pressure then remains fairly constant until bladder capacity is reached. Thereafter, intravesical pressure increases in a linear relationship with volume. Uninhibited voiding contractions are not observed at any time during the procedure in a normally innervated bladder (Fig. 96-1) unless it is infected or irritated by an indwelling catheter.

In the normal child the increase in intravesical pressure in response to the Urecholine supersensitivity test is less than 15 cm H_2O over control. A

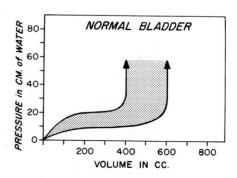

Figure 96-1. A normal cystometrogram.

greater increase provides strong evidence in favor of disease of the sacral spinal cord or the reflex arc, due to the supersensitivity of the ganglionic synapse and the neuromuscular junctions to Urecholine and the enhanced impulse transmission when neurologic disease is present. Thus the denervation sensitivity test is of considerable help in diagnosing autonomous neurogenic, motor paralytic, and sensory paralytic bladders.

Measurement of the *urinary flow rate* may be helpful in the diagnosis of abnormalities of the lower urinary tract. Flow rate is directly proportional to the intravesical pressure and inversely proportional to the intraurethral resistance. Children void into an electric flow meter, while intravesical pressure is recorded by using a small plastic tube inserted into the bladder suprapubically.

This technique permits the simultaneous measurement of intravesical pressure and flow rate, with subsequent calculation of intraurethral resistance.

Sphincter electromyography has been employed in conjunction with cystometry to record the electrical activity of the perineal muscles during micturition. This technique is of value in the delineation of urinary sphincter and urethral dysfunction and diseases of the nervous system.

References

1. Griscom, N. T. Roentgenology of neonatal abdominal masses. *Am. J. Roentgenol. Radium Ther. Nucl. Med.* 93:447, 1965.
2. Lapides, J., Friend, C. R., Ajemian, E. P., and Reus, W. S. Denervation supersensitivity as a test for neurogenic bladder. *Surg. Gynecol. Obstet.* 114:241, 1962.

97. Anomalies of the Upper Urinary Tract   *Alan B. Retik*

Renal hypoplasia and dysplasia, polycystic disease, nephronophthisis, and medullary cystic disease, all congenital diseases of the kidneys, are the subjects of other chapters. In this chapter will be discussed developmental anomalies of the kidneys that are of urologic concern, that is, that may require surgical intervention.

Anomalies of Fusion of the Kidney

Fusion of the kidney is defined as the union of both renal elements, each with its separate collecting system. The most common type of fusion is the horseshoe variety, in which the kidneys are fused at their lower poles. Fusion of the upper poles or of both poles also occurs. The upper pole of one kidney may be fused to the lower pole of the other to produce a sigmoid or L-shaped kidney. The entire kidney substance may be fused into one mass to form the so-called lump kidney.

Prior to the twentieth century, anomalies of fusion were regarded as curiosities and were detected primarily at postmortem examination. With the advent of excretory urography, the incidence and clinical significance of these entities have become better appreciated. The incidence of fusion anomalies, primarily horseshoe kidney, has been estimated from autopsy studies to vary from 1 in 300 to 1 in 1,000 [6, 9, 13]. Clinically the frequency is about 1 : 400 population.

Partial or complete fusion of the kidney results from failure of separation of the metanephrogenic cell mass. Fusion of the primitive renal cell masses occurs at the 5- to 8-mm stage of embryogenesis. It has been theorized [8] that deviation of the point of origin of the umbilical artery may cause primary fusion by interfering with the normal upward growth of the ureteric buds. Ectopia and malrotation are often associated with renal fusion, occur at a later period in embryonic life, and may determine the specific type of renal abnormality.

HORSESHOE KIDNEY

DeCarpi in 1521 was one of the first observers to describe a horseshoe kidney. In 1564 Botallo described the anatomy vividly and illustrated the separate blood supply to the isthmus [7].

Horseshoe kidneys (Fig. 97-1) are composed of two renal segments that are fused across the midline by an isthmus composed usually of renal parenchyma, but occasionally of fibrous tissue. The lower poles of the two kidneys are fused in 90 to 95 percent of cases. The isthmus lies at the level of the fourth lumbar vertebra in 40 percent of cases, just below the origin of the inferior mesenteric artery. In the remaining cases the isthmus is either in the pelvis or lies at the usual level of the lower poles. The isthmus of the horseshoe kidney usually lies anterior to the aorta and vena cava,

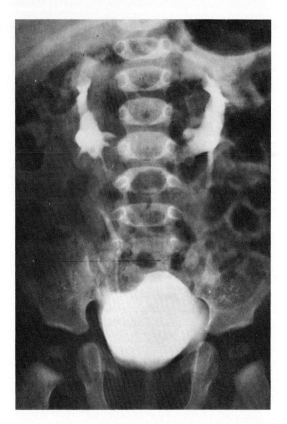

Figure 97-1. Typical horseshoe kidney. Note the medial deviation of the lower poles.

anomalies of other systems of the body. Boatman et al. [3] reported other congenital abnormalities, particularly gastrointestinal, cardiovascular, and anorectal defects, in one-third of 96 patients. Horseshoe kidney is seen not infrequently in children with Turner's syndrome and the Laurence-Moon-Biedl syndrome.

Horseshoe kidney is usually asymptomatic and is *not* a cause of abdominal pain as has been postulated. Many horseshoe kidneys, however, do have malrotated pelves with concomitant urinary stasis leading to urinary infection and calculi. In addition, ureteropelvic obstruction with hydronephrosis is not infrequently seen. These conditions present in adult life, although they may be seen in children.

The diagnosis of horseshoe kidney is usually made from the excretory urogram. On occasion, the isthmus as well as both renal elements can be palpated. The distinguishing features on the excretory urogram are the relatively low level of the renal shadows, downward convergence of the renal axes, medially located and malrotated pelves, and the high insertion of the ureters from the anterior or lateral aspects of the kidney.

Surgery for horseshoe kidney is required only for obstruction. It is sometimes necessary to divide the isthmus at the time of pyeloplasty to provide better drainage.

FUSED PELVIC KIDNEY

Morris [25] in 1901 reported six cases of fused pelvic kidney, which has been described as having a number of different shapes and forms, for example, discoid, lump, sigmoid, or cake kidney. These are irregular masses of renal tissue usually located in the midline, with two separate collecting systems (Fig. 97-2). The ureters are located anteriorly and enter the bladder at the normal location. The blood supply invariably is derived from the aorta, common iliacs, and hypogastric arteries.

Fused pelvic kidney is caused by a developmental arrest following union of the ureteric buds with the renal blastema. This anomaly occurs prior to migration and rotation at approximately the 10- to 14-mm stage of embryogenesis. The anomalies are very rare, being reported by Campbell [7] in 3 of 51,880 autopsies.

Fused pelvic kidney is often detected incidentally on routine physical examination or at the time of exploratory laparotomy for an unrelated disorder. Symptoms may arise from stasis due to malrotation, from hydronephrosis secondary to ureteropelvic obstruction, and from calculus formation. The diagnosis is usually established by palpation

but it has been reported in rare instances to lie posterior to these vessels [16, 23].

The blood supply to a horseshoe kidney is usually multiple and anomalous, and as many as 10 arteries have been reported to supply both kidneys and the isthmus. This is of major importance in surgical management.

Medial fusion of the two nephrogenic blastemas results in the formation of a horseshoe kidney. Fusion occurs when the renal masses are brought into contact as they cross the umbilical arteries during their passage out of the pelvis by the sixth week. Horseshoe kidney is assumed to occur when both kidneys lie at the same level and their inferior poles come into contact. The isthmus of the kidney is formed when the kidneys diverge during ascent. The isthmus is crossed by the inferior mesenteric artery, which prevents further ascent. When fusion precedes renal rotation, as is usually the case, the rotation of the kidneys is prevented and the ureters and pelves are nonrotated or malrotated and anterior. On occasion, when rotation precedes fusion, the pelves are located medially.

Horseshoe kidney occurs twice as often in males as in females, and it is often accompanied by

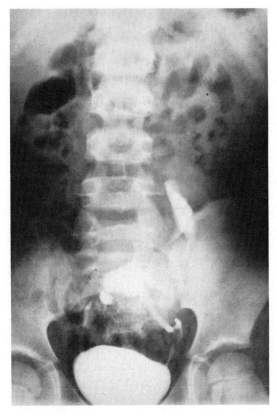

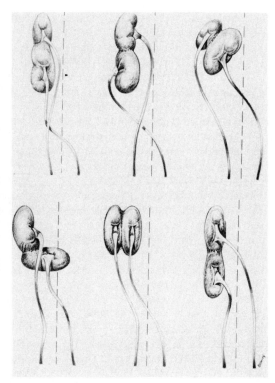

Figure 97-3. Variations of crossed renal ectopia with fusion.

Figure 97-2. A fused pelvic kidney that was detected by palpation on a routine physical examination.

during abdominal examination and by excretory urography.

Treatment. Surgery may be necessary for complications of fused pelvic kidney, such as obstruction or a calculus. Surgical resection of a portion of the fused kidney may be extremely difficult due to the anomalous and bizarre blood supply. These kidneys have been removed unwittingly with the erroneous diagnosis of pelvic tumor.

Ectopia of the Kidney

When the kidney does not lie in its usual position, it is said to be ectopic. Rokitansky (quoted by Campbell [7]) reported the first case of crossed unfused ectopic kidney in 1861. Since that time many series have been published [4, 5, 20, 22, 33, 38]. A *simple ectopic* kidney describes failure of complete ascent of the kidney without crossing the midline; its position may be pelvic, iliac, or lumbar, the first being the most common location. Approximately 10 percent of ectopic pelvic kidneys are solitary.

In *crossed renal ectopia* the kidneys are on the same side of the body, the crossed organ usually lying below and medial to the contralateral one, with the ureters entering normally into the bladder. Of the numerous anatomic variants, the most common is crossed ectopia with fusion (Fig. 97-3). The ectopic kidney usually is smaller than its mate. A number of bizarre shapes caused by growth with fusion have been reported.

In 10 percent of cases of renal ectopia, the two kidneys remain unfused. In rare instances, both kidneys cross to the opposite side; this is known as double crossed ectopia. Several cases of crossed ectopia with solitary kidney have been reported [2, 21, 29].

Rarely, a renal ascent continues into the chest. In this condition, known as *thoracic renal ectopia,* the kidney ascends through a foramen or hernia in the diaphragm. The ectopic kidney has an elongated ureter and may be associated with some degree of malrotation.

The embryogenesis of simple renal ectopia is not clear. It has been postulated that in crossed renal ectopia, the developing ureter induces the formation of a normal kidney on its own side, and that during ascent, this kidney, attached to the trailing kidney, pulls it across the midline. Alternatively, the developing ureter may cross the midline and induce the formation of the kidney from the contralateral nephrogenic blastema. In this situation, the ipsilateral kidney does not form.

The incidence of simple renal ectopia is 1 : 800. If the ectopic kidney is solitary, the incidence is 1 : 1,220 [34]. It is more common in males than in females. Thoracic renal ectopia is rare, about 30 cases being reported in the literature [11, 32].

The incidence of crossed renal ectopia is said to be 1 : 2,000 autopsies [7]. It is slightly more common in males than females, and the left kidney crosses to the right more often than the converse [22].

Many ectopic kidneys are palpable on abdominal examination. The thoracic ectopic kidney may be seen on chest x-ray and confirmed by excretory urography. In the absence of complications, most patients are asymptomatic, but hydronephrosis, infection, or stone formation may occur. Treatment is required only for complications.

Anomalies of Rotation. As the kidney ascends during the first 2 months of embryonic life, the axis of the renal pelvis shifts from its initial anterior position to a medial one. Any deviation from this is called malrotation. There are various degrees of malrotation, including hyperrotation with the renal pelvis facing posteriorly.

Malrotation is seen commonly in children with Turner's syndrome [15]. It does not cause symptoms unless it is associated with severe stasis and urinary infection. Treatment is required only for complications such as ureteropelvic obstruction.

Ureteropelvic Obstruction

Hydronephrosis due to ureteropelvic obstruction, defined as an impediment to urinary flow from the renal pelvis into the ureter, is one of the more common anomalies seen in childhood. Initially there is hypertrophy of the muscle of the renal pelvis, and then there is progressive dilatation of the pelvis and calyces, with subsequent destruction of renal parenchyma and impairment of renal function.

In the series of Uson et al. of 134 hydronephrotic kidneys, ureteropelvic obstruction was found to be intrinsic in two thirds [35]. Adhesions between the upper ureter and pelvis also may be obstructive [17]. Aberrant vessels between the aorta and hilum or lower pole of the kidney have been mentioned as a cause of ureteropelvic junction obstruction. Nixon [27] reported 25 of 78 cases of ureteropelvic obstruction to be secondary to aberrant vessels. The incidence in other reported series [31] is 15 to 20 percent. There is considerable doubt, however, as to the relationship of the vessels to the obstruction. The vessel may very well exacerbate an obstruction secondary to an intrinsic lesion. Simple freeing of these vessels, which may be arteries or veins, usually does not relieve the obstruction.

Hydronephrosis is sometimes seen in the absence of an anatomic obstruction. Murnaghan [26] has shown an interruption of the circular element of the musculature at the ureteropelvic junction and has postulated the failure of transmission of peristaltic waves from the renal pelvis to the ureter.

Valvular mucosal folds have also been implicated as obstructive in a few instances. On rare occasions, polyps at the ureteropelvic junction have been described as an additional cause of ureteropelvic obstruction.

Severe vesicoureteral reflux may cause secondary kinking and tortuosity at the ureteropelvic junction with resultant obstruction. A voiding cystourethrogram confirms this diagnosis. If the obstruction is intermittent and associated with reflux, antireflux surgery rather than surgery at the ureteropelvic junction is indicated. In some children, the ureteropelvic junction obstruction may persist after correction of the reflux, and staged surgery at both ends of the ureter may be necessary.

Ureteropelvic junction obstruction is seen with equal frequency in children of either sex, with a peak incidence in the first 6 months of life. It is frequently seen in ectopic, malrotated, or horseshoe kidneys. Both kidneys have been reported to be obstructed in 10 to 20 percent of the cases [9, 14, 35] (Fig. 97-4). Williams [36] noted a significant incidence of multicystic disease in the contralateral kidney in infants.

The usual presentation of ureteropelvic obstruction in the infant is an asymptomatic mass palpated on routine examination. Occasionally failure to thrive, feeding difficulties, or sepsis secondary to a urinary tract infection will lead the pediatrician to obtain an excretory urogram. In the older child, intermittent flank or upper abdominal pain, sometimes associated with vomiting, are prominent symptoms. Symptoms of upper urinary tract infection are seen in 50 percent of children with ureteropelvic obstruction. The hematuria seen in 25 percent of these children often follows minor abdominal trauma, most probably due to rupture of mucosal vessels in the dilated collecting system.

Severe chronic obstruction may lead to loss of renal function and, if bilateral, to renal failure. With severe stasis and infection, stone formation sometimes occurs.

Although the diagnosis of ureteropelvic obstruction may be suspected clinically, it is confirmed by excretory urography. A distended renal pelvis and calyces are usually seen with an abrupt cutoff at the

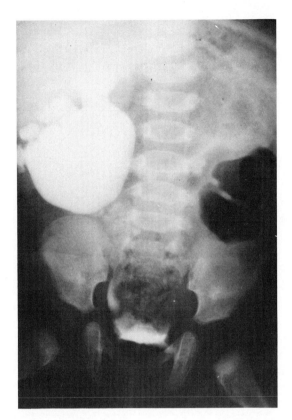

Figure 97-4. Excretory urogram in a 1-month-old boy with bilateral flank masses. Hydronephrosis secondary to ureteropelvic obstruction is present on the right. There is nonvisualization of the left kidney, but a left hydronephrosis was subsequently found, also due to ureteropelvic obstruction.

ureteropelvic junction. It is important to obtain delayed films to determine whether hydroureter is present as well. Significant partial obstruction may be present even though the ureter is visualized beyond the ureteropelvic junction. A retrograde pyelogram performed at the time of surgical correction helps to delineate the anatomic detail of the obstruction as well as the anatomy of the entire ureter. If obstruction is equivocal, it is sometimes worthwhile to obtain a retrograde pyelogram with fluoroscopy to study the mechanics of the ureteropelvic junction. Some patients have intermittent obstruction that is precipitated only by diuresis. They may have normal excretory urograms when asymptomatic. An excretory urogram with induced diuresis should be obtained at the time that the child is having acute symptoms.

As mentioned above, it may be necessary to obtain a voiding cystourethrogram in selected patients to rule out the possibility of ureteropelvic junction obstruction secondary to vesicoureteral reflux.

Ureteropelvic obstruction requires surgical correction. The vast majority of kidneys can be salvaged with pyeloplasty. The most common type of surgical procedure performed is the dismembered pyeloplasty, which is applicable to virtually all types of obstruction. Vessels that are thought to be obstructive are not ligated for fear of causing renal ischemia. In such cases, pyeloplasty may be done by anastomosing the ureter to the pelvis on the other side of the obstructing vessel. Most kidneys do not have a normal postoperative pyelographic appearance, but show some resolution of hydronephrosis. The surgical success rate is greater than 90 percent in most series [19, 31].

Renal clearances and isotopic scans provide information regarding individual renal function and are sometimes helpful in deciding whether or not nephrectomy or pyeloplasty should be performed. If a kidney does not visualize by excretory urography or if the function of the affected kidney is less than 10 percent of total, consideration should be given to nephrectomy. The final decision is made at the time of surgery.

Calyceal Abnormalities
HYDROCALYCOSIS
Hydrocalycosis represents cystic dilatation of a major calyx lined by transitional epithelium with a demonstrable connection to the renal pelvis.

Dilatation of the upper calyx due to obstruction of the upper infundibulum by vessels or stenosis has been described [10, 18]. Hydrocalycosis has also been reported to occur without an obvious etiology [37]. It has been postulated [24, 37] that achalasia of a ring of muscle at the entrance of the infundibulum into the renal pelvis acts as a functional obstruction.

The most common presenting symptom is upper abdominal or flank pain. On occasion a mass may be palpated. Mild upper calyceal dilatation due to partial infundibular obstruction is relatively common but is usually asymptomatic. When stasis is severe, infection may occur.

Hydrocalycosis must be differentiated from multiple calyceal dilatations secondary to ureteric obstruction, calyceal clubbing secondary to pyelonephritis or medullary necrosis, tuberculosis of the kidney, large calyceal diverticula, and megacalycosis. These entities can be differentiated by a combination of excretory urography, findings at surgery, microscopy, and bacteriology.

Hydrocalycosis due to vascular obstruction is usually treated by dismembered infundibulopyelostomy, thus changing the relationship of the infundibulum to the vessel. When the cystic dilatation is due to stenosis of the infundibulum, an intubated infundibulotomy or partial nephrectomy is usually employed. Although clinical improvement is apparent in most instances, the radiologic appearance often is not significantly altered.

MEGACALYCOSIS

Megacalycosis is best defined as nonobstructive distention of calyces due to a malformation of the renal papillae. It was first described by Puigvert in 1962 [28]. The papillary tissue of the renal medulla is thinned out around the hypotonic calyces. The renal pelvis is not dilated nor is its wall thickened, and the ureteropelvic junction is normally funneled without evidence of obstruction. The overall radiographic appearance sometimes simulates ureteropelvic junction or other obstruction and must be distinguished from these conditions. Changes in renal function in children with megacalycosis are not prominent. A mild disorder of concentrating ability has been reported by Gittes and Talner [12].

The child with megacalycosis is usually asymptomatic. The condition most often presents in adult life with complications of urinary stasis, that is, infection, calculi, or hematuria.

CALYCEAL DIVERTICULA

A calyceal diverticulum, first described by Rayer [30] in 1841, is a cystic cavity lined by transitional epithelium that is situated peripheral to a minor calyx to which it is connected by a narrow channel. The cyst or diverticulum may involve one or more calyces, the upper calyx being most frequently involved.

The etiology of the diverticulum has been proposed to be both congenital and acquired. At the 5-mm stage of the embryo some of the ureteral branches of the third and fourth order, which ordinarily degenerate, may persist as isolated branches, resulting in the formation of a calyceal diverticulum. A localized cortical abscess that has opened to drain into a calyx also has been postulated as an etiologic factor. Other proposed etiologies include injury, achalasia, obstruction secondary to stone formation or infection, and spasm or dysfunction of one of the sphincters surrounding a minor calyx. Vesicoureteral reflux has been implicated as an etiologic factor in children.

The majority of cases of calyceal diverticula have been reported in adults. Abeshouse and Abeshouse [1] reviewed 329 cases in the literature and added 16 cases for a total of 345. The sexes are equally affected.

Small calyceal diverticula are usually asymptomatic and are found incidentally at excretory urography. Calyceal distention with urine sometimes causes pain. Infection and stone formation are complications that may produce symptoms. The diagnosis is made by excretory urography; delayed films are helpful in demonstrating calyceal retention of urine. On occasion, retrograde pyelography may be necessary to confirm the precise anatomy and diagnosis.

No treatment is required in asymptomatic cases of calyceal diverticula, although periodic excretory urograms should be obtained. Persistent pain, resistant and persistent urinary tract infections, and calculi are indications for surgery.

References

1. Abeshouse, B. S., and Abeshouse, G. A. Sponge kidney: A review of the literature and report of five cases. *J. Urol.* 84:252, 1960.
2. Alexander, J. C., King, K. B., and Fromm, C. S. Congenital solitary kidney with crossed ureter. *J. Urol.* 64:230, 1950.
3. Boatman, D. L., Kolln, C. P., and Flocks, R. H. Congenital anomalies associated with horseshoe kidney. *J. Urol.* 107:205, 1972.
4. Burford, E. H., and Burford, C. E. Crossed renal ectopia: Report of 9 cases and review of the literature. *Mo. Med.* 54:237, 1957.
5. Caine, M. Crossed renal ectopia without fusion. *Br. J. Urol.* 28:257, 1956.
6. Campbell, M. F. Renal ectopy. *J. Urol.* 24:187, 1930.
7. Campbell, M. F. Anomalies of the Kidney. In M. F. Campbell and J. H. Harrison (eds.), *Urology* (3rd ed.). Philadelphia: Saunders, 1970.
8. Carleton, A. Crossed ectopia of the kidney and its possible cause. *J. Anat.* 71:292, 1937.
9. Culp, O. S. Renal ectopia. *J. Urol.* 52:420, 1940.
10. Fraley, E. E. Vascular obstruction of superior infundibulum causing nephralgia—new syndrome. *N. Engl. J. Med.* 275:1403, 1966.
11. Fusonie, D., and Molnar, W. Anomalous pulmonary venous return, pulmonary sequestration, bronchial atresia, aplastic right upper lobe, pericardial defect and intrathoracic kidney: An unusual complex of congenital anomalies in one patient. *Am. J. Roentgenol.* 97:350, 1966.
12. Gittes, R. F., and Talner, L. B. Congenital megacalyces versus obstructive hydronephrosis. *J. Urol.* 108:833, 1972.
13. Glenn, J. F. Analysis of fifty-one patients with horseshoe kidneys. *N. Engl. J. Med.* 261:684, 1959.
14. Gross, R. E. Ureteropelvic Obstruction. In R. E. Gross (ed.), *The Surgery of Infancy and Childhood.* Philadelphia: Saunders, 1953.
15. Hung, W., and LoPresti, J. M. Urinary tract anomalies in gonadal dysgenesis. *Am. J. Roentgenol. Radium Ther. Nucl. Med.* 95:439, 1965.
16. Jarmon, W. D. Surgery of the horseshoe kidney with a postaortic isthmus: Report of two cases of horseshoe kidney. *J. Urol.* 40:1, 1938.
17. Johnston, J. H. The pathogenesis of hydronephrosis in children. *Br. J. Urol.* 41:724, 1969.
18. Johnston, J. H., and Sandomirsky, S. K. Intra-renal vascular obstruction of the superior infundibulum in children. *J. Pediatr. Surg.* 7:318, 1972.

19. Kelalis, P. P., Culp, O. S., Stickler, G. B., and Burke, E. C. Uretero-pelvic obstruction in children: Experience with 109 cases. *J. Urol.* 106:418, 1971.

20. Lee, H. P. Crossed unfused renal ectopia with tumor. *J. Urol.* 61:333, 1949.

21. Magri, J. Solitary crossed ectopic kidney. *Br. J. Urol.* 33:152, 1961.

22. McDonald, J. H., and McClellan, D. S. Crossed renal ectopia. *Am. J. Surg.* 93:995, 1957.

23. Meek, J. R., and Wadsworth, G. H. A case of horseshoe kidney lying between the great vessels. *J. Urol.* 43:448, 1940.

24. Moore, T. Hydrocalycosis. *Br. J. Urol.* 22:304, 1950.

25. Morris, H. *Surgical Diseases of the Kidney and Ureter.* London: Cassel, 1901. Vol. 1.

26. Murnaghan, G. F. Experimental aspects of hydronephrosis. *Br. J. Urol.* 31:370, 1959.

27. Nixon, H. H. Hydronephrosis in children. *Br. J. Surg.* 40:601, 1953.

28. Puigvert, A. Megacalycosis: Differentiation from hydrocalycosis. *Helv. Chir. Acta* 31:414, 1962.

29. Purponi, I. Crossed renal ectopy with solitary kidney: A review of the literature. *J. Urol.* 90:13, 1963.

30. Rayer, P. F. C. *Traité des Maladies des Reins et des Altérations de la Sécrétion Urinaire.* Paris, 1837–1841. 3 Vol.

31. Retik, A. B., and Jacobs, E. Ureteropelvic obstruction in infants and children. *J. Urol.* In press.

32. Shapira, E., Fishel, E., and Levin, S. Intrathoracic kidney in a premature infant. *Arch. Dis. Child.* 40:86, 1965.

33. Shih, H. E., Sun, W. H., and Chen, H. K. Crossed unfused renal ectopia. *Chin. Med. J.* 75:841, 1957.

34. Thompson, G. J., and Pace, J. M. Ectopic kidney: A review of 97 cases. *Surg. Gynecol. Obstet.* 64:935, 1937.

35. Uson, A. C., Cox, L. A., and Lattimer, J. D. Hydronephrosis in infants and children: I. Some clinical and pathological aspects. *J.A.M.A.* 205:323, 1968.

36. Williams, D. I. Obstructive Uropathy: The Upper Tract. In D. I. Williams (ed.), *Urology in Childhood.* Berlin: Springer, 1974.

37. Williams, D. I., and Mininberg, D. T. Hydrocalycosis: Report of three cases in children. *Br. J. Urol.* 40:541, 1968.

38. Winram, R. G., and Ward-McQuaid, J. N. Crossed renal ectopia without fusion. *Can. Med. Assoc. J.* 81:481, 1959.

98. Abnormalities of the Lower Urinary Tract

*Alan B. Retik and
Myron I. Murdock*

Approximately two-thirds of all urologic anomalies involve the lower urinary tract and external genitalia. An excretory urogram often reveals upper urinary tract changes secondary to lower urinary tract disease. A voiding cystourethrogram will outline the lower tract pathology; it represents the most important single diagnostic tool. New diagnostic techniques, including carbon dioxide cystometrography, external sphincterometry, electromyography of the bladder detrusor and external sphincter, and uroflowmetry, have further elucidated the pathophysiology of lower urinary tract anomalies and have provided methods to evaluate therapeutic modalities.

Treatment of urologic anomalies varies with each individual case. Frequently minor surgical repair is all that is needed. In advanced obstruction, however, diversion may be indicated. Early recognition with prompt diagnosis is of the utmost importance to ensure correct treatment and prevention or resolution of potentially serious complications.

Agenesis and Atresia of the Urethra

Congenital absence or agenesis of the urethra has been reported in 50 infants, predominantly males [43, 128, 154]. Absence of the entire penile urethra implies either failure of the urethral plate or of the pars phallica of the urogenital sinus to develop. Congenital segmental urethral agenesis or atresia is more common. Campbell [30, 32] reported 4 cases of urethral agenesis and 3 of atresia in close to 16,000 autopsies. The level of obstruction is usually at the membranous urethra; however, due to the marked posterior urethral dilatation, the obstruction may appear to be at the bladder neck. Urethral agenesis is usually associated with agenesis of the abdominal wall, sometimes accompanied by a thread of rectum extending toward the bladder (rectal agenesis) [1, 96, 192].

One-third of all affected fetuses are stillborn. Urine secreted in utero distends the bladder, obstructing the umbilical arteries and causing embarrassment to the fetal circulation. Rarely, dystocia may occur. Elevated pressure in the kidney during intrauterine development contributes to upper tract dilatation and renal dysplasia. Unless alternate pathways for the passage of urine are established, the fetus dies. Urachal, cloacal, urethrorectal, urethropenile, urethroscrotal, or vesicovaginal fistulas [118] allow egress of urine and sustain life.

The diagnosis should be considered in a neonate who does not pass urine within 48 hr after birth, has evidence of urinary fistulization, or has anomalies of the external genitalia. Treatment is emergent, with immediate decompression of the upper urinary tract. In the past, most cases of urethral atresia were treated with forage, the forcible creation of a canal through the occluded portion of the urethra using a probe. In selected cases, direct reconstruction of the involved area is feasible.

Congenital Short Urethra

The child with a congenital short urethra may present with varying degrees of urinary incontinence. The functional length of the urethra is short, less than 0.5 cm, or the length is nonexistent. The abnormality is demonstrated by a voiding cystourethrogram and is corroborated by urethroscopy. There are three approaches to treatment: (1) transvaginal plication of the bladder neck accompanied by vesicourethral suspension, (2) retropubic reconstruction of a new urethra by tubularizing either the anterior bladder or trigone, or (3) the use of artificial sphincter devices of a hydropneumatic design. Surgery has been reported to be successful in 40 to 80 percent of cases, depending on the degree of incontinence and the bladder capacity [26, 42, 106, 151, 186].

Congenital Megalourethra

Congenital megalourethra is a term first used by Nesbitt [133] to describe a urethral diverticulum in which there is diffuse anterior urethral dilatation with a generalized defect of the corpus spongiosum. Eleven cases have been reported; we have seen an additional two cases, both associated with hypoplasia of the abdominal musculature. During micturition there is expansion and bulging of the anterior urethra. The penis is huge, lax, and flabby, and there is dribbling following voiding. The anomaly is usually associated with various degrees of agenesis of the abdominal wall musculature [19, 120], or blockage of bladder outflow, or other obstructions [82, 116, 164, 191, 192].

Two forms of anterior urethral dilatation have been described [45]. The saccular form is simply an anterior urethral diverticulum. The diffuse form is the classic megalourethra, and this is further divided into fusiform and scaphoid types [159]. The fusiform megalourethra is the most rare, with only two reported patients, both of whom died, and it is due to defective erectile tissue of both the corpus spongiosum and corpora cavernosa. The penis is extremely distorted with a fusiform urethra on voiding [45, 138, 160]. The scaphoid megalourethra is more common and is

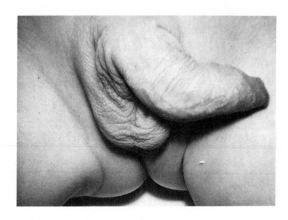

Figure 98-1. *Scaphoid megalourethra in a boy with congenital hypoplasia of the abdominal musculature.*

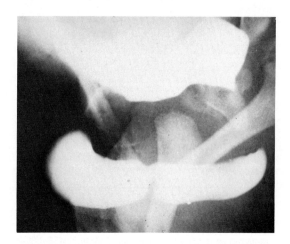

Figure 98-2. *Voiding cystourethrogram in the patient shown in Fig. 98-1 shows marked dilatation of the urethra.*

due to a deficiency only of the corpus spongiosum. The presence of the corpora cavernosa allows erection to occur, but during erection and micturition there is a dorsal curvature with a scaphoid appearance of the penis (Figs. 98-1, 98-2). The distended appearance of the penis during micturition has been mistaken for phimosis, and in one instance, circumcision resulted in a urethrocutaneous fistula [153]. Embryologically there is failure of mesenchyme to surround the penis circumferentially and to differentiate into the specialized erectile tissue.

Treatment of congenital megalourethra is aimed at altering the cosmetic appearance of the penis, reducing urethral caliber, and thereby relieving functional obstruction [133]. If a patient with a fusiform megalourethra should survive, a penile prosthesis would be necessary to permit sexual intercourse.

Congenital Urethral Meatal Stenosis

Allen and associates [2, 3] found that congenital urethral meatal stenosis is rare and is usually seen only in children with abnormal positions of the urethral meatus, such as in hypospadias and epispadias. Lattimer [104] reported identical twins with balanitic hypospadias and extremely tight meatal stenosis.

Rarely a congenital meatal cyst may obstruct the urethral orifice. In most cases of urethral meatal stenosis, the major contributing factor is diaper rash following circumcision. It is extremely unusual for meatal stenosis to cause significant hydroureteronephrosis [30, 32]. Diagnosis is based on symptomatology, inspection of the urethral meatus, and observation of voiding with a narrow, forceful stream. Treatment is urethral meatotomy.

Urethral Duplications

Urethral duplication can occur as true doubling in a complete (double urethra) or incomplete form, or as an accessory urethra in which there is a vestigial duplication [92, 199]. Developmentally both the true and the accessory urethra have a common embryogenesis. The true double urethra anatomically is enclosed within the fascia of the corpus spongiosum and conveys large volumes of urine via each conduit. The accessory urethra conveys little or no urine; if urine is voided, it is usually in an obstructed or incontinent manner.

HISTORY

Aristotle and Versalius described complete duplications in males [68]. During the fourteenth and fifteenth centuries few cases were mentioned; however, by 1797 Baillie [6] described in detail a blind-ending duplication. Taruffi [172] in 1891 proposed a classification of urethral duplications that is still useful today.

Type I. Blind-ending canal opening either on the penile surface or into the urethra, but not both

Type II. Seminiferous cord conveying seminal fluid only and independent of the urethra

Type III. Bifurcation of the urethra or accessory canal that communicates with both the urethra and the penile surface

Type IV. Congenital fistulas that arise from defects of the cloaca

EMBRYOGENESIS

The embryogenesis of urethral duplication is uncertain and may vary with the different types of duplications. In instances in which there is a double urethra and an associated double bladder, a continuous splitting of the urorectal septum probably has occurred [155, 197]; however, this would not explain the situation in which only the urethra is reduplicated [128]. Bifurcation of the urethral gutter [21, 128] or infolding of the lateral mesodermal elements into the urethral anlage explains the latter. The explanation for dorsal accessory urethra is more difficult. Several authors hypothesize, especially concerning accessory urethras extending only from the seminal vesicle areas, that a wolffian duct derivation similar to ectopic ureterocele may be the explanation [158, 159].

SIGNS AND SYMPTOMS

A true double urethra has two meatal orifices associated with diphallus. The incomplete or accessory urethra can produce a double urinary stream, symptoms of urinary obstruction, true incontinence, or bladder symptoms secondary to infection. The two urinary streams need not be equal in size and intensity, since the duplicated urethra may be smaller in caliber than the main urethra. The narrow or blind urethra may enlarge with micturition, causing obstruction of the main urethra [72, 110]. On occasion the point of junction of the channels acts as a valvular flap, obstructing the main urinary conduit [110, 141]; infrequently, total or stress incontinence occurs. Total incontinence is observed when the duplicated urethra does not traverse the sphincteric mechanism. In rare cases the main channel migrates toward the rectum; the patient voids little through the main urethra but voids with good control through the rectum or nearby rectoperineal orifice.

The blind-ending urethra usually causes no symptoms except a purulent discharge. If infected, it may lead to development of a periurethral abscess. This may extend by rupture into the normal urethra or develop into a urethrocutaneous fistula. If the periurethral abscess enlarges, it can obstruct the main channel. If a small communication exists between a pus-filled supernumerary urethra and the main urethra, lower urinary tract infection with its associated symptoms occurs [49]. If the accessory urethral meatus opens on the penile shaft ventrally or dorsally, a pseudohypospadias or epispadias results, frequently with curvature of the penis mimicking chordee.

DIAGNOSIS

Diagnosis of urethral duplication is made by inspection, noting the multiple urethral meatal openings, multiple urinary streams, penile swelling and purulent discharge, and, rarely, the diphallic state. Voiding cystourethrography and retrograde urethrography demonstrate the duplication and the anatomy of each urethra.

TREATMENT

Most patients with urethral duplication are asymptomatic and require no treatment. With symptoms of obstruction, incontinence, or infection, however, treatment is indicated. Blind-ending vestigial accessory urethras can be electrocoagulated or sclerosed with 5% sodium moruate. Other accessory urethras can be excised. On occasion a retropubic approach is necessary if the accessory urethra enters below the pubic arch.

In true duplications the second urethra frequently cannot be excised or sclerosed without risk of injury to the main urethra. Destruction of the septum between the urethras by excision or electrocoagulation has been done, but the results are unsatisfactory. Recently, with urethroplasty techniques, both urethras have been marsupialized, the intervening septum destroyed, and secondary urethral reconstruction performed [5, 59, 68, 149, 176].

Anterior Urethral Diverticula and Valves

Anterior urethral diverticula are not uncommon, although they are seldom discussed in the literature. They may be congenital or acquired. Anterior urethral valves, which usually are associated with diverticula of the anterior urethra, are uncommon. Both must be considered in the differential diagnosis of lower urinary tract obstruction. With increasing use of voiding cystourethrography, these entities have been discovered more frequently [41, 76, 195].

Diverticula are classified as follows:

A. Congenital diverticulum, with or without associated valves
  1. Wide mouth
  2. Narrow neck
B. Acquired diverticulum
  1. Secondary to proximal urethral obstruction
  2. Secondary to perforation

CONGENITAL DIVERTICULA

Forty percent of anterior urethral diverticula are congenital, and all occur in males [30, 32, 61, 95, 180, 182]. The wide-mouthed variety is the most common form and is usually found in the bulbous urethra proximal to the penoscrotal junction. The distal lip of the diverticulum acts as a valvular flap, obstructing the urethra only as the diverticulum distends with micturition, causing the lip to press against the dorsal urethra.

Narrow-necked diverticula are less common,

are not associated with valves, and therefore are not obstructive. This type is usually found in the bulbous urethra with a narrow neck and small spherical sac. The cavity drains poorly and therefore is prone to infection and stone formation.

Many theories as to the etiology of congenital anterior urethral diverticula have been proposed. Watts [185] thought that intrauterine obstructive urethral lesions, such as preputial adhesions, phimosis, meatal stenosis, or strictures, predisposed to formation of diverticula. Some state that diverticula are due to incomplete closure of the ventral aspect of the urethra [166]. Others suggest that this entity represents a residual paraurethral cyst or duct whose lumen enters the ventral urethra [81, 88, 165], although the diverticulum may be due to faulty union of the penile and glandular urethra. It also has been proposed that an abortive urethral duplication may result in diverticula formation.

One-half of children with anterior urethral diverticula present prior to 2 years of age. The most common signs and symptoms are those of lower urinary tract obstruction, with overflow incontinence, diminished urinary stream, and postvoiding dribbling. Occasionally children with nonobstructive diverticula present with irritative symptoms. Rarely acute urinary retention occurs. A swelling at the base of the penis during or after voiding is sometimes noted by the parents. Physical examination reveals a penoscrotal ventral swelling that causes meatal dribbling when compressed. Bladder distention occasionally is observed.

The diagnosis is made by voiding cystourethrography, which characteristically shows a diverticulum that has a sharp, valvular distal lip leading to a narrow distal urethra (Fig. 98-3). Cystoscopy confirms the diagnosis. The intravenous pyelogram may show some degree of hydroureteronephrosis [182, 194].

Nonobstructive diverticula are excised, and the urethra is closed primarily. Obstructive diverticula are treated similarly; however, the valvular flap is also excised, and closure may be staged to avoid formation of strictures. In the unusual situation in which the obstruction is minimal and the diverticulum is small, the valve can be resected transurethrally, allowing the diverticulum to drain adequately. The results of surgery are excellent.

ACQUIRED ANTERIOR URETHRAL DIVERTICULA

Sixty percent of anterior urethral diverticula are acquired [180]. They are usually secondary to long-standing indwelling catheterization, especially with traction. The ventral urethral wall is

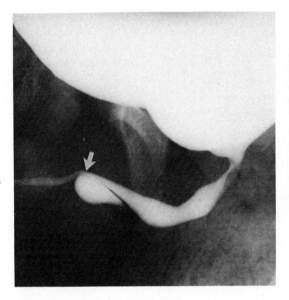

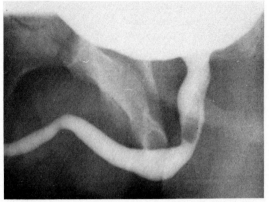

Figure 98-4. *A prolapsing posterior urethral polyp is shown by cystourethrography in a 5-year-old boy with hesitancy and an intermittent urinary stream.*

Figure 98-3. *Voiding cystourethrogram in a 2-year-old boy who entered the hospital with urinary retention due to an anterior urethral diverticulum. The distal lip of the diverticulum (arrow) can be seen compressing the urethra.*

injured at the penoscrotal junction, with resultant pressure necrosis or paraurethral abscess formation or both. Direct urethral trauma, hypospadias, and surgery for urethral stricture may also lead to the same condition. In addition, distal obstruction may contribute to diverticular formation.

Signs, symptoms, and diagnosis of acquired anterior urethral diverticula are the same as for the congenital form; however, urethrography shows an irregular ventral margin due to granulation tissue, rather than the smooth outline seen in the congenital form.

ANTERIOR URETHRAL VALVES WITH NO DIVERTICULUM

Most characteristically, anterior urethral valves are associated with wide-mouth diverticula. A similar situation can occur in a partial duplication of the anterior urethra with a subsequent flap valve and obstruction. Rarely, urethrography in a boy with symptoms of obstruction or irritation shows valvular folds and proximal dilatation with no diverticulum. These can be resected easily endoscopically [15, 37, 114, 173].

Congenital Urethral Polyps

Thirty-five cases of congenital urethral polyps have been reported in the world literature [25, 44, 47, 52, 98, 128, 163, 193]. The majority oc-

cur in the posterior urethra in close relationship to the verumontanum (colliculus seminalis) [8, 22]. They are usually 1- to 2-cm pedunculated, polypoid tumors consisting of a fibromuscular stroma but occasionally containing glandular tissue, smooth muscle, and nervous tissue. In contrast, adult urethral polyps are small, nonobstructing mucosal inflammatory lesions.

The most common symptoms of congenital urethral polyps are those related to obstruction, infection, and irritation. In addition, diurnal enuresis and rarely urinary retention may occur. Williams [191] reported three cases with associated vesicoureteral reflux. Diagnosis is established by voiding and retrograde urethrography, which demonstrates a polypoid filling defect of the posterior urethra (Fig. 98-4). Cystoscopy confirms the diagnosis.

Most polyps can be resected easily transurethrally. In some instances, open excision of large, broad-based polyps is necessary. The results are excellent.

Congenital Posterior Urethral Valves

Posterior urethral valves have been recognized with increased frequency in recent years. Attempts to estimate the incidence of this pathologic entity have caused a great deal of controversy, probably because there is a spectrum of disease [71] ranging from minimal, nonobstructive lesions to marked obstruction with advanced hydrouretero-nephrosis and uremia [24, 34, 71, 119, 144, 179, 181, 187, 191, 192, 194, 196].

INCIDENCE

Posterior urethral valves are a disease of males; however, there are several reports of cases in females and masculinized females [7, 69, 117, 132]. In 1935 Landes and Rall [100] reported 125 cases, most of whom were in the neonatal age group but including one patient who was 89 years old. The majority of patients present during the first year of life, with one-third to one-half given medical assistance within the first 3 months [24, 34, 119, 144, 191].

HISTORY
According to Munger [130], posterior urethral valves were first described by Morgagni in 1769. Thereafter there is no mention of this entity until 1802 [99]. In 1872 Tolmatschen [174] described the disease in detail. Young [202] in 1919 demonstrated the valves cystoscopically and performed the first valvulectomy. His classification is still used today.

EMBRYOLOGY
The embryologic explanation of posterior urethral valves is uncertain and unsatisfactory. No one theory can explain the various types described in the literature, especially type III (see under Pathology). Explanations suggested include persistence and overdevelopment of posterior urethral folds that develop early in utero [174, 184], remnants of the urogenital membrane [10], anomalous junction of the ejaculatory ducts with the prostatic utricle [111], fusion of the epithelial colliculus with the roof of the posterior urethra [135], and persistence of the wolffian ducts [158].

PATHOLOGY
Posterior urethral valves, as described by Young [202], have been grouped classically into three types (Fig. 98-5):

Type I. Valves pass from the verumontanum to the anterolateral urethral wall

Type II. Valves pass from the verumontanum toward the bladder neck

Type III. A diaphragmatic valve is located at the level of the verumontanum

Folds proximal and distal to the verumontanum do occur normally but do not project into the posterior urethra. Maximal development of these occurs in the 100 mm-sized fetus. Why these folds become exaggerated and obstructive is unknown [89]. Type I posterior urethral valves are most common (80 to 90 percent) [34, 55, 58, 144], and in fact Williams [191] believes that types II and III do not exist. Type II valves are thought to be nonobstructive and probably represent hypertrophied urethral folds secondary to distal urethral obstruction. Type III diaphragms, according

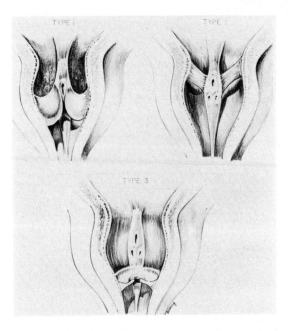

Figure 98-5. The three types of posterior urethral valves. (From H. H. Young et al., J. Urol. 3:289, 1919.)

to Williams, are in reality congenital urethral strictures [191]. Cass and Stephens [34], however, considered 21 percent of 113 valves to be of the type III variety.

Posterior urethral valves have been described arising from the anterior wall of the posterior urethra rather than the posterior wall, unilateral rather than bilateral, and arising from the midverumontanum to the lateral walls (modified type I). They may have the structure of an iris diaphragm with a pinhole opening, hemidiaphragm, partial diaphragm, or wind-sock membrane [60]; they may be associated with urethral atresia.

The effects of valvular obstruction vary according to the severity of the lesion. The back pressure of mild obstruction may be minimal, although this usually is not the case. The posterior urethra is dilated, but in mild cases this may be observed only during micturition. With progression of disease, posterior urethral dilatation becomes fixed and permanent. The verumontanum as well as the normal posterior urethral folds become prominent. The bladder neck and detrusor musculature hypertrophy and thicken. Even though the bladder neck appears and may be obstructive, it may also be wider than normal due to the relatively dilated posterior urethra. The bladder is trabeculated and sacculated, with thick walls. Umbilical fistulas occur but are rare. Transudation of urine through small bladder perforations may cause urinary ascites, which may also occur through renal forniceal extravasation of urine [22, 63, 64, 94].

The ureters are dilated in 70 percent of the cases of posterior urethral valves [34], and they may drain nonfunctioning hydronephrotic sacs. Functional obstruction at the ureterovesical junction can occur secondary to a thickened detrusor. Dysplasia of the kidney may coexist with obstructing urethral valves [12, 40, 126, 135, 194]. Whether this is due to obstruction during early renal development or to a metanephric bud developmental anomaly is still unknown [158].

Other renal anomalies are not common in patients with posterior urethral valves; however, vesicoureteral reflux has been reported to occur in 45 percent of cases, unilaterally in 17 percent [34, 144]. Unilateral reflux may lead to marked asymmetry of the hydronephrosis and impairment of renal function and ureteral drainage. Reflux, especially when associated with urinary tract infection, contributes to more rapid failure of the kidney.

SIGNS AND SYMPTOMS
The majority of patients with posterior urethral valves present in the first year of life, especially in the first 3 months, with failure to thrive (40 percent), sepsis, or an abdominal mass (53 percent) [97, 144]. Respiratory distress secondary to an enormously distended urinary tract or to urinary ascites may be the presenting symptom [94]. Rarely, neonates may be anuric, especially if there is associated urethral atresia or bilateral renal dysplasia. Physical examination often reveals a palpable bladder, kidneys, and, in some cases, ureters. The distended prostatic urethra can sometimes be felt on rectal examination.

After the first year the symptoms vary. Disturbances in micturition predominate, including frequency, diurnal and nocturnal enuresis, hesitancy, and strangury.

DIAGNOSIS
The diagnosis of posterior urethral valves is made by voiding cystourethrography and confirmed by cystourethroscopy [67, 86, 89]. Elongation and marked dilatation of the posterior urethra are present, with a sharp cutoff distal to the verumontanum and a narrowed distal urethral segment (Fig. 98-6). High-dose excretory urography reveals severe hydroureteronephrosis in more than 90 percent of patients less than 1 year of age [103]. In older children, upper urinary tract dilatation is not as common (10 percent) [144].

TREATMENT
In the severely ill infant presenting with posterior urethral valves, therapy is aimed at alleviating ob-

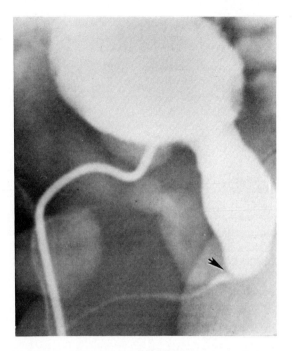

Figure 98-6. *Posterior urethral valves (arrow) in a 1-month-old boy who presented with failure to thrive and urinary infection. Note the marked dilatation of the prostatic urethra.*

struction, correcting fluid and electrolyte imbalance and other metabolic disturbances, and treating infection. In addition, drainage of the obstructed urinary tract is necessary. In most instances renal function will improve and stabilize within a week. The valves are then fulgurated transurethrally.

There are a few infants in whom the upper urinary tract is not decompressed after bladder drainage. They remain severely septic or uremic and require urgent urinary tract decompression, preferably with high bilateral cutaneous ureterostomies or with bilateral nephrostomies [71]. The valves are then resected electively. Ureteroneocystostomy is performed for reflux or ureterovesical obstruction, and the loop cutaneous ureterostomies are closed at a later date.

Over a period of years, most children with posterior urethral valves thrive, have gradual resolution of hydroureteronephrosis, and are able to void satisfactorily with a sterile urine. Bladder neck hypertrophy usually resolves following valve resection, and it rarely necessitates surgery. Occasionally a nephrectomy is indicated for a nonfunctioning, infected, and perhaps dysplastic kidney.

PROGNOSIS
Survival in patients with posterior urethral valves is approximately 60 percent in infants less than 3

months of age, and it depends upon the presence or absence of renal dysplasia and the degree of renal insufficiency. Over this age mortality is less than 10 percent. Approximately 20 percent of deaths are attributed to extraurinary tract causes, often congenital cardiac disease. Bilateral renal dysplasia has been reported in 5 percent [194]. In the children who survive, urinary incontinence may be a problem [188], although improvement usually occurs as the prostate develops at puberty.

Bladder Neck Obstruction

Bladder neck anatomy and physiology as well as the pathology of this area is extremely controversial and is one of the most debated subjects in pediatric urology. It was previously thought that bladder neck obstruction was primarily responsible for urinary infection and vesicoureteral reflux. It is now thought that this entity rarely if ever exists [156, 190].

ANATOMY AND PHYSIOLOGY OF THE BLADDER OUTLET

The anatomy and physiology of the bladder outlet and posterior urethra, and their relationship to the detrusor, are not completely understood; however, Woodburne [198], Hutch [78, 79], Tanagho and associates [169–171], Elbadawi and Schenk [54], and Krane and Olsson [93] have attempted to define the functional anatomy of this area.

The internal sphincter is no longer thought to maintain continence by tonic contraction only at the bladder neck. No clear-cut ring has been demonstrated histologically, and surgery in this area does not produce incontinence. Woodburne [198] showed that the bladder neck fibers were continuous with the detrusor and that voiding was the result of the detrusor fibers pulling the bladder neck open and at the same time shortening the urethra.

Hutch [78, 79] described a "base plate" composed of circular fibers surrounding the bladder neck. Sandwiching these fibers is an inner and outer longitudinal layer of muscle that extends down to the urethra. In the relaxed state, the base plate is flat so that the circular fibers form a series of rings around the bladder neck, which is then closed. Micturition "breaks" the base plate, changing it from a flat to a conical shape by the action of the longitudinal fibers pulling the bladder neck open. Once the plate is conical, the circular fibers no longer close the bladder neck but assist in evacuation of urine.

Tanagho and associates [169–171] also believe that the detrusor and posterior urethral musculature is one continuous structure; however,

they contend that the circularly oriented muscle fibers are the ones responsible for the closure mechanism in urinary continence. Elbadawi and Schenk [54] have demonstrated histologically the parasympathetic and alpha-sympathetic innervation of the bladder neck region; their findings are corroborated clinically by Krane and Olsson [93]. Alpha-sympatholytic drugs such as phenoxybenzamine open the bladder neck region in neurogenic bladder dysfunction.

ETIOLOGY AND PATHOLOGY

Proponents of vesical neck obstruction base their diagnosis upon the following findings: (1) residual urine in the absence of neurogenic bladder dysfunction, (2) decreased rate of voiding, (3) increased intravesical voiding pressure, (4) endoscopic visualization of bladder neck stenosis and bladder trabeculation, (5) palpation of the rigid bladder neck, and (6) certain findings on voiding cystourethrography (Fig. 98-7). These criteria

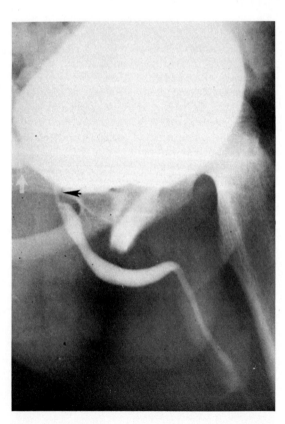

Figure 98-7. Voiding cystourethrogram in a 7-year-old boy with urinary dribbling and a diminished stream reveals marked narrowing at the bladder neck (black arrow). Note the small bladder diverticulum (white arrow).

have been challenged by numerous authors during the past several years [156].

Leadbetter and Leadbetter [107] believe that congenital bladder neck obstruction results from a fault in dissolution of bladder neck mesenchyme with replacement by various connective tissues, giving rise to three histologic varieties: (1) hypertrophic muscle tissue that may be secondary to distal obstruction or neurogenic bladder dysfunction; (2) increased amounts of fibrous tissue producing an inelastic posterior urethra and subsequent obstruction, as described by Bodian and Presman et al. [16, 140]; and (3) chronic inflammatory tissue.

SYMPTOMS

Symptoms of bladder neck obstruction include straining, crying on urination, intermittency, post-voiding dribbling, and urinary retention. Campbell [30, 32] reported a case of an infant with urinary retention from birth. Most patients present in early childhood with obstructive symptoms, enuresis, or secondary symptoms of infection. In less severe cases, patients may reach the second or third decade prior to detection.

DIAGNOSIS

The diagnosis of bladder neck obstruction is very rare in girls (we have never seen a case) and is very uncommon in boys. It is suggested by the symptoms described above and is made by voiding cystourethrography, which shows a rigid, narrow bladder neck that never widens during voiding; a normal urethra distal to the bladder neck; a trabeculated bladder that does not empty completely; and, on occasion, bladder diverticula and vesicoureteral reflux. Cystourethroscopy confirms the diagnosis.

Problems that often mimic a true bladder outlet contracture must be ruled out. Neurogenic bladder dysfunction with vesicosphincter dysynergia can be excluded by performing cystometrography with simultaneous sphincter-detrusor electromyographic studies. Bladder neck hypertrophy secondary to urethral obstruction, such as posterior urethral valves, urethral stenosis, or stricture, must be considered. Children with severe vesicoureteral reflux may develop bladder decompensation with resultant urinary retention. This was previously thought to be secondary to bladder neck obstruction, but actually it results from detrusor failure. Mac-Gregor and Williams [112] have shown that chronic pyuria in young girls without reflux may produce residual urine and even retention. Occult neurogenic bladder dysfunction must be excluded

[75]. Megalocystis may also mimic bladder outlet obstruction. In this condition the bladder is large, but it contracts normally and empties completely. Cystometrography shows a bladder of large capacity with normal pressure relationships. Finally, the bladder outlet may be obstructed by extrinsic masses, such as posterior bladder diverticula, fecal impaction in chronic constipation, and tumors.

TREATMENT

The clinical management of true congenital bladder neck contracture is surgical widening of the bladder neck. This may be done by open bladder neck surgery or by transurethral resection in boys [56]. Preliminary drainage by indwelling catheter or cystotomy may be necessary in patients with advanced renal disease or detrusor muscle failure. Stewart [160] has suggested a cold-punch transurethral technique. All of these techniques will effectively open the bladder neck; however, post-operative retrograde ejaculation and mild stress incontinence may occur in future years. For these reasons transurethral bladder neck incision may be advisable [161, 190].

In patients with secondary bladder neck obstruction or neurogenic bladder dysfunction, primary surgery on the bladder neck is not indicated because the hypertrophy will usually resolve following correction of the underlying disorder. Phenoxybenzamine [93] has been highly effective in decreasing bladder neck resistance in such patients.

MARION'S DISEASE

Marion's disease is a specific form of bladder neck obstruction defined as an idiopathic functional muscular disorder of the internal sphincteric area in which neurogenic bladder dysfunction, distal urethral obstruction, megacystis, and vesicoureteral reflux have been excluded [115]. In addition, there must be evidence of bladder outflow obstruction and hypertrophy of the bladder neck musculature.

BODIAN'S DISEASE
(URETHRAL FIBROELASTOSIS

Bodian's disease is a specific form of bladder outlet contracture that affects boys [16, 140]. The prostate is abnormal due to a thick sheath of fibroelastic tissue surrounding the entire posterior urethra, extending from the bladder neck to the bulbous urethra. This sheath prevents normal posterior urethral distention during micturition, leading to subsequent urinary obstruction and secondary bladder neck hypertrophy. This entity was thought by Bodian to be the major cause of bladder neck obstruction in boys [16]. Most cases have been treated with Y-V bladder neck plasty, occasionally supplemented by internal urethrotomy.

Agenesis of the Bladder

Agenesis of the bladder is very rare in infants, most commonly being seen in nonviable monsters with multiple congenital anomalies [139]. Campbell [30, 32] found 7 cases in 19,046 autopsies. Two were anencephalic, and in each of the others serious anomalies were found, including renal and ureteral agenesis in 5; absence of the cervix and vagina, malformed uterus and tubes, and imperforate anus in 1; penile agenesis in 1; and polycystic liver and kidneys, meningocele, polydactylism, split tongue, cor biloculare, and sigmoid diverticulum in 1. Overall there have been 32 cases reported, of which only 7 were in viable infants [136, 177]. Other reports citing severe degrees of hypoplasia, exstrophy, and contracted bladder have been falsely grouped into this category.

The embryologic defect in bladder agenesis lies in the ventral portion of the cloaca, the cranial aspect of which develops into the bladder and urachus at approximately the third week. It is assumed that with the absence of the allantoic diverticulum, the umbilical vessels also are absent. Boulgakow [19], however, reported a fetus with abnormal but functional umbilical vessels in the absence of the ventrocranial urogenital sinus. Allantoic deficiencies, with rare exceptions, are lethal. The ureters, if present, enter the trigone (embryologically different than the remainder of the bladder) or take the same course as ectopic ureters, entering either the posterior urethra [109], vagina [125], vestibule [66], or rectum [109]. In most cases the trigone and urethra are absent [136].

These ectopic ureters often are obstructed, resulting in hydronephrosis; their location in most cases leads to urinary incontinence. In one case the ureters entered the posterior urethra and, by means of musculofibrous sphincteric tissue around the ureteral orifices, acted as a hydronephrotic reservoir, preventing incontinence [30, 32]. Glenn [66] described a 3½-year-old girl whose ureters entered the vestibule, producing urinary incontinence and hydronephrosis that required diversion. Urinary diversion should be instituted in these patients to prevent progressive hydronephrosis.

Megacystis Syndrome

Megacystis syndrome, described by Williams [191, 192] and expounded upon by Paquin, Marshall, and McGovern [137], is defined as a refluxing thin-walled, unobstructed bladder of large capacity that empties completely.

ETIOLOGY

The etiology of megacystis syndrome is unexplained; however, Paquin, Marshall, and McGovern [137] concluded that the primary defect is in trigonal development with associated thin musculature. Stephens [158] states that this is a congenital disorder of the ureteric bud that, by incorporation of the common excretory bud within the trigone, produces a hyperexpansion of the bladder. Other proposed etiologies include: (1) pituitary diabetes insipidus [33] (however, the enlarged bladder is probably secondary to polyuria); (2) occult neurogenic bladder (however, cystometrograms in megacystis syndrome have a normal configuration; (3) congenital obstruction [96] (however, obstructed bladders are trabeculated and do not empty); (4) aganglionosis of the bladder [167] (this theory has not been borne out by Leibowitz and Bodian [108]); and (5) congenital reflux causing a postvoiding residual urine, decompensation, and dilatation of the bladder (this may well be a contributory etiologic factor in a large number of cases).

INCIDENCE

Megacystis characteristically is seen in childhood, at an average age of 7.6 years [137]. Eighty percent develop symptoms at less than 3 years of age. Williams [191, 192] found no sex predominance; however, Paquin reported 22 males and 5 females [137].

SIGNS AND SYMPTOMS

Children with the megacystis syndrome present with symptoms of infection. Most patients void large quantities of urine infrequently. Interestingly enough, many are toilet-trained at an early age. Uncommonly, a child may present in urinary retention as a result of bladder decompensation in association with severe vesicoureteral reflux. On physical examination the bladder may be palpable.

DIAGNOSIS

The diagnosis of megacystis is established by excluding neurogenic or obstructive disorders of the lower urinary tract. Most patients have bladders that extend as high as the fifth lumbar vertebral space [87]. Voiding is complete with minimal to no residual urine. Neurologic evaluation is normal. Sensation and proprioception are intact. Cystometrography demonstrates a large capacity, normal pressure bladder. Flow studies are normal, and bethanechol chloride hypersensitivity is not present. The characteristic finding at cystoscopy is a smooth, nontrabeculated, thin-walled bladder; the trigone is two to three times normal size with lateral incompetent ureteral orifices. Sacculation and diverticula are not present. Excretory urography may show varying degrees of hydronephrosis and pyelonephritis, depending upon the severity of vesicoureteral reflux and infection [137]. Reflux invariably is demonstrated by voiding cystourethrography.

Other disorders that must be considered in the differential diagnosis of a large-capacity bladder include myogenic failure, chronic constipation, and psychogenic urinary retention.

TREATMENT

The treatment of the megacystis syndrome is the treatment of vesicoureteral reflux. Many children require antireflux surgery for persistent, severe reflux and recurrent urinary tract infection. The prognosis, in general, is good, but it depends on the severity of the underlying disorder. These children usually develop normally, and megacystis is not a disorder incompatible with long life.

Congenital Bladder Divisions

A simple classification of congenital bladder divisions has been proposed [1, 152].

A. Sagittal or longitudinal divisions
1. Complete duplication of the bladder (vesica duplex)
2. Incomplete duplication of the bladder (vesica biparta)
3. Complete sagittal septum
4. Incomplete sagittal septum
B. Frontal or transverse divisions
1. Complete duplication
2. Frontal septum
a. Complete
b. Incomplete
3. Hourglass
C. Multilocular bladders

SAGITTAL OR LONGITUDINAL DIVISIONS

Complete Duplication. Complete duplication of the bladder is part of an anomaly involving the entire caudal end of the body, including the colon, rectum, anus, female internal and external genitalia, and vertebral column [36]. Several reviews have revealed 40 cases [1, 92]. There are two separate bladders, each with its own muscularis and common adventitial sheath (Fig. 98-8). Each bladder has its own ureter and urethra with a distinct urethral meatus. In two cases the bifid bladder was in an ectopic position.

Other findings include duplication of the colon

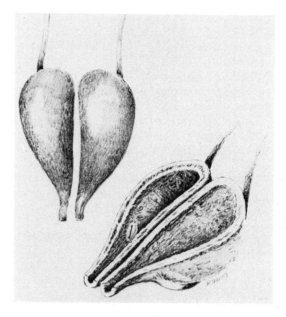

Figure 98-8. Complete duplication of the bladder.

in 50 percent [143], duplication of the anus in 25 percent, duplication of the external genitalia in 90 percent, double penis in 86 percent, double or septate vagina in 80 percent, double spine in 10 percent, and meningomyelocele or spina bifida in 15 percent. There are two cases in which only the urethra was doubled [17, 148]; in two others, the clitoris was bifid [17, 168].

Incomplete Duplication. In incomplete duplication, two bladders lie side by side but at the base have a common bladder neck and urethra [27]. It is less serious due to its infrequent association with other congenital anomalies.

Complete Sagittal Septum. The bladder is divided into two portions by a sagittal septum obstructing half the bladder. This septum is muscular or contains two layers of mucosa. Externally the bladder may have a groove. If the obstructed portion is supplied by a ureter and kidney, the kidney is usually dysplastic, but it may be markedly hydronephrotic. The obstructed half of the bladder may displace and obstruct the functional half, producing contralateral hydronephrosis and consequent renal failure. Colonic anomalies often are associated [142, 143].

Incomplete Sagittal Septum. This anomaly has been reported eight times, and it is usually asymptomatic. Rarely, duplication of the bowel is seen [122].

The *embryogenesis* of sagittal divisions of the bladder is related to duplication of the caudal anlage. This may include a double notochord or may be related only to division of the vesicoure-thral anlage. Associated rectal anomalies suggest splitting after division of the cloaca by the urorectal septum.

These conditions are often diagnosed at birth by inspection. Symptoms may arise due to rectal fistulas [178], bladder exstrophy [35], rectal atresia [102], and ectopic ureter [11].

Treatment of incomplete sagittal septum is individualized. Hydronephrosis and blind-ending duplications must be drained. Genitalia should be reconstructed. Diseased segments or obstructing septa are removed. Rarely, ureteroneocystostomy may be performed to save a kidney.

FRONTAL OR TRANSVERSE DIVISIONS

Complete Duplication. Complete duplication in an anteroposterior plane has been reported by Bowie et al. [20] in a 17-year-old girl in whom the anterior bladder drained into a normal urethra. The posterior bladder drained into the vagina and received a ureter that branched from the normal left ureter.

Frontal Septum. This anomaly is more frequent. Complete partitioning is rare; incomplete partitioning has been described eight times. Genital and rectal doubling is uncommon. Although a septum may be incomplete, it is sometimes long enough to obstruct one ureteral opening.

Hourglass Bladder. Zellermayer and Carlson [203] reviewed the 23 cases of bladders with ring-like constrictions. For all practical purposes, the ringlike constriction is probably not a congenital anomaly but represents either a wide-mouthed bladder diverticulum or urachal maldevelopment. A muscular constriction divides the bladder into an upper and lower chamber; both halves contract normally. The upper chamber is larger; the ureters usually enter the lower chamber; and the opening between the chambers varies from 1 to 6 cm in diameter. Megaureter and hydronephrosis were found in a case described by Berariu et al. [13].

There is no adequate embryologic explanation for frontal partitions. Possibly intrauterine undistended folds or rugae contact each other and fuse to form a partition [183].

Incomplete septa produce no symptoms unless there is bladder neck obstruction. There is usually no difficulty in the retrograde passage of catheters or endoscopic instruments. The symptoms of complete septa are due to obstruction of the associated kidney. Hourglass bladders are associated with recurrent cystitis and painful micturition. Diagnosis is made by voiding cystourethrography and cystoscopy.

Vesical Diverticula

Bladder diverticula are relatively uncommon in the pediatric age group [32, 95]. Ninety-five percent of cases are male [9], and the peak age of presentation is in children from 3 to 10 years. In contrast to adults, in whom bladder outlet obstruction is the primary cause, the etiology of vesical diverticula in children is far from clarified.

ETIOLOGY

Hinman [73] thought that there were three causes for the development of vesical diverticula—anatomic, pathologic, and mechanical (lower urinary tract obstruction). Others [87, 95] state that embryologic malformations are the primary cause; however, in the reported cases diverticula did not form until the distal obstruction became evident. Miller [124] postulated that with outlet obstruction, vesical muscle hypertrophy occurs in an uneven fashion, eventually developing outpouchings in an area of relative weakness. MacKellar and Stephens [113] proposed that congenital hypomuscularization of the bladder, particularly around the ureteral orifices, results in a diverticulum. More recently, Bauer and Retik [9] and others [65, 127, 147, 191] have reported vesical diverticula in children with no evidence of outlet obstruction or increased vesical pressure. This corroborates the theory of Williams and Eckstein [194], who proposed that diverticula develop from congenitally weak areas of the detrusor.

Other intrauterine conditions have been postulated to cause vesical diverticula, including urinary retention in the fetus due to transient occlusion of the urethral mucosa [57], overabundance of embryonic tissue in the bladder wall, supernumerary ureteric buds, patent urachus (the possible cause of all cases found on the dome), and abnormal fusion of the wolffian and allantoic elements leading to areas of weakness. The latter theory is quite reasonable, since greater than 90 percent of all diverticula in children are found at the posterior angles of the trigone points, where trigone-detrusor continuity is weak. [9].

PATHOLOGY

One of the major pathologic criteria for true congenital diverticula is the presence of muscle fibers in the walls, a point of differentiation from acquired obstructive diverticula. Diverticula are usually multiple, rounded or oval, and vary in size. Ninety percent are located near the trigone and in close relationship to the ureteral orifices. When the orifice is in continuity with the diverticulum, reflux usually occurs [9, 159] (Fig. 98-9). The

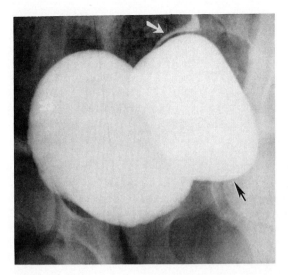

Figure 98-9. Cystogram demonstrates large bladder diverticulum (black arrow) and left vesicoureteral reflux (white arrow).

diverticulum may obstruct the ureteral orifices. Frequently the size of the diverticulum is greater than the bladder capacity. Posterior diverticula may obstruct the bladder neck and proximal urethra during voiding. Five percent of the patients develop calculi, occasionally in a dumbbell configuration.

SIGNS AND SYMPTOMS
Most patients with vesical diverticula present with symptoms of urinary tract infection. In rare situations, acute urinary retention occurs when a fully distended diverticulum compresses the prostatic urethra and elevates the bladder neck [9]. Acute urinary retention may also occur in a very large capacity, elastic diverticulum in which the majority of the bladder urine is displaced into the diverticulum rather than into the urethra [191].

DIAGNOSIS
The diagnosis of bladder diverticula is readily made by voiding cystourethrography and cystoscopy, although intravenous pyelography may suggest the nature of the abnormality. At endoscopy, the ureteral orifices usually can be seen in close approximation to the diverticular mouth; with filling of the bladder, they may disappear into the diverticulum.

Four conditions should be distinguished from true vesical diverticula: (1) In males less than 6 months old there may be transitory bladder pouches anterior to the inguinal rings, which Allen and Condon [4] call "bladder ears." These have no necks. (2) In girls there may be a posterior lateral saucer-shaped depression due to poor musculature, producing a bulge during micturition. (3) A lobulated bladder with normal musculature can be confused with a wide-mouthed diverticulum. (4) A pseudodiverticulum occasionally forms after urinary extravasation from the bladder [157].

TREATMENT
The treatment of bladder diverticula is correction of any obstructive lesions and excision of the diverticulum. If the ureteral orifice is closely associated with the diverticulum, reimplantation of the ureter is necessary.

Anomalies of the Urachus
The failure of the urachus to regress fully results in the following types of anomalies: (1) the bladder is located at the level of the umbilicus with a wide-open umbilicovesical fistula; (2) the bladder is located below the umbilicus with (a) patent urachus, (b) urachal diverticulum (proximal portion opens into the bladder), (c) urachal sinus (distal portion is patent and opens into the umbilicus), or (d) urachal cyst (both ends are closed).

ANATOMY
The urachus is 3 to 5 cm long, is located between the peritoneum and transverse fascia, and is attached to the bladder proximally [14]. In the fetus, and occasionally in the newborn, it has its own mesentery (mesourachus) [69]. Not uncommonly the vesical end of the urachus contains transitional epithelium surrounded by smooth muscle. In 50 percent of children the urachus is continuous with the bladder.

EMBYOGENESIS
The urachus is derived wholly from the ventral cloaca and is formed by the failure of this structure to enlarge. The descent of the bladder attenuates the urachal attachments. When the bladder is distended by obstruction, this descent does not always take place and the urachus may remain open. Thus anomalies of the urachus are thought to be due to failure of obliteration of the urachal lumen. Schrech and Campbell [150] question this obstructive etiology except in patients with the prune-belly syndrome, in half of whom urachal fistulas also occur [105, 137].

INCIDENCE
Patent urachus is very rare, occurring in 3 per 200,000 to 1 million individuals [134, 175]. Males are affected twice as often as females. Ura-

chal diverticula frequently are first found at autopsy, since they are usually asymptomatic. A proximal urachal lumen is not rare. Urachal sinuses are quite uncommon, coming to the physician's attention only when infected [74]. Small urachal cysts usually produce no symptoms and are found in one-third of all cadavers [200]. Larger, clinically important cysts are much less common (3 per 12,500 urologic hospital admissions) [201].

PATHOLOGY

The transitional epithelium of the normal urachus is nonsecretory; however, if metaplasia occurs, mucinous material and cellular debris are produced. This occurs in urachal cysts, which may be as large as 52 liters. Dystocia secondary to extremely large cysts has also been described [50, 145, 162]. Intestinalization of the lining occurs with papillae resembling intestinal villi [175].

Urachal cysts usually form in the lower third of the urachus. Infection, stones [48], and malignant and benign tumors have been reported as complications. Abscess formation and rupture into the peritoneal cavity may occur, mimicking an acute abdominal crisis [51]. Carcinoma usually forms in the intravesical portion [62]. Eight sarcomas have been reported, all in children [29, 189]. A dermoid cyst also has been reported [30, 32].

SIGNS AND SYMPTOMS

The obvious sign of a patent urachus is urine appearing at the umbilicus. Associated with this may be an umbilical protrusion or mucosal prolapse. Pain and erythema indicate associated infection.

Urachal diverticula are usually asymptomatic. A urachal cyst is frequently small and asymptomatic; however, if the cyst is larger, symptoms may include a tender subumbilical mass, irritative urinary symptoms, intestinal disturbances, or fetal dystocia [50, 145, 162]. Systemic signs of infection together with an increasingly tender, reddened subumbilical mass are highly suggestive of secondary infection of a cyst, or a pyourachus. The cysts eventually rupture, draining pus onto or into the umbilicus or bladder. In rare instances they may rupture into the peritoneal cavity.

DIAGNOSIS

After the characteristic signs and symptoms of urachal anomaly are noted, the umbilical discharge should be tested for urine. A urachal sinus or patent urachus must be differentiated from a patent vitelline (omphalomesenteric) duct or umbilical granuloma. Sinography may be necessary. Intravenous pyelography and cystography demon-

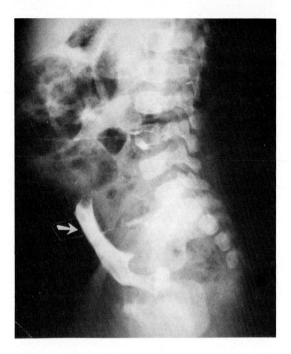

Figure 98-10. A lateral film during cystography shows a urachal diverticulum (arrow). Note extension toward umbilicus.

strate the urinary tract continuity of a patent urachus (Fig. 98-10). Biopsy shows transitional epithelium in urachal anomalies and columnar epithelium in the vitelline duct.

Symptomatic cysts may be shown by cytography to compress the bladder. Rarely the cyst is calcified [84].

TREATMENT

Extraperitoneal excision of the umbilicus, patent urachus, sinus, or cyst is necessary, frequently including a cuff of bladder. Umbilical herniorrhaphy may also be necessary.

A pyourachal cyst, which can mimic appendicitis or other intraabdominal inflammatory problems, should be marsupialized and drained. Excision is usually necessary at a later date.

Congenital Anomalies of the Periurethral Glands, Paraurethral Glands, and Cowper's Glands

Anomalies of the juxtaurethral glandular elements, including the periurethral glands, paraurethral glands, and Cowper's glands, can occur along the entire length of the urethra. The pathogenesis is due to occlusion of ductal structures. In addition, cyst formation occurs from inclusion of an epithelial cell mass consequent to incomplete closure of the urethral fold. This congenital urethral cyst may cause obstruction. Sixteen congenital cysts have been described from Cowper's glands [1, 38, 57, 77]. The cystic lesions rarely occur at the meatus [30, 32]. These cystic dilatations may become infected and subsequently rupture into the urethra or onto the skin, resulting in a fistulous communication (urethrocutaneous fistula) or blind sinus (accessory urethra).

Diagnosis is by palpation, voiding cystourethrography, retrograde urethrography, and urethroscopy. Treatment is usually accomplished by transurethral fulguration of the cyst. Surgical excision may be necessary if the cyst is large.

Anomalies of the Utricle
(Uterus Masculinus)
The utricle is the most distal fused segment of the müllerian ducts, entering the posterior urethra within the verumontanum. In more marked degrees of hypospadias and in some female pseudohermaphrodites, the utricle may be enlarged and more prominent endoscopically [77]. When the enlargement is more pronounced, it is called a utricular diverticulum [121]. If this diverticulum obstructs or becomes distended with accumulated debris, a utricular cyst forms [39, 43]. These utricular cysts rise out of the pelvis and impinge upon the posterior urethra and bladder neck to cause irritative and obstructive symptoms [103] and, rarely, urinary retention. The cysts are usually filled with cloudy or chocolate-colored viscous fluid. A soft midline cyst is often palpated by rectal examination and, if very large, may be felt in the midhypogastrium. Urethrography will usually show the pathology.

Treatment may be difficult and consists in transurethral unroofing of the cyst or excision through a perineal or retropubic approach.

Anomalies of the Prostate
ABSENCE OF THE PROSTATE
Absence of the prostate is associated with other urogenital maldevelopments, such as testicular agenesis, bilateral cryptorchidism, exstrophy of the bladder, epispadias, and pseudovaginal hypospadias. It also occurs in some female hermaphrodites. We have seen its absence in the prune-belly syndrome.

HYPOPLASIA OF THE PROSTATE
Congenital isolateral hypoplasia of the prostate is associated with unilateral anomalies of the urinary tract, including renal agenesis. Severe, generalized prostatic hypoplasia is found chiefly in hypopituitary sexual infantilism.

CONGENITAL PROSTATIC CYSTS
Congenital prostatic cysts are rarely observed in the pediatric age group. They are due to failure of communication between the wolffian ducts and vesicourethral anlage. Isolateral ureteral-renal anomalies almost always coexist. Symptoms include obstruction and secondary infection. Treatment is by transurethral or perineal excision.

References
1. Abrahamson, J. Double bladder and related anomalies: Clinical and embryological aspects and a case report. *Br. J. Urol.* 33:195, 1961.
2. Allen, J. S., and Summers, J. L. Meatal stenosis in children. *J. Urol.* 112:526, 1974.
3. Allen, J. S., Summers, J. L., and Wilkerson, J. E. Meatal calibration of newborn boys. *J. Urol.* 107:498, 1972.
4. Allen, R. P., and Condon, V. R. Transitory extraperitoneal hernia of the bladder in infants (bladder ears). *Radiology* 77:979, 1961.
5. Atherton, L., Atherton, L. D., and Sexter, M. A method of correcting double urethra in a man. *J. Urol.* 98:99, 1967.
6. Baillie, M. *The Morbid Anatomy of Some of the Most Important Parts of the Human Body* (2d ed.). London: J. Johnson, 1797.
7. Bakker, N. J. Valves in the female urethra. *Urol. Int.* 6:187, 1958.
8. Baldridge, R. R. A case of congenital hypertrophy of the verumontanum. *N. Engl. J. Med.* 213:46, 1935.
9. Bauer, S. B., and Retik, A. B. Bladder diverticula in infants and children. *Urology* 3:712, 1974.
10. Bazy, P. Rétrécissement congénital de l'urètre chez l'homme. *Presse Med.* 1:215, 1903.
11. Beach, P. D., Brascho, D. J., Hein, W. R., Nichol, W. W., and Geppert, L. J. Duplication of the primitive hindgut of the human being. *Surgery* 49:779, 1961.
12. Beck, A. D. The effect of intra-uterine urinary obstruction upon the development of the fetal kidney. *J. Urol.* 105:784, 1971.
13. Berariu, T., Scheau, M., and Popse, E. Eine seltene Anomalie der Harnblase: Die Blase in Sanduhrform (hour-glass bladder). *Z. Urol.* 58:35, 1965.
14. Blichert-Toft, M., Koch, F., and Nielsen, O. V. Anatomic variants of the urachus related to clinical appearance and surgical treatment of urachal lesions. *Surg. Gynecol. Obstet.* 137:51, 1973.
15. Blumberg, N., and Maletta, T. J. Anterior urethral valve: Complications and treatment. *J. Urol.* 108:486, 1972.
16. Bodian, M. Some observations on the pathology of congenital idiopathic bladder-neck obstruction (Marion's disease). *Br. J. Urol.* 29:393, 1957.
17. Boissonnat, P. Two cases of complete double functional urethra with a single bladder. *Br. J. Urol.* 33:453, 1961.
18. Boissonnat, P., and Duhamel, B. Congenital diverticulum of the anterior urethra associated with aplasia of the abdominal muscles in a male infant. *Br. J. Urol.* 34:59, 1962.
19. Boulgakow, B. The effect of non-development of

the allantois as illustrated by a case of sympodia. *J. Anat.* 63:253, 1929.

20. Bowie, C. W., Garvey, F. K., Boyce, W. H., and Pautler, E. E.   Supernumerary urinary bladder and ureter, spiral deformity of the ureter, ureteral diverticulum, hypoplasia of the kidney and bicornate uterus: A case report. *J. Urol.* 71:293, 1954.

21. Bramwit, D. N., and Ziter, F. M., Jr.   Accessory urethral channel. *Radiology* 94:359, 1970.

22. Britt, D. B., Bucy, J. G., and Robison, J. R.   Urinary ascites in the neonate. *South. Med. J.* 64:399, 1971.

23. Brody, H., and Goldman, S. F.   Metaplasia of epithelium of prostatic glands, utricle and urethra of fetus and newborn infant. *Arch. Pathol.* 29:494, 1940.

24. Bueschen, A. J., Garrett, R. A., and Newman, D. M.   Posterior urethral valves: Management. *J. Urol.* 110:682, 1973.

25. Bugbee, H. G., and Wollstein, M.   Surgical pathology of the urinary tract in infants. *J.A.M.A.* 83:1887, 1924.

26. Burkholder, G. V., and Williams, D. I.   Epispadias and incontinence: Surgical treatment of 27 children. *J. Urol.* 94:674, 1965.

27. Burns, E., Cummins, H., and Hyman, J.   Incomplete reduplication of the bladder with congenital solitary kidney: Report of a case. *J. Urol.* 57:257, 1947.

28. Burns, E., Ray, E. H., Jr., and Morgan, J. W.   Bladder neck obstruction and associated lesions in children. *J. Urol.* 77:733, 1957.

29. Butler, D. B., and Rosenberg, H. S.   Sarcoma of the urachus. *Arch. Surg.* 79:724, 1959.

30. Campbell, M. F.   *Pediatric Urology.* Philadelphia: Saunders, 1951.

31. Campbell, M. F.   Submucous fibrosis of the bladder outlet in infancy and childhood. *J.A.M.A.* 94:1373, 1930.

32. Campbell, M. F., and Harrison, J. H.   *Urology* (3rd ed.). Philadelphia: Saunders, 1970.

33. Carter, R. D., and Goodman, A. D.   Nephrogenic diabetes insipidus accompanied by massive dilatation of the kidneys, ureters and bladders. *J. Urol.* 89:366, 1963.

34. Cass, A. S., and Stephens, F. D.   Posterior urethral valves: Diagnosis and management. *J. Urol.* 112:519, 1974.

35. Chytilova, M., and Fintasjslova, O.   Exstrophy of the bladder with duplication of the bladder and the urethra. *Acta Chir. Plast. (Praha)* 4:250, 1962.

36. Cohen, S. J.   Diphallus and duplication of colon and bladder. *Proc. R. Soc. Med.* 61:305, 1968.

37. Colabawalla, B. N.   Anterior urethral valve: A case report. *J. Urol.* 94:58, 1965.

38. Cook, F. E., Jr., and Shaw, J. L.   Cystic anomalies of the ducts of Cowper's glands. *J. Urol.* 85:659, 1961.

39. Culbertson, L. R.   Müllerian duct cyst. *J. Urol.* 58:134, 1947.

40. Cussen, L. J.   Cystic kidneys in children with congenital urethral obstruction. *J. Urol.* 106:939, 1971.

41. Daniel, J., Stewart, A. M., and Blair, D. W.   Congenital anterior urethral valve—diagnosis and treatment. *Br. J. Urol.* 40:589, 1968.

42. Dees, J. E.   Congenital epispadias with incontinence. *J. Urol.* 62:513, 1949.

43. Deming, C. L., and Berneike, R. R.   Müllerian duct cysts. *J. Urol.* 51:563, 1944.

44. Dewolf, W. C., and Fraley, E. E.   Congenital urethral polyp in the infant: Case report and review of the literature. *J. Urol.* 109:515, 1973.

45. Dorairajan, T.   Defects of spongy tissue and congenital diverticula of the penile urethra. *Aust. N.Z. J. Surg.* 32:209, 1963.

46. Dourmashkin, R. L.   Complete urethral occlusion in living newborn; report of 5 cases. *J. Urol.* 50:747, 1943.

47. Downs, R. A.   Congenital polyps of the prostatic urethra: A review of the literature and report of two cases. *Br. J. Urol.* 42:76, 1970.

48. Dreyfuss, M. L., and Fliess, M. M.   Patent urachus with stone formation. *J. Urol.* 46:77, 1941.

49. Durrani, K. M., Shah, P. I., and Kakalia, G. R.   Interurethral fenestration for a case of double urethra with hypospadias. *J. Urol.* 108:586, 1972.

50. Easton, L.   Obstructed labour due to foetal abdominal distention. *J. Obstet. Gynaecol. Br. Commonw.* 67:128, 1960.

51. Edeiken, S., Hutchinson, H., and Grimm, G.   Ruptured urachal cyst abscess complicating pregnancy: Report of a case. *Obstet. Gynecol.* 27:338, 1966.

52. Edwards, A. T.   Congenital hypertrophy of the verumontanum causing bladder-neck obstruction. *Br. J. Urol.* 31:60, 1959.

53. Eigenbrodt, K.   Ein Fall von Blasenhalsklappe. *Beitr. Klin. Chir.* 8:171, 1891–92.

54. Elbadawi, A., and Schenk, E. A.   A new theory of the innervation of the bladder musculature: 3. Postganglionic synapses in uretero-vesical-urethral autonomic pathways. *J. Urol.* 105:372, 1971.

55. Ellis, D. G., Fonkalsrud, E. W., and Smith, J. P.   Congenital posterior urethral valves. *J. Urol.* 95:549, 1966.

56. Emmett, J. L., and Simon, H. B.   Transurethral resection in infants and children for congenital obstruction of the vesical neck and myelodysplasia. *J. Urol.* 76:595, 1956.

57. Englisch, J.   Über angeborene Verschleissungen und Verengerungen der männlichen Harnröhre. *Arch. Kinderheilkd.* 2:85, 1880–81.

58. Ericsson, N. O.   Congenital urethral obstructions. *Acta Urol. Belg.* 30:316, 1962.

59. Fellows, G. J., and Johnston, J. H.   Incomplete urethral duplication and urinary retention. *Br. J. Urol.* 46:449, 1974.

60. Field, P. L., and Stephens, F. D.   Congenital urethral membranes causing urethral obstruction. *J. Urol.* 111:250, 1974.

61. Firlit, C. F., and King, L. R.   Anterior urethral valves in children. *J. Urol.* 108:972, 1972.

62. Fisher, E. R.   Transitional-cell carcinoma of the urachal apex. *Cancer* 11:245, 1958.

63. France, N. E., and Back, E. H.   Neonatal ascites associated with urethral obstruction. *Arch. Dis. Child.* 29:565, 1954.

64. Garrett, R. A., and Franken, E. A., Jr.   Neonatal ascites: Perirenal urinary extravasation with bladder outlet obstruction. *J. Urol.* 102:627, 1969.

65. Gertz, T. C.   Vesical diverticula in childhood. *Dan. Med. Bull.* 6:190, 1959.

66. Glenn, J. F.   Agenesis of the bladder, *J.A.M.A.* 169:2016, 1959.

67. Griesbach, W. A., Waterhouse, R. K., and Mellins,

H. Z. Voiding cystourethrography in the diagnosis of congenital posterior urethral valves. *Am. J. Roentgenol.* 82:521, 1959.

68. Gross, R. E., and Moore, T. C. Duplication of urethra; report of 2 cases and summary of literature. *Arch. Surg.* 60:749, 1950.

69. Hammond, G., Yglesias, L., and Davis, J. E. Urachus, its anatomy and associated fasciae. *Anat. Rec.* 80:271, 1941.

70. Harris, A. Congenital vesical neck obstruction in a female child due to cup-valve formation: Open operation, complete recovery. *Am. J. Surg.* 20:64, 1933.

71. Hendren, W. H. Posterior urethral valves in boys: A broad clinical spectrum. *J. Urol.* 106:298, 1971.

72. Higgins, C. C., Williams, D. I., and Nash, D. F. E. *The Urology of Childhood.* London: Butterworth, 1951.

73. Hinman, F. The etiology of vesical diverticulum. *J. Urol.* 3:207, 1919.

74. Hinman, F., Jr. Urologic aspects of the alternating urachal sinus. *Am. J. Surg.* 102:339, 1961.

75. Hole, R. Residual urine in young girls—a hydrodynamic study. *Br. J. Urol.* 39:602, 1967.

76. Hope, J. W., Jameson, P. J., and Michie, A. J. Diagnosis of anterior urethral valve by voiding urethrography: Report of two cases. *Radiology* 74:798, 1960.

77. Howard, F. S. Hypospadias with enlargement of prostatic utricle. *Surg. Gynecol. Obstet.* 86:307, 1948.

78. Hutch, J. A. The internal urinary sphincter: A double-loop system. *Trans. Am. Assoc. Genitourin. Surg.* 62:30, 1970.

79. Hutch, J. A. A new theory of the anatomy of the internal urinary sphincter and the physiology of micturition: II. The base plate. *J. Urol.* 96:182, 1966.

80. Johnson, F. P. Homologue of prostate in female. *J. Urol.* 8:13, 1922.

81. Johnson, F. P. Diverticula and cysts of the urethra. *J. Urol.* 10:295, 1923.

82. Johnston, J. H., and Coimbra, J. A. Megalourethra. *J. Pediatr. Surg.* 5:304, 1970.

83. Johnston, J. H., and Kulatilake, A. E. The sequelae of posterior urethral valves. *Br. J. Urol.* 43:743, 1971.

84. Jonathan, O. M. Mucinous urachal cyst; report of a case and review of the subject. *Br. J. Urol.* 28:253, 1956.

85. Jones, B. W., and Headstream, J. W. Vesicoureteral reflux in children. *J. Urol.* 80:114, 1958.

86. Jorup, S., and Kjellberg, S. R. Congenital valvular formations in the urethra. *Acta Radiol.* 30:197, 1948.

87. Judd, E. S., and Scholl, A. J. Diverticulum of the urinary bladder. *Surg. Gynecol. Obstet.* 38:14, 1924.

88. Kayman, C. *Verletzungen und Krankheiten der Männlichen Harnroehre und des Penis.* Stuttgart: Enke, 1886.

89. Kjellberg, S. R., Ericsson, N. O., and Rudhe, U. *The Lower Urinary Tract in Childhood.* Chicago: Year Book, 1957.

90. Kohler, H. H. Septal bladder with multiple genitourinary anomalies and uremia. *J. Urol.* 44:63, 1940.

91. Kook, H., Kamhi, B., and Hermann, H. B. Trigonal curtain obstruction in a female child. *J. Urol.* 73:1026, 1955.

92. Kossow, J. H., and Morales, P. A. Duplication of bladder and urethra and associated anomalies. *Urology* 1:71, 1973.

93. Krane, R. J., and Olsson, C. A. Phenoxybenzamine in neurogenic bladder dysfunction: II. Clinical considerations. *J. Urol.* 110:653, 1973.

94. Krane, R. J., and Retik, A. B. Neonatal perirenal urinary extravasation. *J. Urol.* 111:96, 1974.

95. Kretschmer, H. L. Diverticula of urinary bladder; clinical study of 236 cases. *Surg. Gynecol. Obstet.* 71:491, 1940.

96. Kruger, R. Uber die RiesenKloake ("Vesica gigantea"). *Z. Urol. Chir.* 32:330, 1931.

97. Kumar, M. M., Shroff, N., and Bhat, H. S. Posterior urethral valve: Problems in management of the upper urinary tract. *Br. J. Urol.* 44:486, 1972.

98. Kuppusami, K., and Moors, D. E. Fibrous polyp of the verumontanum. *Can. J. Surg.* 11:388, 1968.

99. Lagenbeck, C. J. M. Ueber eine einfache und sichere Methode des Steinschmittes mit einer Vonnede von Dr. Johann Barthel Seibold. Wurrzburg: Stahel, 1802.

100. Landes, H. E., and Rall, R. Congenital valvular obstruction of the posterior urethra. *J. Urol.* 34:254, 1935.

101. Landes, R. R., and Ransom, C. L. Müllerian duct cysts. *J. Urol.* 61:1089, 1949.

102. Lange, M. Ueber complete Verdoppelung des Penis, combinirt mit rudimentärer Verdoppelung der Harnblase und Atresia ani. *Beitr. Z. Pathol. Anat. (Jena)* 24:223, 1898.

103. Lanman, T. H., and Mahoney, P. J. Intravenous urography in infants and in children. *Am. J. Dis. Child.* 42:611, 1931.

104. Lattimer, J. K. Similar urogenital anomalies in identical twins. *Am. J. Dis. Child.* 67:199, 1944.

105. Lattimer, J. K. Congenital deficiency of the abdominal musculature and associated genitourinary anomalies: A report of 22 cases. *J. Urol.* 79:343, 1958.

106. Leadbetter, G. W., Jr. Surgical correction of total urinary incontinence. *J. Urol.* 91:261, 1964.

107. Leadbetter, G. W., Jr., and Leadbetter, W. F. Diagnosis and treatment of congenital bladder-neck obstruction in children. *N. Engl. J. Med.* 260:633, 1959.

108. Leibowitz, S., and Bodian, M. A study of the vesical ganglia in children and the relationship to the megaureter, megacystis syndrome and Hirschsprung's disease. *J. Clin. Pathol.* 16:342, 1963.

109. Lepoutre, C. Sur un cas d'absence congénitale de la vessie (persistance du cloaque). *J. Urol. (Med. Chir.)* 48:334, 1939–40.

110. Liban, E. Rare malformation of urethra as a cause of congenital obstruction of lower urinary tract. *Am. J. Dis. Child.* 84:340, 1952.

111. Lowsley, O. S. The development of the human prostate gland with reference to the development of other structures of the neck of the urinary bladder. *Am. J. Anat. (Phila.)* 13:299, 1912–13.

112. MacGregor, M. E., and Williams, C. J. Relation of residual urine to persistent urinary infection in childhood. *Lancet* 1:893, 1966.

113. MacKeller, A., and Stephens, F. D. Vesical di-

verticula in children. *Aust. N.Z. J. Surg.* 30:20, 1960.

114. Malhoski, W. E., and Frank, I. N.   Anterior urethral valves. *Urology* 2:382, 1973.

115. Marion, G.   *Traité d'Urologie* (4th ed.). Paris: Masson, 1940.

116. Masih, B. K., and Brosman, S. A.   Megalourethra. *J. Urol.* 109:901, 1973.

117. Matheson, W. J., and Ward, E. M.   Hormonal sex reversal in a female. *Arch. Dis. Child.* 29:22, 1954.

118. May, F.   Ein Fall von kongenitalem Verschluss der Urethra membranacea. *Z. Urol.* 42:245, 1949.

119. McCrea, L. E.   Congenital valves of posterior urethra. *J. Int. Coll. Surg.* 12:342, 1949.

120. McGovern, J. H., and Marshall, V. F.   Congenital deficiency of the abdominal musculature and obstructive uropathy. *Surg. Gynecol. Obstet.* 108:289, 1959.

121. McKenna, C. M., and Kiefer, J. H.   Congenital enlargement of prostatic utricle with inclusion of ejaculatory ducts and seminal vesicles. *Trans. Am. Assoc. Genitourin. Surg.* 32:305, 1939.

122. Menten, M. L., and Denny, H. E.   Duplication of vermiform appendix, large intestine and urinary bladder; report of a case. *Arch. Pathol.* 40:345, 1945.

123. Miller, A.   Cystourethroscopy of enuretic children. *Proc. Roy. Soc. Med.* 49:895, 1956.

124. Miller, A.   The etiology and treatment of diverticulum of the bladder in children. *Br. J. Urol.* 30:43, 1958.

125. Miller, H. L.   Agenesia of urinary bladder and urethra. *J. Urol.* 59:1156, 1948.

126. Milliken, L. D., Jr., and Hodgson, N. B.   Renal dysplasia and urethral valves. *J. Urol.* 108:960, 1972.

127. Mininberg, D. T., and Pearl, M.   Congenital vesical diverticulum. *N.Y. State J. Med.* 71:681, 1971.

128. Mogg, R. A.   Congenital anomalies of the urethra. *Br. J. Urol.* 40:638, 1968.

129. Morgagni, G. B.   *The Seats and Causes of Disease Investigated by Anatomy* (B. Alexander, translator). New York: Hafner, 1960.

130. Munger, H. V.   Bladder hypoplasia. *Urol. Corresp. Club Letter,* Aug. 5, 1960.

131. Mustard, W. T., Ravitch, M. M., Snyder, W. H., Welch, K. J., and Benson, C. D.   *Pediatric Surgery* (2d ed.). Chicago: Year Book, 1969.

132. Nesbit, R. M., McDonald, H. P., Jr., and Busby, S.   Obstruction valves in the female urethra. *Trans. Am. Assoc. Genitourin. Surg.* 55:21, 1963.

133. Nesbitt, T. E.   Congenital megalourethra. *J. Urol.* 73:839, 1955.

134. Nix, J. T., Menville, J. G., Albert, M., and Wendt, D. L.   Congenital patent urachus. *J. Urol.* 79:264, 1958.

135. Osathanondh, V., and Potter, E. L.   Pathogenesis of polycystic kidneys: Type 4 due to urethral obstruction. *Arch. Pathol.* 77:502, 1964.

136. Palmer, J. M., and Russi, M. F.   Persistent urogenital sinus with absence of the bladder and urethra. *J. Urol.* 102:590, 1969.

137. Paquin, A. J., Jr., Marshall, V. F., and McGovern, J. H.   The megacystis syndrome. *J. Urol.* 83:634, 1960.

138. Pollock, D.   Developmental megalourethra in a monovular twin. *Clin. Pediatr.* 4:612, 1965.

139. Potter, E. L.   *Pathology of the Fetus and the Newborn.* Chicago: Year Book, 1952.

140. Presman, D., Ross, L. S., and Nicosia, S. V.   Fibromuscular hyperplasia of the posterior urethra: A cause for lower urinary tract obstruction in male children. *J. Urol.* 107:149, 1972.

141. Purcell, H. M.   Another cause of urinary obstruction. *J. Urol.* 62:748, 1949.

142. Ravitch, M. M.   Hind gut duplication; doubling of colon and genital urinary tracts. *Ann. Surg.* 137:588, 1953.

143. Ravitch, M. M., and Scott, W. W.   Duplication of the entire colon, bladder, and urethra. *Surgery* 34:843, 1953.

144. Retik, A. B., and Burke, C.   Urethral Valves. In J. Libertino and L. Zinmer (eds.), *Reconstructive Urologic Surgery (Lahey Clinic Symposium).* Baltimore: Williams & Wilkins, 1977. Pp. 287–293.

145. Rosenberg, M. Y.   Fetal dystocia due to urachal cyst and ascites: Report of a case. *Obstet. Gynecol.* 16:227, 1960.

146. Santulli, T. V.   The treatment of imperforate anus and associated fistulas. *Surg. Gynecol. Obstet.* 95:601, 1952.

147. Schiff, M., Jr., and Lytton, B.   Congenital diverticulum of the bladder. *J. Urol.* 104:111, 1970.

148. Schinagel, G.   Bifurcated female urethra. *Urol. Cutan. Rev.* 40:398, 1936.

149. Schmidt, J. D.   Congenital urethral duplication. *J. Urol.* 105:397, 1971.

150. Schrech, W. R., and Campbell, W. A. 3d   The relation of bladder outlet obstruction to urinary-umbilical fistula. *J. Urol.* 108:641, 1972.

151. Scott, F. B., Bradley, W. E., Timm, G. W., and Kothari, D.   Treatment of incontinence secondary to myelodysplasia by an implantable prosthetic urinary sphincter. *South Med. J.* 66:987, 1973.

152. Senger, F. L., and Santare, V. J.   Congenital multilocular bladder; a case report. *Trans. Am. Assoc. Genitourin. Surg.* 43:114, 1951.

153. Shiraki, I. W.   Congenital megalourethra and urethrocutaneous fistula following circumcision: A case report. *J. Urol.* 109:723, 1973.

154. Silvestri, E.   Imperforazione dell'uretra femminile. *Arch. Ital. Urol.* 29:255, 1956.

155. Slotkin, E. A., and Mercer, A.   A case of epispadias with a double urethra. *J. Urol.* 70:743, 1953.

156. Smith, D. R.   Critique on the concept of vesical neck obstruction in children. *J.A.M.A.* 207:1686, 1969.

157. Smith, T. W., Madden, J., and Gillenwater, J. Y.   Gigantic traumatic vesical pseudodiverticulum. *Urology* 1:464, 1973.

158. Stephens, F. D.   Idiopathic dilatation of the urinary tract. *J. Urol.* 112:819, 1974.

159. Stephens, F. D.   *Congenital Malformations of the Rectum, Anus and Genito-Urinary Tracts.* Edinburgh: Livingston, 1963.

160. Stewart, C. M.   Congenital bladder neck obstruction: Diagnosis by delayed and voiding cystography and surgical removal by use of a new, cold, crush-cutting punch. *J. Urol.* 83:679, 1960.

161. St. Martin, E. C., Pasquier, C. M., and Campbell, J. H.   Transurethral incision of median bar formation in selected male children. *J. Urol.* 85:318, 1961.

162. Strickland, C. E., and Bowes, J. E.   Dystocia caused

by anomalies of the fetal urogenital tract; report of two cases. *Obstet. Gynecol.* 9:571, 1957.

163. Stueber, P. J., and Persky, L.   Solid tumors of the urethra and bladder neck. *J. Urol.* 102:205, 1969.

164. Stuppler, S. A., Naranjo, C. A., and Kandzari, S. J.   Megalourethra, uterus didelphys, and double vagina. *Urology* 2:660, 1973.

165. Suter, F.   Ein Beitrag zur Histologie und Genese der congenitalen Divertikel der männlichen Harnrohre. *Arch. Klin. Chir. (Berlin)* 87:225, 1908.

166. Sweetser, T. H., Jr.   Congenital urethral diverticula in the male patient. *J. Urol.* 97:93, 1967.

167. Swenson, O., MacMahon, H. E., Jaques, W. E., and Campbell, J. S.   A new concept of the etiology of megaloureters. *N. Engl. J. Med.* 264:41, 1952.

168. Swenson, O., and Oeconomopoulos, C. T.   Double lower genitourinary systems in a child. *J. Urol.* 85:540, 1961.

169. Tanagho, E. A., and Smith, D. R.   The anatomy and function of the bladder neck. *Br. J. Urol.* 38:54, 1966.

170. Tanagho, E. A., and Smith, D. R.   Mechanism of urinary continence: I. Embryologic, anatomic and pathologic considerations. *J. Urol.* 100:640, 1968.

171. Tanagho, E. A., Smith, D. R., and Meyers, F. H.   The trigone: Anatomical and physiologic considerations. 2. In relation to the bladder neck. *J. Urol.* 100:633, 1968.

172. Taruffi, C.   Sui canali anomali del pene. *Bull. Sci. Med. (Bologna)* 2:275, 1891.

173. Texter, J. H., and Engel, R. M.   Anterior urethral valve as cause for urinary obstruction: A case report. *J. Urol.* 107:316, 1972.

174. Tolmatschen, M.   Ein Fall von Semilunaren: Klappen der Harnröhre und vergrossenter vesicular prostatien. *Virchows Arch. [Pathol. Anat.]* 49:348, 1872.

175. Trimingham, H. L., and McDonald, J. R.   Congenital anomalies in the region of the umbilicus. *Surg. Gynecol. Obstet.* 80:152, 1945.

176. Tripathi, V. N., and Dick, V. S.   Complete duplication of male urethra. *J. Urol.* 101:866, 1969.

177. Vakili, V. F.   Agenesis of the bladder: A case report. *J. Urol.* 109:510, 1973.

178. Volpe, M.   Dell'asta doppia. *Policlinico* 10:46, 1903.

179. Waldbaum, R. S., and Marshall, V. F.   Posterior urethral valves: Evaluation and surgical management. *J. Urol.* 103:801, 1970.

180. Warren, J. W., Jr.   Congenital diverticulum of the urethra. *Am. Surgeon* 21:385, 1955.

181. Waterhouse, K., and Hamm, F. C.   The importance of urethral valves as a cause of vesical neck obstruction in children. *J. Urol.* 87:404, 1962.

182. Waterhouse, K., and Scordamaglia, L. J.   Anterior urethral valve: A rare cause of bilateral hydronephrosis. *J. Urol.* 87:556, 1962.

183. Watson, E. M.   Developmental basis for certain vesical diverticula. *J.A.M.A.* 75:1473, 1920.

184. Watson, E. M.   Structural basis for congenital valve formation in the posterior urethra. *J. Urol.* 7:371, 1922.

185. Watts, S. H.   Urethral diverticula in the male with report of a case. *Johns Hopkins Hosp. Rep.* 13:49, 1906.

186. Wendel, R. M., and King, L. R.   The treatment of total urinary incontinence. *J. Pediatr. Surg.* 5:543, 1970.

187. Whitaker, R. H.   The ureter in posterior urethral valves. *Br. J. Urol.* 45:395, 1973.

188. Whitaker, R. H., Keetson, J. E., and Williams, D. I.   Posterior urethral valves: A study of urinary control after operation. *J. Urol.* 108:167, 1972.

189. Whittle, C. H., Coryllos, E., and Simpson, J. S., Jr.   Sarcoma of the urachus. *Arch. Surg.* 82:443, 1961.

190. Williams, D. I.   Bladder neck obstruction. *Proc. R. Soc. Med.* 51:957, 1958.

191. Williams, D. I.   *Pediatric Urology.* London: Butterworth, 1968.

192. Williams, D. I.   Discussion on lower urinary obstruction. *Arch. Dis. Child.* 37:132, 1962.

193. Williams, D. I., and Abbassian, A.   Solitary pedunculated polyp of the posterior urethra in children. *J. Urol.* 96:483, 1966.

194. Williams, D. I., and Eckstein, H. B.   Obstructive valves in the posterior urethra. *J. Urol.* 93:236, 1965.

195. Williams, D. I., and Retik, A. B.   Congenital valves and diverticula of the anterior urethra. *Br. J. Urol.* 41:228, 1969.

196. Williams, D. I., Whitaker, R. H., Barratt, T. M., and Keeston, J. E.   Urethral valves. *Br. J. Urol.* 45:200, 1973.

197. Wilson, A. N.   Complete dorsal duplication of the male urethra as an isolated deformity presenting as glandular epispadias. *Br. J. Urol.* 43:338, 1971.

198. Woodburne, R. T.   The sphincter mechanism of the urinary bladder and the urethra. *Anat. Rec.* 141:11, 1961.

199. Wrenn, E. L., Jr., and Michie, A. J.   Complete duplication of the male urethra. *Ann. Surg.* 145:119, 1957.

200. Wutz, J. B.   Ueber Urachus und Urachuscysten. *Arch. Pathol. Anat. (Berlin)* 92:387, 1883.

201. Yoerg, O. W.   Cysts of the urachus. *Minn. Med.* 25:496, 1942.

202. Young, H. H., Frontz, W. A., and Baldwin, J. C.   Congenital obstruction of the posterior urethra. *J. Urol.* 3:289, 1919.

203. Zellermayer, J., and Carlson, H. E.   Congenital hourglass bladder. *J. Urol.* 51:24, 1944.

99. Agenesis of the Abdominal Musculature

George T. Klauber

Agenesis of the abdominal musculature describes a congenital defect, usually symmetrical, that is characterized by a variable degree of absence of the musculature of the abdominal wall. The prune belly or triad syndrome applies to males with agenesis of the abdominal musculature and is associated with bilateral cryptorchidism and multiple defects and malformations of the urinary tract. Most characteristic of the abnormalities of the urinary tract are (1) areas of massive dilatation or narrowing, or both, at any point between the renal calyces and the external urethral meatus, and (2) dysplasia of the kidney.

Historical Aspects

Fröhlich [3] is credited generally with the first reported case of agenesis of the abdominal musculature. Parker [14] first noted the association of absent abdominal muscles with urogenital anomalies. In the case he reported, thoracopulmonary abnormalities were also present. The term *prune belly* was suggested by the wrinkled, flabby, dried prunelike appearance of the weakened abdominal wall. This term, incorrectly ascribed to Osler [12], only recently has appeared in the medical literature.

Etiology and Pathogenesis

The cause of the deficient abdominal musculature and associated abnormalities is unknown. All chromosomal studies to date have been normal with the exception of two siblings with a 16-chromosome deletion [4]. The condition was reported in twins on six occasions; in only one set were both siblings affected [7, 15]. Welch and Kearney encountered a patient who was one of homozygous triplets [18]. A simple mendelian recessive or sex-linked recessive condition, therefore, is highly improbable, but numerous polygenetic influences are possible.

Many theories have evolved to explain the coexistence of abnormalities of the abdominal wall and the urinary tract. Early theories implicated either a primary abnormality of the abdominal wall [12] or a primary obstruction of the urinary tract [6, 16]. Incongruities with these theories prompted the embryologic theory of Nunn and Stephens, who carried out careful necropsy dissection and histologic examination of pathologic material before reaching their conclusions [11] (see below).

It has been suggested that passive dilatation of the bladder develops in response to an absence of the abdominal wall or accessory muscles of micturition [12]. In opposition to this theory is the fact that gross urinary tract anomalies seldom accompany other abdominal wall deficiencies, such as those found in exomphalos. Similarly, the passive dilatation theory fails to explain associated findings such as renal dysplasia, dilatation of the urethra, and occasionally a normal urinary tract in children with agenesis of the abdominal musculature.

The obstruction theory presumes that urinary tract dilatation is secondary to distal obstruction [6, 16]. In other words, atrophy and laxity of the abdominal wall are the result of intraabdominal distention of the dilated urinary tract. The absence of demonstrable urinary outflow obstruction in the majority of reported cases does not support this theory [2, 11]. Further evidence opposing an etiology primarily obstructive in nature is the fact that defects in the abdominal wall are not associated with the most severe forms of bladder outflow obstruction, such as posterior urethral valves or urethral stricture.

The variety and complexity of the developmental abnormalities usually found in three or four organ systems in agenesis of the abdominal musculature appear incompatible with a single mechanical cause. Nunn and Stephens concluded, therefore, that the triad syndrome resulted from a primary embryologic defect [11]. An insult occurring between the sixth and tenth week of gestation, which would affect the various mesenchymal components of the abdominal wall, the developing ureteric bud, the renal blastema, and the testes, could explain the combination and variation of pathologic findings in this condition. In the abdominal wall, the same stimulus could result in arrest of the delamination process and dysplasia of the muscle cells. Defects of the muscularization and malformation of the entire urinary tract also can be explained by the embryologic theory. Thus the anatomic and histologic evidence presented by Nunn and Stephens is convincing.

Incidence

Agenesis of the abdominal musculature is quite rare; only about 300 cases have been reported in the English literature to date, and no exact incidence has been reported. Agenesis of the abdomi-

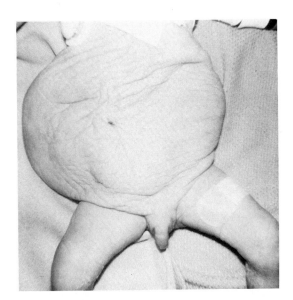

Figure 99-1. Newborn with agenesis of the abdominal musculature.

nal musculature is extremely rare in females, only 10 cases having been reported; in males it is invariably part of the triad syndrome.

Clinical Manifestations

The defect of the abdominal wall is obvious in agenesis of the abdominal musculature, and the coexistence of bilateral cryptorchidism helps to confirm the diagnosis (Fig. 99-1). The umbilicus moves upward upon contraction of the abdominal wall. The prune belly syndrome presents a varying clinical picture according to the severity of the renal dysplasia: (1) the most severe cases are either stillborn or result in neonatal death, (2) less severe cases present as emergencies in infancy, and (3) children who maintain good kidney function may present at a much later age [19].

NEONATAL PRESENTATIONS

Neonates lacking abdominal musculature may be stillborn and are characterized by complete or almost complete obstruction at the prostatomembranous level of the urethra. The bladder, posterior urethra, and ureters are usually extremely dilated. The kidneys are hypoplastic, dysplastic, and cystic. Complete urinary tract obstruction produces oligohydramnios in the mother, which can produce pressure defects in the limbs and Potter facies in the child.

EMERGENCIES DURING INFANCY

Children with little or no abdominal musculature present during the first few weeks of life with uremia, urosepsis, or failure to thrive. Occasionally the bladder outflow is obstructed, in which case the urachus remains patent. Abdominal distention may reach gigantic proportions, usually due to the enormous dilatation of the ureters. Renal hypoplasia and dysplasia are severe; unilateral aplasia or complete unilateral ureteric obstruction is common.

LATE PRESENTATIONS

Although the diagnosis of agenesis of abdominal musculature should be made at birth, these children may present much later to the urologist or nephrologist. Such children usually have maintained good kidney function and require little or no therapy. Despite the radiologic findings, kidney function is often surprisingly good. Children rarely present with voiding difficulties in spite of huge bladders and dilated urethras. Urinary infections and slowly progressive renal failure or bilateral cryptorchidism may be the presenting features. It should be noted that infections often are first introduced as a result of instrumentation or surgery.

Pathology

Agenesis of the abdominal musculature is usually associated with anomalous development of the entire urinary tract and frequently with severe abnormalities of other organ systems as well.

KIDNEY

The kidneys invariably demonstrate some degree of dysplasia in agenesis of the abdominal musculature, usually associated with hypoplasia. In the most severe forms there is cystic dysplasia with embryonic tubules and cartilage similar to that found in multicystic kidneys [11]. Marked renal dysplasia is associated with cases in which fibrous collagen deposition in the ureters is maximal [13]. Hydronephrosis with dilated, irregular, or isolated calyces is often present in association with hydroureter. The amount of normal renal parenchyma is quite variable, with the number of functional glomerular units reduced below normal in all cases [11].

URETERS AND BLADDER

Radiographically, bilateral dilatation, elongation, and tortuosity of the ureters are the most characteristic features of agenesis of the abdominal musculature. The gross and microscopic abnormalities of the ureters are usually more pronounced distally than proximally. Areas of complete atresia occasionally are present, and great variation in size and contour is found from side to side and from patient to patient.

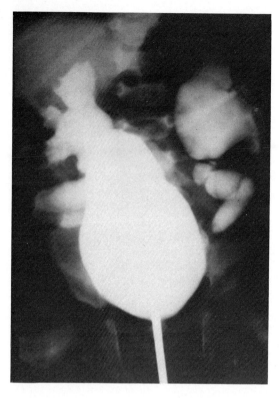

Figure 99-2. Cystogram demonstrating bilateral vesico-ureteral reflux and bilateral hydroureteronephrosis with marked tortuosity of the ureters.

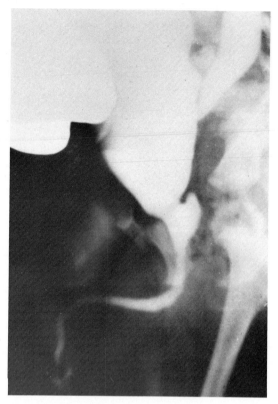

Figure 99-3. Expression cystourethrogram demonstrating posterior urethral diverticulum and prostato-membranous urethral disproportion.

The bladder is usually of very large capacity and is smooth and nontrabeculated (Fig. 99-2). On lateral cystography it sometimes appears to lie anteriorly due to the lack of abdominal support. A patent urachus or a diverticulum at the dome of the bladder suggesting a urachal remnant is frequently present [8].

Abnormalities of the ureterovesical junction are the rule rather than the exception in agenesis of the abdominal musculature. Vesicoureteral reflux is demonstrated in the majority of patients, whereas ureterovesical junction obstruction has been reported in some. The histologic structure of the ureters and bladder is similar, with patchy or total absence of muscle fibers and intrusion of a fibrous collagenous deposit. Some areas of ureter and bladder wall may be composed of epithelium covered by fibrous and hyaline tissue alone. In other areas where muscle fibers are present, differentiation into layers may be deficient [13].

No abnormality of innervation or lack of ganglion cells compared to the normal has been found in agenesis of the abdominal musculature [9, 11]. Light and electron microscopy suggest a congenital or ongoing healing process. The mitochondria of

the muscle fibers are abnormal, and a loss of coherence of the Z bands and glycogen granules is apparent [10].

URETHRA

Typically the bladder neck is wide open and the entire prostatic urethra is dilated in agenesis of the abdominal musculature. The membranous urethra is usually of normal caliber, but the discrepancy in size compared to the prostatic urethra may give the erroneous impression of a urethral stricture or posterior urethral valves (Fig. 99-3). Posterior urethral diverticula, probably utricular in origin, are common. Prostatic tissue and periurethral smooth muscle are both greatly reduced or absent. Absence of the corpus spongiosum urethrae, with resultant megalourethra, is sometimes seen.

ABDOMINAL WALL AND
OTHER PATHOLOGY

The wrinkled abdominal wall remains the most distinguishing external feature of agenesis of the abdominal musculature (see Fig. 99-1), although the degree of involvement is variable. The lower rectus muscles are more severely affected than the upper, and oblique muscles may or may not be affected. A spectrum exists from complete absence of the muscles of the abdominal wall through focal absence, diminution, or dysplasia of the muscle cells. Arrest of the delamination process in the abdominal wall resulting in a single facial layer also has been observed [11]. Innervation is normal. Cryptorchidism, characteristic of the prune belly syndrome, is almost invariably bilateral; the testicles are found in the abdominal cavity overlying the ureters [2]. Orthopedic abnormalities are frequently seen, the most common being talipes equinovarus [19]. Malrotation of the middle and hindgut is a fairly common finding [8].

Treatment

Preservation of kidney function is the primary goal in the management of agenesis of the abdominal musculature. Great care should be taken, therefore, to avoid introducing infection, which, if present, must be eradicated. Urinary obstruction should be relieved to prevent the effects of back pressure and to decrease or eliminate urinary stasis, but treatment should not be directed toward the correction of abnormal radiologic findings, no matter how bizarre. Urosepsis is the only indication for emergency surgical intervention.

A child who in the newborn period demonstrates urinary obstruction has already had such obstruction for many months prenatally. Some urologists believe that surgical intervention is indicated for all children [5, 17]. Most believe that it should be done for very specific indications [1, 19].

A neonate whose condition remains stable and uninfected can be evaluated adequately by means of intravenous urography, serial urinalysis, measurement of blood urea nitrogen or creatinine, or estimation of the glomerular filtration rate. Radioisotope renography may be helpful. Cystoscopy should be performed only if and when surgery is contemplated [19].

If kidney function continues to be satisfactory and the urinary tract remains uninfected, surgical reconstruction is not advised. The urinary tract and especially the ureters in these children are developmentally abnormal; this must be considered before initiating surgery such as tapering and reimplantation of the ureters.

Children who develop progressive loss of renal function, especially with rapid onset of uremia, may require urgent urinary diversion. Peristalsis in the abnormal and dilated ureters is usually poor, so high diversion by cutaneous pyelostomy or ureterostomy is advisable. Routine diversion by nephros-

tomy, as recommended by some [17], should be considered carefully, since the risk of intractable infection is great.

With time some children attain a stabilized condition with an improved although permanently impaired level of kidney function [19]. Permanent urinary diversion may be indicated in such cases, either by perpetuating a ureterostomy or by constructing a pyelointestinal urinary conduit. Some children ultimately will become candidates for staged urinary tract reconstruction, although caution is urged in view of the intrinsic abnormalities of the urinary tract. When severe renal dysplasia is present, little or no improvement of kidney function is likely.

Prognosis

The prognosis in agenesis of the abdominal musculature is related to the level of kidney function. The prognosis for children with severe bilateral renal dysplasia is hopeless. For those with moderate to severe impairment the prognosis is guarded, providing infection can be avoided. Recent studies suggest an excellent prognosis for children with good kidney function (Fig. 94-4) [1, 19]. Operative procedures may add little to the ultimate survival of these children in the absence of definite urinary tract obstruction.

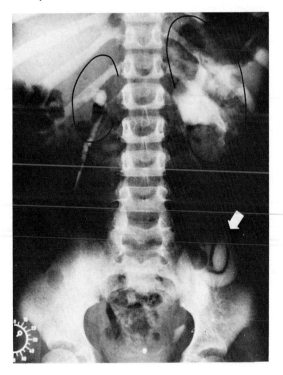

Figure 99-4. Intravenous urogram of 10-year-old child with normal kidney function. Note discrepancy in kidney size and marked tortuosity of the left ureter.

References

1. Burke, E. C., Shin, M. H., and Kelalis, P. P.   Prune belly syndrome: Clinical findings and survival. *Am. J. Dis. Child.* 117:668, 1969.
2. Burkholder, G. V., Williams, D. I., and Parker, R. M.   The prune belly syndrome. *J. Urol.* 98:244, 1967.
3. Fröhlich, F.   Der Mangel der Muskeln insbesondere der Seitenbauchmuskatir. Dissertation, Wurzburg, 1839.
4. Harley, L. M., Chen, Y., and Rattner, W. H.   Prune belly syndrome. *J. Urol.* 108:174, 1972.
5. Hendren, W. H., III.   Restoration of Function in the Severely Decompensated Ureter. In J. H. Johnston and R. J. Scholtmeijer (eds.), *Problems in Pediatric Urology.* Amsterdam: Excerpta Medica, 1972. Chap. 1, p. 1.
6. Housden, L. G.   Congenital absence of the abdominal muscles. *Arch. Dis. Child.* 9:219, 1934.
7. Ives, E. J.   The abdominal muscle deficiency triad syndrome—experience with ten cases. *Birth Defects* (Original Article Series 10, No. 4):127, 1974.
8. Lattimer, J. K.   Congenital deficiency of the abdominal musculature and associated genitourinary anomalies: A report of 22 cases. *J. Urol.* 79:343, 1958.
9. McGovern, J. H., and Marshall, V. F.   Congenital deficiency of the abdominal musculature and obstructive uropathy. *Surg. Gynecol. Obstet.* 108:289, 1959.
10. Mininberg, D. T., Montoya, F., Okada, K., Galioto, F., and Presutti, R.   Subcellular muscle studies in the prune belly syndrome. *J. Urol.* 109:524, 1973.
11. Nunn, I. N., and Stephens, F. D.   The triad syndrome: A composite anomaly of the abdominal wall, urinary system and testes. *J. Urol.* 86:782, 1961.
12. Osler, W.   Congenital absence of abdominal muscles with distended and hypertrophied urinary bladder. *Bull. Johns Hopkins Hosp.* 12 (128):331, 1901.
13. Palmer, J. M., and Tesluk, H.   Urethral pathology in the prune belly syndrome. *J. Urol.* 111:701, 1974.
14. Parker, R. W.   Case of an infant in whom some of the abdominal muscles were absent. *Trans. Clin. Soc. Lond.,* 28:201, 1895.
15. Petersen, D. S., Fish, L., and Cass, A. S.   Twins with congenital deficiency of abdominal musculature. *J. Urol.* 107:670, 1972.
16. Stumme, E. G.   Uber die symmetrischen kongenitalem Bauchmuskeldefekte und die Kombination derselben mit anderen Bildungsanomalien des Rumpfes. *Mitt. Granzgeb. Med. Chir.* 11:548, 1903.
17. Waldbaum, R. S., and Marshall, V. F.   The prune belly syndrome: A diagnostic therapeutic plan. *J. Urol.* 103:668, 1970.
18. Welch, K. J., and Kearney, G. P.   Abdominal musculature deficiency syndrome: Prune belly. *J. Urol.* 111:673, 1974.
19. Williams, D. I., and Parker, R. M.   The Role of Surgery in the Prune Belly Syndrome: In Review. In J. H. Johnston and W. J. Goodwin (eds.), *Pediatric Urology.* Amsterdam: Excerpta Medica, 1974. P. 229.

100. Vesicoureteral Reflux

Alan B. Retik

Vesicoureteral reflux is a condition commonly seen in children in which there is a backward flow of urine from the bladder to the ureter. This entity has caused more controversy than almost any other subject in pediatric urology. It appears to be the most common predisposing factor in the production of chronic pyelonephritis in childhood.

Historical Aspects

Graves and Davidoff [18] in 1924 demonstrated vesicoureteral reflux in 86 percent of normal rabbits. Gruber [19] in 1929 showed experimentally that the trigone is poorly developed and the intravesical ureter is short in those animals susceptible to reflux. The significance of vesicoureteral reflux was not truly appreciated, however, until the early 1950s, when Hutch [27] demonstrated pyelographic changes in patients with reflux and neurogenic bladder dysfunction.

Genetics and Epidemiology

The incidence of vesicoureteral reflux is 1 to 2 per 1,000 population [11, 80]. It is primarily a dis-

order of Caucasians, rarely being described in blacks [37], and it is five times more common in females than males. This figure may be somewhat misleading, however, because the short female urethra predisposes to urinary tract infection and thus to an increased investigation for and detection of reflux.

Although vesicoureteral reflux is thought of as a disorder of childhood, it is not uncommonly seen in adults [2, 3, 44]. Sixty percent of adults studied by McGovern and Marshall [44] gave clear histories of urinary symptoms in childhood. As increasing numbers of patients with end-stage renal failure become candidates for transplantation, investigation of the lower urinary tract has uncovered a significant incidence of previously undetected severe vesicoureteral reflux.

During the past few years a number of authors have reported reflux to occur in families and have commented upon the hereditary aspects of primary or congenital reflux. Seventy-nine families in whom reflux has been identified in more than one member, with a total of 146 individuals, have been reported [1, 5, 9–11, 46–48, 61, 70, 73, 80]. Included in the reports are four pairs of monozygotic twins. No families have been described in blacks. Heale [21] and Little [41] have provided evidence that vesicoureteral reflux may be inherited either as an autosomal recessive trait or as an autosomal dominant of variable expression. Miller and Caspari [46] noted an increased incidence of reflux in studies of pedigrees of 10 families. Although the distribution of affected individuals suggested a dominant gene, the fact that the affected offspring were more frequently detected in families of two nonaffected parents contradicted this assumption, and a dominant gene with incomplete expression was proposed.

Reflux in two consecutive generations has been reported in 15 families [39]. Mother-to-daughter transmission occurred in 8 families, mother-to-son in 3 families, and father-to-daughter in 4 families. Lewy and Belman [39] recently reported father-to-son transmission and noted that several generations of the involved family had reflux. Its occurrence in four of seven offspring was consistent with a pattern of autosomal dominant inheritance. Burger and Burger [10], however, have suggested a polygenic mode of inheritance in which males require a greater number of predisposing genes. It is generally agreed that in families with one member with reflux, all members with urinary tract symptoms or history of urinary tract infection should be evaluated. In families with two or more involved members, strong consideration should be given to evaluation of other family members, even if asymptomatic.

Etiology and Pathogenesis

A number of studies have shown that reflux does not occur in the urinary tract of normal man. Kjellberg et al. [35] found no reflux in the evaluation of 101 normal children. Lich and associates [40] in 1964 found no reflux in 24 of 26 newborns undergoing voiding cystourethrography; the 2 with reflux had urinary tract infection. Suprapubic puncture and subsequent voiding cineradiography were performed in 56 normal premature infants by Peters et al. [50]. Reflux was absent in all subjects, as it was also in 50 children studied by Politano [52]. Jones and Headstream [31] reported on 100 children ranging in age from 14 days to 14 years admitted consecutively for urologic investigation. They only found reflux in one 4-month-old male, who also had urethral obstruction.

A number of factors are responsible for the prevention of reflux in normal individuals. In the normal urinary tract the ureter tunnels obliquely through the bladder wall to insert on a well-developed trigone in such a way that the intravesical portion of the ureter is compressed between the mucosa and bladder musculature. The angle of the passage through the bladder wall, the intravesical portion of the ureter, and the competency of the musculature together constitute a valve mechanism that normally does not permit retrograde flow. The prevention of reflux may be due to active muscle contraction or to passive valvular action. Both mechanisms probably are operative. Stephens and Lenaghan [70] stated that the active contraction of the longitudinal fibers crossing the roof of the intravesical ureter compresses the ureter and closes it after ureteral efflux has occurred. Most authors [12, 28] stress the length of the intravesical portion of the ureter as the most important factor in the prevention of reflux.

A number of circumstances can compromise the valvular efficiency and result in reflux (Fig. 100-1). These include infections and anatomic variations.

Infection. Reflux can be detected in 30 to 70 percent of children undergoing urologic investigation for recurrent urinary tract infections. Infection renders the ureteral orifice incompetent mainly by causing edema of the mucosal portion or roof of the intravesical ureter, so that it cannot function as a flap valve. King et al. [34] found that 44

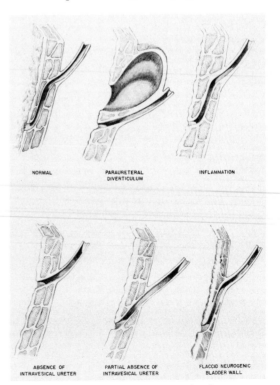

Figure 100-1. Causes of vesicoureteral reflux.

of 50 children spontaneously lost their reflux after acute urinary infection had been controlled. These findings have been substantiated by a number of other investigators [20, 64]. Radiologic evaluation of a child with urinary tract infection should be delayed, therefore, until the urine has been sterile for 4 to 6 weeks, to allow reflux secondary to inflammatory changes to disappear.

A Short Intravesical Ureter. The intravesical ureter is much shorter in the infant than in the older child or adult [28], the average length in the newborn being only 5 mm, compared to that of the adult, which varies from 11 to 18 mm with an average of 13 mm. Vesicoureteral reflux is more likely to occur in the young subject, therefore, due to the short intravesical ureteral segment.

Deficient Muscular Support of the Intravesical Ureter. The hiatus in the detrusor muscle of the bladder may be large enough to allow the mucosa of the ureter to herniate posterolateral to the ureteral orifice, with the resultant formation of a paraureteral (Hutch) saccule or diverticulum. The intravesical ureter in such instances is not backed by sturdy detrusor muscle and therefore permits reflux. Such a condition also may be acquired, the resultant reflux being secondary to back pressure from distal obstruction. The most common cause of this in children is posterior urethral valves, bladder neck obstruction being far less frequent. Children with neurogenic bladder dysfunction and exstrophy of the bladder also may have reflux due to impaired musculature.

Ectopic ureters terminating in the region of the bladder neck show a significant incidence of reflux. The caliber of such ureters is wide, their muscles are deficient, and their intramural courses are not submucosal but are within the muscle and adventitia.

Iatrogenic reflux results from surgical procedures done at the ureterovesical junction or trigone. A ureteral meatotomy or incision of a ureterocele invariably leads to reflux. Extensive dissection of the trigone may lead to reflux, which will usually disappear following healing.

Clinical Features

Vesicoureteral reflux is usually detected in infants and children presenting with urinary tract infection. Others present with symptoms of acute pyelonephritis—high fever and abdominal or back pain—in addition to irritative symptoms of the lower urinary tract. Infants may be septic or may present with failure to thrive. A small but significant percentage of asymptomatic children have been found to have infected urine and vesico-

ureteral reflux during the course of a school or camp examination. [54].

Although reflux may *result* from inflammatory changes in the bladder, it also may *predispose* to infection by leading to continuous residual urine in the bladder. During the past decade, vesicoureteral reflux has been found in an increasing number of patients with chronic pyelonephritis. In our series of children with radiologic evidence of chronic pyelonephritis, vesicoureteral reflux was demonstrated by voiding cystourethrography in greater than 90 percent. In the remaining children a definite anatomic abnormality of the ureteral orifice was seen cystoscopically, leading to the assumption that reflux had been present in the past and had subsided or that these orifices refluxed intermittently. These conclusions have been shared by Williams [74, 75], Hodson [24], Hutch et al. [29], and Scott and Stansfield [63].

There are many children with reflux and infection without chronic pyelonephritis. King et al. [33], in a recent review of 329 patients with reflux followed nonoperatively, demonstrated no evidence of progressive renal scarring or significant impairment of renal function; however, reflux may be the cause of ascent of organisms from the infected bladder to the kidney. It has been shown that the higher the grade of reflux, the more likely is a patient to show progressive renal damage [15, 55]. Development and progression of clubbing and scarring have been reported by a number of authors [14, 15, 23, 38, 63, 66, 69, 76, 79] (Fig. 100-2), Blank [7, 8] being the lone dissenter. Filly et al. [15] demonstrated that infection and reflux appeared important in the development of these changes and that it sometimes took up to 2 years for clubbing and scarring to become maximally evident.

Although it is generally agreed that mild to moderate degrees of reflux without infection are not harmful to the kidney, there is mounting evidence to suggest that severe sterile reflux may on occasion form the basis of renal scarring seen with chronic atrophic pyelonephritis. Several authors have reported impaired renal growth [25] or progressive renal scarring [58, 68] associated with sterile reflux in children and in animals [26]. Sterile reflux associated with chronic pyelonephritis has also been observed in hypertensive children [71, 72]. On the other hand, Ross and Thompson [59] and King and Idriss [32] produced reflux in dogs and found no evidence of scarring or change in renal function over a 22-month period, if infection did not supervene. Thus the entire question of sterile reflux and its relationship to chronic

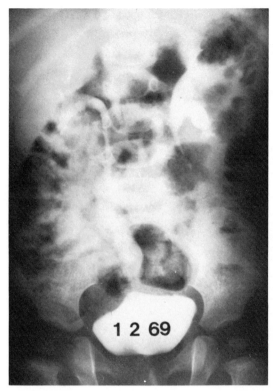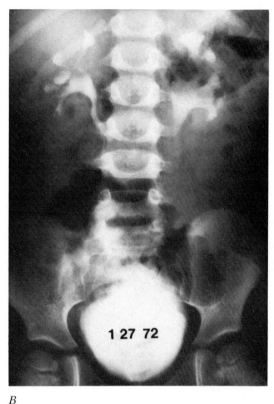

A   *B*

Figure 100-2. A. Excretory urogram in a 4-year-old boy with one documented urinary tract infection. Normally cupped calyces are seen. A voiding cystourethrogram revealed bilateral grade IIb reflux. B. Excretory urogram 3 years later reveals changes consistent with bilateral chronic pyelonephritis. The boy had several infections during the 3-year period.

pyelonephritis and renal growth needs to be clarified.

Rolleston et al. [57] showed "intrarenal reflux" to occur in some children under age 4 years with severe reflux and chronic pyelonephritis, the mechanism appearing to be pyelotubular backflow. Of the kidneys in which intrarenal reflux was observed, 65 percent showed focal renal damage that corresponded exactly to those parts of the kidney in which intrarenal reflux had been observed.

It has been suggested that renal growth is inhibited in the presence of reflux [42, 53]. In our series, however, preoperative measurements of refluxing kidneys without pyelonephritis did not vary significantly from normal. Although reflux may inhibit renal growth in selected instances, very small kidneys with reflux alone and no pyelonephritic scarring more likely represent maldevelopment of the entire ureteral-renal unit. Faulty development of the ureteral bud may account for an incompetent ureterovesical junction with hypopla-

sia and dysplasia of the renal parenchyma [6, 67]. It appears, therefore, that for reflux to cause impaired renal growth, it must be associated with infection leading to pyelonephritis [45, 60].

Evaluation and Treatment

Although the findings on the excretory urogram may lead one to suspect that vesicoureteral reflux is present, the definitive diagnostic study is the voiding cystourethrogram. As mentioned above, neither radiologic study should be done during or soon after an acute infection in order to avoid demonstrating transient abnormalities caused by the infection rather than important underlying abnormalities that are causative [13, 16, 25, 49].

On the voiding cystourethrogram, the degree of reflux is graded from I to IV (Fig. 100-3). The radiologic study helps to define the etiology and mechanics of the disorder and to designate whether reflux is primary (congenital) or secondary to distal obstruction. By cystoscopy the presence of ure-

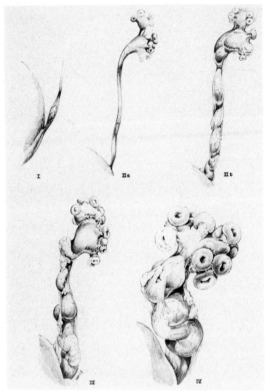

Figure 100-3. Grades of reflux. In grade I, reflux is confined to the ureter. Grade IIa reaches the kidney but does not distend the renal pelvis and calyces. Grade IIb represents ureteral and pelvocalyceal filling with mild calyceal blunting. Grade III involves more significant distention of the pelvis, calyces, and ureter. In grade IV reflux there is hydronephrosis and hydroureter.

thral or bladder outlet obstruction can be verified, saccules and diverticula can be detected, the characteristic appearance of the neurogenic bladder may be noted, and the double ureteral orifices associated with renal duplication may be seen. Of utmost importance are the degree of development of the trigone and the location and configuration of the ureteral orifices. With a calibrated catheter one can probe the ureteral orifice, and, by observing a ripple caused by the catheter lip as it traverses the bladder wall, one can estimate the length of the intravesical ureter. These features are important in deciding whether or not surgery should be performed and in determining the prognosis.

In a small number of children, severe reflux may cause extreme tortuosity and kinking at the ureteropelvic junction, thus in effect producing a secondary ureteropelvic obstruction. It is therefore important to obtain voiding cystourethrograms in all children with ureteropelvic obstruction to ensure that surgery will be performed at the correct portion of the ureter.

It is well known that many children tend to lose their reflux over a period of years [4, 30, 36, 58, 65, 68, 74]. In the study of Dwoskin and Perlmutter [14], 49 percent of 114 girls with various degrees of reflux who were not operated upon lost their reflux. Of the 84 ureters in which reflux ultimately stopped, 65 percent did so within 2 years and 78 percent within 3 years. As the severity of reflux increased, the percentage of ureters that stopped refluxing decreased. In our experience, virtually all grade I and approximately 60 percent of grade IIa reflux will eventually subside. With greater degrees of reflux, there is less likelihood that this will happen; however, most observers have noted the occasional patient, especially the infant, with ureteral dilatation and moderately severe reflux that subsides over a period of years.

The likelihood of reflux disappearing is related to the appearance and position of the ureteral orifice [43], the length of the intravesical ureter [34, 55], as well as the degree of reflux [14, 55]. Thus it would be highly unlikely for grade III reflux to subside in the presence of a gaping, laterally placed ureteral orifice with a very short submucosal tunnel. Recovery of normal physiologic function of the ureterovesical junction has been reported to occur by healing of a chronically inflamed area [34] or by growth and maturation, as described by Hutch [28], who showed a gradually increasing length of the intravesical segment of the ureter with age. Reflux has been reported to subside in 25 to 45 percent of cases following relief of distal obstruction [33, 34, 56, 75].

Treatment of vesicoureteral reflux must be individualized; factors such as duration of disease, age, onset, number of infections, and ease with which they are controlled should be considered in deciding whether or not surgery should be performed. As mentioned above, it is generally agreed that reflux in the absence of infection in most children does not cause renal damage. Therefore, if it is decided to pursue a nonoperative program, I consider it imperative that continuous chemotherapy be employed as a prophylactic measure against infection as long as reflux persists. Urine cultures with colony counts are obtained at 2-month intervals, and excretory urograms and voiding cystourethrograms are repeated at 6- to 12-month intervals. Other measures designed to reduce urinary stasis and infection should be encouraged, including adequate hydration, attention to proper perineal hygiene, and a frequent voiding schedule.

The ultimate goal of nonoperative management is the cessation of reflux. With grade I reflux and normal ureteral orifices seen cystoscopically, the reflux will virtually always disappear with time. Grade IIa reflux will subside in approximately 50 to 60 percent of the cases, especially if it is associated with minor abnormalities at the ureteral orifice, such as a moderately short intravesical tunnel. Surgery must be more strongly considered in grade IIb reflux, of which only 30 percent of cases will subside with time, although most children are given a considerable trial of nonoperative therapy. Decisions for surgery may be made even earlier in instances of grade III reflux, less than 10 percent of which will subside, and in grade IV, in which subsidence of reflux is rare.

In each child, the radiographic picture must be correlated with the clinical course as well as the cystoscopic findings. The indications for antireflux surgery that we have employed are (1) recurrent urinary tract infections despite adequate continuous antibiotics, (2) persistent reflux with a basic anatomic abnormality at the ureterovesical junction, or (3) severe reflux with pyelonephritis. In the application of these criteria, individualization must again be stressed. For example, one might consider a fourth indication for surgery to be persistence of reflux of any appreciable degree in a postpubertal female. The stasis associated with reflux compounds the tremendous dilatation of the urinary tract in pregnancy; the likelihood of pyelonephritis becomes great.

Nephrectomy is indicated only if the involved kidney contributes less than 10 percent of total renal function. It has been our policy in general to preserve renal parenchyma in children, since the involved kidney may function as a life-sustaining organ if the contralateral kidney were ever to be removed.

A number of antireflux operations have been described. The one that appears to be most widely employed and is used in our institution is the Politano-Leadbetter procedure. The purpose of surgery is to lead the ureter through a new submucosal tunnel in the bladder wall. This tunnel should be of sufficient length and placement between mucosa and detrusor so that the mechanical requirements of a functioning flap valve are met, and it should be approximately five times the diameter of the ureter. In very dilated ureters it is necessary to narrow the caliber of the ureter to achieve an adequate tunnel and to permit more effective ureteral peristalsis.

Antireflux surgery has been reported to be successful in more than 90 percent of cases [22, 55, 62, 76]. In our recent series of 342 ureters reimplanted in 223 children, the surgical success rate was 99 percent (elimination of reflux without creating ureteral obstruction).

The postoperative infection rate is generally reported to be between 10 and 30 percent [22, 51, 77]. In our series the incidence of infection after surgery was 21 percent, and the infection was clinically confined to the bladder in most cases. The vast majority of postoperative infections occurred in girls (45 of the 175 females), but only 3 (1.7 percent) had pyelonephritis. It is believed that girls are reinfected because of anatomic and physiologic factors peculiar to the lower urinary tract of the female, rather than to the presence of old pyelonephritis. Boys rarely developed a postoperative infection, the protective effect of the longer male urethra probably accounting for this finding. The incidence of postoperative infection was related neither to the preoperative urographic appearance nor to the grade of reflux. Our findings and conclusions are shared by others [17, 62, 75].

There has been recent interest in the effect of surgery on renal growth [42, 45]. Our studies [78] have shown that all kidneys grow at rates equal to or greater than normal following antireflux surgery.

References

1. Amar, A. D. Familial vesico-ureteral reflux. *J. Urol.* 108:969, 1972.
2. Amar, A. D., Singer, B., Lewis, R., and Nocks, B. Vesico-ureteral reflux in adults: A twelve-year study of 122 patients. *Urology* 3:184, 1974.
3. Ambrose, S. S. Reflux pyelonephritis in adults secondary to congenital lesions of the ureteral orifice. *J. Urol.* 102:302, 1969.
4. Baker, R., Maxted, W., Maylath, J., and Shuman, I. Relation of age, sex, and infection to reflux: Data indicating high spontaneous cure rate in pediatric patients. *J. Urol.* 95:271, 1966.
5. Baker, R., Maxted, W., McCrystal, H., and Kelly, T. Unpredictable results associated with treatment of 133 children with ureterorenal reflux. *J. Urol.* 94: 362, 1965.
6. Beck, A. D. The effect of intra-uterine urinary obstruction upon the development of the fetal kidney. *J. Urol.* 105:784, 1971.
7. Blank, E. Caliectasis and renal scars in children. *J. Urol.* 110:255, 1973.
8. Blank, E., and Girdavy, B. R. Prognosis with vesicoureteral reflux. *Pediatrics* 48:782, 1971.
9. Burger, R. H. Familial and hereditary vesico-ureteral reflux. *J.A.M.A.* 216:680, 1971.
10. Burger, R. H., and Burger, S. E. Genetic Determinants of Urologic Disease. In L. R. King (ed.), *Symposium on Pediatric Urology. Urol. Clin. North Am.* 1 (3):419, 1974.
11. Burger, R. H., and Smith, C. Hereditary and familial vesico-ureteral reflux. *J. Urol.* 106:845, 1971.
12. Castro, J. E., and Fine, H. Passive antireflux mecha-

nisms in the human cadaver. *Br. J. Urol.* 41:559, 1969.

13. Dunbar, J. S., and Nogardy, B. M. Excretory urography in the first year of life. *Radiol. Clin. North Am.* 10:367, 1972.

14. Dwoskin, J. Y., and Perlmutter, A. D. Vesico-ureteral reflux in children: A computerized review. *J. Urol.* 109:888, 1973.

15. Filly, R., Friedland, G. W., Govan, D. E., and Fair, W. R. Development and progression of clubbing and scarring in children with recurrent urinary tract infections. *Radiology* 113:145, 1974.

16. Goldman, H. S., and Freeman, L. M. Radiographic and radioisotopic methods of evaluation of the kidneys and urinary tract. *Pediatr. Clin. North Am.* 18:409, 1971.

17. Govan, D. E., and Palmer, J. M. Urinary tract infections in children: The influence of successful antireflux operations on morbidity from infection. *Pediatrics* 44:677, 1969.

18. Graves, R. C., and Davidoff, L. M., II. Studies on the ureter and bladder with especial reference to regurgitation of the vesical contents. *J. Urol.* 12:93, 1924.

19. Gruber, C. M. I. A comparative study of the intravesical ureters in man and in experimental animals. *J. Urol.* 21:567, 1929.

20. Harrow, B. B. Ureteral reflux in children, concepts for conservative versus surgical treatment. *Clin. Pediatr.* 6:83, 1967.

21. Heale, W. F. Chronic pyelonephritis in the adult. *Aust. N.Z. J. Med.* 3:283, 1971.

22. Hendren, W. H. Ureteral reimplantation in children. *J. Pediatr. Surg.* 3:649, 1968.

23. Hodson, C. J. The radiologic diagnosis of pyelonephritis. *Proc. R. Soc. Med.* 52:669, 1959.

24. Hodson, C. J. Obstructive atrophy of the kidney in children. *Ann. Radiol.* 10:273, 1967.

25. Hodson, C. J., and Edwards, D. Chronic pyelonephritis and vesico-ureteric reflux. *Clin. Radiol.* 11:219, 1960.

26. Hodson, C. J., McManamon, P. J., and Lewis, M. A New Concept of the Pathogenesis of Atrophic Pyelonephritis. In Abstracts of the 5th International Congress of Nephrology, Mexico City, 1972. Abstract 598.

27. Hutch, J. A. Vesico-ureteral reflux in the paraplegic: Cause and correction. *J. Urol.* 68:457, 1952.

28. Hutch, J. A. Theory of maturation of the intravesical ureter. *J. Urol.* 86:534, 1961.

29. Hutch, J. A., Smith, D. R., and Osborne, R. Summary of pathogenesis of a new classification for urinary tract infections. *J. Urol.* 102:758, 1969.

30. Jones, B., Gerrard, J. W., Shokeir, M. K., and Houston, C. S. Recurrent urinary infections in girls: Relation to enuresis. *Can. Med. Assoc. J.* 106:127, 1972.

31. Jones, B. W., and Headstream, J. W. Vesico-ureteral reflux in children. *J. Urol.* 80:114, 1958.

32. King, L. R., and Idriss, F. S. Effect of vesico-ureteral reflux on renal function in dogs. *Invest. Urol.* 4:419, 1967.

33. King, L. R., Kazmi, S. O., and Belman, A. B. Natural History of Vesico-ureteral Reflux—Outcome of a Trial of Nonoperative Therapy. In L. R. King (ed.), *Symposium on Pediatric Urology. Urol. Clin. North Am.* 1 (3):441, 1974.

34. King, L. R., Surian, M. A., Wendel, R. M., and Burden, J. J. Vesico-ureteric reflux. *J.A.M.A.* 203:169, 1968.

35. Kjellberg, S. R., Ericsson, N. O., and Rudhe, U. *The Lower Urinary Tract in Childhood.* Edinburgh: Livingstone, 1957.

36. Kunin, C. M. Tendency of Vesico-ureteric Reflux to Disappear Coincident with Specific Antimicrobial Therapy. In P. Kincaid-Smith and K. P. Fairley (eds.), *Renal Infection and Renal Scarring.* Melbourne: Mercedes Publishing Services, 1970.

37. Kunin, C. M., Deutscher, R., and Paquin, A., Jr. Urinary tract infections in children: Epidemiologic, clinical, and laboratory study. *Medicine* 43:91, 1964.

38. Lebowitz, R. L., and Colodny, A. H. Urinary tract infection in children. *Crit. Rev. Clin. Radiol. Nucl. Med.* 4:457, 1974.

39. Lewy, P. R., and Belman, A. B. Familial occurrence of nonobstructive, noninfectious vesico-ureteral reflux with renal scarring. *J. Pediatr.* 86:851, 1975.

40. Lich, R., Homerton, L. W., Goode, L. S., and Davis, L. A. The uretero-vesical junction of the newborn. *J. Urol.* 92:436, 1964.

41. Little, P. J. Gross Vesico-ureteric Reflux—A Preventable Cause of Renal Failure. In Abstracts of the 5th International Congress of Nephrology, Mexico City, 1972. Abstract 577.

42. Lyon, R. P. Renal arrest. *J. Urol.* 109:707, 1973.

43. Lyon, R. P., Marshall, S., and Tanagho, E. A. The ureteral orifice: Its configuration and competency. *J. Urol.* 102:504, 1969.

44. McGovern, J. H., and Marshall, V. F. Reflux and pyelonephritis in 35 adults. *J. Urol.* 101:668, 1969.

45. McRea, C. V., Shannon, F. T., and Utley, W. L. F. Effect on renal growth of reimplantation of refluxing ureters. *Lancet* 1:1310, 1974.

46. Miller, H. C., and Caspari, E. W. Ureteral reflux as a genetic trait. *J.A.M.A.* 220:842, 1972.

47. Mobley, D. F. Familial vesico-ureteral reflux. *Urology* 2:514, 1973.

48. Mulcahy, J. J., Kelalis, P. P., Stickler, G. B., and Burke, E. C. Familial vesico-ureteral reflux. *J. Urol.* 104:762, 1970.

49. Nogrady, M. B., and Dunbar, J. S. The Technique of Roentgen Investigation of the Urinary Tract in Infants and Children. In H. J. Kaufman (ed.), *Progress in Pediatric Radiology.* Chicago: Year Book, 1970. Vol. 3.

50. Peters, P., Johnson, D. E., and Jackson, J. R. The incidence of vesicoureteral reflux in the premature child. *J. Urol.* 97:259, 1967.

51. Politano, V. A. One hundred reimplants in five years. *J. Urol.* 90:696, 1963.

52. Politano, V. A. Uretero-vesical junction. *J. Urol.* 107:239, 1972.

53. Redman, J. R., Schriber, L. J., and Bissada, N. K. Apparent failure of renal growth secondary to vesico-ureteral reflux. *Urology* 3:704, 1974.

54. Retik, A. B. Unpublished data, 1974.

55. Retik, A. B. Urinary reflux in children: An approach to management. *Hosp. Pract.* 9:125, 1974.

56. Retik, A. B., and Burke, C. Urethral Valves. In J. Libertino and L. Zinman (eds.), *Reconstructive Urologic Surgery* (Lahey Clinic Symposium). Baltimore: Williams & Wilkins, 1977. Pp. 287–293.

57. Rolleston, G. L., Maling, T. M. J., and Hodson, C. J. Intrarenal reflux in the scarred kidney. *Arch. Dis. Child.* 49:531, 1974.

58. Rolleston, G. L., Shannon, F. T., and Utley, W. L. F. Relationship of infantile vesico-ureteric reflux to renal damage. *Br. Med. J.* 1:460, 1970.

59. Ross, G., and Thompson, I. M. Relationship of non-obstructive reflux and chronic pyelonephritis. *J. Urol.* 90:391, 1963.

60. Savage, D. C. L., Howie, G., Adler, K., and Wilson, M. I. Controlled trial of therapy in covert bacteriuria of childhood. *Lancet* 1:358, 1975.

61. Schmidt, J. D., Hawtrey, C. E., Flock, R. H., and Culp, D. A. Vesico-ureteral reflux: An inherited lesion. *J.A.M.A.* 220:821, 1972.

62. Scott, J. E. S. Results of antireflux surgery. *Lancet* 2:68, 1969.

63. Scott, J. E. S., and Stansfield, J. M. Ureteric reflux and kidney scarring in children. *Arch. Dis. Child.* 43:468, 1968.

64. Shopfer, C. E. Vesico-ureteral reflux: Five year re-evaluation. *Radiology* 95:637, 1970.

65. Smellie, J. M. Medical aspects of urinary infection in children. *R. Coll. Physicians* 1:189, 1967.

66. Smellie, J. M. Acute urinary tract infection in children. *Br. Med. J.* 4:97, 1970.

67. Stecker, J. F., Rose, J. G., and Gillenwater, J. Y. Dysplastic kidneys associated with vesicoureteral reflux. *J. Urol.* 110:341, 1973.

68. Stephens, F. D. Urologic aspects of recurrent urinary tract infection in children. *J. Pediatr.* 80:725, 1972.

69. Stephens, F. D. Preliminary Follow-up Study of 101 Children with Reflux Treated Conservatively. In P. Kincaid-Smith and K. F. Fairley (eds.), *Renal Infection and Renal Scarring*. Melbourne: Mercedes, 1970.

70. Stephens, F. D., and Lenaghan, D. The anatomical basis and dynamics of vesico-ureteric reflux. *J. Urol.* 87:669, 1962.

71. Stickler, G. B., Kelalis, P. P., Burke, E. C., and Segar, W. E. Primary interstitial nephritis with reflux: A cause of hypertension. *Am. J. Dis. Child.* 122:144, 1971.

72. Still, J. L., and Cottom, D. Severe hypertension in childhood. *Arch. Dis. Child.* 42:34, 1967.

73. Tobenkin, M. I. Hereditary vesico-ureteral reflux. *South Med. J.* 57:139, 1964.

74. Williams, D. I. The ureter, the urologist, and the pediatrician. *Proc. R. Soc. Med.* 63:595, 1970.

75. Williams, D. I. Vesico-ureteric Reflux. In D. I. Williams (ed.), *Urology in Childhood*. Berlin: Springer, 1974.

76. Williams, D. I., and Eckstein, H. B. Surgical treatment of reflux in children. *Br. J. Urol.* 37:13, 1965.

77. Willscher, M. K., Bauer, S. B., Zammuto, P. J., and Retik, A. B. Renal growth and urinary infection following antireflux surgery in infants and children. *J. Urol.* 115:722, 1976.

78. Willscher, M. K., Bauer, S. B., Zammuto, P. J., and Retik, A. B. Infections of the urinary tract after antireflux surgery in infants and children. *J. Pediatr.* 89:743, 1976.

79. Winberg, J., Larson, H., and Bergstrom, T. Comparison of the Natural History of Urinary Tract Infection in Children with and without Vesico-ureteric Reflux. In P. Kincaid-Smith and K. F. Fairley (eds.), *Renal Infection and Renal Scarring*. Melbourne: Mercedes, 1970.

80. Zel, G., and Retik, A. B. Familial vesico-ureteral reflux. *Urology* 2:249, 1973.

101. Neurogenic Bladder Dysfunction or the Neuropathic Bladder

George T. Klauber

Neurogenic bladder dysfunction is best considered in terms of functional status. This approach is especially suited to dysfunction coexistent with neurospinal dysraphism, which is the most common cause of neuropathic bladder in children. I use the terms *neuropathic bladder* and *neurogenic bladder dysfunction* rather than neurogenic bladder which, embryologically, is incorrect.

The neuropathic bladder continues to be one of the least understood areas in urology; management, therefore, is frequently less than optimal. Confusion arises in part due to the lack of standardization of nomenclature and classifications that explain pathophysiology in terms of anatomic pathology. In this chapter, a brief, simplified introduction will precede a discussion of dysfunction associated with the neuropathic bladder.

Normal bladder function depends upon an adequate storage capacity and an ability to empty completely at will, with a satisfactory flow rate. Such function depends upon (1) intact innervation of the bladder and of the muscles contributing to the bladder outflow resistance, and (2) the inherent properties of the bladder itself, which are independent of the central nervous system: tonus and rhythmic detrusor contractility [43].

Urinary continence requires that the forces of urinary retention, or the bladder outflow resistance, exceed intravesical pressure, which, in turn, is produced by the interaction of the bladder muscle and the bladder contents. The normal bladder musculature withstands stretch without undue rise in pressure until the stretch threshold has been reached [54].

The components of bladder innervation may be thought of as basic spinal reflexes that are modified by facilitative and inhibitory pathways from higher centers. The spinal micturition center is located in the second through fourth sacral segments. Sensory nerve endings for pain, temperature, and proprioception are found throughout the bladder [19]. Sensory impulses travel through the pelvic nerves, reaching the spinal cord via the dorsal root or the afferent limb of the spinal micturition reflex arc. The efferent or motor limb of the reflex arc is predominantly parasympathetic and also travels in the pelvic nerves.

Afferent sensory nerve endings impinge upon the pudendal nuclei in the ventral horns of the spinal cord, initiating inhibitory impulses to the striated muscle of the external sphincter and the pelvic diaphragm. Thus detrusor contraction normally is accompanied by relaxation of the extraurethral sphincteric muscles. Similarly, dilatation of the posterior urethra induces reflex bladder contractions—the so-called Barrington reflex.

Bradley and associates [6] define four basic central nervous system "circuits" or pathways concerned with innervation of the detrusor muscle and urethra. One circuit, between the frontal cortex and the pontine-mesencephalic reticular formation, is concerned primarily with normal volitional control of micturition. This circuit presumably is inoperative at birth. A second circuit between the pontine-mesencephalic reticular formation and the sacral gray matter is concerned with producing a coordinated and prolonged detrusor contraction that produces complete bladder evacuation. Damage to nerve fibers involved in this loop will result in uncoordinated and ineffectual detrusor contractions, commonly seen with myelomeningocele. A third circuit between the motor cortex and the pudendal nuclei results in volitional control of the striated muscle portion of the urethral sphincter. This latter circuit can override the pelvic and pudendal nuclei that comprise the fourth circuit, the spinal reflex arc mentioned previously. In early childhood, bladder emptying comes under voluntary control, and all four circuits are actively concerned with control of micturition. More detailed accounts of normal urodynamics can be found elsewhere [2, 4, 33].

Etiology and Pathogenesis

Table 101-1 outlines the etiology of neuropathic bladder dysfunction in 200 patients presenting consecutively from January, 1973, to November, 1974, at the University of Connecticut Pediatric Urology Service at Newington Children's Hospital.

NEUROSPINAL DYSRAPHISM
Of the 200 children in this series, 84 percent presented with some form of neurospinal dysraphism.

Table 101-1. Etiology of Neuropathic Bladder in 200 Patients*

Etiology		Number	Percent
1. Neurospinal dysraphism		168	84
Myelomeningocele	152		
Sacral agenesis	6		
Myelomeningocele plus sacral agenesis	5		
Miscellaneous (lipoma, dermoid sinus, diastematomyelia)	5		
2. Trauma		15	7.5
Spinal cord injury	14		
Surgical	1		
3. Tumor		5	2.5
Astrocytoma	2		
Neuroblastoma	2		
Miscellaneous extraspinal	1		
4. Miscellaneous		12	6
Cerebral palsy	3		
Multiple sclerosis	2		
Spinal stenosis (achondroplasia)	2		
Abscess, etiology unknown	1		
External sphincter, dyssynergia	1		
Flaccid diaplegia	1		
Hemophilia	1		
Transverse myelitis (infective)	1		
		200	100

* Classification of neuropathic bladder in 200 patients presenting at the Department of Urology, Newington Children's Hospital, from January 1973 to November 1974.

According to Brocklehurst [8], the two major theories of the pathogenesis of this condition were originally advanced by von Recklinghausen and Morgagni. Von Recklinghausen theorized that the pathogenesis of spina bifida is due primarily to a failure of closure of the neural tube during embryologic development, whereas Morgagni believed that rupture of the neural tube with damage to the overlying mesoderm and ectoderm was primarily responsible for the development of dysraphism.

Myelomeningocele
Myelomeningocele is the most common type of neurogenic bladder dysfunction seen, and thus it is the single most common cause of neurogenic bladder dysfunction in children. A spectrum of bladder dysfunction accompanies myelomeningocele and best exemplifies the need for a functional classification of the neuropathic bladder. In myelomeningocele, by definition, elements of the spinal cord and spinal nerves are incorporated into the cystic deformity to a greater or lesser extent. With regard to bladder innervation and function, the lesion invariably is mixed with elements of bladder hypertonicity and hypotonicity. The de-

fect may result in interruption of the reflex arc between the spinal cord and the bladder or external sphincter in any of three different ways: (1) by loss of continuity of spinal efferent nerve fibers, (2) by loss of continuity of spinal afferent nerve fibers, or (3) by damage to the cord itself at the S2 to S4 level.

Continuity of any elements of the sacral reflex arc associated with interruption of the corresponding long spinal tracts will produce spasticity of muscle fibers innervated by the afferent limb of the arc. Muscle fibers lacking efferent spinal innervation are flaccid and unresponsive to central control. Muscle fibers that receive afferent nervous stimuli may be responsive, providing they have not been overstretched due to loss of the integrated regulatory mechanism of the intact reflex arc.

The myelomeningocele lesion usually is symmetrical, so that efferent and afferent nerve fibers are similarly involved. Asymmetrical myelomeningocele lesions affecting only one limb of the arc and sparing the other are seen occasionally.

Either the detrusor muscle or the external sphincter or both can be flaccid or hypertonic. The combinations used to classify neurogenic bladder dysfunction in myelomeningocele patients are (1) flaccid bladders with either low or high outflow resistance, and (2) hypertonic bladders with low or high outflow resistance [52].

Sacral Agenesis
Various degrees of sacral agenesis exist, from partial absence of one or more sacral elements to complete absence of all sacral elements, in addition to absence of one or more lumbar vertebrae. With complete absence of the sacrum, the iliac bones articulate with each other or with the lumbar vertebrae. White and Klauber [55] were unable to find a single case of sacral agenesis unassociated with neurogenic bladder dysfunction, although this has been reported by others. Postmortem dissections suggest that the innervation of the lower urinary tract may be partially lacking in these patients [51]. Many children with sacral agenesis have an associated myelomeningocele or imperforate anus; surgical correction of the latter may increase neurogenic bladder dysfunction. Lack of spinal efferent nerve impulses to the bladder and urethral sphincter result in flaccidity of detrusor or sphincteric musculature or of both. Most of these children are incontinent, with large residual bladder urine volumes or overflow incontinence.

Miscellaneous Spinal Dysraphism
This pathologic group includes diastematomyelia, spinal cord tethering, paravertebral lipomas, and dermoid sinuses extending into the spinal canal. Bladder neuropathy typically develops some time during the postnatal growth period. Tethering bands, bony spikes, or a lipoma within the spinal canal damage the cord or filum terminale by preventing the relative upward movement of the spinal cord during growth of the vertebral column.

TRAUMA
Neurogenic bladder dysfunction resulting from spinal cord injury is relatively uncommon in the pediatric age group, especially when compared to young adults. Cord transections are usually incomplete, but, unfortunately, the higher cord lesions resulting in quadriplegia appear to predominate. Bladder dysfunction varies with the level of the injury. Lesions above the spinal cord at S2 result in detrusor hypertonicity unless there is infarction of the cord below the level of injury [3]. Injuries to the spinal cord at the level of micturition center or below result in detrusor hypotonicity. Immediately following the initial injury there is usually a period of spinal shock, with detrusor hypotonicity lasting from days to months.

Neurogenic bladder dysfunction resulting from surgical trauma in childhood usually is associated with reconstructive surgery for imperforate anus. Excision of sacrococcygeal teratomas or tumors of the sympathetic chain also may result in damage to the pelvic nerves.

SPINAL CORD TUMORS
Spinal cord tumors, such as astrocytoma, are rare; extradural metastases, classically from neuroblastoma, appear to be more common. Such extradural metastases may cause spinal cord compression. Directly or indirectly, a spectrum of neurologically induced abnormalities similar to neurospinal dysraphism may be encountered.

MISCELLANEOUS CONDITIONS
Other conditions affecting the central nervous system, either directly or indirectly, may produce neurogenic bladder dysfunction. Infections are uncommonly etiologic; however, when present, the type of dysfunction depends upon the level of involvement. In our series we found no case of neuropathic bladder caused by spinal meningitis, although transverse myelitis was seen.

Extradural abscesses from spinal tuberculosis or osteomyelitis are now uncommon due to the near-extinction of these diseases in North America. They must be considered when neurogenic bladder develops in the presence of chronic infectious disease. Other causes of neuropathic bladder are hemophilia with intraspinal hemorrhage, which produces a type of paraplegia similar to that seen following traumatic lesions. The spinal stenosis seen in achondroplasia can cause a hypertonic type of bladder dysfunction; most cases involve the spinal cord at a much higher level than the spinal micturition center. Multiple sclerosis, when present in the pediatric age group, usually is very severe and rapidly progressive.

Pathology

The majority of children with neuropathic bladders have neurospinal dysraphism. Wilcox and Emery [56] found an incidence of 29 percent of renal abnormalities in children with myelomeningocele as compared with 5.3 percent in children having no central nervous system deformity. Apart from dilatation, no intrinsic abnormalities in the ureters have been described.

Pathologic findings in the bladder are those of detrusor hypertrophy or lack of development of the bladder muscle. Various degrees of bladder trabeculation may be visualized. Replacement fibrosis and chronic inflammatory changes may be found. The pathophysiology of the neuropathic bladder depends upon the extent and location of the neurologic abnormality.

Urinary stasis, infection, and relative bladder outflow obstruction and reflux are all interrelated causes of the complications and sequelae of neurogenic bladder dysfunction. Urinary stasis encourages the development of infection and urolithiasis, and relative bladder outflow obstruction causes stasis and overflow incontinence. Bladder filling occurs until intravesical pressure exceeds bladder outflow resistance, irrespective of detrusor tonicity. High intravesical pressures, with or without detrusor hypertonicity or hyperreflexia, cause relative ureterovesical obstruction in some patients and vesicoureteral reflux in others. Both conditions produce back-pressure on the kidney, possibly enhancing the development of pyelonephritis or interstitial nephritis.

Urinary infections may cause fibrosis and contracture of the bladder and bladder neck, enhancing both stasis and relative bladder outflow obstruction. Infection itself may produce upper tract dilatation and vesicoureteral reflux, ultimately leading to pyelonephritis, formation of infective calculi, and renal failure.

Reflux, when present, is either primary or secondary to infection or increased intravesical pressure. With reflux, the protective mechanism of the ureterovesical junction is lost; both intravesical pressures and bacteria are transmitted directly to the kidneys, causing dilatation, pyelonephritis, and interstitial fibrosis.

Clinical Manifestations

One should anticipate and look for a neuropathic bladder in the presence of neurospinal dysraphism, trauma, tumors, or other conditions involving the spinal cord as well as in any neurologic disease. Clinical examination provides much information; however, in the infant evaluation of a neurologic lesion is difficult. The presence of a good urinary stream, either spontaneous, in response to cold or pressure in the suprapubic region, or in response to anal dilatation, indicates an active detrusor muscle sufficient to overcome bladder outflow resistance.

A bladder that is palpable and easy to express is abnormal and indicates a low bladder outflow resistance; a palpable bladder with dribbling urine or a bladder that is difficult to express indicates a normal or relatively high bladder outflow resistance [26].

The presence of residual urine should be established; in small children this can be done by rectal examination. An empty bladder suggests satisfactory emptying by whatever means utilized. The presence of enlarged, hydronephrotic kidneys can be ascertained clinically.

The absence of a normal buttock cleft and the presence of skin dimpling are seen in sacral agenesis (Fig. 101-1). Severe scoliosis, swelling, or a tuft of hair over the lower spine all suggest the presence of spinal defects, with the possibility of bladder involvement.

On neurologic examination, anal sphincter tone and perianal sensation are indicators of probable

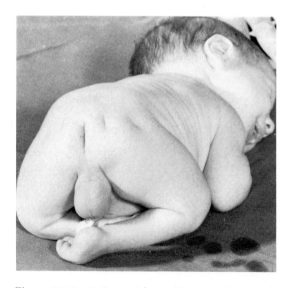

Figure 101-1. Patient with complete sacral agenesis, demonstrating loss of intergluteal cleft and characteristic skin dimpling.

neurogenic bladder dysfunction. Laxity of the anal sphincter and perianal anesthesia are always associated with a neuropathic bladder; however, the reverse is not true. A normal anal sphincter may be associated with normal bladder innervation, although an excessive bladder outflow resistance may be present [26]. A paralyzed bladder may coexist with normal skin sensation, especially when the neural defect is associated with sacral anomalies [51]. A bulbocavernosus reflex indicates that a complete spinal reflex arc is present. This is of use in identifying the type of neurologic deficit. It is also useful in follow-up of patients with traumatic paraplegia. Other modes of presentation are skin ulceration and breakdown due to poor urinary control and the symptomatology of urosepsis or urolithiasis.

Investigations

URINE

Repeated examinations of the urine at regular intervals are essential because most complications of a neuropathic bladder are associated with infection. This is especially important if vesicoureteral reflux is present. Recent tests using fluorescent antihuman globulin antibodies [25] may prove useful in localizing urinary tract infection. The presence of persistent pyuria in a child on antibiotic therapy should alert one to the possibility of urolithiasis or obstruction.

RADIOLOGIC STUDIES

Excretory Urography

This study is the best single investigation for visualizing the entire renal tract, as well as an essential method in the initial evaluation and follow-up of all children with neurogenic bladder dysfunction. Urinary calculi as well as the extent of bony abnormalities can be seen from examination of the scout film. Changes associated with chronic pyelonephritis and hydronephrosis should be noted.

Examination of the bladder outline and filling may provide useful information that is otherwise overlooked. The persistently filled bladder often provides the earliest signs of future upper collecting system decompensation and may suggest the need for improving bladder drainage (Fig. 101-2). One may also learn from this study the size

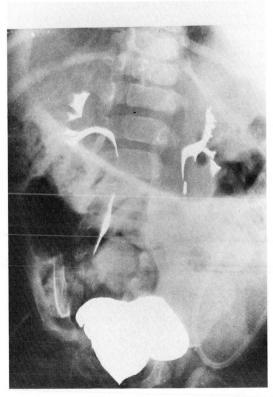
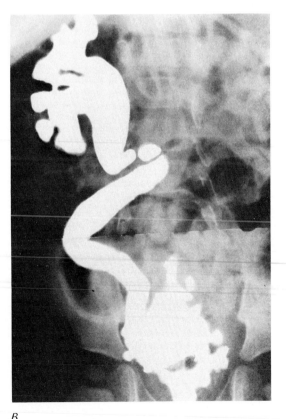

A *B*

Figure 101-2. A. Initial intravenous urogram in infant with lumbosacral myelomeningocele, demonstrating distended bladder. B. Cystogram 8 months later demonstrates massive low pressure vesicoureteral reflux on the right and bladder trabeculation (composite film).

and shape of the bladder and the configuration of the bladder neck and proximal urethra.

Excretory urography should be performed as soon after birth as possible, or as soon as the diagnosis of neuropathic bladder is suspected [26]. Structural abnormalities of the upper urinary tract, such as hydronephrosis or bladder outflow obstruction or both, may be demonstrated and treated promptly. Renal growth can be studied with serial urography [22].

Problems arising from excessive exposure of patients to radiation should be considered; such children invariably require numerous radiologic studies other than those concerned with the urinary tract. Isotope renography may offer a viable alternative to serial radiologic studies [13].

Cystography

Intravenous urography often produces inadequate visualization of the bladder because of incomplete filling or dilution of contrast by residual urine. Cystography is essential, therefore, for a complete evaluation of the lower tract and to confirm the presence or absence of vesicoureteral reflux. Vesicoureteral reflux, commonly associated with myelomeningocele, significantly affects the urologic management [41].

Gross bladder trabeculation, bladder diverticula (see Fig. 101-2B; Fig. 101-3), and the presence of a postvoiding or postexpression residual urine are best demonstrated by cystography. Bladder expression during cystography helps to delineate the lower urinary tract and is especially useful for demonstrating a wide open, incompetent bladder neck and the obstructing external urethral sphincter.

Unfortunately, cystography requires urethral catheterization or instillation of contrast medium by suprapubic puncture; both are potentially hazardous in that they may introduce infection or cause extravasation. The dangers of urethral catheterization are greatest in children with reflux or bladder outflow obstruction, both of which require cystography for accurate delineation. Thus routine cystography, which I advocate, is not recommended universally [12].

Other Radiologic Studies

Loopography is useful for follow-up of children with certain types of urinary diversion if contrast refluxes into the ureters. In conjunction with isotope renography, loopography gives sufficient information for follow-up of these patients, obviating the need for other urographic investigations or renal function tests. Failure to reflux in patients who previously did so suggests urinary obstruction

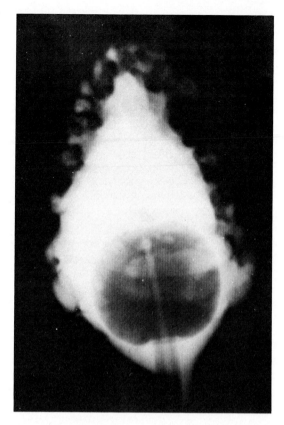

Figure 101-3. Cystogram of so-called Christmas-tree bladder in a 6-year-old girl with lumbar myelomeningocele and neuropathic bladder.

and indicates the need for antegrade urography. Myelography is vital for the diagnosis of spinal dysraphism and confirms the presence or absence of a bony spur in diastematomyelia. Tomography of the spinal cord also may be useful.

ISOTOPE RENOGRAPHY AND CYSTOGRAPHY

Isotope renography and cystography do not give anatomic details comparable to those in excretory urography, but they are useful in demonstrating differential renal function and intrarenal dynamics [13]. Radiation is less than that with uroradiologic studies. Sequential isotope renography studies in conjunction with loopograms or cystograms are particularly useful in children with urinary diversions or reflux. Isotope cystography sometimes demonstrates vesicoureteral reflux that was missed by conventional cystography [11].

URODYNAMIC STUDIES

These studies include cystometry, electromyography, uroflowmetry, and urethral pressure profile.

Cystometry

Cystometry is a technique limited to the evaluation of detrusor muscle function. The precise determination of abnormalities of micturition requires supplemental methods of investigation, including concurrent recording of detrusor and urethral function as well as of urinary flow [48].

The denervation supersensitivity test of Lapides et al. [37] is useful in determining the presence of abnormal bladder innervation as well as the end of the so-called spinal shock phase following spinal cord injury. In children with neuropathic bladder, the cystometer used routinely provides a crude indication of bladder capacity, bladder sensation, and a determinant of the presence or absence of detrusor contraction. Cystometry with anal or periurethral striated muscle electromyography delineates the character of detrusor activity [46].

CYSTOSCOPY

Cystoscopic examination of the neuropathic bladder in children is of little practical use, apart from detecting the presence or absence of vesical calculi and visualizing the trigone and ureteric orifices in children with vesicoureteral reflux. Gross bladder trabeculation, cellule and diverticulum formation, and the appearance of the bladder neck usually can be ascertained by cystography. Determination of bladder capacity under anesthesia sometimes is useful.

Differential Diagnosis

Physical examination usually will differentiate neurogenic bladder dysfunction from other forms of bladder or voiding dysfunction. The bethanechol chloride (Urecholine) supersensitivity test is particularly useful in this regard. Intravenous urography and cystography will demonstrate anatomic causes of urinary incontinence.

Enuresis can be differentiated by an accurate history, physical examination, and cystometrogram unless uninhibited activity is found. Bladder outflow obstruction due to external sphincter dyssynergia can be demonstrated by concomitant cystometrogram and anal sphincter electromyography.

The subclinical or occult neurologic bladder is found in boys with a history of chronic constipation. The cystometrogram may or may not suggest neurogenic bladder dysfunction [57]. Central nervous system examination is entirely normal.

Course of Neuropathic Bladder

Infection develops in the majority of patients, and if untreated, ultimately leads to fibrosis and bladder contracture. Infection can also cause vesicoureteral reflux, upper tract dilatation, and ulti-mately, pyelonephritis and renal failure. Intensive antibiotic therapy may reverse such upper tract dilatation [59].

Over time, an increasing number of children develop relative bladder outflow obstruction [53]. The hypothesis that, in the absence of infection, upper tract deterioration is due primarily to poor drainage is confirmed by that fact that upper tracts show improvement with improved drainage by diversion, catheterization, or diminished bladder outflow resistance.

Renal failure in adults with traumatic neuropathic bladder is an important cause of morbidity and mortality. In children, however, this is not as well defined. Eckstein found only 31 of 373 children with myelomeningocele and hydrocephalus to have died as a result of renal failure [15].

Management

The two goals in the management of the neuropathic bladder are (1) to preserve renal function, and (2) to retain or achieve urinary control. Preservation of renal function depends upon prevention or elimination of urinary infection, reduction or elimination of residual urine, and prevention of the effects of back-pressure from bladder to kidney. All these factors are important from birth onward.

Acquisition of urinary control is a later objective in the management of neuropathic bladder, with a view to achieving success by the time the child starts school. Unfortunately, some school systems will admit only continent children to regular classes. No single plan can be suggested for all children because of the variable functional and pathologic status of the urinary tract and motor and intellectual handicaps. Parental motivation, availability of follow-up care, and the psychological needs of the child must be considered in the selection of an appropriate treatment plan.

BLADDER EXPRESSION

Correct selection of patients for bladder expression is the most important aspect of this form of treatment. Less important are the methods of applying pressure in the suprapubic area to achieve bladder emptying [42]. A bladder consistently empty by clinical examination obviously will not benefit by being expressed. High intravesical pressure, associated with residual urine is a definite contraindication to bladder expression. The presence of vesicoureteral reflux is another absolute contraindication to expression, since the excessively high intravesical pressures produced during expression are transmitted directly to the kidney (Fig. 101-4). A large residual urine volume fol-

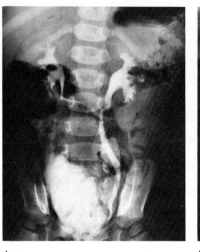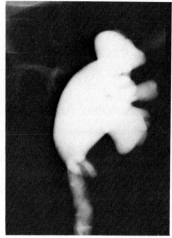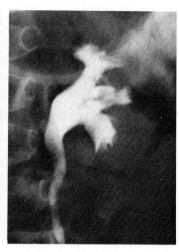

A   *B*

Figure 101-4. A. Intravenous urogram of a 30-month-old girl with sacral myelomeningocele. B. Cystogram showing low pressure reflux on right and acute hydronephrosis on left produced by suprapubic pressure.

lowing expression, when the abdominal wall is relaxed, usually indicates bladder outflow obstruction and also contraindicates bladder expression.

DRUG TREATMENT

Drugs cannot replace loss of innervation. Bladder function may be improved by medication, however, and thus drugs may make possible acceptable urinary control [10].

Urecholine (bethanechol chloride) may be useful in reducing residual urine and thus in controlling urinary infection. Imipramine has been found to increase functional bladder capacity and to obviate the need for urinary diversion for the purpose of continence [10]. Anticholinergics such as methanthelene bromide (Banthine) or propantheline bromide (Pro-Banthine) can increase functional bladder capacity. Oxybutynin chloride [14] has been documented as being useful in overcoming uninhibited contractions and in increasing functional bladder capacity, thus producing continence. Functional bladder neck obstruction may be relieved by the use of alpha-sympatholytic agents such as phenoxybenzamine. Minor degrees of stress incontinence may be improved by alpha-stimulating agents such as phenylephrine [31, 32]. Imipramine, Banthine, or oxybutynin chloride may be used in conjunction with intermittent catheterization. Infection may reduce functional bladder capacity; this can be reversed by appropriate antibiotic therapy.

CATHETER DRAINAGE

Continuous catheter drainage should be used only as a temporary expedient to divert urine in patients with decubiti or undergoing orthopedic surgery, to control persistent infection, to rapidly decompress the upper urinary tract, or when reflux is present. The long-term problems of indwelling catheter drainage are well known.

The use of sterile intermittent catheterization from the time of injury is a well-established and effective approach to the management of patients with acute spinal cord injuries. This procedure should be initiated as soon as possible in all patients with neuropathic bladder dysfunction secondary to spinal cord trauma [20].

Clean intermittent catheterization [35, 36] is the treatment of choice for selected patients with neurogenic bladder dysfunction. Its use in over 125 children at Newington Children's Hospital from October, 1972, to the present time has resulted in a declining incidence of severe urinary infections and a significant increase in the number of continent children.

An increasing number of patients benefit from intermittent catheterization by either increasing the functional bladder capacity or increasing the bladder outflow resistance. This may be achieved in selected patients by the use of drugs or surgery. Surgery designed to tighten the bladder neck, to augment the size of the bladder, or to create a suprapubic catheterizing vesicostomy await the test of time. The psychological aspects of repeated catheterization are an important though still undefined factor.

After a trial of intermittent catheterization, many boys benefit from surgery to create a perineal urethrostomy [44]. The advantages of the transperineal route of catheterization are that it reduces trauma and permits the use of a larger catheter, important in small boys. A short, rigid catheter permits one-handed catheterization, an important factor in children who have neuromuscular impairment of the lower extremities and who require one hand for balance or support. The older child may sit or stand over a toilet bowl. A perineal urethrostomy is completely reversible and is similar to a first-stage urethroplasty.

URINAL

No suitable external collecting device has been developed for females. In larger boys, a condom-type appliance attached to a leg bag affords adequate urinary control if the phallus is of adequate size. Satisfactory light-weight pediatric urinals have been devised [21, 28b] employing a condom-type appliance pressed against the suprapubic area and some are modified with an interposed karaya gum seal [29]. A suspensory applies external pressure to ensure a good seal. The disadvantage of wearing a cumbersome apparatus is obvious. A urinal is suitable for males who have a small bladder residual volume and who do not have excessive bladder outflow resistance. The advantages are that diversionary surgery may be avoided and continence achieved.

INFECTION AND REFLUX

Infection of the urinary tract is usually an indication that some sort of drainage procedure is required to eliminate stasis. A loaded rectum may prevent complete bladder emptying, either spontaneously or by expression. Stasis, the most common etiologic factor in infection of the intact urinary tract, may require intermittent catheterization or bladder outlet surgery to improve drainage. Urinary tract calculi should be removed if possible.

The role of antireflux surgery in children with neurogenic bladder dysfunction is controversial. Some urologists believe that standard reflux-preventing procedures have little place in the management of reflux in these children [16]. Minor degrees of reflux can be improved by reducing bladder outflow resistance through urethral dilatation or internal urethrotomy. Other urologists, including me, believe that antireflux surgery often is successful, especially when intravesical pressure is low. Bladder expression then can be instituted or intermittent catheterization utilized, thereby avoiding more drastic surgical procedures to achieve continence [27].

HIGH BLADDER OUTFLOW RESISTANCE

Relative bladder outlet obstruction may cause both renal functional impairment and urinary incontinence. The site of obstruction in most cases is at the level of the external urinary sphincter. Johnston and Kathel [28] recommend urethral dilation for infants with persistently distended nonexpressible bladders. They found that 12 percent of 219 newborns required this treatment. In infant boys the proximal urethral sphincter may be approached through a perineal urethrostomy. Urethral dilation may be useful in older girls, but it is likely to be successful only before changes in the urethra, bladder, and upper urinary tract have become fixed (Fig. 101-5).

Transurethral sphincterotomy is a very satisfactory method of reducing bladder outflow obstruction due to external sphincter hyperactivity [30]. Infant resectoscopes have made transurethral resection possible even in male neonates. The external sphincter may be approached through the perineum; the urogenital diaphragm and external sphincter then can be incised directly [37]. This method avoids disturbing the integrity of the urethral mucosa and the possible development of a urethral diverticulum.

Bladder neck resections or YV-plasties to enlarge the bladder outflow have a very limited place in the management of the obstructed neuropathic bladder, because the obstruction invariably is distal to the bladder neck [26]. Pudendal neurectomy has been advocated by some investigators with the rationale of dividing the sphincteric muscle innervation [50]. The operation is much more difficult technically than sphincterotomy and, if successful, results in future impotence.

Excessive lowering of the bladder outflow resistance may induce incontinence in children who otherwise might be continent by means of bladder expression, raising intraabdominal pressure, or intermittent catheterization. Surgical procedures to lower outflow resistance, therefore, are best reserved for the boy with a small bladder capacity who will become a candidate for a urinal or condom type of urinary collecting device.

LOW BLADDER OUTFLOW RESISTANCE

Various methods have been employed to increase functional bladder capacity by increasing the bladder outflow resistance. Drugs, reconstructive surgery, electrical stimulation, and artificial sphincters have all been utilized for this purpose. Imipramine has been found to increase bladder outflow resistance. Surgical reconstruction of the bladder neck, if successful, will usually require subsequent intermittent catheterization for satisfactory emptying of the bladder.

Some success with an implantable stimulator has been reported in children with congenital neu-

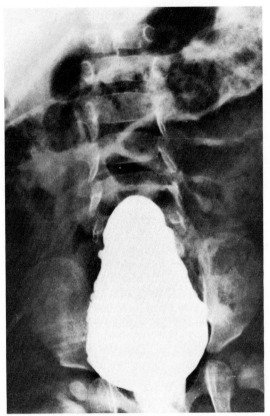
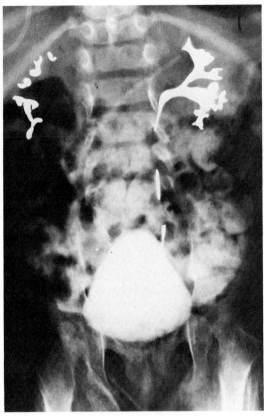

A   *B*

Figure 101-5. A. Cystogram in same patient as in Figure 101-2 14 months later, after urethral dilatation. B. Intravenous urogram.

rogenic bladder dysfunction [9]. Complications appear to be excessively high, with mechanical problems such as fracturing of wires and physical problems such as seromas, adductor muscle spasms, and infection. Growth in children necessitates replacement or revision of wiring, and the long-term effects of continual muscle stimulation are uncertain. An anal plug with circular electrodes [23] does not require any surgical procedure and functions in the same way as the implanted stimulator.

Fair success with the Scott artificial sphincter has been reported [47]. Use of this device may emerge as a suitable long-term method for achieving urinary control; however, insertion of these devices should be limited to a relatively few experienced centers. The long-term effects of tissue compression by the inflated sphincter have not yet been reported. Caution is advised with respect to children who will require revision or replacement of components to allow for growth.

SMALL BLADDER CAPACITY

The functional bladder capacity can be enlarged directly, in addition to the indirect methods of increasing bladder outflow resistance [1, 10]. Intestinal augmentation cystoplasties have been described, and short-term success has been reported [24]. I have used the bowel to enlarge a neuropathic bladder in a few children, utilizing intermittent catheterization to empty the bladder, and children with competent ureterovesical valves and adequate bladder outflow resistance have been treated successfully. Ureteroileocecal cystoplasty for correction of vesicoureteral reflux as well as for bladder augmentation has been less successful; however, the procedure can be converted to a ureterocecal urinary conduit at a later date if necessary [28a].

ELECTRICAL STIMULATION OF BLADDER MUSCLE

Attempts at electrical stimulation of the detrusor muscle to produce a voiding contraction are based on the erroneous assumption that bladder evacuation is effected by means of a simple mass contraction. This explains the lack of success of such devices [5].

URINARY DIVERSION

Urinary diversion may be indicated for progressive upper tract dilatation in children with neurogenic bladder dysfunction and for incontinence in children who cannot be managed by methods outlined earlier.

Vesicostomy

Vesicostomy [34] is a simple procedure technically, but long-term results have been disappointing. Unfortunately, stomal stenosis and prolapse are common, residual urine is not eliminated, and fitting of appliances is difficult in children and worse in adults. Temporary vesicostomy in infants is more satisfactory prior to permanent supravesical diversion [39] or onset of clean intermittent catheterization.

Cutaneous Ureterostomy

Cutaneous ureterostomy is the simplest form of supravesical urinary diversion without intubation, provided that the ureters are permanently dilated. The ureters can be brought to the skin separately, as a double-barreled stoma in the midline, or together as a Y-shaped ureterocutaneous diversion. Drainage is satisfactory, and bowel resection is avoided [58]. Stomal problems are common, but they can be minimized by incorporating skin flaps into the stoma.

Supravesical Ureterointestinal Urinary Diversions

The ileal conduit was popularized by Bricker [7] for urinary tract diversion in bladder malignancy and as an alternative to ureterosigmoidostomy. Early success of this procedure encouraged its adoption in the management of neurogenic bladder dysfunction, first in adults and later in children. Since then, the ileal conduit has become the most popular urinary diversion for the neuropathic bladder, especially in females with a totally incontinent small bladder. In boys, however, the procedure is often questionable [17].

Because the prognosis for children undergoing intestinal diversion is best if the diversion is performed prior to the onset of upper urinary tract changes, very early urinary diversion has been advocated [53]. Pyelographic and functional improvements have been seen in many children who have undergone such urinary diversion [15]. The question remains, however, whether such improvements could have been achieved simply by relieving the bladder outflow obstruction and improving drainage.

The complexity of the diversion procedure lends itself to numerous modifications and techniques. Current techniques utilize a small, isolated segment of bowel, either ileum or sigmoid colon [40], interposed between the ureters and skin. Ureteroileal anastomoses usually reflux. Antireflux procedures may be incorporated into ureterocolonic anastomoses. The stoma usually is situated in the lower abdomen.

Psychological factors should be considered when planning a urinary diversion. Early diversion—before school age—has the advantage of easier acceptance. An older child or adolescent who decides to undergo the procedure will be gratified to achieve urinary control.

Aside from psychological aspects, the morbidity from urinary diversion is exceedingly high. Early complications include bowel obstruction, anastomotic leaks, wound dehiscence, wound infection, conduit necrosis, and acute pyelonephritis. Later complications include chronic pyelonephritis, progressive renal functional deterioration, urolithiasis, electrolyte imbalance, stomal problems (especially stenosis), ureterointestinal stenosis, pyocystis, and malodor [45].

A 10-year follow-up of patients at the Boston Children's Medical Center revealed that only 13.2 percent of children remained free of complications following urinary diversion [49]. The high morbidity associated with urinary diversion procedures has caused a decline in the frequency of these procedures in favor of simpler forms of treatment such as intermittent catheterization.

Prognosis

The prognosis in neurogenic bladder dysfunction in children, unlike that in adults, may be unrelated to the urinary tract [38]. Renal failure was a major contributing cause in less than 10 percent of children who died from myelomeningocele [18]. The prognosis in children is related more to spinal stability and associated pulmonary reserve. Nevertheless, the prognosis for children who have progressive upper tract dilation, infection, and calculus disease, with or without urinary diversion, is guarded and is dependent upon the potential reversibility of these changes.

References

1. Ambrose, S. S., and Swanson, H. S. The hypertonic neurogenic bladder in children: Its sequelae and management. *J. Urol.* 83:672, 1960.
2. Bors, E., and Comarr, A. E. *Neurological Urology.* Baltimore: University Park Press, 1971. P. 31.
3. Bors, E., and Comarr, A. E. *Neurological Urology.*

Baltimore: University Park Press, 1971. Chap. 6, p. 182.

4. Boyarski, S. (ed.). *The Neurogenic Bladder*. Baltimore: Williams & Wilkins, 1967.

5. Bradley, W. E., Timm, G. M., and Chou, S. N. A decade of experience with electronic stimulation of the micturition reflex. *Urol. Int.* 26:897, 1971.

6. Bradley, W. E., Timm, G. W., and Scott, F. B. Innervation of the Detrusor Muscle and Urethra. In J. Lapides (ed.), *Symposium on Neurogenic Bladder. Urol. Clin. North Am.* 1 (1):3, 1974.

7. Bricker, E. M. Substitution for the urinary bladder by the use of isolated ileal segments. *Surg. Clin. North Am.* 36:117, 1950.

8. Brocklehurst, G. The pathogenesis of spina bifida: A study of the relationship between observation, hypothesis, and surgical incentive. *Dev. Med. Child Neurol.* 13:147, 1971.

9. Caldwell, K. P., Martin, M. R., Flack, F. C., and James, E. D. An alternative method of dealing with incontinence in children with neurogenic bladders. *Arch. Dis. Child.* 102:625, 1969.

10. Cole, A. T., and Fried, F. A. Favorable experience with imipramine in the treatment of neurogenic bladder. *J. Urol.* 107:44, 1972.

11. Conway, J. J., Belman, A. B., King, L. R., and Filmer, R. B. Direct and indirect radionuclide cystography. *J. Urol.* 113:689, 1975.

12. Cooper, D. G. Urinary tract infections in children with myelomeningocele. *Arch. Dis. Child.* 42:521, 1967.

13. Cudmore, R. E., and Zachary, R. B. The renogram and the renal tract in spina bifida. *Dev. Med. Child Neurol.* (Suppl. 22) 12:24, 1970.

14. Diokno, A. C., and Lapides, J. Oxybutynin: A new drug with analgesic and anticholinergic properties. *J. Urol.* 108:307, 1972.

15. Eckstein, H. B. Urinary control in children with myelomeningocele. *Br. J. Urol.* 40:191, 1968.

16. Eckstein, H. B. Neuropathic Bladder. In D. I. Williams (ed.), *Urology in Childhood*. Berlin: Springer, 1974. Chap. S, p. 258.

17. Eckstein, H. B. Urinary diversion in children. *Dev. Med. Child Neurol.* 7:167, 1965.

18. Eckstein, H. B., Cooper, D. G., Howard, E. R., and Pike, J. Cause of death in children with myelomeningocele or hydrocephalus. *Arch. Dis. Child.* 42: 163, 1967.

19. Elbadawi, A., and Schenk, E. A. A new theory of the innervation of the bladder musculature: Part 1. Morphology of the intrinsic vesical innervation apparatus. *J. Urol.* 99:585, 1968.

20. Guttman, L. Statistical survey on one thousand paraplegics and initial treatment of traumatic paraplegia. *Proc. R. Soc. Med.* 47:1099, 1954.

21. Hill, M. L., and Shurtleff, D. B. A device for collecting urine in incontinent male children. *Am. J. Dis. Child.* 116:158, 1968.

22. Hodson, C. J., Drewe, J. A., Karn, M. N., and King, A. Renal size in normal children: A radiographic study during life. *Arch. Dis. Child.* 37:616, 1962.

23. Hopkinson, B. R. Electrical treatment of incontinence. *Ann. R. Coll. Surg. Engl.* 50:92, 1972.

24. Hradec, E. Beiträge zur chirurgischen Behandlung neurogener Störungen der Harnblase. *Z. Urol.* 57:97, 1964.

25. Jones, S. R., Smith, J. W., and Sanford, J. P. Localization of urinary tract infections by detection of antibody coated bacteria in urine sediment. *N. Engl. J. Med.* 290:591, 1974.

26. Johnston, J. H. The neurogenic bladder in the newborn infant. *Paraplegia* 6:157, 1968.

27. Johnston, J. H., and Farkas, A. Practicalities and possibilities in conservative management. *Urology* 5:719, 1975.

28. Johnston, J. H., and Kathel, B. L. The obstructed neurogenic bladder in the newborn. *Br. J. Urol.* 43: 206, 1971.

28a. Klauber, G. T. Combined Surgery and Intermittent Catheterization for Neurogenic Bladder Dysfunction in Children. In *Urinary System Malformations in Children*. Proceedings of the International Pediatric Urological Seminar. New York: Alan R. Liss, Inc., 1977.

28b. Klauber, G. T., and Evans, A. I. Pubic pressure urinal for the incontinent male adult and child. *Urology* 9:562, 1977.

29. Klauber, G. T., and Lund, S. T. New pediatric male urinal. *Pediatrics* 55:134, 1975.

30. Koontz, W. W., Jr., Smith, M. J., and Currie, R. J. External sphincterotomy in boys with myelomeningocele. *J. Urol.* 108:649, 1972.

31. Krane, R. J., and Olsson, C. A. Phenoxybenzamine in neurogenic bladder dysfunction: Part 1. A theory of micturition. *J. Urol.* 110:650, 1973.

32. Krane, R. J., and Olsson, C. A. Phenoxybenzamine in neurogenic bladder dysfunction: Part 2. Clinical consideration. *J. Urol.* 110:653, 1973.

33. Lapides, J. (ed.). *Symposium on Neurogenic Bladder. Urol. Clin. North Am.* 1(1):45, 1974.

34. Lapides, J., Ajemian, E. P., and Lichtwardt, G. R. Cutaneous vesicostomy. *J. Urol.* 84:609, 1960.

35. Lapides, J., Diokno, A. C., Lowe, B. S., and Kalish, M. D. Follow-up on unsterile intermittent self-catheterization. *J. Urol.* 111:184, 1974.

36. Lapides, J., Diokno, A. C., Silber, S. J., and Lowe, B. S. Clean intermittent self-catheterization in the treatment of urinary tract disease. *J. Urol.* 107:458, 1972.

37. Lapides, J., Friend, C. R., Ajemian, E. P., and Reus, W. S. Denervation supersensitivity as a test for neurogenic bladder. *Surg. Gynecol. Obstet.* 114:241, 1962.

38. Lorber, J., and Lyons, V. H. Arterial hypertension in children with spina bifida cystica and urinary incontinence. *Dev. Med. Child Neurol.* (Suppl. 22) 12:101, 1970.

39. Lytton, B., and Weiss, R. M. Cutaneous vesicostomy for temporary urinary diversion in infants. *J. Urol.* 165:888, 1971.

40. Mogg, R. A. Treatment of neurogenic urinary incontinence using the colonic conduit. *Br. J. Urol.* 37: 681, 1965.

41. Nergardh, A., Ericsson, N. O., Hellstrom, B., and Rudhe, U. The urinary tract in neonates with myelomeningocele: Neurological and radiological correlative study. *Dev. Med. Child Neurol.* (Suppl. 25) 13: 125, 1971.

42. Perkarovic, E., Robinson, A., Zachary, R. B., and Lister, J. Indications for manual expression of the neurogenic bladder in children. *Br. J. Urol.* 42:191, 1970.

43. Plum, F. Autonomous urinary bladder activity in normal man. *Arch. Neurol.* 2:497, 1960.
44. Rabinovitch, H. H. Bladder evacuation in child with myelomeningocele. *Urology* 3:425, 1974.
45. Retik, A. B., Perlmutter, A. D., and Gross, R. E. Cutaneous uretero-ileostomy in children. *N. Engl. J. Med.* 277:217, 1967.
46. Scott, F. B., Bradley, W. E., and Timm, G. W. Sphincter Electromyography. In J. Lapides (ed.), *Symposium on Neurogenic Bladder. Urol. Clin. North Am.* 1 (1):69, 1974.
47. Scott, F. B., Bradley, W. E., and Timm, G. W. Treatment of urinary incontinence by an implantable prosthetic urinary sphincter. *J. Urol.* 112:75, 1974.
48. Scott, F. B., Quesada, E., and Cardus, D. Studies of the dynamics of micturition: Observations on healthy men. *J. Urol.* 92:455, 1965.
49. Shapiro, S. R., Liebowitz, R., and Colodny, A. H. Fate of 90 children with ileal conduit urinary diversion a decade later; analysis of complications, pyelography, renal function and bacteriology. *J. Urol.* 114:289, 1975.
50. Smart, P. J. Spasm of the external urethral sphincter in spina bifida. *Br. J. Urol.* 37:574, 1965.
51. Smith, E. D. Congenital Sacral Defects. In F. D. Stephens (ed.), *Congenital Malformations of the Rectum, Anus and Genitourinary Tracts.* Edinburgh: Livingstone, 1963. Chap. 5, p. 82.
52. Smith, E. D. *Spina Bifida and the Total Care of Spinal Myelomeningocele.* Springfield, Ill.: Thomas, 1965.
53. Smith, E. D. Follow-up studies on 150 ileal conduits in children. *J. Pediatr. Surg.* 7:1, 1972.
54. Tang, P. C., and Ruch, T. C. Non-neurogenic basis of bladder tone. *Am. J. Physiol.* 181:249, 1955.
55. White, R. I., and Klauber, G. T. Sacral agenesis: An analysis of twenty-two cases. *Urology* 8:521, 1976.
56. Wilcox, A. R., and Emery, J. L. Deformities of the renal tract in children with myelomeningocele and hydrocephalus, compared with those of children showing no such central nervous system deformities. *Br. J. Urol.* 42:152, 1970.
57. Williams, D. I., Hirst, G., and Doyle, D. The occult neuropathic bladder. *J. Pediatr. Surg.* 9:35, 1974.
58. Williams, D. I., and Rabinovitch, H. H. Cutaneous ureterostomy for the grossly dilated ureter of childhood. *Br. J. Urol.* 40:696, 1968.
59. Zachary, R. B., and Lister, J. Conservative Management of the Neurogenic Bladder. In J. H. Johnston and R. J. Scholtmeijer (eds.), *Problems in Pediatric Urology.* Amsterdam: Excerpta Medica, 1972. Chap. 5, p. 121.

102. Hypospadias

Alan D. Perlmutter

Of the developmental anomalies affecting the penis, hypospadias is by far the most common. The word *hypospadias* derives from the Greek words *hypo* (under) and *spadon* (rent or fissure) and indicates that the urethral meatus opens on the undersurface of the penis, proximal to its normal location within the glans (see Fig. 102-1). The prepuce is absent ventrally and is hooded and flaplike dorsally. The skin of the ventral shaft tends to be tion within the glans (see Fig. 102-1). The preventral curvature (chordee) becomes more apparent during erection, and when severe, intercourse is difficult or impossible. The distal urethra lacks a surrounding corpus spongiosum. Fibrous tissue splaying out distally on the ventral shaft beyond the meatus and sometimes extending proximally, deep to the urethra, contributes to or creates the chordee in most cases.

As is typical of all congenital malformations, hypospadias has a spectrum of severity ranging from a slightly dystopic meatus still within the glans and with no associated chordee, to extreme genital ambiguity with a hypoplastic phallus, a bifid scrotum, and a scrotal or perineal meatus.

States of intersex with genital ambiguity will not be discussed in this chapter.

History

Ancient writings demonstrate a fascination with genital disorders and anomalies, but it was not until the first two centuries A.D. that the Alexandrian surgeons Heliodorus and Antyllus first described a surgical approach for treatment of male hypospadias. To relieve chordee and permit coitus, they described "resection," an amputation of the glans penis, followed by shaping of the tip of the penile stump with a hot cautery to simulate a glans. During the Middle Ages, in the eleventh century A.D., Albucasis described an incision into the glans to reshape the hypospadiac meatus and glans. During the Renaissance, Lusitanus created a glandular urethra by penetrating the glans and distal penile shaft with a silver cannula and waiting for healing to occur. Ambroise Paré recognized the nature of chordee and described cutting the "ligament" to relieve penile curvature.

It was not until the late nineteenth century, however, that the modern era of hypospadias reconstruction began with the evolution of staged surgical procedures to correct chordee and then to reconstruct a distal urethra. Duplay and Ombré-danne described the use of local skin flaps for ure-thral reconstruction, and Nove-Josserand utilized an inlay skin graft to extend the urethra. In 1913 Edmunds was the first to transfer the prepuce ventrally at the time of chordee release for use in urethroplasty at a later stage. The many procedures and refinements that have evolved over the years all stem from the fundamental contributions of these surgical pioneers [16, 33].

Classification and Incidence

Although a number of systems for classifying hypospadias have been proposed, a simple, clinically useful classification [15] is based on the position of the urethral meatus: glandular or coronal, distal penile, proximal penile, penoscrotal, and perineal (Figs. 102-1, 102-2). In addition to the location of the meatus, classification includes a description of the location and severity of the chordee: chordee of the glans; mild, diffuse chordee of the shaft; and severe, diffuse chordee. The more extreme degrees of hypospadias are also associated with a bifid scrotum and small penile size. In these severe cases, a variable degree of penoscrotal transposition exists, and in the most marked form, the scrotal compartments fuse cephalad to the penile shaft.

The incidence of hypospadias has been reported to be from 1.0 to 3.3 per 1,000 live births [5, 31, 36, 38]. Although the frequency of various degrees of hypospadias varies somewhat from series to series, partly because of differences in classification, in all series the frequency decreases with increasing severity. The vast majority of cases are

coronal or distal penile, and less than 10 percent are perineal [36, 38].

Counterclockwise torsion of the penile shaft is present in a minority of cases of hypospadias. Ventral skin webbing alone occasionally creates chordee. In rare cases curvature results from asymmetric growth of the corpora cavernosa [38].

Congenital ventral curvature (chordee) also occurs in the presence of a normal meatus and prepuce. Although this condition does not strictly conform to the definition of hypospadias, congenital ventral curvature is generally included in a discussion of hypospadias, since the embryogenesis of chordee, the anatomic findings, and the surgical treatment all bear some relationship to typical hypospadias. Chordee without hypospadias comprises up to 10 percent of cases in most series [9, 39].

Horton and Devine [14] have described three degrees of isolated chordee. In the most severe form, the corpus spongiosum is deficient in the area of chordee, with a thin, membranous urethra beneath the skin and dense fibrous tissue deep to the urethra causing the chordee. In the intermediate form, the corpus spongiosum surrounding the urethra is normally developed, but thickening and fibrous tissue involving the dartos and Buck's fasciae contribute to the curvature. In the mildest form, only the dartos fascia is fibrous and abnormally developed lateral to the urethra. Some authors consider a congenitally short urethra to be one cause of isolated chordee [27, 29, 30], and some report that deficient skin alone occasionally produces this abnormality (with or without hypospadias [24, 35].

Embryology

By the fourth week of development (Fig. 102-3*a*) the cloacal membrane is surrounded by a thickening of mesenchyme, representing ingrowth of mesoderm between the layers of ectoderm and entoderm. As development progresses, this thickening splits into a medial urethral or genital fold on each side—the future anterior urethra in the male and labia minora in the female—and a more lateral genital swelling—the future scrotum of the male and the labia majora of the female. Cranially, a more localized thickening of mesenchyme on each side coalesces to form a central genital tubercle.

By the sixth to seventh week the cloaca is divided into the ventral bladder and dorsal rectum by the descent of the urorectal fold, which also divides the cloacal membrane into the urogenital and anal membranes (Fig. 102-3*b*). At 7 weeks the urogenital membrane ruptures, forming the urogenital sinus. The genital tubercle grows out-

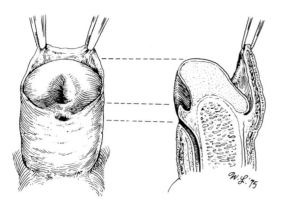

Figure 102-1. Typical hypospadias showing ventral meatus, blind glandular pit, and hooded prepuce that is deficient ventrally. Chordee is not demonstrated in this drawing.

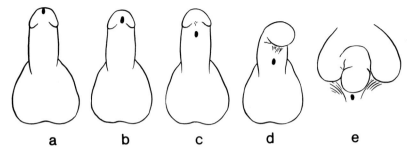

Figure 102-2. Degrees of hypospadias. a, *Normal meatus;* b, *coronal or glandular;* c, *distal shaft;* d, *proximal shaft;* e, *perineal, with bifid scrotum and penoscrotal transposition. (Penoscrotal hypospadias is not depicted).*

ward and elongates into a definitive phallus. An extension of entodermally derived urogenital sinus tissue, called the urethral plate, is drawn out between the urethral folds and becomes the roof of the definitive anterior urethra.

Both male and female fetuses progress through phases of identical development, termed the *indifferent stage,* until about the tenth week. At this time (Fig. 102-3c) in the male there is elongation of the phallus and its ventral urethral groove, progressive fusion of the urethral folds from proximal to distal, and posterior migration of the scrotal swellings (Fig. 102-3d). As the scrotal swellings meet caudally, they fuse to form the definitive scrotum and the scrotal raphe.

During the outgrowth of the phallus, differentiating mesenchyme forms the two erectile bodies (corpora cavernosa) and the unpaired erectile tissue (corpus spongiosum) surrounding the urethra. By the fourteenth week, the urethra has closed to the base of the glans and temporarily has

no external opening. The urethral plate tissue at the depth of the urethral groove extends into the glans as a solid core of tissue. The tip of the glans at this time is still uncovered and is identified by an epithelial tag [4, 8, 38].

There is disagreement as to the precise origin of the glandular portion of the urethra, but more than simple fusion of urethral folds is involved. Arey [4] states that canalization of solid epithelium internally from the urethral plate, plus a trough formation externally, produces a tube extending the urethra to the top of the glans. Glenister [12] believes that canalization occurs from ingrowing ectoderm. The differing origin of the glandular urethra, as contrasted with the progressive, outward fusion of urethral folds for the penile portion, may explain the frequent finding of a blind urethral sinus or pit within the groove of the glans or coronal margin, distal to the termination of a hypospadic meatus.

The prepuce arises during the third month from

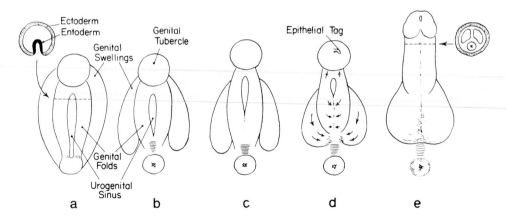

Figure 102-3. Normal embryology of penis. a, b. *Indifferent stage at 4 and 6 weeks.* c. *Early masculinization at 10 weeks.* d. *Progressive growth of phallus, fusion of urethral folds, and posterior migration of scrotal swellings.* e. *Newborn with completed genital development. Cross section of the penis depicts the well-developed erectile bodies and corpus spongiosum surrounding the urethra. Penile skin and fascia are distinct from deeper structures.*

a heaping up of skin dorsally at the base of the glans. This fold of skin overgrows the glans, flowing over it dorsally, then laterally, and finally ventrally, to cover the glans. The ventral coalescence of the prepuce forms a frenulum [17].

From the description of normal embryogenesis, it is apparent that hypospadias can result from any delay or arrest in the normal sequence of external genital development, causing the urethra to open proximally and the prepuce to be incomplete ventrally. Maleness is an induced phenomenon, and lack of a sufficient stimulus to male development will result in a more female form of phallic development, with in-curving beyond the hypospadic meatus. Fibrosis of the urethral plate distal to the hypospadias and associated failure of the ventral mesenchyme to differentiate into corpus spongiosum and Buck's and dartos fasciae results in a fibrous layer ventrally, causing chordee. In more severe forms of hypospadias, decreased or failed migration of the scrotal swellings, with a posteriorly dislocated primordial genital tubercle in the most extreme cases, gives rise to a variable degree of bifid scrotum and penoscrotal transposition.

Ventral penile curvature, or chordee without hypospadias, can occur when the urethra forms fully but there is some degree of failed mesenchymal differentiation. In the most severe example of hypospadias there is absence of the corpus spongiosum and fibrous coalescence of the anlage of the corpus spongiosum and Buck's and dartos fasciae; with lesser cases there is development of corpus spongiosum but with coalescence of Buck's and dartos fasciae ventrally; in the mildest form there is fibrosis only of the dartos fascia superficial to the urethra. Figure 102-4 diagrams fascial planes in a normal penis, in moderate chordee without hypospadias, and in typical hypospadias.

Ventral curvature of the phallus is a normal stage of embryogenesis [12, 19]. In a study of 46 fetuses, Kaplan and Lamm [23] noted ventral curvature in 41 and observed that it persisted longer than previously thought, well into the third trimester in some fetuses. On histologic study, none had abnormal ventral fibrous tissue. They proposed that some clinical cases of isolated chordee may be a simple arrest of normal embryologic development, without defective mesenchymal differentiation. If the persistent chordee is due to differential growth of the dorsal and ventral portions of the corpora cavernosa, it is correctable by mobilization of the ventral skin alone or by plication of the dorsal tunica albuginea.

Detailed discussion of the embryogenesis of the ventral penile integument to explain deviations of the penile raphes, torsion of the penis, and congenital urethral fistula is beyond the scope of this review, and interested readers are referred elsewhere [38].

Absence of the fetal testes results in phenotypically female external genitalia; impaired fetal testicular function results in altered development of the male external genitalia with hypospadias [20, 21]. Although progestational agents ingested by the mother in early pregnancy have resulted in hypospadias [1], such agents are now rarely used. Some severe forms of hypospadias are associated with clinically obvious hypogonadism and sexual ambiguity, but gonadal defects are not apparent in milder cases. In a study of plasma testosterone in human fetuses, Abramovich [2] observed that values in the males remained high from 12 to 18 weeks of gestation, coincident with the critical stage of the formation of the urethra. He proposed that some cases of human hypospadias might be caused by an androgen defect. A decrease in hu-

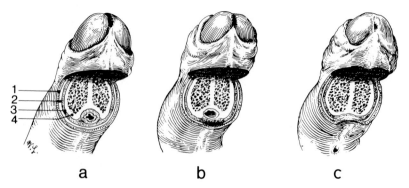

1
2
3
4

a   b   c

Figure 102-4. a. *Cross section of the normal penis.* 1, *Skin;* 2, *dartos fascia;* 3, *Buck's fascia surrounding the corpora cavernosa and corpus spongiosum;* 4, *tunica albuginea (capsule) of corpora cavernosa.* b. *Cross section of chordee without hypospadias. In this depiction the corpus spongiosum is absent and the Buck's and dartos fasciae are fused ventrally.* c. *Cross section of typical hypospadias with chordee distal to meatus. Buck's and dartos fasciae are fused ventrally, and the midline skin is adherent and thin.*

man chorionic gonadotropin during this stage similarly would decrease the stimulus to male external genital development, although this hypothesis is unproved. Roberts and Lloyd [32] identified a cyclic pattern in the incidence of hypospadias and proposed a seasonal variation in maternal gonadotropin production as a cause. Data regarding the seasonal incidence of hypospadias is conflicting, however, and a seasonal variation has not been well documented [5, 31, 32, 37].

Genetics

Most hypospadias presents as an isolated abnormality not associated with anomalies outside the genitourinary tract. Chromosomal studies in patients with hypospadias have revealed normal karyotypes [22], although there are some exceptions [26]. Chen and Woolley [7] studied 26 patients with hypospadias and detected 3 with abnormal karyotypes; each of these had other anomalies. They concluded from their own series and from other reports in the literature that they could not establish a relationship between specific chromosomal abnormalities and hypospadias. Hypospadias occurs occasionally as one manifestation of multiple phenotypic defects; long-arm "Q" chromosome deletions of 5, 13, or 21 have been implicated [25].

Simple hypospadias occurs in families [7], with a risk to male siblings, excluding twins, of about 10 percent. Chen and Woolley [7] calculated the heritability of hypospadias and determined it to be 74.1 percent, with a standard error of 12.6 percent.

Associated Genitourinary Findings

Meatal stenosis is commonly found in association with hypospadias. Inguinal hernias have been reported in up to 30 percent and undescended testes in up to 60 percent of patients [18, 38]. Most series of hypospadias, however, report 10 to 15 percent with unilateral or bilateral undescended testes [38]. The incidence of these associated anomalies rises sharply with increasing severity of the hypospadias [18] and supports the concept that hypospadias is related to decreased androgenic stimulation during a critical phase of embryogenesis.

Voiding cystourethrographic studies will outline an enlarged prostatic utricle (vestigial vagina) in the more extreme forms of hypospadias, but significant utricular enlargement also occurs sporadically in hypospadias of lesser severity [38].

The older literature suggests an increase in urinary tract abnormalities with simple hypospadias [11, 34, 40]. However, critical review of these series reveals the findings to be of dubious impor-

tance, such as ureteral dilatation, "bladder neck obstruction," and renoureteral duplication. More recently, Cendron [6] reported a 10 percent incidence of pyelographic abnormalities similar to that expected in a normal population. McArdle and Lebowitz [28] reviewed excretory urograms of 200 patients with uncomplicated hypospadias and found upper urinary tract anomalies in only 3 percent. None required treatment.

Clinical Manifestations

Hypospadias has a very characteristic appearance, with a proximal meatus on the ventral shaft, a hooded prepuce, and a ventrally curved penis distal to the hypospadic meatus. A blind urethral pit is often present. The degree of chordee is easily underestimated. Compressing the corpora cavernosa in the perineum engorges the penile shaft. Additional compression of the base of the penis will further fill it, simulating a degree of erection adequate to assess the severity of chordee. Children with mild degrees of simple hypospadias are normal, aside from the frequent finding of meatal stenosis. In more extreme forms of hypospadias, the child must sit to void; as he gets older this becomes a source of embarrassment and anxiety.

Urinary tract infection is uncommon in the untreated state, but it may occur postoperatively due to stricture or formation of a diverticulum within the neourethra. Children with an enlarged utriculus masculinus also are more prone to postoperative urinary infections.

Treatment

The objectives of surgical correction of hypospadias are to straighten the curved penis, to move the meatus distally, and to improve the cosmetic appearance of the genitalia. Recommendations regarding the optimal age for starting reconstructive surgery vary, but most authors agree that this should not be attempted during infancy, but should be completed before starting school. The Section on Urology of the American Academy of Pediatrics recently reported that, for technical and psychological considerations, the optimal time for elective surgery on the genitalia is during the fourth year [3]. Figure 102-5 shows diagrammatically a typical one-stage chordee release and urethroplasty, using preputial skin to reconstruct the urethra and to resurface the ventral penis [13].

Prognosis

The surgical prognosis for correction of simple hypospadias is good. The major complications are

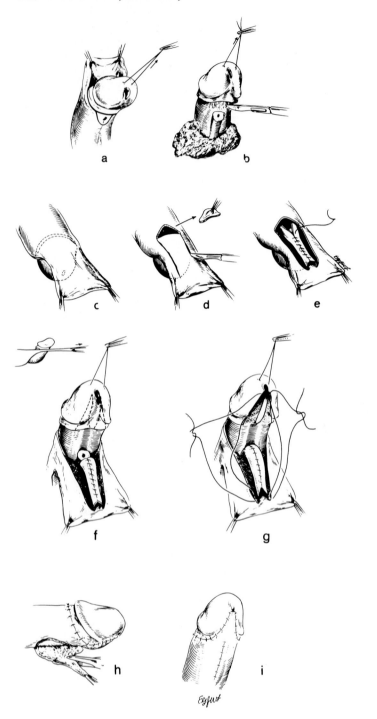

Figure 102-5. Example of a one-stage hypospadias repair. Steps include penile degloving, chordee release with retraction of the urethra, and transfer of the prepuce, with development of a cutaneous urethral tube.

development of a cutaneous fistula from the neo-urethra, stricture, and inadequate release of the chordee. All of these complications are treatable with additional surgery. The most extreme forms of hypospadias require a series of more complex, staged procedures for correction; even after correction the phallus is likely to be smaller than average in size. After a good repair, however, most patients should have the potential for normal urinary and sexual function. Nevertheless, in a series of young adults with repaired hypospadias reviewed by Farkas and Hynie [10], 32 percent of patients refrained from intercourse, another 26 percent rarely attempted intercourse, and only 35 percent married.

To minimize psychological problems after hypospadias surgery, correction should be completed in the preschool period and by a skilled surgeon. Adequate attention to the emotional needs of the patient and his family is essential.

While the fertility of patients with repaired hypospadias has not been studied extensively, patients with coronal and distal penile hypospadias usually have normal fertility [38]. Occasional patients are sterile after reconstruction because the ejaculate remains partially sequestered within the reconstructed urethral skin tube. In extreme hypospadias, penoscrotal or perineal hypogonadism is often present and fertility is diminished.

References

1. Aarskog, P. Clinical and cytogenetic studies in hypospadias. *Acta Paediatr. Scand.* [Suppl. 203] 59:1, 1970.
2. Abramovich, D. R. A possible cause of glandular hypospadias in man. *Arch. Dis. Child.* 49:66, 1974.
3. Action Committee Report, Section on Urology, American Academy of Pediatrics. The timing of elective surgery on the genitalia of male children with particular reference to undescended testes and hypospadias. *Pediatrics* 56:479, 1975.
4. Arey, B. L. *Developmental Anatomy* (7th ed.). Philadelphia: Saunders, 1965.
5. Campbell, H., Newcombe, R. G., and Weatherall, J. A. C. Epidemiology of simple hypospadias. *Br. Med. J.* 3:52, 1973.
6. Cendron, J. Treatment of hypospadias. *Proc. R. Soc. Med.* 64:125, 1971.
7. Chen, Y. C., and Woolley, P. V., Jr. Genetic studies on hypospadias in males. *J. Med. Genet.* 8:153, 1971.
8. Devine, C. J., Jr. Embryology of the Male External Genitalia. In C. E. Horton (ed.), *Plastic and Reconstructive Surgery of the Genital Area.* Boston: Little, Brown, 1973.
9. Dickie, W. R., and Sharpe, C. Crypto-hypospadias—a review of 38 cases. *Br. J. Plast. Surg.* 26:227, 1973.
10. Farkas, L. G., and Hynie, J. After effects of hypospadias repair in childhood. *Postgrad. Med.* 47:103, 1970.
11. Felton, L. M. Should intravenous pyelography be a routine procedure for children with cryptorchism or hypospadias? *J. Urol.* 81:335, 1959.
12. Glenister, T. W. The origin and fate of the urethral plate in man. *J. Anat.* 88:413, 1954.
13. Hodgson, N. B. A one-stage hypospadias repair. *J. Urol.* 104:281, 1970.
14. Horton, C. E., and Devine, C. J., Jr. Chordee without Hypospadias. In C. E. Horton (ed.), *Plastic and Reconstructive Surgery of the Genital Area.* Boston: Little, Brown, 1973.
15. Horton, C. E., and Devine, C. J., Jr. Hypospadias: Introduction. In C. E. Horton (ed.), *Plastic and Reconstructive Surgery of the Genital Area.* Boston: Little, Brown, 1973.
16. Horton, C. E., Devine, C. J., Jr., and Baran, N. Pictoral History of Hypospadias Repair Techniques. In C. E. Horton (ed.), *Plastic and Reconstructive Surgery of the Genital Area.* Boston: Little, Brown, 1973.
17. Hunter, R. H. Notes on the development of the prepuce. *J. Anat.* 70:68, 1935.
18. Hynie, J. The sexuological aspects of hypospadias. *Acta Chir. Plast.* (Praha) 8:232, 1966.
19. Jirasek, J. E. *Development of the Genital System and Male Pseudohermaphroditism.* Baltimore: Johns Hopkins, 1971.
20. Jost, A. Problems of fetal endocrinology: The gonadal and hypophyseal hormones. *Recent Progr. Horm. Res.* 8:379, 1953.
21. Jost, A. Hormonal factors in development of the fetus. *Quant. Biol.* 19:167, 1954.
22. Juberg, R. C., Jewson, D. V., Taylor, M. B., and Moore, V. L. Chromosome studies in patients with hypospadias. *Pediatrics* 43:578, 1961.
23. Kaplan, G. W., and Lamm, D. L. Embryogenesis of chordee. *J. Urol.* 114:769, 1975.
24. King, L. R. Hypospadias—a one-stage repair without skin graft based on a new principle: Chordee is sometimes produced by the skin alone. *J. Urol.* 103:660, 1970.
25. Lewandowski, R. C., Jr., and Yunis, J. J. New chromosomal syndromes. *Am. J. Dis. Child.* 129:515, 1975.
26. Lupo, G., Lupo, M., Magnani, C., and Bergamaschi, M. A chromosome abnormality in hypospadias patients. *Br. J. Plast. Surg.* 26:235, 1973.
27. MacKinney, C. C., and Uhle, C. A. W. Congenital chordee without hypospadias. *J. Urol.* 84:343, 1960.
28. McArdle, R., and Lebowitz, R. Uncomplicated hypospadias and anomalies of the upper urinary tract. *Urology* 5:712, 1975.
29. Moore, C. A. Surgical repair of chordee without hypospadias: Report of three cases. *J. Urol.* 93:389, 1965.
30. Nesbit, R. M. The surgical treatment of congenital chordee without hypospadias. *J. Urol.* 72:1178, 1954.
31. Record, R. G., and Armstrong, E. Epidemiology of simple hypospadias. *Br. Med. J.* 3:233, 1973.
32. Roberts, C. J., and Lloyd, S. Observations on the epidemiology of simple hypospadias. *Br. Med. J.* 1:769, 1973.
33. Rogers, B. O. History of External Genital Surgery. In C. E. Horton (ed.), *Plastic and Reconstructive Surgery of the Genital Area.* Boston: Little, Brown, 1973.
34. Smith, B. J. Hypospadias and associated anomalies of the genitourinary tract. *J. Urol.* 82:109, 1959.
35. Smith, D. R. Repair of hypospadias in the pre-

school child: A report of 150 cases. *Trans. Am. Assoc. Genitourin. Surg.* 58:15, 1966.

36. Sorensen, H. R. *Hypospadias with Special Reference to Aetiology.* Copenhagen: Munksgaard, 1953.

37. Theander, G. Seasonal distribution of births of boys with anomalies of the urethra. *Scand. J. Urol. Nephrol.* 4:1, 1970.

38. van der Muelen, J. C. H. M. *Hypospadias.* Springfield, Ill.: Thomas, 1964.

39. van der Muelen, J. C. H. M. Hypospadias and cryptospadias. *Br. J. Plast. Surg.* 24:101, 1971.

40. Willis, C., Brannan, W., and Ochsner, M. Hypospadias and associated anomalies. *South. Med. J.* 60: 969, 1967.

103. Exstrophy and Epispadias

Alan D. Perlmutter

Exstrophy and epispadias are the most typical manifestations of a spectrum of related congenital genitourinary tract anomalies that are classified as the exstrophy-epispadias complex [22]. This chapter will be limited to a presentation of the three most clinically important forms of exstrophic anomalies: exstrophy of the bladder, epispadias, and exstrophy of the cloaca.

EXSTROPHY OF THE BLADDER (ECTOPIA VESICAE)

Classical exstrophy of the bladder consists of an anteriorly everted bladder and urethra. The open bladder bulges outward whenever abdominal pressure rises. The umbilicus is abnormally caudad, located on the upper margin of the everted bladder. The lower abdominal wall is abnormally developed; the linea alba is broadened, and the rectus muscles diverge on either side of the exstrophic bladder to insert on widely separated pubic bones. In the male, the penis is stubby, broad, and turned upward. Complete epispadias is present as an open urethra consisting of a strip of mucosa from a dorsally grooved glans, extending along the dorsal penis and continuous with the bladder exstrophy. The scrotum is flat and wide (Fig. 103-1). In the female, exstrophy and epispadias are associated with a double clitoris, widely separated labia, and an unusually anterior vaginal opening (Fig. 103-2). In both sexes the perineal structures are flattened and the anus is more anterior than usual due to the widening of the ventrally separated pelvic ring.

EPISPADIAS

Epispadias without exstrophy represents an embryologic fault more limited in degree than exstrophy of the bladder (Fig. 103-3). Here, too, the penis tends to be short and stubby, with a dorsal chordee, although the changes are less extreme than when associated with exstrophy. The dorsal urethral defect rarely may involve the glans alone; usually it extends a variable distance along the shaft of the penis, at times including the vesical neck, through which bladder mucosa can prolapse —a form of mild exstrophy with urinary incontinence. In the female, too, the urethral defect is of variable degree and is flanked by a bifid clitoris.

In both sexes, separation of the pubic bones is an inconstant feature; when present it is generally less extreme than with exstrophy, correlating with the severity of the epispadias [26, 40].

EXSTROPHY OF THE CLOACA (VESICOINTESTINAL FISSURE)

Cloacal exstrophy is a more extensive deformity than exstrophy of the bladder and is characterized by a central field of intestinal mucosa flanked on either side by an exstrophic hemibladder. The cranial margin of the exstrophic defect is contiguous with an umbilical hernia or omphalocele. The phallus in either sex, when present, is duplicated and tends to be small and vestigial. The functioning intestine terminates in the ileocecal region, and the terminal ileum opens onto the upper margin of the bowel field. An opening on the lower margin leads to a short, blind segment of large bowel. The anus is imperforate (Fig. 103-4). Other anomalies frequently are present.

Epidemiology

The exstrophic anomalies are relatively uncommon; exstrophy of the bladder has an incidence generally estimated at 1 : 30,000 to 40,000 live births [22, 26], although during one period in Liverpool an incidence of 1 : 10,000 was observed [28]. Boys are afflicted about twice as often as girls. Of the various manifestations of the exstrophy-epispadias complex, classic exstrophy of the bladder is the most common [21] (Fig. 103-5). In one series of 79 exstrophic anomalies, 44 were cases of classical bladder exstrophy, 4 were

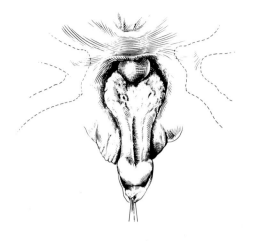

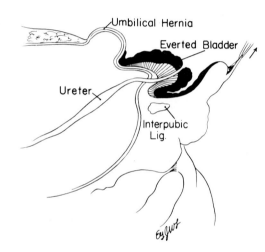

Figure 103-1. Classical exstrophy of the bladder in a male.

examples of cloacal exstrophy, and 26 were varieties of epispadias—8 without incontinence. The remaining 5 cases were variants of the complex, with minor clinical manifestations [22].

History

Prior to the mid-nineteenth century, the exstrophic anomalies attracted considerably less attention than hypospadias, perhaps because of the relative rarity of the lesions and the hopelessness of typical exstrophy. An Assyrian clay tablet from about 2000 B.C. probably described exstrophy; scattered accounts appeared in the sixteenth and seventeenth centuries, and the first thorough description was recorded in the mid-eighteenth century [19, 22].

During the middle of the nineteenth century, surgical efforts were directed at providing coverage by flaps of skin, with a view to reducing local discomfort from the wet, exposed, and tender bladder

surface [19]. In the late nineteenth century reports of treatment by internal urinary-intestinal diversion began to appear, first as a fistula between the trigone and the rectum [38], then as trigono-rectal anastomosis [3, 39], and finally by uretero-sigmoid anastomosis [7, 35]. Ureterosigmoidostomy remained the treatment of choice until the technique of external diversion by ileal conduit was published in 1954 [4].

Around the turn of this century, Trendelenburg attempted to achieve continence in three patients by sacroiliac disarticulation and closure of the bladder and abdominal wall, but all remained incontinent [37]. The first successful bladder closure with continence is credited to Young in 1942 [44]. Since then, and at this writing, despite improvements in surgical technique and the advent of chemotherapy, success with bladder closure has remained limited. Two divergent approaches to the management of classical exstrophy have emerged, with those who prefer primary internal or external diversion and cystectomy on the one hand, and those who attempt primary reconstruction, at least in selected patients, on the other.

Embryology

In contrast to hypospadias, which represents an *arrest* of embryogenesis, exstrophy and its variants result from *faulty* embryogenesis; none of the lesions in the exstrophy-epispadias complex mimics a normal stage of development [21].

In the early embryo, the cloacal membrane, a bilaminar ectodermal-entodermal structure, comprises the lower abdominal wall below the umbilical cord. Progressive ingrowth of mesoderm separates the two layers of the membrane, incrementally limiting its relative size. The mesoderm, which ingrows, fuses, and expands in the subumbilical midline, is the precursor of the musculoskeletal structures of the lower abdomen and anterior pelvis, as well as of the musculature of the anterior bladder wall. At the cephalic end of the cloacal membrane, paired mesodermal masses coalesce to form the genital tubercle, which develops into the definitive phallus. When the cloacal membrane normally ruptures at the 15- to 16-mm stage, the future abdominal wall is intact and the opening is into the urogenital sinus, entirely subphallic, in the area to become the future perineum.

Studies by Muecke [25] suggest that the basic abnormality common to the various forms of the exstrophy complex is an excessively large cloacal membrane, which, for the first 6 weeks of development, acts as a barrier to the migration of mesoderm, delaying or preventing midline ingrowth and fusion in the subumbilical area. Thus the

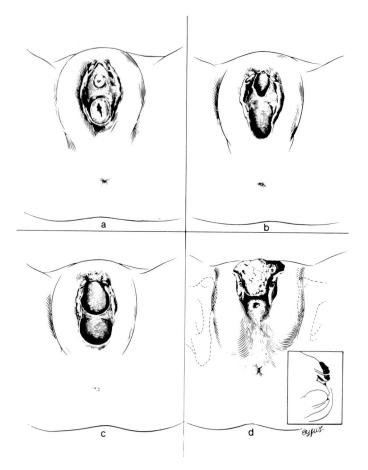

Figure 103-2. Degrees of epispadias and exstrophy in the female. a. Patulous urethra, bifid clitoris. b. Epispadias with incontinence. There is a short, wide urethra that is defective ventrally. c. Subsymphyseal epispadias. Urethral defect extends into the bladder neck. The area of the mons is deficient. d. Classical exstrophy of bladder in a female. Vaginal opening is ventral to the normal position and is stenotic.

bladder wall, the developing muscular elements of the lower abdominal wall, and the skeletal elements of the ventral pelvis are held apart. When the abnormally large cloacal membrane dehisces, the anterior bladder wall is unformed, thus allowing the open bladder to evert and resulting in the defect of classic exstrophy.

During early embryogenesis a transverse fold, the urorectal septum, descends to divide the primitive cloaca into a ventral bladder and dorsal rectum. If the abnormal cloacal membrane dehisces prior to the full descent of the urorectal septum, eversion of the undivided or partially divided cloaca will occur. A central bowel field will arise from the derived dorsal cloaca, flanked on each side by a hemibladder derived from the ventral cloaca—the condition of cloacal exstrophy. Interference with developing hindgut derivatives by their early involvement in the exstrophy explains

why the ileocecal region opens onto the exstrophic bowel field and why large bowel structures are inadequate or absent.

The early disruption of a large infraumbilical membrane also prevents coalescence of the paired precursors of the genital tubercle, leading typically to diphallia, usually with poorly developed or vestigial phallic tissue or even no gross phallic tissue at all. Early interference with the developing cloacal structures may similarly interfere with müllerian duct fusion in the female, resulting in genital anomalies such as uterine, cervical, or vaginal duplication or agenesis.

The abdominally directed extension of the abnormal infraumbilical membrane causes the originally paired genital tubercle to fuse below the membrane, so that when dehiscence occurs the urogenital sinus lies on the dorsal penis, represented by an open strip of urethra and prostate that

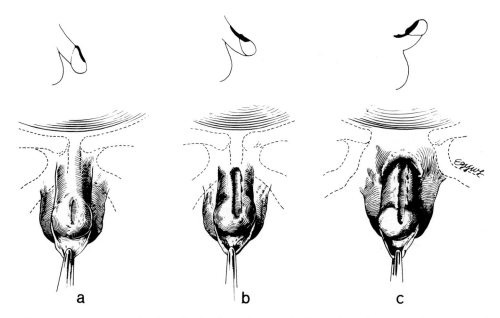

Figure 103-3. Degrees of epispadias in the male. a, *Balanic or glandular;* b, *penile;* c, *penopubic.*

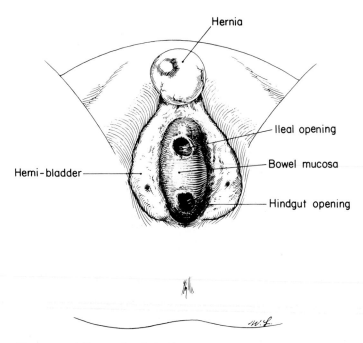

Figure 103-4. Exstrophy of the cloaca.

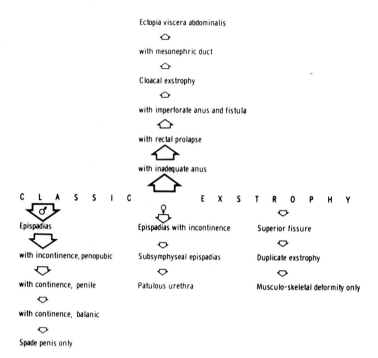

Figure 103-5. Relationships within the exstrophy-epispadias complex. The degree of deformity increases from nearly normal at the bottom to rarer and more severe degrees of abnormality at the top. Classic exstrophy is the most common; the sizes of the arrows and the type indicate the relative frequency of the various anomalies. (From V. F. Marshall and E. C. Muecke, J. Urol. 88:766, 1962 [21]. Copyright © 1962, The Williams & Wilkins Co., Baltimore.)

is continuous with the exstrophic bladder. Occasionally a double penis is encountered with typical exstrophy. In the female, the paired genital tubercles almost always fail to fuse, leading to a double clitoris.

In epispadias without exstrophy, the initial relationship of the abnormal cloacal membrane to the paired genital tubercles is as described for exstrophy; however, mesoderm successfully invades the upper layers of the membrane, forming, to a variable degree, the lower abdominal wall, anterior pelvic ring, anterior bladder wall, and urethral sphincter mechanism. When the remaining inferior portion of the membrane disrupts, its abnormal location on the dorsal penis or dorsal to the paired clitoris gives rise to a degree of epispadias.

The reader is referred elsewhere for additional details of disordered embryogenesis and its relation to other rare forms of the exstrophy complex [19, 22].

Genetics

The exstrophic anomalies appear to be isolated errors of embryogenesis. Familial occurrence is rare and sporadic, and most victims are born into families without a history of urogenital malformations [22].

Clinical Findings and Pathology

EXSTROPHY OF THE BLADDER

The exstrophic bladder varies in size from a small, platelike disc to a large and pliable structure of nearly normal size that can be inverted into the abdomen by external pressure. Although the surface of the bladder is covered by normal-appearing mucosa at birth, the exposed membrane soon undergoes inflammatory changes [8, 11], with the appearance of bullous edema, vascular congestion, friability, ulceration, and squamous metaplasia (which has been observed by 2 weeks of age). Other mucosal changes include acute ulcerations and cystitis cystica, follicularis, and glandularis. These histologic changes may persist for years following bladder closure [29], and metaplastic areas resembling colonic mucosa can also be found [11, 19]. The untreated exstrophic bladder is also likely to develop some degree of thickening and fibrosis of the muscular wall; this is more marked in older patients [19].

Ultrastructure studies of the exstrophic mucosa have shown changes similar to those of transitional carcinoma [6]. The exstrophic bladder is susceptible to malignant change, and adenocarcinoma is the most frequent epithelial tumor, in contrast to the more common transitional tumors arising in normal bladders [17, 19]. A few neoplasms have also occurred after bladder closure, including rhabdomyosarcoma and adenocarcinoma [19, 31]. While the incidence is not high enough to preclude reconstruction, this hazard must be considered.

The upper urinary tracts usually are normal in exstrophy of the bladder, and with proper care of the exposed bladder, they can remain so indefinitely. The inflammatory changes of the bladder mucosa and wall can involve the ureteral orifice and intramural ureteral segment, however, resulting in obstruction, progressive hydronephrosis, and ascending pyelonephritis [22]. A voiding cystourethrogram should be part of any preoperative evaluation of epispadias. In one series, 9 of 10 epispadiac patients, including both sexes, had vesicoureteral reflux; 3 of these also had atrophic pyelonephritis [1].

The epispadiac penis is short, stubby and upturned; its length is taken up by its crura, which arise from the widely separated ischiopubic rami, resulting in a very short segment of fused corpora cavernosa. Despite the penile deformity, sensation and erectile potential are intact. At the dorsal angle of the penile base is an open but otherwise normal prostatic urethra. The ejaculatory mechanism is functional unless it is damaged during reconstructive surgery [15]. Indirect inguinal hernias and undescended testes are relatively frequent [16, 19, 22].

Just deep to (underneath) the exstrophic bladder neck, a fibrous intersymphyseal band that connects the separated pubic bones is palpable. Because of the outward displacement of the pelvis, the acetabula and femoral heads are externally rotated, and the children tend to walk with a waddling gait. This causes no disability, however, and treatment is not required; the pelvis is stable, and with growth the abnormal gait becomes less marked. The separated pelvis also causes flattening of the pelvic diaphragm, with incomplete anterior supports, and the anus often is lax. As a result, rectal prolapse is common, especially in infancy; this is exacerbated by episodes of tenesmus from the inflamed and sore bladder. The prolapse is easily reducible; recurrences cease as growth continues [19, 22]. Occasionally exstrophy is associated with an imperforate anus.

In the female, the anteriorly displaced vaginal orifice tends to be narrow and fibrotic, often requiring vaginoplasty in adolescence. The vaginal barrel is usually normal, although somewhat short. With severe exstrophy, duplication of the uterus, cervix, and vagina may be present (see Embryology).

EPISPADIAS

In either sex, epispadias may be associated with normal urinary control or with stress or total incontinence. The degree of impairment correlates with the extent of the epispadias. In the male, epispadias is classified as balanic or glandular, penile, or penopubic [22] (see Fig. 103-3). The balanic type, which involves only the dorsal glans, is the mildest form and is the least common. In the penile type, the entire dorsal shaft is grooved, and penile shortening, dorsal chordee, and symphyseal separation are evident. Urinary control is usually but not invariably adequate. In the penopubic type, which is the most common, the epispadic fissure extends subsymphyseally to involve the external sphincter and prostatic urethra and can also include the vesical neck to a varying degree.

In the female, similar degrees of involvement occur, although mild cases may not come to clinical attention. Such lesions may escape detection when urinary control is adequate and there is little separation between the halves of a double clitoris. The more severe forms are readily apparent, with widely separated phallic bodies and labia minora, a wide, short, and anteriorly directed urethra, and a flattened intersymphyseal area (see Fig. 103-2).

EXSTROPHY OF THE CLOACA

The cloacal form of exstrophy fortunately is extremely rare. In addition to the exstrophic intestine and flanking hemibladders and the contiguous superior omphalocele, more than half of these infants have vertebral anomalies, and almost one-half have a myelocele or myelomeningocele.

Upper urinary tract anomalies are found in about half the patients, including unilateral or bilateral renal agenesis or dysplasia, multicystic kidney, and hydronephrosis and hydroureter. In addition to duplication or agenesis of the phallus and duplication of the vagina, genital anomalies include a single opening of the ureter and vas deferens as a persistent mesonephric duct and undescended testes. The sex may be indeterminate, and external genital structures can be entirely absent [34, 36].

Treatment and Prognosis
EXSTROPHY OF THE BLADDER
Treatment of exstrophy of the bladder can be divided into an early phase of initial evaluation and management, and a subsequent phase of definitive treatment by single or staged operative procedures. There is no ideal therapy for classic exstrophy; all have drawbacks and limitations. As a result, no consensus has evolved among the centers treating these unfortunate children. Two

general approaches are prevalent, with different philosophies and goals. One is cystectomy and urinary diversion; the other is an attempted functional reconstruction of the bladder, bladder outlet, and urethra.

Initial Management

Once the exstrophic bladder mucosa is exposed after birth, it is subject to continued inflammation, with congestion, easy bleeding, edema, and exquisite tenderness. Until progressive, squamous change decreases vesical sensitivity; the inflammation and soreness can be minimized by proper care. A thin layer of fine-mesh, petroleum jelly gauze applied to the bladder surface provides excellent protection. Frequent diaper changes and bathing of the abdominal and perineal skin will minimize rash and ammonia dermatitis caused from continual contact with urine.

Although the upper urinary tracts are usually free of anomalies, a baseline excretory urogram should be obtained during the neonatal period, since subsequent hydronephrosis and hydroureter are not uncommon, especially if the exposed ureteral orifices become edematous and thickened [22]. Any undue swelling of the orifices and trigone is an indication for follow-up excretory urography. Radiograms should be obtained every 6 months in infancy and yearly thereafter. In the unoperated patient without significant obstructive changes, pyelonephritis is uncommon and renal function can be expected to remain normal.

Repeated rectal prolapse, especially common in infancy, is reduced manually. Crying and severe straining enhance recurrence; protection of the exposed bladder mucosa (as described above) minimizes tenesmus, which can be treated also with anticholinergic agents. Inguinal hernias should be repaired when diagnosed in order to avoid incarceration or strangulation.

The objectives of definitive treatment vary, depending upon whether urinary diversion with cystectomy or functional bladder reconstruction is elected; in either event, proper management includes ultimate cosmetic and functional correction of the genital defects.

Urinary Diversion

Internal Urinary Diversion. Ureterosigmoidostomy to accomplish internal urinary diversion in exstrophy developed from implantation of the trigone into the rectum by Maydl in 1894 (cited in [4a]) and remains the preferred approach at many centers. Ureterosigmoidostomy suffered a period of disfavor several years ago because of appreciable

associated morbidity and mortality [22]; however, the procedure currently is regaining favor as a result of more recent experience. Internal urinary diversion offers the advantage of enabling the child to be appliance-free, without the stigma of an external stoma. The procedure itself is not technically difficult. The method uses a physiologic sphincter, the anus, to provide continence, with periodic evacuation of feces and urine through a single natural orifice.

Retrospective reviews of several series, as summarized by Marshall and Muecke [22], have demonstrated a significant morbidity and mortality rate in ureterosigmoidostomy over the years, with progressive pyelonephritis and ultimate renal failure. Despite these problems, with modern antireflux techniques of ureteral anastomosis, increasing numbers of healthy, long-term survivors are now being reported. In 1962 Higgins [16] reported on 158 patients, with 99 surviving for up to 30 years. In 1966 Spence [33] described a series of 31 cases, with only 7 failures requiring further surgery and 3 deaths. The longest follow-ups were 19, 30, and 42 years. He concluded that an acceptable result could be expected in two-thirds of patients, and that one-third would need further surgery, including another form of diversion. He pointed out that although ureterosigmoidostomy is "a major compromise with normal physiology . . . as in any operation for exstrophy the results must be viewed in the light of the gruesome condition it is designed to correct." In 1973 Bennett [2] reported on 94 children followed from 5 to 35 years. Nine had died, but of the 34 patients operated on since 1954, using more precisely defined criteria for selection and management, 33 were still alive; in 5, the diversion was converted from ureterosigmoidostomy to ileal conduit (3 because of an abnormal pyelogram and 2 because of rectal incontinence). In short, despite significant problems, by judicious selection and careful management, good long-term results can be achieved in a substantial majority of patients.

In ureterosigmoidostomy, each ureter is implanted into the rectum or sigmoid by means of mucosal anastomosis and an antireflux muscle tunnel. Although Spence [33] has favored early operation (3 to 6 months of age), others have preferred to wait until rectal continence is established and the child can be encouraged to "void" at timed intervals, to minimize urinary resorption [19]. Patients undergoing ureterosigmoidostomy should have normal upper urinary tracts and an anal sphincter that is adequate to retain a test load of fluid, such as cooked farina. Anal prolapse, a weak anal sphincter, segmental pyelonephritic changes, and ureteral dilatation are all contraindications to ureterosigmoidostomy.

Because internal diversion places a large surface of intestinal mucosa in contact with urine for varying periods of time, considerable modification of urinary composition may occur. With normal renal function and with regular, timed bowel evacuation, clinically important biochemical abnormalities can be avoided; however, chronic pyelonephritis and impaired renal function are associated with hyperchloremic, hypokalemic acidosis [20]. As a result of urinary loss following ureterocolic anastomosis, depletion of whole body potassium can occur, even in asymptomatic patients [42]. Elixirs containing organic salts of potassium can be used to prevent or correct acidosis and potassium depletion.

In the past, unacceptable morbidity and mortality resulted from progressive upper tract deterioration and other inevitable complications following surgery for calculi and anastomotic obstructions. It is now recognized that when such difficulties begin, prompt conversion to external diversion before advanced changes occur will reduce morbidity and improve survival [2, 33].

To overcome problems with ureterosigmoidostomy, various modifications have been used. An isolated rectal bladder with separate sigmoid colostomy has the obvious disadvantage of external fecal diversion. An isolated rectal bladder with implantation of the sigmoid colon into the external anal sphincter creates a double-barrelled anus, separating the fecal and urinary streams. Despite sporadic successes, the latter procedure has not achieved great popularity due to its technical difficulty and because of complications such as injury to the sphincter that causes incontinence and retraction of the septum between the two anal orifices, allowing the urinary and fecal streams to mix.

A few cases of adenomatous polyp and adenocarcinoma of the rectosigmoid arising at the site of ureteral implantation have been reported, with a mean latent period of 15 years after operation [14, 41]. Therefore, proctosigmoidoscopy and radiographic studies of the large bowel should be performed periodically after ureterosigmoid diversion.

External Urinary Diversion. The ileal conduit [4], and more recently the sigmoid conduit [24], are forms of *external urinary diversion.* An isolated segment of bowel is interposed between the ureters and the abdominal wall. Despite a lessened risk of metabolic imbalance because of continuous emptying, this form of surgery is more extensive than ureterosigmoidostomy and has a higher incidence of later intestinal obstruction. The child is reminded continuously of his deformity by the external urinary nipple and collecting appliance. Late pyelonephritis, calculus formation, and ureteral or stomal obstruction commonly occur. Late upper urinary tract deterioration from a variety of causes after ileal conduit is being seen in increasing numbers [10, 12, 13, 22, 27, 30, 32]. Although it is too soon for long term results, early experiences [15a] with a nonrefluxing sigmoid conduit show that the upper tracts are better protected than with a refluxing ileal conduit—it is technically easier to do an antirefluxing ureteral implant into colon than small bowel. The choice between primary ureterosigmoidostomy and ileal or sigmoid conduit is a difficult one, and the controversy between groups favoring one or the other procedure remains unresolved.

Cystectomy and repair of the lower abdominal wall is done at the time of diversion or as a separate procedure; epispadias repair is best postponed until after 3½ or 4 years of age. Most authors agree that posterior iliac osteotomy enhances the ability to close the abdominal defect without the need for fascial flaps [19, 22]. Although the penile crura become less distracted, with closure the pubis rotates inferiorly and there is no effective increase in penile length. Because osteotomy is a major procedure, it should be done as a separate procedure, 3 to 7 days before cystectomy. In general, there is a tendency to some degree of pubic reseparation over a period of months, even with postoperative castings.

Functional Reconstruction of the Bladder

The ultimate objective in repair of exstrophy should be to have a child with a normal bladder capacity and perfect urinary control. Because this objective is met with great difficulty and only in a minority of children with exstrophy, the surgeon is faced with an uncomfortable dilemma: Is he justified in proposing a series of difficult, staged procedures with an appreciable rate of complication? The overall rate of success in the literature is about 22 percent; some series have had success in achieving continence in 30 to 50 percent, mainly following staged procedures [19, 22]. Jeffs has recently reported the best results to date: Continence was achieved in 60 percent of 53 patients selected for a staged repair [18]. Not all exstrophic bladders are suitable for reconstruction, however; the small, rigid, platelike bladder cannot be closed.

In a staged repair, the goal of the first step is to close the detrusor without any attempt at providing continence [18, 23]. This procedure arrests the progressive alterations of the bladder mucosa and stops the pain and tenesmus these infants suffer. Closure during the neonatal period permits easy approximation of the abdominal defect and pubis without a preliminary posterior iliac osteotomy, since the sacroiliac points are still mobile at that age [19]. After neonatal closure, however, there is a high rate of partial dehiscence [18].

The next stage involves ureteral reimplantation and reconstruction of the bladder neck and posterior urethra-sphincter area. Repair of the epispadias is the final step, done during the preschool age period. Since every stage in repair increases the likelihood of complications, it is not surprising that many of these children require interval procedures as well [18, 43].

Continence following single-stage or multiple-stage bladder closure is not achieved immediately, and ultimate success is greater in females [18, 19]. The risks of bladder reconstruction include upper tract dilatation and deterioration from reflux or obstruction, renal or bladder calculi, bladder outlet obstruction, and damage to the ejaculatory ducts. When urinary diversion is necessary for a failed reconstruction, consideration is given to simultaneous or interval cystectomy because of the recognized histologic abnormalities in these bladders (see under Clinical Findings and Pathology) and because of a high incidence of pyocystis in a defunctionalized and previously operated bladder [32].

EPISPADIAS

In boys with epispadias with continence or epispadias remaining after treatment of exstrophy, cosmetic and functional reconstruction of the urethral fissure and associated penile deformity is required. All patients with isolated epispadias should have an excretory urogram preoperatively, although upper tract anomalies are uncommon. All (except perhaps the balanic group) should have a voiding cystourethrogram because of the high incidence of vesicoureteral reflux, which may increase in severity and complicate management following urethral and sphincteric surgery (the correction of reflux is justified as a part of the reconstructive procedure [1]). In epispadias with incontinence, the voiding cystourethrogram will demonstrate a widened symphysis and a short and wide posterior urethra, usually with an incompetent vesical neck.

Treatment for the occasional case of balanic epispadias is simply closure of the urethral defect and reapproximation of the dorsal edges of the glans. The more common and more extensive cases

of penile and penopubic epispadias have a degree of penile shortening and dorsal chordee that make simple urethral repair inadequate. A variety of one-stage and two-stage procedures are available to release the chordee and to fashion a urethra. Division of the urethral strip is required in order to release the dorsal chordee and to elongate the penis. When necessary the dissection can be carried along the dorsal crura, partially detaching them from the rami to gain additional penile length. Skin from the shaft can be interposed to fill the gap created by the divided urethra, and a second-stage urethroplasty can be performed after several months. Alternatively, the ventral prepuce can be transferred dorsally, and a urethra can be created from a pedicle of prepuce interposed at the time of chordee release. Figure 103-6 depicts diagrammatically one approach to chordee release and urethroplasty for epispadias.

The urinary incontinence present in the majority of boys with epispadias adds an additional dimension to therapy, namely, surgery of the bladder neck and posterior urethra, either at the time of repair of the epispadias or at a separate stage. Here, too, a number of technical procedures that are beyond the scope of this review have been described. Nevertheless the principles are similar: to increase the length of the bladder neck and posterior urethra, using the local smooth muscle to create a pliable tube. The procedure increases the resting tonus of the bladder neck and posterior urethra, thereby preventing a column of urine from directly impinging against an attenuated and underdeveloped external striated sphincter. The overall effect is to dampen the urethral transmission of sudden changes in vesical pressure. The success rate for achieving continence in this group of patients approximates 60 percent, but additional improvement in urinary control appears after puberty, apparently as a result of prostatic growth and enlargement [5, 9, 19].

In the absence of injury to the prostate and ejaculatory ducts during reconstructive stages, sexual function and fertility should be intact [15]. Sexual performance can be affected adversely, however, by the psychological stigma of the deformed genitalia and by mechanical factors related to an inadequate phallus or its incomplete surgical correction.

In the girls with epispadias and incontinence, the techniques of bladder neck and urethral reconstruction are similar. Cosmetic correction of the genital defect is optional and usually is not required when the separation of the clitoris is inconspicuous, as sexual function is not altered by the cleft phallus. For a markedly depressed mons

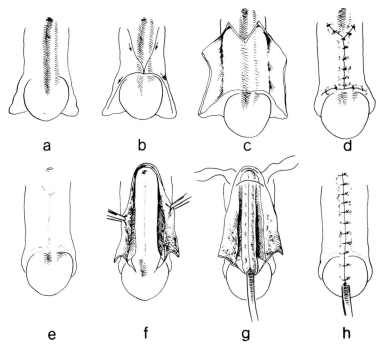

Figure 103-6. *A two-stage epispadias repair.* a *through* d. *Steps in chordee release and dorsal penile resurfacing.* e *through* h. *Steps in formation of a penile urethra several months after the first stage.*

pubis and widely separated clitoral duplication, however, monsplasty and clitoral anastomosis are easily performed.

EXSTROPHY OF THE CLOACA

The most complex and severe of the exstrophic anomalies, cloacal exstrophy, is attended by a high mortality rate. Most babies with this disorder are born prematurely. The congenital ileostomy is associated with a short bowel syndrome, resulting in profuse water and electrolyte loss [19, 36]. The rare presentation of one of these multiply afflicted newborns raises profound philosophic and ethical issues regarding appropriate treatment, as the ultimate result will be one of extreme, permanent disability. Johnston and Kogan [19] have stated "that in some instances . . . these unfortunate children have been treated with more enthusiasm than judgment and common sense," especially when the underlying anomaly is attended by other severe disabilities, such as spina bifida cystica, and severe genital deformities in the male.

Initial management is directed to the problems of prematurity and excessive intestinal fluid loss. Many of these children die in the first days or weeks of life. Tank and Lindenauer [36] emphasize that operative reconstruction is not an emergency and that these infants must first be given the opportunity to survive and to have adequate evalu-

ation of the nervous and cardiovascular systems. An excretory urogram is essential because of the frequent occurrence of upper tract malformations. A barium swallow will define the length of and transit time through the small bowel.

When operative reconstruction is attempted, the omphalocele is closed first, avoiding the use of prosthetic flaps. Because of the absence of normal neuromuscular tissue in the perineum, an anoplasty is to be avoided since it would create an incontinent perineal ileostomy. Instead, for fecal diversion the bowel exstrophy is separated from the hemibladders and is either tubularized to create an abdominal cecostomy or is excised, with establishment of an abdominal ileostomy. For external urinary drainage, the hemibladders are joined to create a bladder exstrophy. After infancy, when prolonged survival is likely, an ileal conduit and cystectomy is done. Although the double penis has been successfully sutured together to form a single midline organ, in most cases the vestigial nature of the hemistructures precludes an adequate result; amputation with conversion to a female phenotype may be preferred when phallic tissue is inadequate [19, 36].

As for all children undergoing various forms of urinary tract diversion or extended reconstruction, lifelong follow-up, including periodic urine cultures and urograms, is essential.

References

1. Ambrose, J. S. Epispadias and vesicoureteral reflux. *South. Med. J.* 63:1193, 1970.
2. Bennett, A. H. Exstrophy of the bladder treated by ureterosigmoidostomies: Long-term evaluation. *Urology* 2:165, 1973.
3. Bergenhem, B. Ectopia vesicae et adenoma destruens vesicae, exstirpation of blasen; implantation of ureterena i rectum. *Eira* 19:268, 1895.
4. Bricker, E. M. Bladder substitution after pelvic evisceration. *Surg. Clin. North Am.* 30:1511, 1950.
4a. Campbell, J. *Clinical Pediatric Urology.* Philadelphia: Saunders, 1951.
5. Cendron, J. L'epispadias: 70 cas. *Urol. Int.* 27:291, 1972.
6. Clark, M. A., and O'Connell, K. J. Scanning and transmission electron microscopic studies of an exstrophic human bladder. *J. Urol.* 110:481, 1973.
7. Coffey, R. C. Physiologic implantation of the severed ureter or common bile duct into the intestine. *J.A.M.A.* 56:397, 1911.
8. Culp, D. A. Histology of the exstrophied bladder. *J. Urol.* 91:538, 1964.
9. Culp, O. S. Treatment of epispadias with and without urinary incontinence: Experience with 46 patients. *J. Urol.* 109:120, 1973.
10. Dretler, S. P. Urinary tract calculi and ileal conduit diversion. *Am. J. Surg.* 123:480, 1972.
11. Engel, R. M. E. Bladder exstrophy: Vesicoplasty or urinary diversion? *Urology* 2:20, 1973.
12. Genster, H. G. Changes in the composition of the urine in sigmoid loop bladders. *Scand. J. Urol. Nephrol.* 5:41, 1971.
13. Genster, H. G., and Skjoldborg, H. Changes in the composition of the urine after ileal loop urinary diversion. *Scand. J. Urol. Nephrol.* 5:37, 1971.
14. Haney, M. J., and McGarity, W. C. Ureterosigmoidostomy and neoplasms of the colon. *Arch. Surg.* 103:69, 1971.
15. Hanna, M. K., and Williams, D. I. Genital function in males with vesical exstrophy and epispadias. *Br. J. Urol.* 44:169, 1972.
15a. Hendren, W. H. Nonrefluxing colon conduit for temporary or permanent urinary diversion in children. *J. Pediatr. Surg.* 10:381, 1975.
16. Higgins, C. C. Exstrophy of the bladder: Report of 158 cases. *Am. Surg.* 28:99, 1962.
17. Jakobsen, B. E., and Olesen, S. Bladder exstrophy complicated by adenocarcinoma. *Dan. Med. Bul.* 15:253, 1968.
18. Jeffs, R. D. Functional Closure of Bladder Exstrophy: Review of Method, Patient Selection and Results. Presented at the Annual Meeting of the American Urological Association, Miami, Fla., May 11–15, 1975.
19. Johnston, J. H., and Kogan, S. J. The Exstrophic Anomalies and Their Surgical Reconstruction. In M. M. Ravitch (ed.), *Current Problems in Surgery.* Chicago: Year Book, August, 1974.
20. Lapides, J. Mechanism of electrolyte imbalance following ureter-sigmoid transplantation. *Surg. Gynecol. Obstet.* 93:691, 1951.
21. Marshall, V. F., and Muecke, E. C. Variations in exstrophy of the bladder. *J. Urol.* 88:766, 1962.
22. Marshall, V. F., and Muecke, E. C. Congenital Abnormalities of the Bladder. In *Encyclopedia of Urology.* Vol. VII/1, *Malformations.* Berlin: Springer, 1968.
23. Megalli, M., and Lattimer, J. K. Review of the management of 140 cases of exstrophy of the bladder. *J. Urol.* 109:246, 1973.
24. Mogg, R. A., and Syme, R. R. A. The results of urinary diversion using the colonic conduit. *Br. J. Urol.* 4:434, 1969.
25. Muecke, E. C. The role of the cloacal membrane in exstrophy: The first successful experimental study. *J. Urol.* 92:659, 1964.
26. Muecke, E. C., and Currarino, G. Congenital widening of the pubic symphysis: Associated clinical disorders and roentgen anatomy of affected bony pelves. *Am. J. Roentgenol. Radium Ther. Nucl. Med.* 103:179, 1968.
27. Retik, A. B., Perlmutter, A. D., and Gross, R. E. Cutaneous ureteroileostomy in children. *N. Engl. J. Med.* 277:217, 1967.
28. Rickham, P. P. The incidence and treatment of ectopia vesicae. *Proc. R. Soc. Med.* 54:389, 1961.
29. Rudin, L., Tannenbaum, M., and Lattimer, J. K. Histologic analysis of the exstrophied bladder after anatomical closure. *J. Urol.* 108:802, 1972.
30. Schwarz, G. R., and Jeffs, R. D. Ileal conduit urinary diversion in children: Computer analysis of followup from 2 to 16 years. *J. Urol.* 114:285, 1975.
31. Semerdjian, H. S., Texter, J. H., and Yawn, T. H. Rhabdomyosarcoma occurring in repaired exstrophied bladder: A case report. *J. Urol.* 108:354, 1972.
32. Shapiro, S. R., Lebowitz, R., and Colodny, A. H. Fate of 90 children with ileal conduit urinary diversion a decade later: Analysis of complications, pyelography, renal function and bacteriology. *J. Urol.* 114:289, 1975.
33. Spence, H. M. Ureterosigmoidostomy for exstrophy of the bladder: Results in a personal series of 31 cases. *J. Urol.* 38:36, 1966.
34. Spencer, R. Exstrophia splanchnica (exstrophy of the cloaca). *Surgery* 57:751, 1965.
35. Stiles, H. J. Epispadias in the female and its surgical treatment. *Surg. Gynecol. Obstet.* 13:127, 1911.
36. Tank, E. S., and Lindenauer, S. M. Principles of management of exstrophy of the cloaca. *Am. J. Surg.* 119:95, 1970.
37. Trendelenburg, F. Treatment of ectopia vesicae. *Ann. Surg.* 44:281, 1906.
38. Tuffier, T. *Traite De Chirurgie.* Paris: S. Duplay and P. Ruclus, 1892.
39. Wallace, D. M. Maydl's operation. *Proc. R. Soc. Med.* 54:383, 1961.
40. Weiss, G., Becker, J. A., Berdon, W. E., and Baker, D. H. Epispadias. *Radiology* 90:85, 1968.
41. Whitaker, R. H., Pugh, R. C. B., and Dow, D. Colonic tumors following ureterosigmoidostomy. *Br. J. Urol.* 43:562, 1971.
42. Williams, R. E., Davenport, T. J., Burkinshaw, L., and Hughes, D. Changes in whole body potassium associated with uretero-intestinal anastomoses. *Br. J. Urol.* 39:676, 1967.
43. Williams, D. I., and Keeton, J. E. Further progress with reconstruction of the exstrophied bladder. *Br. J. Surg.* 60:203, 1970.
44. Young, H. H. Exstrophy of the bladder. *Surg. Gynecol. Obstet.* 74:729, 1942.

104. Disorders of the Testis

Edward S. Tank

The male gonad is responsible for the production of spermatozoa. Its presence in utero is essential for the development of the ipsilateral ductal system. As an endocrine organ, the testis influences the development of the prostate and external genitalia. Both aspects of its functional state, germinal and endocrine, must be operative for fertility. Agenesis, dysgenesis, and torsion with vascular compromise, if bilateral, interfere with both functions. Maldescent and inflammatory processes influence spermatogenesis. Testicular tumors, although rare in infants and children, may threaten the life of the patient.

Development

At age 28 to 30 days after ovulation, corresponding to an embryonal crown–rump length of 5 mm, a thickening of the coelomic epithelium overlying the mesonephros is visible. Primordial germ cells originating in the yolk sac migrate to this area of proliferating mesothelium and underlying mesenchyme, causing projection of the primitive, sexually indeterminate gonad into the coelomic cavity. Male gonadal differentiation begins at 42 days, or 20 mm crown–rump length. The central cells arrange themselves in cords and ultimately converge at the hilus to form the seminiferous tubules. In the peripheral zone, the primordia of the tunica albuginea are represented by small, closely packed cells. Precursors of the straight and rete tubules are located near the mesorchium.

At 55 days the Leydig cells become apparent. The primordial tunic cells become differentiated and assume the character of loose connective tissue. At this point the wolffian duct structures are appropriated and develop into the epididymis, ductus deferens, and seminal vesicles under the influence of the ipsilateral testicle. The müllerian primordia at this point regress. In the absence of the testicle the müllerian structures continue to develop, and internal genital ductile development becomes phenotypically female. At the end of the seventh month of intrauterine life, the testes and epididymids are completely formed and ready for descent into the scrotum.

Agenesis and Dysgenesis

Bilateral testicular agenesis or severe dysgenesis is rare. Congenital anorchia is always associated with a male phenotype and masculine differentiation of the external genitalia. The phallus is normal. Wolffian development is usually normal, but absence has been reported. Müllerian ducts are never present. At puberty these males remain eunuchoid because of the absence of testosterone normally produced by the testes. Surgical and autopsy findings usually consist of a normal vas deferens with a sclerotic, mesodermal mass at its termination. Since the vas deferens is present and the external genitalia are phenotypically male, the testes must have been present during fetal development and then lost, perhaps by some intrauterine accident. Congenital anorchia can be differentiated from bilateral undescended dysgenetic testes by endocrine testing; surgical confirmation is unnecessary.

The most common form of bilateral testicular dysgenesis is Klinefelter's syndrome, which affects one in every 500 newborn males. These patients have a normal sized phallus with small, firm testes. Biopsy of the gonads reveals hyalinized, sclerotic tubules and clumped Leydig cells. The chromosomal constitution of these patients varies, but most commonly it is XXY. Less common forms of dysgenesis are seen in male Turner's syndrome and in the Sertoli-cell–only syndrome (del Castillo syndrome). Males with the Turner syndrome have the typical somatic stigmata of Turner syndrome and usually have genital underdevelopment; however, their buccal smear is almost always negative, and their karyotype is 46XY. Their testicular biopsies show varying degrees of germinal dysgenesis as compared to Sertoli-cell–only patients, who have complete germinal cell aplasia. Those children who present at birth with ambiguous external genitalia and severe dysgenesis of one or both testes are called dysgenetic male pseudohermaphrodites. When the testes are so dysgenetic that they can barely be recognized, with only a few hilar cells in the gonadal streak, the term *mixed gonadal dysgenesis* is more appropriate [4].

On occasion no testis or vas deferens is found at the time of exploration for cryptorchidism. The diagnosis of anorchia can be made only after complete retroperitoneal and intraperitoneal surgical exploration. The absence of both urinary and genital structures suggests an early developmental aberration.

Maldescent

Maldescent of the testis is the most commonly seen condition of the male gonad, affecting approximately 3.5 percent of full-term infants [12]. The incidence increases to over 30 percent in premature infants. The condition most commonly affects the right side, and it is bilateral in 25 percent of the cases. In the full-term infant 1 percent of testes remain undescended at 12 months of age. If truly undescended at this time, the testis is unlikely to descend spontaneously. It is probable that most cases of "spontaneous descent" occur in retractile testes with an overactive cremasteric reflex, rather than in true maldescent. As the testis enlarges, either with growth or with the administration of chorionic gonadotropin, its weight overcomes the cremasteric muscle and the testis remains in the scrotum.

The undescended testis may be ectopic, due to pulling by a gubernacular band in a direction other than toward the scrotum. Most frequently the ectopic location is in the groin above the external oblique muscle, where the testis has exited through the external inguinal ring. More rarely, the testis may be located in the suprapubic, femoral, or perineal region. In these circumstances the spermatic cord usually is of sufficient length so that the testis, which is histologically normal, can be placed in the scrotum surgically.

There seems to be no question that the gubernaculum, named by Hunter, plays a major role in the proper positioning of the testis in the scrotum. It is a tissue of mesenchymal derivation, approximately twice the size of the gonad, which forms at its lower pole. Its presence prior to the complete development of the musculature of the abdominal wall produces an oblique tunnel in the groin for later passage of the gonad. The major portion of the cremasteric muscle is derived from this structure. When the embryo has a crown–rump length of 40 mm, a small peritoneal protrusion, the future processus vaginalis, forms just below the gubernaculum. The gonad now lies just above the internal ring as a result of cranial degeneration and caudal differentiation of the urogenital ridge, as well as differential rates of growth of the fetus. The peritoneal recess subsequently deepens and the gubernaculum expands and changes its consistency, thus dilating the inguinal canal and scrotum and allowing the testis and the epididymis with its gradually lengthening vessels and vas deferens to descend into the scrotum. After passage through the external ring, the testis changes to a more globular shape and the external ring becomes relatively smaller, preventing reentry into the inguinal canal. The processus vaginalis subsequently obliterates, and descent is complete.

Maldescent, if untreated, impairs fertility [5–7, 11]. Men with untreated bilateral cryptorchid testes uniformly are sterile. If both testes are brought into the scrotum surgically prior to puberty, the overall fertility rate rises to 43 percent.

The presence of one normally placed testis does not ensure fertility; only 33 percent of males with untreated unilateral cryptorchidism are fertile, and evidence is accumulating that the apparently normal contralateral testis may also be defective. If the unilateral undescended testis is brought into the scrotum, the fertility rate rises to 75 percent. Even though properly treated, these patients have consistently smaller testes and lower sperm counts than normal subjects. In males with unilateral cryptorchid testes that have been brought down into the scrotum by orchiopexy, mean sperm density was only one-third that of control subjects 20 years after surgery.

Histologic comparison of normal testes, scrotally placed mates of undescended testes, and cryptorchid gonads provides evidence of the adverse effects of maldescent [2, 3, 9, 10]. No difference between the gonads can be detected from birth to 6 months of age. During this period the Leydig cells previously stimulated by maternal hormones regress. From 6 months to 2 years of age a resting phase occurs, with a decrease in mean tubular diameter seen in all groups. Starting at 18 to 24 months, the undescended testis shows a significant decrease in spermatogonia, atrophy of the Leydig cells, and a lack of tubular growth. In the normal gonad the growth phase continues until 8 years of age. If the testis remains undescended, this period of growth is completely inhibited, and germinal activity is absent after puberty. During the twelfth to seventeenth year, spermatogenesis is uniformly established in the normal testis. During this period the scrotal mate of the undescended testis shows dysgenetic changes microscopically, although appearing normal grossly. No active cell division is apparent. Whether these changes are inherent or an effect referrable to the undescended testis is not known.

Since the evidence is unequivocal that surgical placement of unilateral and bilateral undescended testes in the scrotum is essential to ensure maximum fertility, the only question is the optimal time for surgical intervention. Although 4 years of age was once considered the best time for operative treatment, recent evidence suggests that the time of orchiopexy should be as early as 2 years of age, although the increased likelihood of fertility must be balanced against the increased technical difficulties of performing the operation on structures of smaller size.

The cryptorchid testis has an increased potential for malignant degeneration, ranging from 20 to 30 times that of the normal organ [1, 8]. Even if the testis is brought into the scrotum, periodic examination is mandatory, since the potential for neoplastic degeneration is not changed by proper positioning of the gonad.

Torsion of the Testis

The patient with torsion of the spermatic cord and testicular infarction characteristically experiences a sudden onset of pain, often associated with physical activity. This incident may have been preceded by periodic transient pain, suggesting prior incomplete torsion. Physical examination reveals groin pain associated with testicular swelling and scrotal edema. Accurate diagnosis may be difficult because of a reactive hydrocele.

Torsion of the testis may occur in utero or in the neonatal period. It is more common, however, in older children and young adults. The predisposing anatomy is often bilateral, and surgical detorsion should be accompanied by fixation of the opposite testis.

The differential diagnosis includes torsion of the spermatic cord, torsion of the appendix testis or epididymis, epididymo-orchitis, incarcerated inguinal hernia, and testicular tumor. Careful history and physical examination often establish the correct diagnosis. If the diagnosis is in question, it can be made with certainty only by surgical exploration.

The history and symptomatology of torsion of the appendix testis or epididymis are the same as torsion of the testis. Treatment of all three conditions is surgical.

Inflammatory epididymo-orchitis may result from urinary tract infection, which can be diagnosed by appropriate examination of the urine. Viral orchitis complicates mumps in approximately 18 percent of adult males, but it is rare prior to puberty. Diagnosis is made by its association with the other clinical features of mumps. Surgical decompression by incision of the tunica albuginea should be reserved for cases of severe unilateral or bilateral involvement.

An incarcerated inguinal hernia can be ruled out by careful physical examination. Although the presence of a testicular tumor may be confused by the frequent association of a reactive hydrocele or by the history of recent trauma, a high index of suspicion will result in early operative intervention.

References

1. Campbell, H. E. The incidence of malignant growth of the undescended testicle: A reply and re-evaluation. *J. Urol.* 81:663, 1959.
2. Charny, C. W. The spermatogenic potential of the undescended testis before and after treatment. *J. Urol.* 83:697, 1960.
3. Farrington, G. H. Histologic observations in cryptorchidism: The congential germinal-cell deficiency in the undescended testis. *J. Pediatr. Surg.* 4:606, 1969.
4. Federman, D. D. *Abnormal Sexual Development.* Philadelphia: Saunders, 1968.
5. Hansen, T. S. Fertility in operatively treated and untreated cryptorchidism. *Proc. R. Soc. Med.* 42:645, 1949.
6. Hecker, W. C., and Hienz, H. A. Cryptorchism and fertility. *J. Pediatr. Surg.* 2:513, 1967.
7. Lipshultz, L. I., Caminus-Torres, R., Greenspan, B. A., and Synder, P. J. Testicular function after orchiopexy for unilaterally undescended testis. *N. Engl. J. Med.* 295:15, 1976.
8. Marin, D. C., and Menck, H. R. The undescended testis: Management after puberty. *J. Urol.* 114:77, 1975.
9. Mengel, W., Hienz, H. A., Sippe, W. G. II., and Hector, W. C. Studies on cryptorchidism: A comparison of histological findings in the germinative epithelium before and after the second year of life. *J. Pediatr. Surg.* 9:445, 1974.
10. Robinson, J. N., and Engle, E. T. Some observations of the cryptorchid testis. *J. Urol.* 71:726, 1954.
11. Scott, L. S. Fertility in cryptorchidism. *Proc. R. Soc. Med.* 55:1047, 1962.
12. Scorer, C. G., and Farrington, G. H. *Congenital Deformities of the Testis and Epididymis.* London: Butterworth, 1971.

105. Nephroblastoma (Wilms' Tumor)

Edward S. Tank

Nephroblastoma, or Wilms' tumor, constitutes up to 30 percent of malignant solid abdominal tumors in children and is second only to neuroblastoma in frequency. There are approximately 450 new cases per year in the United States. Sex distribution is equal. Although this neoplasm occurs at all ages, the mean age at the time of diagnosis is 2 years. Unequivocal Wilms' tumors have been documented in the newborn, but many questions have been raised about the true character of most renal tumors presenting in the first year of life. Many of these tumors are believed to be benign and have been called fetal renal hamartomas, or congenital mesoblastic nephromas [1, 2, 4, 5, 11, 14]. The predominant cell type is either a fibroblastic or smooth muscle cell. It is the general consensus that these lesions are usually cured by nephrectomy alone; only rarely do mesoblastic nephromas extend beyond the capsule and require postoperative radiotherapy and chemotherapy.

Wilms' tumor has an increased incidence in children with aniridia and congenital hemihypertrophy of parts of the body [15, 21, 23, 27]. Bilateral nephroblastoma occurs in 3 to 10 percent of the cases [3, 12, 17, 19, 25]. Whether this bilaterality represents separate primary growths or metastases from one kidney to the other is difficult to ascertain. In 65 percent of patients with bilateral involvement, tumor in both kidneys is apparent at the time of diagnosis. Appearance of tumor in the opposite kidney has been reported, however, as long as 10 years after discovery of the first lesion.

Clinical Manifestations

An abdominal mass is the initial manifestation of nephroblastoma in 80 to 90 percent of children. The size of the tumor often belies its sudden appearance, especially when the child has been examined recently by a physician. Rapid increase in size or the onset of abdominal pain may reflect hemorrhage into the tumor precipitated by central ischemic necrosis. The mass lesions are usually smooth and do not cross the midline. Pain is the second most common symptom of nephroblastoma, occurring in 20 to 30 percent of patients. Fever, nausea, and anorexia are frequent. Hypertension may be present if the tumor causes renal vascular distortion.

Diagnosis

An abdominal mass may represent pathology of the urinary tract, nervous system, or alimentary tract of either benign or malignant character. An intravenous pyelogram is essential in the differential diagnosis of nephroblastoma. The scout film may reveal calcification in the tumor, which is most common in neuroblastoma but is also seen in nephroblastoma. In neuroblastoma evidence of bony metastasis is present in more than half the patients, and bone marrow involvement is frequent. Nonvisualization of the upper urinary tract on the side of the mass suggests a multicystic kidney or Wilms' tumor with renal vein involvement or, rarely, intrapelvic extension. Delayed films (up to 12 to 24 hr after injection of the contrast material) may show limited function in a severely hydronephrotic kidney. Displacement of an otherwise normal collecting system usually results from adrenal or sympathetic chain neuroblastoma. Gross distortion of the collecting system is characteristic of Wilms' tumor.

Sonography will often define and differentiate fluid-filled lesions, such as multicystic kidney and hydronephrosis, from solid tumors, such as neuroblastoma and Wilms' tumor (see Chap. 11). If the tumor is large or if the involved kidney is nonfunctional, an inferior venacavogram is carried out to determine the presence of extension of tumor from the renal vein into the cava. A liver scan is done if there is a question of hepatic metastasis. A chest film and bone survey complete the radiologic evaluation.

Treatment

If the nephroblastoma is extensive or bilateral, preoperative treatment with chemotherapy and irradiation may be indicated. Since the tumor is usually well encapsulated, preoperative treatment is not often necessary in spite of extensive size. Surgical approach is by a transverse abdominal incision crossing the breadth of both rectus muscles and extending across the lateral muscles on the side of the tumor. This type of incision permits extension into the chest, if necessary, for removal of upper pole tumors. Attention is immediately directed toward control of the renal vein and artery, and both are divided as the initial step, if possible. Great care must be taken to be assured that there is no tumor extending into the renal vein prior to its division. If there is extension into the cava, control of the vessel above and below the tumor and of the opposite renal vein is mandatory. The cava is then opened and the tumor extracted prior to division of the renal vein. If the liver or colon is involved by direct extension in continuity, resection of portions of these structures is done. Ipsilateral regional lymph node dissection is carried out. The contralateral kidney is always examined directly by opening Gerota's fascia.

Staging of tumors is essential to postoperative management and for prognosis. Staging is as follows:

Stage I Tumor is limited to the kidney and is completely resected.

Stage II There is local extension beyond the kidney or to local lymph nodes that is completely resected.

Stage III Residual gross or microscopic tumor remains following surgery, but is confined to the abdomen, or there is spill of the tumor during surgery.

Stage IV Hematogenous metastases are present.

Stage V There is bilateral renal involvement.

Children more than 1 year of age with stage I tumors are given postoperative chemotherapy with actinomycin D and vincristine but are not subjected to irradiation therapy. Actinomycin D is given in courses, each consisting of 15 μg/kg body weight/day for 5 days. The first course is given on the day of surgery, prior to or during the operative procedure. Subsequent courses are given 6 weeks later and every 3 months thereafter over a 15-month period. Vincristine is injected intravenously in doses of 1.5 mg per square meter, with a maximum single dose of 2 mg. The drug is given once weekly for 8 weeks, starting on the day of surgery. Beginning 3 months later, two doses are given a week apart, every 3 months, over a 15-month period.

Patients with stage II or III nephroblastomas receive irradiation therapy postoperatively in addition to the chemotherapy described for stage I tumors. Patients with stage IV tumors are treated similarly. If pulmonary or hepatic metastases do not resolve and are amenable to complete resection, they are treated aggressively. Patients with bilateral involvement receive chemotherapy prior to an attempt at surgical resection. Irradiation therapy is best reserved for the postoperative treatment of residual tumor, but if no substantial response is apparent with chemotherapy, 1,500 rad to the entire abdomen and 300 rad to the most affected kid-

ney is administered. Two to three weeks after completion of this protocol, surgical exploration is carried out with an attempt made to preserve as much uninvolved renal parenchyma as possible. Optimally bilateral heminephrectomies can be done, but more usually nephrectomy and contralateral heminephrectomy is necessary. Bilateral nephrectomy and subsequent allotransplantation may be dictated by extensive involvement. De Lorimier et al. [9] reported five such cases with two survivors. Only one of the three deaths was the result of metastatic disease; the other two were from complications of treatment of the tumor and subsequent immunosuppressive therapy. These authors believe that bilateral nephrectomy should be performed immediately if chemotherapy and irradiation therapy fail to control the tumors.

Prognosis

There has been a decline in mortality from nephroblastoma of 75 percent during the past 50 years. Surgical treatment alone produced a survival rate of slightly less than 20 percent prior to the 1920s. Between 1920 and 1957, with the addition of radiotherapy, the survival rate doubled [16]. The advent of single-agent chemotherapy (actinomycin D) by Farber in 1957 resulted in an increase in survival to 70 percent [10, 18, 20, 22, 24]. Subsequently multiple-agent chemotherapy and extended chemotherapy now produce overall survival rates in the 80 to 90 percent range [7, 25].

The most recent data from the National Wilms' Tumor Study [8] reveal that 2 years after diagnosis, 83 percent of children classified initially as stage I and 81 percent of children classified as stage II or III were disease-free 2 years after diagnosis. In children with stage I tumor who were below 2 years of age at the time of diagnosis, this figure increased to 89 percent.

References
1. Beckwith, J. B. Mesenchymal renal neoplasms of infancy. *J. Pediatr. Surg.* 5:405, 1970.
2. Beckwith, J. B. Mesenchymal renal neoplasms of infancy, revisited. *J. Pediatr. Surg.* 9:803, 1974.
3. Bishop, H. C., and Hope, J. W. Bilateral Wilms' tumors. *J. Pediatr. Surg.* 1:476, 1966.
4. Bogdan, R., Taylor, D. E. M., and Mostofi, F. K. Leiomyomatous hamartoma of the kidney. A clinical and pathological analysis of 20 cases from the kidney tumor registry. *Cancer* 31:462, 1973.
5. Bolande, R. P., Brough, A. J., and Izant, R. J. Congenital mesoblastic nephroma of infancy. *Pediatrics* 40:272, 1967.
6. Cassady, J. R., Tefft, M., Filler, R. M., Jaffe, N., Paed, D., and Hellman, S. Considerations in the radiation therapy of Wilms' tumor. *Cancer* 32:598, 1973.
7. D'Angio, G. J. Management of children with Wilms' tumor. *Cancer* 30:1528, 1972.

8. D'Angio, G. J., Evans, A. E., Breslow, N., Beckwith, B., Bishop, H., Feigl, P., Goodwin, W., Leape, L. L., Sinks, L. F., Sutow, W., Tefft, M., and Wolff, J. The treatment of Wilms' tumor: Results of National Wilms' Tumor Study. *Cancer* 38:633, 1976.

9. De Lorimier, A. A., Belzer, F. O., Kountz, S. L., and Kushner, J. H. Simultaneous bilateral nephrectomy and renal allotransplantation for bilateral Wilms' tumor. *Surgery* 64:850, 1968.

10. Ehrlich, R. M., and Goodwin, W. E. The surgical treatment of nephroblastoma (Wilms' tumor). *Cancer* 32:1145, 1973.

11. Favara, B., Johnson, W., and Ito, J. Renal tumors in the neonatal period. *Cancer* 22:845, 1968.

12. Fay, R., Brosman, S., and Williams, D. I. Bilateral nephroblastoma. *J. Urol.* 110:119, 1973.

13. Fraumeni, J. F., Jr., and Glass, A. G. Wilms' tumor and congenital aniridia. *J.A.M.A.* 206:825, 1968.

14. Fu, Y., and Kay, S. Congenital mesoblastic nephroma and its recurrence. *Arch. Pathol.* 96:66, 1973.

15. Haicken, B. N., and Miller, D. R. Simultaneous occurrence of congenital aniridia, hamartoma and Wilms' tumor. *J. Pediatr.* 78:497, 1971.

16. Klapproth, H. L. Wilms' tumor: A report of 45 cases and an analysis of 1,351 cases reported in the world literature from 1940 to 1958. *J. Urol.* 81:633, 1959.

17. Leen, R. L. S., and Williams, I. G. Bilateral Wilms' tumor: Seven personal cases and observations. *Cancer* 28:802, 1971.

18. Lemeule, J., and Donaldson, S. S. Wilms' tumor: Current concepts in diagnosis, prognosis and treatment. *Pediatr. Ann.* 1:220, 1972.

19. Martin, L. W., and Kluecke, R. J. Bilateral nephroblastoma (Wilms' tumor). *Pediatrics* 28:101, 1961.

20. Margolis, L. W., Smith, W. B., Wara, W. M., Kushner, J. H., and De Lorimier, A. A. Wilms' tumor: An interdisciplinary treatment program with and without dactinomycin. *Cancer* 32:618, 1973.

21. Meadows, A. T., Lichtenfeld, J. L., and Koop, C. E. Wilms' tumor in three children of a woman with congenital hemihypertrophy. *N. Engl. J. Med.* 291:23, 1974.

22. Perez, C. A., Kaiman, H. A., Keith, J., Mill, W. B., Vietti, T. J., and Powers, W. E. Treatment of Wilms' tumor and factors affecting prognosis. *Cancer* 32:609, 1973.

23. Pilling, G. P. Wilms' tumor in seven children with congenital aniridia. *J. Pediatr. Surg.* 10:87, 1975.

24. Swenson, O., and Brenner, R. Aggressive approach to the treatment of Wilms' tumor. *Ann. Surg.* 166:657, 1967.

25. Tsunoda, A., Ishida, M., and Ohmi, K. Bilateral Wilms' tumor: A case report and a survey of nineteen cases in Japanese literature. *Acta Paediatr. Jpn.* 11:1, 1969.

26. Wolff, J. A., D'Angio, G., Hartmann, J., Krivit, W., and Newton, W. A., Jr. Long-term evaluation of single versus multiple courses of actinomycin D therapy of Wilms' tumor. *N. Engl. J. Med.* 290:84, 1974.

27. Woodard, J. R., and Levine, M. K. Nephroblastoma (Wilms' tumor) and congenital aniridia. *J. Urol.* 101:140, 1969.

106. Neoplasms of the Lower Urinary Tract

Edward S. Tank

Urothelial Tumors

Since 1950 only 12 cases of epithelial tumors of the bladder in children under 15 years of age have been reported [2, 3, 9], with a 2 : 1 predominance of males over females. The presenting symptom in each case was hematuria. All lesions were papillomatous.

Since all bladder papillomas are considered grade I carcinomas, these tumors must be considered malignant. They are removed by transurethral resection or open wedge resection; recurrence has not been recorded.

Urachal Carcinoma

In 1970 only 78 cases of urachal carcinoma had been reported in patients of all ages [1], with only 1 patient less than 15 years of age [5]. Radical operative extirpation, including en bloc removal of the umbilicus and bladder, is mandatory. The fact that local recurrence occurred in more than one-third of the patients treated with partial cystectomy suggests that incomplete resection was at fault. Total cystectomy and intestinal urinary diversion is recommended as the treatment of choice.

Rhabdomyosarcoma

The majority of vesical and prostatic neoplasms in children are rhabdomyosarcomas. This very malignant embryonal sarcoma may occur in any part of the body; 15 percent arise within the urogenital tract.

The predilection of rhabdomyosarcomas for the trigone of the bladder, the prostate, vagina, and the paratesticular tissues suggests an origin in the mesenchymal cells of the mesonephros. Some authorities prefer to call these neoplasms embryonal sarcomas, emphasizing the lack of evidence of maturation toward skeletal muscle [8]. Others justify the term *embryonal rhabdomyosarcomas* by stressing the similarity between these lesions and developing embryonic and fetal skeletal muscles [10]. The fact that extensive submucosal growth within the wall of a hollow viscus often produces nodular protrusions into the lumen that resemble bunches of grapes had led to the use of the term *sarcoma botryoides*. This is a poor term, since it describes only the gross characteristics of some tumors.

The high mortality rate that was associated with rhabdomyosarcomas of the bladder and prostate in the past suggested a rapidly invasive tumor with early distant metastases. These tumors, however, are initially locally invasive and spread to distant sites only late in their course. Unfortunately they grow in such a way that they infrequently cause mucosal ulceration with resultant hematuria.

In most instances the age of the patient and his inability to relate bladder symptoms to his parents cause the child to be admitted with urinary retention secondary to bladder outlet obstruction. In 13 patients with vesical and prostatic rhabdomyosarcoma treated at the University of Michigan Hospital [6], 12 presented with urinary retention; only 1 presented with hematuria. In more than half the patients the suprapubic tumor mass is palpable, and in most cases this mass is initially thought to be a distended bladder. The average age of children with bladder lesions is 4 years. Patients with prostatic rhabdomyosarcoma fall into an older age group, with the average age being 9 years. Males predominate over females, probably because of the incidence of prostatic involvement.

In the past, pelvic exenteration was believed to offer the only chance for survival in patients with rhabdomyosarcoma. In spite of this ultraradical surgical approach, however, long-term survival was limited to scattered cases. Cure rates in large series ranged from zero to 20 percent. The use of postoperative chemotherapy and irradiation therapy proved only palliative. Recently the use of triple drug therapy (actinomycin D, vincristine, and cyclophosphamide) preoperatively, conservative surgery limited to organs directly involved, and postoperative chemotherapy and irradiation has dramatically increased the survival rate. Two-year survival rates ranging from 30 to 75 percent are now being reported [4, 6]. Since occult submucosal extension is often present, complete cystectomy and urethrectomy is essential.

References

1. Beck, A. D., and Gaudin, H. J. Carcinoma of the urachus. *Br. J. Urol.* 42:555, 1970.
2. Castellanos, R. D., Wakefield, P. B., and Evans, A. T. Carcinoma of the bladder in children. *J. Urol.* 113:261, 1975.
3. Chandy, P. C. X., Pai, M. G., Budihol, M. R., and Kaulgud, S. R. Carcinoma of the bladder in young children. *J. Urol.* 113:264, 1975.
4. Clatworthy, H. W., Jr., Braven, V., and Smith, J. P. Surgery of bladder and prostatic neoplasms in children. *Cancer* 32:1157, 1973.
5. Cornil, C., Reynolds, C. T., and Kickham, C. J. E. Carcinoma of the urachus. *J. Urol.* 98:98, 1967.
6. Ghavimi, F., Exelby, P. R., D'Angio, G. J., Whitmore, W. F., Jr., Lieberman, P. H., Lewis, J. L., Jr., Mike, V., and Murphy, M. D. Combination therapy of urogenital embryonal rhabdomyosarcoma in children. *Cancer* 32:1178, 1973.
7. Mardsen, H. B., and Steard, J. K. (eds.). *Recent Results in Cancer Research: Tumors in Children.* New York: Springer-Verlag, 1968. P. 198.
8. Patton, R. B., and Horn, R. C., Jr. Rhabdomyosarcoma: Clinical and pathological features and comparison with human fetal embryonal skeletal muscle. *Surgery* 52:572, 1962.
9. Ray, B., Grabstald, H., Ezelby, P. R., and Whitmore, W. F., Jr. Bladder tumors in children. *Urology* 2:426, 1973.
10. Tank, E. S., Fellmann, S. L., Wheller, E. S., Weaver, D. K., and Lapides, T. Treatment of urogenital tract rhabdomyosarcoma in infants and children. *J. Urol.* 107:324, 1972.

107. Tumors of the Testis

Thomas O. Robbins

The group of childhood testicular and paratesticular tumors includes a variety of neoplastic entities that must be considered separately to be understood and to be properly treated. They are relatively rare; only 2 to 5 percent of all testicular tumors occur under age 15 [25]. Few large series have been reported, and the literature, although substantial, contains a predominance of case reports. As a result, the special features of these neoplasms have been obscured, and they have frequently not been adequately differentiated from the more common adolescent and adult testicular tumors. Perhaps the most confusion has resulted from a failure to appreciate the nature of the infantile embryonal carcinoma and its morphologic and behavioral differences from the embryonal carcinoma of adults. In recent years, sufficient numbers of cases have been reviewed and analyzed to provide an adequate basis for classification of testicular and paratesticular tumors in children, but questions concerning proper management remain incompletely resolved.

Epidemiology

Epidemiologic studies of children's testicular tumors in the United States demonstrate a small, narrow peak of mortality at age 2 and a much higher peak that begins at age 15 and extends into adulthood [37]. The early peak is mainly due to the infantile embryonal carcinomas. These are the most common tumors, and 75 percent of them occur in the first 2 years of life. Most of the other types of tumor are distributed more evenly throughout childhood.

Testicular tumors are relatively rare in blacks of all ages. In the United States the mortality rate for testicular tumors in children age 0 to 4 is 1.04/million/year among whites and 0.36/million/year in blacks. A survey of all fatal childhood testicular tumors in the United States from 1960 to 1967 (excluding Louisiana and Missouri from 1965 to 1967) recorded 127 deaths, including 117 whites, 8 blacks, 1 Hawaiian, and 1 American Indian [37]. Most, if not all, of this difference between black and white children is due to the rarity of testicular germ cell tumors in blacks. A survey of the literature in 1965 of all reported childhood testicular tumors with adequate documentation of the tumor morphology included 221 cases [25]. Only seven of these children were known to be black. These tumors in black children included 1 embryonal carcinoma, 3 interstitial cell tumors, 1 gonadal stromal tumor, and 2 lymphomas. No other racial differences are known, although testicular tumors are not rare in Japanese children, judging from the large series of cases reported from Japan [30, 60, 70].

The geographic distribution of deaths from testicular tumors in children appears to be random in the United States, and incidence rates have been stable over the past 35 years [37]. The latter observation is of interest, since the incidence of testicular tumors in adults has been increasing in recent decades in the United States, Great Britain, and Denmark [37, 49].

Clinical Manifestations

The majority of testicular tumors are hormonally inactive and present as painless scrotal masses.

They are frequently misinterpreted as hydroceles [15], an error that may lead to unfortunate delays in treatment. In this regard it should be emphasized that these neoplasms are often associated with hydroceles, which may transilluminate, further supporting the clinical misimpression [19, 55].

Less commonly the tumors are hormonally active and present with precocious sexual development and/or gynecomastia. When such cases are not associated with a palpable scrotal mass, thermography may be successfully utilized to identify the involved testis [57].

The increased incidence of testicular neoplasms in cryptorchid testes, which has been repeatedly confirmed in adults [32, 46, 49], has not been clearly demonstrated in children. Occasional cases have been reported, however, and have included a teratoma in an abdominal testis of a 2-month-old child [22], an infantile embryonal carcinoma in an abdominal testis of a 9-month-old [74], an infantile embryonal carcinoma in the inguinal testis of a 13-month-old [74], and a rhabdomyosarcoma in a 14-year-old whose testis had remained undescended until hormonal treatment at age 6 [37]. While these and other scattered reports [2, 72] suggest a possible weak association between childhood tumors and maldescent, the clear relationship noted in adults has not been demonstrated. The reasons for this difference are unknown, although the studies by Altman and Malament of testicular neoplasms occurring in patients who had previous surgical correction of a maldescended testicle are probably germane [5]. In their review of the literature they found 45 patients whose age at the time of orchiopexy was known. In all but 2 the surgery was performed at age 11 or older, and none was under age 5. The implication seems clear that hormonal or other factors that become operational at or around the time of puberty must interact with the cryptorchid testis in its abnormal environment to produce changes that predispose it to neoplasia.

There is no convincing evidence to support a familial or genetic role in this disease. In a review of testicular tumors reported in siblings, Hutter et al. in 1967 found five sets of twins and four nontwin brothers with these neoplasms [29]. All of the cases of known age were in adults. The only pediatric case they found was in a pair of 6-year-old monozygotic phenotypic females with an XY karyotype and bilateral gonadoblastomas [16]. In the 1960–1967 national survey of testicular tumors in children, only one testicular tumor in a relative, a 55-year-old granduncle, was reported [37].

Table 107-1. Testicular and Paratesticular Neoplasms in Children

Histologic Type	Number of Patients	Percent of Total
Germ cell tumors	157	88.2
Infantile embryonal carcinomas	118	66.3
Teratomas	38	21.3
Seminomas	1	0.6
Non-germ cell tumors	7	3.9
Leydig cell tumors	2	1.1
Sertoli cell tumors	5	2.8
Paratesticular tumors	10	5.6
Embryonal rhabdomyo-sarcomas	7	3.9
Other sarcomas	3	1.7
Secondary tumors	3	1.7
Leukemia or lymphomas	3	1.7
Miscellaneous	1	0.6
Benign cyst	1	0.6
Total	178	100.0

Sources: Compiled from references 2, 7, 9, 30, 48, 70.

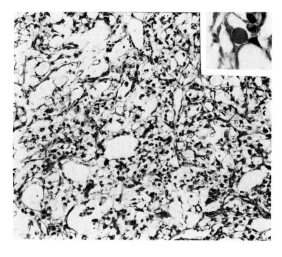

Figure 107-1. Infantile embryonal carcinoma, right testicle, in a 1-year-old male. The loose anastomosing glandular pattern alternating with sheets or nests of vacuolated cells is characteristic. Insert shows typical example of the eosinophilic, periodic acid–Schiff-positive hyaline bodies, which have been shown to contain α-fetoprotein. (×90, insert ×360.)

Classification

Table 107-1 shows the classification of pediatric testicular tumors. The incidence figures are compiled from six large, well-studied series. The advantage of using such series to compare the distribution of tumor types is that the pathologic diagnoses tend to be more accurate than in sporadic case reports, and the bias in favor of the exotic and unusual is avoided. These large series have their own potential bias, however, because they originate from centers where particularly difficult therapeutic problems tend to aggregate, and they may thus have overrepresentation of more aggressive tumors.

GERM CELL TUMORS

Virtually all pediatric testicular germ cell tumors are infantile embryonal carcinomas, teratomas, or mixtures of the two. Seminomas and choriocarcinomas have been reported rarely, but almost all of these occurred in children over age 10. The occurrence of the adult embryonal carcinoma in childhood is difficult to substantiate, because many authors have failed to distinguish adult from infantile embryonal carcinoma. The adult embryonal carcinomas probably occur only rarely, if ever, in children [52].

Infantile Embryonal Carcinoma

Synonyms for infantile embryonal carcinoma include juvenile embryonal carcinoma, yolk sac tumor, Teilum tumor, entodermal sinus tumor, clear cell adenocarcinoma, and orchioblastoma (Fig. 107-1). This is the most common testicular tumor in children and accounts for 40 to 85 percent of the tumors in large reported series [2, 7, 9, 30, 48]. In the collected series shown in Table 107-1, 66.3 percent of all tumors and 76.6 percent of germ cell tumors were infantile embryonal carcinomas. More than three-fourths are discovered during the first 2 years of life (Fig. 107-2).

The infantile embryonal carcinoma has been clearly recognized only in the last 20 years. In 1956 Magner et al. reported a series of seven tumors in infants from the Canadian Tumor Registry under the name testicular adenocarcinoma with clear cells. They recognized the tumor to be distinctly different from adult embryonal carcinoma [39]. Numerous subsequent articles confirmed the tumor's distinctive morphology and suggested a relatively favorable prognosis [26, 52, 66]. Arguments over concepts of histogenesis and over the importance of minor morphologic variations, however, resulted in a profusion of suggested names and doubts about the homogeneity of the group. These questions were subsequently resolved in an elegantly persuasive series of articles by Teilum and others [26, 62–64], demonstrating patterns within these tumors that show remarkable similarity to both human extraembryonic vascular mesoderm and to intraplacental structures in rodents known as the endodermal sinuses of Duval. The latter struc-

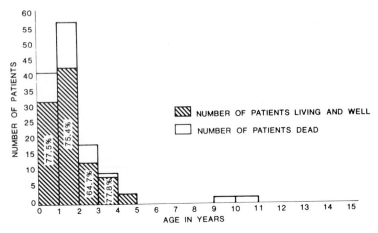

Figure 107-2. Infantile embryonal carcinoma of the testis: frequency distribution and survival by age. (Data are compiled from 127 cases collected from references 30, 31, 34, 39, 52, 73, and 74.)

tures apparently are diverticula of the rodent's yolk sac. These observations provided evidence that the infantile embryonal carcinoma is a specific type of malignant tumor of germ cell origin with maturation toward extraembryonic yolk sac structures [42, 51, 62, 63].

Infantile embryonal carcinoma may originate in locations other than the testis. It has been identified in all of those midline sites where other germ cell tumors are found: paratesticular tissues [36], the pelvis [27, 67], the sacrococcygeal area [11, 12, 27], the retroperitoneum [36, 74], the anterior mediastinum [11, 27], the pineal gland, and the suprasellar region of the cranium [3, 11]. It has been reported in the liver [23], the vagina of infants [4, 50], the ovaries of children and young adults [28], and in adult testes [52, 73]. It frequently occurs in association with other germ cell tumors [52]. When significant numbers of cases have accumulated to allow evaluation of the prognosis, the tumor has been found to be extremely aggressive and usually rapidly fatal in all of these locations. There is no known explanation for the more favorable prognosis when it occurs in children's testes.

The infantile embryonal carcinoma is virtually always unilateral, although one case of questionable bilaterality has been reported [74]. In general, the clinical stage of childhood cases tends to be relatively favorable, although few reports provide sufficient information to evaluate the extent of disease. In the series of Young and associates, 11 of 13 tumors (85 percent) were confined to the scrotum at the time of diagnosis [74]. Forty-nine of 62 (79 percent) of the cases reported from Japan by Ise et al. had no evidence of metastases at the time of the initial diagnosis [30].

Tumor spread may occur by direct extension or by vascular and lymphatic routes. Metastases are found most often in retroperitoneal lymph nodes, lungs, bones, and liver [34]. In advanced disease metastases may involve the homolateral kidney, the brain, and the meninges [73]. New metastases are noted only rarely after the second postoperative year, and children living 3 years with no evidence of metastatic disease apparently have a very high probability of cure [44, 66, 73]. It is, of course, at least theoretically possible that chemotherapy may prolong the interval before the appearance of metastases.

Pierce et al. emphasized the importance of age in the prognosis [52]. They combined their series of cases with those of Magner et al. [39], Teoh et al. [66], and Houser et al. [25] for a total of 31 cases with adequate data. Only 2 of 22 treated prior to age 2 died, while 8 of 9 over age 2 succumbed to their disease. While these figures are indeed striking and may reflect a true difference in prognosis according to age, they suggest a much greater disparity than probably actually exists. In the series of Ise et al. [30], 7 of 44 (16 percent) children under age 2 died of their disease, while 4 of 18 (22 percent) over this age died. Young and colleagues [74] had 5 of 14 (35.5 percent) deaths in the first 2 years of life and only 1 of 4 (25 percent) with evidence of recurrent disease in older children. In the series of Woodtli and Hedinger [73], 6 of 15 (40 percent) of infants under 2 died, while 1 of 4 (25 percent) of older children proved to have fatal disease. These figures suggest that if the age of the patient does indeed have prognostic implications, it is not sufficiently striking to justify either a casual attitude toward these tumors in the first 2 years of life or despairing therapeutic nihilism in older children.

One of the most interesting and important recent advances in the study of infantile embryonal carcinoma is the discovery of its tendency to manufacture and secrete α-fetoprotein [64, 65, 69]. This provides further evidence of the yolk sac differentiation of this tumor, since most α-fetoprotein in the normal human embryo is manufactured in the yolk sac and liver [20] and 70 to 80 percent of hepatomas are also associated with high serum concentrations of α-fetoprotein [35]. The development of a sensitive radioimmunoassay promises to provide clinicians with a valuable adjunct for staging these lesions after orchiectomy. The percentage of patients with positive tests in the presence of metastatic disease has not yet been precisely determined for children, but elevated levels were found in 19 of 23 adult nonseminomatous testicular tumors with metastases. Levels in children may be expected to be even more frequently elevated [35, 64, 69]. It must be remembered, of course, that the test should not be performed for several days after removal of the testicular tumor and that liver disease may cause false-positive results.

Teratomas

Teratomas are complex neoplasms that show evidence of differentiation toward more than one germ cell layer, with tissue foreign to the organ in which they arise. The pure teratomas are benign in children, but they may be mixed with other malignant germ cell tumors. It is imperative, therefore, to sample them thoroughly at the time of pathologic examination. Particular attention should be paid to areas of hemorrhage, necrosis, and mucoid softening, for these are most likely to represent infantile embryonal carcinoma.

Teratomas are rarely bilateral [2]. The most useful classification subdivides the teratomas into three groups: mature teratomas, immature teratomas, and mixed germ cell tumors with teratoma. The term *teratocarcinoma* is often used but is ambiguous, since it has been variously applied to the differentiating teratoma, which in children is benign, and to the mixed germ cell tumors with teratoma, which are malignant.

Mature Teratoma. (Differentiated Teratoma). These tumors contain only mature somatic tissues, frequently in an organoid arrangement. They tend to occur in somewhat older children than the immature teratomas [2]. In children they are uniformly benign [2, 15, 19, 33]. Since approximately one-third of such tumors do metastasize in adults, however, patients with mature teratomas that occur after puberty should be evaluated carefully. Nevertheless, it must be emphasized that meta-

stases occur very rarely, if ever, in patients under age 16.

Keratin-filled, squamous-lined cysts occur occasionally in the testes of children and adults and are known as epidermoid cysts. If they are unaccompanied by scar tissue or teratomatous elements, they are benign in both children and adults [54].

Immature Teratoma (Differentiating Teratoma). These tumors contain immature somatic tissues, with or without accompanying mature elements. The immature tissues most often consist of cellular mesenchymal or neural tissues with variable mitotic activity (Fig. 107-3). These tumors are usually found in younger children, and in this group the clinical course is uniformly benign [2, 15, 25]. It is important to note, however, that four of five such tumors proved fatal in a group of patients age 16 to 19, suggesting that immature testicular teratomas occurring after puberty should be considered as at least potentially malignant [1].

Mixed Germ Cell Tumors with Teratoma. This group contains tumors with mature or immature teratomatous areas associated with other germ cell tumor patterns. In children the second pattern is almost always that of the infantile embryonal carcinoma. Seminomas, adult embryonal carcinomas, or choriocarcinomas may be seen after puberty.

These tumors should be considered malignant. While insufficient numbers of cases have been evaluated to assess the prognosis in children, there is no doubt that they have the ability to metastasize [31, 73].

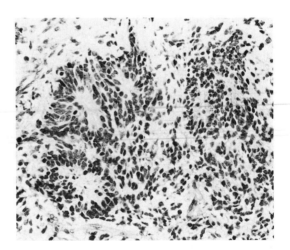

Figure 107-3. Immature neuroepithelial tissue within a right testicular immature teratoma from a 22-month-old boy. This pattern should be carefully distinguished from the infantile embryonal carcinoma pattern of a mixed teratoma. ($\times$360.)

NON-GERM CELL TUMORS

These tumors arise from either specialized gonadal stroma (Sertoli or Leydig cells or their precursors) or supporting tissues (connective tissue, blood vessels, nerves, etc.).

Tumors of Specialized Gonadal Stroma

Leydig Cell Tumors (Interstitial Cell Tumors). Of an estimated 170 interstitial cell tumors recorded in the literature, 40 occurred in children [25]. The age distribution appears to be bimodal, with a peak at age 5 to 10 and a second peak at 30 to 35 years [17]. The incidence in blacks and whites is almost the same.

In children, Leydig cell tumors virtually always present clinically as pseudoprecocious puberty,* with enlarged penis, facial and pubic hair, acne, and deepening voice. There may be impressive skeletal and muscular development and awakening sexual awareness [53]. These masculinizing symptoms are, in a small percentage of cases, paradoxically accompanied by gynecomastia [17]. The hormonally induced manifestations are usually accompanied by a palpable testicular tumor. Urinary 17-ketosteroids are usually elevated [13, 25, 44]. Patients may present after puberty simply with a scrotal mass, but 20 to 25 percent have accompanying gynecomastia and feminization [17, 57].

These neoplasms are usually unilateral, but bilateral tumors are found in 5 to 9 percent of the cases. The presence of bilateral tumors should suggest the possibility of adrenogenital syndrome with Leydig cell hyperplasia [49].

Somewhat less than 10 percent of Leydig cell tumors have proved to be malignant. All of these malignant cases, however, have been in adults, and there is to date no documented example of a malignant Leydig cell tumor in a child [17, 25, 40]. Regression of secondary signs and symptoms is reported to occur in 80 percent of patients after removal of the tumor [17].

Sertoli Cell Tumors (Androblastoma or Undifferentiated Gonadal Stromal Tumors). Sertoli cell tumors may show varying degrees of histologic differentiation, from primitive, undifferentiated stromal tissue to well-formed tubules lined by Sertoli cells. Mostofi prefers to refer to those with no evidence of differentiation simply as "primitive gonadal stromal tumors" [49]. Occasionally Sertoli cell tumors show a pattern closely resembling granulosa-theca cell tumors, which are, of course, the major tumor of ovarian gonadal stroma [49].

* The term pseudoprecocious puberty refers to the premature development of secondary sex characteristics without associated formation of mature sperm.

In 1974 Weitzner and Gropp reviewed 23 childhood cases of Sertoli cell tumors from the English and Western European literature [72]. Over two-thirds occurred in the first year of life. Two were bilateral, and 1 was found in an undescended testis. One 7-month-old showed evidence of sexual precocity, and 3 children had gynecomastia. Only 1 case proved malignant. This was a huge, 10-cm tumor in an 8-year-old black male with retroperitoneal lymph node metastases. The patient was alive 2 years after surgery, radiotherapy, and chemotherapy [56].

The criteria of malignancy have not been clearly delineated, since only a few malignant Sertoli cell tumors have been reported in children or adults. Extension of the tumor outside the testicle, high mitotic rates, and invasion of vascular and lymphatic spaces have been suggested as indicative of malignancy, but at this time only the presence of metastases can be accepted as proof [72]. Metastases are usually first noted in iliac and paraaortic lymph nodes [59].

Tumors of Nonspecialized Gonadal Stroma and Paratesticular Tumors

Tumors of nonspecialized gonadal stroma in the testes of children are very rare and include a variety of miscellaneous lesions such as fibromas, hemangiomas, and retinal anlage tumors [25]. Their major significance lies in the confusion they cause in differential diagnosis.

Paratesticular tumors are more common. The most frequent tumor found in this location in children is the tiny adrenal rest, which is usually an incidental finding at the time of a hydrocelectomy. It has no clinical significance. The relatively common adenomatoid tumors of the spermatic cord found in adults occur only rarely in children [71].

The most important childhood paratesticular tumor is the embryonal rhabdomyosarcoma (Fig. 107-4) [6, 8, 24, 38, 41, 49, 60]. It usually presents as a painless scrotal mass adjacent to the testicle. It may transilluminate and may therefore be misdiagnosed as a hydrocele, leading to delays in therapeutic intervention [10, 60]. Such delays are unfortunate, because the tumor is clinically aggressive with a tendency to metastasize widely by both vascular and lymphatic routes.

A recent review of 80 paratesticular rhabdomyosarcomas in children and adolescents showed a 35 percent 1-year survival [19]. Seventy-one percent of children under age 5 survived 1 year, but only 8 percent of 11- to 15-year-olds were alive after 1 year. The review by Brosman et al. of 45 cases from the English literature, however, offered a

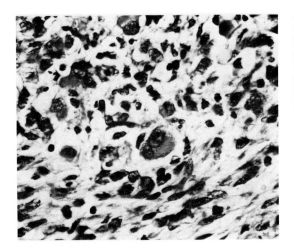

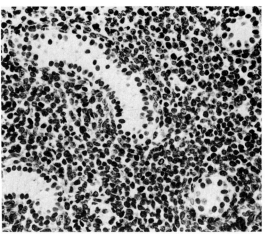

Figure 107-4. *Spermatic cord embryonal rhabdomyosarcoma from a 4-year-old boy. Cells with abundant eosinophilic cytoplasm help confirm the diagnosis when they are found in a poorly differentiated spindle cell tumor. No cross striations were identified.* (×360.)

Figure 107-5. *Acute stem cell leukemia, left testicle, from a 5-year-old boy. Diffuse stromal infiltration by immature cells with orderly separation of seminiferous tubules is characteristic of leukemia and lymphoma.* (×230.)

more hopeful prognosis [10]. Thirty-five (74 percent) of these patients with paratesticular embryonal rhabdomyosarcoma survived 2 years. The authors advocated aggressive therapy, including radical orchiectomy, lymph node dissection, radiation therapy, and chemotherapy. They reported that all 13 patients treated in this way were alive at 2 years despite the initial presence of retroperitoneal lymph node metastases in 10 of them.

A variety of other benign and malignant tumors may be found rarely in a paratesticular location. These include fibromas, hemangiomas [47], retinal anlage tumors [14, 75], fibrous histiocytomas [45], and extratesticular infantile embryonal cell carcinomas [36].

Metastatic Tumors
The most common secondary tumors of the testes in children are the leukemias and lymphomas (Fig. 107-5). Leukemic infiltrates are frequently noted in the testes at autopsy, but involvement is seldom detected clinically [21]. In one study of 163 male leukemic children, 13 (8 percent) developed testicular enlargement [58]. These 13 children had 19 such episodes, 9 unilateral and 10 bilateral. In the majority of cases there was complete bone marrow remission at the time of the testicular enlargement, suggesting that the testes may have served as a "sanctuary" that protected the leukemic cells from chemotherapy. In this series 140 children had acute undifferentiated or lymphoblastic leukemia, and 10 of them had

testicular involvement. Five of the children, 3 with testicular involvement, had non-Hodgkins lymphomas with leukemic transformation. The remainder had nonlymphoblastic leukemia and had no testicular involvement. Whatever the primary diagnosis, testicular infiltration served as an ominous prognostic sign with a median interval of 9 months from testicular enlargement to death.

Other tumors, such as neuroblastoma and Wilms' tumor, occasionally metastasize to the testes.

Treatment
Most authors agree that the initial approach to a suspected testicular or paratesticular neoplasm should be high inguinal orchiectomy without preliminary biopsy. Subsequent therapy will depend upon the histologic classification of the tumor and the clinical stage. As noted above, mature and immature teratomas, epidermal cysts, Leydig cell tumors, and Sertoli cell tumors are almost invariably benign in children and are best treated, therefore, by careful clinical evaluation of the patient and long-term follow-up to detect the rare patient with asynchronous development of tumor in the contralateral testis and the even more unlikely patient with subsequent metastases.

Infantile embryonal carcinomas (with and without teratomas) are a more difficult therapeutic problem. There are advocates of radical orchiectomy alone, retroperitoneal lymph node dissection, radiation therapy, chemotherapy, and various combinations of these modalities [11, 18, 31, 43, 44, 61]. Most acknowledge that these recommendations are based on small numbers of cases that are frequently not randomized for stage of disease, type of therapy, or follow-up periods. The analyses are plagued by the limitations of retrospective comparisons.

Evaluation of tumor stage is a particularly difficult problem. Its importance can be demonstrated in the series of Ise et al., in which 10 of 13 patients with metastases at the time of initial diagnosis died, while only 1 of 49 without such metastases succumbed to disease [30]. Despite the importance of staging, it is frequently impossible to rely on its accuracy in literature reviews.

The absence of adequate data on which to base recommendations and the rapid advances occurring in the field of pediatric oncology preclude definitive recommendations for therapy of infantile embryonal carcinomas at the present time. Two points should be emphasized, however. The radioimmunoassays for α-fetoprotein should prove a sensitive adjunct to staging and following these patients and, therefore, in deciding which patients require therapy beyond radical orchiectomy [35]. The second point is that many of these patients with metastatic disease have experienced tumor regression and prolonged survival in response to an aggressive therapeutic approach [30, 61, 74].

Rarely, lung metastases have first appeared more than 4 years after the initial diagnosis. This fact emphasizes the need for careful long-term follow-up despite the favorable prognostic implications of prolonged disease-free intervals noted above [66].

Finally, the embryonal rhabdomyosarcoma should be recognized as a highly malignant tumor. In recent years it has been shown to respond dramatically to aggressive therapy, even in the presence of metastases [7, 8]. New and more effective approaches to this tumor are being developed constantly and would probably quickly render obsolete any specific recommendations. It seems enough to emphasize that the previous pessimistic outlook for patients with embryonal rhabdomyosarcoma is no longer justified [10, 31].

References

1. Abell, M. R., and Holtz, F. Testicular neoplasms in adolescents. *Cancer* 17:881, 1964.
2. Abell, M. R., and Holtz, F. Testicular neoplasms in infants and children: I. Tumors of germ cell origin. *Cancer* 16:965, 1963.
3. Albrechtsen, R., Klee, J. G., and Møller, J. E. Primary intracranial germ cell tumors including five cases of endodermal sinus tumor. *Acta Pathol. Microbiol. Scand.* [A] [Suppl. 233] 80:32, 1972.
4. Allyn, D. L., Silverberg, S. G., and Salzberg, A. M. Endodermal sinus tumor of the vagina: Report of a case with 7-year survival and literature review of so-called "mesonephroma." *Cancer* 27:1231, 1971.
5. Altman, B. L., and Malament, M. Carcinoma of the testis following orchiopexy. *J. Urol.* 97:498, 1967.
6. Arlen, M., Grabstald, H., and Whitmore, W. F., Jr. Malignant tumor of the spermatic cord. *Cancer* 23:525, 1969.
7. Bhargava, M. R., and Reddy, D. G. Tumors of the testis: II. Tumors of the testis in children. *Cancer* 19:1655, 1966.
8. Bissada, N. K., Finkbeiner, A. E., and Redman, J. F. Paratesticular sarcomas: Review of management. *J. Urol.* 116:198, 1976.
9. Boatman, D. L., Culp, D. A., and Wilson, V. B. Testicular neoplasms in children. *J. Urol.* 109:315, 1973.
10. Brosman, S. A., Cohen, A., and Fay, R. Rhabdomyosarcoma of testis and spermatic cord in children. *Urology* 3:568, 1974.
11. Carney, J. A., Thompson, D. P., Johnson, C. L., and Lynn, H. B. Teratomas in children: Clinical and pathologic aspects. *J. Pediatr. Surg.* 7:271, 1972.
12. Chretien, P. B., Milam, J. D., Foote, F. W., and Miller, T. R. Embryonal adenocarcinoma (a type of malignant teratoma) of the sacrococcygeal region. *Cancer* 26:522, 1970.
13. Cook, C. D., Gross, R. E., Landing, B. H., and Zygmuntowicz, A. S. Interstitial cell tumor of the testis: Study of a 5-year-old boy with pseudoprecocious puberty. *J. Clin. Endocrinol. Metab.* 12:725, 1952.
14. Eaton, W. L., and Ferguson, J. P. A retinoblastic teratoma of the epididymis (case report). *Cancer* 9:718, 1956.
15. Fraley, E. E., and Ketcham, A. S. Teratoma of the testis in an infant. *J. Urol.* 100:659, 1968.
16. Frasier, S. D., Bashore, R. A., and Mosier, H. D. Gonadoblastoma associated with pure gonadal dysgenesis in monozygous twins. *J. Pediatr.* 64:740, 1964.
17. Gabrilove, J. L., Nicolis, G. L., Mitty, H. A., and Sohval, A. R. Feminizing interstitial cell tumor of the testis: Personal observations and a review of the literature. *Cancer* 35:1184, 1975.
18. Gangai, M. P. Testicular neoplasms in an infant. *Cancer* 22:658, 1968.
19. Giebink, G. S., and Ruymann, F. B. Testicular tumors in children: Review and report of three cases. *Am. J. Dis. Child.* 127:433, 1974.
20. Gitlin, D., Perricelli, A., and Gitlin, G. M. Synthesis of alpha-fetoprotein by liver, yolk sac, and gastrointestinal tract of the human conceptus. *Cancer Res.* 32:979, 1972.
21. Givler, R. L. Testicular involvement in leukemia and lymphoma. *Cancer* 23:1290, 1969.
22. Hansen, J. L. Tumor of undescended testicle in an infant. *J.A.M.A.* 199:944, 1967.
23. Hart, W. R. Primary endodermal sinus (yolk sac) tumor of the liver: First reported case. *Cancer* 35:1453, 1975.
24. Holtz, F., and Abell, M. R. Testicular neoplasms in infants and children: II. Tumors of non-germ cell origin. *Cancer* 16:982, 1963.
25. Houser, R., Izant, R. J., Jr., and Persky, L. Testicular tumors in children. *Am. J. Surg.* 110:876, 1965.
26. Huntington, R. W., Jr., and Bullock, W. K. Endodermal sinus and other yolk sac tumors, a reappraisal.

Acta Pathol. Microbiol. Scand. [Suppl. 233] 80:26, 1972.

27. Huntington, R. W., Jr., and Bullock, W. K. Yolk sac tumors of extragonadal origin. *Cancer* 25:1368, 1970.

28. Huntington, R. W., Jr., and Bullock, W. K. Yolk sac tumors of the ovary. *Cancer* 25:1357, 1970.

29. Hutter, A. M., Jr., Lynch, J. J., and Shnider, B. I. Malignant testicular tumors in brothers. *J.A.M.A.* 199:1009, 1967.

30. Ise, T., Ohtsuki, H., Matsumoto, K., and Sano, R. Management of malignant testicular tumors in children. *Cancer* 37:1539, 1976.

31. Johnson, D. E., Kuhn, C. R., and Guinn, G. A. Testicular tumors in children. *J. Urol.* 104:940, 1970.

32. Johnson, D. E., Woodhead, D. M., Pohl, D. R., and Robinson, J. R. Cryptorchism and testicular tumorigenesis. *Surgery* 63:919, 1968.

33. Kedia, K., and Fraley, E. E. Adult teratoma of the testis metastasizing as adult teratoma: Case report and review of literature. *J. Urol.* 114:636, 1975.

34. Klugo, R. C., Fisher, J. H., and Retek, A. B. Endodermal sinus tumors of the testis in infants and children. *J. Urol.* 108:359, 1972.

35. Lange, P. H., McIntire, K. R., Waldmann, T. A., Hakala, T. R., and Fraley, E. E. Serum alpha fetoprotein and human chorionic gonadotropin in the diagnosis and management of nonseminomatous germcell testicular cancer. *N. Engl. J. Med.* 295:1237, 1976.

36. Leaf, P. N., Tucker, G. R., III, and Harrison, L. H. Embryonal cell carcinoma originating in the spermatic cord (case report). *J. Urol.* 112:285, 1974.

37. Li, F. P., and Fraumeni, J. F., Jr. Testicular cancers in children: Epidemiologic characteristics. *J. Natl. Cancer Inst.* 48:1575, 1972.

38. Littmann, R., Tessler, A. N., and Valensi, Q. Paratesticular rhabdomyosarcoma: A case presentation and review of the literature. *J. Urol.* 108:290, 1972.

39. Magner, D., Campbell, J. S., and Wiglesworth, F. W. Testicular adenocarcinoma with clear cells, occurring in infancy. *Cancer* 9:165, 1956.

40. Mahon, F. B., Gosset, F., Trinity, R. G., and Madsen, P. O. Malignant interstitial cell testicular tumors. *Cancer* 31:1208, 1973.

41. Malek, R. S., Utz, D. C., and Farrow, G. M. Malignant tumors of the spermatic cord. *Cancer* 29:1108, 1972.

42. Marin-Padilla, M. Histopathology of the embryonal carcinoma of the testis. *Arch. Pathol.* 85:614, 1968.

43. Matsumoto, K., Nakauchi, K., and Fujita, K. Radiation therapy for embryonal carcinoma of testis in childhood. *J. Urol.* 104:778, 1970.

44. McCullough, D. L., Carlton, C. E., and Seybold, H. M. Testicular tumors in infants and children: Report of five cases and evaluation of different modes of therapy. *J. Urol.* 105:140, 1971.

45. Meares, E. M., Jr., and Kempson, R. L. Fibrous histiocytoma of the scrotum in an infant. *J. Urol.* 110:130, 1973.

46. Miller, A., and Seljelid, R. Histopathologic classification and natural history of malignant testis tumors in Norway 1959–63. *Cancer* 28:1054, 1971.

47. Miningberg, D. T., and Harley, D. P. Scrotal wall hemangioma in an infant. *J. Urol.* 106:789, 1971.

48. Mostofi, F. K. Infantile testicular tumors. *Bull. N.Y. Acad. Med.* 28:684, 1952.

49. Mostofi, F. K. Testicular tumors: Epidemiologic, etiologic, and pathologic features. *Cancer* 32:1186, 1973.

50. Norris, H. J., Bagley, G. P., and Taylor, H. B. Carcinomas of the infant vagina. *Arch. Pathol.* 90:473, 1970.

51. Pierce, G. B., and Abell, M. R. Embryonal Carcinoma of the Testis. In S. C. Sommer (ed.), *Pathology Annual.* Vol. 5. New York: Appleton-Century-Crofts, 1970.

52. Pierce, G. B., Bullock, W. K., and Huntington, R. W., Jr. Yolk sac tumors of the testis. *Cancer* 25:644, 1970.

53. Pomer, F. A., Stiles, R. E., and Graham, J. H. Interstitial-cell tumors of the testis in children: Report of a case and review of the literature. *N. Engl. J. Med.* 250:233, 1954.

54. Price, E. B., Jr. Epidermoid cysts of the testis: A clinical and pathologic analysis of 69 cases from the testicular tumor registry. *J. Urol.* 102:708, 1969.

55. Ravich, L., Lerman, P. H., Drabkin, J. W., and Noya, J. Embryonal carcinoma of testicle in childhood: Review of literature and presentation of two cases. *J. Urol.* 96:501, 1966.

56. Rosvoll, R. V., and Woodard, J. R. Malignant Sertoli cell tumor of the testis. *Cancer* 22:8, 1968.

57. Selvaggi, F. P., Young, R. T., Brown, R., and Dick, A. L. Interstitial cell tumor of the testis in adults: Two case reports. *J. Urol.* 109:436, 1973.

58. Stoffel, T. J., Nesbit, M. E., and Levitt, S. H. Extramedullary involvement of the testis in childhood leukemia. *Cancer* 35:1203, 1975.

59. Talerman, A. Malignant Sertoli cell tumor of the testis. *Cancer* 28:446, 1971.

60. Tanimura, H., and Furuta, M. Rhabdomyosarcoma of the spermatic cord. *Cancer* 22:1215, 1968.

61. Tefft, M., Vawter, G. F., and Mitus, A. Radiotherapeutic management of testicular neoplasm in children. *Radiology* 88:457, 1967.

62. Teilum, G. Endodermal sinus tumors of the ovary and testis. *Cancer* 12:1092, 1959.

63. Teilum, G. *Special Tumors of Ovary and Testis: Comparative Pathology and Histological Identification.* Philadelphia: Lippincott, 1971.

64. Teilum, G., Albrechtsen, R., and Nørgaard-Pedersen, B. The histogenetic-embryologic basis for reappearance of alpha-fetoprotein in endodermal sinus tumors (yolk sac carcinoma) and teratomas. *Acta Pathol. Microbiol. Scand.* [A] 83:80, 1975.

65. Teilum, G., Albrechtsen, R., and Nørgaard-Pedersen, B. Immunofluorescent localization of alpha-fetoprotein synthesis in endodermal sinus tumor (yolk sac tumor). *Acta Pathol. Microbiol. Scand.* [A] 82:586, 1974.

66. Teoh, T. B., Steward, J. K., and Willis, R. A. The distinctive adenocarcinoma of the infant testis: An account of 15 cases. *J. Pathol. Bacteriol.* 80:147, 1960.

67. Thiele, J., Castro, S., and Lee, K. D. Extragonadal endodermal sinus tumor (yolk sac tumor) of the pelvis. *Cancer* 27:391, 1971.

68. Tiltman, A. J. The racial incidence of testicular tumors. *S. Afr. Med. J.* 43:97, 1969.

69. Tsuchida, Y., Saito, S., Ishida, M., Ohmi, K., Urano, Y., Endo, Y., and Oda, T. Yolk sac tumor (endodermal sinus tumor) and alpha-fetoprotein: A report of three cases. *Cancer* 32:917, 1973.

70. Tsuji, I., Nakajima, F., Nishida, T., Nakanoya, Y., and Inoue, K.   Testicular tumors in children. *J. Urol.* 110:127, 1973.

71. Viprakasit, D., Tannenbaum, M., and Smith, A. M. Adenomatoid tumor of the male genital tract. *Urology* 4:325, 1974.

72. Weitzner, S., and Gropp, A.   Sertoli cell tumor of testis in childhood. *Am. J. Dis. Child.* 128:541, 1974.

73. Woodtli, W., and Hedinger, C.   Endodermal sinus tumor or orchioblastoma in children and adults. *Virchows Arch. [Pathol. Anat.] Histol.* 364:93, 1974.

74. Young, P. G., Mount, B. M., Foote, F. W., Jr., and Whitmore, W. F.   Embryonal adenocarcinoma in the prepubertal testis: A clinicopathologic study of 18 cases. *Cancer* 26:1065, 1970.

75. Zone, R. M.   Retinal anlage tumor of epididymis: A case report. *J. Urol.* 103:106, 1970.

Index

Index